Oxford Textbook of

Palliative Care
for Children

Oxford Textbook of
Palliative Care for Children

Edited by

Ann Goldman
Consultant in Paediatric Palliative Care, Great Ormond Street Hospital, London, UK

Richard Hain
Senior Lecturer in Paediatric Palliative Care, University of Wales College of Medicine, UK

Stephen Liben
Associate Professor of Pediatrics, McGill University, Canada

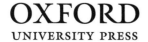

OXFORD
UNIVERSITY PRESS

OXFORD

UNIVERSITY PRESS

Great Clarendon Street, Oxford OX2 6DP

Oxford University Press is a department of the University of Oxford.
It furthers the University's objective of excellence in research, scholarship,
and education by publishing worldwide in

Oxford New York

Auckland Cape Town Dar es Salaam Hong Kong Karachi
Kuala Lumpur Madrid Melbourne Mexico City Nairobi
New Delhi Shanghai Taipei Toronto

With offices in

Argentina Austria Brazil Chile Czech Republic France Greece
Guatemala Hungary Italy Japan Poland Portugal Singapore
South Korea Switzerland Thailand Turkey Ukraine Vietnam

Oxford is a registered trade mark of Oxford University Press
in the UK and in certain other countries

Published in the United States
by Oxford University Press Inc., New York

British Library Cataloguing in Publication Data

Data available

Library of Congress Cataloging in Publication Data

Data available

Typeset by Newgen Imaging Systems (P) Ltd., Chennai, India
Printed in Italy
on acid-free paper by Lito Terrazzi

ISBN 0–19–852653–9   978–0–19–852653–7

10 9 8 7 6 5 4 3 2 1

Preface

Fortunately death in childhood is uncommon, but for those families who have to live with the knowledge of their child's impending death and confront the problems of caring for them throughout their illness, the emotional and practical burdens are great. For the health care workers too, dealing with the particular problems of the dying child and their family, as well as acknowledging their own sadness, can lead to considerable stress and anxiety.

It has taken many years for society, including healthcare workers, to acknowledge the problems of dying patients. Perhaps because death in childhood is uncommon, it is only now becoming clear that children with life-limiting conditions and their families have special needs that are often not recognized or met. The adult hospice movement, focusing on the care of those dying from cancer has been established since the 1960s but palliative care in paediatrics, with its broader approach, is newer and only began in the 1980s. Although this is partly related to the relatively small numbers involved it is also reflects the discomfort most of us feel when facing the certain death of a child.

In comparison with other aspects of paediatrics there is only a small research and literature base to palliative care. Although we can learn from the growing literature of the adult hospice movement the problems are not identical and children need to be considered in their own right.

The aim of this book is to gather together the best and most up-to-date information about current knowledge and clinical practice in paediatric palliative care, with contributions from many of the pioneers in the field from a wide variety of disciplines, around the world. We hope this will provide a practical and informative text, which will promote a model of care that is sufficiently flexible to address the complex and multifaceted needs of children with life-threatening illnesses and their families, across many countries and continents. The book focuses on children with chronic disease and the specific issues of sudden infant death, accidental death and suicide are not included.

Every child and family facing death has their own unique, complex and varied problems. There can be no single 'right' way of providing care. In this text we consider a wide range of issues including medical, psychological and practical aspects of caring for terminally ill children and their families and provide diverse resources from which we hope readers will be able to draw out what is useful to them, in their particular circumstances. The different authors have chosen to use a combination of approaches in the text reflecting both the differing needs of the topics and their own personal writing styles. We hope this approach will also meet the individual needs and preferences of the readers. However, some important common themes that reflect our underlying beliefs will thread throughout the book. These are:

- the need for care to be child and family centred

- the need for care to be flexible and individualized for each child and family

- the need for care to be based on teamwork between the child, family, professional of all disciplines and non-professional carers.

- the need for our practice to be reflective and evidence based as much as possible.

The book begins with a section we have called 'Foundations of care', in which the first two chapters give a background and overview of paediatric palliative care and the groups of children who may benefit from it. These are followed by discussions about communication and ethics, which are core issues at the centre of all aspects of our work.

In the second section, 'Child and family care', we have started with a chapter looking at society's perceptions of death in children. We then have a wide range of chapters looking at different aspects of psychological, social and spiritual care, both for the sick child, adolescent and also their family. We look at the ways children view death, the ways in which they express themselves and the roles of play and school. These chapters cover both the time course of the illness and also the time immediately following death and finally support for the family through bereavement.

'Symptom care' is the focus of the third section in which a number of broad-based chapters cover symptom assessment, the use of medications and symptoms at the end of life. These are complemented by more specific and detailed exploration of individual symptoms and their management. We have encouraged the authors to take a holistic view and discuss both pharmacological and non-pharmacological approaches, and also to recognize the importance, especially to families, of including the role of complementary medicine.

In the fourth section we have brought together themes related to the 'Delivery of care'. There are chapters relating to the practical issues involved in care in a range of different environments such as home care, children's hospices, hospital wards and intensive care units. We have also tried to look at the way children's palliative care is developing (or not yet happening) in some of the different countries around the world with their contrasting physical, geographic and financial environments. Teamwork, which is such an essential part of paediatric

palliative care is explored as are the responses and needs of healthcare professionals working in this difficult field. The book ends with an eye towards the future examining quality assurance, education, training and research.

We hope this book will be of help to paediatricians in particular but also to all those professionals and volunteers who may be involved in the care and management of a dying child. We hope it will help them to look after the children with skill and confidence, and work with and support the family so the children can die in peace and with dignity wherever they are cared for.

October, 2005

A. G.
R. H.
S. L.

Contents

List of contributors

Trygve Aasgaard Oslo University College, Oslo, Norway

Thomas Attig Professor Emeritus, Department of Philosophy, Bowling Green State University, Bowling Green, Ohio, USA

Nigel Ballantine Birmingham Children's Hospital NHS Trust, Birmingham, UK

Muriel Barber Claire House Children's Hospice, Wirral, UK

Sandra Bertman Graduate School of Social Work, Boston College, Boston, MA, USA

Myra Blubond-Langer Department of Anthropology, Center for Children and Childhood Studies, Rutgers University, New Jersey, USA

Lynda Brook Royal Liverpool Children's Hospital, Liverpool, UK

Erica Brown Head of Research and Development, Acorns Children's Hospice, Birmingham, UK

John J. Collins Pain and Palliative Care, Children's Hospital at Westmead, Sydney, Australia

Nancy Contro Lucile Packard Children's Hospital, Stanford University Medical Center, Palo Alto, CA, USA

David L. Coulter Department of Neurology, Children's Hospital, Boston, MA, USA

Finella Craig Consultant in Paediatric Palliative Care, Great Ormond Street Hospital for Children, London, UK

Betty Davies Professor, Family Health Care Nursing, University of California San Francisco School of Nursing, San Francisco, CA, USA

Dawn Davies Medical Director, Pediatric Palliative Care Program, Capital Health; Assistant Professor, Department of Pediatrics, University of Alberta, Edmonton, Canada

Amy DeCicco Center for Children and Childhood Studies, Rutgers University, New Jersey, USA

Deborah deVlamin Program Coordinator, Pediatric Palliative Care Program, Capital Health; Professional Practice Lead, Children's Team Homecare, Capital Health; Edmonton, Canada

Frances Dominica Helen and Douglas House, Oxford, UK

Gwyneth Down Great Ormond Street Hospital, London, UK

Russ Drake Paediatric Palliative Care Service, Starship Children's Hospital, Auckland, New Zealand

Veronica Dussel Research Associate, Pediatric Advanced Care Team, Department of Pediatric Oncology, Dana Farber Cancer Institute, Boston, MA, USA

Nicola Eaton Director of Children's Palliative Care Research, Centre for Child and Adolescent Health, Bristol, UK.

Kate W. Faulkner Kid Care Consultants, Dover, MA, USA

Linda Ferguson Professor of Nursing, University of Saskatchewan, Saskatoon, Saskatchewan, Canada

Nicki Fitzmaurice Birmingham Children's Hospital NHS Trust, Birmingham, UK

Susan Fowler-Kerry Professor of Nursing, University of Saskatchewan, Saskatoon, Saskatchewan, Canada

Gerri Frager Medical Director, Pediatric Palliative Care Services, IWK Health Care, Halifax, Nova Scotia, Canada

Brother Francis, OSB Clinical Nurse Specialist in Paediatric Oncology and Related Palliative Care, The Children's Hospital, Brighton; Monk, Worth Abbey, UK

Ann Goldman Consultant in Paediatric Palliative Care, Great Ormond Street Hospital, London, UK

Robert Graham Attending Physician, Division of Critical Care Medicine, Department of Anesthesiology, Perioperative and Pain Medicine, Children's Hospital, Boston, Boston, MA, USA

Richard Hain Senior Lecturer in Paediatric Palliative Medicine, Children's Hospital for Wales, Cardiff, UK

Jim F. Hammel US-UK Fulbright Program, University of Oxford; Department of Psychiatry, Harvard Medical School, Boston, MA, USA

Anne Hunt Senior Research Fellow—Children's Palliative Care, Department of Nursing, Faculty of Nursing, University of Central Lancashire, Preston, UK

Jenny Hynson Consultant Paediatrician, Victorian Paediatric Palliative Care Program, Royal Children's Hospital, Melbourne, Australia

Marek W. Karwacki National Research Institute of Mother and Child; Warsaw Hospice for Children, Warsaw, Poland

Leora Kuttner Departement of Pediatrics, University of British Columbia, Vancouver, Canada

Satbir S Jassal Rainbows Children's Hospice, Loughborough, UK

Vic Larcher Consultant in General Paediatrics and Clinical Ethics, Great Ormond Street Hospital, London, UK

Judith Leet Chestnut Hill, MA, USA

Simon Lenton Consultant Paediatrician, Community Child Health Department, Bath, UK

Mary Lewis Centre for Child and Adolescent Health, University of the West of England/University of Bristol; Senior Nurse, The Lifetime Service, Bath, UK

Stephen Liben Associate Professor of Pediatrics, McGill University, Canada

Victoria Lidstone Locum Consultant in Palliative Medicine, Prince Charles Hospital, Merthyr Tydfil, Wales, UK

Tom Lissauer Consultant Neonatologist, St Mary's Hospital, London, UK

Anita MacDonald Consultant Dietician in Inherited Metabolic Disorders, Birmingham Children's Hospital, Birmingham, UK

Erica Mackie Consultant Paediatric Oncologist, Southampton General Hospital, Southampton, UK

Rodica Matusa Presedinte, Asociatia Speranta, Constanta, Romania

Renee McCulloch Oxford Radcliffe NHS Trust; Helen House Children's Hospice

Marie-Louise Millard Consultant Paediatrician, St Mary's Hospital, Portsmouth, UK

Debbie Norval Consultant in Palliative Care, Johannesburg, South Africa; Hospice Association of the Witwatersrand; Hospice Palliative Care Association of South Africa

Bernadette O'Hare Consultant Paediatrician, Cardiff and Vale NHS Trust, Children's Hospital in Wales, Cardiff, UK

Danai Papadatou Professor of Psychology, Faculty of Nursing, University of Athens, Greece

Michelle Rogers Research Assistant, Judith N. Miller Integrative Medicine Initiative, Children's Memorial Hospital, Chicago, IL, USA

Susan Scofield Lucile Packard Children's Hospital, Stanford University Medical Center, Palo Alto, CA, USA

Harold Siden Canuck Place Children's Hospice; BC Children's Hospital, Vancouver, Canada

Jean Simons Great Ormond Street Hospital, London, UK

Jo Sims Rainbows Children's Hospice, Loughborough, UK

Barbara M. Sourkes Palo Alto, CA, USA

David Southall OBE Honorary Medical Director, Child Advocacy International; Professor of Paediatrics, University of Keele; Consultant Paediatrician, University Hospital of North Staffordshire

David M. Steinhorn Associate Professor of Pediatrics, Pediatric Pulmonary and Critical Care Medicine, Northwestern University Feinberg School of Medicine; Medical Director Judith N. Miller Integrative Medicine Initiative; Medical Director, Pediatric Palliative Care Program, Children's Memorial Hospital, Chicago, IL, USA

Paul B. Thayer Child Life and Family Studies, Wheelock College, Boston, MA, USA

Angela Thompson Associate Specialist Paediatrics, Palliative Care Lead Paediatrician, North Warwickshire PCT, Warwickshire, UK

Michael Towne Coordinator, Child Life Department, University of California San Francisco Children's Hospital, San Francisco, CA, USA

Jan Vickers Royal Liverpool Children's Hospital, Liverpool, UK

Suellen M. Walker Children's Hospital, Westmead, Sydney, Australia; Institute of Child Health, London, UK

Joanne Wolfe Assistant Professor, Department of Pediatrics, Harvard Medical School; Medical Director, Pediatric Advanced Care Team, Department of Pediatric Oncology, Dana Farber Cancer Institute/Children's Hospital Boston, Boston, MA, USA

Isabel Wood Canuck Place Children's Hospice, Vancouver, Canada

List of abbreviations

AACN	American Association of Colleges of Nursing		DIC	Disseminated Intravascular Coagulation
Ach	Achetylcholine		DMD	Duchenne Muscular Dystrophy
ACT	Association for Children with Life-threatening or Terminal Conditions and their Families		DNA	Deoxyribonucleic Acid
			DNAR	Do Not Attempt Resuscitation
AIDS	Acquired Immunodeficiency Syndrome		DNR	Do Not Resuscitate
ALL	Acute Lymphoblastic Leukaemia		DOH	Department of Health
APA	American Psychiatric Association		DREZotomy	Dorsal Root Entry Zone-otomy
ARV	Anti-Retroviral Drug		DRG	Dorsal Root Gangtion
ASICI	Acid Sensing Ion Channels		DRV	Dietary Reference Value
BAE	Bronchial Artery Emboligation		DSM	Diagnostic and Statistical Manual
BANS	British Artificial Nutrition Survey		DZ	Dopamine
BAPEN	British Association for Enteral and Parenteral Nutrition		EAPC	European Association for Palliative Care
BCCAA	Branched Chain Amino Acids		EB	Epidermolysis Bullose
BCL	B-cell Leukemia		EBV	Epstein Barr Virus
BDNF	Brain Derived Neurotrophic Factor		EEG	Electrodencephalogram
BiPAP	Biphasic Positive Airway Pressure		ELNEL	End-of-Life Nursing Education Consortium
BMA	British Medical Journal		EOL	End of Life
BMT	Blood and Marrow Transplant		EPA	Eicosapentanoic Acid
BTx	Botulinum Toxin		ESPR	European Society for Pediatric Research
CAI	Child Advocacy International		EXQOL	Exeter Quality of Life Scale
CAM	Confusion Assessment Method		FDA	Food and Drug Administration
CAM	Complementary and Alternative Medicine		FEVI	Forced Expiratory Volume in 1s
CAMP	Cyclicadenosine Monophosphate		FHSSA	Foundation for Hospice in sub-Saharan Africa
CBT	Cognitive Behavioural Therapy		FVC	Forced Vital Capacity
CD	Compact Disc		GABA	Gamma Amino Butyric Acid
CDI	Children's Depression Inventory		GDNF	Glial Derived Nuratrophic Factor
CDRS-R	Children's Depression Rating Scale-Revised		GET	Gastric Emptying Time
CF	Cystic Fibrosis		GFAP	Glival Fibrillary Acidic Protein Hyphenation
CFR	Code of Federal Regulations		GFR	Glomerular Filtration Rate
CFS	Children Fatigue Scale		GH	Growth Hormone
CF-TON	Cystic Fibrosis Therapeutics Development Network		GI	Gastrointestinal
CGRP	Calcium Gene Related Peptide		GMC	General Medical Council
CHD	Coronary Heart Disease		GORD	Gastro Esophageal Reflux Disease
CHI-PACC	Children's Hospice International Programme for All-Inclusive Care for Children and their Families		H	Histamine
			HBV	Hepatitis B Virus
CINRG	Cooperative International Neuromuscular Research Group		HIV	Human Immunodeficiency Virus
CLIPPS	Children Int. Proj Palliative Services		HPOA	Hypertropic Pulmonary Ostecarthopathy
CML	Chronic Myelogenous Leukemia		HPV	Human Papilloma Virus
CNS	Central Nervous System		HRQ	Health Related Quality of Life
COG	Children's Oncology Group		HTLV	Human T-cell Leukemia Virus
CONSORT	Consolidated Standards of Report Clinical Trails		IASP	International Association for the Study of Pain
CP	Cerebral Palsy		ICH	Idiopathic Chronic Hiccup
CPAP	Continuous Positive Pressure		ICP	Increased Intracranial pressure
CQI	Continuous Quality Management		ICU	Intensive Care Unit
CRF	Corticotropin Releasing Factor		ID	Intellectual Disability
CSF	Cerebrospinal Fluid		IL	Interleukin
CSM	Committee on the Safety of Medicines		IPPC	Initiative for Paediatric Palliative Care
CTZ	Chemoreceptor Trigger Zone		IQ	Intelligence Quotient
CVAD	Central Venous Access Device		IRB	Investigation Review Board
DHA	Docose Hexanoic Acid		ITT	Intention-to-Treat

IV	Intravenous		PKC	Protein Konase C
JCAHO	American Joint Commissioner for Accreditation of Health		PKU	Phenylketouria
	Care Organization		PML	Promyelocytic Leukemia
KHD	Kinky Hair Disease		PMN	Polymodel Nociceptor
LLC	Life Limiting Condition		PNET	Primitive Neuroectodermal Tumor
LLT	Life Limiting Illnesses		PR	Per Rectum
LST	Life Sustaining Treatment		PRISM	Pediatric Risk of Mortality
LTR	Long Terminal Repeats		PRO	Peer Review Organization
MA	Magestrol Acetate		PVS	Persistent Vegetative State
MA	Marketing Authorisation		PYY	Polypeptide
Mach	Muscasiric Acetyl Choline		QA	Quality Assurance
MAPK	Mitogen Activated Pinae		QI	Quality Improvement
MCA	Medicines Control Agency		QOL	Quality of Life
MDD	Major Depressive Disorder		QUEST	Quality of End-of-Life Care and Satisfaction with Treatment
MDR	Multiple Drug Resistance		RCPCH	Royal College of Pediatrics and Child Health
MFO	Mixed Function Oxidase		RCT	Randomized Controlled Trials
MGLUR	Metabotrophic Receptor		RGC	Retrograde Giant Contraction
MHRA	Medicine And Healthcare Products Regulatory Agency		SC	Subcutaneous
MI-E	Mechanical Insuffocation-Exsuffocation		SEIQOL	Schedule of the Evaluation of Individual Quality if Life
MPS	Mucopoly Sacehari Diesease		SEP	Somatory–Sensory Evoked Potential
MSAS	Memorial Symptom Assessment Scale		SIDS	Sudden Infant Death Syndrome
MTD	Maximum Tolerated Dose		SIOP	Societe International O' Oncologie Pediatrique
MVV	Maximum Voluntary Ventilation		SL	Sublingal
N&V	Nausea and Vomiting		SMA	Spinal Muscular Atrophy
NACWOLA	Association of Women Living with AIDS		SP	Substance P
NCCAM	National Centre for Complementary and Alternative		SSRI	Selective Serotonin Reuptake Inhibitor
	Medicine		STAIC	State-trait Anxiety Inventory for Children
NCI	National Cancer Institute		STAS	Support Team Assessment
NGf	Nerve Growth Factor		SUDEP	Sudden and Unexpected Death in Epilepsy
NGT	Nasogastric Tube		SVC	Superior Vena Cava
NHS	National Health Services		SVCO	Superior Vena Cava Obstruction Syndrome
NICE	National Institute of Clinical Excellence		TCA	Tricylic Anti Depressant
NICHD	National Institute of Chile Health and Human Development		TCM	Traditional Chinese medicine
NICU	Neonatal Intensive Care Unit		TIME	Toolkit of Instruments to Measure End-of-Life Care
NIPPV	Non-invasive Positive Pressure Ventilation			Attached
NK	Neurodegenerative Life-threateneing Illness		TNF	Tumour necrosis factor
NMB	Neuromuscular Blockers		TOP	Termination of Pregnancy
NMD	Neuromuscular disease		TQM	Total Quality Management
NMDA	N Methyl D Asparate		TREND	Transparent Reporting of Evaluations with
NPY	Neuropeptide Y			Non-Randomized Designs
NSCLC	Non-small Cell Lung Cancer		TRKA	Tyrosine Kinase A
NT-3	Neurotrophin 3		TV	Tidal Volume
NTS	Nuclear Tractus solitarus		UCP	United Cerebral Palsy Research and Education Foundation
OCD	Obsessive Compulsive Disorder		UDPGT	Uridine Diphosphate Glucuronyl Transferase
ORS	Oral Rehydration Solution		UKCCSG	United Kingdom Children's Cancer Study Group
PAPAS	Pain, Palliative Care and Support Care		UNCRC	United Nations Convention on the Right of the Child
PCA	Patient-Controlled Analgesia		VAS	Visual Analogue Scale
PCRF	Parvicellular Reticular Formation		VC	Vomiting Center
PEDSQL	Pediatric Quality of Life Inventory		VGSC	Voltage Gated Sodium Channel
PEG	Percutaneous Endoscopic Gastronomy		VIP	Vasoactive Intestinal Peptide
PeGL	Polyethylene Glycol		VRI	Vanilloid Receptor 1
PGI	Patient Generated Index		VRLI	Vanilloid Receptor Like Protein Subtype 1
PICU	Paediatric Intensive Care Unit		WEEFIM	Functional Independence Measure
PIM	Paediatric Index of Mortality		WHO	World Health Organization
PKA	Protein Kinase A		WMA	World Medical Association

Section 1

Foundations of care

1 Development and epidemiology

Simon Lenton, Ann Goldman, Nicola Eaton, and David Southall

Introduction

All over the world children are living with and dying from life-threatening illnesses in a wide variety of social, economic, and health environments. Paediatric palliative care with its broad approach to symptom management, psychosocial, spiritual, and practical care has the potential to help enormously in the care and relief of suffering of these children and their families, particularly as it is relatively inexpensive and 'low tech'. However the vast majority of those children who die do so in the less developed countries where palliative care, as yet, has had almost no impact on their management. Even in the industrialised countries where palliative care is emerging as a new specialty, the provision of care is still extremely uneven, both between different countries and within each country individually. On the other hand, considering the modern concept of paediatric palliative care, or hospice care as it is often called in the United States, was unknown before the 1970s, it is remarkable how widely it has developed in less than 30 years and how much contribution it is already making.

The development of palliative care in paediatrics

Looking back in the literature the need to consider the problems for children with life-threatening and terminal illness seems to have become apparent synchronously to a number of different people, including both innovative health care workers and also individuals who had been affected personally [1–8]. It's not easy to trace the origins of an idea and exactly why a particular time was right for its development. A combination of factors seem to have been involved. One major influence must have been awareness of the growing strength and benefits of the adult palliative care movement, particularly following the opening of St Christopher's Hospice in 1967. Further

less tangible factors seem to have been the changing attitudes to health care and to the relationship between health care professionals and patients, particularly in the developed countries. Here society has been taking a more active interest in holistic approaches to health care and also there has been a trend away from a patriarchal and all-powerful health care system with increasing emphasis on personal autonomy. This shift has enabled families to express their wishes and needs (such as to care for their dying child at home) more clearly, and also the nurses and doctors have been more willing to listen and respond than in the past.

Many of the earlier paediatric palliative care projects were inspired by individuals with a powerful commitment relating to a personal experience of a child with a life-threatening illness, often combining the complex desire to improve the situation for the future and also to provide a lasting memorial to their loved one. Some families took a very active role and channelled great energy and commitment into developing projects through charitable funding. Helen House and many of the other children's hospices are named after particular children, as is the Edmarc programme in the United States [9,10]. Professionals too describe personal stories influencing their work in the field [11].

Offering a realistic choice to families of where they provide palliative care for their child and providing support and care in these different environments has been one of the core themes in paediatric palliative care. In the resource rich countries, a range of models of home care programmes are working towards this, supplemented by the development of children's hospices, respite care services, hospital-based initiatives, and bereavement programmes. In the developing countries, the provision lags far behind with local resources, priorities, and geography influencing the possibilities of providing palliative care. Those programmes that are beginning to develop are through community and home-based paediatric initiatives or in association with an established adult palliative care programme.

Home care

The earliest reported programmes developed in the United Kingdom and the United States. Specialist cancer services were among the first to recognize the need for palliative care [12–15]. The majority of services developing for children with malignant diseases were hospital based, originating in oncology units, depending often on specialist nurses, and in some more multidisciplinary teams. They offered palliative care support to families from a range of different services (Table 1.1).

In the United Kingdom palliative care for oncology patients was from the time of diagnosis, whereas in the United States the structure of their health care and insurance systems resulted in teams tending to focus on children with later stage and terminal illnesses. In contrast with adult palliative care, many home care programmes recognised, from very early on, the importance of including children dying from a wide range of illnesses, not just cancers [10,16–20]. The teams with a brief to care for all children with all life-limiting and terminal illness had more diverse origins than the oncology teams. Some began from a hospital-based oncology focus and then extended their role [16]. Others were community [10,18,20] or hospital [17,19] based.

As paediatric palliative care has expanded, so the range of models of care has also extended, to fit in with local ideas, clinical need, resources, cultures, and health care systems. Teams have in common the basic principles of providing expertise in symptom management, psychosocial, spiritual, and practical support, but vary in aspects of day-to-day operation such as size, staffing, funding, links with hospital and community, and links with children or adult hospices. The literature has many descriptions of individual teams and their approaches. In addition many more are established and are providing care are but are not formally described. There has still been very little evaluation and comparison between the different types of home care teams.

Table 1.1 Different components of palliative care

Outreach nursing care
Liaison
Support for community health care professionals
Expert advice
Direct hands-on care
24-h on-call
Bereavement follow up

Inpatient care

Only one hospital with a dedicated inpatient paediatric palliative care service is reported in the early literature [17,21]. This was established at St Mary's Hospital in New York in 1985 as part of a wider programme for children with all life-threatening illnesses, and also included home care. It was initiated at a time when AIDS was emerging as a major problem. Interestingly, although the hospital continues to have a strong commitment to palliative care and an outpatient and home care programme, their inpatient unit was closed in the late 1990s [11]. A combination of factors are cited for this change including negative perceptions of the unit within the hospital and community, intensity of emotions for staff, parents, and children, and the changing outlook for patients with AIDS. Palliative care is now provided by their multidisciplinary teams throughout the hospital.

Much more recently, three hospitals in the United States have reported dedicated paediatric hospice beds [22] but no details are given. Others have initiated programmes, special rooms, and family facilities to bring the hospice philosophy to relevant patients and families in their units [23,24].

Most hospital-based teams have chosen to adopt a consultative role rather than develop specific inpatient facilities. Some, like the oncology outreach teams, already had a close link to a particular diagnostic group of patients and are involved with them both in hospital and at home. Others have a wider range of diagnostic groups under their care. They may offer only inpatient care and help co-ordinate discharge but many combine this with a home care programme after discharge.

These generic hospital-based services are increasingly common in well-resourced countries. They vary in size and multidisciplinary constitution, but tend to have a nursing core with medical input and contributions from a wide range of other professionals (e.g. psychologists, social workers, play therapists, chaplains, physiotherapists, occupational therapists, pharmacists, art and music therapists). The reasons for referrals within the hospital are often complex, relating to difficult ethical decisions, communication problems, and staff support as well as the expected symptom management, family support, and discharge planning.

An emerging theme is the potential for valuable co-operation between palliative care teams and paediatric intensive care units [25]. This provides the opportunity to work together with families exploring the type of care that will be in the best interest of their child at the end of life. This is especially helpful for those with progressing prolonged illnesses and previous intensive care unit admissions. This close mutual relationship between palliative care and intensive care interest is also reflected by the intensive care background of a number of the paediatric palliative care physicians.

Children's hospices

Helen House was the first freestanding children's hospice facility and opened in the United Kingdom in 1982. It provides an attractive eight-bedded home-from-home unit, with play rooms, gardens, and family accommodation and staffed by a multidisciplinary team [7,9,26,27]. It has always been available to children with all life-limiting illnesses but found that most of the children admitted have longer-term illnesses such as metabolic or neurodegenerative diseases. Although a proportion of their patients receive terminal care the majority of admissions are for respite care. Families including siblings are supported throughout the illness and their bereavement. Helen House is a voluntary organisation and funded independently from charitable donations but works alongside the National Health Service.

The initial response to Helen House was ambivalent both from the paediatric establishment [28–30] and from adult palliative care [31]. Even Frances Dominica, the founder, herself felt that the need for more children's hospices was unlikely [27]. However, there are now 23 children's hospices open and 15 more planned in the United Kingdom as well as those that have now open or are being planned in Australia, Germany, Canada, Holland, and the United States.

Helen House has been a model for most of these children's hospices, but each has developed its own particular character and strengths with some now having close links with an adult hospice, some with links to local children's hospitals, and others with outreach and home care teams or day care facilities. Recently, hospices focusing specifically on the needs of adolescents and young adults have opened.

Parents value the standard of care and support, staff commitment, and the environment of the children's hospices [32,33], but the financial costs are considerable and concern has been expressed that children's hospices will face challenges as they move beyond the pioneering phase to become embedded in regular health and social care structures [34,35].

Adult palliative care

Paediatric palliative care sits in the overlap between the two much larger and more established fields of paediatrics and of adult palliative care (Figure 1.1). Its boundaries are distinct but should not be impermeable. From this central position children's palliative care stands to gain from the knowledge and experiences of both and also to contribute to both. Working in close co-operation should be to everyone's mutual benefit. However, in this situation, particularly, whilst paediatric palliative care develops and clarifies its role and as its voice strengthens, there can also be some difficulties, with confusion about its particular expertise. Some paediatricians do not understand the contribution that palliative care can make to their patients and others can fail to recognise their own limitations in providing it. Adult palliative care professionals may not acknowledge the special needs of children and families and the changes in practice needed for this. These special needs are being acknowledged both by those in paediatric palliative care [36,37] and also by adult palliative care teams with some familiarity caring for children [38,39].

The common features for both adult and children's palliative care include:

- Threat to life
- Impact of symptoms on activities of daily living
- Emotional impact
- Distress to families
- Need for a co-ordinated multi-agency approach.

There are, however, significant differences:

- Death in childhood is relatively rare in well resourced countries.
- The range of illnesses is different—wide range, often rare, often genetic, serious learning difficulties are common, varied time course, and crises can be rapid and unpredictable.
- Developmental factors influencing physiology and pharmacokinetics—fluids, nutrition, choice of medication, doses, side effects.
- Developmental factors influencing cognitive and emotional understanding—special skills in communication, assessment, art, music, play, education.
- Family care—working alongside parents as primary care givers, parent education, parent support, siblings, grandparents.

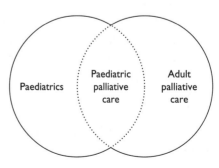

Fig. 1.1 Paediatric palliative care between paediatrics and adult palliative care.

- Ethical issues—child's developing autonomy, parents' role, professionals' role, decisions, respecting parents whilst including children.
- Grief in parents and siblings may be more severe.
- Multiple professionals and sites of care—teamwork, communication, home, hospital, hospice, school.
- Emotional strain and difficulty with boundaries for staff especially those not used to caring for dying children.

Those familiar with adult palliative care are likely to find the least differences working with families when a child is dying from malignant disease, especially with older children. With other illnesses such as metabolic and neurodegenerative diseases and with infants the differences are greater. Adult palliative care teams will need to work closely alongside paediatricians to manage the day-to-day care of a child with profound physical and developmental disability, with fluctuating health problems over long periods, possible behavioural difficulties, and the need for respite care. Care at home is, by its nature, child and family orientated and adult home care teams can accommodate their roles relatively easily to work with families here. In contrast, adult inpatient hospice care may be less easily adapted with difficulties arising both for the children and families, the hospice staff, and the other adult palliative care patients.

In many countries, especially those with a large geographic area and a small population, the only realistic way children will be able to receive palliative care will be through a co-operation of paediatric and adult health care professionals. Good communication and recognition of each other's roles become essential. This joint approach is currently widespread and is likely to be the only way children have access to paediatric palliative care in many parts of the world in the foreseeable future.

Definitions in paediatric palliative care

When starting to develop palliative care services, it is important for individuals and agencies involved to have a shared understanding of what they want to achieve. They, therefore, need to define what palliative care is and the children and families who might benefit.

What is paediatric palliative care?

Traditional, adult orientated, definitions of palliative care which have been used are:

Palliative care is the active total care of patients whose disease is not responsive to curative treatment. Control of pain, of other symptoms and of psychological, social and spiritual problems is paramount. The goal of palliative care is achievement of the best possible quality of life for patients and their families [40]

Palliative care is active total care offered to a patient with a progressive illness and their family when it is recognised that the illness is no longer curable, in order to concentrate on the quality of life and the alleviation of distressing symptoms within the framework of a co-ordinated service [41]

These definitions presume that curative treatment is an option, but for many children their conditions have no curative options. Neither does the term 'progressive illness' fit comfortably with children's palliative care, where many of the children have non-malignant life-threatening conditions that may not in themselves be progressive, but are likely to limit the child's life.

The definition of children's palliative care is evolving with time. The most frequently quoted definitions are:

Palliative care is an active and total approach to care, embracing physical, emotional, social and spiritual elements. It focuses on enhancement of quality of life for the child and support for the family and includes the management of distressing symptoms, provision of respite, and care following death and bereavement [42]

The goal of palliative care is the achievement of best quality of life for patients and their families, consistent with their values, regardless of the location of the patient [43]

At one level, these broader definitions cover the care that most clinical practitioners would strive to achieve for all the children and families they are involved with, regardless of their diagnoses, threat to life, or other circumstances. However, where the survival of the child is limited with a life-threatening condition, there is a greater emphasis on the emotional and spiritual well-being of all family members throughout the child's life.

Which children will benefit from palliative care?

The ACT definition above does not specify which children should benefit from palliative care. Because it assumes that palliative care starts when a diagnosis of a life-threatening condition is made, rather than the terminal phase as in adults, there is inevitably a degree of prognostic uncertainty for a substantial number of children. The largest group where there is uncertainty is of those with static neurological conditions, mainly quadriplegic cerebral palsy, who quite frequently deteriorate during the increased demands of adolescence and early adult life. Further work still needs to be undertaken to determine more accurately the life expectancy for this group of children and young people, within different societies/health care systems [44–47].

The four broad groups of children which have been delineated [42] are those with:

(1) life-threatening conditions for which curative treatment may be feasible but can fail. Children in long term remission or following successful treatment are not included (e.g. cancer, organ failures);

(2) conditions where premature death is inevitable, where there may be long periods of intensive treatment aimed at prolonging life and allowing participation in normal activities (e.g. cystic fibrosis);

(3) progressive conditions without curative treatment options, where treatment is exclusively palliative and may commonly extend over many years (e.g. Batten disease, mucopolysaccharidoses);

(4) Irreversible but non-progressive conditions causing severe disability leading to susceptibility to health complications and likelihood of premature death (e.g. cerebral palsy).

Issues which need to be addressed for planning clinical service delivery

Definitions of childhood. Definitions range from conception to 21 years through to birth to 14 years. Many children with non-malignant life-threatening conditions have associated learning difficulties and consequently attend special schools up to the age of 19 years. An upper limit of 19 years, therefore, seems appropriate in the United Kingdom as school health services continue to be involved. A definition of childhood needs to be considered when establishing a clinical service.

Duration of threat to life. Definitions tend to assume long-term conditions and fail to take into account conditions that are life-threatening for a limited period, for example, extreme prematurity, injuries, or acute diseases such as meningitis. For a short time, these conditions may pose a serious threat to life and the needs of these families may be similar to those who have a child with a longer-term illness. Hence, there needs to be clarity about the inclusion of acute illness or injury in the service plan.

Degree of threat to life. Children with diabetes are not usually considered as having a life-threatening illness, however, life expectancy is normally reduced and there is a threat to life during periods of poor control. However, the actual risks are relatively small and with good control life is not significantly shortened, even though some families may perceive the risks as significant. An estimate of the degree of threat to life needs to be included.

Death in childhood. Many definitions suggest that death should occur in childhood despite the fact that prediction of death is so difficult. Increasingly, many conditions that were universally fatal in childhood are now not causing death until early adulthood. Cystic fibrosis, Duchenne muscular dystrophy, and some cardiac conditions are all examples. Death in childhood is not essential for children to be included within a service.

Most parents presume to die before their children, and examining patterns of age at death, there is a nadir around 40 years of age by when most young people with fatal conditions, starting in childhood, have died. Therefore, the term 'premature death' in the definition, meaning expected to die before their parents, rather than stating death by a specific age is preferable.

Changing prognosis. Seventy per cent of children with leukaemia now survive; cystic fibrosis used to be a fatal condition within childhood, but estimates of average survival are ever increasing and have now almost reached 40 years [48]. Likewise, HIV/AIDS used to be a fatal diagnosis, but with early treatment with anti-retrovirals and effective treatment of intercurrent infections, HIV is beginning to be seen as a long-term infectious disease rather than a fatal disease in developed countries. In any definition of children's palliative care an estimate of probability of death or life expectancy should be considered, recognising that this may change over time.

Condition based definition. Definitions that are based on diagnoses are unhelpful due to the clinical variability of individual conditions, so some may, and others may not, be life-threatening. Occasionally a life-threatening illness is recognised, but no formal diagnosis is possible. An entirely condition/diagnosis-based approach to definition is unhelpful, rather a non-categorical approach based on life expectancy is recommended [49].

Severity/impact on daily living. There are many children and young people with multiple complex disabilities whose life expectancy is not appreciably shortened, yet their condition has a profound impact on their lives and on family functioning, for example, classical autism. On the other hand, boys with Duchenne muscular dystrophy may have a long period of life without a very significant disability and yet their prognosis in terms of years of life may be worse than the child with the severe but static neurological condition. Levels of support/input to the family will be more related to impact on quality of life and morbidity than the duration of the condition, so severity/impact does not influence the definition, but does significantly impact on service provision.

Severe mental health diagnoses. It can be argued that severe anorexia nervosa or depression associated with suicidal behaviour, also have a high probability of death and should therefore be included as life-threatening conditions. However, because of their need for specialist psychiatric services, they are normally excluded from the definition of palliative care for children.

Technology dependent children. Technology-dependent children are those children: 'who need both a medical device to compensate for the loss of a vital bodily function and substantial and on-going nursing care to avert death or further disability' [50,51].

Included would be children requiring mechanical ventilation, parenteral nutrition, and peritoneal dialysis. These children are dependent on technology for survival, and using this technology they may not be expected to die prematurely. Many children who have life-threatening illnesses are also dependent on technology to improve the quality of their lives, for example, gastrostomies for feeding, night-time ventilation for children with neuromuscular conditions. Technology dependence *per se* does not determine whether palliative care is needed.

Preventability/treatability of conditions. Millions of children die worldwide from starvation and infectious disease; their death is inevitable, often uncomfortable and lonely, but they are not perceived as needing palliative care. On the other hand, hundreds of thousands of children die from AIDS, often through starvation and infectious disease, and yet these children are perceived as requiring palliative care. The definition of palliative care should exclude children with easily treatable or preventable conditions.

Bereavement care. This is an integral part of the work of the palliative care team. However, those children who die acutely and never reach a hospital, for example, victims of house fires or road traffic accidents, or those who die in emergency departments or intensive care units, generally, receive their on-going care from the team involved at the time. A decision needs to be made as to whether the palliative care team should be involved with those families where the child was not known to the team before death. This often depends on whether there is an adult bereavement service already in existence, and how comfortable they feel with the specific issues around the deaths of children.

In conclusion, defining the role for palliative care needs to be society and health service specific and recognise that resources are not unlimited. In some situations, greater health gain could be achieved with alternative investment strategies, which may mean focusing on prevention rather than intervention, in other situations, focusing and management of symptoms and supportive care will benefit a much larger number of children than introducing expensive interventions for a few. Transplantation for organ failure may be an option in some countries, but not in others, likewise, access to life-giving technology will not necessarily be universally available, or indeed culturally acceptable.

Each service therefore needs to develop a clear definition based on factors discussed above and the resources available, and then to inform parents and other professionals of the criteria for referral to the service. For example the following definition used for referrals to one community-based palliative care team in the United Kingdom, is pragmatic, clear, and has clinical relevance to those making referrals [13].

A life-threatening condition [in childhood] is any illness or condition developed in childhood (before the age of 19 years) whereby the child is likely (a probability of greater than 50%) to die prematurely (before the age of 40 years), or any condition developed in childhood that without major intervention (which itself carries a significant mortality) will result in the child dying prematurely. Short term/acute illness/injury and mental health diagnoses are excluded.

Epidemiology of life-threatening conditions

Definitions in epidemiology

Classical epidemiology studies the incidence and prevalence of diseases or conditions in the population and their association with either causal factors or outcomes. Clinical epidemiology considers the effectiveness of tests, investigations, and interventions and when combined, the two epidemiological approaches complement one another to determine need (the ability to benefit from services) and the 'burden of disease' in society.

Incidence is the number of new cases occurring in a defined population over a specified period of time. It can also be applied to the number of deaths in a defined population over a specified period of time. It is particularly useful for acute illnesses or events, for example, meningitis or sudden infant death syndrome.

Prevalence is the number of cases in a defined population over a specified time period. It is particularly relevant to long-term conditions.

> *point prevalence* is the number of cases in a defined population at one moment in time
>
> *period prevalence* is the number of cases in a defined population over a defined period of time.

Prevalence cannot be derived from incidence, unless length of life is known. Generally, more children are surviving, and for longer periods of time, so the incidence of death in childhood is decreasing, and prevalence of children needing palliative care increasing.

In the absence of an agreed international definition of a life-threatening condition it is not possible to provide comparative figures on a global basis for children who require palliative care. Review of a global perspective of palliative medicine for adults is included in the *Oxford Textbook of Palliative Medicine* [52].

Global epidemiology of mortality

Children living in poorly resourced countries today, face problems similar to children now living in the well-resourced nations in previous centuries, often with the additional burden of tropical diseases and armed conflict. In many developed nations, infant mortality is now below 10 per 1000 births compared to many developing countries where it is still above 100 per 1000 births. These gains in life expectancy are due primarily to a decrease in deaths from infectious diseases. Consequently, health services in developed countries have shifted their focus to longer-term conditions as the predominant causes of morbidity and mortality [53].

There are approximately 1.5 billion children in the world and 85% live in poorly resourced countries. Approximately, 11 million children will die before they reach the age of five. Sixty per cent lack sanitation, 30% lack safe water, and 20% have no access to health care. Malnutrition affects around a third of children under 5 years of age and is implicated in more than 50% of the deaths [54,55].

It is estimated that 63% of these deaths could have been prevented with a few simple, affordable, and effective health interventions. For example 26% of the world's children go without immunisations, 28% receive no oral rehydration therapy, 40% receive no antibiotics for pneumonia, 58% are not breast-fed for the first 4 months, and 32% do not have access to sufficient iodine [56–59].

Poverty is the largest remediable cause of excess mortality. A total of 1.3 billion people live on less than one dollar a day while the world's 358 richest individuals have a combined wealth equivalent to the annual income of the poorest 2.3 billion people (nearly half the world's population), or alternatively, the richest 1% of the world's richest population have a combined income equivalent to 57% of the world's poorest [60–62].

More worryingly, in the poorest countries there has been very little improvement in wealth over the last decade. These inequalities are becoming greater over time, with Europe's per capita income now being 13 times greater than Africa's, which represents a fourfold increase over the last century. Indeed, overall measures of 'human development' have fallen in 21 countries during the last decade [57–59].

The effects of war and conflict are a major cause of mortality and morbidity in children. In the ten years before 1998 two million children were killed by war, 4 million children were permanently disabled, 1 million children orphaned and 12 million children displaced [63].

Every year over half a million women die from pregnancy-related causes, leaving one million motherless children, who will then often be more vulnerable to disease. Girls in Sudan are ten times more likely to die in pregnancy than complete primary school education [64].

Worldwide 2 billion people are currently infected with hepatitis B, causing 1 million deaths per year. A further 2 billion people are infected with tuberculosis, with 300,000 new cases each year. Over 36 million adults were estimated to be living with AIDS at the end of 2000 and 1.3 million children worldwide are living with HIV. In 2001, there were 3 million deaths from HIV/AIDS-related infections; in Kenya alone, 700 people die each day from HIV/AIDS. Many long-term viral infections are associated with an increased risk of cancer, for example, HIV and Kaposis sarcoma, herpes and cervical carcinoma, or hepatitis B and hepatocellular carcinoma, all further adding to morbidity and burden of disease.

Epidemiology in developed nations

Estimates of incidence from death certification

There are no systematic reviews, equivalent to those in the adult literature [65], examining the need for palliative care in childhood. Horrocks *et al.* [66] reviewed UK data for non-malignant disease and concluded that current literature was inadequate and recommended systematic research to accurately identify children with specified life-threatening conditions.

All reported incidence studies are based on the incidence of death rather than diagnosis, as information systems do not exist to reliably identify children with life-threatening illnesses at the time of diagnosis.

In one of the earliest UK estimates, based on an extrapolation of 1986 mortality data of 0–16 year olds, Thornes [67] suggested that there were 5400 children with life-threatening diseases. These figures suggest a prevalence of 4.9 children per 10,000, with 1.46 per 10,000 deaths per annum. Using OPCS data on child deaths over a 5-year period (1987–1991). While [68] calculated the incidence of deaths (all causes) for children aged 1–17 years in England and Wales as 10 per 100,000 per annum.

Jones studied all deaths over a 2-year period in New Zealand and of a total of 2122 deaths during the study period, 348 cases (16%) were assessed as potentially having required palliative care, giving a rate of 1.14 per 10,000 children per year. Thirty seven per cent of these deaths were due to cancer, 24% congenital anomalies, 11% cardiac conditions, and 28% other conditions. Twenty-nine per cent of these children died in hospital [69].

In the United States approximately 55,000 children aged 0–19 years died in 1999. Seventy per cent of these deaths are from illnesses but data is not available for assessing how many of these might have benefited from palliative care [70].

Dastgiri [71] studied infants born with congenital anomalies and found that 12% had died by the age of 5 years. Death secondary to chromosomal abnormalities was approximately 50% by 5 years.

Cancer in children differs from cancer in adults. Leukaemias account for 30%, brain tumours 20%, lymphomas 10%, and neuroblastomas for 8% of all new child cancer cases. Cancer incidence has remained relatively constant over time. In Canada, the incidence of cancer derived from mortality data between 1984 until 1994 was 14.7 per 100,000 children per year. The crude average annual incidence of cancer in Australian children under the age of 15 years was 13.8 per 100,000 [72]. These rates are 20–30% higher than those of most developing countries, which are lower, for reasons of both higher mortality from acute conditions and under-recognition. Any variation in international cancer rates reflects differences in case ascertainment as well as genetic susceptibility and environmental exposure to carcinogens; HIV exposure is likely to increase the numbers of people with Kaposi's sarcoma and lymphoma.

Estimation of incidence from hospital-based studies

If all children with a life-threatening condition died in hospital, studies based on hospital admissions/deaths would be a good proxy for the incidence of death in these conditions. However, increasingly children are dying at home, for example, an increase from 21% to 43% over the period from 1980 to 1998, especially in more affluent areas in developed countries [73,74]. Also conditions surviving into adulthood would be under-represented, as would children who died unexpectedly at home or died in hospitals remote from their local hospital. Determining population denominators for hospital-based studies is also often problematic because specialist children's hospitals are often remote from the place of residence of the children.

Prevalence of life-threatening conditions in the United Kingdom

Prevalence is very dependent on definition of a life-threatening condition—some studies are limited to those children who died in childhood, some exclude malignancies while others do not clearly state the population studied. Estimates of prevalence can either be derived from use of services, or specially designed population surveys. In addition communities where there is a high incidence of intra-familial marriage have a greater prevalence of recessive genetic disorders, and therefore local figures need to be derived taking account of conditions specific to ethnic minority groups and local populations.

Some examples include:

- A local Chichester (UK) evaluation by Wallace and Jackson [18] identified children with life-threatening conditions from a district-wide special needs register and estimated a prevalence of 8.57 per 10,000 in 0–16 year olds.
- Nash [75] estimated a prevalence of 10 per 10,000 children in Cornwall, excluding malignancies.
- A National Health Service Executive review of a number of Department of Health funded local projects for children with life-limiting conditions (all causes) suggested a prevalence of 10–13 children per 10,000 population, but no age range was specified [76].
- A population-based survey by Lenton *et al.* [77] in Bath (UK) suggested a prevalence of non-malignant life-threatening illness to be 1.28 per 1000, while simultaneously the prevalence of malignant disease was 0.65 per 1000 children aged 0–19 years. This study excluded children in hospital with acute conditions either in the neonatal period or secondary to acute illness or injury. Mental health diagnoses which were life-threatening were also excluded.
- ACT reviewing the UK data suggests that there are at least 12 per 10,000 children with life-limiting conditions in need of palliative care. [36]
- The Association of Children's Hospices (ACH) in the UK estimates that the number of children actively using hospice services is currently 3000 per annum. The growth in numbers of hospices catering for children may increase demand to 4000–4500 children in the next 5 years [78].

Non-malignant life-threatening disease profile

The Bath (UK) study indicates that cystic fibrosis is the commonest single diagnosis, but neurological conditions as a group are the commonest case of premature death [77]. The authors acknowledge that children with severe disabilities, mainly severe learning difficulties associated with cerebral palsy, are probably underestimated as clinicians rarely perceive or label them as life-threatening during early childhood (see Table 1.2).

Associated morbidity

Assessment of associated morbidity is difficult, largely because of the wide range of impairments, and absence of a clinically relevant assessment scale that is applicable to all types of disability. The Bath (UK) study assesses functioning derived

Table 1.2 Diagnostic groups of children with non-malignant life-threatening disease

Organ category	% total	Diagnoses
Respiratory	22.0	Cystic fibrosis Atypical tuberculosis Bronchopulmonary dysplasia
CNS abnormality	20.3	Cerebral palsy Microcephaly Birth asphyxia Spina bifida Arachnoid cyst (inop) Von Hippel–Lindau Hydrocephalus
CNS degeneration	8.1	San Philippo Hurler Scheie Niemann–Pick Unknown degenerative Multiple sclerosis
Cardiovascular	14.6	Complex congenital heart disease Cardiomyopathy
Syndromes	6.5	Unknown syndrome Retts syndrome Nagers syndrome Cockaynes syndrome Chromosome deletion Cornelia de Lange Edwards syndrome
Renal failure	4.1	Bilateral ureterocoeles Multiple abnormalities Neuropathic bladder Post urethral valves Post transplant
Neuromuscular degeneration	12.2	Duchenne muscular dystrophy Spinal muscular atrophy Other muscular dystrophy Progressive neuropathy
Metabolic	4.1	Atherosclerosis 3 MGA Mitochondrial disorder Tyrosinaemia type 2 Metabolic—unknown
Other	3.3	Gastroschisis/shortgut Severe osteogenesis imperfecta Epidermolysis bullosa
Liver	4.9	Biliary atresia Alpha 1 antitrypsin deficiency Other liver disease
Total	100	

from a British Association for Community Child Health publication [79]. The impact on everyday activities was assessed according to whether additional help was required. The results of this UK study also indicated high levels of psychological distress, significant effects upon employment and relationships, and a family environment characterised by low expressiveness, cohesion, and high conflict. Differences between mothers and fathers were found on a number of variables, for example, 53.8% of mothers and 30.0% of fathers were identified by the General Health Questionnaire [80] as having significant mental health problems. Length of time since diagnosis, level of family cohesion, and sex of parent, significantly predicted parental mental health status [81]. Almost 24% of healthy siblings were identified by the Rutter Questionnaire (1970) as having some degree of emotional or behavioural problems. A finding confirmed in a review of the literature by Williams *et al.* [82] in studies of siblings of a child with a chronic illness, where the majority (60%) were negatively affected, for 30% there was no impact, and in 10% there was improved functioning.

Summary

In developed countries, children requiring palliative care fall into two groups, those with malignant conditions and those with non-malignant conditions. The majority of malignant conditions are now curable, though a significant minority will have a terminal phase requiring palliative care. In contrast, the majority of non-malignant conditions are not curable. Non-malignant conditions fall into two groups—those with neurological conditions where there is a profound impact on everyday living through severe learning difficulty or impaired sensory/motor skills, and those without neurological conditions who often have intensive therapy regimes (for example, cystic fibrosis, renal dialysis, or cardiac disorders) to maintain life. Both groups of conditions impact on quality of life for the child and his/her family in different ways.

The best estimate of prevalence, allowing for methodological flaws, under-ascertainment, and likely trends, is 1.5/1000 children and young people from birth to 19 years likely to die prematurely from non-malignant life-threatening conditions. The annual incidence of death from these conditions is 1 : 10,000 and slowly decreasing over time.

References

1. Sahler, O.J.Z. (ed.) *The Child and Death*. St Louis: CVB Mosby, 1978.
2. Chapman, J.A. and Goodall, J. Dying children need help too. *BMJ*, 1979;1:593–4.

3. Chapman, J.A. and Goodall, J. Helping a child to live whilst dying. *Lancet* 1980;April 5:753–6.

4. Corr, C.A. and Corr, D.M. (eds.) *Hospice Approaches to Paediatric Care*. New York: Springer, 1985.

5. Corr, C.A. and Corr, D.M. Paediatric hospice care. *Pediatics* 1985; 76:774–80.

6. Lauer, N.E., Mulhern, R.K., Hoffmann, R.G., and Camitta, B.M. Utilisation of hospice/home care in paediatric oncology. *Cancer Nurs* 1986;9(3):102–7.

7. Dominica, F. The role of the hospice for the dying child. *Br J Hospital Med.* 1987;October:334–43.

8. Baum, J.D., Dominica, F., and Woodward, R.N. *Listen My Child has a Lot of Living to do*. Oxford: Oxford University Press, 1990.

9. Worswick, J. *A House called Helen*. 2nd edn. Oxford: Oxford University Press, 2001.

10. Sligh, J.S. An early model of care. In A. Armstrong-Daley, S.Z. Goltzer, eds. *Hospice Care for Children*. New York: Oxford University Press, 1993, pp. 219–30.

11. Grebin, B. Palliative care in an in-patient hospital setting. In A. Armstrong-Daley and S. Zarbock, eds. *Hospice Care for Children* (2nd edition). New York: Oxford University Press, pp. 313–22.

12. Martinsen, I.M., Armstrong, G.D., Geis, D.P., Anglim, M.A., Gronseth, E.C., MacInnis, H. *et al.* Home care for children dying of cancer. *Pediatrics* 1978;62:106–113.

13. Lauer, M.E., and Camitta, B.M. Home care for dying children: a nursing model. *Pediatr* 1980;97:1032–5.

14. Goldman, A., Beardsmore, S., and Hunt, J. Palliative care for children with cancer—home, hospital or hospice. *Arch Dis Child* 1990;65:641–3.

15. Curnick, S. Domiciliary nursing care. In J.D. Baum, F. Dominica, and R.N. Woodward, eds. *Listen My Child has A Lot of Living To Do*. Oxford: Oxford University Press, 1990, pp. 28–33.

16. Martin, B.B. Home care for terminally ill children and their families. In C.A. Corr and D.M. Corr, eds. *Hospice Approaches to Paediatric Care*. New York: Springer, 1985, pp. 56–86.

17. Lombardi, N. Palliative care in an in-patient hospital setting. In A. Armstrong-Daley and S.Z. Goltzer, eds. *Hospice Care for Children*. New York: Oxford University Press, 1993, pp. 248–65.

18. Wallace, A. and Jackson, S. Establishing a palliative care team for children. *Child Care, Health Dev* 1995;21:383–85.

19. Kopecky, E.A., Jacobson, S., Prashant, J., Martin, M., and Coren, G. Review of a home based palliative care programme for children with malignant and non-malignant diseases. *J Palliat Care* 1997;13(4):28–33.

20. Lewis, M. The lifetime service: a model for children with life-threatening illnesses and their families. *Paediatr Nurs* 1999; 11(7):21–2.

21. Wilson, D.C. Developing a hospice programme for children. In C.A. Corr, and D.M. Corr, eds. *Hospice Approaches to Paediatric Care*. New York: Springer, 1985, pp. 5–29.

22. Field, M.J. and Behrman, R.E. (eds.) When children die, improving palliative and end of life care for children and their families. *Committee on Palliative and End of Life Care for Children and their Families, Board on Health Sciences Policy*. Washington: National Academies Press, 2003, p. 208.

23. Levetown, M. Pediatric care: The in-patient/ICU perspective. In B.R. Ferrel, and N. Coyle, eds. *Textbook of Palliative Nursing*. New York: Oxford University Press, 2001, pp. 570–81.

24. Catlin, A. and Carter, B. Creation of a neonatal end of life palliative care protocol. *J Perinat* 2002;22(3):184–95.

25. Craig, F. and Goldman, A. Home management of the dying NICU patient. *Semin Neonatal* 2003;8(2):177–83.

26. Dominica, F. Helen House a hospice for children. *Mat Child Health* 1982;7:355–9.

27. Burne, S.R., Dominica, F., and Baum, J.D. Helen House—a hospice for children: Analysis of the first year. BMJ 1984;289:1665–8.

28. Editorial. On children dying well. *Lancet* 1983;April:966.

29. Chambers, T.L. Hospices for children. Editorial, *BMJ* 1987;294: 1309–10.

30. Moncrieff, M.W. Life-threatening illness and hospice care. *Arch Dis Childhood* 1990;65:468.

31. Saunders, C. In D. Clark, ed. *Cecily Saunders (Letters 1959–1999)*. Oxford: Oxford University Press, 2002, p. 192.

32. Stein, A. and Woolley, H. An evaluation of hospice care for children. In J.D. Baum, F. Dominica, and R.N. Woodward, eds. *Listen My Child Has a Lot of Living to Do*. Oxford: Oxford University Press, 1990, pp. 66–90.

33. Davies, B., Collins, J.B., Steele, R., Pipke, I., and Cook, K. The impact on families of a children's hospice programme. *J Palliat Care* 2003; 19(1):15–26.

34. Robinson, C. and Jackson, P. *Children's Hospices. A Lifeline for Families? National Children's Bureau*. London 1999.

35. Sheldon, F. and Speck, P. Children's hospices: organisational and staff issues. *Palliat Med* 2002;16:79–80.

36. A guide to the development of children's palliative care services. *Report of a Joint Working Party of the Association for Children with Life-Threatening or Terminal Conditions and their Families (ACT) and the Royal College of Paediatrics and Child Health (RCPCH)* (2nd edition), 2003, Published ACT.

37. Hynson, J.L., Gillis, J., Collins, J.J., Irving, H., and Trethewie, S.J. The dying child: How is care different. *Med J Aust* 2003;179(6):S20–22.

38. Finlay, I. and Webb, D. Paediatric palliative care: the role of an adult palliative care service. *Palliat Med* 1995;9(2):165–6.

39. McKeogh, M.M. and Evans, J.A. Paediatric palliative care: The role of an adult palliative. *Palliat Med* 1996;10:51–4.

40. National Council for Hospice and Specialist Palliative Care Services. Specialist palliative care: A statement of definitions. *National Council for Hospice and Specialist Palliative Care Services*. London, 1995.

41. Standing Medical Advisory Committee (SMAC) and Standing Nurse and Midwifery Advisory Committee. The principles and provision of palliative care. *Joint Report of SMAC and Standing Nurse and Midwifery Advisory Committee*. London, 1992.

42. A guide to the development of children's palliative care services. *Joint Working Party of the Association for Children with Life-Threatening or Terminal Conditions and their Families (ACT) and the Royal College of Paediatrics and Child Health (RCPCH)*. London: ACT/RCPCH, 1997.

43. World Health Organization (WHO), WHO Definition of Palliative Care, 1998. http://www.who.int/ cancer/palliative/definition/en/

44. Strauss, D.J., Shavelle, R.N., and Anderson, T.W. Long term survival of children and adolescents after traumatic brain injury. *Arch Phys Med Rehabil* 1998i;79:1095–1100.

45. Strauss, D.J. Life expectancy of children with cerebral palsy. *Lancet* 1988ii;349:283–4.

46. Grossman, H.J. and Eyman, R.K. Survival estimates of severely disabled children. *Paediatr Neurol* 1998;19(3):243–4.

47. Hutton, J.L., Cooke, T., and Pharoah, P.O.D. Life expectancy in children with cerebral palsy. *BMJ* 1994;309:431–5.

48. Doull, I.J. Recent advances in cystic fibrosis. *Arch Dis Childhood* 2001;85(1):62–6.

49. Stein, R.E. and Jessop, D.J. What diagnosis does not tell: The case for a non-categorical approach to chronic illness in childhood. *Soc Sci Med* 1989;29(6):769–78.

50. Kirk, S. and Glendenning, C. Supporting parents caring for a technology dependent child in the community. Research Report, National Primary Care Research and Development Centre, University of Manchester, 1999.

51. Glendenning, C., Kirk, S., Guiffrida, A., and Lawton, D. Technology dependent children in the community: Definitions, numbers and costs. *Child Care Health and Dev* 2001;27(4):321–24.

52. Stjernsward, J. and Clark, D. Palliative medicine—a global perspective. In D. Doyle, G. Hanks, N. Cherney, and K. Calman. *Oxford Textbook of Palliative Medicine*, 2003, pp. 1199–1224.

53. Seale, C. Changing patterns of death and dying. *Soc Sci Med* 2000; 51(6):917–19.

54. Alloo, F., Arizpe, L., *et al*. Bellagio declaration: Overcoming hunger in the 90s. *Lancet* 2003;362(9387):915.

55. WHO (World Health Organization). Bridging the gaps. *World Health Report*. Geneva, WHO, 1995.

56. Anonymous. The world's forgotten children. *Lancet* 2003i; 361(9351):1.

57. Anonymous. The Bellagio study group on child survival. Knowledge interaction for child survival. *Lancet* 2003ii;362:323–7.

58. Bryce, J., Arifeen, S., Pariyo, G., and Lanata, C. Reducing childhood mortality: Can public health deliver. *Lancet* 2003;362(9378):159.

59. Jones, G., Steketee, W., Black, R.W., Bhutta, Z.A., and Morris, S.S. The Bellagio study group on child survival. How many child deaths can we prevent this year. *Lancet* 2003;362:65–71.

60. Haines, A. and Smith, R. Working together to reduce poverties damage. *BMJ* 1997;314:529.

61. United Nations Development Programme. *Human Development Report*. New York: Oxford University Press, 1996.

62. United Nations Annual Human Development Report. http://www.undp.org/hdr2003/

63. Plunkett, M.C.B. and Southall, D.P. War and children. *Arch Dis Childhood* 1998;78:72–7.

64. UNICEF. *The state of the world's children*, 2004.

65. Franks, P.J., Salisbury, C., Bosanquet, N., Wilkinson, E.K., Lorentzon, M., Kite, S., *et al*. The level of need for palliative care: A systematic review of the literature. *Palliat Med* 2000;14(2):93–104.

66. Horrocks, S., Somerset, M., and Salisbury, C. Do children with non-malignant life-threatening conditions receive effective palliative care? A pragmatic evaluation of a local service. *Palliat Med* 2002;16(5):410–16.

67. Thornes, R. Working party on the care of dying children and their families: Guidelines from the British Paediatric Association. Birmingham NAHA: King Edward's Hospital Fund for London, 1998.

68. While, A., Citrone, C., and Cornish, J. A study of the needs and provisions of families caring for children with life-limiting incurable disorders. King's College London: Department of Nursing Studies, 1996.

69. Jones, R., Trenholme, A., Horsburgh, M., and Riding, A. The need for paediatric palliative care in New Zealand. *N Z Med J* 2002;115(1163):U198.

70. Field, M.J., and Behrman, R.E. (eds.) When children die: Improving palliative and end of life care for children and their families. *Committee on Palliative and End of Life Care for Children and their Families Board on Health Sciences Policy*. Washington: National Academies Press, 2003.

71. Dastgiri, S., Gilmour, W.H., and Stone, D.H. Survival of children born with congenital anomalies. *Arch Dis Childhood* 2003;88:391–4.

72. McWhirter, W.R., Dobson, C., Ring, I. Childhood cancer incidence in Australia. *Int J Cancer* 1996;65:34–8.

73. Feudtner, C., Silveira, M.J., and Christakis, D.A. Where do children with complex chronic conditions die? Patterns in Washington State 1980–1998. *Pediatrics* 2000;109(4):656–60.

74. Higginson, I.J. Children and young people who die from cancer: Epidemiology and place of death in England. *BMJ* 2003;327 (7413):478–9.

75. Nash, T. Summary report and recommendations of Department of Health Funded project for children's hospice South West. Development of a model of care for children suffering from life-limiting illness other than cancer and leukaemia and their families in the South West. University of Exeter, 1998.

76. National Health Service Executive Review of Department of Health Funded Projects for Children with Life-limiting Conditions, 1998.

77. Lenton, S., Stallard, P., Lewis, M., and Mastroyannopoulou, K. Prevalence of non-malignant life-threatening illness. *Child: Care Health and Dev* 2001;27(5):389–97.

78. ACH (2001) Joint briefing—Palliative Care for Children www.childhospice.org.UK/download/paediatricleaflet.pdf.

79. British Association for Community Child Health. Disability on childhood: Towards nationally useful definitions. British Paediatric Association, London.

80. Goldberg, D. The manual of the general health questionnaire. Windsor: Berks, 1978.

81. Mastroyannopoulou, K., Stallard, P., Lewis, M., and Lenton, S. The effects of childhood non-malignant life-threatening illness on parent health and family function. *J Child Psychol Psychiatr*, 1997; 38(7):823–9.

82. Williams, P.D. Siblings and paediatric chronic illness: A review of the literature. *Int J Nurs Studies* 1997;34(4):312–23.

2 The child's journey: Transition from health to ill-health

Jenny L. Hynson

Introduction

A distinctive feature of paediatric palliative care is the diagnostic diversity encountered within the patient population. Children die from a range of conditions [1] and unlike the patient population encountered in the palliative care of adults, it has been estimated that less than half of children with palliative care needs have a malignant condition [2]. The remainder have a range of conditions including neurodegenerative diseases, congenital anomalies, and chromosomal disorders [3]. The ways in which children move from health to ill-health are myriad but may be broadly categorised into distinct illness trajectories, each with particular implications for children and their families, the health professionals caring for them and the broader community. The transition may be abrupt or gradual and it is not always possible to identify a point at which the focus of treatment becomes exclusively palliative.

The idea that palliative care begins when curative treatment fails is outdated. The World Health Organization [4] and the American Academy of Pediatrics (AAP) [5] both now advocate an integrated model of palliative care that 'is applicable early in the course of illness, in conjunction with other therapies that are intended to prolong life'. [4] Perhaps more than their colleagues in adult medicine, paediatricians have been forced to think of an integrated approach to palliative care because of the diagnostic diversity they encounter, the often protracted nature of the many illness trajectories, and the developmental needs of children and their families. The AAP defines an integrated model of palliative care as one 'in which the components of palliative care are offered at diagnosis and continued throughout the course of the illness, whether the outcome ends in cure or death' [5,6].

A mixed model of care in which facets of palliative care and cure-oriented or life-prolonging treatment are married together is a helpful way of approaching the management of many children with life-threatening or life-limiting illnesses [7,8]. In this way, a child might participate in a Phase One trial or be placed on the list for organ transplantation while receiving optimum symptom management and support in living with uncertainty and the possibility or probability of death. The family is assisted to 'hope for the best but prepare for the worst'. One of the major challenges is balancing hope with reality but it has been demonstrated that it is possible for families to balance dual goals simultaneously [9]. Indeed, it is important for children and families to know what options are available to them so that they can make informed decisions. They need reassurance that palliative care is an active approach and that care does not end when cure is no longer possible.

Transition from health to ill-health: Illness trajectories

In the palliative care setting, children can be understood to move from health to ill-health in four distinct ways:

1. The child has a potentially curable illness but treatment fails.

2. Intensive treatment can be expected to prolong and enhance life but the child is likely to die prematurely.

3. The child is diagnosed with a progressive condition for which no curative treatment exists.

4. The child has a non-progressive condition but is vulnerable to early death as a result of general debility and complications such as respiratory infection etc. [10].

An understanding of the various ways in which children move from health to ill-health provides a foundation on which to build a flexible and responsive service system for children with palliative care needs and their families. It is important to remember however that the existence of multiple other variables means that the circumstances for each individual child and family are unique. These include the particular features of the child's condition (e.g. histology, genetic determinants, extent of disease, response to treatment etc.), the age and developmental stage of the child, the structure of the family, relationships within the family, educational background, social supports, geographic location, the health professionals involved and the service systems available. This means that for reasons that are at times unclear, two children with the same diagnosis can experience quite different outcomes.

Children and their families may make multiple transitions during the course of the same illness. The goals of care should be regularly discussed and renegotiated so that they reflect the child's changing circumstances. Take for example a 2-year old boy diagnosed with Duchenne muscular dystrophy after a delay in his gross motor development is noted. Although he is otherwise quite well, a major transition has occurred. He is no longer a well child who has taken a little longer to learn to walk. He is a boy with a life-limiting illness for which no cure exists. His parents know that early intervention will optimise his quality of life and they focus on this, hopeful that in the next few years a cure will be found. Over time, he makes the transition from being able to being disabled but he attends and enjoys school and is socially active. During adolescence, his lung function deteriorates and hospitalisations become more frequent. He becomes more and more dependent on his family for basic needs and is no longer able to attend school. During these years he becomes increasingly aware of his lack of independence and is concerned about body image and what his peers think of him. His family's hopes for a cure fade. Non-invasive ventilation is commenced but the burdens of intervention begin to outweigh the benefits and a decision is made not to progress to more invasive forms of ventilation. The transition to the terminal phase of the illness is made and therapy aimed at minimising respiratory distress initiated. Yet another transition is made when the young person dies and the family is bereaved.

Conditions for which potentially curative treatment fails

Case Frederic, aged ten, was found to have a tumour of his left frontal lobe following a generalized seizure. A diagnosis of glioblastoma multiforme was made and the family was informed that the prognosis was poor although effective surgical resection offered hope of survival. The lesion was surgically removed with good clearance. Frederic received chemotherapy and radiotherapy but

the tumour recurred a few months later and was again resected. Despite further chemotherapy, a small nodular recurrence was noted 6 months later. The family elected to participate in an investigational Phase One trial but the tumour continued to progress and the child's condition deteriorated until his death 11 months after diagnosis.

For most children with malignant conditions, cure is a probability or possibility at the time the diagnosis is made. In this situation, children and their families are dealing with a life-threatening illness and move into the treatment phase with a prospect of cure. Whatever the ultimate outcome, malignancy is a dangerous condition with the ever present possibility of death as a consequence of infection or other complications. Children and families need support in dealing with this uncertainty. This has been referred to as 'upstream palliative care' in which the seriousness of the condition is revisited and discussed at regular intervals during the child's illness [1]. Many clinicians are concerned about raising such issues when the child is relatively well but for most families such thoughts are never far away and many are grateful for an opportunity to address them. Knowing that care will continue if cure is not achieved may be very reassuring [1]. Unhappily for some, curative treatment fails and there is a clear transition to palliative treatment which may or may not include chemotherapy or radiotherapy. For others, the transition is less clear with ongoing use of experimental therapies (Figure 2.1). The transition to palliative care may come after

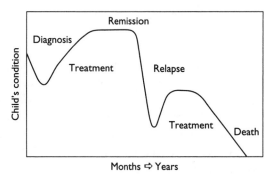

Fig. 2.1 Example of an illness trajectory for a potentially curable malignancy: early treatment causes the child's condition to deteriorate temporarily. Subsequent recovery and remission is followed by relapse. Further treatment is partially successful but the child's condition deteriorates and the child dies. (Adapted from Committee on Palliative and End-of-Life Care for Children and Their Families, Institute of Medicine (2002). In M.J. Field, R.E. Behrman, eds. *When Children Die: Improving Palliative and End-of-Life Care for Children and Their Families.* © 2003 by the National Academy of Sciences. Courtesy of the National Academies Press, Washington, D.C. Reprinted with Permission.)

years of treatment. The child may have survived a number of life-threatening complications and there may be a sense that he or she could 'pull through' again.

Conditions in which intensive treatment can be expected to prolong and enhance life but premature death is likely

Case Kylie was diagnosed with cystic fibrosis at the age of three but remained well until her tenth birthday. At that time, she began to suffer recurrent chest infections which increased in frequency and severity over the next 2 years. There was a substantial decline in her lung function over that time. Kylie spent long periods in hospital receiving intravenous antibiotics and no longer wanted to see her school friends. The option of lung transplantation was explored and her parents decided to pursue this. They asked that their daughter not be told about her prognosis. Appropriate investigations were carried out and Kylie was placed on the list of patients awaiting transplantation. She suffered recurrent episodes of severe respiratory deterioration requiring intensive care and her parents were told to prepare for her death on a number of occasions. Kylie recovered each time but became increasingly withdrawn and angry. She started refusing medications and physiotherapy. One night she confided to the nurse caring for her that she was frightened of dying but did not want to upset her parents by talking about this. The next day, the social worker met the family and helped Kylie express her fears and wishes. Her parents asked what she wanted to do and she explained that she was tired and did not want to return to intensive care. She asked to see her friends. Kylie's requests helped guide her parents and doctors in their decision-making. She died in the ward two days later.

Cystic fibrosis is a condition in which early recognition and intensive treatment significantly prolongs and enhances life (Figure 2.2). Premature death occurs, however, not infrequently during childhood or adolescence. Respiratory failure in cystic fibrosis is characterised by periods of severe deterioration which the child very often survives with the help of intravenous antibiotics and intensive chest physiotherapy. Families, health professionals, and patients are very reluctant to forego these interventions as they are perceived to pose relatively little burden with the potential benefit of a period of survival. In this way, the palliative care of a child with cystic fibrosis is quite different to that of a child with terminal cancer. There may be no clear transition to palliative care but rather a mixed approach to management as outlined earlier. Indeed, the care of children and young people with cystic fibrosis who are at the end of life has been described as an 'amalgam' of three types of care: therapeutic (e.g. intravenous antibiotics), palliative (e.g. opioids for dyspnoea), and preventive (e.g. the

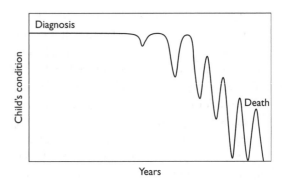

Fig. 2.2 Example of an illness trajectory for cystic fibrosis: disease-modifying treatment maintains the child's condition for a number of years. The advanced stages of disease are characterised by severe exacerbations. (Adapted from Committee on Palliative and End-of-Life Care for Children and Their Families, Institute of Medicine (2002). Reprinted with permission from M.J. Field, R.E. Behrman, eds. *When Children Die: Improving Palliative and End-of-Life Care for Children and Their Families.* © (2003) by the National Academy of Sciences. Washington DC: National Academy Press.)

continuation of enzyme replacement to prevent malabsorption) [11]. Children and young people with cystic fibrosis frequently die in the hospital setting [11]. Outdated concepts of palliative care as mutually exclusive from active therapeutic endeavours may mean important aspects of care are not adequately addressed. If health professionals wait until they are certain that death is imminent before initiating conversations with families about death and dying, this important intervention may never occur [12].

Parents and health professionals are forced to make an impossible choice when aspects of support, such as interventions directed to cure and those directed to comfort, are presented as a mutually exclusive dichotomy. [13]

One of the features of the terminal phase of cystic fibrosis is uncertainty. Episodes of acute deterioration may see the patient, their family, and the staff caring for them prepare for imminent death on numerous occasions before it actually occurs. While lung transplantation now offers hope for some sufferers of cystic fibrosis, there are numerous barriers to the success of this intervention such as strict criteria for being placed on the list, limited organ availability, and the rigours of surgery and the post-operative phase [12,14].

Progressive conditions where treatment is exclusively palliative from the time of diagnosis

Case Max, aged 4 years, fell from his bed and complained of a sore knee. There was no swelling and Max remained ambulant so his parents managed the situation expectantly. Complaints of knee pain persisted and after one week, the local doctor was consulted.

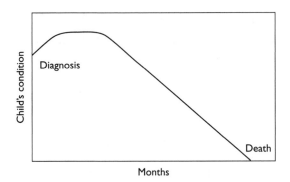

Fig. 2.3 Example of an illness trajectory for incurable cancer: palliative chemotherapy and/or radiotherapy improve the child's condition but there is a subsequent deterioration. (Adapted from Committee on Palliative and End-of-Life Care for Children and Their Families, Institute of Medicine (2002). Reprinted with permission from M.J. Field, R.E. Behrman, eds. *When Children Die: Improving Palliative and End-of-Life Care for Children and Their Families.* © (2003) by the National Academy of Sciences. Washington DC: National Academy Press.)

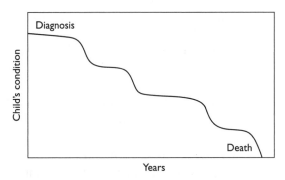

Fig. 2.4 Example of an illness trajectory for incurable neurodegenerative disease: the child is relatively well at diagnosis but slowly deteriorates. There is a stepwise progression towards death. (Adapted from Committee on Palliative and End-of-Life Care for Children and Their Families, Institute of Medicine (2002). Reprinted with permission from M.J. Field, R.E. Behrman, eds. *When Children Die: Improving Palliative and End-of-Life Care for Children and Their Families.* © (2003) by the National Academy of Sciences. Washington DC: National Academy Press.)

Examination and imaging revealed no abnormality of the knee and the family was reassured. Weeks later, following the development of pallor and weight loss, Max was diagnosed with advanced metastatic Ewing's sarcoma of the hip. There was no possibility of cure and he died at home 3 months later.

A child may be diagnosed with a condition which will be fatal within a short period of time and for which no curative treatment is available (Figure 2.3). Examples of such conditions include central nervous system tumours considered inoperable at the time of diagnosis or certain forms of solid tumour with widespread metastatic disease noted at the time of presentation. Chemotherapy or radiotherapy may be utilised as a means of controlling symptoms and increasing longevity but the child will die within months. In this way, treatment is palliative from the time of diagnosis. These children and their families must assimilate such devastating news in a short time.

The illness trajectory associated with incurable illness is not always so short. More often in children, the prognosis is one of slow deterioration over many years (Figure 2.4). Children in this group account for a substantial number of those requiring palliative care. Many have neurodegenerative conditions. Although individually rare, degenerative conditions of the central nervous system comprise a significant proportion of the patient population in paediatric palliative care. Indeed, the experience of paediatric hospices in the United Kingdom has been that children with neurodegenerative disorders comprise 41% of their patient group [15]. Patterns of deterioration and symptomatology vary according to the disease process. Care is generally provided by parents in a community setting and children may have little contact with tertiary centres. While something is known of the needs of families caring for

children with malignant conditions, relatively little attention has been paid to understanding the palliative care needs of children with neurodegenerative conditions.

Case John, aged 2 years, was still unable to walk. He was otherwise a bright and engaging child whose other developmental skills were age-appropriate. A neurologist diagnosed Duchenne muscular dystrophy and over two sessions with John's parents, described what was likely to evolve over the following years. John would learn to walk and later lose that skill such that he would be wheelchair-bound by about the age of 8 years. For a time, he would be able to attend and actively participate in school and other activities. Weakness of the upper limbs would follow and John would become increasingly dependent during his teenage years. Later, respiratory failure would occur and John would probably die in late adolescence or early adulthood.

In some circumstances children present early in life with symptoms which may not necessarily lead parents to suspect a life-threatening condition. Indeed the child may be quite well apart from developmental delay, regression, or unsteadiness. In this context, parents must learn that their child has a condition which will cause progressive neurological deterioration and ultimately death. For some, a relatively accurate prognosis may be given and information provided about the nature of the condition and the anticipated rate of decline. For others, the condition is so rare, that little information is available and the prognosis cannot be predicted with certainty. Circumstances occasionally arise in which, despite exhaustive tests, only a broad diagnosis can be made. The clinical course will guide prognosis. Children may be very well in infancy and early childhood with gradual and variable deterioration. The subsequent clinical course is often protracted with long periods of severe disability necessitating intensive nursing care. This has important implications for parents who generally assume the role of direct caregiver. Children in the later stages of neurodegenerative disease experience problems with communication, mobility, and feeding. Respiratory difficulties occur in many children secondary to reduced mobility, weakness, aspiration, and spinal deformities. Excessive secretions may also be problematic and for some patients, suctioning is required around the clock [16]. Central nervous system involvement in these conditions may result in seizures and irritability as well as an inexorable decline in intellect and communication making the assessment of symptoms very difficult.

Many children experience recurrent episodes of severe, acute deterioration which appear life-threatening. The family may be told that death is near and relatives are called to say farewell. The child then recovers. This phenomenon has been termed Lazarus Syndrome [17]. Families describe the emotions that accompany these episodes as intense and exhausting. The child could die at any time but might also live for months or even years...a situation which has been referred to as 'certain death at an unknown time' [18]. Some parents harbor a secret wish that it would all be over but feel afraid or guilty to share this with even their closest relatives and friends.

Although relatively little attention has been given in the literature to the palliative care needs of children with neurodegenerative conditions, something has been written about respiratory care in the advanced stages of conditions like Duchenne muscular dystrophy and spinal muscular atrophy. Parents are now faced with difficult decisions in these situations particularly in relation to the question of ventilatory support [19] (see also Chapter 27, Respiratory symptoms). This raises the complex interaction between children with life-limiting illnesses and medical development. As the child makes various transitions over time so too does the health care system and its capacity to offer new therapies and modes of support. In the past, boys with Duchenne muscular dystrophy and their families expected death to occur in late adolescence or early adulthood. More recently, various forms of ventilatory support have become available. Non-invasive forms of ventilation used overnight may have an important role in managing the daytime symptoms of respiratory failure thereby enhancing quality of life. More invasive or continuous forms of ventilatory support do not offer a cure for the underlying condition, but offer the prospect of increased longevity [20]. In this way, what was once an anticipated and expected transition to the terminal phase of a progressive illness has become blurred by advances in technology.

Non-progressive conditions which result in an increased susceptibility to complications and premature death

Case Lisa was diagnosed in the first year of life with infantile spasms, spastic quadriplegia, and developmental delay. At age 7, her oral intake was inadequate and a gastrostomy was placed percutaneously. At age 12, she was unable to walk and her ability to communicate was minimal. Each winter and autumn, she would be admitted frequently (at least monthly) to hospital with respiratory infections and protracted seizures. There had been numerous occasions when her parents had been asked to prepare for her imminent death. Each time, Lisa had recovered. Her father felt her quality of life was extremely poor and believed care should be limited to pain and symptom control. Her mother had seen Lisa recover from life-threatening complications and did not want to 'give up'. She believed care should include intravenous antibiotics, intubation, and ventilation.

Children with severe spastic quadriplegia are vulnerable to premature death as a result of respiratory infection or intractable seizures. Although their condition is not progressive they share many features with children who have neurodegenerative disorders including the uncertainty surrounding their prognosis. This case highlights the difficulties encountered in circumstances where the prognosis in terms of time is unclear and families are reluctant to forego interventions which have been successful in the past.

While a particular condition may be non-progressive, changing developmental needs mean that a child's quality of life may be viewed quite differently at various points in time. Similarly, the burdens and benefits of any particular intervention are measured differently according to the child's stage of development and by different people involved. Consequently, the goals of care need to be re-evaluated and renegotiated over time.

Special circumstances

Perinatal diagnosis of a fatal condition

In developed countries, birth defects constitute one of the commonest causes of neonatal death and infant mortality [1,21]. Antenatal screening and advances in diagnostic imaging and genetic testing mean that parents may be aware of a lethal congenital condition affecting their child from quite early in the pregnancy. Some families will elect to terminate the pregnancy but others will continue albeit knowing their child will die soon after birth. In the past, such abnormalities would have led to unexpected neonatal death and there has been a growing literature on the impact of this on parents, in particular on mothers. Now, parents may know that their child will die for months before this actually occurs. The sophistication of the technology which allows prenatal diagnosis has not necessarily been matched by understanding regarding the optimal way of managing such a pregnancy. While there is a paucity of medical literature to guide practice in this area, some writers have advocated a model of care for these families known as 'perinatal hospice' [22]. In this way, the fundamental principles of palliative care are applied to families who find themselves in this situation. These principles include regarding the family as the unit of care, ensuring pain and other symptoms are controlled, considering the emotional, social and spiritual elements of care, and providing support from diagnosis through death and into bereavement. Parents who elect to terminate a pregnancy after receiving a diagnosis of fetal abnormality can also be expected to benefit from ongoing care in the period leading up to and following this difficult decision.

Case A male fetus is diagnosed with megalencephaly, aqueduct stenosis, and severe hydrocephalus at 18 weeks gestation. There is evidence of only residual cortex and the prognosis is extremely poor. The family elect to continue the pregnancy and are informed that the infant will probably die in the first few days of life. Provision is made for the child to be cared for on the neonatal ward and the parents are assisted to make decisions regarding the nature of the care provided. The infant is delivered by elective Cesarean section at 37 weeks gestation and survives the first few days of life. His head circumference begins to enlarge rapidly and the insertion of a ventriculoperitoneal shunt is considered as a way of managing what is emerging as a major practical problem. The child begins experiencing episodic apnoea and the insertion of a shunt is no longer considered appropriate. The family members suddenly decide that they wish to care for him at home but no supports have been arranged. In the absence of other services and in their own time, a nurse and a doctor from the hospital visit the family at home and support them through apnoeic episodes until two days later, the infant dies. The parents feel positive about having been able to care for their child at home and are supported by family and friends during bereavement.

Effective palliative care involves anticipating potential symptoms and other eventualities and planning for these in advance. In this case, the infant survived longer than was anticipated so community supports were not established. Although the family's wishes were ultimately accommodated, there was a delay and hospital staff were required to visit the child at home some distance away. Families may feel committed to a certain plan of care early in their child's illness but often change their minds suddenly or as circumstances change. Even a short period of time at home may help parents feel that they have brought their baby home and may allow them to create important memories and spend time with family and friends. The service system requires flexibility and preparation so it can respond quickly to requests such as the one described above. This case also provides an important reminder that prognostication is an inexact science and one should prepare for both the expected and the unexpected.

Familial conditions

Case Inisha was diagnosed with renal medullary cystic disease at age five. Her younger sister was also found to have the disease. Management aimed at slowing the progression of renal insufficiency was initiated for both the girls and dialysis commenced some years later. Inisha underwent renal transplantation but suffered severe rejection. A second transplant was also complicated by rejection and the family asked that Inisha be discharged home from the intensive care unit after it became clear she was dying. She spent 12 hours at home where her sister was well-informed about and very involved in Inisha's care. A palliative care team was involved at short notice and she died peacefully. Both her doctor and family were concerned that the situation be managed carefully to enable Inisha's sister to continue her treatment and cope with the heightened awareness of the life-threatening nature of her condition.

Some families find themselves in the devastating situation of having more than one child affected by a genetically determined life-limiting condition. Little has been written on the experience of such families but their circumstance requires special mention as there are significant implications for both parents and siblings. The guilt commonly experienced by parents who have children with genetically determined conditions is compounded as are the physical, emotional, and financial burdens associated with caring for a sick and dying child. Younger siblings witness the progression of an illness that they know they have and future challenges are played out on a daily basis. Such a complex scenario requires careful management with particular attention to the principles of honesty and trust. Many familial conditions begin with subtle signs such as developmental delay, regression, or unsteadiness. Where genetic testing is unavailable, families describe watching healthy siblings intently for early signs of illness. Those able to access prenatal diagnosis face the prospect of terminating a pregnancy and the subsequent grief and guilt associated with such a difficult decision.

Organ transplantation

Organ transplantation has become an option for some children with life-threatening conditions. These include various cardiac anomalies and cystic fibrosis. While this intervention offers hope to children who would in the past have certainly died, there are no guarantees. Criteria for acceptance onto the transplant list may be narrow, donor organs may be difficult to obtain and survival rates post-transplant may be poor. Families and those caring for them are faced with the difficult task of balancing the hope of cure with the probability or possibility of death. In this way, they are asked to 'hope for the best and prepare for the worst'. Although the transition may not be clear, elements of palliative care can sit comfortably along side active efforts to pursue cure including 'listing' a child for transplant. Children and their families can be supported through the uncertainty that they face and the child's symptoms can be carefully managed. A mixed model of care, as described earlier, is an appropriate approach to this sort of a situation [7,8].

The effects of transition and the meaning of illness

Ask not what disease the person has, but rather what person the disease has. (attributed to) Sir William Osler. [23]

The experience of illness involves numerous transitions for children and their families: from healthy to sick, from person to patient, from home to hospital, from parent to 'nurse'. There are also numerous points of transition along the illness trajectory…from a worrying symptom complex to a diagnosis, from the diagnosis of a potentially curable illness to an incurable illness, from life to death. For children with neurodegenerative conditions, these transitions may be less clear and less predictable, their families live with chronic uncertainty never knowing which episode of deterioration will be the last.

The child

The transition from health to ill-health has important implications for the child, their parents, the wider family, and the community. For the child, the transition to ill-health is experienced differently at various stages of development. In addition to physical symptoms, the infant or toddler may experience separation from key attachment figures and the home environment as well as the disruption of routines. Parents of sick toddlers may also be more protective at a time when the child is needing to develop a sense of autonomy and self [24]. They often have difficulty setting and enforcing limits.

Preschoolers have distinct characteristics which impact upon their experience of illness. Their tendency to think magically may mean they view illness and procedures as punishment for wrongdoing. The development of peer relationships may be impaired by illness and the capacity to master new skills may also be compromised by pain and disability.

School-aged children develop increasing independence and become more reliant on peers for support. There may be a strong desire to be like other children. School represents a significant part of the child's life and is more than a place of learning.

Cognitive ability influences the way in which children conceptualise illness, but their understanding changes over time as they develop and acquire information and experience. Children are known to be very proactive in seeking information about their condition. In addition to the information provided by parents and health professionals, they learn from other children with similar illnesses on the ward and in the outpatient clinic and they watch the progression of disease in their peers. In this way, a 6-year-old child with a chronic illness may know more about illness and death than a healthy 9-year old. Sick and dying children have been found to have a more sophisticated understanding of their illness and prognosis than previously thought and those dying of malignant conditions have been shown to progress through five consecutive stages of understanding [25].

Stage 1	I am seriously ill
Stage 2	I am seriously ill but will get better
Stage 3	I am always ill but will get better
Stage 4	I am always ill and will not get better
Stage 5	I am dying

The final stage is characterized by a preoccupation with death in conversation and play, oppositional behaviour in relation to procedures and medication, and a reluctance to discuss events in the future.

The transition from health to ill-health occurs at the time of another important transition for the adolescent: the transition from child to adult. Serious illness has the potential to disrupt or delay some of the major developmental tasks of adolescence [26]. As well as a growing sense of autonomy, adolescents develop a greater capacity for understanding likely outcomes and are therefore able to participate more fully in decision-making. They gain a sense of future in terms of long-term relationships, child bearing, and employment and therefore come to know what it is they will lose. The experience of this loss of the future is highlighted in the following vignette.

Case Jennifer was a 13-year old with cystic fibrosis admitted for a severe exacerbation of her illness. In discussing the uncertainty over what could happen over the next while, she expressed her wishes to live long enough to achieve some of her life goals including becoming a marine biologist and having children of her own. When asked if there was anything she might like to do sooner just in case things didn't go as well as everyone hoped, Jennifer expressed her wish to hold and feed a baby. A staff member with

2 THE CHILD'S JOURNEY

a young baby agreed to help and Jennifer spent some time cuddling and feeding the infant and pictures were taken for her family. (Personal Communication: Dr. Gerri Frager, Medical Director, Pediatric Palliative Care Service, IWK Health Centre, Halifax, Nova Scotia, Canada with gratitude to the family of Jennifer Rozee.)

Illness increases the adolescent's sense of dependence at a time when they are striving to achieve independence. Consequently, they may feel a loss of control at a time when they are learning to exert control over some elements of their lives. The physical effects of illness and treatment (alopecia, amputation, weight loss or gain) occur at a time of acute awareness of body image and may be a source of great distress to the adolescent. Peer relationships may also be disrupted at a time when they are needed most and opportunities for sexual expression and experimentation may be curtailed. Rates of depression have been found to be higher in adolescents with life-threatening illness [27].

The adolescent (see Chapter 9, Adolescents and young adults) faces particular challenges when confronted with terminal illness and their needs are quite distinct from those of children and adults [28]. One of the added complexities faced by this group is the need to make the transition from paediatric to adult services. Advances in the management of conditions like cystic fibrosis mean children are now surviving into adulthood with life-limiting conditions not frequently encountered in the adult sector. Until recently, sufficient expertise has not been available within that service system and this has created a barrier to this important transition [28].

The parents

The diagnosis of fatal illness in a child strikes at the very core of what it is to be a parent. The role of parent as nurturer and protector is fundamentally challenged by the development of a condition over which they have no control.

For parents, the child's transition to ill-health may be viewed as a loss...the loss of the healthy child and all the hopes, dreams, and aspirations that go with it. In this way, much of what is experienced by families at this time may be seen as grief with all the reactions and experiences associated with this phenomenon. Families may experience shock and disbelief, confusion, anger, sadness, fear, and despair [17,29]. Some describe feeling numb or overwhelmed. When children become ill, parents very often look for some act or omission that may have caused their child's illness. They may believe that they or someone else should have recognised the problem earlier [30]. Self blame or blaming others may be a major part of the reaction. In circumstances where the condition is inherited, parents may feel directly responsible for passing the

condition on to their child. Many parents also describe fearing for the health of their other children.

As is the case with the grief that follows bereavement, the reactions of shock, denial, anger, and sadness do not occur in a predictable order. Many reactions may be present simultaneously and some that were apparent initially may fade and reappear at a later time. This is particularly true of children who relapse or suffer a marked deterioration in their condition. Reactions experienced at the time of initial diagnosis are experienced time and time again [31]. Families cope in different ways depending on the nature of the illness, their previous experience with trauma, their coping strategies, culture, social supports, and family dynamics [32].

Families need time to adjust to new information and a sudden shift in thinking should not be expected. The existence of significant discrepancies between physicians and parents in regard to prognosis has been documented [33]. In one study, the parents' understanding of the child's prognosis lagged significantly behind the physician's understanding by more than 3 months [9]. Importantly, in cases where both the physician and the parent recognised the child had little chance of cure early, elements of palliative care were more likely to be integrated into the child's care.

Parents of children with life-threatening illnesses have been described as having a variety of needs which may be broadly divided into two categories: conscious and unconscious (see Table 2.1) [29]. Unconscious needs are often more significant but are less likely to be articulated by parents. They are therefore much more difficult for staff to identify. This has significant implications for practice. Health professionals need to be aware that many of the things that concern, and in some cases preoccupy, parents remain unspoken.

Table 2.1 Parents of children with life-threatening illnesses have a variety of needs: conscious and unconscious [29].

Conscious needs	Unconscious needs
• Cope with the terminal disease	• Understand changes in family dynamics
• Cope with the child's imminent death	• Understand what is likely to occur in the final stage of the disease
• Cope with social stigma	• Describe feelings regarding funeral
• Cope with the ill child	• Discuss what home will be like after the child dies
• Prepare family members for the child's death	
• Discuss fears	

There are many other losses incurred as a consequence of illness...loss of a way of life, loss of income if one or both parents cease work, loss of friends, loss of privacy, and loss of control. Most importantly for some families, there is a loss of naivety that comes with the realisation that this is not something that happens to others. That life is not just. There is a loss of the certainty which makes daily life possible. For the child there is a loss of confidence in his or her own body. Things that were once taken for granted can no longer be. The desire for normalcy may be intense but illness brings with it the potential for significant disruption to family life and interactions. Special occasions, holidays, and daily activities are constantly threatened by the unpredictability of the child's condition.

The transition to ill-health brings significant changes to the life circumstances of the family. In one study, 73% of parents of children with a non-malignant life-threatening illness described significant effects on their employment status with at least one parent leaving work to care for the child [34]. Reduced income and increased expenditure on travel, medications, and equipment conspire to compromise the family's financial status [30]. The physical effort involved in caring for a sick and disabled child is immense and many need to learn new technical skills such as suctioning, managing nasogastric feeds, maintaining central venous lines, and even operating a ventilator. For parents who take on such 'nursing tasks' there may be a difficulty in reconciling to the role of parent as nurturer and protector and the role of nurse [35]. Many families find that they are unable to maintain regular contact with family and friends and this places them at risk of social isolation. Mothers and fathers appear to cope very differently. Mothers are more likely to be emotionally expressive. Fathers tended to withdraw and focus on practical issues and often feel a sense of helplessness [34]. The risk of mental health problems is increased among women and members of less cohesive families [34].

Families also make important transitions between care settings. Much of the early care may occur in a tertiary paediatric centre. This involves settling into a new context, meeting new people, and learning about the disease, its treatment, and the service system. Many lose confidence and feel a loss of control. Some find the acquisition of information slow and demanding. Much of it comes from other parents [36]. Later in the disease when home care becomes a priority for the child, and therefore the family, there is a shift back to what may now seem a less secure environment. Families leave a setting and group of individuals with whom they have become very familiar and secure [35]. They may feel that the health professionals caring for them are the only ones who can understand their predicament. When a family goes home, community-based staff need to be introduced and a whole new service system negotiated. Some children also move to a hospice setting thus adding another range of staff and another context to understand.

Chronic illness is always associated with an element of uncertainty and it is this aspect that many families find most difficult to cope with [18]. There may be periods of relative calm interspersed with exacerbations of illness and intense anxiety. There is always a sense that stability cannot and will not be sustained. During periods of calm, parents may be able to contain anxiety regarding prognosis but they are always waiting for the next decline. Deterioration in the child's condition upsets the delicate equilibrium and sends the family into uncertainty again. Some have likened this to living on the side of an active volcano [37]. For many children the illness trajectory is not a smooth downward trend but rather a stepwise progression towards death. Families have been found to expend much energy in maintaining the child in the best possible physical condition in an effort to avoid the next step down [18]. They grieve anew each time their child's condition deteriorates. Such anticipatory grief may mean that exhausted parents concerned about the suffering of their child are wishing it would all end. Death may come as something of a relief.

The transition to bereaved parent is associated with multiple losses...loss of the living child, loss of the future, loss of identity. Parents may however, experience other less obvious losses. They may lose a way of life and contact with significant individuals upon whom they have relied heavily for support. For some, the care of the child has required turning, suctioning, feeding, and the administration of medication around the clock. For others, there will have been long hospital stays and frequent outpatient visits. Death brings a sudden end to these tasks and leaves a vacuum many find hard to fill in the short term. Contact is lost with staff members and other parents who have seen the family through the intense highs and lows of chronic illness. Social isolation is a real risk.

Much can be said about the devastating impact that life-threatening illness has upon a family but for some there are positive aspects. Parents may find courage and skills that they had not previously recognised and many go on to support others in similar circumstances.

Case Steven, aged 15 years, sustained serious head injuries in a motor vehicle accident. He was left severely disabled. During his multiple hospital admissions, Steven experienced attitudes and practices which he believed were unhelpful and should be addressed. With the help of his doctor, he and his mother became involved in educating medical staff about how patients experience interactions with their doctors. His mother commented that she would never have imagined herself in such a role prior to the accident and had discovered a previously unrecognized strength of personality.

Some children and families are able to make meaning out of their situation and view it as an opportunity for personal growth [18]. They talk of meeting people, learning things, and achieving goals that they could not have achieved if their child had not become ill. For others there is a sense that they have been able to appreciate their child's life in a way they may not have done if they had not been faced with fatal illness. They talk of saying things and doing things which families without such pressures do not. While much has been written about the negative impact of chronic illness on family relationships, some families find their relationships strengthened by the adversity they face [30]. Parents have described having a greater appreciation of life and a better understanding of what is really important as a consequence of their child's illness and death. For some there is a sense that they have survived the very worst that life can offer [38]. Grief is a normal human reaction and although the death of a child represents a profound loss, the achievements of surviving family members may effect positive social changes through advocacy and the fruits of individual careers [39].

The siblings

The siblings of an ill child also experience loss and grief. Their sick brother or sister and their parents may become physically and emotionally unavailable to them for long periods. Life as they knew it is changed forever. Siblings who are not adequately informed and included may misunderstand the nature of the illness and its treatment [40]. This may cause them to fear for their own health and the health of others. Siblings frequently experience anxiety and social isolation [41]. They may feel different or even embarrassed as a result of their brother's or sister's illness. They may also feel jealous of the attention the sick child receives and then feel guilty about having such negative feelings. Very often they are torn between friends and family. Siblings often feel unable to share their concerns with already burdened parents and may express their distress indirectly. Developmental regression, academic failure, and social withdrawal may be signs of difficulty [31,42].

The health professional

Supporting a child through a lengthy illness can be physically and emotionally exhausting for parents as they lurch from one crisis to another, never knowing which deterioration will be the last. Chronic illness can also take its toll on health professionals and burnout is a possibility. Families sometimes fear abandonment and the steadfast and supportive presence of a familiar team can provide a sense of security in such uncertain times. The fear of abandonment is very real. The death of a child is a relatively unusual event and the modern paediatrician is more familiar with cure and prevention than with death and dying. While advances in medicine have led to happier outcomes for the majority of children, there remains a group for whom cure is impossible. The relative infrequency with which death occurs in childhood has implications for those caring for this group of children. Health professionals may feel a sense of failure and impotence. A lack of exposure to dying children may also leave them feeling ill-equipped to support a child and family through this phase of their care. Particular challenges can arise when children and families 'hit out' at members of the team caring for them. It is important to understand that episodes of aggression and anger are usually not personal. Indeed, the capacity of the family to ventilate negative emotions may reflect the safety of the therapeutic environment in which they find themselves. Doctors, nurses, and allied health professionals may also become very attached to the child and family and experience their own grief. All of these responses are normal but in the absence of adequate self-awareness and support, health professionals may, over time, become 'burnt out'.

Burnout is 'the progressive loss of idealism, energy and purpose experienced by people in the helping professions as a result of the conditions of their work' [43]. This may manifest as excessive cynicism, a loss of interest in work, and a sense of 'going through the motions' [44]. Other features include fatigue, difficulty concentrating, depression, anxiety, insomnia, irritability and the inappropriate use of drugs or alcohol. The consequences for families are significant as staff affected in this way may:

- avoid families or blame them for difficult situations
- be unable to help families define treatment goals and make optimal decisions
- experience physical signs of stress when seeing families.

The quality of care may be compromised and families may become disenchanted with the health professional and seek help elsewhere, sometimes from inappropriate sources.

Supporting children and families through transition

A key function of the health professional is to offer ongoing support through all the phases of the child's illness and all the transitions that the family makes. Reliability and dependability are highly valued by families experiencing such immense change.

Information

Children are endlessly curious and filled with wonder about things great and small. How remarkable it would be if their wonder and curiosity were to halt abruptly only when they were terminally ill.[45]

When faced with a crisis, an almost intuitive human response is to try and better understand one's situation. Children seek information just as adults do but they may be protected from 'bad news' by those around them. Through the work of Bluebond-Langner and others it has become clear that even quite young children very often know a great deal about their illness and its prognosis even when parents and staff go to great lengths to conceal such information [25,46,47]. They may not reveal what they know however, for fear of upsetting their parents. The anxiety generated by misinformation is potentially more harmful than any arising from the truth. Children may have all sorts of fantasies and worries, many of which an adult might not expect. Information presented in a developmentally appropriate way and at a pace determined by the child has the potential to reduce misunderstandings and feelings of isolation.

The amount of information desired by parents varies, but in general, they appreciate honest, accurate information presented in a sympathetic way. Information allows them to understand their situation better but it needs to be presented carefully and at a pace determined by them so as not to over-whelm a shocked and potentially disbelieving family. Repeating information on a number of occasions, writing it down, and even recording it can be helpful as can having a family member or friend present. Opportunities to ask questions and explore certain aspects in more detail are invaluable. Time invested in generating a trusting relationship early in the illness creates a solid foundation on which to face the challenges of palliative care later. Many parents will access a range of resources to better understand their child's condition. These might include books, journals, and information available through the internet. Some of this will be accurate and helpful, some will be confronting, and some will be inaccurate. Families may need help in sorting through what can be a vast array of information.

Parents often talk of losing control of their lives. Providing families with information, including them in case conferences, and viewing them as key partners in the child's care help to increase their sense of control [48].

It is important to be aware that what parents are able to articulate as their needs represents only a small proportion of what is really concerning them. Awareness of some of the unconscious needs described earlier allows health professionals to proactively address them with families where appropriate. Framing questions in ways that normalise negative feelings can help put parents at ease. For example, 'Some parents have told me they worry a lot about what will happen close to the time of death but feel they shouldn't be thinking of such things. Have you had any of those sorts of worries and is there anything you would like to ask me?'

Parents might also seek guidance as to how best to support their child and how they should inform siblings and other members of the family.

For many parents, key information and support comes from other parents who have lived through what they are currently experiencing. Likewise, older children may find sharing experiences with peers comforting and helpful. Health professionals involved in supporting families should make themselves aware of the various support groups and agencies in their local community so that they can make this information available to families.

Consider the impact on siblings and broader family

In a hospital setting, health professionals are very aware of the needs of the unwell child and their parents. It is easy to forget the other, less visible, members of the family who may be equally affected by the development of serious illness in the child. Siblings and grandparents often benefit from an opportunity to ask questions of medical and nursing staff and this simple intervention may avoid misunderstandings at home.

Listen

As families struggle to make sense of a world gone awry, they may wish to spend time sharing their concerns, fears, hopes, and expectations. Doctors, nurses, and social workers often feel families expect them to be wise and to 'fix the problem'. Health professionals may also expect this of themselves. Parents would obviously wish that someone could cure their child but most know the reality and what they seek is support. Health professionals may feel that they have nothing to offer if they can't cure an illness or solve a difficult situation. On the contrary, by listening to the concerns of parents, providing guidance, affirming their skills and resources, and staying with them through it all, health professionals can make a major difference to how a family copes.

Home care

Minimizing time spent in hospital reduces the stress placed on a family at the time of transition. Many describe the overall experience of caring for their child at home as a positive one [49,50]. In the familiar and private surrounds of home, children and parents feel more in control and are subject to fewer interruptions and intrusions [35,51]. Parents are better able to attend to the needs of siblings, and friends and family may be more accessible. Encouraging and facilitating family outings, holidays, and ongoing attendance at school (e.g. by sensitively timing admissions and treatments) can also be helpful. One of the central tenets of palliative care is affirming life...encouraging life to go on. While home care is desirable for many families, it is important to remember that this is not true for all. Some children and families feel safer in a hospital environment.

School

The school environment represents a significant part of a child's life. Interventions aimed at supporting the child's return to school can significantly enhance the child's ability to participate in school activities and maintain social relationships. Helpful interventions include renegotiating the goals of school attendance, working with and informing the child's teacher (with the family's permission), and providing a clear plan for emergencies. Children unable to attend school might benefit from ongoing contact with peers through email, home visits, and telephone conversations. School attendance is also very important for siblings. It provides a point of relative constancy and predictability in a world disrupted by change.

Spirituality

There is more to spirituality than religion. Indeed, it has been said that 'all human beings are essentially spiritual' [52]. Spirituality has been described as 'relating to the search for existential meaning within any life experience' [53]. Assisting a family to find meaning in what might seem a tragic and unjust situation may enhance their capacity to manage the many transitions they face. This might involve providing access to pastoral care workers, exploring the spiritual dimensions of patients, and encouraging families to seek out spiritual leaders and resources. Health professionals who care for dying children and their families may also need spiritual support.

Planning and coordination

Families very often move between care settings such as home, hospital, and hospice. In each setting, families interface with a number of individuals from a range of disciplines and there is the potential for intrusion, confusion, and unnecessary replication of services. The transition between places of care and the coordination of the individuals and many agencies involved may be facilitated by the early inclusion of community-based care providers and the appointment of a key worker. This individual might be a general practitioner, a paediatrician, a nurse, or a social worker [54]. Medical care management is important in its own right as children with long illness trajectories often have a range of subspecialists involved in their care. It is important that one of these individuals take overall responsibility for the care of the child to ensure that families are not exposed to a range of conflicting and confusing opinions. Regular communication between those involved is essential.

A proactive approach to care planning may avoid families lurching from one crisis to another [13,55]. Anticipating the development or exacerbation of symptoms allows decisions and plans for treatment to be made ahead of time. Families feel more secure if they know who to call or where to go. Discussions with families about these issues necessarily includes informing them about what is likely to happen and helping them make decisions regarding the extent and nature of the care to be provided.

Care into bereavement

The time at which the child dies represents a major point of transition for the family. Depending on their circumstances, families may feel anything from relief to overwhelming sadness. Much of their life has been invested in the care of the child and the time of death can mean the end of a way of life. Families who have spent long periods in the hospital leave behind staff members and other families who have formed an important source of social contact and support. The various tasks involved in caring for a sick and dependent child suddenly cease. Some parents find themselves socially isolated and unoccupied. Continuity of care at this time can be very important and is achieved by offering the family a follow-up appointment with the doctor and an opportunity to visit the staff on the ward. Recognition of anniversaries is also important.

Research

Families seek and benefit from accurate information regarding their child's prognosis. They describe uncertainty as one of the most difficult aspects they have to cope with and yet, in most circumstances, prognostication remains an inexact and inadequate science. To date, efforts to enhance our capacity to predict with certainty a particular child's outcome, have met with meager rewards. Data collection, research, and collective thinking are required to better understand the various illness trajectories and clinical indicators of physical decline.

Conclusion

Children with life-threatening or life-limiting conditions make the transition from health to ill-health in a variety of ways. This transition may be sudden or gradual and although the various illness trajectories can be broadly categorised, other variables mean that the individual circumstances for each child and family are unique. Furthermore, children and families make multiple transitions during the same illness: from a child with a symptom complex to a child with a diagnosis; from a child with a potentially curable illness to a child with an incurable and fatal illness; from life to death. The impact of illness is such that children must make the transition from person to patient, home to hospital, and able to disabled. Their body image changes too and this may be of special concern to older children and adolescents. Parents are also forced to make transitions. Fatal illness strikes at the very core of what it is to be a parent. The 'protector' and 'nurturer' must witness the ravages of a disease they cannot control. In order to fulfil their child's wish to be at home, parents may need to take on what they see as 'nursing tasks' which may conflict directly with their role as a parent. Their social, financial, and employment status may change significantly. Parents are thrust into a new world in which they must meet new people and learn about the disease, its treatment, and the service system. Much of what is experienced by these children and their families can be viewed as grief in response to a series of losses. For some however, there are significant gains. They uncover personal strengths they did not know they had and are able to appreciate their child's life at a level others do not. The health professional caring for families in these circumstances also has an opportunity to make an important transition as the following account describes.

In my office adjacent to the medical intensive care unit, I have a growing file of letters from relatives of patients we have treated, thanking us for our care. But the majority of these letters are not from families of patients who survived. Rather, most come from people who have lost a loved one, from the bereaved survivors of patients who died in our intensive care unit (ICU). Yet they are deeply grateful for what we did. At first, I found these letters ironic and odd. I expected and basked in appreciation for lives saved. But the ones about lives we could not save—those I had trouble understanding. I read the letters over and over, wondering what the writers meant to me ... Saving deaths, I have come to realize, is as important and rewarding as saving lives. [56]

The face of paediatrics is changing. Many previously fatal conditions of childhood can now be either prevented or cured. However, advances in technology also mean that children who once died early of congenital anomalies and other conditions now live for longer periods in high states of dependency. Much of the early thinking in paediatric palliative care has focused on children with malignancies but the patient group encountered in paediatric palliative care is far more diverse than this. This diagnostic diversity and the prognostic uncertainty encountered in paediatric palliative care means that an integrated approach is required.

There is more to palliative care than terminal care. Many of the principles and fundamental tenets of palliative care can be applied early in the course of chronic conditions to help families live better with a fatal disease. Opportunities for professional development and liaison with experienced palliative care providers can assist paediatric health professionals who deal with children and parents at various points in the illness trajectory so that the experience of care is improved for all concerned. The early establishment of effective communication, trust, and a supportive therapeutic environment inclusive of community providers facilitates effective palliative care later on. A key function of the health professional is to offer ongoing support through all the phases of the child's illness and all the transitions that the family makes. Reliability and dependability are highly valued by families experiencing such immense change.

References

1. Committee on Palliative and End-of-Life Care for Children and Their Families, Institute of Medicine. In M.J. Field, and R.E. Behrman, eds. *When Children Die: Improving Palliative and End-of-Life Care for Children and Their Families.* Washington, DC: National Academy Press, 2002.

2. Jones, R., Trenholme, A., Horsburgh, M., and Riding, A. The need for paediatric palliative care in New Zealand. *N Z Med J* 2002;Oct 11:115(1163):U198.

3. Association for Children with Life Threatening or Terminal Conditions and their Families and the Royal College of Paediatrics and Child Health. A guide to the development of children's palliative care services. London: Association for Children with Life Threatening or Terminal Conditions and their Families, 1997.

4. National Cancer Control Programs. Policies and Managerial Guidelines (2nd edition). Geneva: World Health Organization, 2002.

5. American Academy of Pediatrics. Palliative care for children. *Pediatr* 2000;106:351–7.

6. Frager, G. Palliative care and terminal care of children. *Child Adolesc Psychiatr Clin N Am* 1997;6:889–909.

7. Glare, P. and Virik, K. Can we do better in end of life care? The mixed management model and palliative care. *Med J Aust* 2001;175:530–6.

8. Committee on Care at the End of Life, Institute of Medicine. In M.J. Field, and C.K. Cassel, eds. *Approaching Death: Improving Care at the End of Life.* Washington, DC: National Academy Press, 1997.

9. Wolfe, J., Klar, N., Grier, H.E., *et al.* Understanding of prognosis among parents of children who died of cancer. *JAMA* 2000; 284:2469–75.

10. Goldman, A. ABC of palliative care: Special problems of children. *BMJ* 1998;316:49–52.

11. Robinson, W.M., Ravilly, S., Berde, C., and Wohl, M. End-of-life care in cystic fibrosis. *Pediatrics* 1997;100:205–9.

12. Mitchell, I., Nakielna, E., Tullis, E., and Adair, C. Cystic fibrosis: End-stage care in Canada. *Chest* 2000;118:80–4.

13. Frager, G. Pediatric palliative care: Building the model, bridging the gaps. *J Palliat Care* 1996;12:9–12.

14. Warner, J.O. Heart-lung transplantation: All the facts. *Arch Dis Child* 1991;66:1013–17.

15. Hunt, A. and Burne, R. Medical and nursing problems of children with neurodegenerative disease. *Palliat Med* 1995;9:19–26.

16. Hunt, A.M. A survey of signs, symptoms and symptom control in 30 terminally ill children. *Dev Med Child Neurol* 1990;32:341–6.

17. Stevens, M.M. Care of the dying child and adolescent: Family adjustment and support. In D. Doyle, G.W.C. Hanks, and N. MacDonald, eds. *Oxford Textbook of Palliative Medicine* (2nd edition) Oxford: Oxford University Press, 1998.

18. Steele, R.G. Trajectory of certain death at an unknown time: Children with neurodegenerative life-threatening illnesses. *Canadian J Nurs Research* 2000;32:49–67.

19. Miller, J.R., Colbert, A.P., and Osberg, J.S. Ventilator dependency: Decision-making, daily functioning and quality of life for patients with Duchenne muscular dystrophy. *Dev Med Child Neurol* 1990;32:1078–86.

20. Hilton, T., Orr, R.D., Perkin, R.M., and Ashwal, S. End of life care in Duchenne muscular dystrophy. *Pediatr Neurol* 1993;9:165–77.

21. The Consultative Council on Obstetric and Paediatric Mortality and Morbidity. Annual report for the year 1999, incorporating the 38th survey of perinatal deaths in Victoria. Melbourne (Australia), 2001.

22. Hoeldtke, N.J. and Calhoun, B.C. Perinatal hospice. *Am J Obstet Gynecol* 2001;185:525–9.

23. Sachs, O. *An anthropologist on Mars.* New York: Knopf, 1995.

24. Perrin, E.C. and Gerrity, P.S. Development of children with a chronic illness. *Pediatr Clin North Am* 1984;31:19–31.

25. Bluebond-Langner, M. *The Private Worlds of Dying Children.* Princeton, NJ: Princeton University Press, 1978.

26. Carr-Gregg, M.R.C., Sawyer, S.M., Clarke, C.F., and Bowes, G. Caring for the terminally ill adolescent. *Med JAust* 1997;166:255–8.

27. Kashani, J. and Hakami, N. Depression in children and adolescents with malignancy. *Can J Psychiatry* 1988;227:474–7.

28. Joint Working Party on Palliative Care for Adolescents and Young Adults, Association for Children with Life-threatening or Terminal Conditions and their Families. In Elston S, editor. *Palliative care for young people aged 13–24.* National Council for Hospice and Specialist Palliative Care Services: Scottish Partnership Agency for Palliative and Cancer Care: United Kingdom; 2001.

29. Jefidoff, A. and Gasner, R. Helping the parents of the dying child: An Israeli experience. *J Pediatr Nurs* 1993;8:413–5.

30. Sloper, P. Needs and responses of parents following the diagnosis of childhood cancer. *Child Health Care Dev* 1996;22:187–202.

31. Sabbeth, B. Understanding the impact of chronic childhood illness on families. *Pediatr Clin North Am* 1984;31:47–57.

32. Barakat, L.P., Sills, R., and La Bagnara, S. Management of fatal illness and death in children or their parents. *Pediatr Rev* 1995;16:419–23.

33. Mulhern, R.K., Crisco, J.J., and Camitta, B.M. Patterns of communication among pediatric patients with leukemia, parents, and physicians: Prognostic disagreements and misunderstandings. *J Pediatr* 1981;99:480–3.

34. Mastroyannopoulou, K., Stallard, P., and Lewis, M., and Lenton, S. The impact of childhood non-malignant life-threatening illness on parents: Gender differences and predictors of parental adjustment. *J Child Psychol Psychiatr* 1997;38:823–9.

35. Darbyshire, P., Haller, A., and Fleming, S. 'The Interstellar Cold'. Parents' experiences of their child's palliative care. Report prepared for the South Australian Health Commission, Palliative Care Program—Statewide Projects. Adelaide (Australia), 1997.

36. Sach, S. When a child dies. In *Caring for Children with Life-Threatening Conditions.* Palliative Care Service Development Series, Department of Human Services, Victoria: Melbourne Australia, 1997.

37. Kleinman, A. *The illness narratives: Suffering, healing and the human condition.* New York: Basic Books, 1988.

38. Wheeler, I. Parental bereavement: The crisis of meaning. *Death Stud* 2001;25:51–66.

39. Kellehear, A. Grief and loss: Past, present and future. *Med J Aust* 2002;177:176–7.

40. Cairns, N.U., Clark, G.M., Smith, S.D., and Lansky, S.B. Adaptation of siblings to childhood malignancy. *J Pediatr* 1979;95:484–7.

41. Stallard, P., Mastroyannopoulou, K., Lewis, M., and Lenton, S. The siblings of children with life-threatening conditions. *Child Psychol Psychiatr Rev* 1997;2:26–33.

42. Sourkes, B.M. Siblings of the pediatric cancer patient. In J. Kellerman, ed. *Psychological aspects of childhood cancer.* Springfield (USA): C.C. Thomas, 1980.

43. Edelwich, J., and Brodsky, A. *Burn-out: Stages of disillusionment in the helping professions.* Springer: New York, 1980.

44. Stein, A., and Woolley, H. An evaluation of hospice care for children. In J.D. Baum, F. Dominica, R.N. Woodward, ed. *Listen My Child Has a Lot of Living To Do.* Oxford: Oxford University Press; 1990.

45. Attig, T. Beyond pain: The existential suffering of children. *J Pall Care* 1996;12:20–3.

46. Waechter, E.H. Children's awareness of fatal illness. *Am J Nurs* 1971;71:1168–72.

47. Clunies-Ross, C. and Lansdown, R. Concepts of death, illness and isolation found in children with leukaemia. *Child Health Care Dev* 1988;14:373–86.

48. Contro, N., Larson, J., Scofield, S., Sourkes, B., and Cohen, H. Family perspectives on the quality of pediatric palliative care. *Arch Pediatr Adolesc Med* 2002;156:14–19.

49. Sirkia, K., Saarinen, U.M., Ahlgren, B., and Hovi, L. Terminal care of the child with cancer at home. *Acta Paediatr* 1997;86:1125–30.

50. Lauer, M.E., and Camitta, B.M. Home care for dying children: A nursing model. *J Pediatr* 1980;97:1032–5.

51. Vickers, J.L. and Carlisle, C. Choices and control: Parental experiences in paediatric terminal home care. *J Pediatr Oncol Nurs* 2000;17:12–21.

52. Sneiders, S.M. *New Dictionary of Theology.* Dublin: Gill and MacMillan; 1987.

53. Speck, P.W. Spiritual issues in palliative care. In D. Doyle, G.W.C. Hanks, N. MacDonald, eds. *Oxford Textbook of Palliative Care.* Oxford: Oxford University Press, 1993.

54. Woolley, H., Stein, A., Forrest, G.C., and Baum, J.D. Cornerstone care for families of children with life-threatening illness. *Dev Med Child Neurol* 1991;33:216–24.

55. Ashby, M.A., Kosky, R.J., Laver H.T., *et al.* An enquiry into death and dying at the Adelaide Children's Hospital: A useful model? *Med J Aust* 1991;154:165–70.

56. Nelson, J.E. Saving lives and saving deaths. *Ann Intern Med* 1999;130:776–7.

3 Communication

Gwynneth Down and Jean Simons

An understanding of the concept of paediatric palliative care may be familiar to readers with a specific clinical background or personal interest. Such understanding may not however, be shared by all health care professionals, and we therefore wish to define the territory being described in this chapter with the following:

Palliative care for children and young people with life limiting conditions is an active and total approach to care embracing physical, emotional, social and spiritual elements. It focuses on enhancement of quality of life for the child and support for the family and includes the management of distressing symptoms, provision of respite and care through death and bereavement. [1]

This definition, formulated a decade ago refocuses away from a purely clinical care model to a promotion of patient centred, family needs led, joined up care; the values now promoted in the modernising culture within the National Health Service (NHS) and incorporated into the Children's National Service Framework [2]. For these values to be translated into practice, professionals need to find ways of working with children and families that transcend traditional models of biomedical care. Embracing the psychological, social, and spiritual aspects of their experience requires a focus both on the relationship between professionals and families, and on the skills and attitudes needed. In this chapter then, we will focus on various aspects of communication between children with life limiting conditions, their families, and health care providers. We will suggest that the skills that professionals need when caring for a family in the terminal phases of illness are an extension of those needed for caring for all ill children and thus important for professionals in all fields of health care.

What is meant by communication?

Communication between patients, families and health care professionals has received significant attention in the professional literature. It has been suggested that important patient outcomes such as adherence to treatment, patient knowledge, physical functioning, satisfaction, and health status are all influenced by doctor–patient communication [3–7]. Psychological adjustment and quality of life may also be profoundly affected by communication between health care professionals, patients and relatives [8].

The term 'communication', as used in relation to professionals and families in health care, is often associated with specific points on the patient journey such as 'breaking bad news', or 'obtaining informed consent'. That is, communication is seen as task oriented and often centred on biomedical concerns, rather than as an opportunity for the exploration of psychosocial and emotional issues.

In paediatric palliative care, however, there is a strong emphasis on all aspects of communication with the ill child; the child's understanding of illness and death, what the child is told about the type of illness, or prognosis, whether they are enabled to explore their concerns and worries, and whether the child and family are able to communicate openly about these issues [9–11]. Communication *within* families facing illness has, however, traditionally been assumed to be the domain of psychotherapeutically trained professions, rather than that of other health care disciplines. Within family therapy and other psychological fields, there is a growing body of literature about families and illness [12–14]. This encompasses both the practical, social, financial, and relational *impact* of illness on families, and the ways in which families may act as a *resource* to the ill person and to each other, both in practical and emotional domains. There has been a marked change in emphasis in this literature from potential causes of adverse outcomes in children and families to which factors promote resilience in the face of adversity [12,15].

Relationships between health care providers and families as a context for communication

Policy and practice in the United Kingdom

Both from within the health care field and on a governmental policy level, relationships between patients and providers have been undergoing scrutiny and culture change. There is a move to change from a service provision orientation to a focus on a user led service, and to rebalance the traditional patriarchal model of health care, in favour of 'partnership' with patients and families [16]. The expertise of patients is being recognised as a cornerstone of government policy for management of chronic illness; an important context for recognising the expertise both of young people with prolonged illness and parents in the case of the young child patient [2].

Changing culture and focus in favour of service users clearly requires different types of involvement: 'Patients must be at the centre of the NHS, and thus the patient's perspective must be included in the policies, planning, and delivery of services at every level' [17]. The need to consult with children and young people and to provide them with 'an opportunity to influence decisions and policies' has also been recognised [18]. However, it is important to note that currently much of the work on consultation with young people focuses on the views of well children about potential health care provision.

Models of care in both paediatric medicine and nursing have evolved in accordance with the culture change in health care. There is some evidence that these models have diverged in their emphasis, with that of medical literature being on 'patient centred medicine' [19], and that of nursing on 'family focused' care [20]. As Doherty [21] has suggested, however, 'every individual patient intervention in health care is simult- aneously a family intervention' (p. 131). This is particularly true in paediatric palliative care, where the quality of relationships within each dyad of child, siblings, parents, and professionals will reciprocally affect the others [22]. There is then a strong argument for using family centred approaches to paediatric palliative care [23].

However, despite the changing rhetoric in the NHS [24] communications at all levels in the health service have been critically scrutinised in recent years as a result of service failings. Major inquiries with particular relevance to paedi- atrics. The Redfern report [25], and the Climbie Inquiry [26] have, all, within their own contexts, reported systemic commun- ication failures within health care settings. Communication difficulties between health care professionals and patients

and families were particularly highlighted in the first two reports, which focused on particular specialist paediatric settings, but were acknowledged to represent issues across the NHS.

The widespread nature of these problems is also con- firmed by evidence from parents and patients in the fields of disability and palliative care. This consistently reveals gaping inadequacies in the basic provision of services, in 'joined up' working, and in the required level of psychosocial and emo- tional support and communication which families say they need. Voices for Change [18], quotes a parent of a child receiv- ing palliative care 'It feels like I am fighting a battle all by myself without any training or preparation for this. I sometimes feel like screaming, but no one would listen anyway . . .'

That parents and patients have found a say at all is often through the work of voluntary agencies, especially the condition-specific support groups or charities. Sadly, qualitative 'evidence' of this type has often been dismissed as 'merely anecdotal' and therefore less reliable, so that govern- ment policy and the attitude of many health care professionals have been slow to recognise a widespread need.

Parent to parent support, especially in the area of paediatric palliative care and bereavement support, has increasingly confirmed dissatisfaction with the availability or quality of professionally led services. Self-help or parent led services such as the Child Death Help Line, Compassionate Friends or the FSID befriending scheme are examples of families' need for empathic mutual support and communica- tion with others who have experienced a similar situation for themselves. These services represent a positive choice for parent to parent volunteer support, separate from professionally delivered, clinical model, counselling. Condition-specific support groups often accessed through umbrella organisa- tions such as ACT or Contact a Family, provide a family needs led service through the provision of specific information or help lines. Other support services exist for children and young people to derive support directly from one another—usually led by professionals or adult volunteers, such as Winston's Wish for bereaved children.

Relationships in the care domain

In the field of psychotherapy, the quality of relationship between therapist and client has consistently been found to outweigh the relative benefits of model-specific techniques or skills, for positive outcome. It is not a surprise then, that the quality of relationships between families and professionals is also central to the experience of living with a chronic illness [27]. Positive relationships may provide hope, physical and emotional support and contribute to family resilience [28–30].

Positive relationships may be achieved by the development of certain skills and attitudes. Knafl *et al.* [28] suggested that although parents valued the expertise and technical behaviours of professionals, they placed more emphasis on interactional skills. While they needed and valued the expertise of professionals, this was best communicated in a compassionate and respectful manner. Professionals who were able to develop the parents confidence *and* interact effectively with the ill child were also seen as particularly helpful. By contrast, Hunt *et al.* [18] found that parents perceived lack of understanding or empathy on the part of health care professionals as a real barrier to providing care for their children. Some parents felt that staff may actually be unwilling to empathise with their situation, thus leaving them feeling less supported in the most difficult times that families may have to experience.

Maguire [31] notes that 'most doctors and nurses . . . have been alerted to the importance of giving psychological support and alleviating psychological distress yet they will not be able to do this unless they can first establish a dialogue (engage with) patients and identify their true concerns'. His work has consistently shown that health professionals avoid eliciting patient's emotional reactions and views of their current situation for fear of opening up areas that they feel unable to help with [32]. Many doctors and nurses fear that if they 'clarified how a dying patient was feeling they could unleash strong emotions like despair and anger that they could not contain' and 'to seek psychological problems by active enquiry might overload them . . .'. Maguire concluded [33] that the cost of engaging emotionally with a child or family, often without appropriate support within their own work context, might make professionals fearful for their own psychological survival.

Professionals commonly use a variety of 'distancing tactics' with patients, which serve a consistent and important function of (self) protection from the impact of the work. These 'tactics' may be outside of their awareness, but will be picked up by patients and families. Work by Heaven and Maguire [34] showed that adult hospice patients revealed a greater or lesser degree of information about their psychological concerns to nurses whom they perceived as stronger or less fragile as opposed to those who they saw as 'vulnerable'. These 'serious barriers have to be overcome if communication is to be effective' [31]. This is a crucial point; it is often incorrectly assumed that being aware of what is needed and drawing up a practice standard or guideline will somehow enable the job to be done, without commensurate training and support for the carer's competence.

Therefore, in order for staff to engage with the pain and difficulties that families experience when a child has a life-threatening illness, they also need to feel supported emotionally (and their work valued). This may be achieved in many ways, including regular supervision, 'debriefing meetings', and working in dedicated multidisciplinary teams. Whichever way support is provided, it is crucial that all staff recognise the impact of the work on themselves and each other and do not perceive the need for support as a weakness, but as an integral part of the work of the multidisciplinary team.

Patient and family relationship to professionals

Consideration of *only* the professional issues that influence positive relationships does not, of course, address the reciprocity of influences from *both* professionals and families. Family members will have their own history of relationships with authority figures, beliefs about the involvement of others in 'family business', and patterns of boundaries that allow for more or less connection with professionals.

As children develop, families naturally have to allow their boundaries to be more flexible and permeable, allowing for others (such as teachers, or children's friends), to come and go, bringing in new information. When a child becomes ill, the family boundaries may have to become very permeable indeed, to accommodate physical and emotional involvement, and often personal disclosures and evaluations [32]. In chronic illness and in the later stages of palliative care, the family may have to struggle to keep a sense of their integrity, whilst allowing professionals to be involved in appropriate levels of care and support.

Friedson [36] wrote that the 'differing perspectives' of the partners (to the interaction) must be taken into account and it must be noted that '. . . the doctor and patient come from different worlds—those of the professional and the layman— which possess divergent values and beliefs'. Friedson was somewhat ahead of his time when he acknowledged the importance of examining '. . . the dynamics of interpersonal relationships; it is also important to look at roles within their social context and to take into account the influence of extraneous social and other variables . . .'

Thorne and Robinson [18] conducted multiple interviews with families having either an adult or child with a chronic illness. Their results suggested that relationships with health care professionals evolve through three stages that they named 'naive trust, disenchantment and guarded alliance'. In the first phase of the chronic illness, families described believing that professionals would share their own perspectives and experiences of the illness. They implicitly trusted that 'all health care professionals would act in what the family viewed as the sick member's best interests, and they waited passively for this to happen' ([18], p. 297). However, in retrospect, all the families felt these were naive assumptions. Their own expectations of what was in the sick person's best interest conflicted with that of professionals, and they often felt that their own knowledge and experience was disregarded. In the 'disenchantment' stage the families often became more assertive or aggressive in their attempts to influence the care provided and their fear, frustration and dissatisfaction was often expressed as anger. This adversarial position is very difficult to sustain because of the need for a working relationship with professionals. Consequently, there was another phase of relationship, named as 'guarded alliance' in which trust was rebuilt 'on an informed, rather than naive, level and enabled cooperative caring that accommodated both the family perspective and the professional medical perspective' ([18], p. 298).

Being aware of the family's previous experiences of health care and relationships with providers can promote understanding and encourage a different response to their anger and distress. While this can also be comprehended (often rightly) as part of necessary emotional adjustment, or even a normal grieving process, it could also be taken as an invitation to professionals to consider their own roles in relation to the family. In order to work in partnership with patients or to provide family centred care, it is necessary first to ascertain and understand families' values and expectations. Wherever possible, care should then be provided according to child and family values, rather than those of the professionals or institutions.

The family and communication

Using the term 'family' may suggest that all of the individuals within it will have the same views and feelings, which of course is often not true. Being able to engage with all family members and recognise their individual needs is a skill that many professionals need to develop. However, the needs of each individual should always be considered within the context of the relationships and connections between them rather than in isolation. It is important to realise that an intervention with one person will also impact on others within the family and that this might be either positive or negative. An example of this might be the ill child being offered individual counselling. While this may offer the child an opportunity to share worries and anxieties, it has the potential to undermine parents' belief in their ability to care for their child's emotional needs, unless opportunities for family discussion are also offered.

Understanding some common themes and dimensions of family life during illness may be helpful to professionals in trying to assess the need for and potential impact of their interventions.

Some of these themes will be around relationships and dynamics prior to the illness: whether the child has had a chronic illness that has meant many previous challenges, the developmental stages of different family members, and the beliefs and meanings that they each give to the illness.

Lifecycle stages

All families need to achieve a balance between stability and change. Family life can provide essential continuity and consistency for family members, allowing them to use the security that this provides to branch out and develop new skills and relationships [37]. However, roles and relationships also need to adapt and change to accommodate developments in the physical, social or emotional life of the family members, thus, all families can be seen to have 'stages' of development in which major adjustment takes place. In considering the impact of a terminal illness on families, it can be helpful to professionals to consider what 'lifecycle stage(s)' [38] the family is in currently. The interrelationship between the stage of family development, and the particular demands of the illness can inform staff about the particular struggles faced by all family members.

Case John, aged 15 years had a relapse of leukaemia, after 4 years in remission. Over the intervening years, he and his parents had negotiated a path between his developing wish to be independent, and his parents' wish to monitor his wellbeing and protect him. The relapse and increasing realization that the treatments were unsuccessful, led to renewed tension between himself and his parents. He wanted to continue as long as possible to lead the rest of his life as a teenager, spending time with friends and attending school. His parents however wanted to spend as much time with him as possible and to protect him from activities that might be harmful to him.

In this example, the family is negotiating the lifecycle stage of adolescence which in itself requires them to balance the need for protection and independence. The illness further exacerbates this tension and pulls family members in two directions, potentially exacerbating the sense of loss for all the family.

At other lifecycle stages, such as the family having a much younger child with illness, the physical and emotional requirements of the illness may be less incongruent—it is more usual for a family to be very closely connected, protective, and inward looking when they have a small child, but this style needs to change to accommodate the independence needs of an adolescent. Thus the need to adapt family roles and relationships because of an illness may be part of the losses experienced by the family.

Relational styles and communication

Developmental stages experienced by children and families will influence their communication patterns and styles of relationships, but all individuals and families will have their favoured modes of connecting with others and preferred levels of closeness and distance with others.

On one end of a notional spectrum of relationships, family members may be so close to each other that they may feel that they know what each other, is feeling and thinking without needing to speak about it. This style provides a high level of protection and emotional connection that may be very supportive, particularly in 'crisis' stages of an illness. However, a disadvantage may be that in more chronic phases of illness, a child's independence is discouraged or the possibility of different views and ideas being expressed is limited. Thus parents may find it very hard to accept that their child is expressing worries or fears to staff of which they are unaware. Staff may perceive parents as 'overprotective' and wish to separate the child from them, to address their fears. It is however very important that the staff support the family's strong connections, rather than moving in to 'rescue' the child. Helping parents to talk appropriately with their children may provide a better long-term solution where the child is able to express his or her feelings to those closest to him or her.

While some families appear very close, others place a higher premium on autonomy and independence. They will find it easier for children to express different views and to have their individual styles recognised—adolescents with unusual hairstyles, clothes and piercings may be very acceptable. In the extreme, however, families with this style may find it harder to connect emotionally, to give and receive support under times of enormous stress and may even pull further apart.

Case A 16 year old boy was waiting for the results of a biopsy which would confirm the spread of cancer to his bones. His mother asked that he be told this separately from her as she felt that he dealt better with things on his own.

Patterns of cutting-off emotionally from each other, or indeed of forging deeper connections during times of immense stress, may each be part of repetitive 'scripts' in families [37]. Our 'scripts' for how *to be* in relationships, when loss is threatened, are influenced by previous family generations, although some may make a conscious effort to change relationship patterns if they have not been helpful in the past. While few families will

have had to negotiate the pathway to a child's death before, they may use signposts from other experiences to help them.

The challenge for the family is how to allow professionals to support the child and themselves, and yet keep a sense of privacy and family integrity [35]. When the child dies, the family's losses will include the relationships with professionals who the family may have known for many years. As with all other interventions, it is important to ascertain the family's own wishes in relation to connections with professionals after a child's death, and which rituals, if any (memorial services, cards, phone calls) would be experienced as helpful. It is important for health care professionals to consider how their own particular styles affect how they may judge family relationships.

Family beliefs and meanings

The experience of illness will always be mediated by the meanings that are attached to it [39], as will the family responses [40]. The values and meanings attached to illness can be very powerful factors in a family's adaptation to the illness and child's death. Parental coping and family resilience have, for example, been linked to the ability to see beneficial aspects of a child's illness, such as the family becoming closer or positive aspects of the child's personality being highlighted [41].

Understanding the meaning that different family members attach to the child's illness is crucial to developing a partnership between the family and helping professionals, yet this is an area of potential difficulty for professionals who may not feel that they have the skills to elicit views about illness. In usual medical consultations, individual or family beliefs are seldom explored, rather professionals often focus on the physical aspects of the patient's story and do not feel confident or skilled enough to address other areas [42,43].

Although families will have received information from professionals about the illness, this may be very different to their own views or beliefs about it. It is important to elicit their understanding of what the illness is, how it arose, and what course they think it will take; not only in medical terms but in its connection to family history, spiritual, or societal meanings.

The value given to talking about illness and death, for example, may highlight different levels of meaning. In many Western developed countries, the professional community now largely holds the belief that open disclosure to child and family is usually the right course. This, however, constitutes a major change in practice from 20 to 30 years ago when a poor prognosis (or even the diagnosis) was withheld from patients. Stories within families of how the illness of older family members was managed historically may influence how *they* think about their current situation. Some may fear that telling the ill child or their siblings that they have a serious illness will frighten them, make them give up on life, or will somehow jinx the situation so that death will happen sooner. For others, talking with relatives about their illness may have brought them closer, and enabled past relationship difficulties to be overcome.

Some illnesses have negative cultural/societal meanings; HIV being a commonly cited example [44]. Family members may not wish their child to know the diagnosis, both to protect them from emotional distress, and from the potential harm of stigma on them and other family members [45].

Illness may also impact on how family members think about their own roles and relationships. A strongly held belief in most societies is that parents (or other adults) should protect children from harm, and a life-threatening illness challenges this role in the most fundamental way. Parents may often feel guilty and in some way responsible for the child's illness—that there is something they should have done, or not done, to prevent it. When there are genetic factors in an illness, the risk of guilt may increase, and covert or overt blaming by others may occur. There is a very human need to find an answer to the question 'why?' and to find an outlet for anger at the unfairness of the child's illness.

For some a focus on what (or who) caused the illness may even be a way of feeling in control—if they can reverse the '*cause*', perhaps they can cure the illness.

Case A mother appeared frantic in her attempts to prevent her daughter expressing any 'negative' emotions, such as anger, distress, or fear. While staff initially understood this as the mother attempting to protect herself from her daughter's feelings, it become clearer one day when she told a nurse that she believed that her acrimonious divorce from the child's father had caused her daughter's cancer; that negative feelings had become cancerous, and were therefore dangerous.

Gender may also be an important context for considering how family members react to illness, and how they communicate with both professionals and each other. Men, women, and boys and girls are brought up with different messages about the expression of emotions, roles in childcare, and styles of relationships. If this context is ignored, there is a danger of family members being pathologised for reactions that might otherwise be seen as normal. An example of this would be the tendency for mothers sometimes to be seen as 'over involved' and fathers, perhaps, as disengaged [46].

The culture of the family (and that of professionals) will also profoundly affect both communication and experience of illness and health care [47]. There is a need for professionals to be aware of their own culturally informed aspects of belief and practice, and to develop culturally sensitive practice towards people who have different beliefs to their own. It is likely to be unhelpful to view certain ethnic groups as holding particular health beliefs, as this may only contribute to stereotyped (and perhaps mistaken) assumptions. However, the use of skills advocated throughout this chapter in identifying needs and values and negotiating care, are a necessary part of culturally sensitive practice.

For families who do not speak English, or have it as a second language, the regular and consistent provision of interpreters is essential. Even when a child is in his or her last few days of life, interpreters may be used only for special meetings and not provided as part of routine care. How communication can be truly effective or supportive in these circumstances is difficult to understand.

Communication, children, and young people

When considering communicating with children and young people about life-threatening illness, many will immediately think of the issues of disclosure about diagnosis and prognosis. Strong feelings are often aroused, guided by personal and professional beliefs about the relative value of open communication and the need to protect children from potentially devastating news. Fredman [48] has commented that alongside strong professional beliefs about the need for children and families to discuss illness and death, paradoxically, the death taboo in Western society provides a strong injunction against talking about it.

Over the last 20 years, evidence of the benefits of talking with children openly about illness is increasing. Sharing information in chronic illness has been linked to less depression in ill children, and increased social competence in siblings [49]. An open approach to disclosure in childhood leukaemia was also shown to enhance psychological adjustment in children and their families [50,51]. 'Not telling' did not reduce stress in the children, but may have increased their isolation and anxiety [50].

In some illnesses, such as HIV-related conditions, diagnostic disclosure presents many complex ethical, medical, social and psychological implications [52]. These are dimensions that professionals and families struggle with in many illness situations, and individual negotiation with each family should still be undertaken.

Children's cognitive and emotional understanding of illness and death is linked to their cognitive developmental level and to their own exposure to these experiences [53,54]. Kane [55] identified approximate ages at which children develop components of a mature concept of what death means, including irrevocability, universality, causality, and the effects of death on appearance and function. Lansdown [9] has suggested guidelines for stages that children may go through in their developing understanding of their own life-threatening illness, ranging from the understanding that they are ill, through the realisation that their type of illness can cause children to die, to the realisation that they themselves are going to die. Bluebond-Langner [54] has proposed that even very young children may reach this understanding if they have themselves experienced bereavement or are suffering a life-threatening illness.

In addition to cognitive developmental approaches, others have described phases of emotional processes that are experienced by dying or grieving people [56,57]. While all of these models may help to guide professionals in communicating with children and families, Fredman [48] cautions against using them as normative views of the way that dying or grieving should be 'done'. She suggests that 'such theories and policy has dominated helpers' relationships with clients' and suggests considering that many professionals have different *personal* beliefs that should alert them to the myriad ways that it is possible to die or grieve 'well'.

While many of the same issues arise in communication with children as with adults (e.g. the need to elicit their understanding, views and wishes), there will be a greater reliance on nonverbal communication with younger children or those with specific communication difficulties or learning disabilities. Ill children and their siblings may experience a range of feelings in the face of serious illness, including fear, anger, shame and distress about body changes, resentment of others who are well or getting more attention, and the wish to protect and be protected. These feelings may be exhibited through general behaviour and play rather than being verbalised directly.

***

Case A 6-year-old child (Lucy) undergoing a second course of chemotherapy for leukaemia, showed her distress about the side-effects by angrily chopping the hair from her favourite doll.

***

Providing opportunities for children to use play or drawing can be important ways for them to show their feelings. This can be as important for siblings as for the ill child. While staff need to be alert to the meaning contained within play, it is important to ask the child, or to suggest comments tentatively rather than to 'interpret' what they have done.

***

Case Lucy (above), had two brothers, one aged 10 (Tom) and the other age 4 years (Ricky). Whilst they were all in the playroom of the treating hospital, Lucy drew lots of shapes on the page. When the play specialist tentatively suggested that they looked like blood cells, Lucy beamed and said that she was drawing leukaemia. Tom became very interested in this and said 'my friend at school says you can die of leukaemia'. As he said this, all three

children looked at the play specialist to see how she would respond.

***

The regular provision of opportunities for play with a trusted adult can enable children to express feelings, thoughts, and questions. As in this example, children may 'test out' what it is possible to say to professionals, as also to their own family members. They are often very adept at picking up emotional nuances and avoid areas that may upset others.

***

Case (contd.) The play specialist gave an honest answer to their 'question' saying that this did sometimes happen, and asked them what they thought and felt about this. Lucy was able to say that she didn't mind dying, as she would see her aunties and grandparents in heaven. She was however, worried about how her parents would manage without her. Ricky however, asked when he would get leukaemia.

***

This example illustrates that even young children may have thought a lot about their illness without adults necessarily being aware of this. Lucy had known two other children who had died of leukaemia and this linked with her brother's information from his peers. It is important to note that we cannot assume we know what children's anxieties about death will be, as Lucy's fears were less for herself at that time and more for her parents. The example also shows that siblings may have worries or fears that also need to be explored. In this case Ricky had donated bone marrow to his sister and linked the operation to 'catching leukaemia'. Other children may believe that they have caused the illness in some way—one 5-year-old child, in-patient in hospital, was told that another child had died of something wrong with his tummy. Later he commented anxiously that he had tickled the other boy's tummy. He was then reassured that he had not caused the problem.

***

Case (contd.) The play specialist was concerned to know what to do with the information she had about the children's anxieties and worries, and discussed this with a nursing colleague. She was then able to go back to the children, ask them if their parents were aware of what they had discussed and get their agreement to tell the parents. She chose to tell the parents on their own in private. The mother immediately burst into tears, and was comforted by her partner.

***

Professionals may be concerned about how much of children's anxieties to share with their parents, if they were obtained separately. Asking the children's views is one way of going forward. It may be important to talk to parents separately, to allow them time to react and adjust away from the children. It may be that this can then facilitate all family members to talk together more openly, depending on their style of communication.

While exploring anxieties about open conversations ('talking about talking'), it is crucial that professionals respect families' style and do not push them into situations in which they cannot sustain their support because of their own beliefs about the 'right' way to do things.

Families may also communicate their knowledge and feelings to each other with stories, metaphors and play situations [48]: a dying child asked his mother what she would do if he became 'a little bird who pecked at her window'. She responded that she would be 'delighted to see him' and 'would give him food and water every day'. Without mentioning dying directly they were communicating about this very effectively, and within their own spiritual belief system.

Young people

Adolescents will of course, have different needs to those of young children. The increasing need for privacy, control, and independence in adolescence, may contrast strongly with the physical dependency of illness. In this context, limit testing behaviour, often seen as a normative task of adolescence in western societies, may extend to relationships with health care staff and affect adherence to treatments. Whereas conflictual relationships at this 'life cycle stage' are seen as almost normative in the west, they may be particularly painful for all concerned when death is also in mind.

While peer and sexual relationships may also be strongly in focus for healthy young people, those with life-threatening illness may be more isolated and depend on family and professionals for social support and companionship. Experience in hospices and voluntary organisations suggests that bringing young people together for treatment or recreation can be helpful in providing mutual support [58]. As many ill or disabled young people have extra concerns about their body image at a time when this is developmentally perceived as crucial, this may also help alleviate that particular stress.

Young people may have a fuller understanding of their illness, and how their family and friends are affected by it, than younger children. While they may be preoccupied with concerns about their own life and future, they may wish to protect their loved ones from their pain and anxiety and thus be left alone with these worries. As with younger children then, it is important that opportunities are given for adolescents to discuss and explore their feelings. It may also be very helpful to comment to the family and young person together that the process of mutual protection is very common and normal, which may paradoxically allow them to overcome this barrier.

Siblings

While the child and parent(s) may be the focus of professional attention, siblings can often be sent to other relatives or friends to be cared for. They may then lose parental attention and closeness at the time when their own anxieties may be at their highest and they may not feel that they can express their own concerns or issues for fear of upsetting other family members. One study suggested that nearly half of well siblings did not talk to anyone about the life-threatening illness, while only 38% talked to their parents [59]. Grandparents or other trusted adults may be able to take up this role.

Professionals may need to facilitate parents' consideration of the siblings' needs, as there is a tendency for them to under-estimate the effect that the illness is having on them [59].

Siblings may receive less information about the illness partly because they are not around to hear the less formal conversations that take place in health care settings over time, as also because they are considered as not so much in need by family or professionals. A study of the siblings of children who died of cystic fibrosis reported that many had no idea about the seriousness of the illness, sometimes until death actually occurred [60]. Even where the seriousness is known, siblings have their own needs and may show great resentment towards the ill child, creating tension with their parents ('how could he be so awful when she's so ill?') complicating their reaction when death occurs. Others may take the role in the family of the 'joker', who does something cute when family stress is too high, or may deny their own emotional needs and sink into the background.

Professionals need to try to hold the entire family in mind, assessing all members' needs both individually and as an interacting unit [61].

Interactive communication skills training

All health care staff who treat children . . . should also be trained in communicating with young people and parents. [17]

'Learning from Bristol (ibid)' recommends broadening the notion of professional competence to include non-clinical aspects of care in the key areas of education, training and continuing professional development, including a key skill in 'communicating' with patients and with colleagues '. . . there should be more opportunities than at present for multi professional teams to learn, train and develop together'.

Humphrey [62] concluded that 'there is relatively little detailed advice or recommendations specifically about the

provision of psychosocial support or counselling for
parents . . . except in the context of life-threatening illness or
bereavement'. It is in this field, especially in hospices or in
oncology units, that many 'communication studies' have
been based. Medical sociologists have also extensively examined communication issues between health care professionals and patients. Friedson [36] confirms a widespread
assumption that communication problems between a doctor
and a patient were often to do with the fact that the doctor
was usually a highly educated male and the patient often
was not.

He concluded: 'It is my thesis that the separate world of
experience and reference of the layman and the professional
worker are always in potential conflict with each other.'

Studies of nurse/patient communications have examined
attitudinal issues revealing more of what patients expect and
appreciate in terms of the characteristics of a 'good nurse'.
Bailey and Wilkinson [63] found that almost all patients valued a 'kind, caring attitude' but overall, the study found that
nurses lacked the skills to elicit and address the (oncology)
patients' main concerns, many of which were not disclosed to
the nurses in the study.

Heaven and Maguire [34] have also found that health care
professionals made assumptions about patients' concerns
which 'if not discussed or checked out with the patients may
lead to an overestimate or underestimate of the true situation'.

Recent guidelines from the Department of Health (DOH),
Kings Fund and elsewhere collated in the BMJ [64] indicate
that better communication could be achieved by giving more
information in several media.

Of course giving accurate, honest information is a very
important aspect of communicating effectively with any
patient, but in order to effectively engage in realistic shared
decision-making, information from the patient also has to
be elicited and included in the discussion. Coulter [65]
writes'. . . shared decision making at the clinical level is the
foundation stone in which all the other efforts to promote a
more patient centred health service must rest . . .'.

Research on aspects of health care professional's communication and interactive skills has shown that in the case
of information giving it is rare for health care professionals
to be able to check effectively the patient's understanding
and adapt their own discursive style accordingly. What very
often happens is that information is repeated, perhaps in
even greater detail than previously if the patient appears to
fail to understand. A nurse quoted in the Nursing Times
[66] said, 'if a patient does not understand a procedure you
get the surgeon to speak to them again. . . . .' Other studies
consistently show that, when giving information, health
care professionals tend to do most of the talking leaving

little time for listening to patients' views and eliciting their
understanding.

Shared decision-making with children may be even more
problematic. Even if their views are expressed they may not be
respected or understood, as it is difficult for many to acknowledge childrens' own experiences and to respect their
judgement. The assumption that children are too young to
make their own decisions until they reach the somehow 'magic
birthday' of 16 years is still a prevalent idea. Lansdown's work,
[9] illustrating a grid of possibilities for shared decision-
making with children and young patients, offers an important
tool for paediatric palliative care. It respects the important
knowledge that, in the case of children who have themselves
experienced serious illness and bereavement or who are
undergoing their own illness process, such children form a
mature competence and understanding at a much earlier age
than health care professionals would normally consider
appropriate. Sanz [67] found the same issue on the topic of
preventative medicine'. . . children up to eleven years old
seldom attach a preventive value to drugs and they find it hard
to understand why someone should take drugs when not
actually being ill. [But] quite a different picture is drawn by
children with asthma. . . .' 'Children as young as seven years
old were able to give clear explanations about their disease, the
drugs used and their main characteristics, how they work,
when they should be taken and at which doses.' Sanz goes on to
discuss research showing that 'there is much room for
improvement for doctors direct communication with
children'. He concludes that achieving concordance with
children is 'demanding, but most rewarding, and requires
stamina and flexibility from health professionals. . . .'.

ACT (Ibid), in their study, recognised that when young
people felt most ill they were not really capable of truly shared
decision-making with the health care staff '. . . When I was in
the hospital, I would have valued my mum being there as I
constantly had to explain many different things; this took a lot
out of me whilst feeling so ill. . . .' Young patients receiving
palliative care, like all people 'who are seriously debilitated
by chronic or life limiting illness, may find themselves disem-
powered and excluded'. In this field '. . . user's views have generally been represented by voluntary groups rather than
directly . . .' [68].

The entire issue of health care professionals' communication with patients of any age is bedevilled by the debate as to
what constitutes 'communication skills'. Much is made of the
fact that medical students now undergo communication skills
training at under-graduate level, but teaching is still patchy
and inconsistent across all medical schools. Boohan [69]
showed that there was still a very wide range of interpretation
of the communication skills curriculum ranging from an

integrated course over the 5 years of study at some medical schools to lectures in the final year, probably from a psychosocial professional on breaking bad news, in some other centres. Her study also revealed a lack of consistent communication skills training once doctors qualified and graduated into postgraduate medical education. Maguire [70] found when looking at the interviewing skills of recently qualified doctors, that though most of them could give simple information on diagnosis and treatment, there were virtually no attempts made to obtain patients' views or to 'check whether a patient had understood what had been said or to categorise the information given'. Maguire stated that '. . . unfortunately the doctors were weakest on the techniques that have been found to increase patient satisfaction and improve their compliance with medical advice and treatment'. These techniques include discovering the patients' own views of their illnesses and their expectations of treatment and, sadly, also 'the doctors reluctance to discover the patient's views of their predicaments and to mention prognosis parallel their tendency to avoid asking them about social and psychological aspects'. Maguire concludes that when these doctors were medical students they had not learnt 'to communicate effectively and sensitively with patients'.

A common assumption is that this issue of 'communication' is confined to 'breaking bad news' or bereavement care. Communication is of course often focused around these issues in acute health care settings, and many authors have written extensively about the skills required in order to break bad news effectively [71]. However, the concept of the patient journey in paediatric palliative care provides a useful illustration that the two specific points of the diagnosis and eventual need for bereavement support are certainly not the only times when communication skills are required.

It is obvious that there is a need to communicate all through the patient's life cycle, from the shock and grief of diagnosis, through financial and lifestyle changes, family relationship dynamics, the child patient's understanding, sibling issues, patient autonomy issues, acute hospital admissions, operations, transition episodes, disease exacerbations, time of death and terminal care decisions.

Even though in paediatric palliative care professionals and many families assert that bereavement begins at diagnosis, it is also clear that the focus on death or impending death, even though it may be inevitable, is certainly not an appropriate one for the majority of families, who for large tracts of the child's life wish to normalize their situation

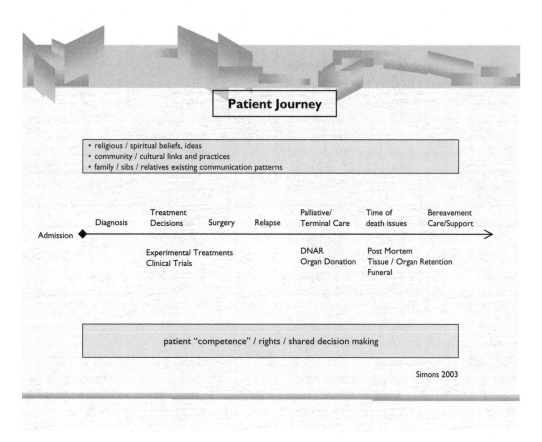

Fig. 3.1

or try to minimise the negative aspects of the child's condition [73].

Numerous personal communications indicate that professionals confuse the term 'palliative' with 'terminal', and assume therefore that someone who is skilled or qualified in bereavement counselling needs will best meet the families' communication. This qualification in itself may be seen as the province of a psychosocial member of the health care team. Doctors, nurses, and others in the health care team who do not normally have such qualifications may often feel deskilled in what might be a very appropriate desire to engage with the patient in discussion of time of death or bereavement issues. Personal communication again has revealed several instances of nurses who have been supporting a family successfully for months or even years, who, when the child has become terminally ill felt that they have needed to introduce another professional into the family in order to engage in the activity of 'pre-bereavement counselling'.

Because of a professional wariness around the topic of bereavement nurses have often said that they don't feel qualified or confident to engage in this apparent extension of their role. This is a great pity as a recent study [74] concludes that the preferred key supporter is the person or team they have known best and with whom they feel the greatest rapport, because of their years caring for the child. This need not mean a professionally qualified person but may be a volunteer.

It is important to recognise that families have consistently said they value 'continuing support in their bereavement'. If this is not forthcoming then naturally families may feel abandoned and isolated in their grief. It may be a mistake, however, to construe their request as a need for 'bereavement support' *per se*. A careful assessment of the family's individual needs should be undertaken by a key worker and ongoing support needs agreed upon. Dent and Stewart [75] propose that nurses, midwives, and health care professionals should have the basic communication skills required to meet the needs of newly bereaved parents and families. Their work focuses on babies and young children who have died a sudden death, but the principles addressed are entirely relevant in paediatric palliative care. The authors discuss what they call 'considerations for practice', and do not recommend any particular qualification or indeed method of assessment or support work, but emphasise that the health care professional engaged in the support must have the interactive skills to be able to assess accurately with the family the meaning that they attach to the illness and death of the child according to their own beliefs, culture and life cycle factors. The authors make an

important point, however, that is, crucial to communication in paediatric palliative care. They acknowledge that professionals and lay people alike may actually be frightened of engaging with patients and families when a child is dying. A health visitor [75] said that many in her profession are 'hugely ill prepared and consequently dread' the job of supporting bereaved families.

The benchmarking of best practice currently underway in nursing to establish an appropriate level of what are called interpersonal skills for nurses states that 'all health care personnel demonstrate effective interpersonal skills when communicating with patients and carers. Further it says appropriate and effective methods of communication are used actively to promote understanding between patients and carers and health care personnel'. The benchmark goes on to identify detailed examples of what the appropriate and effective methods of communication may be and laudably details the kinds of issues that the health care professional must consider and 'address', but there is little concrete guidance on how to evince these skills in practice. There remains a gap between recommendations for practice and competence in the delivery of care. The skills must be identified, learnt, and practiced, not merely theorised. The key is always appropriate engagement with patients; no shared decision-making can happen without a confident use of evidenced 'interactive communication tools'. Without these tools, the issues that block appropriate communication with adult patients are emphasised when attempting to engage with children, even many paediatricians and children's nurses find it hard to assess children's competence, engage in informed consent, promote the child's best interests, or truly encourage the child's voice in shared decision-making. Many instead take refuge in distancing tactics, or in a false apprehension of the legal status of their professional obligations, for example, the child doesn't have to be engaged in a discussion about consent if he or she is under 16.

Real engagement with the issues raised by the Children Act 1989, the UN Convention on the Rights of the Child, or indeed the Children's National Service Framework (NSF) and its recommendations for joined up working across health care, social care, and education remain hollow without a real commitment to the training and application in the tools of real engagement.

Faulkner, Maguire, Heaven, and others have examined communication competencies in several settings and evidenced consistent issues: what health care professionals do, what they fail to do, and the effects of their actions.

Approaches that enhance communication include:

- hearing and recognising patients' cues

- asking open questions, particularly psychologically or emotionally focused ones, to elicit the patient's feelings and concerns

- reassuring appropriately only after the patient's problems have been explored

- negotiating and clarifying the conversational agenda.

These result in the patients feeling that they have been sympathetically heard and respectfully treated. None of this is new, all of it is recognisable as good, effective 'listening skills'.

Conversely, approaches that compromise communication include:

- distancing tactics

- blocking tactics

- false reassurance

- premature solution finding

- changing the subject

- ignoring patient's cues

- sticking to discussion of physical as opposed to psychological or emotional topics

- making assumptions about patients views, feelings, and concerns, rather than exploring them actively.

Maguire [33] suggests that it is appropriate to view people as 'robust and capable of working through difficult predicaments' albeit with appropriate help, rather than as 'fragile and susceptible to harm'. This is an important point in relation to the alleged paternalistic attitudes revealed during the Bristol Royal Infirmary (BRI) inquiry and in the debate about organ retention. Parents from the Bristol Children's Heart Action Group were very angry at what they reported as the paternalism of the cardiologists and surgeons in keeping from them the real risks of proposed operations. Similarly parents said, 'I would probably have agreed if I had been asked', (to allow organs to be retained for research), but the assumption that parents would find it too difficult to engage in discussion about their own child's post mortem angered and disgusted many.

Maguire concludes that active exploration of patients' cues, feelings, and concerns is more effective than encouragement to give their story with few interruptions. He concludes that guesswork about concerns, whether gleaned from non-verbal cues or unexplored verbal cues, is often inaccurate;

that when distress is shown, it is inappropriate to assume the cause of distress, and reassure before the nature of the distress has been properly explored. Furthermore, an 'empathic understanding' manner does not lead to more disclosure, only active elicitation of feelings as a response to cues achieves this.

Summary

Although there has been emphasis in this chapter and elsewhere on the types of skills needed to improve communication between professionals, patients, and families, it is important that such skills are viewed as contributing to, but not synonymous with, relationships between these groups. In addition, it is important to recognise that *all* behaviour is communication—it is impossible for us not to communicate even if we say or do nothing [76]. When professionals feel lacking in confidence to engage with families facing the deaths of children, their avoidance of them is a communication, as is the ability of some staff to be with a child or family without speaking, or carrying out unnecessary tasks. Questions that we ask or don't ask of children and families reveal a great deal about our feelings and beliefs. We are constantly communicating, in ways that may be outside of our conscious awareness.

References

1. Report of the Joint Working Party of the Association for Children with Life-Threatening or Terminal Conditions and their Families and the Royal College of Paediatrics and Child Health (1997). *A Guide to the Development of Children's Palliative Care Services.* London: ACT, Bristol and RCPH.

2. Department of Health. The Children's National Service Framework, 2001b.

3. Ley, P. Satisfaction, compliance and communication. *British Journal of Clinical Psychology* 1982;21:241–54.

4. Green, L.W. Determining the impact and effectiveness of health education as it relates to federal policy. *Health Education Monographs* 1978;6(supp 1):28–66.

5. Hall, J.A., Roter, D.L., Katz, N.R. Correlates of provider behaviour: a meta-analysis. *Medical Care* 1988;26:657–75.

6. Wooley, F.R., Kane, R.L., Hughes, C.C., Wright, D.D. The effects of doctor-patient communication on satisfaction and outcome of care. *Social Science and Medicine* 1978;12:123–8.

7. Wartman, S.A., Morlock, L.L., Malitz, F.E., Palm, E. The impact of divergent evaluations by physicians and patients of patients' complaints. *Public Health Reports* 1983;98:1414–15.

8. Faulkner, A., and Maguire, P. Talking to cancer patients. Oxford Medical Publications, 1994.

9. Lansdown, R. Communicating with Children. In Goldman, A. (ed) *Care for the Dying Child*. Oxford: Oxford University Press, 1994.

10. Committee on Paediatric Aids, American Academy of Pediatrics. *Disclosure of Illness* Status to Children and Adolescents with HIV Infection. *Pediatrics* 1999;103(1):164–6.

11. Melvin, D., and Lukeman, D. Bereavement: A Framework for Those Working with Children. *Clin Child Psychol Psychiatr* 2000;5(4): 521–39.

12. Eiser, C. *Growing up With a Chronic Illness*. London: and Bristol; Jessica Kingsley Publishers, 1993.

13. Rolland, J. *Families, illness, and disability. An integrative treatment model*. New York: Basic Books, 1994.

14. McDaniel, S.H., Hepworth, J., and Doherty, W.J. *Medical Family Therapy. A Biopsychosocial Approach to Families with Health Problems*. New York: Basic Books, 1992.

15. Walsh, F. The Concept of Family Resilience: Crisis and Challenge. *Family Process* 1996;35(3):1–22.

16. Smith, R. Preparing for Partnership. *BMJ* 2003;326:1–3.

17. *The Report of the Public Inquiry into children's heart surgery at the Bristol Royal Infirmary 1984–1995*. Learning from Bristol. COI Communications, The Stationary Office, England.

18. Hunt, A., Elston, S., Galloway, J. *Voices for Change. Current perceptions of services for children with palliative care needs and their families*. Association for Children with Life-threatening or Terminal Conditions and their Families, 2003.

19. Laine, C. Patient-centered Medicine. A Professional Evolution. *JAMA* 1996;275(2):152–6.

20. Hutchfield, K. Family-centred care: A Concept Analysis. *J Adv Nurs* 1999;29(5):1178–87.

21. Doherty, W.J. Family intervention in health care. *Family Relations* 1984;34:129–37.

22. Blanchard, C.G., Ruckdeschel, J.C., and Albrecht, T.L. Patient-Family Communication with Physicians. In L. Baider and G.L Cooper: A. Kaplan De-Nour, *Cancer and the Family*. John Wiley & Sons, 1996.

23. Deeley, L., Stallard, P., Lewis, M., and Lenton, S. Palliative care services for children must adopt a family centred approach. *BMJ* 1998;317(7153):284–5.

24. Klein, R. The new politics of the NHS (3rd edition). London. Longman, 1995.

25. Report of the Joint Working Party of the Association for Children with Life-Threatening or Terminal Conditions and their Families (ACT), National Council for Hospice and Specialist Care Services and Scottish Partnership Agency for Palliative and Cancer Care (SPAPCC) (2001). Palliative Care for Young People Aged 13–14 years.

26. Lord Laming. *The Victoria Climbie Inquiry*, Summary and Recommendations. England. Crown Copyright, 2003.

27. Thorne, S.E. *Negotiating Health Care: the Social Context of Chronic Illness*. Sage Publications, London, 1993.

28. Knafl, K.A., Breitmayer, B., Gallo, A., and Zoeller, L. Parents' views of health care providers: An exploration of the components of a positive working relationship. *Children's Health Care*, 1992;21: 90–5.

29. Rousseau, P. Hope in the Terminally Ill. *West J Med* 2000;173: 117–18.

30. Patterson, J.M. Family Resiliences to the Challenge of a Child's Disability. *Pediatr Ann* 1991;20:491–9.

31. Maquire, P. Barriers to the care of the dying. *Br Med J* 1985;291: 1711–13.

32. Maguire, P. Barriers to psychological care of the dying. *BMJ* 1985;291:1711.

33. Maquire, P. Improving Communication with Cancer Patients. *Eur J Cancer* 1999;35(10):1415–22.

34. Heaven, C.M. and Maguire, P. Disclosure of concerns by hospice patients and their identification by nurses. *Palliat Med* 1997:283–290.

35. Cohen, M.S. *Families Coping with Childhood Chronic Illness: A Research Review. Families, Systems and Health* 1999;17(2): 149–65.

36. Friedson, E. Dilemmas in the doctor patient relationship, Cox C. & Mead A.A. *Sociology of Medical Practice*, Collier-Macmillan, London, 1975, pp. 285.

37. Byng- Hall, J. *Rewriting Family Scripts. Improvisation and Systems Change*. New York, London; The Guildford Press, 1995.

38. Carter, B. and McGoldrick, M. eds *The Changing Family Life Cycle: Framework for family therapy* (2nd edition). Boston, Allyn& Bacon, 1989.

39. Kleinman, A. *The Illness Narratives: Suffering, Healing, and the Human Condition*. New York: Basic Books, 1988.

40. Patterson, J., and Garwick, A. Annals of Behavioural Medicine, *The Impact of Chronic Illness on families: A family systems perspective*. 1994;16(2):131–42.

41. Patterson, J.M. and Leonard, B.J. Caregiving and children. In E. Kahana, D.E. Biegel, and M. Wukle eds *Family caregiving across the lifespan*. Newbury Park, CA: Sage, 133–158.

42. Ley, P. Satisfaction, compliance and communication. *British Journal of Clinical Psychology* 1982;21:241–54.

43. Wilkinson, S., Roberts, A., and Aldridge, J. Nurse–patient communication in palliative care: an evaluation of a communication skills programme. *Palliat Med*, 1998;12:13–22.

44. Sontag. *Illness as Metaphor and Aids and its Metaphors*. Harmondsworth: Penguin, 1991.

45. Lester, P., Chesney, M., Cooke, M., Whalley, P., Perez, B., Petru, A., Dorenbaum, A., and Wara, D. Diagnostic Disclosure to HIV-Infected Children: How Parents Decide When and What to Tell. *Clinical Child Psychology and Psychiatry* 2001;7(1):85–99.

46. Altschuler, J. *Working with Chronic Illness. A Family Approach*. Macmillan Press, Ltd., 1993.

47. Ferguson, W.J. and Candib, L.M. Culture, Language and the doctor-patient relaionship. *Family Medicine* 2002;34(5):353–61.

48. Fredman, G. Death Talk. *Conversations with Children and Families*. Karnac Books, 1997.

49. Evans, C.A., Stevens, M., Cushway, and Houghton, J. Sibling response to childhood cancer: A new approach. *Child Care Health and Dev* 1992;18(4):229–44.

50. Clafin, C.J., and Barbarin, O.A. Does 'telling' less protect more? Relationships among age, information disclosure, and what children with cancer see and feel. *Journal of Pediatric Psychology* 1991;16:169–91.

51. Katz, E., and Jay, S. Psychological aspects of cancer in children, adolescents and their families. *Clin Psychol Rev* 1984;4: 525–42.

52. Lipson, M. What do you say to a child with AIDS? *Hastings Center Report* 1993;23:6–12.

53. Spinetta, J., Rigler, D., and Koron, M. Anxiety in the dying child. *Pediatrics* 1973;52:841.

54. Bluebond-Langer, M. *The Private Worlds of Dying Children.* Princeton University Press, NJ, 1978.

55. Kane, B. Childrens conceptions of death. *J Genet Psychol* 1979;134: 141–53.

56. Kubler-Ross, E. *On Death and Dying.* New York: Macmillan, 1970.

57. Parkes, C.M. *Bereavement: Studies of Grief in Adult Life.* New York: Pelican, 1972.

58. Thornes, R. *Palliative Care for Young People Aged 13–24.* Joint Working Party on Palliative Care for Adolescents and Young Adults, 2001.

59. Stallard, P., Mastroyannopoulou, K., Lewis, M., Lenton, S. The siblings of children with life-threatening conditions. *Child Psychol Psychiatry Rev* 1997;226–33.

60. Fanos, J. *Sibling Loss.* New Jersey: Lawrence Erlbaum Associates, 1996.

61. Elston, S. *Assessment of children with life-limiting conditions and their families.* Association for Children with Life-threatening or Terminal Conditions and their Families, 2003.

62. Humphrey, C. *Support and Counselling for Parents in Acute Healthcare Settings.* Unpublished briefing paper for the BRI inquiry. (*The Report of the Public Inquiry into children's heart surgery at the Bristol Royal Infirmary 1984–1995.* Learning from Bristol. COI Communications, The Stationary Office, England.)

63. Bailey, K. and Wilkinson. Patient's views on nurses' communication skills: Apilot study. *Int J Palliat Nurs*, 1998;4(6):300.

64. British Medical Journal. Most young doctors are bad at giving information. 1986;292:1576.

65. Coulter, A. Whatever happened to shared decision-making? *Health Expectations*, Vol. 5. Blackwell Science Ltd, 2002, pp. 185–6.

66. *Nursing times*, 2002;98(16):14.

67. Sanz, E.J. Concordance and children's use of medicines. *BMJ* 2003; 327:858.

68. Small, N., and Rhodes, P. *Palliative and Community Care, To Ill to Talk?* London & NewYork: Routledge, 2000.

69. Boohun, M. Teaching communication to medical undergraduates— are we advancing? Forum of medical communication, Royal Society of Medicine, 1998.

70. Maguire, P. Most young doctors are bad at giving imformation. *BMJ* 1986;292:1576.

71. Buckman, R. How to break bad news. Papermac, 1992.

72. Simons, J. Internal document. Great Ormond Street Hospital for Children Trust, 2003.

73. Bluebond Langner, K. In the shadow of illness: Parents and Siblings of the Chronically Ill Child. Princeton University Press, 2000.

74. *A Guide to the Development of Children's Palliative care Services.* Update of a report by The Association for Children with Life-threatening or Terminal Conditions and their Families. The Royal College of Paediatrics and Child Health. Second edition, ACT, 2003.

75. Dent, A. and Stewart, A. *Sudden Death in Childhood: Support for the Bereaved Family.* Butterworth Heinemann, 2004.

76. Watzlawick, P. and Beavin, J. *Pragmatics of Human Communication: A Study of Interactional Patterns, Pathologies and Paradoxes.* New York: W.W. Norton, 1967.

4   Ethics

Vic Larcher

The boast of heraldry, the pomp of power
And all that riches, all that wealth e'er gave
Awaits alike the inevitable hour
The paths of glory lead but to the grave [1]

Whatever their own personal religious beliefs or values, health care professionals need little reminding of the frailty and finite nature of human existence in the form that we understand it. Birth and death are inescapable aspects of living. Nevertheless, all professionals as part of their humanity hope that their lives will be as fulfilled, happy and rewarding as possible. They, like the patients they serve, will also hope that advances in medicine and technology will enable them to remain as healthy and as active as possible throughout their lives—to enable them to live lives to the full. We hope, and have come to expect, that our children will grow up to lead the lives to which we aspire. Those who work with children are especially aware of the physical, physiological, psychological, spiritual, and emotional journey that children undertake between infancy and adulthood. They, like others, have a duty to ensure that this journey is accomplished as safely and as freely as possible. However, not all children can, or will, make this journey; their lives are limited by a variety of constraints over which they and their parents may have little control.

This chapter is concerned with the ethical principles, which underpin how our society responds to children whose lives are limited. Not all societies will respond, or have responded in the same way. The Spartans and Romans practiced infanticide for babies who were weak, infirm, had disability, or who were of the wrong gender. Whilst contemporary society largely condemns such practices, and holds respect for human life as a fundamental moral value, ethical difficulties remain. Does all life in all its diversity demand equal respect and carry equal value? What of those with life limiting illnesses (LLI)?

Background considerations

Globally life expectancy of children has improved (as a result of both technological advances and public health measures). Effective treatments have reduced mortality and morbidity of many diseases, including endemic infectious disease, for example, polio, hepatitis B, HIV, etc. Survival rates for many childhood cancers have increased. Patients with chronic illness, for example, cystic fibrosis have increased life expectancy. Organ or marrow transplantation offers hope of survival for children with chronic renal failure or advanced liver disease or such chronic blood disorders as Beta thalassaemia. Gene therapy and xenotransplantation may have future benefits that cannot be quantified at present [2]. There is great public expectation that technology can produce cures in most circumstances and that death in childhood is avoidable. Since childhood mortality in developed countries is low many professionals may have neither experience at managing death nor the morbidity of chronic incurable disease.

The context in which death occurs in children is variable. Death may be sudden in premature babies with catastrophic cerebral bleeds and in child victims of road traffic accidents. In others the dying process is more protracted, for example, multiple relapses in childhood leukaemia or slow decline of child with progressive neuro-muscular disease [3]. The responses of children, families, and professionals to impending death are likely to be as variable as the circumstances in which they occur. It is therefore hardly surprising that management of LLI poses ethical difficulties and practical challenges for all concerned.

There can be, and not infrequently are, actual or potential disputes between all parties as to what values should govern how decisions about management are to be made. We live and practice in a pluralistic multi-cultural, multi-faith society in which individual preferences, beliefs, and values (which govern what actions parties consider as morally appropriate), may vary enormously. There can be particular concerns as to whether adequate account is being taken of the intrinsic value of a child's' life, particularly as some LLIs limit not only the length of life, but also its emotional, psychological, and spiritual content.

Some parents may want active treatment to prolong life to be given to the point of death itself. Others may wish for a speedy and peaceful end to what they perceive as their child's intolerable pain and suffering. Such parents may feel that their own pain compromises their ability to give emotional and physical support to their dying child. Parental feelings of loss, anger, bewilderment, and injustice may further compromise their capacity to make rational choices on behalf of their child.

Professionals, mindful of the developmental potential and resilience of children may frequently give them more chances to recover from their illness than an adult might receive in similar circumstances [4]. This tendency, reinforced by a sense of empathy with the suffering of families may lead to increased efforts to restore the child to health, even in circumstances when this is unlikely. Moreover, professionals may feel that they must respect the beliefs, preferences, and values of families—with which they may not concur—as part of their perceived moral duty in contemporary society.

Approaches to ethical issues

Care of children with LLI raises dilemmas, that cannot be addressed or answered by appeal to scientific fact alone. Their resolution involves value judgements about what ought to be done rather than what is technically possible. Professionals facing these moral dilemmas may find that published guidance is either too prescriptive or too vague to be helpful [5].

The traditional analytical ethical approach has been the application of classical moral theories or principles (discussed in more detail below) to deduce whether a proposed course of action is morally acceptable. But there are occasions when conflicting moral principles may be present.

Clinicians tend to approach problems in a different fashion, working from the facts of a given case towards the general medical and nursing principles that might apply. Ethical examination of cases can also follow a similar pattern starting from the features of the particular case and seeking to recall similar cases, which might provide assistance in obtaining the resolution to the case in hand [6]. In dealing with a 15-year old who has refused further chemotherapy which his or her doctors recommended we might examine how similar cases were resolved and what ethical principles were relevant to them.

Other application of ethics may be concerned with what the practitioner (good doctor/nurse) would do in similar circumstances. Another would be to focus on the primacy of the patient's story and also take into account the narrative of others (e.g. professionals, parents) and how professionals might respond to it (narrative ethics) [6].

Consequentialist/utilitarian moral theory
(for general references on specific ethical theory see ref 7)

For consequentialists the rightness or wrongness of an action is determined by its actual or likely consequences in maximising benefits and minimising harms. Some kind of formal calculation of risks and benefits is necessary and as such it justifies reflective, evidence-based, audited practice. The principle of utility states that the rightness of any action is determined by its contribution to the happiness of everyone affected by it. An action is morally correct if it maximises welfare or individual preferences—'the greatest good for the greatest number'.

Effective palliative care satisfies the principle of utility in that it provides benefits for children and families alike. Clinicians may themselves derive immense personal benefit from practice of palliative care, but failure to involve others who could also benefit the child would not be justified. Moreover excessive altruism on part of the clinician, in so far as it may lead to burn out and an inability to provide care for others, may paradoxically lead to adverse consequences.

It is not clear as to the extent that a child's preferences might count, when compared to those of adults, so that difficulties can arise because of this conflict of interest. For example, should children be forced to have treatment that they do not want because adults want them to have it? Some applications of the principle of utility can cause psychological unease. What if the consequences of allowing the death of a child with severe developmental delay and physical disability can be calculated as maximising welfare in a particular society? This could be used as a moral justification for active euthanasia, albeit in a humane way, which many would find psychologically repugnant.

Although the application of the principle of utility requires a potentially difficult calculation of the effects of uncertain consequences, this does not differ from any other exercise that involves balancing value judgements.

Inevitably there are concerns that the principle of utility takes insufficient account of individual preferences and may lead to subjugation of these to the preferences of the majority. This may not provide sufficient protection for the interests of the weak and vulnerable or of those who are felt to have limited capacity or those whose life is limited.

However, some form of utilitarian calculus is inherent in delivering health care to populations and to the allocation of scarce resources.

Deontology (for general references see ref 7)

A problem with consequential theories is that consequences cannot always be controlled even though they may be foreseen. Deontological theory is based on a doctrine of moral obligation or duty. To be moral is to do one's duty, or intend to do it, regardless of the consequences, because intention and motive are subject to an individual's control and determination. To do one's duty involves obeying moral rules, which can be derived by rational consideration or discovery in the same way as natural laws, for example, the law of gravity can be deduced from physical events. Moral rules must be universal (apply to everyone), unconditional (no exceptions) and imperative (obligatory or absolutely necessary). Moral principles, for example, beneficence, non-maleficence, respect for autonomy, and justice underpin moral rules and establish prima facie duties. It follows that in deontological theory some obligations are deemed right regardless of consequences, for example, truth-telling.

To be moral requires the ability of rational consideration to discern rules. It also requires the ability of self-determination (autonomy), that is, the ability to formulate and carry out plans and govern conduct by rules and values. Finally, a free choice must be available. Rational, autonomous beings have their own intrinsic value and are worthy of respect. They may not be used as means to further the ends of others, however laudable these may be. Thus, if we wish to eliminate a disease in society by mass immunisation programmes, but do not obtain informed consent from subjects, we use them as means to achieving our ends without respecting their intrinsic worth. The extent to which children are regarded as rational, autonomous agents who are worthy of respect has been contentious. Children vary enormously—as do adults—in their possession of these characteristics. Moreover autonomy may be affected by LLI, its treatments, or by moods. Finally, children go through a process of developing autonomy. As well as respecting autonomy, clinicians have a duty to enhance the development of autonomy. This involves giving enough information to enable a free choice to be made and encouraging some participation in decision-making.

As with consequential theory, there are some difficulties. For example, we may decide that both truth-telling and doing no harm to humans are absolute duties. If this is the case then there will certainly be circumstances in breaking bad news to children and families when truth-telling produces harm. Suppose the parents do not want their child to be told about their illness because of harms they fear may be caused. There remain difficulties in deciding which of the prima facie moral principles might take precedence. Inherent in deontology is the notion that only rational autonomous decision-making is of moral worth. Yet this feels psychologically unreal because other factors are involved. Indeed an absolute freedom of decision-making may be practically impossible because culture, law, or psychological make-up all condition decisions. The notion of autonomy emphasises the notion of individual choice when other societally derived rights and obligations may also be important. Finally, deciding between competing moral duties is difficult without taking some account of the consequences or likely consequences of actions.

Moral theory and children

One particular problem with 'classical' moral theories is the extent to which they serve the best interests of the weak and vulnerable in general, and children in particular, without unjustifiable paternalism. Of course, such theories tend to reflect the values and standards of the societies that formulated them and it is only relatively recently that we have been particularly concerned with paying due regard to the views of children [8]. Moreover, many jurisdictions that frame legislations concerning children have traditionally been concerned with their age rather than their experience or capacity.

Children in general and those with LLI in particular may lack the capacity to express their views and such views as they have may not count sufficiently in the utilitarian calculus. If morality is a function of rationality and the will, children may be thought to lack the capacity for autonomy and as such their moral status may not be sufficiently respected. Some children with LLI may not live long enough to develop autonomy, for example, an infant with a brain stem tumour; others may not achieve physical autonomy because of disability, for example, muscular dystrophy; whilst others do not develop cognitive ability for self-determination, for example, severe microcephaly, spastic quadriplegia. Yet paradoxically some children with LLI develop more insight into life and its meaning than many adults, precisely *because* of their experience of living with LLI. If moral capacity develops by experience and practice there is no reason why many children cannot develop the capacity earlier than one might expect.

Rights, duties, and responsibilities

Children's rights

There has been increased global acceptance of the role of rights as providing status and protection for individuals (UN Declaration of Human Rights 1948 [9], UN Convention of Rights of the Child 1989 [10]). Dworkin has suggested that rights are necessary to protect individuals from the utilitarian calculus [12]. Similarly rights confer status on those who are thought to lack capacity or rationality.

Rights are justified moral claims made on behalf of individuals, which confer duties (action, or forbearance), on others. Positive rights, requiring action by others, include welfare, institutional, and legal rights and are established by social contract and may change as our society changes. They include rights to information and to the best available health care. Negative rights entail an obligation by others not to infringe them and may be characterised as natural or liberty rights. They include freedom of movement, speech, of practice of religious beliefs, and usually take precedence over positive rights. Special rights exist because of special relationships, for example, parent/child, professional/patient. However, a child's right not to be harmed may take precedence over the rights to family life when the latter cannot be maintained without abuse or neglect.

Holders of positive rights are justified in asking others to act to allow them to exercise their rights, but even these claims may be difficult to fulfil in practice. For example the family of a child with LLI could justifiably ask for effective and appropriate palliative care to enable them to care for their child at home. But if neither local resources nor expertise exists for them to do this then their just claims may be difficult to meet.

Rights, including those of beneficence, non-maleficence, respect for autonomy and justice, are often regarded as being derived from fundamental moral principles which then provide an established basis for health care ethics (Beauchamp and Childress). [7] In turn these principles may be divinely given, derived from natural law or based on social contract. Possession of rights enables individuals to seek redress if their rights are infringed and those who infringe the rights of others without due cause may be subject to ethical or legal censure.

In health care a child's right to the highest attainable standard of health confers upon others the obligation to deliver it. But it is unclear whether such a right is unconditional and, if it is not, what morally relevant considerations should apply. Some consideration of justice or fairness is involved in deciding such issues especially in circumstances when resources are finite. For example do children with LLI have the right to life sustaining treatment in all circumstances and, if they do not, what circumstances are morally relevant and acceptable? Are those in whom fertility is compromised by their own actions, such as promiscuity, less deserving of infertility treatment than those in whom fertility is compromised by LLI or its treatment?

The UN Convention of Rights of the Child sets out rights of children in a series of articles which member states need to ratify and implement [10]. Whilst the UN Convention applies to all aspects of a child's life, the World Medical Association (WMA) [11] has codified those rights pertaining to health. Both endorse the development of a rights-based, child-centred health care system.

A fundamental principle asserts that any decision or action concerning children as individuals or a group must have their best interests as a primary consideration. The Convention also affirms that a child who is capable of forming views on issues including treatment has a right to express them freely. Moreover their view should be given due weight in accordance with their age and maturity. Applied to medical practice this confers obligation to consult children about treatment decisions and their implications. These are particularly important in the many types of LLI where cognitive ability is unimpaired, for example, CF, cancer, renal failure, etc. Other articles confirm the right of freedom of expression (A13), the highest attainable standards of health care, and rehabilitation from illness (A24), privacy (A16), freedom from discrimination (A2), and the right to family life and to hold religious beliefs. Additionally there are obligations to provide families with the necessary support, advice, and services in caring for their children.

The WMA document emphasizes a child's right to child centred health care and encouragement to achieve full potential [12]. It also affirms a child's right to choose how much they should be involved in decision-making and how much information they wish to receive. Children should receive help and support in decision-making but have the right to delegate others to make decisions on their behalf. Importantly they should also have the right to confidentiality and to an explanation of reasons why their preferences cannot be met.

Arguments exist concerning the extent to which children should be allowed to exercise their rights for themselves and the extent to which others might do so on their behalf [13]. Whilst it would be wrong to underestimate a child's capacity it would also be wrong to assume that it was necessarily equal to that of an adult. Nonetheless, adults, be they parents, professionals, or advocates, make decisions from an adult perspective and, in their understandable desire to protect children, may act to their detriment. A teenage child with learning difficulties or muscular dystrophy who is prevented from mixing with the opposite sex may have his or her potential for personal choice restricted. Children with chronic conditions might be so over protected that their development into autonomous individuals is compromised. Some children may be unable to make a big choice, for example, as to *whether* they will have a particular treatment but can decide on aspects such as *where* they will have it.

Children's rights do not exist in isolation and the claim of a right is often more appropriately the beginning, rather than a trump card, of a moral argument. Rights may conflict, for example, the right to life as opposed to freedom from inhuman and degrading treatment. Rights possessed by various parties may constrain each other, for example, parental vs professional rights; children vs parental rights. A rights-based approach may be inherently adversarial. Enactment of rights-based legalisation may lead to re-examination of legal principles involving end of life decision-making (see below). It is not clear as to whose rights take precedence and it may be that children's interests are no better served by a rights-based approach than by application of other moral theories. Nevertheless, highlighting these issues continues to raise questions about the moral status of children and hence the way in which they are treated in our society. Such a debate is likely to have beneficial rather than adverse consequences, especially in the context of LLI.

Traditional moral theory has been concerned with how we should treat persons who are able to think and act autonomously. Although the past 20 years have seen no change in the criteria that we might use to define such individuals, there have been increasing recognition that some children do possess these qualities. Even when they do not, consideration of their rights leads to the obligation to provide them with information they can comprehend, to consult them, and to respect their wishes to the extent that is compatible with their best interests [14].

Moral duties and responsibility of health care clinicians

Clinicians have a special moral relationship with their patients, which imposes particular obligations upon them. Their primary duty is to serve their patients' good by placing their best interests as paramount. This involves two, sometimes, conflicting moral duties [15].

The first duty is to respect life and the health of patients by preserving life, restoring health and preventing disease; to perform these duties to an acceptable standard and to do so fairly and justly. Thus, there is a requirement for practice which is based on best evidence and to keep knowledge and skills up-to-date. Any proposed treatment should confer maximum benefit at the expense of minimal harm. Analysis of harms and benefits should include not only clinical factors but also emotional, psychological, and social factors in relation to the patient and their family.

The second duty is to respect patients' autonomy. This, as we have seen, involves respecting their right to as much self-determination as they are capable of and respecting known or ascertainable wishes, beliefs, preferences, and values. Since it is only an individual who can know what his or her best interests are, clinicians should not manipulate, coerce, or deceive patients into doing what they believe is in their patients' best interest.

Inevitably circumstances arise when a clinician feels that his obligation to benefit a patient is compromised by duty to respect their wishes. This is especially so in relation to children whose moral status may be unclear. In these circumstances clinicians will look to others who have power and responsibility to act on the child's behalf [14].

Parental responsibilities, rights, duties, and power

Although the impact of contemporary, sociological, and legal thinking has been to empower children by encouraging their involvement in decision-making, there remain circumstances in which children cannot or will not express their views. There may be sociological or cultural constraints that limit some children from expressing their own views. For example, cultures where children are expected 'to be seen, but not heard' still exist. Where children do lack the capacity to express their views because of age, developmental, psychological, or other factors, others have ethical and legal authority to make decisions on their behalf.

In most cultures, religions, and legal systems parents have this responsibility. The UK Children Act defines parental responsibility as 'all the rights, duties, power, responsibilities and authority which by law a parent of a child has in relation to the child and his property' [16]. Although much ethical theory does not consider the matter specifically it is clear that parents, by reason of their special relationships with their children, are expected to take a moral responsibility for their upbringing. Parents would be expected to know their child best and hence determine his or her best interests until he or she is able to do so for themselves. The UN Convention acknowledges parental obligation to promote and enhance autonomy and their right to be supported in this task [10].

Application of both moral theory and law supports the autonomy of parents to rear their children in accordance with their own values provided they act in the child's best interests.

A family's concept of their child's best interests is likely to be determined by their own ethical framework or the kinds of duties, rights, and principles outlined above. Social, cultural, and spiritual influences also shape an individual's moral framework. A family's religious beliefs, political and cultural attitudes, peer pressure, religious groups, neighbours, life experiences, and outside influences, for example, media reports, all shape its collective value judgement systems. These may not coincide with those of professionals from different social-economic backgrounds and matters are compounded by power imbalance inherent in the professional/patient (child)/parent relationship. A further conflicting variable may be a child's burgeoning need to make his or her own decisions, which may not coincide with professional or parental choices.

If palliative care focuses on providing the best quality of life for patients and relatives [16] then some way of resolving potential conflicts over what constitutes best interests and who decides them must be found.

Moral arguments in favour of palliative care

Against the background of moral theory, professional, and parental responsibility, it is easy to see that provision of palliative care or symptom relief for children with LLI is as morally justified, as it is clinically important. If health is the absence of physical and mental disability that results from disease then the use of palliative care to alleviate the effect of illness and disabilities is entirely consistent with a duty to restore health or alleviate suffering. It enables the child to sustain his or her capabilities for as long as possible. Good palliative care maximises a child's potential within the constraints of his or her illness and as such achieves the duty to respect and promote such autonomy as the child is capable. Since palliative care supports parents and carers it satisfies the utilitarian calculus. As palliation aims at symptom relief irrespective and independently of any intention to provide curative or life-sustaining treatment (LST) then its use from early on in LLI is mandatory. Some elements of palliative care are a moral requirement of any treatment, but they are especially so in children with LLI and those in whom overall prognosis remains in doubt.

There are also some circumstances where it is neither morally nor legally acceptable or necessary to continue to provide LST because it is no longer in the patients' best interest

to do so [18,19]. There may be little or no likelihood of clinical benefit or the child may have a life which is so severely limited that further prolongation of existence is more than can be borne. However, a decision to change the goals of treatment from cure to palliation can only be ethically justified if there is adequate and appropriate palliative care, which must include support for the family [20].

Formally changing the goals of care from cure to palliation poses intellectual and emotional challenges. Inherent to the process is a frank discussion of the child's condition and prognosis and a decision to forego some aspects of LST. Both the process of initiating such discussions and their timing require skill and sensitivity. It is important to consider at what stage in the context of a child's LLI that the future provision of LST is no longer ethically or legally justified. Since an essential prerequisite is the ability to provide effective palliative care it is highly likely and appropriate that those health care workers responsible for providing that care should be involved in the discussions.

Discussions not to prolong life can raise self doubt in clinicians and introducing the topic may lead to conflict between all parties involved especially when there are serious moral questions about sustaining life [21]. It is recommended that those who participate in discussions that precede decision-making understand the ethical and legal principles involved. Such understanding enables a proposal to limit, withhold, or withdraw LST to be discussed in as open, constructive and sensitive fashion as possible. In addition clinicians require qualities of empathy, sympathy, and team work in managing children with LLI and their families. Particularly important are good communication skills, which are highly valued by families.

Moral argument against provision of LST

Decisions not to provide LST are made on a regular basis in clinical medicine [22–24] and at first sight this seems to run contrary to the clinician's duty of care. In most circumstances protecting and saving lives is in the patients' best interests because they can benefit from medical treatment [18,19]. Decisions 'to let nature takes its course' can only be justified if it is no longer in the patients' best interests to intervene against nature.

It is important to consider the circumstances and contexts in which the objective interests of patients as human beings are not served by prolonging their lives, because in such circumstances offering LST imposes burdens which are not commensurate with benefits. Put another way, we need to consider the circumstances in which it is more in the interests of the child with LLI to allow him or her to die rather than to institute or continue treatments to prolong life. Such circumstances are particularly likely to arise when a child is permanently unable or becomes no longer able to engage minimally with some sense of sustained self-awareness and well-being in any of the activities that uniquely characterise human life [18,19].

In practice there are a range of circumstances in which a child's best interests might be compromised by continued existence. One situation might be when a child is so close to death or so physically and emotionally weak that he or she cannot initiate any coherent action for his or herself. Another would be when there is such severe brain damage that a child has minimal actual or foreseeable capacity to reason, choose, or plan ahead and develop or have any meaningful conversation or interaction. Such interactions are fundamental to an individual's understanding of themselves and the world in which they live and their absence may seem to compromise all that is valued in life. In contrasting circumstances patients may have all the attributes of autonomous beings but decide, because of either physical, emotional, or psychological limitations resulting from their illness, that life does not have enough sustained purpose (despite appropriate clinical intervention) for them to wish to continue it. They may decide for themselves that LST is a greater burden than benefit.

In all these circumstances it may be argued that life has limited value to the extent to which certain qualities maybe lacking or diminished. The relevant qualities include the ability for self-development or following ones own preference expressed through choices, a sense of happiness or well-being and a sense of interaction with others in society. Scales to quantify values of life exist and have been used to quantify the value of health care interventions. However, it has been argued that quality of life is multifactorial and the factors involved are incommensurable, so that attempts to produce some form of utilitarian calculus to influence decision-making are likely to fail [25,26].

Nonetheless, clinicians may conclude that it is morally and professionally unacceptable to strive to prolong the lives of patients by medical means. If ongoing treatment is no longer in a patient's best interests then deciding to override this by appeal to the sanctity of life principle is just as much a breach of professional duty as failure to intervene when it is in a patient's interests to do so [27].

It may be difficult to apply these arguments to children, especially when age, communication problems, and developmental factors limit the capacity for the kinds of interaction described. There may be more uncertainty about the likely prognosis for a small child than there is for an adult with a comparable condition. Uncertainties about the potential

for an infant's developing cognitive capacity can only be clarified as time passes. Part of the moral justification not to provide LST is that the pain and suffering imposed by LLI can be effectively relieved by palliative care. However palliative care should not be identified with acute non-treatment decisions but rather with the moral obligation to relieve pain and suffering of those with LLI both before and after such decisions. Ability to provide palliative care may help relatives and other carers to come to a decision which is in the best interests of the child rather than prolonging of life at all costs. The legal justification for such decision-making is discussed below.

Legal considerations
The role of courts in end-of-life decision-making

Whilst ethics debates what should be done the law decrees what shall or shall not be done. Care for children with LLI must therefore be delivered within the framework established by law.

In general the law provides

- A framework in which to resolve difficult ethical issues
- Safeguards in response to controversial issues
  absolute prohibition, for example, active euthanasia
  procedural hurdles—regulation, for example, withdrawal of treatment in PVS
- Mechanisms for resolving intransigent disputes
- Protection for the weak and vulnerable.

Law provides that the courts are the agents of the law and have a number of powers and functions that include:

- Interpretation and application of existing statute, criminal, and case law
- Creation of new precedents depending on the level of court
- Provision of an impartial, fair, and transparent system to resolve competing claims.
- Ultimate definition of the best interests of incompetent individuals and decision-making on their behalf.

Depending on the nature of the jurisdiction different emphasis may be placed on the rights of the family as opposed to the rights of individual children.

General legal considerations
(for general references on legal principles see ref 28)

Although certain aspects of criminal law, for example, the prohibition of murder are clear there has been a lack of clarity with regard to the extent to which clinicians must provide LST for children with LLI, especially when they do not believe that the treatment is ethically justified.

Clinicians who take no action to save the life of patients whose death is foreseeable, may face prosecution because they have knowingly and deliberately acted in direct contravention to their duty of care. However, clinicians who give treatments that a patient has rationally and competently refused, for example, blood transfusion to an adult Jehovah's witness have technically committed an assault and have infringed their patient's physical autonomy. Even if they do not find themselves criminally liable the patient may sue for damages produced by non-consensual treatments provided that they are able to satisfy the legal criteria for negligence. In practice clinicians are more likely to worry that they may face criminal charges if they fail to provide LST.

Although the general legal principles given below are likely to have wide application the details will vary in jurisdiction outside the United Kingdom, and readers will need to obtain advice germane to their own country.

Before 1989 the only English legal precedent on which to base decision-making related to a child with Down's syndrome and duodenal atresia whose parents had not wanted the child to undergo surgery. The judgement in this case suggested that if an infant had such a 'demonstrably awful life' that no reasonable person would want to live it, then it might be appropriate to let them die without medical intervention [29]. The criteria for what constitutes such a life were not enunciated but the presumption was that a level of disability greater than that associated with Downs' syndrome was envisaged. In the United States a series of contemporary judgements seemed to establish that on balance, infants should continue to receive treatment directed to prolong their lives even when they had significant disability.

In the 1990s, a further series of cases, mainly involving infants with disabilities, were brought before English Courts. Although in strict terms the judgements refer only to the individual cases themselves, their outcomes have been used to define circumstances in which the non-provision of LST might be legally justified. The overriding principle enunciated in all judgements was that such treatment should be in the best interests of the patient. Courts have tended to take a broader view of best interests than that defined by an analysis of purely clinical outcomes.

Courts have determined that the provision of LST is not in the best interests of patients in the following circumstances:

• An infant who was imminently and irreversibly close to death as a result of hydrocephalus and cerebral malformation [30].

• An infant with severe spastic quadriplegia, deafness, blindness, and a limited capacity to feel pain. Although not close to death, the baby had such severe disabilities that he would never be able to engage in any form of self-directed activity [31].

• A baby with severe brain damage as a consequence of microcephaly and cerebral palsy. Although his mother wanted active treatment the clinician's decision not to provide it was upheld. The principle established here was that clinicians cannot be forced to administer LSTs that they believe are not in the best interests of the child, even when the parents insist [32].

• A young adult in PVS was dependent on tube feeding for survival. The Court held that in these circumstances tube feeding was medical treatment and could be withdrawn because it conferred no clinical benefit and was not in his best interests. The Court also held that there was no legal distinction between withdrawing and withholding LST. [33] A concern is that withholding treatment from patients may mean that they do not receive treatment that might produce some, albeit, limited benefit. No cases involving withdrawal of tube feeding in infants or children have subsequently come to Court in the United Kingdom. In consequence, the legality of withdrawal of fluids from children who are not close to death remains unclear and many professionals have ethical concerns about it.

• In both adults and children it has been held that non-provision of cardiopulmonary resuscitation was acceptable in circumstances of very severe brain damage [34].

• Adults who are competent to do so may request that LST be withdrawn, especially if they face continuation of life they regard as being worse than death. This was the case with Miss B, a 43-year-old woman who had suffered bleeding into an upper spinal cord haemagioma and was quadriplegic and ventilator dependent [35]. In contrast, the request by a women with advanced motor neurone disease to have her life ended by her partner in what was effectively assisted suicide or active euthanasia has been rejected by English Courts [36].

Whilst courts appear to be unwilling to condone practices which require active intervention by others which would normally be regarded as unlawful they may condone what has been termed passive euthanasia [36,37]. Such judgements serve to flesh out what may be considered a 'demonstrably awful life' and are essentially moral in nature.

It is not clear in the United Kingdom as to what effect that enactment of Human Rights Legislation might have on the outcomes of the judgements described above. However it does seem that Courts are prepared to accept that there are circumstances in which the continued provision of LST has limited clinical benefit and no longer serves the broader concept of best interests. It has been argued that they would be unlikely to have reached this position without the availability of high quality, effective palliative care.

Practical aspects of decisions to withhold LST

Consideration of ethical and legal principles discussed above leads to a number of specific issues in relation to children.

- In what kind of circumstances might it be in the best interests of a child to change goals of care from cure to palliation?

- What should be the underlying process for such a change, so as best to represent the interests of all concerned?

- If changing goals of treatment requires consent who is able to do so?

- To what extent should children be involved in decision-making and what weight should their views carry?

Circumstances in which goals of care may be changed

Decisions to change goals of care may be dictated by clinical circumstances, for example, when death is imminent, whatever action is taken. In others the child's clinical condition *per se* is not determinative, for example, a child with moderate/severe learning difficulties who develops renal failure requiring dialysis or transplantation.

In 1997 and 2004 the Royal College of Paediatrics and Child Health (RCPCH) published an ethical and legal framework within which decisions to withhold or withdraw LST might be made [18]. Other bodies have since published guidance but the RCPCH identified five situations in which withholding or withdrawing LST might be discussed. These were:

1. *Brain stem death.*

2. *Persistent vegetative state.*

3. The '*no chance*' situation when LST would only marginally delayed death without alleviating suffering.

4. The '*no purpose*' situation when prolonging survival is possible but only at the cost of physical or mental impairment, which it would be unreasonable to expect the child to bear. It was envisaged that such a child would never be capable of sufficient self-directed activity to make decisions for themselves.

5. The *intolerable* situation where prolonging survival was again possible but, in the face of progressive and irreversible illness, the child and/or family believe that further treatment is more than the child and/or family can endure with any acceptable degree of human fulfilment. This situation clearly includes children with and without mental impairment.

The situation envisaged in 1 and 2 above arouse little controversy although some may not accept brain stem death on religious grounds [39,40] and diagnosis of PVS in young children may pose practical problems. Equally few would contest withdrawal of LST where clinical benefit is impossible, for example, in an 18 month child with meningococcal septicaemia, tissue gangrene, and multiple organ failure.

The situations envisaged under the 'no purpose' and 'intolerable' headings are more controversial essentially because they raise issues and conflicts which surround the focus of the duty of care (to child or parent), about what might constitute best interests and who might decide them.

The no purpose situation envisages that the outcome for the child might be so severe in terms of physical or developmental damage that it would be unreasonable for them to be expected to bear it. Such a child might already have, or regress to, minimal self-awareness and capacity for social inter-reaction. Such an example might be provided by the ongoing care of an extremely premature baby following severe intraventricular haemorrhage or a child with neurodegenerative disease, for example, Tay Sachs, Batten's disease, who develops respiratory failure.

In the intolerable situation the infants and children may have a wide range of cognitive abilities. The burden of repeated clinical intervention may here be considered to be too great in terms of clinical benefit, for example, a child with some intellectual impairment, renal dysplasia, and chronic renal failure who ultimately requires dialysis. Similar cases might involve a child with sufficient experience or maturity to refuse further treatment, for example, heart/lung transplantation in an 11-year old with cystic fibrosis in which the family supports the child's decision not to undergo transplant surgery.

Some children in this situation may be able to express their feelings about their disabilities or illness and its impact on their lives, such as, inability to attain certain goals, which they have set or peer groups achieve. This level of awareness may be sufficient to generate feelings of anger and frustration that may be increasingly difficult to alleviate. In these circumstances continued provision of LST is increasingly questionable for children, parents, and carers. Recognising when this stage is reached and knowing how to broach the subject requires particular clinical and humanitarian skills. At all events consent is required.

Consent in children with LLI and palliative care

All health care intervention requires the valid consent of patients or those empowered to make decisions on their behalf [28]. All persons have an ethical and legal right to decide what shall be done to them. Consent grants the clinician the permission to do something which would otherwise be unethical or unlawful. Consent is therefore more than mere acquiescence or the 'symbolic' signing of a form. Rather it is a dynamic process embodying information sharing and understanding, expression of preferences and choices over what treatment an individual shall receive and satisfies the professional obligation to confer benefit and to respect autonomy.

Although consent involves exercising a right of choice over treatment options, it does not create a right to demand treatments, even when these may prolong life. Some parents, and indeed some children with LLI, may be willing to accept treatments which carry high risks but little likelihood of prolonging life, even for a short time. However, clinicians cannot be expected ethically to provide treatment which would cause overall harm, neither does the law compel them to do so. It follows that agreement to undertake investigations or treatment is a dynamic decision made in partnership between children, families, and clinicians. Such partnerships are justified because they establish a relationship of trust and are associated with better health care outcomes [41]. A valid consent should be sufficiently informed, given by a competent person, and obtained without coercion or threat.

Information

To make choices children and families need information about their diagnosis, prognosis, and treatment options, which in this situation may be sad or unpleasant. Clinicians have traditionally been unwilling to present such information to children on the grounds that it may cause harm, but if the clinician/child/parent relationship is to become one of trust then there has to be increasing openness about what treatment can and cannot achieve [42]. Research shows that children can benefit from knowing potentially unpleasant facts about their parents' health care and from being given truthful explanations [43]. There is a tendency for clinicians to underestimate a desire for information but overestimate a desire for participation in all decision-making [44]. Competent children and adults may elect that others make decisions on their behalf although their views may change with deepening experience of LLI.

Since parents are the key decision-makers for children who lack competence it is important that they have sufficient information to make decisions which are in their child's best interests. As well as information they need sufficient support and help to understand the meaning of what is discussed and also the opportunity to acknowledge their own feelings. For older children, and those who have developed understanding by their experience of LLI, imparting sufficient information which is unlikely to cause harm is important. Parents may have difficulty with this and may want unpalatable or unpleasant facts to be kept from their child. However, they may not understand that their child with LLI knows that they are dying but does not want to upset their parents by letting *them* know this.

Imparting information requires effective communication skills, which are highly regarded by patients and relatives in the adult end of life decision-making. However they should not be used to coerce or manipulate children or parents to do what clinicians regard as being in the patient's best interests.

Quantification of information given requires thought. Previous 'professional standards'—the information that a reasonable professional might disclose—may spare both clinicians and patients from the effects of distressing information, but may not provide enough information for reasonable choice, and hence fail to respect autonomy. A more acceptable standard is the amount of information a reasonable parent or child might wish to have in similar circumstances. It is difficult to know to what extent children with LLI may conform to this standard. Some experienced, competent patients may want more information, whilst in others what can be imparted will be limited by cognitive ability or circumstance. There may be cases, albeit rare, in which children are genuinely harmed by receiving information, which a reasonable child might want.

Information given to the extent that a particular parent or child might want provides maximum respect for autonomy at the expense of being time consuming. But neither parents nor children may disclose preferences, and say precisely what they *do* want. Spending time trying to achieve this standard may be at the expense of time spent in providing necessary care for others in whom there might be greater chances of clinical benefit.

In practice it seems that truth-telling and information sharing is important but the quantum depends on the harms/benefits calculus [45].

Although the above standards refer to rational adults who are assumed competent to consent, children also have the right to receive information at a pace and in a form which they can comprehend.

Without prior information, a child's capacity for understanding can only be assessed in abstract and they will have little chance to develop specific capacity for the task in question. If it is a professional duty to enhance a child's competence then they should receive the information that will enable them to achieve this. Children with LLI will vary enormously in respect of their information requirements. The principle of justice requires that we treat those with differing needs fairly but in accordance with morally relevant differences which exclude discrimination on purely social, religious, or ethnic grounds or indeed of disability itself.

Adults may waive their right to make an adequately informed choice on their own behalf, but may still accept (or reject) a treatment which clinicians believe to be in their best interests. It is more arguable as to whether parents may waive this right in respect of children who are unable to make informed choices for themselves. Accepting a treatment for another without due deliberation may fail to take that person's best interests seriously and may lead to clinicians making unquestioning, paternalistic judgements. Where there is doubt that parents, for whatever reason, are acting in the best interests of their child or not taking them seriously, then it may be necessary to obtain legal advice.

Competence

Competence is the ability to undertake the task in question, in this case to make a decision about treatment options. It is contextually and culturally dependent. Patients may be temporarily incompetent by reason of confusion, diminution of consciousness or pain and similar constraints apply to children. Equally, families who face difficult decisions may feel that they lack the emotional competence to make them.

In legal terms competence involves the following abilities [46]:

(1) to understand relevant information;

(2) to believe that it applies to oneself;

(3) to retain information for long enough to deliberate upon it;

(4) to use information to make a decision;

(5) to communicate the decision.

These abilities are not necessarily a function of age, also children may be competent in one area, for example, choosing what to eat, but lack competence to make major decisions about treatment options. Different legal ages for competencies, for example, driving, drinking, reflect a society's desire both to protect the vulnerable as well as itself [14]. In English law a child's capacity with respect to consent to treatment is a function of his or her ability to understand fully the nature and purpose of the procedure, its complications and the impact of their choice upon their family [47].

When the decisions faced are important and the impact on the child and family is great it has been argued that the barriers to granting a child his or her wish should be greater [48]. This does not mean that a child's views should not be sought. If his or her views are not accepted, he or she should be told the reasons why.

Even children who are competent may elect that others make choices for them. The general ethical and legal duty to enhance and develop competence of patients applies as much to children with LLI as any others, to an extent commensurate with their abilities. Clearly some children with LLI lack the capacity to develop self-directed activity irrespective of age. Others will do so, albeit at a slower rate than their peers. Others may have sufficient capacity for self-determination, but may be perceived to lack capacity because of physical disabilities, for example, severe movement disorder as a result of cerebral palsy or severe disfigurement may lead to a false assumption of incompetence. Children with Duchenne muscular dystrophy may be thought to have a poorer quality of life than they themselves acknowledge.

Voluntariness

Adult patients should not be coerced or manipulated by clinicians into accepting treatment that they have not chosen on the basis of information received. In order that choices for children are as freely given as possible, consent givers should receive a rational balanced presentation of benefits, harms, and risks of treatments. When confronted by distressing information, failure to provide adequate time for reflection and questioning is also coercive. Children with LLI, even if they have developed competence, may be vulnerable because of the circumstances of their illness. Their parents may seek to prevent them from receiving distressing information in order to protect them. Such manoeuvres, whilst understandable, may limit free choice and create mistrust. The power imbalance between professionals, parents, and children may also threaten voluntary choice. Attempts should be made to minimise all these factors.

Collusion

Contemporary health care depends on partnership which is based on mutual trust and understanding. Patients make informed choices about health care with the help and support of their clinicians. The situation is more complex in paediatrics where children, especially those with LLI, may lack the capacity to make informed choices and where parents have ethical and legal responsibility for decision making. The WHO definition of palliative care includes the care of relatives, emphasising their significance [17].

In practice the ideal of partnership may be difficult to achieve because of power imbalances between professionals, children, and parents/carers. Understandably parents and carers may wish to control the flow of information to their child, whether the latter is competent or not. However, this approach is potentially both paternalistic and parentalist and may not be in the best interests of the child [54]. It may lead to collusion between professionals and parents so that children are excluded from receiving information which others deem harmful or distressing. In turn this compromises a child's capacity for choice and adversely affects his or her potential to develop capacity. Collusion is also likely to inhibit the duty of confidentiality, which is owed to a child, and may exist independently of their capacity. One way of overcoming this is for professionals to share information with both children and parents in a sensitive, appropriate, and timely fashion, enabling both parents and children to ask questions which they may have [54].

Secrets between parents and professionals, for example, the withholding of the fact that a child's prognosis is poor, may be difficult to keep from children, especially when they have gained experience of their illness and may be able to recognise uncomfortable body language which adults may subconsciously exhibit in these circumstances. Collusion between parents and professionals can also be used to force the children to have treatment that they do not want but which adults in similar circumstances can refuse [14,54].

Recognition of collusion and how to tackle it requires tact and skill. For competent children, adults have no specific rights to control the flow of information, unless it is likely that harm to others will result. Despite this, parents do need information in order for them to fulfil their role as carers in as humane and efficient manner as possible.

Children may also share information with clinicians which they do not want their parents or others to know. By and large such confidences should be respected because they are essential to the relationship of mutual trust and respect between patients and clinicians. However, in case where failure to share such information potentially compromises the ability of parents and others to provide care for the child, then it should be shared on a need to know basis.

Conflicting views between parents, children, and clinicians

Demands for continuing LST by parents

Sometimes parents may demand that clinicians continue to provide LST in circumstances where intervention will neither significantly prolong life nor confer clinical benefit. Such claims may stem from genuinely held parental (social, religious, or cultural) values and beliefs, which may not be shared by the clinicians. Although parents may have a right to

make decisions on behalf of their child, this does not confer the right that demands for treatment must be met.

The best interests of the child remain the clinician's primary ethical and legal duty. Some moral duties are owed to parents but related to relief of their pain and distress and the provision of support and guidance [20]. They should be helped with sensitivity and compassion to understand the nature and prognosis of their child's illness and given clear reasons as to why continuing LST is not in the child's best interests. This approach is time consuming, may be difficult, and may arouse conflicts. Ethical problems also arise when views of parents and children have not been fully ascertained.

Resolution of conflict requires negotiation, communication, consensus building, and avoidance of potential areas of misunderstanding. Deferring to requests for benign or uncomplicated treatments may be helpful, for example, antibiotics but not ventilation in a child with severe cerebral palsy and respiratory failure due to a chest infection. It must be emphasised that withdrawal of LST does not mean withdrawal of care. Taking a second opinion, involving other family members, religious advisers, and advocacy services may all be helpful. Family conferences with or without formal ethical support, for example, from a clinical ethics committee may also be valuable [49].

Despite these approaches, which can be used in any type of ethical dispute, parents may continue to demand LST. In these circumstances they should be advised that it is their right to seek judicial review, should be told what this entails, how they may approach it, and if necessary be helped to do so. Despite the impact that such a decision to seek legal advice may have on clinicians the parents should continue to receive support and not be engaged in adversarial conflict or debate.

Refusal of LST by parents or children

Some children with LLI may have a personal experience of life which, in so far as it is ascertainable, is terrible and may be able to express feelings of pain, anger, frustration, and sadness at the effect of LLI on their aspirations and hopes. Although some of these feelings may be alleviated by palliative care there may come a time when continuing LST becomes questionable for children, parents, and carers. Further treatment may extend life but confers greater burdens. In response to these situations some parents may feel that the life of their child is now so limited that further treatment is not in their best interests. Recognition of when this stage has arrived and how to discuss it is part of 'the art of medicine'.

Clearly some children may be able to decide for themselves that they do not want further LST and by and large their views should be respected, especially if the clinicians concur. For those who lack competency it seems likely that, as long as clinicians and parents agree, LST may be lawfully withheld. However, if parents continue to disagree with the clinicians and an agreement cannot be found by the use of the techniques outlined above, referral to the Courts may be necessary.

A rather uncomfortable situation for clinicians may arise. It is possible to envisage a scenario in which two children with very similar clinical conditions may or may not continue to receive LST depending on their contrasting parental views. The logical conclusion is that respect for parental autonomy or rights overcomes the best interests of the child. The moral justification for this, in the absence of a clearly expressed view from the child, is that it would be wrong to force the beliefs and values of the clinical team on parents who disagree with them, though there clearly are other circumstances, for example, child abuse, where this occurs. However, it is the parents, not professionals, who will have to live with the consequences of whatever decisions they have made. In these circumstances a utilitarian calculus may trump the professional duty of care.

Whatever alternative is chosen the duty to provide relief of suffering for the child and family remains and will fall to the palliative care team.

The extent to which children should be involved in decision-making

Children are actively developing their personalities through inter-reactions and relationships with peers, parents, and other adults. As they mature they acquire the skills and confidence to carry out tasks and are deemed competent to do so. Their emotional well-being is in part dependent upon their self-satisfaction with these dynamic evolving achievements [50]. Interference with this process of developing capacity by denying children the right to be involved in decision-making may result in the loss of self-esteem and the lack of confidence. Balanced against this is the duty to protect children from making harmful choices when they may not fully understand the implications and consequences of their choices.

'Good parenting [and clinical care] involves giving minors as much rope as they can handle without the unacceptable risk that they will hang themselves' (Lord Donaldson in Re W [51]). Finding a proper balance between the harms produced by over-protection and those produced by too little can be complex and difficult in the clinical care of children [13].

There is both an ethical and legal obligation to consult children about their feelings thoughts, and preferences to an extent commensurate with their maturity and understanding [10,16]. This is not to say that a child's views should or will prevail. The extent to which it might do so is determined by

the importance of the decision in hand and its impact on the family in a way that is not required for adults—provided that an adult can show that they are competent as previously defined and they are free to make choices about their treatment that clinicians may regard as irrational and dangerous.

It is logical to argue that if a child is deemed competent to consent to treatment then he or she should be able to refuse it—even LST in the context of LLI. There are strong moral arguments, founded on a duty to respect a young person's autonomy and upon the adverse consequences of forcing unwanted treatment on them, as to why this might be so. Because children with LLI may be vulnerable and physically weakened by their condition, it is all the more important that unwanted treatment is not forced upon those who are competent to refuse it. As we have seen the child's experience of LLI confers a degree of competence that other children of similar ages simply do not have. Indeed it is widely accepted that a competent child's decision to refuse treatment which is not essential to prolong life or avoid serious ill-health should be respected [14].

However, in practice, clinicians have difficulties in honouring a child's choice to forego LST, especially when they do not believe that it is in their best interests to do so. It is in these difficult circumstances, as in other disputes, which cannot be resolved by application of procedures previously described, that judgement of Courts may be requested.

Courts and the role of law

Courts are the ultimate arbiters in matters concerning the definition of best interests in circumstances of disagreement. In determining best interests Courts have taken a broader perspective of best interests than that provided by analysis of purely clinical benefits and harms. The welfare checklist includes ascertaining the wishes of children and families, their cultural, social, and religious backgrounds along with other factors.

In general, Courts have accorded great weight to clinicians' views of best interests and have been reluctant to force clinicians to give treatments, which they believe are futile and burdensome. Thus, they have over-ruled parental demands (made on the basis of strong religious beliefs) to provide LST for a child with spinal muscular atrophy. They have also been reluctant to allow parents to refuse LST for their children in circumstances when clinicians felt it was in the child's best interests to treat. However this is not invariable, in that parental right to refuse liver transplantation for their child with chronic liver disease was upheld on the basis that their views of their child's best interests overrode the clinical view [14].

Courts have been equally reluctant to sanction a child's refusal of LST, even in circumstances where their consent would be lawful. Thus, although children over 16 years, or those who are competent to do so, may consent under English Law, in practice they may not be able to refuse LST until they are over 18 years. Thus a boy with leukaemia, who was a Jehovah witness, was deemed unable to refuse blood transfusion, which was in his clinical best interests [52]. Courts have also sanctioned heart transplantation in a teenager with acute cardiomyopathy, despite her reasoned refusal, on the grounds that she did not understand the consequences for her family [53].

Thus English Courts have defined circumstances in which both parental and children's wishes may be overcome, although it is not clear what force these judgements might have in other jurisdictions.

Resuscitation

In the United Kingdom all establishments that face decisions about attempting resuscitation are required to have policies relating to these decisions. These should respect patients' rights, be understood by all relevant staff, and be accessible to those who need them [55]. Resuscitation is potentially life saving and there is a general presumption that it will be attempted unless specific agreement to the contrary exists in the form of a Do Not Attempt Resuscitation (DNAR) Order. The outcome of resuscitation attempts will depend upon the nature and severity of underlying disease process.

Attempts at resuscitation may not be in the child's best interests because

(1) they are unlikely to be successful;

(2) because there will be no material benefit in restarting the heart because of likely duration of survival or high risk of severe side effects;

(3) any expected benefits are likely to be outweighed by burdens.

The issuing of DNAR orders may result in limitation, withdrawal or withholding of LST. Families may find it difficult to agree to a DNAR because they may have unrealistic expectations of the likely success of resuscitation, poor knowledge of complication rates, and poor perception of the processes involved. They may have difficulty in accepting withdrawal of treatment for cultural, psychological, and religious reasons. However, they may be able to accept some limitation of treatment [23].

There is considerable variation of practice as to how the decisions to issue DNAR orders are made with families. Such variability doubtless results from differing views as to whether such discussions are appropriate in the context of terminal illness [56]. The view that discussions should not take place is based on the paternalistic notion that discussions cause more pain and distress than likely benefit, and may reinforce false expectations and hopes in the likely outcome of resuscitation. The contrary view is that families are more likely to suffer harm and have less trust in their doctors if they do not have such discussions and, as unpleasant as they may be, they are essential for informed choice. Some support for the latter view comes from studies of bereaved parents in the United Kingdom, where the parents felt that they had made the decision to withdraw or withhold LST and they needed to feel that their decision in retrospect was the right one [57]. There seems no reason why children with LLI should not be sensitively involved in discussions provided they have sufficient maturity, understanding, and insight and provided they receive appropriate help and support to the extent they require it.

Euthanasia

The term euthanasia is most commonly reserved for the compassion-motivated deliberate rapid termination of the life of someone afflicted with an incurable and progressive disease [58]. It may be regarded as voluntary if the dying person requests it and involuntary if they do not or can not. Respecting autonomy of patients allows them to decide the timing and manner of their own death [59].

Treatment given with the intention to alleviate pain and suffering in children with LLI is clearly consistent with the moral purpose of medicine, even when it can be reasonably foreseen that such treatment will not prolong life and may even be associated with some shortening of life. If a literal meaning of euthanasia is 'a peaceful gentle death' then the aim of palliative care is to achieve this.

In contrast, treatment given or omitted with the intention to shorten life is a criminal offence, even if a patient or parent of a child with LLI requests it. Clinicians have a duty not to kill their patients. Thus it could be argued that any omission, for example, by not providing LST, is a breach of that duty. The law in the United Kingdom and many other jurisdictions does not permit euthanasia or assisted suicide.

Arguments continue over the validity of accepting the intention of a clinician as a criterion for the moral and legal validity for an action or omission which may be followed by the death of a patient [60]. Those who accept intention as a valid argument consider that there are actual, experiential, conceptual, moral, and legal distinctions between foreseeing that an action will kill a patient and intending that it does so.

This is consistent with the doctrine of double effect where the beneficent intention of an action outweighs its unintended but foreseeable adverse consequences. In the circumstances of LLI it is the consequences of the illness that is responsible for the death of the patient and not the action of the clinician. The counter argument runs that the moral validity of an action should be based on the best interests of patients rather than the moral character of clinicians. As we have seen there may be circumstances in which the provision of LST is no longer in the best interests of children with LLI. If this is the case then some would say an action which results in the death of the patient, even if intended, may be justified.

It has been argued that the effect of the recent series of judgements in UK Courts and professional guidance is ethically incoherent since passive euthanasia—that is death produced by withholding, withdrawing, or limiting LST—is permitted but active euthanasia (as defined above) is not. An alternative view is that Courts are prepared to grant a great deal of discretion to the intention and professional integrity of clinicians in these intensely personal, emotional, and spiritual matters while respecting the right to punish individuals who flout or abuse their moral responsibilities. In so doing Courts recognise the difficulties facing clinicians who wish to provide compassionate palliative care but who wish to do so without the threat of prosecution [61]. However, the issue of euthanasia is likely to remain a matter of moral indeterminacy and continuing debate in adults, let alone children with LLI.

Sex and sexuality

The acknowledgement of adults' sexuality and their freedom to express it are important aspects of personal autonomy which should be respected in so far as they do not cause harm to others [62]. When adults' capacity is impaired the focus of Law is to protect them from particularly abusive relationships [63].

Children with LLI increasingly survive into adolescence and early adulthood. Although the Law defines the age at which they may enter into sexual relationships their desire to explore sexual feelings and discover their sexuality evolves before this. This is especially challenging for those with physical rather than cognitive disabilities who have the same rights as adults to protection, advice, and confidentiality. Specific concerns which need to be addressed are the voluntariness of sexual relationships, peer pressure, and vulnerability [64].

Sexual education

Children with LLI may be physically or emotionally vulnerable and as such their educational needs relating to sexual development may not be met. School curricula may cover biological aspects of sex education but omit to explore the moral tensions or develop the personal skills needed to cope with the emotional aspects and sexual experience of adolescence, especially when a child has cognitive and physical disabilities. Neither school nor parents may discuss issues such as masturbation and homosexuality. It is possible that the relationship of professionals with young people with LLI means that they are the most appropriate persons to broach them. However professionals may feel uneasy about this because of their own values and uncertainties and in the face of possible parental disapproval. But young people who are experimenting sexually may not practice safe sex and may not approach parents for advice. In these circumstances denying young people information about sex and sexuality also denies them the opportunity for protection against unwanted pregnancy and sexually transmitted diseases [65].

The scope of professional duty should be limited to education, counselling, and information sharing. This may pose problems in those adolescents who have physical disabilities and who may wish to express their sexuality, but who lack the physical ability to do so. To what extent should professionals assist them? Some form of professional assistance could be defended by appeal to the principles of beneficence and maximising respect for autonomy, for example, by helping them acquire sexually explicit videos. But it could be argued that some levels of involvement, for example, masturbation would be potentially harmful for the professional/patient relationship in that it extends it to a far more emotional level than many would feel comfortable with.

Contraception

Provision of contraception advice without parental knowledge can be given in England to those below the legal age of consent provided that they fulfil specific criteria and are able to understand fully the issues involved and the impact on their family [47]. Ethically, this satisfies the right of a competent child to make decisions and to have their confidentiality respected.

A young person with learning disabilities should be able to experience aspects of life from which they may formerly have been excluded, for example, romantic and sexual relationships. However, there is no justification for providing contraception—especially if given by invasive means—if the young person shows no interest in sexual activity. Provision of contraception is lawful if there is proxy consent or in the case of over 18 years old in England if it is in their best interests. The least invasive means to get the best possible results should be used and where dispute persists Court action should be taken [64].

Abortion

If contraception fails or is not used the question of termination of pregnancy (TOP) may arise in young people with LLI. Such children may be competent to consent and TOP may be indicated on grounds of detriment to mental or physical health [64].

Confidentiality should be respected, but the young person needs to be aware of the potential emotional and psychological sequelae of abortion, and have access to counselling. Requests for confidentiality can be over-ridden if the young person is subject to a Court order or it there are good grounds to suspect exploitation or abuse [64,66].

Conclusion

This chapter has sought to consider the ethical and legal principles that underpin end of life decision-making and the provision of palliative care in children with LLI. However, defining and applying principles cannot always relieve ethical uncertainty or perplexity. Clinicians, parents, and children will continue to disagree at times on what constitutes a child's best interests, who should determine them, and how they might be addressed [67,68].

Differing personal, social, and religious values and beliefs between parties will fuel such disagreements. The latter include such issues as the sanctity of life, the ability of children to make decisions, the extent to which children might be forced to accede to adults' wishes, and the balance to be struck between competing rights of individuals.

Those who expect ethical analysis to provide definitive solutions to such disputes will be disappointed. However, focusing on what principles should be involved, in deciding what should be done, and the reasons for it optimises the rationality of the decision-making process [69]. Acknowledging that decision-making is hard, emotionally draining, and accepting that protagonists in the moral debate are all worthy of empathy and support, is procedurally important. In these circumstances transparency, rigour, and fairness of the decision-making process is, perhaps, ultimately more important that its outcome. It is important that the power imbalance between professionals and parents and children is minimised, as difficult as this may be for professionals. Fairness demands that due attention is paid to the narrative of the key participants and that the focus remains on the child. It is possible that Clinical Ethics Committees can provide an objective, independent forum for such discussion [49].

Perhaps the most important factor is the empathy, care, and concern of professionals in reaching out to families.

In adult medicine decisions to withdraw LST are normal in the palliative care setting and are commonly reached by mutual agreement between patients and clinicians. When a choice to withdraw LST is made, helping the patient to achieve a 'good' death is a legitimate and ethically acceptable goal of health care [70]. From a patient's perspective the key considerations are adequate management of symptoms, avoidance of inappropriate prolongation of dying, achieving a sense of control and strengthening relationship with loved ones [71]. There is no ethical reason why similar principles should not apply to the management of children with LLI.

Whatever the outcome of the complex, often harrowing, emotionally draining, and sometimes contentious ethical and legal discussions which occur, clinicians have a fundamental duty to provide high quality, compassionate palliative care for children with LLI and their families. It is no less than they need and no more than they deserve.

References

1. Gray Thomas. Elegy in a Country Churchyard. In *Oxford Book of English Verse*. Oxford: Oxford University Press.
2. Nuffield Council on Bioethics *Animal to human transplants: The Ethics of or xenotransplantation*. London, Nuffield Council on Bioethics, 1996.
3. Association for children with life threatening or terminal conditions and their families *A Guide to the Development of Children's Palliative Care Services*. London Royal College of Paediatrics and Child Health, 1997.
4. Nelson, L.J., Rushton, C.H., Cranford, R.E., Nelson, R.M.,and Glover, J.J., Forgoing medically provided nutrition and hydration in paediatric patients. *J Law Med Ethics* 1995:23, 33–46.
5. Doyal, L., Larcher, V. Drafting guidelines for the withholding or withdrawing of life-sustaining treatment in critically ill children and neonates. *Arch of Dis Childhood. Fetal and Neonatal edition* 2000; 83; F60–63.
6. Jones, A.H. Narrative in Medical Ethics. *Br Med J;* 1999; 318: 253–6.
7. Raphael, D.D. *Moral Philosophy*. Oxford: Oxford University Press, 1981, pp. 34–42; Gillon, R. *Philosophical Medical Ethics* (2nd edition). Chichester Wiley, 1994.; Beauchamp, T.L. and Childress, J.F. (1994). *Principles of Biomedical Ethics* (4th edition). Oxford: Oxford University Press, 1994.
8. Lansdown, G. Implementing children's rights in healthcare. *Arch Dis Childhood* 2000;83:286–8.
9. United Nations Association. *Universal Declaration of Human Rights*. General Assembly of the United Nations, New York, 1948.
10. *United Nations Convention on the rights of the Child*. General Assembly of the United Nations Convention on the rights of the Child (1989). The Stationery Office London, 1996.
11. Dworkin, R. *Taking Rights Seriously*. Oxford: Oxford University Press, 1981.
12. World Medical Association. *Declaration of Ottawa on the rights of the Child to Health Care*. 50th World Medical Assembly, Ottawa, October, 1998.

13. Kurtz, Z. Do children's rights to healthcare in the UK ensure their best interests? *J Royal College Phys Lond* 1985;29:508–16.

14. Chantler, C. and Doyal, L. Medical ethics: The duties of care in principle and practice. In M. Powers and N. Harris, eds. *Clinical Negligence*. London: Butterworths,2000.

15. British, Medical Association. *Consent Rights and Choices in Health Care for Children and Young People*. London: BMJ Books, 2001.

16. The Children Act. London Her Majesty's Stationery Office, 1989.

17. World Health Organisation. *Cancer, Pain Relief and Palliative Care Report of a WHO Expert Committee Report series No. 804*. Geneva a World Health organization, 1990.

18. Royal College of Paediatrics and Child Health. *Withholding or Withdrawing Life Saving Medical Treatment in Children: A framework for practice*. London: Royal College of Paediatrics and Child Health, 1997, 2004.

19. British Medical Association *Withholding and withdrawing life-prolonging medical treatment* (2nd edition) London: BMA books, 2001.

20. Trapp, A. Support for the family. In A. Goldman, ed. *Care of the Dying Child* Oxford: Oxford University Press, 1998, pp. 76–92.

21. Way, J., Back, A.L., and Randall-Curtis, J. Withdrawing life support and resolution of conflicts with families. *BMJ* 2002;325:1342–5.

22. Balfour-Lynn, I.M. and Tasker, R.C. Futility and death in paediatric intensive care. *J Med Ethics* 1996;22:279–81.

23. Goh, A.Y.T., Lum, L.C.S., Chan, P.W.K., Bakar, F., and Chong, B.O. Withdrawal and limitation of life support in paediatric intensive care. *Arch Dis Child* 1999;80:424–8.

24. Roy, R., Narendra, A., Costeloe, K., and Larcher, V. Modes of death in a tertiary neonatal intensive care unit. *Fetal Neonatal Ed* 2004;89:F527–30.

25. Downie, R.S. The value and quality of life. *J Royal College Phys Lond.* 1999;33:378–81.

26. MacNaughton, R.J. Numbers, scales and qualitative research. *Lancet* 1996;347:1099–1100.

27. Levetown, M. Ethical aspects of paediatric palliative care. *J Palliat Care* 1996;12:35–9.

28. Montgomery, J. *Health Care Law*. Oxford: Oxford University Press, 2002, pp. 227–48; Kennedy, I. and Grubb, A. *Medical Law Text and Materials*. London: Butterworths, 2000.

29. Re B. (1981) 1 WLR 1421.

30. Re C. (1989) 2 All ER 782.

31. Re J. (1990) 6 BMLR 25.

32. Re J. (1992) 9 BMLR 10.

33. Airedale NHS Trust v Bland (1993) 1 All ER 821.

34. Re R. (1996) 2FLR 99.

35. Ms B v an NHS Hospital Trust (2002) EWHC 429 (Fam).

36. Pretty v United Kingdom (2002) 35 EHRR 1.

37. Keowan, J. Medical murder by omission? The law and ethics of withholding and withdrawing treatment and tube feeding. *Clin Med* 2003;3:460–3.

38. Montgomery, J. *Health Care Law*. Oxford: Oxford University Press, 2002, pp. 437–39.

39. Inwald, D., Jacobovits, I., and Petros, A. Brain stem death: Managing care when accepted medical guidelines and religious beliefs are in conflict. *BMJ* 2000;320:1266–7.

40. Gatrad, A.R. and Sheikh, A. Palliative care for Muslims and issues before death. *Int J Palliat Care Nurs* 2002;8:526–31.

41. Greenfield, S., Kaplan, S., and Ware, J.F. Expanding patient involvement in care. *Ann Int Med* 1985;102:520–8.

42. Anderlik, M.R. *et al.* Revisiting the truth-telling debate; a study of disclosure practices at a major cancer center. *J Clin Ethics* 2000; 11(3):251–9.

43. Barnes, J., Kroll, L., Burke, O., Lee, J., Jones, A., and Stein, A. Qualitative interview study of communication between parents and children about maternal breast cancer. *BMJ* 2000;321:479–82.

44. Montgomery, A.A. and Fahey, T. How do patients' preferences compare with those of clinicians? *Qua Health Care* 2001;10(Suppl. I):39–43.

45. Campbell, E.M. and Sanson-Fisher, R.W. Breaking bad news 3. Encouraging the adoption of best practice. *Behav Med* 1998;24(2):73–80.

46. Re C. (1994) 1 All ER 819.

47. Gillick v West Norfolk and Wisbech AHA (1986) AC 122 and (1985) 3 All ER 423–24.

48. Lansdown, R. Listening to children: Have we gone too far (or not far enough)? *J Royal Soc Med* 1998;91:457–61.

49. Larcher V. The role of Clinical Ethics Committees in paediatric practice. *Arch Dis Childhood* 1999;81:104–6.

50. Doyal, L. and Gough, I. *A Theory of Human Need*. London: MacMillan, 1991

51. Re, W. (1992) 4 All ER 627.

52. Re, E. (A Minor) (Medical treatment) (1993) 1 FLR 386.

53. Re, M. (Child refusal of medical treatment) (1999) 2 FLR 1097.

54. Alderson, P. and Montgomery, J. *Health Care Choices. Making decisions with Children London*. Institute for Public Policy Research, 1996.

55. Joint statement from the British Medical Association, the Resuscitation Council (UK) and the Royal College of Nursing On Resuscitation and do not resuscitate orders. www.bma.org.uk/ap.ncf

56. Manisty, C., Waxman, J. and Higginson, I.J. Education and Debate: Doctors should not discuss resuscitation with terminally ill patients. *BMJ* 2003;327:614–6.

57. McHaffie, H. *Crucial Decisions at the Beginning of Life. Parents' Experience of Treatment Withdrawal from Infants*. Oxford: Radcliffe Medical Press, 2001.

58. Roy, D. and Lapin, C. Regarding euthanasia, *Eur J Palliat Care* 1994; 1:57–9.

59. Campbell, C., Hart, J., and Matthews, P. Conflict of conscience: hospice and assisted suicide. *Hastings Center Reports* 1995;25(3): 36–43.

60. Doyal, L. and Gillon, R. When doctors might kill their patients *BMJ* 1999;318:1431–3.

61. Sensky, T. Withdrawal of life-sustaining treatment. Patients' autonomy and values conflict with the responsibilities of clinicians. *B M J* 2002;325:175–76

62. Doyal, L. Infertility counselling and IVF. The moral and legal background. In *S. Jennings, ed. Infertility Counselling*. Oxford:Blackwell, 1995, pp.191–204.

63. British Medical Association and the Law Society. *Assessment of mental capacity: Guidance for doctors and lawyers*. London, 1995, pp.56–64 books.

64. British Medical Association. Sensitive and controversial issues. In *Consent Rights and Choices in Health Care for Children and Young People* 2001, pp. 165–173 BMJ Books London.

65. Richardson, J. and Webster, S. The HIV positive adolescent. In Ethical issues in Child Health Care Mosby, London1995; pp. 61–66

66. General Medical Council. *Confidentiality: Protecting and providing information* London GMC 2000.

67. Randolph, A.G., Zollo, M.B., Egger, M.J., Guyatt, G.H., Nelson, R.M., and Sidham, G.I. Variability in physician opinion on limiting pediatric life support. *Pediatrics* 1999;103:c46.

68. Farsides, C.C.S. Autonomy and its implications for palliative care; a northern European perspective. *Palliat Med* 1998;12:147–51.

69. Doyal, L. Medical Ethics and moral indeterminacy. *J Med Ethics* 1990;27(Suppl. II):44–49.

70. Cook, D.J., Giacomini, M., Johnson, and Williams, D. Life support in the intensive care unit: a qualitative investigation of technological purposes. *Canad Med Assoc J* 1999;161:1109–13.

71. Singer, P.A., Martin, D.K., and Kellner, M. Quality end of life care: patients' perspectives. *JAMA* 1999;281:163–8.

Section 2

Child and family care

5 Through the creative lens of the artist: Society's perceptions of death in children

Sandra Bertman and Judith Leet

Introduction

It is difficult
To get the news from poems
Yet men die miserably every day
For lack
Of what is found there.

William Carlos Williams, MD

These words of William Carlos Williams, a doctor and a poet, remind us that medical textbooks, professional journals, and the Internet are not the only sources for data that should inform our practice. Indeed, information alone is not all we need to understand our patients, their families, and ourselves. Sir William Osler once said, "The practice of medicine is an art, not a trade; a calling, not a business; a calling in which your heart will be exercised equally with your head." (Aequanimitas, 1920.) It is not enough for physicians simply to understand the theories and principles that underlie their patients' bodily ailments. Samuel Taylor Coleridge remarked that such doctors "…are shallow animals, having always employed their minds about body and gut, they imagine that in the whole system of things there is nothing but gut and body." (On Doctors, 1796.)

One of the important themes of this textbook is to emphasize the need for an evidence-based approach to our practice of caring for children with life-limiting conditions. Another fundamental principle, however, is that, having taken human experience apart to analyze its problems, we then need to reintegrate it and remember that we are dealing not with just symptoms or diseases but with young human beings and their families.

Patients cannot always articulate their experiences clearly. Simply communicating the presence of physical pain can be problematic enough. Expressing anguish that arises, for example, from emotional or spiritual distress can be even more difficult. Many patients can benefit from the insights, perceptions, and acuity of artists and poets, finding relief and understanding from their words or images.

Artists and poets have at one time or another been patients, parents, siblings, friends, or relatives of patients. Some have used their creative abilities to communicate something of that experience. This chapter provides an introduction to accessing this rich and valuable source of information, and considers how a few representative artists have depicted the dying or death of a child. These artists speak from profound personal experience, having participated in the death either as a family member (like Edvard Munch), as a parent (like Luke Fildes), or sometimes (like William Carlos Williams) as a professional.

Williams' poem is an illustration of the point that this chapter is trying to make. He chooses the medium of poetry to teach us that important information—perhaps *the* most important information—can be gleaned by us as healthcare professionals from what artists create.

Art reflects the way society thinks about death and captures both the times and the timelessness of it. This chapter scrutinizes how society grapples with the meaning of death in children, especially as portrayed in the visual arts and as interpreted in creative literature. Our assumption is that, by studying certain pertinent works of art, we will learn something of value to pediatric palliative care.

Death in children: From commonplace to rarity

While there are many works of art, past and present, dealing with death in children, they tend to be marginalized these days as a "special" subject matter. Art about dying children is now conspicuous by its low visibility, partly because confronting the reality of a dying child negates our culture's most important preoccupations: youth and happy endings. And it is also true that many childhood illnesses and infections (scarlet fever, whooping cough, rheumatic fever, strep throat, etc.) have been largely controlled in the developed world through medical advances and that death of children is not the constant presence and threat it had been in previous centuries. Any walk through a nineteenth-century cemetery will reveal how precarious the existence of children was; several siblings in the same family would have died before the age of 10. Mozart's parents had seven children, yet only two reached adulthood. That Mozart survived childhood was fortunate for all music lovers. Though we take it for granted within the industrialized world, the death of children has moved from a commonplace to a rarity during the last century.

Nevertheless, children continue to die of devastating diseases—cancers, cystic fibrosis, lissencephaly—and they and their families suffer. This chapter raises many questions that those in palliative care struggle with—how best to support the family before their child's death and how to prepare them for life without their child. We will consider various perspectives: the doctor's uneasy role, the sibling's struggle, the father's consolation, the mother's "journey through grief." Their views can provide us with insight.

How society views the death of a child: The creative artist reacts

The heroic doctor as seen by the Victorian painter

Reproductions of one of today's most well-known paintings of a very sick child, a best-selling engraving of the Victorian era, have been used on postage stamps in Britain and the United States, and can still be found on the walls of almost all medical schools (Figure 5.1). The canvas shows a concerned physician portrayed in profile, leaning forward in his chair at the bedside of the dying child upon whom his attention is totally absorbed. Barely visible in the shadowed background are the parents. Gazing at the physician, the father stands helplessly, his hand on the shoulder of the mother, who is seated at a table with her face hidden in her hands. Variously titled "The Doctor," "The Visit," or "The Vigil," the painting says much about our subject: the innocent child lying peacefully, glowing, almost angel-like—the child's figure lit from a lamp on the table, sharing the spotlight and the center of the canvas with the doctor, who has nothing more to offer medically. The doctor can only wait for the passage of time to find out whether the child will recover—or not.

There are differing accounts about the painting's origin; one is that Henry Tate commissioned the fashionable artist

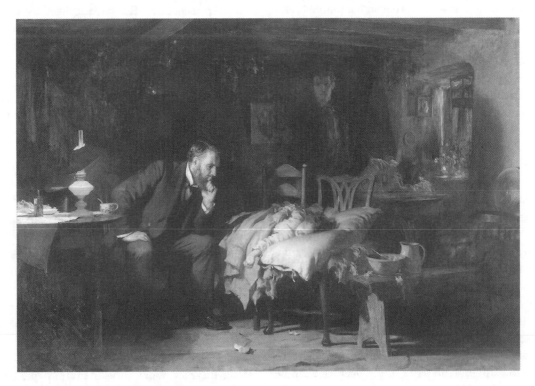

Fig. 5.1 Luke Fildes, The Doctor, 1891. © Tate, London.

Sir Luke Fildes in 1890 to paint a picture, the subject to be of the artist's own choosing, for the new National Gallery of British Art. Fildes' son, in a biography of his father, writes that the painter's inspiration was the memory of the doctor attending his firstborn child, who had died in infancy.

By his presence, the physician seen in the painting is a model of empathy and compassion. One doctor told his students: "A library of books would not do what that picture has done and will do for the medical profession in making the hearts of our fellow men warm to us with confidence and affection."[1] And, of course, for those of us in palliative medicine, what is represented here—not abandoning a patient and family, challenging the stance "nothing more can be done," and attending to the end—makes this painting most relevant.

The image of the ordinary family doctor's quiet heroism became a huge success with the late-Victorian public when it was first exhibited in the 1890s. However, some present-day viewers consider this image as sentimental, maudlin, and simplistic, one that plays into stereotypes: the child as angel-like and innocent; the father as stoic, strong, and nonexpressive; and the sobbing mother emotional and grief-stricken.

Questioned about his intentions for the painting, Fildes answered "At the cottage window the dawn begins to steal in, the dawn that is the critical time of all deadly illness, and with it the parents again take hope into their hearts ... the father laying his hand on the shoulder of his wife in encouragement of the first glimmerings of the joy which is to follow."[2] Doubtless, Fildes envisioned a happy ending for his canvas and intended the child in his painting to recover. We may interpret this painting as the artist's wish fulfillment, fixing in his art something that he wished had happened in real life to his own son.

Through society's lens: Reason, logic, and religion

The core of human identity is the need to make sense of things: to organize somehow all the information we absorb into a cohesive, reasonable whole. The death of a child is unnatural in that it disrupts the life cycle: infancy, childhood, youth, maturity, old age, and finally death. It turns the world upside down: parents are not supposed to outlive their children. It goes against everything that parents, grandparents, caretakers, and society as a whole expect, wish, and fervently desire for each child. Reason and logic provide too few answers to those crushed by a child's death. There is no timely death of a child.

Religion offers concepts not restricted by logic or reason or scientific proof. Many people turn to God and to Scriptures— to the Koran, the Bible, the Torah— for answers to life's great questions, and to faith, belief, heaven, theology, prayer, and ritual.

If God creates all life and if all life ultimately returns to God, shouldn't parents rejoice in their child's reunification?[3] The child can now enjoy immortality in heaven with the angels, as in the words of a folk tune called "Daniel": "You were closer to the angels/That's why they called you home ... They took your tiny hand."[4] But can the faith that a child is with God fully satisfy a grieving parent? No matter how strong or comforting religious beliefs may be, they cannot and should not deny the fact that death of a beloved child is heart-wrenching.

A grieving father in Trollope's *The Claverings*, who has just lost his only son, says to his wife's uncertain reassurances about "God's will" and their child's new home with the angels, "That's all very well in its way, but what's the special use of it now?" The father is able to voice what the mother dares not: that their professed faith is not enough in the face of such pain.

We human creatures recognize certain experiences as almost impossible to bear: one of those is the anguish of seeing a child die slowly of a terminal disease, and knowing that the child is cognizant of his or her impending death. Even if we disagree with the conclusion, we can sympathize with the expression of overwhelming grief felt by the individual who wrote "There is only one thing worse than a dying child—a child that knows he is going to die. This proves that there is no God."[5] Being human involves suffering. No one is immune from it.

Various cultures and religions believe, as some Native American tribes do, that life is complete whether it lasts 2 days or 80 years. The Bible teaches that death can be a blessing (Revelation 14: 13) yet we see Rachel grieving for her massacred children: "A cry was heard in Rama/weeping and great lamenting/It was Rachel weeping for her children/And refusing all consolation because they were no more." (Jeremiah 31: 15–17.)

In addition to consolation provided by the clergy, many therapists are knowledgeable about the emotional roller-coaster trajectories of grief, and can offer understanding of its course. The advent of support groups and chat rooms has also provided comfort to many bereft individuals in their immediate and long-term struggle.

[1] Source: net, The National Archives Learning Curve, Fildes.
[2] Wilson, S. *Tate Gallery: An Illustrated Companion*. London: Tate Gallery Publications, 1990.

[3] Sullivan, E. (2003). Communication with author, September 30.
[4] McClelland, S. Daniel. www.wjffradio.org/FolkPlus/setlists/991120.ntml.
[5] Digital Theatre Dying child is shown Rings film, e-mail response 10 December, 2001, 2:22 PM Dtheatre.com/read.php?sid=1602.

Through the lens of a writer: At a loss for words

Artists use their own medium, whether painting, music, photography, dance, or sculpture, to work out their questions or anguish following the death of a child. But a contemporary American writer, Lisa Schnell, whose medium is language, noted how immediately after the death of her young child, she was totally speechless, wordless—wanting only to be dead.

Lisa Schnell, as a grant recipient of a Project on Death in America Humanities Fellowship, produced her most recent work, *Learning How to Tell* (in press), about the death of her baby daughter and how she slowly regained her ability to find and express herself in words. When her baby, Claire, suffering from the rare and devastating birth defect lissencephaly, died at 18 months, words were not forthcoming to this connoisseur of words—a literary critic, English professor, and writer. Schnell talks of "choking on" her grief, her vocal chords becoming, metaphorically, paralyzed.

Words had turned on me…they were language, a reminder of what Claire would never have; or they were just absent—the core of inarticulateness inside me, my helplessness, my inability to turn my grief and fear into a narrative with a happy ending.[6]

Incapacitated by grief, she wished only to be with her baby daughter: "I just wanted to be dead with Claire. I wasn't suicidal. I didn't want to make myself dead, just be dead." Ultimately, this grieving mother found the words for the "lessons" death had taught her.

Only later did I understand that Claire needed me to live; that her dying—and my not—hadn't been a flagrant violation of some sort of maternal symmetry. I am still Claire's mom.

Moved by Lisa Schnell's writing—and with great trepidation— one of the authors sent her a photocopy of Deidre Scherer's fabric art, "Child" (Figure 5.2) and asked her to fill out a "Visual Case Study," in which we ask participants to have a dialogue with a work of art and respond to it in whatever ways the work suggests to them. We provided a broad "probe question" to guide her: "Please flesh out your reflections on this image with a story, vignette, title, quotation or any commentary."

Schnell responded both to the Scherer image and to how it felt to write about it. Here are her words describing how it felt to do the case study:

I was very struck by one particular part of the incredibly moving image you sent me, but in focusing on that I've tried to get across some of the complexity of my own experience of mothering a dying child…It was good to write it, a more powerful experience than I had anticipated.

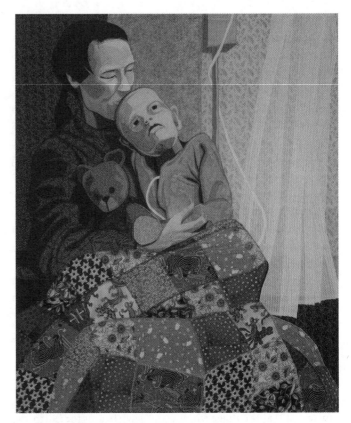

Fig. 5.2 ©Deidre Scherer, Child, 2001. Fabric and thread. (See plate 1.)

And here is Lisa Schnell's response to the Visual Case Study, centering around ordinary plastic tubing but blossoming into something quite extraordinary:

Clear plastic tubing: there was so much of it, and it was stiff and cumbersome in the cold December house at 3 a.m. But the pain of my engorged breasts was greater even than the discomfort of pumping them out in the cold, quiet house. And so I would struggle with all that tubing, hooking up body to bottle to pump…The anxiety stayed inside, cold as the house, inhabiting the questions that rattled around inside my head: Why couldn't she nurse? Why wouldn't she wake up to eat? Why did she twitch all the time? But for a few moments as I felt the warm swoosh of my own milk, I would relish the dark calm of December and imagine that everything would be all right.…

Clear plastic tubing: months after the breast pump had been put away, it reappeared, what seemed like miles of it, stretching from the tiny cannula in her nostrils to the big oxygen machine. It was May now, and the tubing was soft and flexible as we carried her from the living room to the bedroom, and sometimes even outside to the front porch. The gush of milk had long since ceded to the persistent leak of tears; the chill of anxiety was about to be replaced by the everlasting ache of grief. But there was an unmistakable calm in her wide gray eyes as she looked at me, tangled up in all that plastic tubing.[7]

---

6 Schnell, L. The language of grief. *Vermont Quart* 2000; Fall: 25–9, especially p. 26.

7 Bertman, S. Visual case studies: In the beginning was the word. *AAHPM Bull* 2003;5(spring).

Schnell read "voraciously" after her child's death, from Emily Dickinson to Freud, and was especially drawn to those, such as Christopher Noel, who also had taken "a journey through grief."[8] She explains: "all of the writers I was leaning on had learned not just what to tell, but how to tell." Schnell gradually discovered the "redemptive power of language." She was helped both by reading other artists and by writing for herself. "I found the process of writing profoundly enriching; in its simplest formulation I suppose it was a way I could continue to be Claire's mom."[8]

Friedrich Ruckert: Missing a child in 400 poems

Often writers who lose a child turn to their art to explain the loss to themselves, to describe it to others, and to try to struggle toward some understanding that enables them to continue. Friedrich Ruckert (1788–1866), German poet and professor of Oriental languages, wrote over 400 poems on the death of his son Ernst, which affected him as 'an overwhelming emotional upheaval.'[9]

The intense emotions remain in the poetry: "When thy mother enters, her gaze does not go to me but to the spot where your face should be...thou quickly extinguished ray of joy!" Another line: "One tiny lamp went out, my soul's delight." (p.289.)

Gustav Mahler used five of these Ruckert poems as setting for his "Kindertotenlieder" (Songs for Dead Children). He wrote the first three songs as an "artistic challenge," before he was married or had children of his own. His wife Alma was aghast that he could continue to complete the last two songs when he had his own young children playing outside. She later questioned Mahler's choice of text by comparing the two men's artistic motivation: "Ruckert did not write these harrowing elegies out of his imagination; they were dictated by the cruelest loss of his whole life." She had warned Mahler at the time, "For heaven's sake, don't tempt providence" (p. 288). When their oldest daughter died two years later, she was convinced that fate had been tempted.

Emily Dickinson grieves in letters: "Where makes my lark his nest?"

Poet Emily Dickinson lost her eight-year-old nephew Gilbert, her brother's child, who died of typhoid fever in 1883—after only a few days of illness. She felt very close to the boy, who had lived next door, and she grieved for him in her letters, which throughout her life she had made into an art form. As a means of remembering her nephew and expressing her grief

indirectly, each Christmas after his death she wrote his playmates: "Santa Claus still asks the way to Gilbert's little friends— Is Heaven an unfamiliar road? Come sometime with your sled and tell Gilbert's."[10] And to another young friend: "Our Santa is draped this Year, but Gilbert's Little Mates are still dear to his Aunt Emily."[11] For several years, the anniversaries of his birthday and death and Christmas without him troubled her— frequently the case with those who grieve for a loved one.

Writing to one of her own friends 2 years after his death, she wrote: "October is a mighty month, for in it Little Gilbert died. 'Open the door' was his last cry—'the Boys are waiting for me.' Quite used to his Commandment, his little Aunt obeyed, and still two years and many Days, and he does not return. Where makes my Lark his Nest?"[12]

She also wrote a clergyman for clarification of a statement in his letter, in which he wrote, "I can but believe that in such a mysterious providence as the dying of little Gilbert, there is a purpose of benevolence which does not include our present happiness." The clergyman's comment is kindly meant and admits to his own confusion. Like Trollope's character, Dickinson finds his assurances inadequate, and asks him exactly what point he is trying to make, remarking: "We would gladly possess it more accurately." (p. 890.)

Gilbert's mother Susan was Emily Dickinson's close friend as well as her sister-in-law. Though they lived next door, they frequently communicated in written messages. She wrote several letters to Susan after the unexpected, unacceptable death of the boy. Dickinson, struggling with her own sorrow, was able to send a note and a flower to Gilbert's mother attempting to give her support. "Perhaps the dear, grieved Heart would open to a flower, which blesses unrequested, and serves without a sound." (p. 800.)

By her letters, she attempted to console Gilbert's mother while trying to console herself: "No crescent was this creature— He traveled from the full." And she concluded this same letter with a short poem—a message to Gilbert:

> Pass to thy Rendezvous of Light,
> Pangless except for us—
> Who slowly ford the Mystery
> Which thou hast leaped across.
> (p. 799)

The anniversary of death dates and holidays are especially distressing for the family—for many years after the death itself.

---

[8] Christopher, N. *In the Unlikely Event of a Water Landing: A Geography of Grief.* New York: Time Books, 1966.

[9] Gartenberg, E. *Mahler: The Man and His Music.* New York: Schrimer, 1978, p. 288.

[10] Johnson, Thomas, *Letters of Emily Dickinson.* Cambridge, Mass and London: Harvard University Press, 1958 pp. 804–5. Reprinted with permission of the publishers. © 1958, 1986, The President and Fellows of Harvard College; 1914, 1924, 1932, 1942 by Martha Dickinson Bianchi; 1952 by Alfred Leete Hampson; 1960 by Mary L. Hampson.

[11] Johnson, p. 805. Reprinted with permission of the publishers, as above.

[12] Johnson, p. 891. Reprinted with permission of the publishers, as above.

Excellent information regarding bereavement and coping strategies exists in print and on the Internet, and many children's hospitals prepare their own brochures alerting families to this fact.

The early experiences of Edvard Munch: An artist remembers grief

Artists who have themselves suffered an earlier loss, especially of a sibling or a child, often work on—even years later—their response to that loss in their art. The Norwegian painter Edvard Munch experienced a childhood with multiple tragedies: he lost his mother to tuberculosis when he was only 5 years old, at age 14 lost his 15 year-old sister Sophie to the same disease, and saw another sibling afflicted by severe mental illness, perhaps exacerbated by her mother's and sister's deaths.

In 1885, when Munch was a young artist of 22, Sophie's death 8 years earlier presented itself to him as a subject—a source of unresolved emotion—that he wanted to reflect on and wrestle with in his art. His first version was a stunning oil painting, "The Sick Child" (painted around the time that Luke Fildes completed "The Doctor"). He shows the profile of his fragile, frail sister propped on a white pillow, looking steadily toward a window covered with dark drapes, perhaps representing the dark closed mystery of death (Figure 5.3).

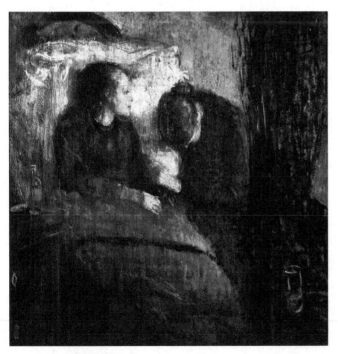

Fig. 5.3 Edvard Munch, The Sick Child, oil, 1885–1886, National Gallery, Oslo. (See plate 2.)

Her back bent over in inconsolable grief, Aunt Karen (the woman who replaced their mother) is unable to look at the stricken girl. The sister and aunt grasp hands, their two hands painted together as one simplified form. Munch worked over the surface for years, scratching the paint, enhancing the color, creating a restless texture—perhaps attempting to capture, as well as to quiet, his inner unease with the subject.

Munch believed that this painting marked a maturation of his art, saying it "provided the inspiration for the majority of my later works."[13] He returned to the theme of his dying sister over the years, painting it five more times in oils, and rendering it also in drypoint, lithograph, and etching. In a lithograph 10 years later, also called "The Sick Child" (Figure 5.4), he concentrates on the profile of his sister's head, with her damp and disheveled reddish hair, as she gazes steadily at the dark window. This time he leaves out Aunt Karen entirely, and eliminates much of the surrounding space—possibly to meditate on his sister's profile, searching for meaning in her unknowable thoughts.

As if he could not escape this theme and had to revisit it periodically, Munch detailed the progression of her illness in his art: the fevers, the medicine bottles, the witnesses, identifiable family members. In "Death in the Sickroom" (1895), the dying Sophie is hidden from view, seated back to the viewer in a wicker chair (Figure 5.5). The focus is on the helplessness of the many relatives: the father is shown praying, a sister bent in sorrow, Munch himself (or his brother) staring out the window, further isolated from the family grouping. One sister, Inger, is standing, seen full face, her weary eyes rimmed with red, drawing the viewer into the silent hopelessness of the scene. Interestingly, the family members are depicted as mature adults, and not at the much younger ages they were (and Munch was) at the time of Sophie's death. Applicable to any family—not just to the habits of Munch's Norwegian family—is the aloneness of grief. No one is touching anyone else. Each is dealing with the grief within. The work depicts an often expressed insight: even in the midst of family and friends, ultimately we grieve alone.

A major difference between Munch and Fildes is that Munch was far more innovative in his painting style—using flat planes, expressive color, and simplified forms. Fildes was a deeply conservative, academic painter who expressed himself largely through the content of the scene, depicting the character of the stymied yet caring doctor. Munch's more avant-garde expressionistic technique requires us to react to his own (and our) intense search for meaning.

[13] Loshak, D. *Munch*. The Mallard Press, 1990, p. 24.

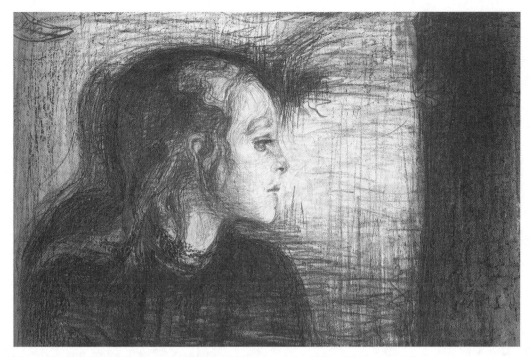

Fig. 5.4 Edvard Munch, The Sick Child, lithograph, Sch 59, Munch Museum, Oslo, 1896, p. 25. (See plate 3.)

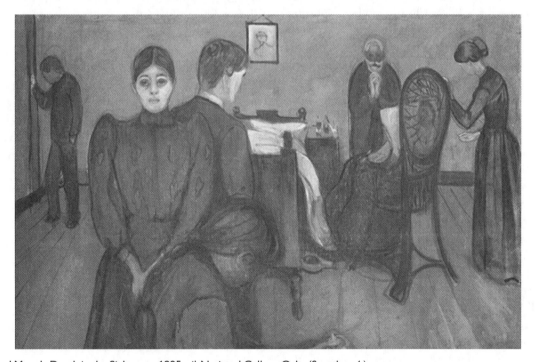

Fig. 5.5 Edvard Munch, Death in the Sickroom, 1895, oil, National Gallery, Oslo. (See plate 4.)

Another artist imagines grief: The psychological probes of Kathe Kollwitz

We can conjecture that Edvard Munch was troubled by his own early experiences and hoped to resolve these tragic memories through his art. More problematic is the case of Kathe Kollwitz, who painted a series of scenes of dead children without having had a life experience that explains her choice of exploring the subject of death. She did many graphics (charcoals, chalks, etchings) on the subject "Woman with a

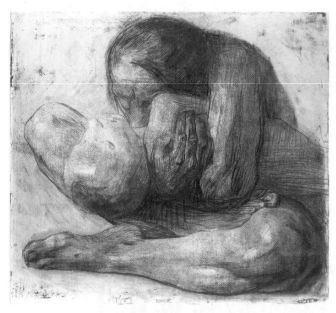

Fig. 5.6 Kathe Kollwitz Woman with Dead Child, 1903, National Gallery of Art, Washington, DC . © 2004 Artists Rights Society (ARS), New York/VG Bild-Kunst, Bonn.

Dead Child" (Figure 5.6) starting in 1903, which had evolved from earlier studies of a Pietà, Christ's mother mourning her son.

Kollwitz often relied on her young son Peter as a model for the dead children, as in "Dead Boy," another work of 1903. Her close friend, Beate Bonus-Jeep—temporarily out of touch with Kollwitz—was shocked at seeing "Dead Boy" in an exhibition. "Can something have happened with little Peter that she could make something so dreadful?" In retrospect Bonus-Jeep concluded: "she is someone to whom it is given to reach beneath the ultimate veils."[14]

Kathe Kollwitz described her working method: "When he [Peter] was seven years old, I made the etching 'Woman with Dead Child.' I drew myself in the mirror, holding him in my arm. That was very tiring, and I moaned. Then his little child's voice said comfortingly, 'Don't worry, Mother, it will be very beautiful.'" She developed the etching in eight different states, and took up the subject again in 1910, as "Death, Mother, and Child," considered "one of the most moving drawings Kollwitz ever made on the theme of death and leavetaking."[14] And again in 1910, she completed "Death and a Woman," where an ago-nized mother, neck strained and wrenched, holds off the skeleton representing death.

Kollwitz's preoccupation with death remains an enigma, having herself suffered no personal loss. Yet she captures the

essence of grief. Why was she drawn to the subject of the dead child, suffering, pain? Perhaps her strong interest in social betterment, her desire to fix the world, explains it in part. Or it might be her desire to express, in her drawings and graphics, deep and extreme psychological empathy. She wrote in her diary entry of April, 1910, "Great piercing sorrows have not yet struck me."[15] The great grief portrayed in her many works struck her eventually. Her son Peter, model for the dead boy, was killed in the First World War at the age of 21, and her grandson, another Peter, was killed in the Second World War.

Picasso in his Blue Period

Picasso, not motivated by the loss of a child but motivated, in fact, by the suicide of his friend Carlos Casagemas, painted with tenderness a monochromatic canvas of a suffering family. During his Blue Period, he conveyed a desolate scene (Figure 5.7). Saturated with cold blue tones, the canvas reflects pathos, bleakness, a pervasive melancholy mood.

Does Picasso's "The Tragedy" hint at the death or impend-ing death of someone not shown? Or is the cloaked woman holding a sick infant in her arms? Or have any of the figures—presumably mother, father, child—received a fatal diagnosis? Is the child excluded from the grief of the parents?

This image distills other essences or truisms of bereave-ment and grief—anticipatory or after the fact.[16] In their suf-fering, the adults clutch their own bodies, turning within themselves, as in Munch's paintings. The "contagion" of grief is clear, as one sees the youngster touching his father's body, reaching out for support and assurance. If the dying (or dead) child not pictured was a sibling, the child's gesture suggests his need for attention and inclusion. Siblings need reassurance that nothing they did or thought caused the death. Their grief needs to be acknowledged and validated. Perhaps the paint-ing's title has less to do with the subject of a death than with the existential insight into the solitariness of grief, the tragedy being the unavailability of one to another.

Though belonging to Picasso's "Blue Period" brought on by the suicide of his best friend, Casagemas, this composition is from the child's-eye view. It is interesting to note that Picasso himself experienced the illness and death of his only sibling, Conchita, a younger beloved sister, who died at age eight when Picasso was age thirteen.[17]

[14] Prelinger, E. *Kathe Kollwitz*, New Haven, CT: Yale University Press. Beate Bonus-Jeep, cited in Catherine Krashmer, *Kathe Kollwitz on Selbstzeugnissen und Bilddokementen* (Reinbek bei Hamberg, 1981), 1992, pp. 42, 160.

[15] *The Diary and Letters of Kathe Kollwitz*. Entry April, 1910, edited by her son, Hans Kollwitz. Chicago, IL: Henry Regnery, 1955.
[16] Bertman, S. Children and death: Insights, hindsights, and illuminations. In D. Papadatou and C. Papadatos, eds. *Children and Death*. New York: Hemisphere, 1991, pp. 311–29.
[17] See discussion of title in Bertman's annotation: http://endeavor.med.nyu.edu/lit-med/lit-med-db/webdocs/webart/picasso87-art-.html.

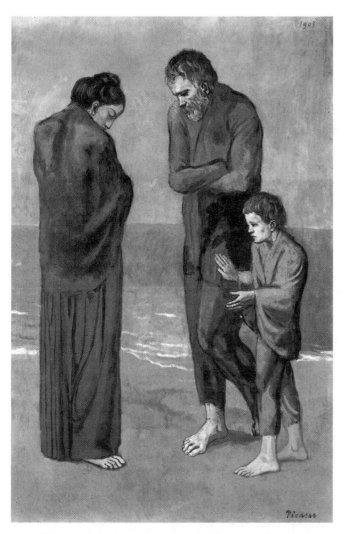

Fig. 5.7 Figure Picasso, The Tragedy. 1903. National Gallery of Art, Washington, DC. © 2004 Estate of Pablo Picasso/Artists Rights Society (ARS), New York.

Through the lens of the professional: The creative physician reacts

Telling it straight

In contrast to the Fildes painting of the dedicated and heroic doctor, we examine a poem written by a contemporary physician, John Graham-Pole, an American/British poet.[18] In the poem "Candor" (1997) he characterizes the doctor as a self-questioning, perplexed, and doubting professional, only rescued by the wit of a dying child.

In the poem, set not in the home as in the Fildes, but in the impersonal doctor's office, the mother wants the physician to

---

[18] Graham-Pole, J. *On the Wings of Spirit*. Bloomingdale, IL: Enhancement Books, 1997, p. 99.

"square" with her 8-year-old child, to inform him that he is dying of his cancer. Graham-Pole is no neophyte physician. He is highly skilled in communication skills, a compassionate, authentic human being: he realizes he can use himself, and is willing to use himself, as part of the medical treatment.

> Candor
>
> At eight years old, the cancer running rampage,
> Joe perches on my office sofa edge
> thigh-to-thigh with mom
> (who has enjoined me: Square with him).
>
> But I beat around the bush a bit,
> then come at last to it: Joey:
> you're going to die, go to heaven—
> words lost in his howl, like a wolf's
>
> the hurling of his body into
> the yellow print dress's recesses.
> Three minutes at least of this, this keening,
> as we eye each other panicked:
>
> Whatever else was right to do this wasn't it.
> Then, as instantly, on a long-drawn-in
> breath's end, he stops, swivels out, flicks a look,
> spots tears on cheeks of mom, dad, nurse, me,
>
> determines he's grieved enough: time to
> lighten up, knowing me at other times a joker,
> a wearer of odd socks, funny noses. He spies
> memos, charts, photocopies, journals,
>
> jetsam of an urgent life, bespattering my carpet,
> and becomes the stand-up comic,
> offers his own joke: Didn't your mom
> teach you to pick up after yourself?

First, we see the many points of view: the doctor, the child, the mother are central figures; the father and the nurse play lesser roles. Then the issue of candor is raised: is it helpful for the doctor to address the child directly about his impending death? When the doctor "squares" with Joey, the child's immediate response is to howl for three minutes, causing the adults inward panic and outward tears. Then we, the readers, experience sudden unexpected relief: the child makes a joke at the doctor's expense. The "happy" ending that many of us long for materializes: the child rescues the physician with his wit, thus making the scene more tolerable.

The complexity of the whole issue is brought up midway by the doctor's outright rejection of his own approach: "Whatever else was right to do this wasn't it." The poem not only highlights the child's pain, but also the pain of the parents and the nurse: "[the child] spots tears on cheeks of mom, dad, nurse, me." Told in the doctor's voice, however, it is his doubts and suffering that are most transparent.

Is there such a thing as a right way to give a child news of this magnitude? There is no "right" way to tell; in fact the notions of right and wrong in this case are irrelevant. What is important is counteracting the child's sense of isolation and fear that results from secrecy and what Glasser and Strauss label "mutual pretense."[19] For often the child intuits the situation. Most contemporary studies posit that the psychologist, parents, and the doctor should take time to determine what is the best, least stressful way to present the situation to the child in order to minimize the damage and to allow opportunities for hope and healing. Of course, this telling has to be individualized to take into account not only the child's developmental stage but also his life experiences. Has the child witnessed other children who died in hospital? Has he been aware of other children's illness trajectories? The results of Bluebond-Langner's research (1978) indicate: "The issue is not 'to tell or not to tell,' but rather what to tell, when to tell, and who should do the telling."[20]

Perhaps the doctor in the poem should have prepared more carefully how he would approach telling the child. He seemingly came up with a plan on the spur of the moment to please the mother. He admits to beating around the bush, and then announcing the unhappy truth in a blunt way that caught the child off-balance and unprepared. But in all fairness there is no template for handling this very difficult situation. One might even argue that the physician's fumbling attempt actually returned the control of the situation to the little boy, who in the end exhibits a sense of self-respect and self-worth that takes the reader by surprise. As a Dr Seuss character in *Horton the Who* tells us, "a person is a person, no matter how small." The poem "Candor" challenges us to become adept at ministering to the grief and stress of very ill children, their families, and the caregiving professionals involved.

It is well accepted that children grow in spurts; this poem is evidence that they also grieve in spurts, and when they cannot bear to grieve any longer, they distract and console themselves by other interests; in this case the child focuses on the messiness of the doctor's office. One physician reading "Candor" wondered if the child's remark at the end of the poem might be intended to symbolize the mess the doctor had made of breaking the news.

It has been observed that children bring a sense of lightness and play even to dying—just as they do to every other aspect of their lives. A very sick child may "play dead" when a parent enters the sickroom as a joke, and wonder why it makes the mother cry rather than laugh. Children in a cancer ward have been known to act out funerals, taking turns being the dead person. One nurse asked a young boy whether he wasn't uncomfortable keeping so still in order that his tubes would stay put, and he replied, "No, I'm practicing for my coffin."[21]

Telling it slant

Criticized by other doctors for his bluntness as described in "Candor," Dr Graham-Pole replied to his colleagues in a later poem titled "Slant" (2002).[22] In "Slant," he tells in verse how one surgeon suggested he (or the doctor in the poem) should be more "soft-hearted" in telling a child and "tell the truth but tell it slant"—the surgeon echoing a well-known line by Emily Dickinson. Dr Graham-Pole defends himself: he'd spoken to please the parents, so "there'd be no conspiracy of silence," but instead there would be trust-building; he also acknowledged in his first poem that he had compressed—not told the whole story. In the later poem, he adds that he had recognized the child already knew the essential. But finally he asks himself in "Slant" whether he had been too outspoken in his first poem:

> Was I too candid?
> They'd thought so. For me, I knew he knew.
> He knew I knew it: straight, no slant in that.[22]

He recognized the child knew the situation, and he went for the truth—straight.

The situation described here is one that pediatric palliative caregivers confront in their practice. Some professionals would argue that the doctor in "Candor" demonstrates the wrong approach; others would defend his attempt to get at the greater good—trust-building, truth, and straight over slant.

The poem that follows, titled "Cancer Pain", is by another physician/poet, Richard Hain.

> Cancer Pain
>
> How many times
> in a twelvemonth stalked and terrorised by a tumour,
> did you ask 'Will I die?'
> And we, smiling into your eyes
> with all the tyranny of tenderness,
> tore up your question
> and threw it away.
>
> How often, when we spoke,
> did we feed you hopes of immortality,
> spoonful by narcotic spoonful,
> to deaden the pain?
>
> The pain we hoped to drug away was never yours.
> Not the simple catch and scratch and smart of cancer
> (we are used to that.

19 Glaser, B. and Strauss, A. Awareness contexts and social interaction. *Am Sociol Rev* 1964;29:669–79.
20 Bluebond-Langner, M. *The Private Worlds of Dying Children*. Princeton, NJ: Princeton University Press, 1978, p. 191.
21 Bluebond-Langner, M. Ibid.
22 Graham-Pole, J. "Slant." In *Quick: A Pediatrician's Illustrated Poetry*. Bloomingdale, IL: Writers Club Press, 2002, p. 90.

We have watched before,
while others did your dying).

The pain was ours.
It was the twist and ache of telling you
and seeing you know,
and watching you
while you watched yourself die
by the count
and the clock
and the calendar.

Our pain eats out our bones and bowels,
and long after the end of your immortality
when we have run out of smiles and other opiates,
our pain will go on.

In this poem, we are not told specifically who, or how old, or even what sex, the patient is. Unlike in Graham-Pole's "Candor" the narrator here chooses at first not to tell the patient the prognosis—that she or he is dying: "How many times ... did you ask, 'Will I die?' And we ... tore up your question/and threw it away."

The doctor is willing to absorb the distress of his choice, postponing until later trying to answer the patient's question: "The pain was ours/It was the twist and ache of telling you."

Like the Graham-Pole poem, the patient eventually knows with certainty the disease is fatal. The doctor is forced to watch the patient "while you watch yourself die." The doctor's pain persists long after the patient—the child—meets death, and what the poet refers to as "hopes of immortality." The reader and the poet together confront the pangs and painfulness of the living who watch someone die, and of the dying passing to the total mystery, which Emily Dickinson evokes as passing to the "Rendezvous of Light."

Medicine is a human art. These poems exemplify how the discipline of art is a resource for palliative caretakers—enabling them to reflect upon these basic questions vicariously and soulfully before, while, or after they face them—and to prepare for forthcoming situations. We hope this brief sampling of three poems demonstrates how art documents the human struggles of medicine, as well as being a catharsis for the physicians, who are able to confront—if not work through—some of their doubts and distress in the act of composing the poem.

Summary: Art as a resource to caregivers and the bereaved

Pediatric palliative professionals can observe, through art, how individuals react to the death of children, and can look to art for many approaches, reflections, suggestions, insights,

questions, distractions—on how to attend to and relieve the suffering of patients and their families. Lisa Schnell, enduring her most painful months, "leaned on" other writers, who offered her their most intense impressions of life and grief. Art is a catharsis for artists, who are fortunate to have their media as an expressive outlet as well as a lasting tribute and memorial. Artists brilliantly teach us about the suffering of others, and demonstrate how others deal with their grief.

Often feeling cut off from others who go about their routine lives, bereaved persons can find suitable companionship with writers and artists who have shaped and ordered their personal anguish. The bereaved only have to find a few ideas, or even one idea, that they can cling to, perhaps latching on to a simple statement such as Lisa Schnell's "I am still Clare's mom," rewriting it to fit their own situation. The palliative caregiver can offer, unobtrusively, or at least have available poems, memoirs, biographies, photographs, paintings, photocopies—even brief quotations—in the hope that a few might be the exactly right prescription for the pain. Painting and poems console us by connecting us to others who have suffered what we've suffered or whose suffering reminds us of our frailties, our own helplessness.[23] Intimating that we are not alone, art offers us lifelines. It enables us to shift lenses, to borrow the lens of an artist and see anew. And so back to newspapers, hard data, music, poetry and paradox. As the philosopher Fredrich Wilhelm Nietzsche puts it, "We have art in order not to die of the truth."

---

[23] Shapiro, A. Some questions concerning art and suffering *Tikkun Jan/Feb 2004.*

6 The spiritual life

Brother Francis, OSB

Introduction

There are only three great puzzles in the world: the puzzle of love, the puzzle of death and, between each of these and part of both of them, the puzzle of God. God is the greatest puzzle [1].

The 'spiritual life' of anyone is an enigma and this is even more so when it comes to children. It will be very different from one person to the next, from one child to the next and from members of one family to the next. However, for all of us, there are common threads. Spirituality is universal, while at the same time, intensely personal and subjective by its very nature.

In paediatric palliative care we come up against the great puzzles mentioned above, every day of our working lives. Sometimes we are expected to know the answers, but in reality we all spend most of our lives trying to work them out. God is, as Williams suggests, perhaps the greatest puzzle of all time and particularly hard for us to make sense of when faced with the care of a dying child and his or her family. When faced with a family whose child or children are dying, or a child coping with an intractable pain or what could be called 'Soul Pain', we are forced to confront the puzzle of God and may feel:

The chill of loss, the draughty air as if the walls of your soul have been knocked down in the night, and you wake to realise that you are living in a vast exposed emptiness . . . [1]

And when a child, for whom you have been caring over several years dies:

you start to wonder if God was ever there at all, or if the puzzle itself was your own invention to excuse the existence of the random and the brutal where they criss-crossed your life[1]

This chapter sets out to define and explore the experience of soul pain in dying children and their families, and complements the study of the scientific aspects of pain. Soul pain is a distinct condition and there is a risk that a child's 'soul pain' may not be properly addressed if this is seen as just the work of the Chaplain.

Spirituality in the context of this chapter refers to 'the inner life of the child or adolescent as the cradle for a construction of meaning'[2]. The chapter will outline some of the diverse views on spirituality, and look at the psychological factors that influence pain in children. It will start to explore the importance of understanding the role of suffering in children's pain, looking at the spiritual needs of children and families and, through a case history, how we as health care professionals may 'help' with this aspect of their care.

The chapter can only be a 'whistle-stop tour' of the territory of the spiritual care of the dying child and the family. It is a territory that has no reliable map; all we have is other people's accounts, their stories and their own experiences of this painful and hard journey.

Spirituality

Spirituality and spiritual care are the proper concern of all who work with dying children and their families. We must recognise that spirituality and religion are very important to a number of people. However, they are two different aspects of care; spirituality is what gives a person's life meaning, how he views, the world he finds, himself in, and this may or may not include a 'God' or religious conviction. Religious care relates more to the practical expression of spirituality through a framework of beliefs, often pursued through rituals and receiving of sacraments.

Nothing in life is black or white, but a thousand shades of grey, and that is the problem in trying to define spirituality in a meaningful way. All people have a spiritual dimension, but not everyone expresses that dimension through formal or traditional religious language or practices. Therefore, all people will have spiritual needs, but trying to define spirituality in a way that is acceptable to everyone is difficult, as it will be different for each and every one of us. For instance, it has been suggested that 'Spirituality may be expressed intra-personally, as connectedness with oneself; inter-personally, as relationships with others and the environment, and trans-personally, in terms of relatedness with the unseen, or greater power' [3].

The literature suggests a 'sacred core' that consists of feelings, thoughts, experiences, and behaviours that arise out of a search for the sacred in our lives, and is an ongoing dynamic process [4, 5].

Spirituality and spiritual care should be found at the core of good paediatric palliative care, but because spirituality, especially in children, can be difficult to understand, we sometimes use the need to tackle the practical needs in palliative care as an easy escape route from spiritual exploration. This way, we can be seen by the family to be 'making a difference', and we ourselves can see that we made a difference. However, if we shy away from spiritual care we run the risk of missing something profoundly important to the child and family.

Symptom control follows a relatively clear and well-defined pathway of thought and actions, looking something like this:

(a) analysis,

(b) problem identification,

(c) choice of a solution,

(d) an outcome and followed by,

(e) review.

In contrast, this is not the case when it comes to either identifying or addressing spiritual issues in a child's care, as it:

(a) defies logical analysis,

(b) is difficult to define the problem, and,

(c) often has no measurable solution.

At a much deeper level it also demands more of us as health care professionals.

Spiritual care is about responding to the uniqueness of the child in front of you. The spiritual questions are perhaps the most important questions that we hear or that are ever asked. Companionship is at the heart of real spiritual support; a person needing it wants the presence of a person, not a theological theory.

Little is really known about children's spirituality: what goes on in their minds and how they express it. We can only know these things by asking the individual child and family. We need to give them the respect they deserve at this time and phase of their journey. We need to allow them the honour of expressing what they think, by just asking them.

It has been suggested that the problem in coming to terms with children's spirituality is not in determining whether or not children are spiritual, but whether they have a chance to develop and express their spirituality. Many authors have suggested that children, far from being less spiritual than their adult counterparts, are already equipped for their spiritual

journey by virtue of a higher level of openness to an awareness of spiritual realities [3–7].

The question is not at what age or developmental level children can understand spiritual concepts, but how the child, at his age and developmental level of understanding, expresses his or her spirituality [8].

Coles, after 30 years of working with and writing about children in different settings, suggests that children possess a great 'spiritual curiosity', and seek both God and the meaning of life. A limitation is that his work dealt mainly with physically well children and not dying children. Even so, he makes the very important point that:

The spiritual needs of children are no different from the spiritual needs of older people. But the expression of their spirituality may be different. The child's 'house has many mansions'—including a spiritual life that grows, changes, responds constantly to the other lives that, in their sum, make up the individual we call by a name and know by a story that is all his, all hers [9].

If we are to address the spiritual needs of dying children and their families, we must first come to terms with our own spirituality [10, 11]. As Somers [10] suggests, we need to ask ourselves what our own assumptions about spirituality and maybe even religion are. How do we see spirituality in our own lives and the psychological influence it has on us?

As Sommer aptly says:

To understand how another person is limited, we must understand our own limitations. To enter into another person's pain, we must identify that pain in ourselves. To help another face death, we must be able to imagine our own death. [10]

Spiritual care needs to be seen in the context of relationship with the child and his or her family. It is about being present to them and about accompaniment on their journey as they travel the road and encounter the puzzle of God [12]. There is no one model or book we can turn to for help when it comes to the spiritual care of the dying child. This is because each child is unique, and there is no room for rigidity or inflexibility when it comes to offering spiritual care. We need to be open, spontaneous and intimate, and to hold in mind that children have a high level of openness and awareness for all things spiritual. Our task is to keep the channels of communication open and unblock them if they are blocked.

There are no ready answers to the questions about children's spirituality and what we might say to a child who asks 'Why am I sick?' or even 'Why does God hate me?'; or to a parent when we are asked 'Why my child?' or 'Why our family?' No book can give the answers to these profound questions that we, the families we work with, or the child we hold in our arms now seek. It has been suggested that spirituality originates in the heart and therefore, spiritual care comes from 'the heart after the head has done its homework' [25]. Children ask questions from the heart (soul); questions that come from the child's heart can only be met with answers that come from the adult's heart (soul).

Spirituality is about how we view the world and how we react within it. In talking about spirituality we need to bear in mind that we all come from different social contexts, that we each have a past, and some have a future. We all have our own form of spirituality. Some may have a religious faith or background, while others may not, and it is out of this setting that our spirituality will manifest itself. It is from this background or setting that the questions and work will come. It is worth noting that before religion was a theology, it was an experience! 'Spirituality is not restricted to those who belong to a religious denomination. Spirituality can do without religion, but the opposite is not true' [25].

Spirituality is central to the care of dying children and their families. If we fail to address these issues, we do the children and families we work with a great disservice.

Children's understanding of death

An important baseline when working with children is knowledge of children's understanding of illness and the concept of death. This is also useful when working with parents, to help them understand just what their child might be thinking and what information they may need [15]. It is very easy for adults to underestimate a child's understanding, and this can be to the detriment of the child and his or her care. Goldman and Christie [13] found that only 19% of families of children dying from malignant diseases mutually acknowledged what was going on. It was felt that 23% of children knew what was happening, but chose not to discuss it. Staff involved in the study tended to overestimate how often discussions took place about the impending death of the child.

Bluebond-Langner [14] demonstrated that children very rarely talk openly about what is happening to them, because of taboos deriving from parents or carers. If they do talk, it tends to be in highly symbolic ways. She also states that the child:

goes through what can often be a long and painful process to discover what it all means. In this process he assimilates, integrates, and synthesises a great deal of information from a variety of sources. With his arrival at each new stage comes a greater understanding of the disease and its prognosis. This leaves him with a great deal to cope with, and it is part of his anticipatory grief process [14].

The above quotation brings together some of the aspects from this and previous chapters to illustrate soul pain in a child. There is a sense of an inner 'journey' the child has to make to find meaning, and this can be a painful process.

Substantial literature is now available on how and when children develop their concepts of death (see also Chapter 7, Children's view of death, Bluebond-Langner). Most of the literature derives from work originally done by Anthony [16] in pre-war London in the late 1930's, and by Nagy [17] in Budapest in the 1940's. These studies have since been replicated, enriched and refashioned as new insights have come to the fore, and as society has changed and developed Bowlby [18], Koocher [19], Swain [20], Bluebond-Langner [21], Kane [22], Lansdown and Benjamin [23], and Clunies-Ross and Lansdown [24].

Most of these studies were undertaken with healthy children. Fewer studies have been done with sick children, or with children living with a life-threatening illness. Clunies-Ross and Lansdown [24] 1988, however, repeated an early study of healthy children carried out by Lansdown and Benjamin [23] in 1985, but this time examined children with leukaemia. This study was very small, involving only 21 children, but no significant differences were found between the two studies.

Lansdown and Benjamin [23] found that out of 105 children aged between 5 and 9 years the following had a complete or almost complete understanding of a concept of death:

- 60% of 5-year-olds
- 70% of 6-year-olds
- 66% of 7-year-olds
- nearly 100% of 8–9 year olds.

They also found that children who were verbally competent would be able to discuss death in a way that was surprising for their respective age group. Kane [22] identified a number of components of a developing concept of death:

1. Realisation   All 3-year-olds
2. Separation   5 years
3. Immobility   5 years
4. Irrevocability   6 years
5. Causality   6 years
6. Dysfunctionality 6 years
7. Universality   7 years
8. Insensitivity   8 years
9. Appearance   12 years

She found that if children under 6 had experiences with death of a relative, this would hasten their understanding of death. However, this was not the case in children over 6.

The journey to the centre

'I will take the ring,' he said, 'though I do not know the way' [26].

The story 'The Lord of The Rings' offers a helpful metaphor. Here we have a group of people on a journey, a journey that covers some very difficult territory and one that has no map. It is a journey that they seem to have very little choice about making, and as much as they would have liked not to make the journey, they find themselves on it. The same can be said for the children we care for, their families and those who work with them.

To help the fellowship in the story make their journey, they have been given a guide and companion. He cannot make the journey for them, but can travel with them, offering support and advice from his past journeys. In many ways this story reflects the interior landscape of the children we care for, our own journey, and the territory of the journey that we will cover together.

For our part it is worth remembering what happened in the story at the council of Elrond:

No one answered. The noon-bell rang. Still no one spoke. Frodo glanced at all the faces, but they were not turned to him. All the Council sat with downcast eyes, as if in deep thought. A great dread fell on him, as if he was awaiting the pronouncement of some doom that he had long foreseen and vainly hoped might after all never be spoken. An overwhelming longing to rest and remain at peace by Bilbo's side in Rivendell filled all his heart. At last with an effort he spoke, and wondered to hear his own words, as if some other will was using his small voice. 'I will take the Ring,' he said, 'though I do not know the way [26].

We have to take the 'ring' even though we don't know the way or where it will lead us.

Tolkein was a profound believer, a devout Christian who knew that the battlefield is the human soul and that storytelling and the imagination were ways into that world. He was a man who took us on an inner journey even when we thought we were exploring the fantasy landscape of his 'Middle Earth'. It is in this land of the imagination that we can make a connection to the children we work with. It is a land of adventure and story-telling.

We can continue the metaphor of a journey. The journey is to the centre, to the heart of the matter (or, as in the Lord of the Rings to 'the mountain of fire in Mordor'). On this journey, we have to engage with the children and families and travel through several stages of trust with them, if we are to get to the 'heart of the matter'. They need to know that we are truly listening to what they are saying and that we are also listening out for what they are not saying: 'Every illness has two diagnoses, one scientific and the other spiritual, which involves meaning and purpose' [27].

To identify both these diagnoses we need to bring 'wide angle' lenses to palliative care, otherwise we may not be able to grasp or see what is being suggested in this chapter, or indeed, by the children we work with. We need to expand our thinking from our purely scientific and practical minds, and try to see with our inner eye and listen with our inner ear.

Dying children and their families find themselves on a journey, a journey that they have had very little choice about making, and as much as they would have liked not to make the journey, they now find themselves making it.

Spirituality is about making a 'journey', and that journey is to the centre, to the heart of the matter, to our 'deep centre', where sometimes we meet our pain, and have to name it.

All sick children will at some time think about what is going on not only in their bodies, but also in their inner worlds [21]. On this journey they need us to be alongside them. They need us to be both their companion and their advocate. Knowing that, the most we can do is to prepare and hold the space where they can start to do the work they need to do for the next stage of their journey, where they can explore their inner-world and where the miraculous may happen.

We need to try and create a safe and secure or 'sacred space', where the child and family can express their inner-world and suffering and know that it is all right to do so, that they will be heard and taken seriously. We can help them best by sitting with them, watching with them, waiting with them and just wondering what may happen next. We can take our lead from them, go with them, try not to direct them, and try to use the language and imagery they present to us.

Sir Luke Fildes depicts this attitude well in his painting 'The Doctor'. (cross reference to this illustration is also being used by Sandra Bertman in Chapter 5). It depicts the doctor, the child and the quality of the relationship between the two of them. The doctor is attending to the child, watching, waiting and wondering. He is there, which is by far the most important thing he can do. However, we must not forget the parents waiting in the shadows of this powerful painting.

Spiritual care is about responding to the uniqueness of the child in front of you and accepting their range of doubts, beliefs and values just as they are. It means responding to their spoken or unspoken statements from the very core of that child as valid expressions of where they are and who they are. It is to be their friend, companion, and their advocate in their search for identity on their journey and in the particular situation in which they now find themselves. It is to respond without being prescriptive, judgmental, or dogmatic, and without preconditions, acknowledging that the child and other members of the family will be at different stages on that very personal spiritual journey [28].

On this journey we are the 'invited guest', we will join them for a part of the journey as a guest and accordingly we should behave like a guest. Sometimes we just want to fix things but we may need to acknowledge that we can't, though we may be able to help. The beginning of wisdom is being able to say, 'I don't know'.

We need to be able to be open to the children teaching us. We need to be prepared to learn from them. It seems that the trick here, as in other aspects of paediatric palliative care, is that we need to be able to understand or 'crack' the child's code. We can start to do this if we just sit with them, if we learn to watch, wait and wonder with them. We can take our lead from them and be responsive to their needs, and not the needs we think they may have or our own needs at this time.

Concepts of soul pain

In this chapter when the word soul is used, it is implied that it is that which we sense to be:

'the essential part of each of us',
'the soul is the world within',
'the world we ignore at our peril'.

'Soul pain' holds the key to the child's world. For me it is a reality in clinical practice. It is on my 'check-list', when I am assessing a child or his or her family who are in 'pain'. This approach is born out of many years of clinical experience of working with children who are either life-threatened or life-limited. I hope that by the end of this chapter, soul pain will be on your 'check-list' of things to look out for, when you are faced with a child or family with 'intractable pain'.

Definitions of soul, psyche, and spirit

In modern Christian culture, the soul is that uniqueness and passion within each human being and the soul is thought to be that part of human beings which gives their lives meaning and essence, conferring individuality and humanity on them.

Our soul has two main functions. First, it must put some fire in our veins, keep us energised, vibrant, living with zest, and full of hope as we sense that life is ultimately worth living. Secondly, it has to keep us together. It has to give us that sense of who we are, where we came from, and where we are going. It is also that part of us that 'holds' memory for us.

One of the hardest words, or concepts, to define is that of 'soul'. Definitions again will depend on the cultural, religious and psychological influences on an individual; the way each person views himself and the world. Some would even say that the concepts of soul and psyche are the same. However, Hillman [29] suggests that people incorrectly use the term psyche and soul synonymously: 'The terms 'psyche' and 'soul' can be used interchangeably, although there is a tendency to escape the ambiguity of the word 'soul' by recourse to the more biological, more modern psyche. 'Psyche' is used more as a natural concomitant to physical life, perhaps reducible to it. 'Soul', on the other hand, has metaphysical and romantic overtones'.

For Hillman the two are quite different. He suggests that 'The spirit has to do with an upward movement [**transcendence**], and the soul relates to a downward movement [**depth**]' [30].

Spirit is about transcendence and soul is about depth. He saw the spirit as the phoenix rising from the ashes. The soul being the ashes from which the phoenix arose.

Or, as Moore [31] has eloquently put it:

'Soul' is not a thing, but a quality or a dimension of experiencing life and ourselves. It has to do with depth, value, relatedness, heart, and personal substance. I do not use the word here as an object of religious belief or as something to do with immortality.

The key words in this definition are '*depth*', '*value*', '*relatedness*', and '*personal substance*'. It is these words that mark some of the differences between soul and spiritual pain. It is in these words that we will begin to find some of our symtomatology of 'soul pain'.

Soul pain can be likened to walking through a labyrinth. We think we are getting closer to the heart of the matter, and then we turn a corner and find that we are even further from the centre. However, we need to remember that a labyrinth, unlike a maze, has a single path that, eventually, takes us to the centre and is not designed to make us lose the way, but paradoxically, to find it.

The Labyrinth (Figure 6.1) is symbolic of our life's journey and that journey is towards the center,—our 'deep centre', where sometimes we meet our pain, and have to name it.

This in turn relates to what hospice is all about. The concept of hospice comes from a monastic background. A hospice was a place run by monks, for sick and tired pilgrims. They were on a journey, like the families we work with and they too can be seen as coming to us for rest and refreshment on their pilgrimage. They have invited us in, to join them on this part of their journey. We are invited guests...Christians walked the labyrinth when they could not make the pilgrimage to the Holy Land.

There is a difference between the concept of 'soul pain' and what is often referred to in the literature as 'spiritual distress'

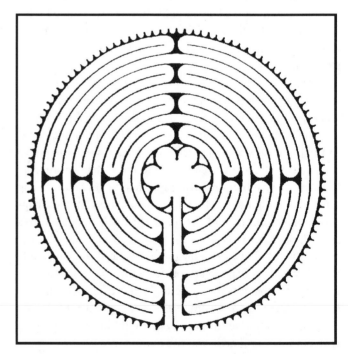

Fig. 6.1 The Labyrinth from Chartres Cathedral in France.

or 'spiritual pain'. The children and families with whom we work demonstrate this difference and the work is clearly 'soul work', as Freud would have called it. I believe that the fundamental difference between the two is that of direction [32]. Spiritual distress may well be one of the symptoms of a child's soul pain, but it could also be a distinct condition needing its own definition.

Both soul and pain have a subjective quality about them that eludes precise definition or even assessment in the scientific sense. It may be that they can only be depicted.

Pain

The experience of pain is very difficult to define, as it will be different for each and every one of us.

Pain is a paradox. It is replete with anomalies and contradictions. It can be creative and destructive; it can ennoble and embitter; it can protect and destroy. Pain can be a warning sign that something is wrong, and yet can diminish the will to live. It can be associated with survival and also with disease and death [33].

We do not doubt the need to be very focused in our work when trying to assess and manage a child's pain, distress or suffering. But sometimes, especially for a child or a family who have an 'intractable pain', we need to expand our focus. We need to take a wider view than the purely scientific, and think more about the experience of the pain for the child and the family.

Patients with intractable pain highlight the complex interaction between pain and suffering, and force us to recognise our medical and psychological limitations [34].

Pain is subjective and has been described as:

an unpleasant sensory and emotional experience associated with actual or potential tissue damage or described in terms of such damage. **International Association for the Study of Pain: Pain [35]**.

It is important to recognise that pain, including children's pain, cannot be predicted solely by the nature of tissue damage. We know and understand that:

The degree of tissue damage is only one factor among many that contribute to the perception of a painful experience [36].

Now we talk about what Dame Cicely Saunders has called 'Total Pain' [37] or what we might call total or persistent suffering. The word pain implies: That which causes the individual to suffer, be it physically, psychologically, spiritually or emotionally.

The cure of physical pain may be analgesia, but the cure for spiritual (*soul*) pain is to be found in the experience of the pain itself. Spiritual (*soul*) pain, then, is not so much a 'problem to be solved', as a 'question to be lived', and thus demands different qualities in health care professionals [38].

The question at this point may be: is it physical pain or is it emotional distress? Regnard and colleagues [39] have looked at identifying pain and distress in adults with profound communication difficulties, and conclude that there is no difference between some of the signs of pain and distress. This work could be applicable to the children we work with. The similarities they found in physical expressions of pain and distress, for example, facial expression and behaviour, make the assessment process very difficult, so we need to keep an open mind as to what we are seeing, and make more enquiries. When trying to assess a child with either profound communication difficulties or poor communication abilities, or even a child with good communication skills, albeit distressed, Regnard suggests we can look to his eyes for some clues to the degree of this distress. Eye contact is usually made when the person is content, while the eyes just stare when distressed. Early distress may be indicated by changes when eye contact is no longer given.

Suffering

'Suffering is not a question that demands an answer; it is not a problem that demands a solution; it is a mystery that demands a presence.' (Anon, quoted in Wyatt J. Matters of Life and Death, Leicester IVP/ CMF 1998).

Suffering is a difficult and poorly understood concept. It is a generic concept, and just as there are many different types of physical pain, so too, there are different types of suffering. Loss is one form of suffering, grief is another, and soul pain in a dying child or the family is another form of great suffering. A number of definitions have been offered:

A loss of wholeness and the distress and anguish that accompany it [40]. Suffering occurs when the impending destruction of the person is perceived [41].

Bringing these together in making a start at conceptualising soul pain, the following is a good working definition:

Soul pain is **the experience** of an individual who has become **disconnected** and **alienated** from the **deepest** and most **fundamental aspects** of himself or herself [42].

The key words here are, '*disconnected*', '*alienated*' and '*fundamental aspects of self*'. It is in these words also that some of the symptomatology of soul pain may be found. 'Soul pain is a deep homesickness having little to do with physical location and everything to do with our longing for the embrace of those who share life with us [in this case, parents and siblings] and our yearning to feel at home in the world' [42].

Soul pain cannot be seen or measured as something that is happening in a child's body, it is about what is happening in his or her soul. It is the difference between 'crying' and 'weeping', a kind of 'malignant sadness'. The truth is, none of us knows what the other is suffering. We must try to remember to use our imaginations and let the children also use theirs.

The following poem, written by a young teenager dying from cancer, is a powerful expression of what I perceive as soul pain. She finds herself unable to talk about either her disease or her dying to the person she loves the most, her mother, or to the people who care for her, her father and her doctor. All three of them have silenced her by their own fears and anxieties: 'Searching For Me' by Gitanjali

> Disillusioned
> Discouraged
> Despair writ
> On his face
> The doctor
> Holds my hand
> Not my attention
> He retreats
> The moment
> I catch his glance
> He hurriedly
> Looks away.
>
> Neither he, nor my daddy
> Can fool me, no way
> It's poor Mom
> Who is lost to the world
> And relies heavily on God
> Little does she realise
> I don't even have
> A lean chance.
>
> I pity her
> And sorry be
> For none is there
> To share
> Her loneliness
> Her pain, and
> longing, for
> only I know
> how she cares.
> She'll go about
> her life, as any
> normal human being
> only it will be her form
> her soul will be searching...
> for me [44].

Responding to soul pain

'The starting premise is that it is impossible for one individual to prescribe for another's soul pain. No matter how well meant and no matter how great the effort, it is not possible for one person to give another person a sense of meaning' [45].

However, being with a child in soul pain is often more important than any other intervention you might make, and small interventions may help start the process of helping a child do the work he or she needs to do.

Case Ben was 7 years old when he was diagnosed with acute myeloid leukaemia, with CNS involvement and spinal cord compression. He is now about 4 years post his treatment. He was treated with intensive chemotherapy and irradiation, over about 6 months, most of which was as an in-patient. He lives with his parents, a 4-year-old brother and a 15-month-old sister.

Ben was, and is, a very bright boy. It did not take him long to work out that all was not well, and that he was very ill. He became very uncertain and frightened about his future, and though he could not always make sense of the little information he was picking up, he was not asking for information.

He feared the future. Each tomorrow was seen as heralding increased sickness and pain in his life. The nausea and vomiting from the chemotherapy were distressing, but no more so than the anticipation of his hair loss, change in body image, and time away from home, school, and his friends. He felt isolated because he was no longer like his friends, and could not do what they were doing at home and at school. At every stage, the treatment as well as the disease was a source of great suffering to him and his family. He suffered from the effects of his disease and its treatment on his appearance and abilities. He also suffered unremittingly from his perception of the future.

Recall Cassell's definition of suffering: 'Suffering occurs when the impending destruction of the person is perceived'.

As a way of working with Ben's mother, I asked her to write down the changes she saw in him, and she listed:

- general sadness/ few smiles;
- withdrawn—avoids eye contact, especially with professionals;
- angry at times—verbally and physically;
- tearful at times;
- concentration span very small;
- regressed to sucking his thumb and using a teddy as a comforter;
- reduced mobility and weight;
- tires quickly and is very lethargic. Needs help with basic things, i.e., toileting, eating and drinking;
- Ben has lost his 'zest for life'. He was a child (and hopefully will be again) with lots of energy both physical and emotional.
- Impatient.

It is an interesting list of symptoms, some of which can be put down to the side effects of the chemotherapy. Others might well be symptoms of his soul pain. She then went on and asked Ben what he thought and he said:

- Everything has changed.
- Doesn't think he will ever get better.
- Desperately wants to go home.

- Angry—not being able to run around with other children, especially his brother and sister.
- Want to be left alone.

It seemed to me, as I cared for Ben, that he had become helpless and powerless, in what was for him, a new experience. This in turn, seemed to have undermined his motivation to go on living. He felt that his distress and the anguish caused by his diagnosis was unrelenting and unending, and that his future was possibly hopeless. This suffering reinforced itself in his passivity. His helplessness and hopelessness combined to paralyse him in his bed, from which he would not get up. He had turned his head away from the world. I came to see this suffering as Ben's 'soul pain'. I was acutely and painfully aware of his disconnectedness from what used to bring value, hope and meaning into his life, and I could see that he had distanced himself from what used to bring him consolation and comfort: namely his parents, family, and friends.

Soul pain is something we come to: 'feel', 'see', and 'sense' in another [42]. It was clear that this child was suffering. His mother gave him the key to open the door by asking him what had changed, and surprisingly, that was all that was needed. Ben demonstrated the change in behaviour and eye contact noted by Regnard and colleagues [39], which was one of the first clues that he was becoming more and more distressed. They were also the first signs that life was improving for him as he started to make sense of how his world had changed.

Having suggested that children may experience some degree of soul pain, some ways in which we may facilitate its expression will now be considered, while remembering, as Coles suggested:

We are not obliged to try knowing all things or being all things to the people we work with [9].

Children of all ages can express their inner-worlds and all that goes to make up these worlds through play, music, art, image work, and dream work [46]. (See also Chapter 10, Children expressing themselves and Chapter 8, Psychological impact of life-limiting conditions on the child). We could start by asking the question Coles asked the children he was working with:

Tell me, as best you can, who you are—what about you matters most, what makes you the person you are. I would then qualify: if you don't want to emphasise any one thing, any one quality or trait or characteristic, then include others...[6].

This can be done in words, pictures, play or music, as it may be too painful for the child to do so in words alone. In this way the child can remain in control, and choose to reveal as much or as little as he can cope with [47].

The child, especially during the years from two or three through adolescence, can communicate a great deal of his emotional life

through drawing. Children often express themselves more naturally and spontaneously through art than through words. Kramer links the freedom of expression inherent in art to that found in imaginative play, where forbidden wishes and impulses can be expressed symbolically. Even when the child draws a picture that symbolically represents thoughts and feelings that might be too painful to express verbally, he is still able to maintain his ego strength. His art work, therefore, may be used as an indication of his thoughts and emotions [48].

Paediatric clinicians can justifiably say that they are not trained or skilled to work in these media. However, we watch children do these things every day of our working lives: 'Play is far more than an arena for motor development. It is a mirror of the child's knowledge of his world' [49].

Paediatric clinicians and carers can use these media as part of an ongoing emotional assessment of the child, and then refer to an appropriate therapist, such as a clinical psychologist, or an art or music therapist, if they feel unable to work with what the child is presenting to them. It is not necessarily a question of being able to interpret what the child is doing; it is more about being with the child as he or she surprises himself or herself by discovering his or her inner-world [50]. Our role may only be to provide the child with a safe environment, in which to express his or her inner-world.

Bluebond-Langner said that 'A child who is terminally ill seldom tells what he knows in ways easy to understand. But when one learns to listen and take cues from him, it is soon realised that the child does know the truth, and this is often more than can be borne' [21].

Axline [51] supports this statement and suggests that play therapy is 'An opportunity which is given to the child to 'play out' his feelings and problems just as, in certain types of adult therapy, an individual 'talks out' his difficulties'.

Providing children with this opportunity to discuss, or play out issues related to their illness or impending death, should not necessarily increase their anxieties. Pinkerton, Cushing and Sepion [52] suggest, in fact, that it decreases them, in that it reduces their sense of alienation and isolation from their parents and carers.

Ibberson [53] describes how a 13-year-old girl came to terms with the death of her sister and prepared herself for her own death through music therapy: '... music became an invaluable source of communication, exploring the anxieties and confusion that Catherine faced as grief and fear came to the fore, while nurturing her innate zest for life.'

Children of all ages need to be given a window of opportunity they can open or close, if they so choose, to communicate about their illness or impending death. This is a short conversation between a child and his mother:

'It's time to take your antibiotic, son.'
'No, it is not, mum, it's time to stop taking it.'

Is this child telling his mother that it is no longer any good taking his antibiotic or that she has got the time wrong? Mothers don't usually get the times wrong for their children's medication.

Hymovich [54] found that children find informal ways of communicating: 'Children choose the people with whom they wish to communicate, as well as control over what they will talk about and when they will talk.'

We need to bear in mind that each child we meet will be different. It cannot be assumed, even knowing that children of different ages have different understandings of illness or death and dying, that all children in a given age group will have the same understanding. They all come from different backgrounds and environments, and have had different life experiences. Their personal experience with illness or death, their cognitive abilities, and their religious and cultural backgrounds will all play a part in their understanding and will form their ways of coping with trauma, loss, grief, death and ultimately, their dying. The problem of identifying what each child understands and feels is amplified when having to rely on non-verbal communication and observations with younger pre-verbal children, children with complex neurological diseases or older children who have become silent because of fear.

The only way to gain this information is through good communication with the individual child, be that through therapeutic play, art, music, dream work, story-telling, creative writing, visualization, guided imagery, straight talking with the older child, or just sitting with the child and waiting, watching and wondering what may happen next. All these media may be used to help distressed children express their inner-worlds, where they may start to discern their meaning and their own hopes [55].

These illustrations indicate that soul pain can be explored in children by understanding how children process information and by being aware of the psychopathology of their soul pain. Moreover, we can help this group of children by facilitating them to find ways in which they feel comfortable in expressing their inner-worlds, even though this is not easy to accomplish.

Paediatric clinicians and carers appear to be committed to the concepts of holistic and family-centred care [56–59]. However, they may be the first to admit, like other groups of clinicians, that they find this dimension of care difficult to address with children, with children from different cultural and religious backgrounds, and children who may be dying [60].

Caring for the soul

'Care of the soul would be those aspects of care that help a person connect with his inner self and find the centre of his being. The difference between spiritual and soul is primarily one of transcendence' [43].

'Care of the soul begins with observance of how the soul manifests itself and how it operates. We can't care for the soul unless we are familiar with its ways' [33].

In order to care for the families we work with, we first need to understand how our own soul manifests itself and how we care for it. Children who are dying will at some time think about the ramifications of their illness for their souls as well as for their bodies. On this journey, we are called to be their companion, guide and advocate and we can only do this if we are at home in our own soul. They need our help, but they don't need us to do the journey for them.

Our role as paediatric clinicians and carers is to work with both the child and the whole family to give them all a feeling of security, so that they can start to do the work they need to do in trying to find meaning in their child's pain, suffering, and death.

'We must recognise that the most we can do is to prepare and hold the space where the miraculous may happen' (cited by Kearney 42).

Preparing and holding a safe and secure or 'sacred space' is what we do when we offer expert and effective care and symptom management, when we help open up blocked channels of communication, and as we work with distressed families who can find no meaning in their child's illness, suffering, or death. If we can find a creative way of responding to the challenge of soul pain, it may open up a path to the very heart of living, even in the shadow of death . . .

When we are mindful observers and respectful listeners to children, we nurture their spirits (souls) and provide an opportunity to connect them fundamentally—to themselves and their experiences [61].

Edwards and Davis [62] have described this role well, and it is reproduced here with consent, as a summary of what has been suggested in this chapter and to give guidelines.

Exploring the child's experiences and understanding

Getting to know children and exploring their experiences of events are perhaps the most important parts of the process of helping.

Exploration of the child's experience or problem:

- is only possible when sufficient trust and openness have been established in the relationship between the child and helper;

- is a prerequisite to enabling a shared understanding of the difficulty and required areas of change/help, and in implementing strategies for helping;

- is important in getting to know the child better and enabling the helper to put the child's difficulties into the context of his life circumstances generally;

- can in itself be of enormous value in facilitating change, by enabling developments in the child's understanding or perception of events;

- has important implications for the development of the relationship between the helper and child, enabling the child to realise that the helper is interested in him or her and not just his or her problem;

- can be facilitated with verbal prompts including open and closed questions, multiple choice responses, facilitative comments, such as empathic responses, and using questions which structure and therefore enable a more coherent and clear account to be given;

- using open questions most frequently enables the child to tell his or her story in his or her own words;

- can use non-verbal modes of expression, including drawings, models/puppets, and play;

- can use more structured forms such as the use of sentence/story completion tasks, books, diaries, rating scales, and exploratory games.

Conclusion

'Professionals who use listening skills to hear what the child is expressing within the limits of the developmental and cognitive stage, and who have the courage and imagination to respond or to refer on appropriately are providing good spiritual care' [63].

'We so often treat children as if we have forgotten what it is like to be a child. These are things we can ill afford to do if we wish to understand what it is like to be a child with terminal illness and to respond appropriately' [40].

When it all gets too hard and you are at a loss as to what to do next, it is well worth remembering that old Indian proverb about God: 'God gave us one mouth and two ears so that we can listen twice as much as we speak.'

The children and their families just need us to be there, watching with them, waiting with them, and wondering with them as they surprise themselves. They need us to be truly 'present' to them, and to be ourselves. This work is about a 'journey', and that journey is to the centre, to the heart of the matter, or, as in the Ring, to 'the mountain of fire in Mordor'. On this journey, we have to engage the child and family, if we are to travel with them, get to the 'heart of the matter,' and help them move on to the next stage of their journey.

References

1. Williams. N. *As it is in Heaven*, London: Picador, 1999.
2. Garbarino J. and Bedard C. Spiritual challenges to children facing violent trauma, *Childhood* 1996;3(4):467–78.
3. Kenny. G. Assessing children's spirituality: What is the way forward, *Brit J Nurs* 1999;8(1):28–32.
4. Larson, B.B., Sayers J.P., and Mccullough, M.E. Scientific Research on Spirituality and Health: A Consensus Report. National Institute for Health Care Research. Rockville, 1997.
5. Meraviglia, M.G. Critical analysis of spirituality and its empirical indicators: Prayer and meaning in life, *J Holist Nurs* 1999;17(1):18–33.
6. Shelley, J.A. *The Spiritual Needs of Children*, USA: Inter-Varsity Press, 1982.
7. Pehler, S.R. Children's spiritual response: Validation of the nursing diagnosis in spiritual distress. *Nurs Diag* 1997;8(2).
8. Doka, K.J. Suffer the little children; the child and spirituality in the AIDS crisis. In B. Dane and C. Levine, eds. *AIDS and the New Orphans*. Wesport: Auburn House, 1994, pp. 33–41.
9. Coles, R. *The Spiritual Life Of Children*, London: Harper Collins, 1992.
10. Sommer, D.R. The Spiritual Needs of Dying Children. *Issues Comprehens Pediat Nurs* 1989;12:225–33.
11. Davies, B., Brenner, P., Sumner, L., and Worden, W. Addressing Spirituality in Pediatric Hospice and Palliative Care. *J Palliat Care* 2002;18(1):59–67.
12. McKivergin, M.J. and Daubernimire. M.L. The Healing Process of Presence. *J Holist Nurs* 1994;12(1):65–81.
13. Goldman, A. and Christie, D. Children with cancer talk about their own death with their families. *Pediatr Hematol Oncol* 1993;10(3):223–31.
14. Bluebond-Langner, M. I Know, do you?, 171–181, In Schoenberg, B. et al. *Anticipatory Grief*, New York: Columbia University Press, 1974.
15. Kubler-Ross, E. *To Live Until We Say Good-Bye*, Chapter 2, 'JAMIE', USA: Prentice Hall, 1985.
16. Anthony, S. *The Child's Discovery of Death*. New York: Brace & Co., 1940.
17. Nagy, M. The child's theories concerning death. *J Genet Psychol* 1948;73:3–27.
18. Bowlby, J. *Attachment and Loss*. London: Hogarth Press, 1980.
19. Koocher, G. Childhood, death and cognitive development. *Developmental Psychology* 1973;9:369–75.
20. Swain H. The concepts of death in children. *Dissertation Abstr Int* 1975;37(2-A):898–9.
21. Bluebond-Langner, M. *The Private Worlds Of Dying Children*, New Jersey, NJ: Princeton University Press, 1978.
22. Kane B. Children's concepts of death. *J Genet Psychol* 1979;134:141–53.
23. Landsdown R. and Benjamin, G. The development of the concept of death in children 5–9 yrs. *Child and Dev* 1985;11:13–20.
24. Clunies-Ross C. and Lansdown R. The concept of death in children with leukaemia. *Child: Care, Health Dev* 1988;14: 373–86.
25. Dom Henry, T. Vaisnava Hindu and Ayurvedic Approaches to Caring for the dying. In M. Solomon, A. Romer, K. Helper, and D. Weilsman eds. *Innovations in End-of-Life Care Practical*

Strategies & International Perspectives. Vol 2. USA: Mary Ann Liebert, Inc. Publications, 2001, pp. 223–30.

26. Tolkien, J.R.R. *The Lord of the Rings*, 284. London: George Allen & Unwin, 1954, p. 284. Reprinted by permission of Harper Collins Publishers Ltd. © Tolkien 1954.

27. Tournier, *A Doctor's Case Book in the Light of the Bible*. London: SCM Press, 1954.

28. Stoter, D. *Spiritual Aspects of Health Care*. London: Mosby, 1995.

29. Hillman, J. *Suicide And The Soul*. Woodstock. USA: Spring Publications, Inc., 1965.

30. Hillman, J. *Re-Visioning Psychology*. New York: Harper & Row, 1975.

31. Moore, T. *Care of the Soul*. New York: Harper Collins Books, 1992.

32. Bettelheim, B. *Freud & Man's Soul*. London: Flamingo, 1983.

33. Autton, N. *Pain: An Exploration*. London: Darton, Longman & Todd, 1986.

34. Cassell, E. J. *The Nature Of Suffering and The Goals of Medicine*. Oxford: Oxford University Press, 1991.

35. International Association for the Study of Pain: Subcommittee on taxonomy. Pain terms: A list with definitions and notes on usage. *Pain* 1979;6:249–52.

36. Hain, R. Pain scales in children: a review. *Palliat Med* 1997;11: 341–50.

37. Saunders, C. and Baines, M. *Living With Dying: The Management Of Terminal Disease*. Oxford: Oxford University Press, 1983.

38. Elsdon, R. Spiritual pain in dying people: The nurse's role. *Professional Nurse* 1995;10(10):641–3.

39. Regnard, C., Matthews, D., Gibson, L., and Clarke, C. Difficulties in identifying distress and its causes in people with severe communication problems. *Int J Palliat Nurs* 2003;9(4):173–6.

40. Attig T. Beyond Pain: The existential suffering of children. *J Palliat Care* 12(No 3):20–23.

41. Cassell, E.J. The nature of suffering and the goals of medicine. *N Engl J Med*, 1982;306(11):639–45.

42. Kearney, M. *Mortally Wounded*. Dublin: Marino Books, 1996.

43. Lane. J.A. The care of the human spirit. *J Professional Nurs* 1987; 3(6):332–7.

44. Badruddin, K. *Poems of Gitanjali*. London: Oriel Press, 1982.

45. Kearney. A Talk Given in London,1998.

46. D'antonio, I.J. Therapeutic use of play in hospitals. *Nurs Clin N Am* 1984;19(2):351–9.

47. Bach, S. *Life Paints Its Own Span: On The Significance Of Spontaneous Pictures By Severely Ill Children*. Switzerland: Daimon Verlag, 1990.

48. McLeavey, K.A. Children's art as an assessment tool. *Pediatr Nurs* 1979;March/April:9–14.

49. Marino, B.L. Studying infant and toddler play. *J Pediatr Nurs* 1991;6(1):16–20.

50. Wilson, K. Kendrick, P., and Ryan, V. *Play Therapy: A Non-Directive Approach For Children And Adolescents*. London: Bailliere Tindall, 1992.

51. Axline, V.M. *Play Therapy*. Edinburgh: Churchill Livingstone, 1989.

52. Pinkerton, C.R., Cushing, P., and Sepion, B. *Childhood Cancer Management*. London: Chapman & Hall, 1994.

53. Ibberson, C. A Natural End: One story about Catherine. *Br J Music Ther* 1996; 10(1):24–31.

54. Hymovich D. The meaning of cancer to children. *Semin Oncol Nurs* 1995;11(1):51–58.

55. Armstrong-Dailey, A. and Goltzer, S.Z. *Hospice Care for Children*. Oxford: Oxford University Press, 1993.

56. Thompson, J. Family centred care. *Nursing Mirror* 1985;Feb 13th: 25–28.

57. Casey, A. A partnership with child and family. *Senior Nurs* 1988; 8(4):8–9.

58. Darbyshire, P. *Living with a Sick Child in Hospital*. London: Chapman & Hall, 1994.

59. Palmer Care of the sick child by parents: A meaningful role. *J Advanced Nurs* 1993;18:185–91.

60. Winkelstein, M, L. *Spirituality and Death of the Child*. In V. B.Carson, ed. *Spiritual Dimensions of Nursing Practice* Chapter 9. London: Saunders Co., 1989.

61. Thurston C. Ryan J. Faces of God: Illness, healing, and children's spirituality. *ACCH Advocate* 1996;2(2):13–15.

62. Edwards, M. and Davis, H. *Counselling Children with Chronic Medical Conditions*. The British Psychological Society Books, 1997.

63. Pfund. R. Nurturing a child's spirituality. *J Child Health* 2001;4(4):143–8.

64. Cobb, M. *The Dying Soul*. Buckingham: Open University Press, 2001.

65. Stoter, D. *Spiritual Aspects of Health Care*. London: Mosby, 1995, p. 8.

66. Goodliff, P. *Care in a Confused Climate: Pastoral Care and Postmodern Culture*. London: Darton: Longman & Todd, 1998.

7 Children's views of death

Myra Bluebond-Langner and Amy DeCicco

Introduction

Did you ever think when a hearse goes by that you may be the next to die? They wrap you up in a big white sheet and then they bury you ten feet deep. The worms crawl in and the worms crawl out. They chew at your gizzard and spit it out. And then you turn a vomit green and the pus rushes out like sour cream. [Children's street rhyme portions dating back to the 18th century].

Death, like sex, is a topic which adults find difficult to discuss with children. Talking about it seems to them to be a painful, confusing intrusion into a child's world. This assumes that death is foreign to a child's usual thoughts, that it is distressing for a child to even consider, and that it is difficult for him/her to grasp. Ideally, thoughts and talk about death should wait for a time of more maturity, both emotional and cognitive.

As we all know, discussions of death are usually forced upon us by the death of a pet, relative, close friend, or even the impending death of the child himself/herself. This leads us to ask whether adult reservations about discussing death with children are well founded. What should we say? What can they understand?

In this chapter, we consider what needs to be taken into account in assessing children's understanding of death, and suggest guidelines for talking to well and ill children about their own dying and the deaths of others. We begin with a review of the literature on well children's views of death and then move into a discussion of terminally ill children's views of death, followed by a brief presentation of the thoughts of well siblings of children with life-threatening and fatal illnesses and how they communicate with their ill siblings.

Children's views of death

The literature on children's views of death is dominated by a developmental perspective, which focuses on the emergence of a "mature concept of death." Scholars have differed about the particular age or stage when a particular view emerges, and

about the prevalence of particulars views at a given age or stage (see Table 7.1). But, prevalent throughout developmental work is the assumption that at points in the maturation process the child casts aside immature notions for the elements of the adult or mature concept of death (see Chart 1). According to developmental thinking, there are five essential components to a mature concept of death: non-functionality (all life functions cease at death); irreversibility (being cannot come alive again); universality (all persons, indeed, all living things, die); causality (causes of death); personal mortality (the individual himself/herself will die) [18]. As children grow up, then, their view of death changes from that of death as a reversible occurrence, not unlike sleep or being transported to a different place, to a view of death as an irreversible and universal event, a consequence of physiological process, aging and disease, something that befalls everyone including oneself. 'Mature' views feature scientific notions and 'immature' ones draw upon fantasy.

In the developmental model, then, the child's understanding of death is seen in terms of a linear process of development linked to age and a definite endpoint. The essential components of the endpoint concept are of a cognitive sort and a particular one at that—what Klatt [19] calls 'a biologized concept of death.' In the age-graded developmental approach not enough attention is given to experience—social, cultural or personal—or to emotional factors like anxiety, and how these impact a person's understanding of death and the meaning death has for them.

Our own view is that people's views of death do not lie neatly on a progression. Young children can show sophisticated understanding of death and adults do not necessarily abandon what developmental researchers regard as childish notions. Research from both developmental and a non-developmental perspective supports this. For example, Candy-Gibbs, Sharp and Petrun [20] did not find correlations between age and concepts of irreversibility. Atwood [21] found that while a majority of kindergartners studied

Table 7.1 Children's views of death: Developmental perspectives

Perception	Stage/age (source)
Death as temporary, not final, reversible	Preoperational, young [1]
	Less than 5 [2]
Continuous with life-diminution of alive	Less than 5 [2]
Life goes on under changed circumstances	Preoperational, young [1]
	Less than 5 [2,3]
Separation of concern	Less than 5 [2,3]
Caused by external forces (violent or	Preoperational, young [1]
accidental)	Between 5 and 9 [2]
Death is personified (skeleton, the dead)	Between 5 and 9 [2]
	Other children, but uncommon
	(Koocher/Kane/Wass) [1,4–6,7]
	Between 6 and 8 [3]
	Adults (Kastenbaum) [8–10]
Personal death can be avoided (e.g. via tricking	Between 5 and 9 [2]
personification)	Between 6 and 8 [3]
Concrete and non-specific ideas about life	Concrete operational, middle childhood
and death	and preadolescent [1]
Death as cessation of functions	Concrete operational, middle childhood
	and preadolescent [1]
	Between 5 and 7 [11–13]
	Between 5 and 8 [14]
	By age 5 [15]
	By age 5 [16]
Death as final/irreversible	Concrete operational, middle childhood
	and preadolescent [1]
	Between 5 and 7 [11–13]
	Between 5 and 10 [15]
Death as universal/inevitable cannot be avoided	Concrete operational, middle childhood
	and preadolescent [1]
	Between 9 and 10 [2]
	Between 5 and 7 [11–13]
	Between 5 and 12 [16]
	Between 5 and 8 (Mahon) [14]
	Between 5 and 6 (Candy-Gibbs et al.) [17]
Causality / Understanding what causes death	Between 5 and 12 [15]
Personal mortality	Between 6 and 8 [15]
	Between 5 and 9 [16]
	Between 5 and 8 [14]
	By age 5 [17]
Sophisticated and abstract philosophies and	Formal cognitive operations
theologies about the nature of death and	(propositional and hypothetical deductive
existence after death	thinking), adolescence [1]

acknowledged that they could die, the sixth-graders did not (reversing the prediction of developmentalism).

Looking at studies of adult views of death, Kastenbaum and Aisenberg [22] reported that adult descriptions of death are replete with macabre images. Personifications of death

(a view of death associated with school-age children) as gentle comforter, gay deceiver, grim reaper, wrinkled old woman are not uncommon—all conceptions associated with a not fully mature view of death. Kubler-Ross's [23] work with terminally ill adults is also relevant in this respect. She demonstrated that even among patients who were able to conceive of themselves as dying, there was a preoccupation with death as the ultimate separation, and a tendency to portray themselves as going on to another life after death. Patients painted themselves in scenes where God takes them into the splendor of heaven. These are views that, in the context of the age-graded, developmental model of concepts of death, are associated with young children at very early stages of cognitive development.

Studies of children's views of death that attend to factors such as children's religious and cultural background, as well as the children's own personal experiences with death and dying, raise serious questions about the saliency, and in some cases even the relevancy, of age in assessing a child's view of death [22,24–26].

Candy-Gibbs et al's [20] study of 114 white children of ages from 5 to 9, from middle income families, found that age was not a significant factor in children's views of the irreversibility and finality of death. 50% of the children who attended Baptist schools held a view of death that included an afterlife. 81% of the Unitarian children saw death as complete, final and irreversible. Religious background also played a role in the children's views of the causes of death. Baptist children saw death as stemming from external catastrophic events. Unitarian children saw death as stemming from internal natural causes.

Also relevant with regard to religion and religious instruction is a study by Anthony and Bhana [27], cited by Kenyon in her extensive review of the literature on children's views of death, where "despite clearly understanding most of the components of death by 6 years of age, religious teachings were reflected in Muslim girls' assertions at all ages, that death was reversible and the dead could return to life". [18]

In Bluebond-Langner's study of religious and ethnic differences in American children's views of death, she and her students found that Jewish American children saw death as the result of natural or medical events, whereas Baptist African-American children and Catholic Hispanic children saw death as the result of catastrophic accidents and violence [28]. April Zweig [29], in a study comparing 10- and 11-year-old African-American children from a poor area of Chicago with Jewish American children of the same ages from a middle class area, found that African-American children usually attributed death to an outside force, usually violent, whereas Jewish American children saw it as a result of a medical or natural event. Unlike the Jewish American children, the African-American children also personified death and did not see death as final. And with a focus on ethnicity, Brent et al [30] found a better understanding of irreversibility and non-functionality in the Chinese children (ages 3–17) than in American children. In short, these are not differences of maturity.

The salience of factors other than age or stage of development in a child's conceptualization of death is given further credence when one considers the findings of those who have studied and compared children from cultures and societies outside the United States with those within the United States. For example, Schonfield and Smilansky [31] found that second grade children in Israel were clearer about finality and irreversibility than second graders in the US. However, the American children were more likely to see death as universal—all living things will die. Schonfield and Smilansky attribute the difference to the children's experiences. The Israeli children are living in the context of war, where they are regularly exposed to the finality of death, and where adults try to comfort children (many of whom have fathers and siblings in the military) by telling them that not everyone dies.

In assessing a child's view of death, one must also consider how the child's view was elicited, by whom and in what context. Some of the contradictions in the literature may be attributable to the variety of methods of study—open-ended interviews, questionnaires, story completions, analysis of drawings. But this still doesn't explain the variations that occur even when a single method is used. For example, in Carol Irizarry-Hobson's study [32] of the views of death of children who experienced the death of a grandparent, she found that what the children told or asked their parents with regard to their grandparent's death was different from what they told her. Further, the 'less mature view' came through with their parents and the 'mature view' with the researcher. For example, one 7-year-old asked his mother when they were packing for a vacation, six months after his grandfather had died, if he would see his grandfather. He also told the researcher, quite clearly, that dead is dead, you don't come back. Or take the 8-year-old who asked her mother if her grandfather had socks in the grave to keep him warm; she gave the researcher a lengthy account of her grandfather's death from a heart attack.[1]

Just as the child's presentation may be affected by who he/she is talking to, so too it may be affected by whether one is asking about death in some abstract sense, or with regard to a stranger, or a family member. For example, Orbach et al [33] asked children of ages 6–11 to answer questions about death, in terms of people they knew, and in terms of strangers. Orbach et al [33] concluded that the stress and other emotional issues that revolve around thoughts of the death of a loved one distorted the children's actual conceptions of death such that children's concept of death when referenced to loved ones was less developed than that referenced to strangers.

---

[1] The need to look at context in assessing child's view is further explored in succeeding sections on ill children and their siblings.

A child's response may also be limited by his verbal ability. He may understand more than he can articulate or explain. Consider how the toddler can follow multi-step directions, but cannot necessarily give multi-step directions. Toddlers and young children are exposed to death (for example, dead animals, sometimes even human individuals) before they can talk about their experiences in any detailed way. Yet, we know from their non-verbal responses that they respond to the experience [22,34].

In sum, as Koocher states [24], "The child's comprehension of death is a complex phenomenon mediated by his own cognitive capabilities, personal experiences, cultural background, and emotional reactivity." Their presentation of their views requires consideration of these factors as well as the context of the discussion about death—who the child is speaking with, where the conversation takes place, as well as how the issue is put forward.

Terminally ill children and death

The need to look beyond an age-graded, developmental model for explanations of children's views of death was dramatically demonstrated for Bluebond-Langner [25] in her research with terminally ill children, when she found that age was not at all predictive of the children's views of death, their awareness of their condition, or the ways in which they communicated that awareness. For example, the 5 year-old concerned with separation who talked about worms eating him, and who refused to play with the toys from deceased children, was the same 5 year-old who knew that the drugs had run out and demanded that time not be wasted. So, too, the 9-year-old who drew pictures of herself on blood red crosses and knew that the medication was damaging her liver she was the same 9-year-old who never mentioned the names of deceased children, and could not bear to have her mother leave her for a moment.

In each of these children we find views that are expected for their age, as well as views one would not expect from children of that age. Yes, to hear a 5-year-old speak about worms eating him, and being concerned about separation, is predictable from the developmental perspective. But discussion of drugs running out is something that, according to these models, would not occur until much later, in middle childhood. Similarly, that a 9-year-old girl could state that drugs were damaging her liver is not terribly surprising, but a taboo on names of deceased children is more problematic in terms of the development model. In short, in both children all of the elements of a 'mature view' of death are there, as well as elements on an 'immature view.'

What is going on here? Why these contradictions? Have these children both gained in wisdom and regressed? We would

suggest that children, like adults, are capable of simultaneously holding several views of death, even seemingly contradictory ones. The particular view that comes out at any one point in time reflects the child's concerns, thoughts, and feelings, not to mention the person the child is speaking to at that point in time.

Of primary concern to terminally ill children is separation: leaving everything and everyone behind. At the same time, they seek to protect those they care about—often their siblings, particularly their parents. For example, Jeffrey was a boy who often yelled at his mother. When asked why he simply replied, "Then she won't miss me when I'm gone." When Bluebond-Langner asked Jeffrey's mother, "Why does Jeffrey yell at you so much?" She replied, "He knows when I can't take it in that room anymore. He knows that if he yells at me I'll leave. He also knows I'll come back" [25]. Displays of anger, banal chitchat, and silence were all distancing strategies, if you will, or, as some staff saw them, rehearsals for the final separation. As folks at St. Christopher's Hospice say, "Withdrawal is not necessarily a hostile act". They also were a part of mutual pretense.[2]

As noted above, death as a separate personality is often present in both adults' and terminally ill children's views. Bluebond-Langner [25] found that the tendency to view death as a separate personality, or more commonly, to identify death with the dead, was notable among the ill children in two significant ways. First, it was through the death of a peer that the children internalized the terminal nature of their illness, which they would then present in conversation through comparisons of the deceased with themselves.

BENJAMIN: Dr Richards told me to ask you what happened to Maria. [Note: Dr Richards had said no such thing.]
MYRA: What do you think happened to Maria?
BENJAMIN: Well she didn't go to another clinic and she didn't go to another hospital or home.
MYRA: No. She was sick, sicker than you are now and she died.
BENJAMIN: She had nosebleeds. I had nosebleeds, but mine stopped [25].

Benjamin went through this conversation with everyone he saw that day. When asked why, he responded, "I want to know who my friends are."

Second, the identification of death with the dead was apparent in their reluctance to mention the names of deceased children, or to play with toys brought by the deceased's parents, or purchased in the child's memory—as if death were somehow contagious. These 'magical fantasy' views may be

---

[2] For further discussion of mutual pretense—particularly with regard to ill children and their parents see Bluebond-Langner 1978. See Section IV for discussion of mutual pretense among ill and well siblings.

coupled with very real scientific views of death, as Tom's conversation with a nurse so dramatically illustrates.

TOM: Jennifer died last night. I have the same thing, don't I?
NURSE: But they are going to give you different medicines.
TOM: What happens when they run out?
NURSE: Well, maybe they will find more before then [25].

In this conversation, we see a notion of death as the time when the drugs (chemotherapies) would 'run out.' Following this interchange, his conversations about drugs and their side effects diminished. The drugs were not the answer that he and his parents once thought them to be. As with other children aware of the prognosis, he made little reference to his condition or progress. What was there to say? There were only indications of further deterioration and closeness to death. For these children, death is the result of a biological and inevitable process marked by steady deterioration. "I just get weaker and weaker and soon I won't even be able to walk."

With dying comes a loss of identity. Children with life-threatening and life-shortening illnesses feel that they are not like other children. For example, Bluebond-Langer [25] noted that the children whom she studied spoke of not getting braces, clothes to grow into, or going to school. What is the identifying marker of childhood if not becoming? Looked at another way, to say these things meant that they knew that they had no future, that death is final. Death marks the end, the future is cut off. They did not mention what they would be when they grew up, and some became angry if others did.

One child who, when first diagnosed, said that he wanted to be a doctor, became angry with his doctor when she tried to get him to submit to a procedure with, "I thought you would understand, Sandy. You told me once you wanted to be a doctor." He screamed back at her, "I'm not going to be anything," and then threw an empty syringe at her. She said, "OK, Sandy." The nurse standing nearby said, "What are you going to be?" "A ghost," said Sandy and turned over [25].

To these children, closeness to death also meant no future; consequently, conversations about the future declined noticeably. The future was limited to the next holiday or occasion. The children knew that holidays and events had a new significance for parents as well. Children would often talk about the way that holidays used to be celebrated and the way in which it was celebrated now that they were ill.

At the same time, the children also tried to rush these holidays or occasions, to bring them closer to the present. For example, one child asked for his Christmas presents in October; another wanted to buy a winter coat in July. In June, several children asked the physicians if they could go back to school in September.

Even doctors who doubted that a young child could know the prognosis without being told regarded these actions as indications that the child was suspicious, and perhaps even probing for how much longer he or she had to live. The child's lack of interest in future plans does not reflect a lack of interest in the passing of time.

Children with chronic life-shortening illnesses are very much concerned about the time that they have left, often pushing themselves to get things done. Bluebond-Langner [25] reported how some became angry when people took too long to remember things, or to answer questions, or to bring things to them. The parents and staff often commented on such behavior. As one staff member commented, "They demand because they know time is short. It's as if they know that if they wait too long, they might be dead by then. They're not just being difficult," the staff person included, "Those children know something.[3]"

Some children verbalized their fear of wasting time directly with phrases like, "Don't waste time," or "We can't waste time." The staff often noted the activity and urgency that followed the death of a peer [25].

Time takes on meaning not usually found in young children. These children are having their time cut short, and they know it. Death and disease are constants in their lives. Images of death and disease fill disease related as well as non-disease-related play and conversations.

Well siblings' views of illness and death

Bluebond-Langner [25] found that death and disease are also constants in the lives of the well siblings of children with chronic, life-threatening illnesses.[4] Their thoughts about the incurability of the disease reach a peak when the complications of the disease (for example, refractory infections, intermittent use of oxygen, development of Burkholderia cepacia, onset of diabetes). At this time the well siblings start to view cystic fibrosis (CF) as a chronic, progressive, incurable disease that shortens the life span.

But I still get worried about my sister. I just know that with CF you could die from it and you get all skinny, and your lungs fill up with mucus, and you can't breath, and you die [35].

Acknowledging a shortened lifespan or a terminal prognosis for persons with CF does not necessarily mean acknowledging

---

[3] For example, Mary was a demanding child who never said anything directly about her prognosis. When she died, a list of all the children who had died, and under what circumstances, was found in a bureau drawer along, with a list of whom she wanted to receive particular belongings.

[4] For a full discussion of the well sibling's views of the ill child's condition, prognosis and death over the course of the illness, see Bluebond-Langner 1996.

that one's own sibling will die at an early age from CF. While well siblings may glibly link incurable and terminal, they do not necessarily internalize it as an outcome for their own brother or sister, at least not in the near future. There is an attempt to distance oneself, one's sibling from the imminence, if not the eventuality of death.

The well siblings' views are sprinkled with conditions and qualifiers.

It's one of the deadliest diseases. You are in the hospital a lot. Your chances of surviving are almost zero. That's a lot, really scary [35].

The disease is a despised enemy to be fought.

My sister has cystic fibrosis and I hate it. I wish there was a miracle; that they could have a medicine for cystic fibrosis [35].

In their eyes, there is still room to do things. As a well sibling, whose sister now required oxygen during hospitalization, said, "There are still things they can do. I'd worry with the oxygen and all, but I know Andrea's a fighter." (N.B. The use of oxygen is a highly charged issue for families. Siblings and parents often refer to the use of oxygen as a "turning point.")

Increased deterioration

In the face of still further and increased deterioration, well siblings find it increasingly difficult to separate the disease and its sequelae from what will happen to 'my brother' or 'my sister.'

She acts like she's gonna grow old some day, and have a real nice car and stuff. (Pause) It would be nice, but sounds impossible. Everybody never makes it, (pause) that far. All of her friends die. She thinks that maybe she'll beat it. I don't, but it's hard to say. Maybe she'll beat it [35].

As the deterioration becomes more marked with the patient more oxygen dependent, activities more restricted, and thought given to the insertion of central lines, many well siblings come to see CF as a chronic, progressive, incurable disease that will claim the life of their own sibling in the near future. There is a quality of hopelessness in their statements. Gone are the conditional tense (for example, 'could die'), the use of qualifiers, (for example, 'chances of survival are almost zero'), the possibility of controlling the disease, the hope for a cure.

They express their views of CF and their sibling's condition in short, declarative statements.

I know they're not going to find a cure. With the lungs filling up you die. Everybody never makes it. All of her friends die. She'll never be O.K. She's got cystic fibrosis. She'll never be O.K. There's no cure for her [35].

There is no doubt about the finality of death, not to mention the cause. As one well brother explained, "My mom always asks me how come I never go down to the hospital to see them [his siblings who have CF]. I don't want to go to the hospital. I don't

want to go down there and see them in the hospital. Not the fact that I don't want to go see them; it's just that I know what's going to happen. You know it's inevitable. You know the progression of the disease will get worse. That's inevitable."

Awareness of the imminence of death comes in the terminal phase of the illness. For some well siblings, the awareness is there earlier than it is for others, as illustrated in this conversation between two well sisters of a recently deceased brother.

ROBERTA: Right up until the end, even with the morphine I didn't quite get it together that Reggie was really going to die then. Sally and the others [other family members] could, even before, but not me. But then I wasn't as close to Reggie as Sally was.

SALLY: I knew he was dying probably before any one else; probably even before my mother, because I talked to Reggie about it [35].

Without speaking, they could maintain distance from the imminence, if not the eventuality, of death. As Roberta continued, "I was afraid to talk to him because I didn't want him to tell me that he was dying. I didn't want to talk to him because of that. So I would go in and he'd be in his room, on oxygen and I would talk to him, but I would never; you know, I didn't want it to get to the point where he would start telling me, 'You know it's going to be over soon.'"

Much as they might want to or even try to avoid the finality of death and its frank irreversibility, they knew otherwise, as is evident in this mother's recollections. Even when Ethan died, Ian [well brother] knelt by the bed and said, "He isn't dead." He knelt by the bed and said, "See, he's still here." Ian would come home everyday after school and say how much better Ethan looked. He'd go, "See how much better he is." I had to shake him and say, "He isn't going to get better." But he knew that. His teacher told me he knew.

Communication

For both well siblings and children with chronic life-threatening illness, communicating with each other as well as with their parents about the illness and death is problematic throughout the course of the illness. Conversation about the illness and death is often shrouded in *mutual pretense*.

In the practice of mutual pretense, each party knows what is happening, but neither wishes to speak or acknowledge it to the other. As outlined by Glaser and Strauss [36], in the context of mutual pretense: dangerous topics are avoided; safe topics dominate the conversation; individuals provide a way for the other party to leave the conversation if it appears that they will break down and the pretense get shattered. Behaviors such as avoiding discussion of the future, display of anger, withdrawal, and banal chitchat so that people will have an excuse for leaving reflect adherence to these rules.

The reasons for the practice of mutual pretense are many, but in case of well and ill siblings, two reasons are primary. First, mutual pretense is in part a means to avoid having to confirm, in no uncertain terms, one's certain knowledge that the disease is terminal, and all that having that knowledge brings in its wake. As one adolescent with CF explained, "It's hard to talk about, to even think about Sid and the others who have died, and still keep doing what you to. And then if you did as much as they wanted you to do, you wouldn't have much of a life in the outside world, which they want you to do too?"

Talking about another's deterioration or death, not to mention one's own, especially when one is beginning to experience some of the complications of the disease, brings the prognosis, of which people with CF are well aware, to the forefront of their minds, where they would rather not have it.

Confirmation is not desired by well siblings, either. One well brother summarized the feelings of many when he said, with regard to not wanting to talk to his mother about his sister's condition, "We don't talk about it. I try to stay away from it, because I don't like to hear it. I already know for a fact what's going on. I know as much as I need to know. I don't care to hear anymore about it. If they come up with a cure that's great. Then I won't have to worry about it all. But they haven't, so we don't talk about it."

To receive confirmation of their sibling's fate and then to talk about it raises a host of problems for well siblings, not least among them the ability to ask for and make demands directly.

Well siblings aware of the chronic, progressive, incurable nature of the disease, not to mention their parents' binds, feel less justified, less able to make some of the demands that they had made earlier in the course of the illness. For example,

The girls [sisters who have CF] are angels, you know, as far as my mom's concerned. And, I'm always spiteful of them. I mean, "Aw, come on. How come they get so much and we [well brothers] . . . You know, like they're going to the shore and stuff. But I'm only saying that because, you know, in a joking manner. You know, I realize what the situation is. How, you know, the disease works and everything. So, I know, she's [mother] just trying to spend as much time with them as she can to make them happy, to keep it out of their minds, you know. It doesn't bother me that much. Every once in a while it will build up and be a big explosion." [35]

A second reason for the emergence of mutual pretense is concern about the impact of such a conversation on the other persons in the interaction: Will they be upset? Will they never want to speak with them again? Will they then even avoid them? As one ill child, in discussing why she didn't talk to her well brother about her condition, remarked,

He worries a lot. He worries about me mostly. I don't know why. Sometimes he talks to me about what he worries about. Sometimes. I wouldn't say much because he doesn't want me to know. He just, well, I can hear it on the phone that he is [worried]. [35]

Well siblings are similarly concerned. As one well sibling said, "I don't think I'd be able to talk about it. I might say something that would get her mad or upset. I'm really scared about what her reactions will be. Maybe something would come up that my parents don't want her to know. I don't want to tell [what I know] because I don't know what is going to happen. I don't know how she is going to react. I don't know if she's just going to say, 'Well, when it happens,' or if she's going to start crying or something like that."

Siblings' reluctance to speak often occurs with full recognition that the ill sibling not only knows the prognosis, but also knows that people are not willing to talk about it. As one 12- year-old sister commented, "I think she sort of feels out in the cold about that we know more about it that what we're telling her. I think she knows, from the people that we have known, who have had CF and died. We haven't said that kid had cystic fibrosis, or anything like that. We sort of say it's a shame and leave it at that. We don't really tell her. But she knew one [who died] and that he had treatment like her."

The struggle over what to say, let alone what to do, remains problematic right up to the moment of death, as seen in this conversation between two sisters recalling the time of their brother's death.

MINDY: Just like before he took it, [the morphine], he asked us. He said um . . . It was just you [Faith] and I there. And he said, "Do you think I'm a real asshole for doing this [taking the morphine, which would bring on respiratory failure and death]?" You wanted to say, "Yea, don't do it." But that would have been for us.

FAITH: And the kid couldn't breath, as it was [he had been on oxygen for quite some time].

MINDY: And I could see you [Faith] were just about to tell him not to do it.

FAITH: Oh God, it was on the tip of my tongue, 'No! No! No!' But I was . . .

MINDY: That was hard.

FAITH: Yea, that was hard. He didn't want us to think he was copping out, like he wasn't a survivor. He couldn't breathe. I mean he was saying good-bye to us and he couldn't even breathe (pause). It was the hardest thing. He didn't want us to think that he was giving up.

MINDY: We knew that he had to do it. And we were all there with him. And we all did get to say good-bye. How many of us will get to say good-bye to everybody before we go? [35]

Guidelines for talking to children about death

Assessment of children's understandings of death, and illness for that matter, must proceed with an awareness of the social, cultural, and emotional factors that are in operation whenever the subject of death or dying is before the child. We must look beyond age and verbal presentations for indications of the child's conception of death and his understanding of chronic, life-threatening illness. In general, we would do better not to look at the concept of the disease or death as fixed, but rather as fluid, in process, and as such, subject to change. From this perspective, several specific suggestions for talking to children about illness and death emerge.

Above all, listen to the child. Take your cues from the child. As you listen as well as when you speak, bear in mind the following: (1) the child has the ability to learn about illness whether or not we choose to tell him; (2) children have fluctuating needs and desires at different points in their illnesses; (3) children can simultaneously hold magical as well as scientific views of death; (4) and most of all, children desire to keep those they care about around them—a desire which leads them to follow the rules we set up. Children are wilful, purposeful, capable individuals aware of their own needs as well as those of others. If the child senses that an individual is uncomfortable talking about death and illness, chances are that he will not pursue the discussion.

The issue is not 'to tell or not to tell', but rather *what* to tell, *when* to tell and *who* should do the telling. Children want to know about illness and death, and will try to figure it out regardless of what we say or do not say. Bluebond-Langner [25] found that all of the ill children whom she studied became aware that they would die, regardless of whether or not they were told. Misinformation is always around, and wrong conclusions are all too easy to draw. Silence teaches that death is taboo, dangerous, and too difficult even for adults to handle. In framing your response to the child's questions, do not simply be guided by the child's age. Very young children can understand or at least have feelings about what it means to die. Bowlby [34] found that very young children can experience a deep sense of loss and mourn. As noted earlier in the chapter, children are capable of talking and thinking about illness in rather sophisticated terms.

Children share different kinds of information with different people at different times. For example, what children say to the minister about death is different from what they want to talk about with the physician, or with their parents. Children may share feelings with friends or teachers, and not with parents, lest they upset them. Discussions about illness and death may proceed rather differently when the child feels the parent wishes to pursue further treatment, but the child does not [37].

Similarly, parents may not wish to discuss various aspects of proposed treatment or death with their child, or have anyone else do it, for that matter. In such situations, it is extraordinarily important, as well as beneficial, for the physician to pursue with the parents why they do not want particular information shared with the child. Bluebond-Langner, Belasco, and Goldman found that in talking with parents about what they don't want the child to know, the physician also became aware of misunderstandings about various care and treatment options, such as prognosis or other issues in the family that may be affecting choice of care [37]. Continued discussions with parents about what they do not want discussed with their child is an opportunity not to be missed.

The physician should open the dialogue with the parents by acknowledging that he/she understands where they are coming from. In the course of conversation, the physician might note that from his/her experience the child knows the likely outcome. The physician might give some examples of the ways in which children indicate their desire to know more from their parents, as well as the cues that children give to indicate what they know, and their desire for more information. He/she might ask the parents what they are most afraid of, if the topic of dying or the efficacy of other treatment alternatives came up. The physician might suggest that perhaps further discussion with the child, either with them present, or with the physician alone, would be helpful for all of them—if not straightaway, then perhaps in the future.

The parents may continue to refuse to have discussions with the child about particular issues, or to even allow the physician to have discussions with the child that would broach, for example, the child's prognosis, side effects or efficacy of various types of treatment. However, the groundwork has been laid for further discussions, and insights have been gained that will serve the physician well in other situations as they arise with the parents and their child.

In discussing illness-related issues with children, remember that what is going on in the child's mind is not always the same as what comes out of his mouth. Children can understand or know more than verbal statements indicate. Tell the child what he wants to know and can understand, in his terms. Use terminology and approaches that the child can understand. Sometimes, it is helpful to ask the child to repeat back what you have said. One can check the child's understanding through statements like, "Now if you were the doctor, how would you explain this"?

Remember that the child's questions are not necessarily yours; his needs are not your needs. Children want to know different things at different times. It takes a long time before children with life-threatening illness or their siblings see the illness as life-shortening, let alone see themselves or their sibling as terminally ill. For this reason it is helpful to elicit as much information as possible about the child's understanding of the disease, and his perception of his condition, before responding to a child's question. For example, embedded in a question, "How does the chemotherapy work?" may be a desire to know not just how the drug attacks various cells or what the side effects will be, but also the proposed efficacy of the treatment. It is important to be concrete when talking to children. Diagrams and pictures are often helpful. For example, draw pictures of body parts in question—lungs, cells, or tumor.

A child's way of expressing loss may be quite different from adults, and from what we would expect. For example, when her brother died, one well sibling said, "Good, now I can have all his toys." Obviously, there was more there than the statement would suggest. Children can be sad one minute and out playing the next—that doesn't mean the child doesn't hurt or doesn't need someone to talk to. We must keep in mind that children are often frightened by adult displays of grief and need reassurance. As dialogue proceeds, try to elicit the child's concerns so that you know what is on his mind.

Children may ask questions that we see as obvious, or in some cases even offensive. For example, "Well, how did they know Grandpa was really dead?" and, "When will you die?" Some children have a real passion for gory, macabre details. Watch children at a wake—given the opportunity, they might touch the corpse, ask about embalming—not necessarily behavior adults would engage in.

Remember that one conversation is not enough. The desire of a child, whether well or ill, to talk about death does not necessarily go away after one discussion. There will be different questions and concerns in the face of different experiences. As various new experiences are processed, the issues that they raise need to be addressed.

Be honest—do not say to a child what you do not believe. This does not mean, however that one needs to be brutal! It is important to reassure the child that he is loved and will be cared for, not abandoned.

Finally, all children will at some point face loss and will grieve. We do not have to, nor should we even try to, fix a child's grief. It is the child's alone, he owns it and must work though it. But children need not and should not do it alone. Let us offer children our support and encouragement in a way that respects their awareness of the situation in which they find themselves.

References

1. Wass, H. (1984). Concepts of death: A developmental perspective. In H. Wass and C. Corr, eds. *Childhood and Death*. New York: Hemisphere Publishing Corp.

2. Nagy, M. The child's theories concerning death. *J of Genetic Psychology* 1948;73:3–27.

3. Lonetto, R. *Children's Conceptions of Death*. New York: Springer Publishing, 1980.

4. Koocher, G.P. Childhood, death and cognitive development. *Dev Psychol* 1973; 9(3):369–75.

5. Koocher, G.P. Conversations with children about death: Ethical considerations in research. *J Clin Child Psychol* 1974;3(2):19–21.

6. Koocher, G.P. Children's conceptions of death. In Bibace and Walsch, eds. *Children's Conceptions of Health, Illness and Bodily Functions*, San Francisco: Jossey Bass Inc, 1981.

7. Kane, B. Children's concepts of death. *J Genet Psychol* (1979);134(1):141–53. Reprinted with the permission of the Helen Dwight Reid Educational Foundation Published by Heldref Publications, 1319 Eighteenth St., NW, Washington, DC 2003 6–1802. Copyright © 1979.

8. Kastenbaum, R. The child's understanding of death: How does it develop? In E.A. Grollman, ed. *Explaining Death to Children*. Boston, MA: Beacon Press,1967.

9. Kastenbaum, R. *The Psychology of Death*, 2nd editon. New York: Springer Publishing Company, 1992.

10. Kastenbaum, R. *Death, Society, and Human Experience*. Boston, MA: Allyn and Bacon, 1998.

11. Speece, M.W. and Brent, S.B. Children's understandings of death: A review of three components of a death concept. *Child Dev* 1984; 55(5):1671–86.

12. Speece, M.W. and Brent, S.B. The 'adult' concept of irreversibility. In J.D. Morgan, ed. *Young People and Death*. Philadelphia, PA: The Charles Press, 1991.

13. Speece, M.W. and Brent, S.B. The acquisition of a mature understanding of three components of the concept of death. *Death Stud* 1992; 16(3):211–29.

14. Mahon, M., Goldberg, E., and Washington, S. Concept of death in a sample of Israel: Kibbutz children. *Death Studies* 1999;23:43–59.

15. Reilly, T.P., Hasazi, J.E., and Bond, L.A. Children's concepts of death and personal mortality. *J Paediat Psychol* 1983;8(1):21–31.

16. Atwood, V.A. Children's concepts of death: A descriptive study. *Child Stud J* 1984;14(1):11–29.

17. Candy-Gibbs, S.E., Sharp, K.C., and Petrun, C.J. The effects of age, object and cultural/religious background on children's concepts of death. *Omega* 1984–85;15(4):329–46.

18. Kenyon, B. Current research in children's conceptions of death: A critical review. *Omega* 2001; 43(1):63–91.

19. Klatt, H.J. In search of a mature concept of death. *Death St J* 1991;15(2):177–87.

20. Candy-Gibbs, S.E., Sharp K.C., and Petrun, C.J. The effects of age, object and cultural/religious background on children's concepts of death. *Omega* 1984–5;15(4):329–46.

21. Atwood, V.A. Children's concepts of death: A descriptive study. *Child Stud J* 1984;14(1):11–29.

22. Kastenbaum, R. and Aisenberg, R.B. *The Psychology of Death.* New York, NY: Springer Publishing Co., 1972.

23. Kubler-Ross, E. *On Death and Dying.* New York: Scribner, 1969.

24. Koocher, G.P. Children's Conceptions of Death. In Bibace and Walsch, eds. *Children's Conceptions of Health, Illness and Bodily Functions,* San Francisco: Jossey Bass, 1981.

25. Bluebond-Langner, M. *The Private Worlds of Dying Children.* Princeton, NJ: Princeton University Press, 1978.

26. Gartley, H. and Bernasconi, M. The concept of death in children. *J Genet Psychol* 1967;110:71–85.

27. Anthony, Z. and Bhana, K. An exploratory study of Muslim girls' understanding of death. *Omega: J Death Dying* 1988–9;19(3):215–27.

28. Bluebond-Langner, M. Meanings of death to children. In H. Feifel, ed. *New Meanings of Death.* New York: McGraw Hill, pp. 47–66, 1976.

29. Zweig, A. and Burns, W. Self-concepts of chronically ill children. *J Gene Psychol* 1980;137:179–90.

30. Brent, S.B., Lin, C., Speece, M.W., Dong, Q., and Yang, C. The development of the concept of death among Chinese and US children 3–17 years of age: From binary to 'fuzzy' concepts? *Omega* 1996; 33(1):67–83.

31. Schonfeld, D.J. and Smilansky, S. A cross-cultural comparison of Israeli and American children's death concepts. *Death Stud* 1989; 13(6):593–604.

32. Irizarry-Hobson, C. *Childhood Bereavement Reactions to the Death of a Grandparent.* Graduate Program in Social Work, Rutgers University Thesis,1988.

33. Orbach, I., Gross, Y., Glaubman, H., and Berman, D. Children's perceptions of various determinants of the death concept as a function of intelligence, age and anxiety. *J Clin Child Psychol* 1986;15(2): 120–6.

34. Bowlby, J. *Attachment and Loss* (Vol. III). New York: Basic Books, 1980.

35. Bluebond-Langner, M. *In the Shadow of Illness: Parents and Siblings of the Chronically Ill Child.* Princeton, NJ: Princeton University Press, 1996.

36. Glaser, B. and Strauss, A. Awareness contexts and social interaction. *Am Soc Rev* 1964;29:669–79.

37. Bluebond-Langner, M., Belasco, J., and Goldman, A. *Talking to children about death.* Presentation at the Yale University Institution for Social Policy Studies, 2003.

8 Psychological impact of life-limiting conditions on the child*

Barbara M. Sourkes

I felt much better because I knew that I had somebody to talk to all the time. Every boy needs a psychologist! To see his feelings!

(six-year-old child) [1, p. 3]

You take what kids feel like off their chests.

(ten-year-old child)

As pediatric palliative care develops into a field of its own, there is a window of opportunity to define the parameters of optimal psychological care for these children. [2,3,4] While the need for "support" is often articulated, the word is overused and under defined. Dictionary definitions of 'support' connote 'holding up' or 'serving as a foundation for' and 'keeping from losing courage'. Yet, these definitions simply indicate that 'support' is the general underpinning—the *given*—of palliative care—as it should be in any clinical care. Support is garnered from the family and from the professional team as a whole. It is not specifically meaningful in terms of psychological intervention for the child, and thus is distinct from the psychological *treatment* that is the domain of pediatric mental-health professionals.

Ideally, the psychological status of each child admitted to palliative care should be evaluated in order to plan for optimal care, in the same way as medical and nursing assessments are carried out. Child psychology and psychiatry as well as other mental-health disciplines, contribute specialized knowledge and skills. The specific and unique interventions include: evaluation of the child's psychological status, diagnosis of psychological/psychiatric symptoms and disturbance, role of psychotherapy and psychotropic medication, consultation to families and the team. The healthy siblings are included within this network of care. Thus, under optimal circumstances, psychological intervention can play a pivotal role in the integration of the child's comprehensive palliative care.

However, the availability of psychological consultation in pediatric palliative care is often limited. While it is true that psychological treatment is not universally necessary, the ability to identify 'high-risk' children and intervene in a timely fashion is often missed. The challenge, under these circumstances, is to provide thoughtful emotional support for the child in a carefully planned manner. One must take into account the child's need and expressed wish for such support beyond the family, as well as the level of comfort that the child has formed in relationships with members of the team (or one particular individual). Emotional support comes in many forms, from an openness to listen and answer questions, to regular visits at expected times, and to creative art and play activities that allow the child, expression of feelings and concerns.

On a cautionary note, there are risks when untrained or inadequately skilled personnel undertake a more profound psychotherapeutic role. These include: opening up too much vulnerability in the child and then not knowing how to contain the emotion; interpreting—beyond simply clarifying—the child's disclosures; promising confidentiality that may set up competition, rather than collaboration, with the parents; and becoming over-involved with the child beyond appropriate boundaries. As a pediatric oncologist stated: "Psychological intervention is no less a professionally skilled phenomenon than giving chemotherapy."

A four-year-old boy coveted the child life specialist's Mickey Mouse watch. He tried it on, inspected it from every angle on his wrist, and

---

* Sections of this chapter have been adapted with permission from the University of Pittsburgh Press from: Sourkes B: *The Deepening Shade: Psychological Aspects of Life-Threatening Illness* and *Armfuls of Time: The Psychological Experience of the Child with a Life-Threatening Illness*.

said: "I like time. I wish I could wear a whole armful of watches." Later that day, in describing the watch to the therapist, he sighed: "I just wish that I had armfuls of time." [5, p. 116]

The metaphorical image of wishing for 'armfuls of time' exemplifies the extraordinary challenges faced by the seriously ill or dying child. These children *live* with many levels of awareness, and their pain and suffering, both physical and psychic, can be great. The following examples attest to these struggles:

The physical:
THERAPIST: If you could choose one word to describe the time since your diagnosis, what would it be?
CHILD: PAIN. [6, p. 275]

And the psychic:
THERAPIST: Are you in any pain? Does anything hurt?
CHILD: My heart. My heart is broken . . . I miss everybody. [6, p. 271]

The child-in-the-family is a unit unto itself, with its own distinctive identity, strengths and vulnerabilities. The child's ongoing struggle to withstand and integrate the trauma of illness unfolds within this framework. His or her ability to cope is greatly influenced by the family—the individual and collective responses of its members. Under optimal circumstances, 'the interior of the family assumes a central role in preserving the patient's psychological integrity.' [7, p. 4] The family affords a refuge in which the child can replenish psychic resources, shielded from the battering assault of the illness. The myth that a child's life-limiting illness, either unites or destroys a family reduces complexity to oversimplification.

I have a closer relationship with my family than most other kids because I've needed them more these last years. (11-year-old child) [5, p. 87]

Most of the children described or quoted in this chapter are (or were) living with cancer, a prototype of a life-*threatening* illness, and wherein cure is a possible outcome. Nonetheless, these children and families live in great uncertainty, experiencing anxiety, and anticipatory grief reactions to the *potential* loss of the child, if not ultimately to the actuality. The clinical issues are, with some variation, relevant for children living with many other chronic life-threatening and life-limiting illnesses as well. The common denominator among what may look like quite disparate disorders (from those characterized by intermittent hospitalizations and disruptions, to those of a more deteriorative course), is their relentless and insistent presence. The threat of separation and death, varies in intensity depending on both the overall time course and the particular phase of the illness.

The children who speak in this chapter articulate concerns that are universal to all those living under the extraordinary stress of illness. This is crucial to bear in mind, especially when working with children who are not, or are no longer verbal, or who are severely developmentally delayed. Regardless of whether the identical form of psychotherapy described here is applicable, the process illustrates how all children, whatever their own developmental level, have to negotiate both the progressive losses of illness and the anticipation of the ultimate loss of life.

Psychological/psychiatric symptoms

Knowledge of normal psychological development is essential in evaluating the impact of illness on the child. Cognitive, affective and social perspectives intersect at every juncture. The child's passage through both Piaget's and Erikson's developmental stages, is challenged to the utmost by the presence of life-limiting illness.

Although many psychological problems of the child with a life-limiting illness may be categorized as adjustment reactions, more severe psychopathology can emerge. This is especially true in the child with pre-existent vulnerabilities, or when there is a prior psychiatric history in the child or a family member. While it is important not to overemphasize pathology in the child, there is also a risk in minimizing or not recognizing it. Furthermore, any psychological response, however benign initially, can freeze into a traumatic reaction under sustained stress. Thus, mental health professional must be able to assess the severity of symptoms, particularly in terms of intensity and duration, relative to the child's current reality.

In addition to knowledge of normal development and psychopathology, the clinician must be well informed of the child's medical status and implications thereof (both symptomatic and prognostic). This latter requirement provides grounding in the child's life situation, and is crucial for accurate and effective diagnosis and intervention.

Psychological symptoms in seriously ill children are often multiply-determined and in flux. Physical pain, metabolic imbalance, neurological dysfunction, infection and the impact of medications are closely linked, if not at times inseparable from psychological distress. Most common are diagnoses in the broad categories of anxiety and depression. Anxiety represents a widely diverse group of developmentally appropriate and pathological coping responses, ranging from pre-existent anxieties exacerbated under the stress of illness, to cumulative generalized anxiety, and even to post-traumatic stress disorder. Yet, sleep deprivation and delirium may present as anxiety and agitation. The psychological and somatic symptoms of depression can be hard to differentiate from the

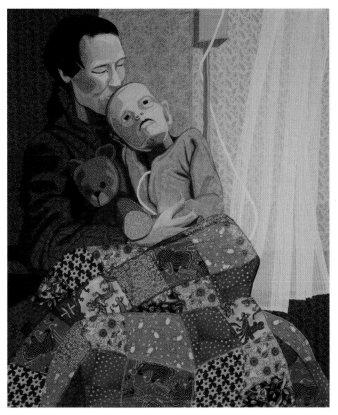

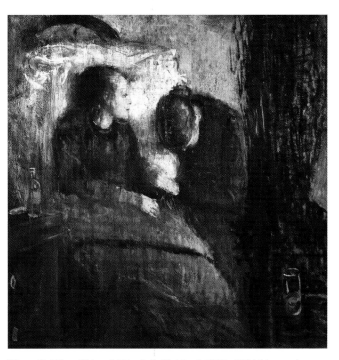

Plate 1 ©Deidre Scherer, Child, 2001. Fabric and thread. All rights reserved.

Plate 2 Edvard Munch, The Sick Child, oil, 1885–1886, National Gallery, Oslo.

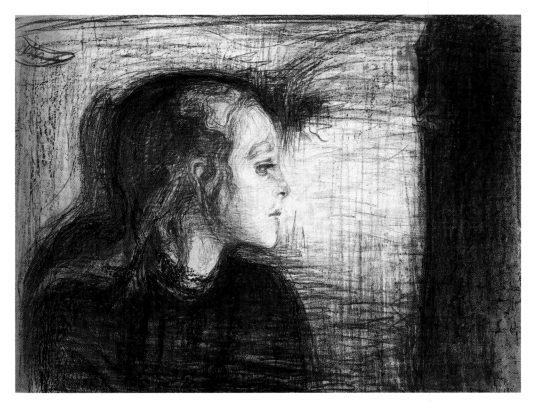

Plate 3 Edvard Munch, The Sick Child, lithograph, Sch 59, Munch Museum, Oslo, 1896, p. 25.

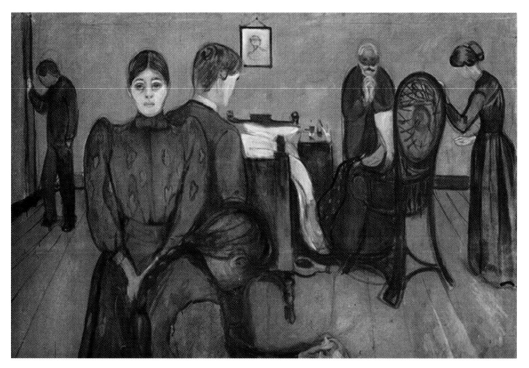

Plate 4 Edvard Munch, Death in the Sickroom, 1895, oil, National Gallery, Oslo.

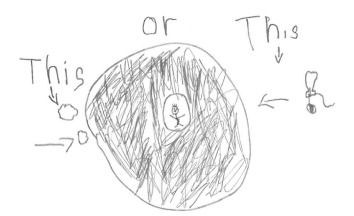

Plate 5 This or This.

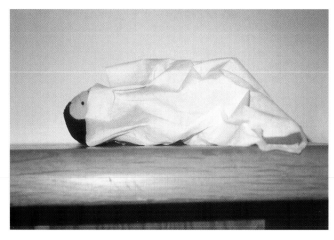

Plate 6 Curious George under a shroud.

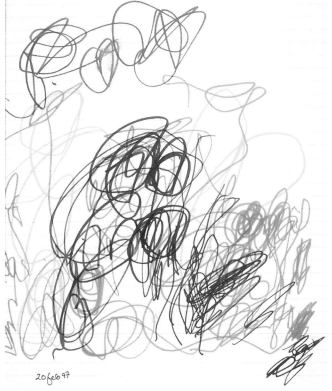

Plate 7 Matthew—Untitled, February 20.

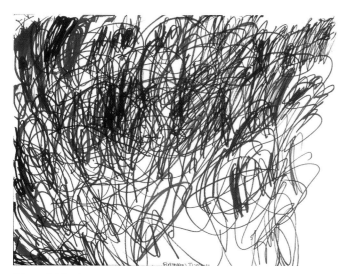

Plate 8 Matthew—Batman Tunnel, March 11.

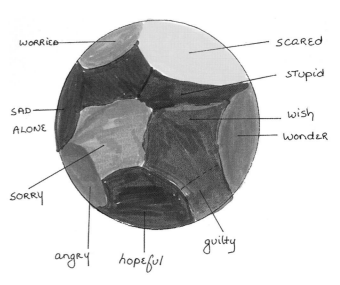

MY MIND

"Sometimes I wonder how it's going to be in the past without my little brother"

Plate 10 Erin—My Mind, March 18.

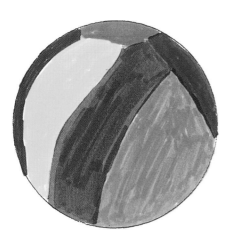

- SAD
- hopeful
- scared
- worried
- strong
- Don't know . . .

THE COLORS OF LIFE

Plate 9 Abby—The Colors of Life, March 18.

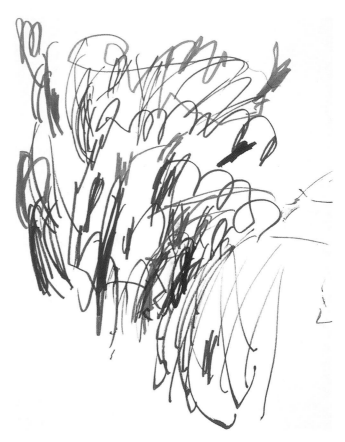

Plate 11 Matthew—Bad Monster, March 25.

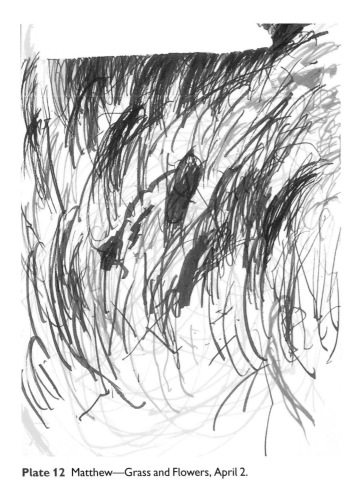

Plate 12 Matthew—Grass and Flowers, April 2.

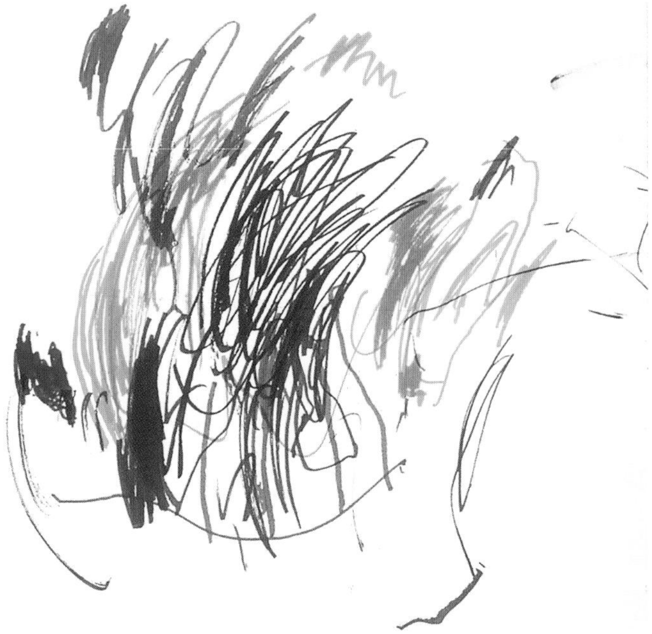

Plate 14 Matthew—I don't know that, June 5.

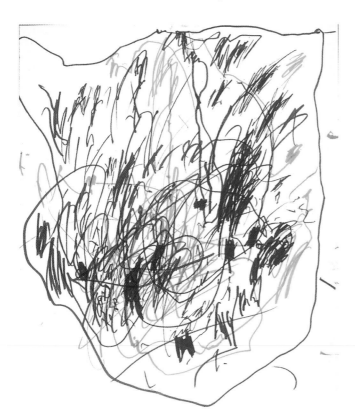

Plate 13 Matthew—Slide, Horses and Boats, May 15.

Plate 15 Matthew—Outside—Yellow Sun and Trees, June 11.

effects of the illness and treatment. Furthermore, there is often confusion between sadness/anticipatory grief and clinical depression: What is a 'normal' response to impending loss versus the 'symptom' of depression that should be treated with psychotropic medication? Psychotic and organic brain syndromes often present with cognitive and perceptual disturbances. Delirium may also present as anxiety or oppositional or aggressive behavior; parents frequently report sensing something is 'different' about their child, but are unable to describe specifically the change.

It is for reasons such as these that definitive psychiatric diagnosis can at times be elusive. As a result of these diagnostic ambiguities, one often proceeds with psychological or psychotropic intervention on the basis of managing specific symptoms rather than treatment of a presumed underlying psychiatric disorder.

Psychotherapy—a conceptual framework

A physician asked a ten-year-old child how she was feeling. She answered: "Medically I'm fine, but psychologically I'm not so fine, but I'll discuss that with my psychologist." [5, p. 11]

THERAPIST: Do you remember what we talked about last time?
CHILD: (without hesitation) About dying... (A few minutes later) If I don't feel like talking about dying today, there will be other days. [5, p. 121]

Psychotherapy for the child with a life-limiting illness can provide the opportunity for the expression of profound grief, and for the integration of all that he or she has lived, albeit in an abbreviated lifespan. Furthermore, even for a young child, considerations about the remaining quality of life may be discussed. Within its framework—through words, drawings and play—the child conveys the experience of living with the ever present threat of loss, and transforms the essence of his or her reality into expression.

In working with a child facing death, the therapist must be able to enter the threat with the child, accompanying him or her down the road toward ultimate separation. The shared 'knowledge' of the fine line that separates living from dying, whether implicit or explicit, becomes the containment of the psychotherapy. The child can derive profound comfort from the safety and "ongoing ness" afforded within its framework. (For a detailed discussion of the psychotherapeutic framework and techniques, see Sourkes.[1,5,6])

The therapist had seen a hospitalized girl for a session just prior to her receiving heavy sedation. When the therapist returned the next day, the girl said: "I've been asleep for a full day. I feel as if you were just here a few minutes ago, although I know it was really yesterday. It's as if you never left!." [8, p. 66]

Most children enter psychotherapy because of the stress engendered by the illness, rather than more general intrapsychic or interpersonal concerns. From a psychological point of view, the majority of the children are well adjusted. Psychopathology is the exception, not the rule. In *The Spiritual Life of Children* [9], child psychiatrist Coles remembers advice offered by Lindemann, a psychoanalyst, during the polio epidemic of the 1950s. Parallels to the child with other illnesses are evident.

These are young people who suddenly have become quite a bit older; they are facing possible death, or serious limitation of their lives; and they will naturally stop and think about life, rather than just live it from day to day. A lot of what they say will be reflective—and you might respond in kind. It would be a mistake, I think, to emphasize unduly a psychiatric point of view. If there is serious psychopathology, you will respond to it, of course; but if those children want to cry with you, and be disappointed with you, and wonder with you where their God is, then you can be there for them. [9, p. 101]

Lindemann thus reminds the therapist to 'bear witness' to the child's extraordinary situation, and to respond within the context of that reality.

The concept of psychic trauma lends itself to understanding the experience of life-limiting illnesses in childhood. Terr, a child psychiatrist, offers the following definition in her book, *Too Scared to Cry* [10]:

Psychic trauma occurs when a sudden, unexpected, overwhelmingly intense emotional blow or a series of blows assaults the person from outside. Traumatic events are external, but they quickly become incorporated into the mind. A person probably will not become fully traumatized unless he or she feels utterly helpless during the event or events.[10, p. 8]

This description certainly relates to the overwhelming sense of loss of control experienced by the seriously ill child: the shock of diagnosis, the indelible imprint of the sustained assault on the body and psyche, and the uncertainty of the outcome. Whereas malevolence of intent characterizes many forms of trauma (e.g. abuse, kidnapping), the culprit in life-limiting illnesses is the inexplicable, impersonal randomness of fate.

Winnicott, the first British pediatrician to become a psychoanalyst, wrote extensively about the developmental processes of childhood, and their implications for psychotherapy. He defined trauma as 'an impingement from the environment and from the individual's reaction to the environment that occurs prior to the individual's development of mechanisms that make the unpredictable, predictable.' [11, p. 44]

While life-limiting illness does not literally originate in the environment, its devastating impact on the child more than qualifies it as trauma. In fact, the illness goes beyond what Winnicott referred to as "unthinkable anxieties" in its *actual* threat of death. Winnicott further stressed the importance for the young child of the "presentation of the world in small doses . . . the preservation of a certain amount of illusion—an avoidance of too sudden an insistence on the reality principle."[11, p. 108] The child with a critical illness can stand unshielded from pain, terror and the ultimate threat of loss of life. In this sense, it is no exaggeration to state that he or she loses a critical aspect of childhood in the moment of diagnosis, or through the trajectory of the illness. This "paradox" of precocious awareness is reflected in a five-year-old child's pensive query: "It takes a lot of days to be grown up, doesn't it? . . ." [11, p. 28]

In child psychotherapy, play is the crucial vehicle of communication. Winnicott stressed that enjoyment of play is an a priori condition of entering into the depth of the psychotherapeutic process. For the child whose very existence is suffused with gravity, such pleasure is intrinsically valuable. The overwhelming nature of the illness cannot be approached by reality alone. Paradoxically, the illusion afforded by play is what allows reality to be integrated. Through play, the child can advance and retreat, draw near and pull away from the intense core. These tentative forays allow the child to contain and master the experience. Illusion is not to be construed as avoidance; on the contrary, play is the essence of a child's expression. Furthermore, illusion is translucent, if not transparent, and thus reality shines through for both the child and the therapist even when not addressed directly by either. Inextricably linked with play is the child's use of symbolic language and graphic images that provide windows into his or her experience.

During the previous night, a six-year-old boy's temperature and blood pressure had dropped precipitously. Although he was revived quickly, he had been blue, hard to rouse, and very cold. In a session the next day, the child reported that: "Poly Polar Bear [one of his stuffed animals] is very sad now because he didn't swim. The water was ice." Through this image, the child reiterated his own traumatic experience of being 'cold.' [5, p. 113]

The child's voice in decision-making

One side of my head says: "Think optimistic." The other side says: "What if this treatment doesn't work?" (eleven-year-old-child) [5, p. 156]

The child is often aware of the diminishing curative or life-prolonging options that he or she faces. It is at this time that the child may ask anxiously: "What if this medicine doesn't work? What will you give me next?" The child experiences a profound sense of loss of control. It is at this time that families are confronted by a series of decisions regarding the nature and intensity of medical interventions that they wish to pursue. This process can be excruciating: they do not want their child to suffer more, yet they cannot often tolerate the thought of 'leaving any stone unturned' in the quest for a cure or prolonged time, however miniscule the chance. The physician's and team's roles shift from leadership in recommending a curative treatment plan to the clarification of experimental and palliative options and consequences. In most instances, the parents make the decision; however, to varying degrees, the child may be involved in such discussions.

During the last decade, there has been increased recognition of the child's participation in making treatment decisions.[12] Crucial to this process is an assessment of the child's ability to appreciate the nature and consequences of a specific medical decision. This becomes particularly complex when the wishes of the child differ from those of the parents. Since actual assessment tools are only in the early stages of development, professionals must rely exclusively on their clinical judgment to assess children's understanding of the contingencies they are facing. This is often a juncture when input from members of the interdisciplinary team can be crucial: children often express their understanding, awareness and thoughts about treatment options and living/dying to individuals other than their parents or primary physician. Very frequently, their most candid disclosures evolve within the context of psychotherapy.

Case A 10-year-old child who had just relapsed drew a picture entitled 'This or This'. (Figure 8.1) On one side of a doughnut she depicted tumor cells, on the other side she drew a needle for spinal taps. In the middle of the doughnut is a little stick figure of a person. At the time of drawing the picture the child said: "I hate needles and spinal taps, but I also don't want my tumor to come back. If I don't have all the needles, then more tumor cells will grow. So, if I don't want them to grow, I have to have all those awful needles. That's why I feel as if I am stuck in the middle of a doughnut."

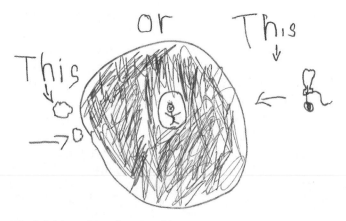

Fig. 8.1 This or This. (See plate 5.)

Reflecting back on the drawing months later, the child elaborated more explicitly:"What I mean by 'I was stuck in a doughnut' is that I had two choices and I didn't want to take either of them. One of the choices was to get needles and pokes and all that stuff and make the tumor go away. My other choice was letting my tumor get bigger and bigger and I would just go away up to heaven....My mom wanted me to get needles and pokes. But I felt like I just had had too much—too much for my body—too much for me....So I kind of wanted to go up to heaven that time....But then I thought about how much my whole entire family would miss me and so just then I was kind of like stuck in a doughnut...."

An 11-year-old child who had been offered radiation therapy for palliative symptom control confided to her therapist:"I'm scared because I'm not so good at making decisions. My parents want me to have radiation, but a little voice in me tells me not to.... My mother always said that if I die, she wants me to die happy and at home. If I had radiation, I'd have to come into the hospital every day. And I don't know if radiation will really help, or if I would die anyway"

This child had been through many remission-relapse cycles, and had been informed and involved in all aspects of her illness and the treatment from the beginning. Nonetheless, her statements highlight the 'burden' of decision-making that children may feel at critical junctures of their illness, particularly at end-stage. Furthermore, despite what had been her clear understanding of the reason for radiation therapy (exclusively for palliative symptom management), her intense emotion and hope have overridden the intellectual as she wonders whether the radiation will help her to live longer ('or would I die anyway?').

Awareness of impending death

In my heart, something is telling me...my heart is pulling me away from earth. It's hard for me. Everyone has a second life. The soul has a second life and it cannot be broken. My first life is starting to break into pieces. (10-year-old child)

During the terminal phase of the illness, the child's awareness of dying becomes more focused. No longer an abstract threat in the distance, death takes on an identity of its own. Rather than being a possible outcome, death is *the* outcome, its time of occurrence the only unknown. Catastrophic images often emerge in the child's language and stories during the terminal phase. Fear, desperation and the sense of disaster are all evident, even if in derivative form. However, references to its proximity can be quite direct and explicit. If an open climate has been established from the beginning of the illness, it will be reflected in how the child talks about death.

An 11-year-old girl commented matter-of-factly: "Some of my friends have died. I wish I could talk to those kids' parents to see what their symptoms were, so that I would know what is happening to me." [5, p. 157]

The awareness may also be expressed symbolically, although no less powerfully, through play.

A 3-year-old boy played the same game with a stuffed duck and a toy ambulance each time he was hospitalized. The duck would be sick, and need to go to the hospital by ambulance. The boy would move the ambulance, making siren noises.

THERAPIST: How is the duck?
CHILD: Sick.
THERAPIST: Where is he going?
CHILD: To the hospital.
THERAPIST: What are they going to do?
CHILD: Make him better.
THERAPIST: Is he going to get better?
CHILD: Yes, better.

During what turned out to be the boy's terminal admission, he played the same game with the duck. However, the ritual changed dramatically in its outcome:

THERAPIST: How is the duck?
CHILD: Sick.
THERAPIST: Is he going to get better?
CHILD: (shook head slowly) Ducky not get better. Ducky die.[5, p. 157]

A 4-year-old child had always done a lot of medical play with a stuffed Curious George monkey, giving him shots and bandages. In a session close to her death, she methodically covered him with tissues and taped the tissues in place. By the end of her play, he appeared to be buried under a shroud. She was very quiet during her activity and made no comment about her play (Figure 8.2).

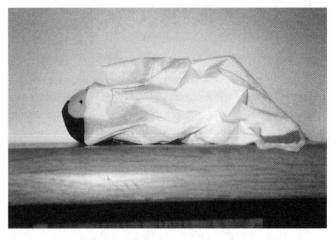

Fig. 8.2 Curious George under a shroud. (See plate 6.)

Anticipatory grief

THERAPIST: What does it mean to be alive?
CHILD: That your family doesn't miss you. They miss
            you if you die. When you're alive, you don't miss
            people because they are right here.[1, p. 37]

Loss of relationships—expressed through fears of separation, absence and death—is paramount in anticipatory grief: "grief expressed in advance when the loss is perceived as inevitable"[13, p. 4]. Anticipatory grief may show itself as the child's increased sensitivity to separation, without any specific reference to death; comments or questions related to death that may be seen as a type of preparation or rehearsal; and the undiluted and unmistakable grief of the end phase of the illness.

In one manifestation of anticipatory grief, the child projects concern about himself or herself onto a significant adult, usually a parent or the therapist. On one level, the child recognizes his or her extreme dependence on the adult, and panics at the thought of something happening to that person. This reaction may be particularly pronounced in the child of a single parent. On another level, the child is expressing fear about his or her own situation through this mirror image. At least initially, the projection is best left untouched, as the child is clearly communicating extreme vulnerability.

After a discussion about his bad dreams, the therapist asked a six-year-old child what else he felt scared about.

CHILD: I am scared of what if my mother dies. Then
            there will be no one to take care of me.
THERAPIST: I know that your mother takes good care of
            herself and is healthy so that she can take good
            care of you.
CHILD: Yes. She is trying very hard to stay alive. She
            eats all the time and she kisses me a lot.
THERAPIST: What else are you scared about?
CHILD: I am scared that when I come back to the hospital, you will not be here.[5, p.142]

The child's grief related to the possibility of his or her own dying may be cloaked in symbolic terms, or in questions about others. As in all other communications, the therapist must stay close to the immediate concern, leaving the child in control of how far to pursue the topic. Often, he or she will make an isolated statement, or pose one question, and then, without further comment, turn to other subjects. The most powerful disclosures are those in which the child makes reference to the possibility of his or her own dying. Whether through the weight of the sadness, or through the actual words or images, the dying child's anticipatory grief is palpable, as he or she lives the intensity of separation in its ultimate form.

As the child confronts impending death, he or she may show signs of preparation. The child's actions or words are often quite matter-of-fact; their significance is not necessarily elaborated.

A seven-year-old girl had a recurrent dream: "In the dream, I want to be with my mother, and I can never quite get to her." The girl recounted the dream in a joint therapy session with her mother. Whereas the mother found the dream "excruciating," her daughter stipulated that "even though the dream is very sad, it's not a nightmare." The dream eventually provided the focal image for mother and child to work through the anticipatory grief process.[1, p. 70]

The distillation of anticipatory grief to its essence marks the imminence of death. At times imperceptibly, at other times dramatically, the child who has been living with the illness is transformed into a dying child. The endpoint of the terminal phase is often marked by a turning inward on the part of the child, a pulling back from the external world. Cognitive and emotional horizons narrow, as all energy is needed simply for physical survival. A generalized irritability is not uncommon. The child may talk very little, and may even retreat from physical contact. Although such withdrawal is not universal, a certain degree of quietness is almost always evident. The child is pulling into himself or herself, not away from others. This behavior is a normal and expectable precursor to death—a form of preparation for the ultimate separation that lies ahead.

Three days before her death, and in what turned out to be her last session, a ten-year-old child said to her therapist: "I am tired and I am very happy. I wanted to tell you more about being happy, but I am too tired to talk anymore." This peaceful disclosure provided the opening for a profound talk with her parents. They reassured her that they understood how tired she was after fighting so hard, that it was all right for her to let go now, and that they would be with her all the way. She listened calmly, smiling, nodding to their words.

Work with parents

From the moment of diagnosis of a life-limiting illness, the relationship between the child and the parents organizes around a pivot of threatened or impending loss. Thus, it is critical that the therapist not intercede as a divisive wedge between them. From the outset, an ongoing alliance between the child's therapist and the parents diminishes this threat, and optimizes the outcome of the work. The nature of the alliance will of course differ depending upon the age of the child. Terr [10] in her work with traumatized children, comes to similar conclusions: "It is almost impossible for a . . .[therapist] to treat a child without providing some access to parents . . . who participate in the child's life" (p. 307). Without the respect of an established alliance, the therapeutic work with the child will be compromised, and during the end-stage of the illness, probably rendered impossible.

The therapist must always be vigilant of the danger of over-involvement with the child. In such circumstances, the parents can begin to feel estranged and supplanted, just at the time when they are desperately trying to "keep" their child. Parents' pervasive guilt about their dying child (whether conscious or unconscious) will only be exacerbated if they feel that the therapist is "better" than they are at achieving closeness with the child, or at eliciting secrets that cannot be shared.

The child may become frightened by an inordinate amount of closeness to the therapist, while simultaneously needing the relationship. During this critical time, a sense of threat arises from the child's guilt at being close to an adult other than the parents. He or she may feel trapped: 'having to choose' between parents and therapist, with the simultaneous fear of alienating either. However, if the child senses a strong alliance between the therapist and parents, he or she can feel secure in the therapeutic relationship.

Case The following case study illustrates many of the themes discussed in the first part of this chapter. Furthermore, it demonstrates how, the confluence of medical and psychological expertise can result in optimally integrated end-of-life care. The clinical material presented here focuses primarily on Matthew, the child who was ill, with reflections by his sisters, Abby and Erin. The psychotherapeutic intervention occurred over a four-month period, from February until Matthew's death in June. Inserted into the clinical material with Matthew are comments to highlight the themes generally applicable to children with a life-limiting illness.

Matthew was a four-year-old child who had been diagnosed with a brain tumor, an ependymoma, at the age of two. Over the course of his illness, he had undergone three surgeries, one course of chemotherapy and one of radiation therapy. He had had one good remission of nine-months duration. In February, just after his fourth birthday, it was decided that there were no further curative treatment options. The parents elected to provide palliative care for Matthew at home, and in fact promised him that he would not return to the hospital again. Thus, he remained at home from February until his death in June.

In the palliative care plan for Matthew, pain management was a foremost concern, particularly relief from headaches. Matthew received increasing doses of morphine, as well as sedation for sleep at night. The parents were taught basic physical therapy techniques and suctioning to relieve the discomfort of excess secretions. Although Matthew initially received tube feeding (he complained about hunger although he would not swallow food), over the course of the months, he began to eat again. However, the tube remained in place as a route for medications, as did his port access. Although Matthew spent most of each day in his parents' bed, surrounded by toys, books and videos, a specially adapted chair and stroller allowed him to sit at the family dinner

table and at the computer, to take baths safely, and to be taken for walks outside. The palliative care physician visited approximately every two weeks, the nurse weekly, and the psychologist (myself) weekly. In addition to these weekly sessions with Matthew, every two to three weeks I met with his two sisters, Abby and Erin, ages ten and eight. They were included and well informed by the parents at every juncture, and remained actively involved with Matthew until his death. My meetings with the parents focused on their concerns about all three children. All the members of the team were available for frequent telephone consultation with the parents.

I saw Matthew weekly for 15 sessions, until the day before his death. Each session lasted 30 to 40 minutes; it had to end exactly at 10:30 AM when his favorite television program began. Matthew's mother came into the sessions occasionally on Matthew's or my request: either for clarification of his speech (his articulation was sometimes slurred), or to discuss an issue that had emerged in the session. All our meetings took place on his parents' bed. Matthew would be comfortably propped up by pillows, surrounded by his toys, and would be ready to draw using a clipboard for support. Although Matthew's pictures may look as if they were hastily drawn, in fact, each was done slowly and methodically, with great (silent) deliberation about his choice of colors.

Psychological intervention with Matthew had important impact on his overall functioning and care. At the time he was referred to palliative care, he was described by the parents as being 'stoic—he can tolerate pain—he never reports distress—we are in awe of his courage.' Matthew's response to most questions by the parents or the care giving team was "I'm OK" or "I'm fine" even when it was obvious that he was not. In fact, his non- or underreporting of symptoms made it difficult for the mother to administer medication effectively. Through a combination of drawing, talking and play, he became increasingly able to express feelings—both positive and negative—and to be an accurate reporter of his physical and emotional state.

- It is not infrequent that parents describe their child as being stoic, or non-complaining. While to a certain extent, this can be a point of pride, it can also be a 'risk signal.' The child may not be reporting symptoms:
  - for fear that he or she will be taken back to the hospital despite assurances to the contrary (as was probably the case with Matthew).
  - with the 'magical thinking' that if he or she doesn't report symptoms, then they are not really there and things are not really getting worse.
  - to protect parents from his or her pain/worsening condition.

An early drawing (Figure 8.3) is light and airy. Matthew told me: "I'm not sick anymore" and adamantly denied any discomfort. This statement was entirely consistent with the 'stoicism' reported by his parents. In that session, I introduced him to a rabbit puppet, which he promptly named Donald Bunny. I used the puppet to model the reporting of symptoms (e.g., Donald Bunny has a headache, his eyes hurt when it is too bright, etc.). Matthew

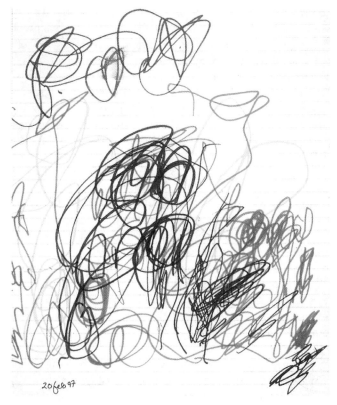

Fig. 8.3 Matthew—Untitled, February 20. (See plate 7.)

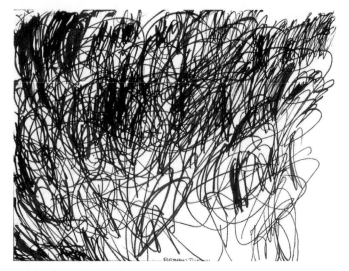

Fig. 8.4 Matthew—Batman Tunnel, March 11. (See plate 8.)

watched and listened with some interest. I left the puppet with him for the week, and at the next session, his mother said that Matthew had begun reporting symptoms attributed 'through the voice' of Donald Bunny. Although Matthew still would not acknowledge that he himself had any of the problems, Donald Bunny's reporting was serving an important purpose.

Matthew's next drawing (Figure 8.4) is dark and threatening. Matthew described it as: "A batman tunnel. It's completely dark, but I wasn't scared." In this drawing is evident, the beginning of a shift away from the rigid denial expressed in "I'm not sick any-more." Matthew allowed for a frightening image ('completely dark batman tunnel') although he then, 'undid' the fear by asserting that *he* was not scared.

- A stuffed animal or puppet may be introduced into the psychotherapeutic process simply as one of the therapist's toys, or with a more focused agenda. In the latter instance, the therapist draws attention to the animal, and discloses that it is being treated for the same illness, or shares some of the same symptoms as the child. Most children are intrigued by this connection (even if skeptical), and question the therapist about the animal's experiences. Through this commonality, an alliance between the child and animal is formed. For a child who is receptive to this form of play, the identification with the animal, and the projective process do not take long to establish. By naming the animal, the child gives it a distinct identity, and simultaneously asserts a definite proprietary sense.

- The progression in Matthew's comments from the first to the second drawings illustrates how, children gradually let down their defenses at their own pace and time. While clinical judgment prevails in each situation, it is often best to allow the unfolding to occur without much direct questioning or commentary.

By the next session, we began a ritual of reviewing what had been good and what had been bad during the week. Although Matthew would not initially mention any of the 'bad', he allowed his mother to list some of his symptoms (headache, pain behind eyes) and he nodded affirmatively to them. He did add—for the first time—"I don't like it when I cough." Matthew's acknowledgment, and even spontaneous reporting of his symptoms, reflected a completely new phase in his candor, and thus in his care.

* * *

At this juncture, Matthew's sisters, Abby (10) and Erin (8) did the following mandalas (Figures 8.5 and 8.6) during individual sessions with me. A mandala is a graphic symbolic pattern or design in the form of a circle. As a projective art therapy technique, an individual is asked to fill in a blank circle to reflect 'how you are feeling now.' In a more structured version developed by the author[5], the therapist defines a topic around which the mandala will be focused, and then presents a set of feelings that are commonly attributed to the experience. The child is asked to think about which feelings 'fit' him or her, and to choose a color to match each feeling. The child then fills in part of the circle to represent each emotion, and the area accorded to each feeling proportionate to its importance. Upon completion, the child gives the mandala a title and explains his or her choices of feelings and colors.

Abby and Erin did their mandalas around the topic: 'How it feels to have a little brother who is sick.' The feelings presented to the girls included *strong, worried, scared, hopeful, sad, guilty* and *helpless*, as well as a category called *other feelings you may have*. Following are their verbatim descriptions, as well as interpretive comments.

Abby (age 10) 'The Colors of Life' (Figure 8.5)

Matthew had some good and bad days this week. I don't sleep well—I need to calm down…I don't feel *guilty* and I don't feel *helpless*—I feel *strong*. I don't feel helpless or weak or *scared* of baby things—I can stand up for myself. *Hopeful* (yellow is pretty)—maybe he'd stop that weird cough—it scared me. I'm not very very *worried* or scared. When I didn't know what was happening I was very *upset*. Now I'm getting used to it. I do feel *sad* and upset sometimes. [Do you worry that he might die?] Yes—I'm trying to get used to it. He acts and feels better. My parents said that there is no cure, that he will not get better, that he's going to die. For a month I was upset and crying. But now I'm *hopeful*—his coughing ended—it did.

Abby's mandala is bold and forthright. *Strong* is the 'largest' feeling, followed by *scared* and *hopeful*. Although *scared* almost bisects/severs the circle, it is flanked by the two positive feelings. *Sad, worried*, and *don't know* are dramatically smaller. Her title, *The Colors of Life*, captures the totality of her experience of the moment.

- Sibling issues highlighted in Abby's statement:
  - siblings' own stress is often expressed in somatic symptoms (e.g. insomnia)
  - pride in their own strength and maturity
  - upset at not knowing/understanding/being included in what is happening
  - 'getting used to' the ill child's condition—or impending death—is an adaptive part of coping, and being informed is the necessary condition for such preparation.
  - the focus of hope fluctuates as symptoms improve with effective palliation. This can cause some confusion in children ('He acts and feels better—his coughing ended.').

Erin (age 8) 'My Mind' 'Sometimes I wonder how it's going to be without my little brother' (Figure 8.6)

I feel *sad* because I love Matthew so much. It was so nice when he was here. Now he doesn't have fun because he is very sick. Blue is for tears. I think I'm *worried*. When he's sick, I don't know what to do. He used to stop Abby and me from fighting. He was the only person who was really nice to me. I don't know what I'll do without him. *Angry* is red—like I feel like killing someone—the color of blood. Abby fights with me. Matthew is crying or screaming because his head hurts. I have nobody to talk to—not even Matthew is there. I chose purple for *hopeful* because it's a good color. *Guilty* (green)—that's the color I feel. Like it's my fault that Matthew is sick because when Abby and

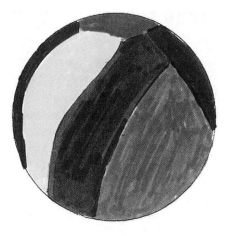

Fig. 8.5 Abby—The Colors of Life, March 18. (See plate 9.)

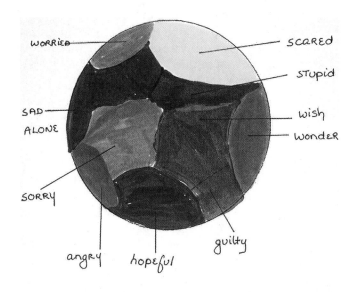

Fig. 8.6 Erin—My Mind, March 18. (See plate 10.)

I fight, the yelling hurts Matthew's head. *Scared*—I think of all the bad things that could happen to me. When he's gone, I'll have nothing to do. With him, it's very fun. Without him here I'm bored. When he's sick it's like he's not even here. *Wonder*—Sometimes I wonder how it's going to be in the past without him. Maybe okay, maybe terrible, maybe good. In my dreams I think about how it's going to be. I never finish my dreams because Matthew wakes up and I have to go get my mother or father. *Alone*—I feel like crying. *Stupid*—Everyone annoys me. When I finally get to talk to my mother, Matthew's beeper goes off. I just want them to be with me a little, not a lot. *Sorry* for him for being sick. *Wish* that he get better. If I had one wish, I would wish for no one in my family to get sick. If I had to choose money or family, I'd choose family. What was the one I skipped? *Hopeful?* There's not really anything to say. *Helpful?* I can't help—sometimes I can—only for little things. [Do you have hope?] That he might just get very better. . . .

Erin's mandala is suffused with anticipatory grief, wherein the tenses of time (past, present and future) and Matthew's presence/absence intermingle. She kept confusing *hopeful* with *helpful*; it was clear that she had trouble holding on to her hope—it eluded her grasp.

- Sibling issues highlighted in Erin's statement:
  - Anticipatory grief figures consciously in the experience of some siblings. It is often felt most intensely by children who are close playmates, and already sense the aloneness that lies ahead—not only in the family constellation, but also in their day-to-day activities.
  - Guilt is a frequent contributor to siblings' distress, although children do not tend to admit to it, spontaneously or easily.
  - Siblings' needs for time and attention loom huge to parents who are overwhelmed with the needs of an ill child; however, the siblings are—more often than not—remarkably reasonable in their demands ("I just want them to be with me a little, not a lot")
  - Hope pervades all, including intense grief.

* * *

By the fourth session, Matthew was able to draw a picture that clearly acknowledged his own vulnerability (Figure 8.7): "A bad monster that scared everybody. He hurts people with his big nails." No longer did he single himself out as being immune to the threat. He now reported pain quite emphatically, as in: "Mummy—go get my pain medicine NOW." He often commented on whether he was having a 'good' or a 'rough' day. ('Rough' was a word that his mother often used.) At this point, there was an exact correlation between his open reporting of his own symptoms and the 'inclusiveness' in his drawing ('monster scared *everybody*').

The following drawing (Figure 8.8) of 'jumping and rolling in the grass and picking flowers like I did last summer' reflected the fact that Matthew's pain was now well controlled and he was

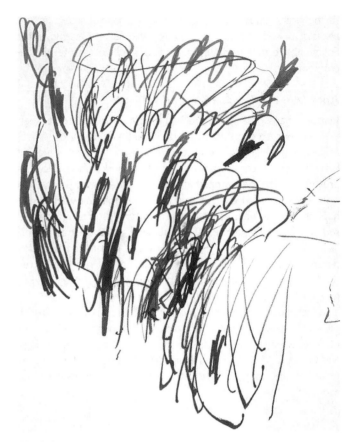

Fig. 8.7 Matthew—Bad Monster, March 25. (See plate 11.)

much calmer. He had begun to eat again, and was sitting up unassisted at the computer. His good-bad list (dictated) was:

bad
the booboo came but it went bye-bye
spitting up a whole bunch of mucus makes me sad
when I hurt, I cry
when birds scream outside, it hurts my head

good
I went downstairs and sat up and nothing hurt
I eat Mummy's soup
I sit up in my blue chair
I watch cartoons on the couch
I play on the computer
me better

At this point, the family and close friends all observed how much more relaxed Matthew was, and that he seemed 'busy' in his life, however restricted. "He's playing again!" reported his parents with pleasure.

- Children generally like to make lists, and if the 'bad' is counterbalanced—even to a limited degree—by the 'good'—they often willingly engage in the activity. Older children enjoy writing the lists themselves, using colored pens, stickers, other

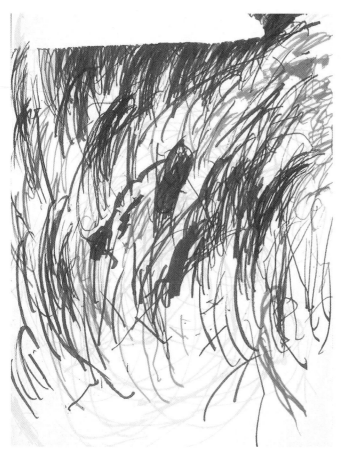

Fig. 8.8 Matthew—Grass and Flowers, April 2. (See plate 12.)

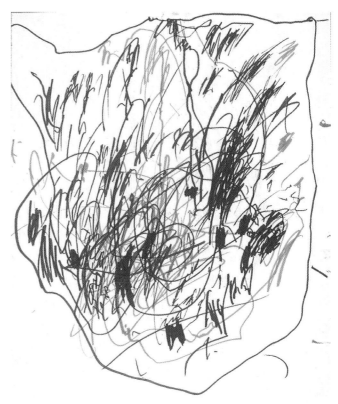

Fig. 8.9 Matthew—Slide, Horses and Boats, May 15. (See plate 13.)

decorative details to make the threatening content more approachable.

• Play and learning define 'quality of life' in childhood. Parents instinctively note their child's involvement (or lack thereof) in play activities as a significant marker of his or her sense of well being.

Over the month of May, Matthew talked more openly about his emotional state. For example, after watching a television program, he talked repeatedly about a cat that went away and didn't see his mother anymore: "He's dead. I don't like that show. It scared me." Through the story of the cat as a vehicle, he was able to express his fears of separation and anticipatory grief. His mother discussed how the cat would see his mother again, but in a different way—an explanation that mirrored her belief in reunion after death, and gave Matthew much comfort. At the same time as he reported that he couldn't ride his bike anymore "because me sick", he talked about wanting to walk again. A picture of: "Sand. Slide coming out of a house. Something to climb—horses and boats" (Figure 8.9) led the mother to realize that he was thinking about the park. As a

result, the parents took him to the park that weekend in his special stroller.

• It is not uncommon that a 'serendipitous' event or trigger (e.g. television program) provides the opening for children to disclose their deepest anxieties, without ever having to identify them explicitly as their own.

• The co-existence of realistic appraisal (not being able to ride his bike) and hope (wanting to walk again) are in constant flux with children; the adults need only follow.

By early June, Matthew's condition was clearly deteriorating. He was having increased levels of pain, as well as more break-through episodes. After completing his picture, I asked him what it was. For the first time, he could (or would) not come up with a title. He said flatly: "I don't know that..." (Figure 8.10) I suggested that perhaps the picture was of his booboo that was hurting; he yelled "NO." In fact, he was expressing a lot of anger: "Why do I have that booboo in my head? What is it in my head?" as well as sadness: "I'm very sad—poor me." His refusal to put a title on his drawing reflected both his physical and emotional vulnerability. Furthermore, the intensity of his anger may have even scared himself (and thus his adamancy about not 'naming' it). However, the security in his parents' presence was intact: "When I feel the booboo hurting

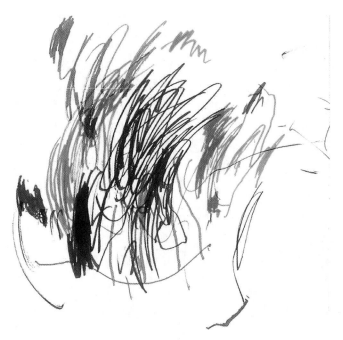

Fig. 8.10 Matthew—I don't know that, June 5. (See plate 14.)

me, Mummy calms me down. I call on the beeper and she and Daddy stay with me."

• The constellation of anger, fear, and sadness/grief is—in one form or another—universal to all children facing death. By providing a "safe" environment for the expression of these feelings (whether it be within the family and/or a psychotherapeutic context and/or another professional relationship), their intensity can be mitigated and contained. The reassurance of family and professionals' ongoing availability and presence allows the child to remain connected even while pulling inward.

Matthew's last drawing was done the day before his death. Although he was very weak and no longer even watched television, when I asked him if he wanted to do a drawing, he gave his usual response: "Sure." He entitled his picture: "Outside—yellow sun and trees." (Figure 8.11) He died peacefully the next morning.

The family was intensely grateful for the months that Matthew was at home, when they, as part of the palliative care team, provided him with optimal care.

Thank you for giving me aliveness. (6-year-old child) [5, p. 167]

Even when life itself cannot be guaranteed, psychotherapy may "give aliveness" to the child for however long that life may last. Through the extraordinary challenges posed by life-limiting illness, the children develop a precocious inner wisdom of life and its fragility. Yet the spirit of childhood continues to shine through both their vulnerability and their resilience.

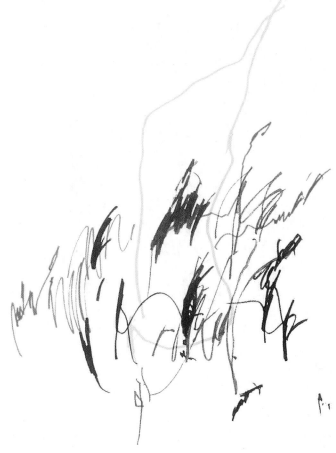

Fig. 8.11 Matthew—Outside—Yellow Sun and Trees, June 11. (See plate 15.)

References

1. Sourkes, B. *The Deepening Shade: Psychological Aspects of Life-Threatening Illness*. Pittsburgh, PA: University of Pittsburgh Press, 1982.

2. Institute of Medicine. *When Children Die: Improving Palliative and End-of-Life Care for Children and their Families*. Washington DC: National Academy Press, 2003.

3. Jelalian, E, Boergers, J., Spirito, A., and Sourkes, B. Psychologic aspects of leukemia and hematologic disorders. In D. Nathan, S. Orkin, D. Ginsburg and A. Lock, (eds.) *Nathan and Oski's Hematology of Infancy and Childhood* (6th edition). Philadelphia, PA: Saunders, 2003, pp. 1671–83.

4. American Psychological Association. Task Force Report on Children and End-of-Life. (in preparation).

5. Sourkes, B. *Armfuls of Time: The Psychological Experience of the Child with a Life-Threatening Illness*. Pittsburgh, PA: University of Pittsburgh Press (Published in Great Britain by Routledge), 1995.

6. Sourkes, B. The child with a life-threatening illness. In J. Brandell, (ed.) *Countertransference in Child and Adolescent Psychotherapy*. New York: Jason Aronson, 1992, pp. 267–84.

7. Rait, D. and Holland, J. Pediatric cancer: Psychosocial issues and approaches. In Wiernik, (ed.) *Mediguide to Oncology*, Vol. 6, 1986.

8. Sourkes, B. Facilitating family coping with childhood cancer. *J Pediatr Psycholt* 1977;2(2):65–7.

9. Coles, R. *The Spiritual Life of Children*. Boston, MA: Houghton Mifflin, 1990.

10. Terr, L. *Too Scared to Cry*. New York: Basic Books, 1990.

11. Davis, M. and Wallbridge, D. *Boundary and Space: An Introduction to the World of D.W. Winnicott*. New York: Brunner/Mazel, 1981.

12. National Hospice and Palliative Care Organization Website. www.nhpco.org. See: ChIPPS 0.8169 Bibliography Summary of the Ethics and Decision-making Subgroup.

13. Aldrich, C.K. Some dynamics of anticipatory grief. In B. Schoenberg, A. Carr, A. Kutscher, D. Peretz, and J. Goldberg, (eds.) *Anticipatory Grief*. New York: Columbia University Press, 1974.

9   Adolescents and young adults

Finella Craig

Young people with palliative-care needs form a distinct group with physical, emotional, psychological, and social needs that are significantly different from those of adults and children. They are neither 'large children' nor 'small adults', but are in a continuum, during which their needs as children are evolving into those of adults. This evolution usually occurs between the ages of 13–24 years.

Better supportive care for conditions that manifest in childhood means that there are increasing number of young people surviving into early adulthood. The prevalence of life-limiting or life-threatening disorder in this group is estimated at 6000–10,000, with an annual mortality of 1.7 per 10,000 [1]. These young people have a wide spectrum of diseases and disorders, some presenting in early childhood (e.g. genetic and congenital conditions) and others apparent later in childhood or adolescence. Many reach a crisis in terms of physical deterioration in adolescence or early adulthood and many die in their late teens or early twenties. Within this group patients demonstrate a range of developmental levels and cognitive abilities, social, and emotional maturity, such that service provision for adolescents is a very distinct area of clinical health care.

Life-limiting and life-threatening conditions affecting young adults

The spectrum of life-limiting and life-threatening disorders encountered in young adults is considerable. While there is overlap with conditions encountered in the paediatric and adult populations, many conditions take on increasing significance in the adolescent years, as a consequence of natural disease progression, because of the physical and emotional changes of adolescence or simply because the child has outlived all expectations.

Most of the conditions encountered fall into one of the four groups identified in Table 1 (based on [1].)

Table 1   Life-limiting and life-threatening conditions affecting young adults

Group	Examples
Conditions where curative treatment is feasible but may fail	Cancer Organ failure for example, kidney, heart, liver
Conditions where there may be long periods of intensive treatment aimed at prolonging life, where premature death is still possible or inevitable	Cystic fibrosis Muscular dystrophies HIV/AIDS Some congenital heart diseases Pulmonary hypertension
Progressive conditions without curative options, where treatment is exclusively palliative	Batten disease Mucopolysaccharidoses Cruetzfeldt–Jakob disease
Severe neurological disability, which may cause weakness and susceptibility to health complications	Severe multiple disabilities following brain or spinal cord injury Severe cerebral palsy

One of the particular challenges of working with young adults is the wide spectrum of cognitive ability encountered. Some will have severe cognitive impairment related to their underlying disease, whereas others, such as those with congenital heart disease or cancer may have no cognitive delay. Those with progressive impairment, such as the young adults with Leigh's disease or Cruetzfeldt–Jakob disease, will have been mentally alert earlier in their lives and may still have some degree of cognitive autonomy, even if it cannot be expressed. These young adults may once have been relatively independent, able to organize parts of their own lives and make decisions regarding their care.

Adolescence as a transition phase

Adolescence is a period of rapid physical, emotional, social, and cognitive change, during which key developmental tasks must be achieved. These include the development of personal value systems and identity, independance from parents, taking responsibility for one's own behaviour, and achieving financial and social independence. Hormonal changes lead to alterations in physical appearance, changing body image, and sexual awakening. Even in the presence of deteriorating health, neurological and/or physical impairment, development will continue in some, if not all, of these areas.

Normal adolescent, development [2,3]

In early adolescence, pubertal changes are usually accompanied by rapid growth, and mood swings. Cognitive skills develop, with improved abstract thought and greater ability to understand consequences and make plans for the future. Alongside these changes is the need to socialize and identify with a peer group.

During middle adolescence there is often an increase in risk-taking behaviour as young people develop autonomy through testing limitations and boundaries imposed by parents and authority figures. This is an essential process through which young people work out who they are and who they want to be, often challenging previously accepted family beliefs and values. As part of this process, the need to identify with a peer group intensifies. Sexual development continues with the emergence of physical needs and for many young people their first sexual experiences.

By late adolescence young adults are defining and understanding their functional roles in life with regard to lifestyles, careers, and relationships. They should have a sense of who they are, who they identify with, and the type of life they want to lead. This is a time of making plans for the future, establishing permanent relationships, developing increased financial independence, and spending time away from the family.

Difficulties of normal adolescent development faced by life-limited young people

For those with life-limiting illness, the complexity of achieving even some of the developmental tasks of adolescence is immense. Acute illness or progressive physical and/or cognitive impairment is often accompanied by increased dependence on parents, a requirement to conform to the values and beliefs of adult carers, and increasing isolation from healthy peers.

Chronic ill health may delay the onset of pubertal changes, including sexual development, and limit the young person's potential for growth, giving them the appearance of being younger than their age. Immediately they become more identifiably different from their peers. Normal adolescent mood swings may be harder to express and less well accommodated. A life limited young person may not have the physical ability to

'storm off' or slam doors as an outlet to their frustrations. Additionally, they often have to spend more time with adults than their peers, and moodiness towards carers or parents can cause considerable tensions, especially when it is interpreted as rudeness.

Many life-limited young people, due to their underlying diagnosis, may not experience the development of cognitive skills that accompanies normal adolescence. Indeed, this may be a time when those with neurodegenerative disorders have an accelerated cognitive decline. Without maturity of abstract thought and the ability to understand consequences, they are less likely be allowed, or to achieve, some of the freedoms and responsibilities of their peers. Even those with mature cognitive development may experience difficulty achieving personal freedoms, perhaps due to the demands of medical care, physical limitations imposed by their disease, or parental involvement [4]. Without such freedoms, opportunities to socialize with peers, to test limitations, and to explore and experience sexuality are limited.

By late adolescence, most young people should have a sense of who they want to be and the lifestyle they want to follow. The freedom to socialize independently, to choose a peer group, to test limitations, and to explore and define sexuality are essential processes in determining who an individual will become. For the majority of life-limited young people adolescent development will have been affected by restrictions and limitations. Physical impairment, cognitive impairment and ill health, rather than individuality and freedom, determine, at least to some extent, who the young person will become. Making plans for the future, in the face of an inevitable early death, may not seem worthwhile or possible.

Developing independence

I am aware that I can never really be independent because I have special needs and cannot get a job. But it's difficult. I don't want to sit at home and watch telly and I can't go on the buses by myself. (Palliative Care for Young People aged 13–24 [1])

Achieving independence and aiming for personal goals can be extremely difficult for life-limited young people. Some, such as those with malignant disease, may have been progressing through normal adolescent development, with increasing independence, prior to receiving a life-limiting diagnosis. Others may have chronic conditions with varying degrees of life-long dependence, or progressive disorders where the changes of adolescence are accompanied by deteriorating physical health and mental ability. Whatever the nature of the underlying condition, the psychological impact of impaired, lost, or potentially unachievable independence can be immense, particularly when the young person sees healthy peers and siblings becoming increasingly independent.

Conflict with parents is not unusual, especially when previously compliant children challenge parental control, and act-out risk-taking behaviour, such as refusing to comply with health-care needs. Achieving autonomy, independence and peer group relationships, the necessities of adolescent progression, can become an increasingly difficult struggle.

For parents, the steps towards independence can be extremely difficult, particularly if they have been heavily involved in all aspects of their child's life. Acknowledging that their child is growing up and could become less dependent is in itself a bereavement—the loss of their child, and a change in their role as parents. Added to this is the anxiety that their child may not manage, that they may not want to be more independent, that they may come to harm or could experience failure and disappointment.

Not all young adults will seek or welcome increasing independence. This may be particularly true if they have been relatively isolated from healthy peers and have become dependent on parents for companionship as well as physical support. Some may feel threatened by the suggestion that they could take part in activities away from the security of their parents. They may also fear failure—it may be better not to try than to prove it is impossible.

All young people, whatever the degree of physical and cognitive dependence, need to be given opportunities to become as independent as possible [5], as a necessary developmental transition from childhood. With good information and support even those with severe physical and cognitive impairment may be able to take over the organization of at least part of their own lives. Others may become fully independent or may be able to live away from home, if provided with an independent carer.

Professionals working with young people and their families must support and facilitate the transition to independence, while at the same time acknowledging difficulties faced by parents and their children. The potential of a young person is developed over a number of years, so the expectation of what may be possible should be introduced early. However, even the most independent young adults have a great need for their parents [1], and it is important to balance a young person's need for independence with encouragement to continue including their parents in at least some aspects of their life and decisions around health care [5].

Physical independence

Within the group of young people with life-limiting disorders the spectrum of physical dependency is wide. Some are heavily dependent on others for physical care, unable to escape from a parent or carer even for short periods. Others may retain considerable independence, becoming physically dependent only for some aspects of care when they are unwell. Whatever the situation, opportunities to maintain and develop independence must be optimized.

All life-limited young people should be assessed for physical aids and housing adaptations. Equipment that enables them to control their own environment (e.g. electric wheelchair, self-operated hoists) may create opportunities for independence and privacy at home, as well as reducing some of the burden for carers. Additionally, parents may feel more able to allow their child some independence, such as time on their own at home, if they are confident that they are using appropriate and safe equipment.

Forward planning is essential if equipment and house modifications are to be in place when needed. This should be possible with knowledge of the natural history of diseases, yet many families still find that equipment provision and replacement is difficult [6]. There may be delays because the young person is about to transfer to adult services, or because they have recently transferred and are now on a waiting list for an assessment. There may also be bureaucratic delays while teams determine whose budget is responsible for adaptations and aids. Good communication and clear budget allocation between the agencies (Health and Social Services in the UK) is essential so that families are not hampered by bureaucracy or forced to rely on crises intervention.

Independence in decision making [4,5,7,8]

Parents often find it difficult to allow their child to take responsibility for their own life. To do this a young person must develop sufficient intellectual maturity to consider choices and the consequence of choices. Some parents may feel, appropriately, that their child does not have the intellectual maturity to make informed choices, particularly if the young person has a disorder associated with intellectual impairment. Other parents may be unable to recognize, or accept, that their child has developed sufficient intellectual maturity to make these choices.

Involving their child in decisions about health care can be particularly difficult, especially if parents have not included them in discussions about their diagnosis, prognosis, treatment, and future management. The young person needs to be given this information in order to make fully informed choices, whereas the parents may want to protect them from a full awareness of their prognosis. Some parents may feel that including the young person in health care decisions would be an unnecessary responsibility that should not be imposed on them. They may also feel that the consequences of decisions about health care are so big that their child, even if capable of autonomy in other areas of their life, should not be given autonomy in this area. Additionally, giving the young person more responsibility and autonomy could represent to the parents a loss of their role as parents and carers, which they are not yet prepared for.

The extent to which young people can be involved in health care decisions will vary within the group. Some will have, or will achieve, the emotional maturity to understand actual and hypothetical concepts and the consequences of possible actions. Others may not achieve, or may lose, the ability to think conceptually or to fully understand consequences. Some will need assistance in understanding the available options, future risks, and consequences of choices. This can be especially true for younger adolescents. Young people with learning difficulty should also be encouraged and enabled to take part in at least some aspects of decision making and it is suggested that they have independent advocates [1] to support them.

Some young adults, although capable of achieving independent decision-making, may have been content to let their parents maintain control in this area of their lives. They may need encouragement to start taking some responsibility for their own lives, as part of a natural and healthy transition to adulthood.

Professionals must be sensitive to the difficulties faced by parents and young adults when the balance of responsibility starts to shift, and should start to prepare them for this transition well in advance. The young person should be given opportunities to become increasingly involved in making decisions about their day-to-day life, as well as health care. The parents should be assisted to view this as a natural progression to independent adulthood, while the young person should be encouraged to continue including their parents in decision-making, although no longer as the sole decision-makers.

Restricting the young adult from participating in decision-making can clearly create unnecessary tension. However, professionals and families should be aware that including the young person in decision-making can also create tensions, particularly if the young person, parents and professionals express differing viewpoints. A young person may make an informed decision to discontinue a particular treatment, against the wishes of their parents, causing considerable family tension and emotional stress if the parents feel their child lacks the emotional or intellectual maturity to understand the consequences of such a decision. Parents may feel at times that their child, however intellectually mature, is making a particular decision for inappropriate reasons, and may fear that health professionals will inappropriately support their child's autonomy. An 'adolescent tantrum', where the best weapon is the refusal of life-prolonging medication, can have dramatic consequences if not handled appropriately. Health professionals must be able to help the young person identify the reasons for making certain choices and ensure that they fully understand the consequences of these choices. Explanation and negotiation, between parents, health professionals, and the young person, is essential.

At one point I decided not to take my calcium tablets—they tasted like chalk. But then the doctor explained the pros and cons and I realized that they were right. I could then evaluate the situation and make a decision. Sometimes this information stage is missed out. (Palliative Care for Young People aged 13–24 years [1])

Financial independence

Financial independence for the young person with life-limiting illness is frequently impossible. While healthy school attenders often find part-time jobs, giving them a small independent income and valuable work experience, such opportunities are rarely available to those with life-limiting illness, especially where there are physical limitations to work access, treatment regimens that need to be accommodated and absences due to ill health. Long-term financial prospects are similarly poor. Interrupted schooling can hinder educational achievement and, in conjunction with a poor attendance record and ill health, limit employability. Access to higher education is difficult and limited and deteriorating physical or mental ability makes many career paths inaccessible. Many young people have high educational aspirations and should be given career advice, vocational training, and assistance to attend school or university. Comprehensive multidisciplinary support should be provided, but is rarely available [1].

Peer group identification

Opportunities for peer group identification are limited when poor health, physical appearance or impaired cognitive function identify a young person as different. At a time when a young person should be experiencing a new independence, the life-limited young adult faces medical treatments, ill health, isolation from their friends, and an increasing dependence on parents. This can be particularly difficult for previously healthy young people, such as those diagnosed with cancer during adolescence. Their appearance and priorities may change, such that they can no longer easily identify a peer group amongst their healthy friends, but identify with a new world of illness, treatment, and death.

It was so much easier to make friends in the hospital than it is anywhere else. (Nicky A, teenager with cancer: Nicky's Story [9])

For many life-limited young adults links with peers are lost through school absence, hospitilization, friends being overwhelmed by the illness, or friends moving on and developing new relationships. Increasing physical dependence further increases social isolation and impairs the young person's opportunities for independent interactions. Family and carers may inappropriately, but almost inevitably, become the young person's main source of social support and companionship. With the majority of carers being female, male companionship is frequently limited, further isolating young men in particular from peer identification.

She wants to be 15 and talk about 15 year-old things. It's not the same doing things with your mum. (Palliative Care for Young People aged 13–24 years [1])

Most young people want to be involved in leisure activities and a social scene, which should be considered as important as health care and education. When a young person is unable to attend school, alternative social (not just educational) provision should be made. Parents should be encouraged to enable their child to take part in independent social activities, with professionals ensuring they have appropriate physical aids to achieve this. Opportunities for group activities with other life-limited young people are important, but interaction with peers of all abilities is also essential to minimize feelings of separateness and isolation [1].

Sexual development

With progressive pubertal development comes the need for physical satisfaction and sexual relationships. Many life-limited young people will develop physical and cognitive sexual maturity alongside their peers, although others may have delayed sexual development as a consequence of chronic ill health. Those with cognitive impairment or impaired motor function may experience sexual maturity with physical needs that they cannot express or satisfy. There are also some young adults with cognitive impairment who reach physical sexual maturity and become inappropriately sexually active as they have insufficient cognitive development to understand that their behaviour is socially inappropriate.

Much normal adolescent activity and discussion is focused on sexual awareness, finding a partner, and sexual activity. Through peer group isolation, young people with life-limiting illness often miss out on this normal adolescent information and discussion, while parents and carers may be unaware or unwilling to accept that a 'child' has sexual feelings. Even when parents and carers are aware of the young person's sexual maturity, the young person may not have the same freedom of discussion that they would with their peers.

Young people who develop sexual maturity alongside their peers may find physical disabilities, or anxieties associated with their disability, in addition to a lack of appropriate social contact and limited independence, impair their opportunity to experience a similar level of sexual activity. Those with delayed sexual development may find it increasingly difficult to fit into their peer group, both in terms of physical appearance and interests. Personal expectations relating to relationships and sexual experiences can become a major concern to the young person, who may have no one with whom they can safely discuss these issues. Some will mourn the fact that they may not live to experience sexual intimacy and others may become overtly sexually active in an attempt to achieve acceptance and normality. Without being able to join in the sexual arena of their friends, many life-limited young people can feel increasingly different and isolated.

Sex education is important for all young people, but especially those who may have limited access to education through school and peers. For several disorders more specific information about sexual activity and fertility is essential—it is not unusual, for example, for young adults with cancer to presume they are infertile. Young people may also want information about masturbation, finding a sexual partner and accessing videos—information that is usually provided by peers. In the absence of peers they may rely on parents and carers to provide this information, or let their questions (and needs) remain unaddressed. Young men may have particular difficulty accessing information of a sexual nature if they have only female carers. Providing opportunities for peer group interaction away from parents, which includes structured sexual education and emotional support, may be one way to address some of these issues.

Relationships with parents and siblings

I tended to push my mum away and shut her out . . . I was scared to admit that I really needed her. (Nicky A, teenager with cancer)

Relationships with parents can be particularly complex for the life-limited young adult. Most are striving for, or have previously experienced, a degree of autonomy with physical and emotional independence. Declining health and/or impaired physical and cognitive ability requires them to need their parents more, for both emotional and practical support. They have to cope with two conflicting realities—the need to be independent of parents and the need to be supported by parents.

Many young people also feel the need to protect their parents [10]. They may not want them to know if they are feeling unhappy, depressed or in pain, and may push them away rather than expose them to how they are feeling.

My mum stayed with me everyday but I would never tell her how I felt and I tended to push her away and shut her out . . . I also thought I was mean for making her watch me get ill. (Nicky A, teenager with cancer)

Encouraging parents and young adults to share their feelings, however, can be helpful.

I remembered my mum saying that's what families were for, to help and support each other when we were ill . . . Now I like it when my mum stays with me because we had a long talk and I realized my mum was also suffering. I also agreed with my mum that I would stop shutting her out . . . now we are closer than ever. (Nicky A, teenager with cancer)

Sibling relationships can be strong, but the burden on a healthy sibling can be tremendous [10]. They may be the main confident of the life-limited sibling, while worrying about their parents coping abilities and the conflicting need to pursue their own life [11]. They may appropriately complain of displacement, deprivation, anger, injustice, loneliness, and vulnerability, as parents have insufficient time for them [10]. Without appropriate support, these feelings can cause resentment and disruption of their relationship with the life-limited sibling.

Professionals caring for young people with life-limiting illness should be aware of, and should prepare the family for, some of the difficulties in family relationships, and dynamics that they may experience. It may be helpful if there is someone the family can talk to who is not part of the clinical team. Parent and sibling groups can also provide opportunities for family members to discuss how they are feeling and to feel less isolated. In the United Kingdom such groups can often be accessed through children's hospice services.

Psychological needs

With limitations in peer group interaction, employability, social and financial independence, and the opportunity to explore sexuality, it is difficult for young people to establish functional roles in life with regard to careers, relationships, and lifestyles. For most young people, the adolescent development of identity and autonomy is accompanied by a sense of immortality and the opportunity to determine and shape their own future. For many with life-limiting illness, mortality is a reality and the future is determined by limitations not possibilities. They cannot develop their own identity and autonomy from the same perspective as their peers, nor can they look to a seemingly endless and purposeful future of their own choosing. As their healthy peers establish permanent relationships, develop increased financial independence, spend time away from their family, and make plans for the future, the life-limited young person can feel increasingly isolated with no sense of purposeful future.

Many young people with life-limiting illness are mentally alert and fully understand their disease and prognosis and the implications for both themselves and their family. They may not, however, have established mechanisms to cope with the anxiety and uncertainty [4]. Feelings of anger and grief at being ill, anxiety about medical procedures, worries about

family members, depression caused by separation from friends and normal activities, and fears of death are not uncommon [4,5,12,13]. A physical appearance that the young person feels, identifies them as different from everyone else may cause feelings of being damaged and deviant in the outside world, further contributing to feelings of low self esteem. At a time when peer group acceptance and support is so important, they may feel increasingly ostracized. Some may grieve future losses, such as having a career and family, or act out risk taking behaviour in their struggle for autonomy or in an attempt to gain peer group acceptance.

It was a big relief that I was going back to hospital . . . everyone is like me and no one looks at me like I am weird or a freak. (Nicky A, teenager with cancer)

Because the emotional demands of young adults are particularly complex, all professionals involved in their care should receive training that enables them to offer appropriate support. In addition to this, clinical psychology should be a core service in all care plans for young adults and should include the needs of parents, siblings, partners, and significant others [1]. Clinical psychologists should routinely work as part of the teams caring for life-limited young adults, offering interventions when needed and working with small groups. Many young adults are capable of discussing their prognosis, and the issues arising from this, but need to set the pace for these discussions. They also need opportunities to explore their feelings without fear of upsetting other members of their own family or professional carers. A neutral professional, who is not part of the clinical team, could take this role and may be someone with whom the young person can most easily voice fears and express anger.

Assessing the psychological needs of young adults with cognitive impairment and/or physical barriers to communication is particularly challenging.

Spiritual needs

As part of the quest to develop their own identity and value systems, adolescence is often a time when young people question the meaning of life and look for reasons for pain and suffering, unfairness, and punishment. With the prospect of an early death, the ideas and concepts of identity and who a person may become, gain increasing significance. Many will want to 'make their mark' on the world, aware that they have limited time, and may be facing increasing physical and/or cognitive decline. Some may express hope for some kind of spiritual continuity, especially if they see little potential to achieve something before death.

Faith and religious belief may have played an important role in parental family values, but the young person may need to explore their own belief system and reasons for their illness and impending death [14]. They need opportunities to discuss and express their beliefs and for these to be acknowledged and respected, even where there is the potential for conflict if they choose to reject parental beliefs. Through this, their sense of individuality, autonomy, value, and continuity can be reinforced. Providing such opportunities for young adults with cognitive disability or physical barriers to communication can be especially difficult, as they may be unable to formulate or express spiritual needs. It is also important to be aware, particularly when working within units based on a specific religious ethic, that some young people may not have the maturity or confidence to refuse what is on offer.

Respite care

Young people living at home usually welcome the opportunity for respite away from the family, with opportunities for peer socialization [1]. Equally, caring for a life-limited young person, particularly with physical limitations and progressively deteriorating health, places a huge demand on parents. Appropriate respite should be available for young people both for scheduled breaks away from their family and in emergency situations. Unfortunately, facilities, for this age group are scarce [15] and for some young people respite may only be available in units that are primarily tailored to the needs of adults with learning disabilities and mental health problems.

Paediatric hospices may be able to offer respite admissions, usually if the young person is under 19 years of age, but this may be inappropriate for a mature young adult, who is, or has been, relatively independent. They may feel uncomfortable being admitted alongside much younger children or those with cognitive impairment, or into an environment with childish decorations, and activities.

Adult hospices can be equally inappropriate, particularly if the young person's cognitive age is below their chronological age, and more suited to a paediatric environment. Additionally, the environment of an adult hospice is unlikely to be geared towards accommodating more active young people, as the majority of users are often middle aged or elderly. Staff may not be aware of the specific needs of the young adult, particularly in relation to social activities, sexuality, privacy, and independence.

Young adults often want to stay up late at night and spend the day in bed. They want to be able to listen to their own music or to be noisy without fear of disturbing younger children or older adults. They want to be able to watch adult films and television programmes, perhaps not appropriate in a paediatric hospice environment. They want personal space and privacy to be alone when they feel like it. They want to be with people of their own age, with things to do in the evenings and weekends, and they want to 'fit in'.

The very specific needs of young adults with regard to respite and hospice care are being increasingly recognized and the number of facilities for this age group is slowly increasing. In the UK, Acorns Hospice in the West Midlands and Helen House in Oxford have now opened units for young adults, having recognized the needs of the maturing paediatric users. Whatever the environment, respite admissions should be co-ordinated to maximize the young adult's opportunities for peer socialization and staff should be trained to support the developing and changing needs specific to this age group.

Terminal care

There is a large gap in the provision of terminal care for young adults. Paediatric teams may lack confidence in the symptom management of older patients, while adult community nurses and palliative care teams may feel less confident with patients who are much younger than they are used to. The adult teams may also feel less comfortable when working in partnership with parents, and may find it particularly difficult working with young adults whose parents have always taken a strong lead in care. Family doctors are also likely to have had little experience in the terminal care of this age group and may not have easy access to specialist support to advise on symptom management and drug doses. These difficulties can be compounded if the young adult is dying from a rare condition, particularly if it is one not usually encountered in adult patients. Where possible, the young adult and their family should be allowed to choose, who should take on the key co-ordination of their care, being able to choose from available paediatric and adult services. For some patients, partnership working between adult palliative care and paediatric teams may offer a solution [16], but such practice is not routinely available.

There are often practical difficulties when caring for young adult patients at home. Parents are often the main carers and may have difficulty with the physical demands of care. Nursing support from adult services may not be available if the young adult is still within the paediatric age range and, if the deterioration has been very rapid, appropriate aids may not be available in the home.

Finding an appropriate hospice to care for a terminally ill young adult can also be difficult, as discussed in the previous section. Even if an appropriate hospice is identified, there may be age restriction to admission, although these may sometimes be relaxed if the young adult is well known to the service. Young adults over the age of 19 years, however, are unlikely to have a first admission to a children's hospice, even if this would be the ideal location both for them and their family. While there are still insufficient hospices dedicated specifically to young adults, many will continue to be admitted to acute hospital wards for terminal care when this cannot be delivered at home.

Transition to adult services [17–21]

The transition to adult services can be incredibly difficult for young people, their families, and the health care teams involved in their care, for many reasons.

Families are likely to have used paediatric services for many years and feel secure in the familiar environment, dealing with professionals who know them well, and have long-term knowledge of the patient, the family, and the condition.

Paediatricians may feel reluctant to allow their patients and families to move to adult services. They may have a degree of emotional attachment, having worked hard for the child over a number of years, and watched them grow up.

It can often be difficult to identify the most appropriate team to take on the continuing care of a young adult. For those with rare disorders, particularly when they have outlived their predicted life expectancy, there may be no adult physicians or community services with sufficient experience and expertise.

Within adult services there is less tradition of a single general physician to oversee care and maintain a holistic quality, which is particularly needed for patients under the care of several different specialists. There is a fear that families are being transferred into new unfamiliar services, without a clear co-ordinator to guide them through and pull all the services together.

Families and paediatricians may perceive adult services to be inadequate, poorly co-ordinated, unsupportive, and impersonal. There is often an anxiety that parents and families will be excluded, as the adult teams will focus on the patient as an individual, rather than within the context of the family dynamic. Parents may feel that their child will be given too much autonomy in an adult service and will be allowed to behave irresponsibly, particularly if they are trying to assert their own identity through contradicting their parents' choices.

Transfer to adult services is usually determined by the age of a young person, not their clinical health. For young adults not expected to live beyond childhood, the transfer to adult services (i.e. an acknowledgement of adulthood) may signify that 'time is running out'. Many will be reaching the end stages of their disorder, sometimes deteriorating as a consequence of the physical and hormonal changes of adolescence. They face deteriorating health in the care of people they do not know, who have the potential to deliver a less well co-ordinated service than they are used to. Many families and health care workers would prefer to 'sit it out' in paediatric services rather than transfer care for what may be a short, but critical, period.

Age does not determine emotional readiness to transfer to adult services. Some young adults, particularly those with cognitive impairment, may not want, or be able, to take on the responsibility of more autonomous interactions with health care staff. They may not feel comfortable in a more adult environment, and may still want the security of the familiar child-oriented surroundings of the paediatric clinic. Additionally, even the most mature young adults may feel that they are being abandoned by the staff they have got to know and may suffer separation anxiety, loss of identity, loss of self esteem, and loss of significant relationships. Transfer can, for many, be a loss that is grieved.

Transition to adult services must be well planned and the young adult should be involved in the timing of the transition. It is essential that preparation for the transition starts well in advance, and that the young adult and their family are supported through the transition on both a practical and emotional basis. The transition should not be a 'black cloud' hanging over their future, or something to be put off in the 'hope' that the young person may die before transfer becomes necessary.

A long transition time is necessary for the family to adjust and look at alternatives to fill some of the gaps between paediatric and adult services. Association for Children with life-threatening or Terminal conditions and their family (ACT) recommends a framework for transition within which there should be scope for individual flexibility [1]. They recommend that a first stage might be identified ranging from 13 to 17/18 years with the goal of transferring to the adult service. Another goal could be set to increase the young person's independence by 25 years. The transition should be planned with the young person and set out for the patient, the family, and all professionals involved. Everyone must have a clear direction as an open-ended process can make it difficult for families and professionals to accept the change.

One useful way of making the transition gradually is to hold joint clinics with paediatric and adult staff, enabling the young person and family to build up confidence in the new team before completely transferring care. They should also be given written information about the adult unit (well in advance of transfer) and an introductory visit to the ward area, accompanied by a member of the paediatric team who knows them. It may be helpful to have a liaison nurse or another professional in a similar position to act as a link between the paediatric and adult teams, as well as joint visits by paediatric and adult nurses and therapists, so that there is a smooth handover and continuity. Psychological support, provided before and during the transfer, should be continued while the young person settles into the new environment.

Developing smooth systems for transfer to adult services should be possible for conditions where a relatively large proportion of paediatric patients reach adulthood. Some adult respiratory physicians, for example, have developed a special interest in the care of young adults with cystic fibrosis [22,23] and there are also specialist clinics for adults with congenital heart disease [24]. The most difficult young people to place in adult services are those with disorders that do not fit easily into a disease–specific or system–specific category. For example, it can be difficult to identify the most appropriate team to take on a young adult with cerebral palsy, gastro-oesophageal reflux, a gastrostomy and deteriorating lung function. They may be transferred to at least three different adult teams, with no obvious physician in overall charge of management. It may be that the family doctor is the most appropriate professional to oversee and co-ordinate the continuing care of these young adults, if they are willing and able to provide the extra time and commitment needed. The family doctor should continue to be supported by paediatric services during the transition.

It can be equally difficult to find an appropriate team to take on young adults with rare disorders, particularly when they have outlived their predicted life expectancy. Because of the relatively small numbers of patients involved it is unlikely that there will be adult physicians or community services with sufficient experience and expertise to manage them confidently. The development of central specialist services for these patients would enable them to receive care locally, with a central service and providing the specialist input to oversee their care [25].

The needs of professional staff and carers [1]

Young adults are a unique group to work with, yet in most countries there is no career structure in medicine, nursing or allied professions specifically for this age group. Professionals and carers may come from a range of back-grounds, with experience of working with children or adults or people with cognitive impairment or mental health problems. Some teams, for example, children's community nursing teams or adult palliative care teams, may only occasionally work with young adults. Where possible, there should be a dedicated member of the team who takes a specific interest in this age group, who can take a lead role in the care of the young person, educating and supporting other members of the team.

Whatever their background, staff working with young adults must have an interest in, and a commitment to, working with this age group, as well as the ability to communicate and empathize. Young people often like to be cared for by young staff, who they may find less threatening and easier to relate to. They also like to have a choice of male or female carers. Young men, particularly if they need assistance in their personal care, often value the availability of male staff.

Staff must have a wide range of basic knowledge and competencies to work with young adults. Recommendations from *Palliative Care for Young People aged 13–24 years* [1] include skills and understanding of:

- The developmental stages of normal adolescence
- The rights of young people, issues around consent, and ethical dilemmas
- The effects of loss and bereavement
- Work with reference to families, partners, and close friends
- The needs of siblings
- Cultural diversity
- Spiritual needs—religious and secular approaches
- Liaison with school and college
- Communication skills, focusing on particular issues, in addition to listening skills and non-verbal communication
- Management of non-adherent behaviour
- Management of emotional involvement
- Counselling
- Advocacy.

Essential experience for those working with young adults, recommended in *Palliative Care for Young People aged 13–24 years* [1], should include:

- Experience in the community, to gain experience of care in different locations, an insight into family problems and the diversity of professionals involved.
- Experience in a specialist unit, providing care for diseases such as muscular dystrophy, cystic fibrosis or cancer, where care is co-ordinated from the hospital.
- Attachment to a children's hospice or an associated primary care team to gain experience of a wide cross-section of life-limiting conditions and to have the opportunity to spend time with the parents.
- An opportunity to acquire counseling and communication skills (e.g. through attachment to psychology or to a palliative care team).
- A training placement to gain knowledge of physical symptom control, perhaps with a paediatric or adult palliative care team.

Individual and team support for those working with young adults is essential. The powerful feelings young people often need to explore, grieving future losses and trying to make sense of their life in the context of illness and premature death, can be emotionally draining for staff, especially if the young person chooses one member of staff to confide in. Staff may find the work raises questions about their own mortality and purpose in life. Young, less experienced staff may find it particularly hard to cope with the emotional demands of caring for this age group and will need regular support and supervision. Self-awareness and maintenance of professional boundaries is essential, to avoid responding to young people as social friends or, in the case of older staff, responding as though the young person was their own child.

Service development [1]

Palliative care strategies should take into account the wide range of disorders encountered in life-limited young adults. Those responsible for planning services should carry out a local needs assessment, specifically including and defining the care of young people with life-limiting conditions when developing their palliative care strategies. Services must be multidisciplinary and multi-agency, but with a clearly identified professional to lead and co-ordinate services.

Each young adult should have a named key worker who has specialist knowledge and training to support their specific needs. This should include addressing the spiritual and psychological issues as well as the practical and medical concerns. The key worker should know what services the young person needs, their availability and how to access them. They should support the young person to be as independent as possible, with the ability to organize their own systems of clinical and social support.

The transition to adult service should be facilitated by early multidisciplinary planning that includes the young person. They should be supported through this transition by their key worker from the paediatric team and passed on to the worker who will maintain this role in the future. While there is a need for central specialist clinics for young adults with conditions rarely seen in adulthood, adult consultant medical physicians also need to develop expertise in the care of these young people. Primary care teams should have opportunities to receive training in palliative care and in supporting the transition to adult services.

Appropriate respite care needs to be more readily available, with clear and easy routes of access. Social opportunities should be provided, both within a respite setting and in the community. Each young person must be assessed and provided with appropriate aids for independence, planned in advance so that these are available when needed. A proper system of purchasing,

maintaining, upgrading, and replacing aids and equipment must be in place and monitored.

Well co-ordinated multidisciplinary and multiagency support to achieve educational goals is essential. This should include career advice and assistance to attend higher education or access employment. Links between further education or employment and occupational therapists could be extremely helpful.

Above all, flexibility and choice in service provision is important, with the young person making decisions whenever possible.

Summary

The transition from childhood to adulthood occurs over a number of years and is characterized by hormonal, physical, emotional, and cognitive change. The purpose of this change is to develop an individual who is autonomous and functions effectively within a community. Even in the presence of life-limiting illness and deteriorating physical and/or cognitive ability many of these changes will continue and must be supported.

For the life-limited young person the transition to adulthood is fraught with difficulty. While cognitive and emotional changes drive them to pursue individuality and independence, their opportunities to experience and achieve this are limited. The adolescent sense of immortality and freedom that shapes one's future is often replaced by increasing dependence and the reality of what will never be achieved. It is important that they are viewed as young people first, and as being unwell second. They need opportunities to take part in 'normal' adolescent activities, with people their own age and to socialize with healthy peers as well as others with life-limiting illness. This is essential to continuing development.

Staff working with young people must be dedicated to working with this age group and should have a wide range of basic knowledge and competencies. They should be able to support the young person through the transition to adulthood and to help them achieve as much autonomy as possible. Transfer to adult services is an important step in this transition, and should be well co-ordinated and planned in advance, identifying appropriate services to smoothly take on the continuing care. Alongside this, young people should be given the opportunity to take an increasing role in responsibility for, and decisions regarding, their own health care, as well as other aspects of their own life. It is important that staff are aware of the difficulties faced in 'normal' adolescence and how life-limiting illness impacts on these, not only for the young person, but also for their family and carers. They must also be aware that many families and carers need support to allow the young person to make the transition to adulthood, recognizing what can be achieved as well as what can not.

Whatever a young person's abilities or potential, the physical and emotional changes of early adulthood must be acknowledged. In the face of life-limiting illness, well co-ordinated multidisciplinary and agency support is essential to help a young person achieve the goals of transition to adulthood, and to support them as they face the reality of goals that cannot be achieved.

References

1. Palliative Care for Young People aged 13–24 years. Report of the Joint Working Party of Association for Children with Life-threatening or Terminal Conditions and their Families (ACT), National Council for Hospice and Specialist Palliative Care Services, Scottish Partnership Agency for Palliative and Cancer Care (SPAPCC).

2. Hamburg, B.A. Psychosocial development. In S.B. Friedman, M.M. Fisger, S.K. Shonberg, E.M. Alderman, eds. *Comprehensive Adolescent Health Care* (2nd edition). St Louis, MO: Mosby; 1998, pp. 38–49.

3. Russell-Johnson, H. Adolescent survey. *Paediatr Nurs* 2000;12(6):15–19.

4. Evans, M. Teenagers and cancer. *Paediatr Nurs* 1993;5(1):14–15.

5. David, R., and Freyer, D.O. Care of the dying adolescent. *Pediatrics* 2004;2:381–8.

6. Glendinning, C. and Kirk, S. High-tech care: High skilled parents. *Paediatr Nurs* 2000;12(6): 25–7.

7. Harrison, C., Kenny, N.P., Sidarous, M., and Rowell, M. Bioethics for clinicians: Involving children in medical decisions. *Can Med Assoc J* 1997;156(6):825–8

8. Weithorn, L.A. and Campbell, S.B. The competency of children and adolescents to make informed treatment decisions. *Child Dev* 1982;53:1589–98.

9. 'Nicky's Story' The personal diary of Nicky Allsop, a teenager with cancer (unpublished). Reproduced with the permission of her family, and in accordance with Nicky's wishes that her diary could be used to help other young adults.

10. Bluebond-Langner, M. *In the Shadow of illness.* Princeton, NJ: Princeton University Press, 1996.

11. Whyte, F. and Smith, L. A literature review of adolescence and cancer. *Eur J Cancer Care* 1997; 6:137–46.

12. Cooper, L.B. Potentially fatal illness. In S.B. Friedman, M.M. Fisher, S.K. Shomberg, E.M. Alderman eds. *Comprehensive Adolescent Health Care* (2nd edition). St Louis, MO: Mosby, 1998, pp. 142–6.

13. Sourkes, B. *The Deepening Shade: Psychological Aspects of Life-Threatening Illness.* Pittsburgh, PA: University of Pittsburgh Press, 1982.

14. Hart, D. and Schneider, D. Spiritual care for children with cancer. *Semin Oncol* 1997;13(4): 263–70.

15. Prewett, B. *Short-Term Breaks. Long-Term Benefit. Family-Based Short-Term Care for Disabled Children and Adults.* Sheffield: University of Sheffield, Institute for Social Service Research, 1999.

16. Edwards, J. A model of palliative care for the adolescent with cancer. *Int J Pall Nurs* 2001;7(10):485–8.

17. Viner, R. Transition from paediatric to adult care. Bridging the gaps or passing the buck? *Arch Dis Child* 1999;81:271–5.

18. Schidlow, D. and Fiel, S. Life beyond pediatrics. Transition of chronically ill adolescents from pediatric to adult health care systems. *Med Clin North Am* 1990;74:1113–20.

19. Blaum, W.R. Transition to adult health care: Setting the stage. *J Adolesc Health* 1995;17:3–5.

20. Sawyer, S., Blair, S., and Bowes, G. Chronic illness in adolescents: transfer or transition to adult services? *J Paediatr Child Health* 1997;33:88–90.

21. Rosen, D.S. Transition from Pediatric to adult-oriented health care for the adolescent with chronic illness or disability. *Adolesc Med* 1994;5(2):241–8.

22. Madge, S. and Byron, M. A model for transition from pediatric to adult care in cystic fibrosis. *J Pediatr Nurs* 2002;17(4):283–8.

23. Nasr, S., Campbell, C., and Howatt, W. Transition program from pediatric to adult care for cystic fibrosis patients. *J Adolesc Health* 1992;13:682–5.

24. Grown-up congenital heart (GUCH) disease: current needs and provision of service for adolescents and adults with congenital heart disease in the UK. Report of the British Cardiac Society Working party. *Heart* 2002;88 (Suppl. 1): i1–14.

25. Somerville, J. *Services for Young People with Chronic Disorders in Their Transition From Childhood to Adult Life.* London: Royal College of Physicians of London.

10 Children expressing themselves

Trygve Aasgaard

Aiding communication between child, family, and carers

It is easy to fall into the trap of thinking of communication, as though it were only one way, from adults to children, with factual content only. In fact it is always two way, for even if an adult gives some information to a child there will be some feedback from the child's response [1].

People caring for children with life-threatening diseases may be more concerned about 'what to say to the child?' than 'what does the child want to say?'. Sometimes the child's questions and comments come 'out of the blue' or at times when carers feel unprepared to answer. Feelings of sadness and powerlessness may complicate mutual communication with the patient (and parents). 'Bedside manners'[2] and withdrawal from the non-task oriented encounters may temporarily protect the carer, but will certainly hinder dialogues and will also easily be noticed by the child patient. The challenge is often simply doing nothing and just being there; the best carers are probably those who are able to concentrate more on listening than saying the 'appropriate' things, and those who, to some extent, have clarified their own relationship with death and dying.

Facing illness and death

Spending enough time with the individual child is a prerequisite for understanding what the child wants to know and is able to understand. The patient's level of awareness can be seen in play activities, drawings, poems, or song-improvisations. Practical and existential concerns are often closely woven together. Even terminally ill children generally focus on living (and life's good or bad sides), rather than on dying. Glazer and Landreth [3] characterize the child's world as "an experiential world of now"; also in cases when the child has come to accept the inevitability of their death. In general, children, having not reached adolescence, are better equipped than adults to face death because they know how to live life to its fullest today, and do not focus on the lost future.

Carers may be toiling with questions as to what patients ought to be told about the progression of their disease, treatment, and future prospects. Quite often it turns out that the child has understood the situation long before any adult person has said anything:

A 5-year-old boy commented, after having been told that his abdominal cancer had "returned", that he knew this already: he had felt the tumour growing inside his belly. There were no visible signs of the tumour that had been detected on a routine control. For the boy, however, this information was seemingly no surprise [4] (translation by T. Aa.).

Fatally ill children become aware of the seriousness of the illness even when others attempt to keep it a secret (Chapter 7, Children's views of death). They may spend much energy, testing and questioning both their parents and hospital staff and trying their honesty and patience. It is not strange that these patients want to control what can be controlled. They may dislike their parents talking to others outside of their sphere of control, they may want to decide who shall be allowed to enter the sick room, and what shall be talked about in their vicinity. As a rule, the patient ought to know what the carers know, but to inform them about all the details is not always necessary. Nor should siblings be shut out of the dying process 'for their own good'. That will only intensify their pain and confuse them [5]. The patient must be allowed to control what she or he wants to know, and carers must respect this. Talking together is most likely to become a real dialogue when it takes place on the child's terms. Lack of language and different interpretations of basic concepts sometimes cause bewilderment or misunderstanding of the message from children's expressions. It is important that carers make sure that their own interpretations are correct.

Glazer and Landreth suggest the following guidelines that can enhance the process of sharing:

• Be open and sensitive to the child

• Allow the child to lead

• Listen with your eyes

- Recognize and accept the child's feelings
- State what you hear verbally and non-verbally
- Allow what the child says or does to be more important than what the adult says
- Recognize that children express grief in different ways (anger, withdrawal)
- Keep responses short and brief
- Don't overwhelm the child with information
- Don't pretend everything is okay [3].

Major threats

One point of departure for approaching the child's potential existential questions is being aware of some of the major threats for children of different ages:

- the first years of childhood: fear of being left alone
- from 4 years old: fear of what might happen to the body
- from 7 years old: fear of losing control
- from about 10 years old: fear of losing self-determination
- teenagers: fear of losing ones life—and future [6].

Children less than 5 years of age seldom are afraid of dying because of their vague conceptions of what it involves to be dead. When younger schoolchildren gradually understand that death is inevitable and strikes all, their fear of death can become intense. Teenagers, like adults, may experience the mentioned threats at different times and without necessarily saying what they think and feel.

Openly expressing one's concerns about illness or death is a right, but not a duty. To acknowledge what is happening does not mean that every subject ought to be talked about. Children and their parents and carers may spend their last days together with a silent, seemingly common understanding of what is going to happen. One cannot claim that the more openly children express their thoughts and feelings, the better their life will become. What is important for carers to know, however, is that their own responses to the children's communicative attempts may influence which thoughts and feelings the child will share with others in the future. Bluebond-Langner [7] discovered that some children did not talk about death because they realised it made the adults around them uncomfortable. Young patients soon learnt how to keep off this taboo subject and rather, tried to cope through being engaged in a mutual pretence. Children often want to protect their parents, and other carers must respect this attitude. I have only met terminally ill children who are constantly blaming or scolding their mother or father at the bedside a couple of times. But children should not be made to feel that

they need to protect adults from pain. If effective mutual communication is to be established, adults must help them to understand that pain and grief are an acceptable part of life, not something to be avoided [3].

Play and artistic activities as normal means of communication

Play, artistic, and musical activities, like different forms of verbal conversations, are all normal elements in children's lives and should, therefore, also be generally encouraged—as long as there is life. Children's first scribbles on paper are the beginnings of their symbol-making capacity, opening the door to emotional expression and representation of images and ideas through graphic means [8]. A human being making any kind of musical sound—improvising, recreating or responding—is expressing intentions that can communicate. The function of music is to enhance in some way the quality of individual experience and human relationships. Man is a musical being from the very beginning. Research on infants' vocal play with their parents shows how they imitate and reciprocate intricately coordinated expressions. Music is much more than just 'non-verbal' or 'pre-verbal', and its use in therapy is based in the life-long human trait of creating companionship with another by structuring expressive time together [9].

Both music and art (here: the creation of images or artefacts), are media for interpersonal, emotional, and aesthetic experiences; they are, however, not only *means* to obtain a specific result, but meaningful activities 'as such'. Creative interactions may be just as marked by *play* fulness as by goal directness and very sick or dying children often surprise their carers through preserving this quality for a very long time. A number of key reports [10, 11] state that specialists in play should be available to children in hospital. Also when terminal care takes place within the home setting, those professionals involved require skills in recognising the play needs of the child and offering appropriate guidance, inspiration or assistance. Encouraging and facilitating playing, according to the age and desire of the patient, even willingness to take part in play (to various degrees), should not only be the realm and responsibility of play specialists, but be in the repertoire of communication for anyone entering the sick room.

Paediatric wards may be abundantly equipped with tools for video-entertainment, PC games and Nintendo. The electronic play-stations are valuable tools for 'killing time', and entertainment for young and old, but as expressive tools alone they are of limited value. Television *can* be used creatively: some paediatric hospitals have their own TV 'stations' where isolated or bed-ridden patients may interact with persons in other parts of the ward/hospital and be socially active if they so please and have the strength.

Because young children are often unable to communicate emotionally meaningful material, solely through verbalisation, the possible emotional pain of the child who is dying may go unrecognised. Through play activities initiated by the patients or their carers those children may be helped to understand and to cope with their life situations, telling their stories, or exploring their questions. Play often seems to make the participants able to see traumatic events and experiences or the here-and-now realities from a little distance, due to its power of altering perspectives. Children use symbolic play, creating an alternative and safe language of self-expression. The use of symbols enables them to transfer anxieties, fears, scary fantasies, and guilt to objects rather than to people [3]. It is, however, important to bear in mind that play is, first of all, many children's natural (and normal) way of interacting with 'the world'—even during hard times when their carers might be overwhelmed by seriousness and powerlessness.

It is particularly challenging trying to meet the expressive needs of teenagers, who are progressively marked by incurable illness. Adolescents, like adults (parents included) may be in great need of playing. How they play is, however, more subtle: they do not simply play, but play football, or date, dance etc. Life in hospital and severe illness restrict activities like that. Finding ways of playing and liberating the *homo ludens* in these patients require carers who, at times, are able to let fantasy take over, to be able to pretend anything 'as if', and just fool about together with these patients. With or without the inspiration from others very sick teenagers momentarily may throw themselves into the playfulness, the childishness, sometimes even the naughtiness of various creative or 'nonsense' activities. Daily life experiences (e.g. related to isolation, bodily problems, or persons in the environment) are often points of departure for slightly crazy or flippant social communication.

Common artistic activities in the sick room may inspire pleasurable *interplay* between the participants. The making of a socially stimulating but secure environment is a prerequisite for the young patients feeling free to express themselves as they wish. At times when patients, as well as their families, are experiencing an extremely insecure and unpredictable life situation, one way of helping the patient is providing room and means for their parents or brothers or sisters to express themselves and even to be involved in playful activities [12,13]. Parents' own attitudes and abilities to play certainly influence how their children find outlets for expression. Observing the inventiveness and readiness for playing that occasionally characterise seriously ill children's families may be a useful experience for professional carers.

On the other hand, the health care team may also act as role models for the sick child and her or his family in 'the art of playing'. Remember that not playing seriously (!) will easily be seen through by any child patient.

Different methods and techniques for aiding expression and understanding including play, music, and art

Carers need to consider which communicative means are at hand, and how the child may be helped to 'say' or to 'do' what he or she wants, and is able to. Because all children are different and constantly developing, and because contexts are changing, there are no standard ways of facilitating expression. Boys employ words and conversations to express problems and feelings less than girls, not least in relation to traumatic experiences. Activity-based conversations may facilitate expression and communication; Dyregrov [14] mentions several possible activities accompanying conversation-like encounters suitable for many boys: for example, playing cards or looking at photo albums during the conversation, telling stories, writing letters on a (portable) PC, or even watching videos. Communication through the arts can usually not replace the use of speech, neither are the artistic codes universal languages, but rather cultural knowledge woven into the children's lives in many ways. In a hospital ward, the presence of toys, musical instruments and art materials counteract an unfamiliar and possibly threatening environment and provide the child with expressive tools always at hand. This is especially helpful, when words are not sufficient while explaining or illustrating events and relationships, expressing feelings, concerns, or dreams. The child artist also gains an important measure of control, as he or she is the creator and foremost expert on his or her own artistic works [8].

Art therapy and music therapy in paediatric palliative care

An interdisciplinary team approach in paediatric palliative care may include the presence of art therapists and music therapists. Since the early 1980s there has been a slowly growing body of literature on the use of art therapy, music therapy, and other creative arts therapies in palliative care. Art therapy with children who have an incurable illness has been documented by relatively few authors [8,15–24]. Music therapy in paediatric palliative care can be divided in two interrelated practices and fields of research: one aiming at reducing specific bodily symptoms, such as pain, nausea or towards having an anxiety reducing effect [25–27], and one mainly focusing on the patient's experiences, spiritual or existential questions, her or his role, communicative and expressive needs [5,28–34]. The patient's *life situation* is just as important here as the symptoms or degree of pathology. Few extensive and systematic research projects on art or music in paediatric care have yet been carried out [35,36].

Basic musical communication

Music therapy interventions with babies or very young children with AIDS, serve to stimulate not only the auditory system but also the tactile. The voice or musical instruments are used to promote sensory stimulation and awareness of the environment—a prerequisite for the development of expressive functions such as independent movements. Rhythm instruments, for example, a triangle or maracas, can be played against the skin to determine preferences and to develop auditory tracking skills. But the most important indication to expose these children to music, during their sometimes very short life span, is the general enjoyment related to musical activities. At the Farano Center, New York, music has also been a means to support caregivers who sometimes feel that they have little to offer the children with AIDS in terms of comfort [31].

Children expressing their concerns through the arts

Free drawings, paintings, or other expressions (ie with no directive given by the therapist) are almost always informative, especially when children reflect their choices of subject and the meaning of artwork [8]. A child's perception of pain may be most accurately expressed through an illustration. Art-based activities and assessments provide information, not only about the patient's feelings about her or his illness, but also about cognitive and developmental maturity, coping styles, and personality. Several specific assessment techniques have been developed [8]. The child may be invited to make, for example, a volcano drawing to understand how she or he manages anxiety. Drawing a bridge may similarly be useful in understanding the child's expectation of the future [37]. Children with cancer symbolically cross many bridges during the course of treatment, and, in some cases from life into death. Councill describes how 'Mike', a 12-year-old boy with leukaemia, made his own pencil drawing of a bridge.

The task was selected to allow him to express how he bridged the gap between the period of his cancer treatment, his life at present, and his hopes for the future. Mike's well-articulated drawing of a bridge shows a past (during initial treatment), full of holes and broken boards, suggesting a very real possibility of falling off the bridge altogether. The middle section, representing the present, appears solid, but the bridge

ends abruptly, leaving the right quarter of the page completely blank. [. . .] His shaky past and relatively solid present make sense in the context of his medical history, but the absence of any future at all is an indication that his expectation of the future—continuing life—may not be possible [8, p. 87].

This reflection of a life between the known and the unknown seems to characterise many drawings by seriously ill children. During the last months of her life a 15-year-old girl creates a drawing of a girl's head where half of the face is hidden in black (see Figure 10.1). The toothed contour of the shadow adds to the uncertainty of whether this blackening describes a static feature or an ongoing process. On the right side of the drawing is written "m m me", an indication of a 'self portrait'? Sometimes, one single picture symbolically presents the child's fatal life situation at the same time as it reflects a search for meaning in the process of illness and death [24].

The use of creative writing techniques encourages older children to verbalize their feelings on paper, such as in poetry [38,39]. Also song—texts written by seriously ill children may be clearly autobiographic, but one should be very careful of uncritically interpreting any art work by a sick person (or any other person), as a personal testimony. Froehlich [40], in her experimental study comparing the effect of music therapy and medical play therapy, on the verbalisation behaviour of 40 paediatric patients, found a significant difference between the two groups. The chi square statistic revealed that music therapy elicited significantly more involved verbalisation about hospitalization, than did the play therapy session. Verbalisation was unrelated to the patient's diagnosis and prior hospitalizations.

Musical improvisation on appropriate instruments may serve both as a *sensorimotor*, concrete form of self-expression, and a highly representational and abstract one. If the child is old and fit enough to use objects to make sounds, instrumental improvisations may both express the physical self and release energy. Occasionally, fatally ill young or old persons become intensely involved in improvisational activities, also at times when their carers believe they lack the required strength to do so. Improvisations can be understood as projections of the patient's inner world or as metaphors for conscious experience [41].

Looking for resources

Working with the arts aiding understanding and expression may start with a defined problem that ought to be looked into or, by contrast, with the patient's healthy sides or interests as points of departure. Being involved with the arts often add new elements to the participants' lives: very sick children may discover and appreciate (unexpected) talents, reach new levels or fields of understanding and experience moments of

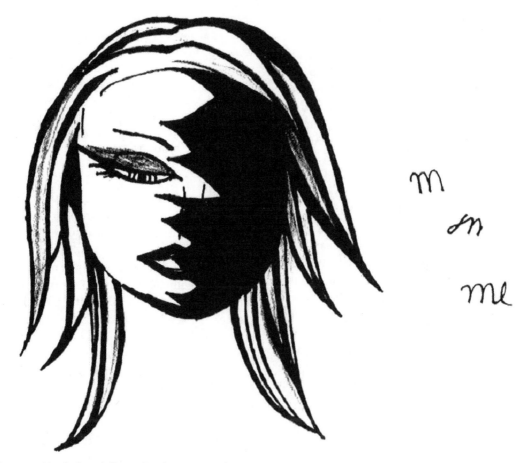

Fig. 10.1 Self portrait: Head of a girl. (Printed with permission.)

pleasure. Carers must enduringly nurture the children's healthy sides but also be brave enough to face up to the harsh realities of these children's lives and their often hopeless, desperate, or utterly pessimistic expressions. Sometimes it is right to challenge the patient's skills—children like to express and show others their normality—even during hard times. Parents may even be surprised to be asked about a seriously ill child's healthy side. One mother commented, after having been asked about her son's resources, this was the first time someone in the paediatric oncology ward had asked what her son was good at!

There are many ways of triggering the patient's expressive resources: for example carers may ask the child if she or he wants to share a song, a game or tell a story. Sometimes it helps the child if this question first, is directed to the accompanying parents.

'Kala', an 8-year-old girl of African origin, has inoperable abdominal metastases and large amounts of ascites that must regularly be removed from her peritoneal cavity. Even though she is bedridden and generally marked by fatigue, Kala has preserved her playfulness and inventiveness. One time, she and her mother teach me (the music therapist) the words and melody of their national anthem. Every new session opens with an examination of my performance of the song: here Kala and her mother are the teachers and me the student. They patiently correct my many mistakes. The patient is given the opportunity to express some of her strengths, and the therapist is being challenged to learn an unfamiliar song.

During the next 2 months Kala's condition deteriorates and her respiration becomes increasingly strenuous, however, she seemingly still appreciates being an active participant in musical activities. One morning I ask her if we should sing *Ba, Ba, Blacksheep*, and Kala insists she will only sing a 'nasty' version (where the sheep is 'farting in a restaurant'). It strikes me that the patient, who is breathing heavily and noisy when talking, sings rather effortlessly. She died 2 weeks later.

What Kala expresses here, is that she still is, in many ways, a normal girl who is having fun and being naughty. Seriously ill children seem to preserve such qualities better than adults. A comprehensive study of song texts created by children and adult patients in cancer care/hospice care, shows that elements of humour are much more predominant in the children and adolescents' songs than in song texts written by adults [36].

Maintaining a sense of humour through times of illness, is a most valuable resource for coping.

'Games' can also be safe outlets for expression. Children with a progressive disease may benefit from taking part in games where they have a fair chance of winning. Pre-school children sometimes enjoy small, improvised competitions with their parents, arranged by the music therapist. Guessing names of familiar songs, or finding the right word, left out in a rhyme or song, may nurture the child's resources and result in pleasurable interactions—particularly when the child is tired and unable to take part in more physically active games. Some children even create and perform their own games, fusing artistic work and elements of play together. Councill gives a vivid account of the *Kingdom of Cancer*, a winding board game created by a 5-year-old girl. The game was drawn on two large sheets of paper and included a very special set of dice. In this case, the rules of the game were made up by the patient herself, then dictated to and written down by her mother. *Kingdom of Cancer* was an impressive dramatization through words, pictures and play of the girl's own experiences of having cancer and she repeatedly invited other patients to play the game with her. Each player endured many hardships, but eventually made it to the birthday party at the end [8].

Artistic achievements as expressive acts

'Expression' and 'achievement' are often the interrelated aims and results from artistic activities, including when the artist is a terminally sick young person. Hilliard [32] describes his work with a 12-year-old boy diagnosed with AIDS and who is referred to music therapy for increased emotional support following his admission into the hospice program. Both his parents have died of AIDS and he now resides with his maternal grandparents. The boy reveals that he has always wanted to play the trumpet in school, but his family was never able to afford instrument rental. He avoids talking about the deaths of his parents and is initially resistant when the subject is broached. The music therapist formulated the following treatment goals: emotional expression and support, grief support, and increased self-esteem. 'Jamahl' gets a trumpet through the hospice foundation and during the first sessions learns the basic techniques of trumpet playing. His grandmother reports that 'Jamahl hasn't been this happy in years!'.

Case In subsequent music therapy sessions, Jamahl systematically learned to play several tunes on the trumpet. During the playing, he would often stop and talk to the music therapist about emotions and events occurring since the previous session. Jamahl developed trust with the music therapist and was able to express his feelings of grief over the loss of his parents. [...](One) session ended with a song writing activity which used a trumpet solo for

introduction followed by a rap Jamahl wrote about his mother and ended with a trumpet solo. The music therapist, therefore, reinforced the positive memories shared by Jamahl through the song-writing and allowed for the expression of grief. [...]Over time, Jamahl was no longer able to play the trumpet due to increased weakness and fatigue associated with the disease progression. [...]The music therapist offered to play guitar and sing for Jahmal, and the grandmother agreed and sang along. She chose several hymns to sing, as well as the songs Jamahl had learned to play on his trumpet [34, p. 131].

It is not uncommon to see very sick children being overwhelmed with presents from their families. This may not be a problem at all, however, at some point, almost no new gifts seem to please some patients. The best entertainment, for these children, often stems from their own active participation and effort. With the assistance of the music therapist patients can be helped to make 'musical gifts' for their loved ones. One mother of a 'spoilt' 8-year-old critically ill girl said, after having received a cassette recording of her daughter's first own song, this event meant much more to her daughter than any gift she had received. A cassette or a CD with songs, made by the child or teenage patient, may serve as a means of communication between the patient and persons outside the sick room at home or in an institution. In my own practice it is the young patient, sometimes assisted by parents or siblings, who always makes the text. Melody and musical arrangement are, most often, the music therapist's task, but the patient may be involved in this process too, and also in charge of designing the CD- cover. A music therapist involved in similar projects must be able to materialise musical ideas fast: this is one arena where the sick child should not need to wait long to see the result. The child may have the strength and interest to sing at the recording, if not, the music therapist serves as a 'preliminary' stand in. Family members are, as a rule, most willing to participate in one or several of the elements in the song creatiing activities, if the child thinks this is a good idea. Friends, or school-mates who receive the musical greetings (at times with texts addressing named persons) often provide feed-back, sometimes in the form of sending *their* home-made cassettes to the patient. Such expressive interactions can help the young patients to dispaly some of their healthy sides and to develop a creative network wider than the patient–therapist dyad.

Case 'Fred', who is 8 years old and becoming gradually more tired and bed-bound because of an inoperable brain tumour, weekly makes one little non-sense and funny song text. On three consecutive Tuesdays Fred's texts instantly get a melody and are performed by the music therapist, other patients, parents and hospital staff during the weekly singsong in the paediatric department entrance hall. The author himself is lying quietly 'all day' on a bench in the hospital school room or on his bed—he can't stand 'noises' any more—but he appreciates very much being told that other children enjoy and sing his songs.

Often, it does not matter much what the texts 'say' (in Fred's case nothing but 'funny rhymes', I believe). Artistic activities may show other children something one is good at. Fred also tells the world that he still can, at least in some respects, take part in enjoyable activities.

Small or big achievements, like those mentioned above, are also related to *hope*. Short-term goals becomes gradually more important as the expected life-span decreases. Carers must help the child finding goals that are realistic and, to a certain extent, measurable. A child needs some boundaries to obtain a feeling of safety; and boundaries may foster hope. When a child between 6 and 16 is no longer called 'pupil', but 'patient' only, both the child and the parents often seem to interpret this as a sign of hopelessness. This detail may be important even when the child is not able to attend normal school programs.

Nurturing fantasy and pleasurable imagination

Even a child with life limiting illness must be given the opportunity temporarily of expanding her or his role repertoire from that of being a patient: a *homo patiens* who suffers and patiently accepts his fate. 'Fantasy' and 'imagination' are key words here. Some carers arrange "fantasy trips" with bed-bound children: they 'leave' the sick room, 'travel' to distant places and do funny things. A pre school teacher may make daily trips with children, may be to 'Barbie-land', 'Fairytale-land', 'Africa', where they create nice objects, read special stories and listen to music. One paediatric oncology nurse–specialist claims that fantasy trips like these seem to have the power of temporarily carrying severely ill children to places where they are everything but patients [4]. A music therapist may use a keyboard (often storing sounds like helicopter, sea waves, telephone bell, steam train etc.) to perform the most far reaching adventures. If the child has the strength and interest, she or he pushes the buttons, sings or plays (more or less) simple phrases on the keyboard or improvise freely. Parents or other persons in the room can also be drawn into these performances that may serve as an opening to verbal dialogues and wishful thinking and act as 'times-out' from the harsh realities.

Music and art therapists often have a variety of communicative means in their *repertoire*. Stories and fairy tales have the quality of providing a form and frame of understanding for the child's own concerns and expressive needs; they can be used alone or in combination with music or art-work. The German music therapist Friederike von Hodenberg illustrates this in a case illustration about the 4-year-old 'Florian'. After all curative cancer treatment has failed and the patient has moved back home, the music therapist continues to visit the critically ill boy. She writes:

From now on I worked with Florian, his mother and other members of his family. Florian never allowed me to play the Lyre again. Whilst he never gave a reason for this decision, I believe that it might have reminded him of his life in hospital. Instead, I decided to tell him the story of *The Little Prince* [42]. Through the dialogue I offered Florian the opportunity to talk about his concepts of dying. It transpired that the important theme was of the Prince being in heaven. In the story, the Prince comes to earth to find friends. When he eventually finds them he returns to heaven. I began to realise that this story mirrored Florian's life and impending death. At one point in the story Florian remarked, *I believe there are more "little humans" in heaven than on earth.* [. . .] During his last days Florian only wanted to hear the beginning of the story. I repeated it at least ten times, concentrating on the tone-quality of my voice as a means to calm and relax him [29, p. 63].

Sometimes the young patients temporarily or permanently lose the strength to say or do much themselves, but they may still appreciate passively taking part in play activities, music making or art work. When this happens, carers who know the patient well can continue similar activities from their bed-side position. As long as the child is awake one can, most often, sense if the ongoing activity appears meaningful and beneficial to the child. An artistically gifted 14-year-old severely anorectic and fatigued girl, who just could whisper a word or two when spoken to, could sit for hours observing how a young nurse was drawing cute rabbits, in various situations, on a sheet of paper. The nurse had seen many of the patient's earlier, humorous drawings, she knew her preferences and style, and now she was able to follow up some of this. The nurse's drawings became a kind of common enterprise for the two of them. A pre-school teacher, play therapist (or any of the health care team) may play, more or less 'alone', with cars or dolls on a blanket in front of the patient in bed.

The 4-year-old boy, Peter, is lying on his side, with closed eyes. His tummy is large, his limbs are very thin. I have placed myself quite close to Peter, improvising very quietly on a pentatonic (five-note scale) lyre. The mother is also in the room. Her tears are flowing. No words are spoken by any of us. After a time, Peter opens one eye and looks at me. I am surprised. He is, perhaps, less unconscious than I have been thinking. Familiar with Peter's musical preferences, I whisper to him: "Shall we sing *Hocus-pocus*"? I believe he is nodding. As softly as I can, I start singing about the jack-in-the-box. Peter interrupts me: "The blanket, the blanket"! I have forgotten to cover his head with a blanket. (In this song the child that is chosen to be the jack-in-the-box is hidden under some kind of cover. The Swedish song ends with the words "come forward!", The jack-in-the-box emerges suddenly, and all bystanders are, of course, highly surprised.) I cover Peter's head halfway with his sheet, sing the song with a brittle lyre accompaniment and remove the sheet most carefully at the end. Peter smiles for a second, but shortly after he closes his eyes again [33].

An ecology of love

If music has been an integral part of the child's life, it can be a significant element to help the transition to death [30]. When a dying child's favourite song is being sung in the sick room, this performance may have a *representative* function of the patient's wishes or dreams and need for expression. In the case of Peter it is difficult to evaluate who benefited most from this very modest play activity: the mother or the child. Who is 'giving' and who is 'receiving' are probably less interesting questions than to search out which *meanings* can be related to these acts or events. Peter's mother's experience was to see that her little boy preserved some 'normality' to the last day of his life. For some moments he was not *just* a child with incurable cancer. The above example tell of a dying child's last expressive act, and other parents' accounts from the last period of their children's lives often focus on similar acts of creativity, playing, their very often simple enjoyments, or simply humorous events. Aspects like those mentioned here give us a more complete picture of the lost child, underlining his or her humanness, childishness, and not the least: the child's preserved healthy sides . . . in the middle of sickness and the process of death.

When people are approaching death the feeling of loneliness can be overwhelming. Singing together certainly helps many experience that they are not alone. Singing together is a strong demonstration of *being* together. At the deathbed of the beloved person the singing together means being active participants. The musical activity can soothe as well as support the mourners and it can promote more or less collective deep and meaningful life experiences. One general aim is to foster an interplay of loving acts between patient, family and professsional carers. We can still discuss 'healing consequences' even when a prolongation of life is out of reach. Healing is done at a variety of levels, not just for the individual, but within an ecology of relationships [43].

References

1. Lansdown, R. *Children in Hospital: A Guide for Family and Carers.* Oxford: Oxford University Press,1996.
2. Jourard, S.M. *The Transparent Self.* New York: D van Nostrand Company,1975.
3. Glazer, H.R. and Landreth, G.L. A developmental concept of dying in a child's life. *J Humanistic Educ Dev* 1993;31: 98–105.
4. Saevig, B.I. *Når barn dør. Psykososial omsorg i terminalfasen.* Oslo: Den Norske Kreftforening, 1999.
5. Froehlich, M.-A. Music therapy with the terminally ill child. In M.-A. Froehlich, ed. *Music Therapy with Hospitalized Children.* Cherry Hill, NJ: Jeffrey Books, 1996.
6. Tamm, M. *Hälsa och sjukdom i barnens värld.* Liber, Stockholm, 1996.
7. Bluebond-Langer, M. *The Private Worlds of Dying Children.* Princeton, NJ: Princeton University Press, 1978.
8. Councill, T. Art Therapy with Pediatric Cancer Patients. In C. Malchiodi, ed. *Medical Art Therapy with Children.* London: Jessica Kingsley Publishers,1999.
9. Trewarthen, C. and Malloch, S.N. The dance of wellbeing: defining the musical therapeutic effect. *Nordic J Music Ther* 2000;9;2:3–17.
10. Department of Health. Hospital Play Staff. Executive Letter EL (92) 42, London,1991.
11. Hogg, C. *Health Services for Children and Young People.* Action for Sick Children, London,1996.
12. Aasgaard, T. Music environmental therapy in hospice and paediatric oncology wards. In D. Aldridge, ed. *Palliative Music Therapy.* London: Jessica Kingsley,1999.
13. Aasgaard, T. A Suspiciously cheerful lady: A study of a song's life in the paediatric oncology ward, and beyond. *Br J Music Ther* 2000;14(2):70–82.
14. Dyregrov, A. *Barn och Trauma.* Lund, Studentlitteratur, 1997.
15. Bach, S. Spontaneous paintings of severely ill patients. *Acta Psychosoma;*8:1–66.
16. Bach, S. Spontaneous pictures of leukemic children as an expression of the total personality, mind and body. *Acta Paedopsychiat* 1975;41 (3):86–104.
17. Perkins, C. The art of life-threatened children: A preliminary study. In: R. Shoemaker and S. Gonick-Barris, eds. *Creativity and the Art Therapist's Identity: The Proceedings of the Seventh Annual Conference of the American Art Therapy Association.* Baltimore, MD: AATA,1997.
18. Bertoia, J. *Drawings from a Dying Child.* London: Routledge,1993.
19. Moore, M. Reflections of self: the use of drawings in evaluating and treating physically ill children. In A. Erskine and D. Judd, eds. *The Imaginative Body.* London: Whurr,1994.
20. Lunn, S., Sattaur, A., and Wood, M.J.M. Working with children at Mildmay Mission Hospital. In *HIV/AIDS no time to waste* London: Barnardo's Publications,1995.
21. Sourkes, B. *Armfuls of Time: The Psychological Experience of a Child with a Life-Threatening Illness.* London: Routledge,1996.
22. Pratt, M. and Wood, M.J.M. eds. *Art therapy in palliative care.* London: Routledge,1998.
23. Malchiodi, C. Understanding Somatic and Spiritual Aspects of Children's Art Expressions. In C. Malchiodi ed. *Medical Art Therapy with Children.* London: Jessica Kingsley Publishers,1999.
24. Wolski, M. Das kindliche Ausdrucksbild in der Bearbeitung der Krebserkrankung. *Kunst + Unterricht* 2000;246/247:79–80.
25. Fagen, T.S. Music therapy in the treatment of anxiety and fear in terminal pediatric patients. *Music Ther* 1982;2(1):13–23.
26. Loewy, J. The Use of Music Psychotherapy in the Treatment of Pediatric Pain. In C. Dielo, ed. *Music Therapy & Medicine: Theoretical and Clinical Applications.* Silver Spring, MD: American Music Therapy Association, Inc,1999.
27. Edwards, J. Anxiety Management in Pediatric Music Therapy. In C. Dielo, ed. *Music Therapy & Medicine: Theoretical and Clinical Applications.* Silver Spring, MD: American Music Therapy Association, Inc,1999.

28. Griessmeier, B. and Bossinger, W. *Musiktherapie mit Krebskranken Kindern*. Gustav Fischer Verlag, Stuttgart,1994.

29. von Hodenberg, F. Music Therapy with Patients Undergoing Radiation and Chemotherapy. In C.A. Lee, ed. *Lonely Waters. Proceedings of the International Conference Music Therapy in Palliative Care, Oxford 1994*. Oxford: Sobell Publications,1995.

30. Lane, D. Songs of love: Music therapy can make a difference in the care of dying children. *Hospice*,1996;6:6–8.

31. McCauley, K. Music Therapy with Pediatric AIDS Patients. In M. Froehlich, ed. *Music Therapy with Hospitalized Children.* Cherry Hill, NJ: Jeffrey Books,1996.

32. Dun, B. Creativity and Communication Aspects of Music therapy in a Children's Hospital. In D. Aldridge, ed. *Music Therapy in Palliative Care: New Voices*. London: Jessica Kingsley Publishers,1999.

33. Aasgaard, T. An Ecology of Love: Aspects of Music Therapy in the Pediatric Oncology Environment. *J Palliat Care* 2000;17(3): 177–181 (+Companion CD-rom segment 6).

34. Hilliard, R.E. Music Therapy in Pediatric Palliative Care: Complementing the Interdisciplinary Approach. *J Palliat Care* 2003;19(2):127–33.

35. Bach, S. *Life Paints Its Own Span*. Einsiedeln: Daimon Verlag,1990.

36. Aasgaard, T. *Song Creations by Children with Cancer—Process and Meaning*. [doctoral dissertation] Aalborg University: Institute of Music and Music Therapy,2002.

37. Hays, R.E. and Lyons, S. The bridge drawing: a projective technique for assesment in art therapy. *Arts Psychother* 1981;8:207–17.

38. Lewis, N. I probably won't have all the luxuries in the world. *J Assoc Care of Children's Health* 1978;8:28–32.

39. Sweeny, L. and Zingher, G. Hospitalization enhances creativity. *J Assoc Care of Children's Health* 1979;7:14–16.

40. Froehlich, M.-A. A comparison of the effect of music therapy and medical play therapy on the verbalization behavior of pediatric patients. *J Music Ther* 1984;21(1):2–15.

41. Bruscia, K.E. *Improvisational Models of Music Therapy*. Springfield, IL: Charles C. Thomas Publisher,1987.

42. de Saint-Exupérym, A. *The Little Prince*. London: Pan Books Ltd,1982.

43. Aldridge, D. *Music Therapy Research and Practice in Medicine: from out of the Silence*. London: Jessica Kingsley Publishers,1996.

11 School

Isabel Wood

Introduction

School plays a unique role in our society, immensely contributing to the social, emotional, aesthetic, and physical development of children. School programmes promote the development of mutual respect, cooperation and social responsibility, and emphasize the worth of each individual. Also the school is the only public institution whose primary role is fostering the cognitive development of young people.

Some might wonder why a child not expected to live beyond the teenage years would bother learning algebra or studying Julius Caesar. Others might question the value of a child with a metabolic disease which limits his ability to communicate or learn how to read and write, being involved in classroom activities. This chapter will look not only at why education can and should play an important role in the lives of children with progressive life-limiting illnesses, but also at the unique challenges faced by educators as they work collaboratively with health care providers to deliver a quality educational experience for these children.

A glossary of terms that are specific to the educational setting is included at the end of this chapter.

Rationale

Why educate children who have progressive life-limiting illnesses?

Every child has a legal right to an education. Numerous influential documents have been released over the past 50 years concerning the education of children with disabilities [1].

- The Universal Declaration of Human Rights, passed by the United Nations in 1948, declared the 'inherent dignity and inalienable rights of all members of the human family', and stated that everyone has the right to a free, compulsory education [2].

- The Convention on the Rights of the Child, adopted in 1989, reaffirmed these rights in Article 23 which states that children with disabilities should not only receive an education but should have effective access to education [3].

- In 1990, the World Declaration on Education for All was ratified by UNESCO, and stated in Article 3 that 'the learning needs of the disabled demand special attention'.

- The guiding principle of the Salamanca Statement of 1994 [4] stated that 'schools should accommodate all children regardless of their physical, intellectual, social, emotional, linguistic or other conditions'.

- The ACT Charter for Children with Life-threatening or Terminal Conditions and their Families states that every child shall have access to education [5].

- National Council for Hospice and Specialist Palliative Care Services states that, 'provision of education to sick children is essential and a legal entitlement'. [6]

Besides being the right of every child, education or going to school is a normal part of a child's life. Going to school for a child could be equated to going to work for an adult. School can provide not only the routines so important to children but can even provide a purpose for daily living. The child has a reason to get out of bed each morning and an important job to do. Besides providing purpose, being involved in this important job can also provide distractions from the worries of illness.

It is important for children to be viewed by themselves and their peers as 'normal'. Children have a strong desire to be like other children and do what other children do. A child who has suffered physical or intellectual losses may not be able to run like other children or read at the same level but he can participate in parallel activities and participate in classroom activities which not only help him to view himself as being normal but help other children to view him as their equal. A child who does not have the energy to stay at school all day may be able to participate in a subject that is important to him, thus enabling him to see that there are still possibilities for learning and growth in his life.

Parents also have a need to see their child participate in the normal routines of life. When parents see their child going to school and participating in the normal activities of childhood, even if in a limited way, the day-to-day coping with their child's illness may seem a bit more purposeful and they may be able to celebrate each milestone, however large or small, in their child's life journey.

Children near the end of life sometimes have an even stronger desire to be a part of school as if trying to compress all their learning into their last days or cling to the small threads still connecting them to the normal world of schooling. They may wish to come to a hospice school to do some math but settle for listening to a story when their energy and attention will not allow them to carry out their desires. They may pursue a frantic quest for information on a particular subject and then die that evening or the next day. Right until the end of life children seek to be connected to the world, and for most children participation in schooling represents normality. By normalizing life, schools prolong living rather than postpone dying [7].

Schools offer opportunities for developing friendships and becoming part of a caring community. Peer relationships have a special role in a child's life, which cannot be filled by adults; they give a child the 'possibility of sharing thoughts on an equal basis' [8]. 'Peers lock you into life' [9]. Close peer relationships enrich a child's life with the normal day-to-day interactions of friends and provide a special support to a child who is sick at home or in the hospital. This also helps the child feel connected to the normal world.

School is a place where children can explore, discover, learn, and create, thus developing their abilities more fully. By participating in activities at which they can be successful, children are able to further develop their abilities and are more likely to develop positive self-esteem. Schools today are mandated to provide opportunities for children to succeed regardless of the academic, physical, or emotional level at which they are working. For the child who is ill, it can be especially rewarding to work on and be successful at achieving goals, whether the goal is completing a specific math problem, completing a science project, or graduating from school with their peers [10].

History

The spectrum of progressive life-limiting illnesses from which a child may suffer encompasses a wide variety of diseases and

conditions. Palliative care may extend for weeks, months, or many years [6]. Children who require palliative care, while of school age, range from those working on regular curriculum with little support, to those working on regular curriculum with adaptations, and to those who require major modifications of curriculum. Some of these children will be non-verbal and physically dependent and will require one-on-one full time individual support at school. Nearly all of the children with progressive life-limiting illnesses will qualify as 'students with special needs'. A clearer understanding of the services available for these children within the school system today can be gained by looking at the history of special education and how it has evolved.

Prior to the mid-eighteenth century in Europe, children with disabilities were often neglected, mistreated, and abused. During the nineteenth century, children with disabilities were often rejected by their parents and put in institutions [11]. Such attitudes still prevail in some cultures today as indicated by a parent who recently arrived in Canada from an eastern European country. At a transition meeting for his daughter, the father said, 'In our country it was assumed that we had done something wrong because we have a child with special needs. Coming to Canada has meant that we can share our sorrow and celebrate our joy.'

There are reports of interventions for children with special needs in Spain in the late sixteenth century, but there are no other reports of special needs education in Europe until the mid-eighteenth century. Several pioneer educators in France: de l'Epée, Periere, Hauy, and Seguin not only established schools for children with special needs but also developed methodologies for working with them. These educators could be said to be the 'founders of special education as we know it today' [10]. Following their lead, several schools for children with hearing impairments were opened in North America in the nineteenth century.

During the early years of the twentieth century in North America, children who were confined to wheelchairs, not toilet trained, or considered 'uneducable' were institutionalized or kept at home where they received no formal schooling. By the 1950s, some parents in North America started to arrange for private education of children with moderate disabilities but, for the most part, children with severe disabilities still received no education [12].

The 1944 Education Act in Britain required local education authorities to identify children who required special education services. 'Physically handicapped pupils' and 'delicate pupils', defined as 'children who by reason of impaired physical condition or health or educational development require a change of environment' were categorized, but children thought to be 'uneducable' were not included in the regular school system. It was not until the Act of 1970 that provisions in the regular education system were made for these children [13].

The civil rights movement in the United States during the 1950s and 1960s brought a growing awareness of the rights and human dignity of all individuals. In 1982, David Smith, Chairman of the Special Committee on the Disabled and Handicapped, wrote:

It is precisely in times of economic, political and social strain that the true humanity of a people is proved. In those times, in these present times, a country decides whether it is a nation which includes everyone, or whether it is an economically segregated society, which includes as full members only those who can pay the full price of admission. [14]

The 1970s and 1980s saw legislation being passed that not only ensured the rights of all children to an education but also ensured their right to an education in a regular school setting. In 1975, in the United States, the Education of All Handicapped Children Act was passed. This was followed by various documents such as the Warnock Report in England in 1978, the 1984 report by the Ministry of Education in Victoria, Australia, and the 1991 policy statement of the New Mexico Department of Education all reiterating the right of all children to be educated with their peers [12].

The United Nations issued a number of documents during the 1980s and 1990s which have influenced special education practices around the world [1]. Of particular note is the Salamanca Statement and Framework for Action on Special Needs Education from the World Conference on Special Needs Education held in Spain in June 1994. This statement was approved by delegates from 92 governments and 25 international organizations. The key statements of belief in this document are:

• Every child has a fundamental right to education, and must be given the opportunity to achieve and maintain an acceptable level of learning.

• Every child has unique characteristics, interests, abilities and learning needs.

• Education systems should be designed and educational programmes implemented to take into account the wide diversity of these characteristics and needs.

• Those with special education needs must have access to regular schools, which should accommodate them within a child-centred pedagogy capable of meeting those needs.

• Regular schools with this inclusive orientation are the most effective measures of combating discriminatory attitudes, creating welcoming communities, building an inclusive society, and achieving education for all [15].

As has frequently happened throughout history, theories and declarations do not always translate into practice. As recently as in 1999 there have been reports from countries in central and eastern Europe of children with special needs being marginalized or even excluded from local schools due to both attitudes and economic reasons [16]. Recent findings indicate that in Thailand 70% of children with disabilities do not attend schools [17]. Contrasting this is the observation that in North America and western Europe current practice has involved merging special education and regular education into one system with a focus on meeting individual learning needs [18].

Service delivery models

Choosing an educational placement for a child with palliative care needs can be a very difficult process for parents and professionals. Sometimes the best choice is very clear. Other times, because of the complex needs of the child, the decision is emotionally a very difficult one. Both parents and educational professionals need to be aware that there is seldom an absolutely perfect placement and that compromises have often to be made. Parents, in consultation with the personnel involved in the decision making process, need to consider the available options and evaluate the pros and cons for their child at that particular time. If, after a reasonable trial period, the placement does not appear to be satisfactory or if the child's circumstances change, then parents or teaching staff need to re-evaluate the suitability of the placement.

Integrated settings

In recent years, many school systems have moved away from segregated settings for children with special needs towards integrated settings for all children, especially in the elementary grades. The goal of inclusive classrooms is for each child to be valued as a unique and special individual. Children learn that differences are a part of life and that everyone has gifts that they bring to the diversity of the children within a classroom. Children are able to work together, help each other, and make friends with those whom they might not otherwise have recognized as possible friends. Skillful teachers can guide and direct relationships and understandings, helping each child discover their individual strengths.

The success of inclusion in an integrated setting is dependent on the support provided in the classroom and its quality [19]. Support personnel might include a special education resource teacher, a special education assistant, and appropriate consultants such as psychologists, speech language pathologists, doctors, nurses, occupational and physiotherapists, social workers, and counsellors.

Regular classroom with no support

A small number of children with progressive life-limiting illnesses will not be designated as having special needs and will have placements in a regular classroom with no additional support. This group might include children following a regular curriculum who have developed a life-shortening condition such as cancer. If no physical or academic adaptations or modifications are required to their educational programme, the teacher, with the help of a counsellor, may be able to meet this child's learning needs.

Regular classroom with support personnel

Most children with progressive life-limiting illnesses will qualify for designation as a student with special needs under a health category. This would result in the child having an Individual Education Plan (IEP) which guarantees collaborative planning by teachers, parents, the child if appropriate, and other appropriate personnel. The educational programme for the child should be discussed thoroughly at an initial IEP meeting. Specific goals for the child, along with support and resources required, would be documented in the IEP. The goals, and progress towards their attainment, would be reviewed and evaluated at subsequent IEP meetings throughout each school year.

Many children with progressive life-limiting illnesses will also have a Care Plan, which would include emergency protocols. If the child has a DNR order all members of the educational team would need to be aware of this and the school would need to know procedures to be followed in an emergency situation. A Care Plan would include personal care details such as seating, lifting, feeding, medication schedules, and physiotherapy requirements. It would also include seizure protocol if applicable, and any pertinent transportation requirements.

When a child with mobility difficulties first registers at a school, a site evaluation by a physiotherapist and occupational therapist would occur. A newer facility should be completely wheelchair accessible but might require some changes. For example, a special desk or work area might be needed and a washroom might require adjustments. An older school might not be wheelchair accessible from streets and sidewalks around the school, and for parking spaces from which a child may be safely dropped off in a wheelchair. Classrooms, playground, drinking fountains, door handles, blackboards, and elevator buttons all need to be wheelchair accessible. In both new and old schools the design of the classroom would be assessed to ensure there is space for the child and the equipment he might require, such as a walker, a standing frame, oxygen, or suctioning equipment. Following this assessment, any necessary adjustments would need to be made.

When applicable the special education assistant or SEA working with the child and a backup staff member would be trained by a physiotherapist and occupational therapist in all

aspects of care particular to that child. This might include feeding, transferring, or seizure management. For a child on a ventilator or who has specialized health care needs the assistant working with the child must have appropriate medical training. In some instances two assistants may be required, one for medical needs and one for educational needs. Ideally one person would have both sets of required skills.

A child on a *regular* programme may need curricular *adaptations* for written output only and may require SEA assistance for only certain types of assignments. An assistant may work in other classrooms for part of the time or may assist other children in the same classroom, depending on the number of assistants and the number of children with special needs at the school.

There are a wide variety of adaptations which may be used with students depending on the difficulties they are experiencing. Adaptations can include:

- using extra thick pencils
- using a specialized device to hold papers or books in a visible position
- using a computer
- scribing by an adult or peer
- using photocopied sheets rather than copying from a book
- reducing amount of written work a child is expected to complete
- breaking assignments into smaller components
- providing alternate ways of presenting assignments such as posters, pictures, audio or video recordings, designing games or puzzles
- scribing tests or allowing the child to record answers onto a tape
- allowing more time for assignments and tests.

Teachers and children will find their own ways of overcoming barriers to successful learning.

With the availability of special adaptations such as track balls, joy sticks, adapted or on-screen keyboards, a computer can often be a key piece of equipment in enabling communication and learning to take place. Word prediction programmes, programmes that use words and symbols, art programmes, and programmes with voice output have all widened the scope of what is possible for children. In some jurisdictions, children will qualify for the loan of adaptive technology through special education technology resource centres. The mandate of such resource centres is to assist children with physical disabilities in reaching their individual potentials with the aid of technological devices.

For a child on a *modified* programme, extensive planning is required to develop age-appropriate activities which parallel those of the regular curricula and allow the child to develop skills at his own level. For instance, if a class were studying Ancient Egypt in social studies, a child at an emerging reading and writing level might be able to participate fully in oral discussions, learn from watching videos, and participate in many cooperative group activities. Concepts that are most readily developed through reading might be approached using sources at a simpler level. Instead of requiring that the child submit a written report he might be able, with assistance, to construct a model of a pyramid to submit as his project.

The classroom teacher, special education resource teacher, and special education assistant would work together to plan age-appropriate activities that allow the child on a modified programme to interact positively with his peers but at the same time take into consideration the types of materials from which he learns best. This is a task that becomes increasingly more complex as the child progresses through the intermediate and secondary grades. As children requiring a modified programme become older, the gap between the development of a child and that of his typical classmates may widen, and more class time tends to be spent on highly academic 'paper and pencil' centred activities. This necessitates even more careful planning to enable the child to attain his educational goals in a regular classroom.

A significant number of children with progressive life-limiting illnesses are *non-verbal*. Some have not developed a system of communication while others have developed communication skills but are losing these because of the progress of their illness. These children will require a thorough assessment by a communication development team specialized in augmented or assistive technology. Such a team often includes an occupational therapist as well as a speech language pathologist. Following an assessment, this team will recommend a communication training programme with either low or high technological equipment depending on the communication level of the child and his motor skills. The team will look at how the child is communicating currently, assess whether the child is able to move to the next stage with practice, and consider which parts of his body the child can move most reliably. Communication devices that can be adapted to operate under the control of almost any muscle group are becoming more widely available. For some children the most reliable body part might be a hand, for others it might be their head, eyes, mouth, feet, or knees. The child may be working at a very basic stage, choosing objects by looking and reaching for them. Others may use eye pointing, looking at objects to make real life choices about the activities they wish to participate in (Figure 11.1). Some children may be developing an understanding of cause

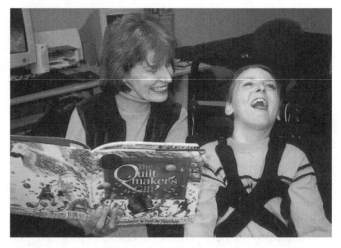

Fig. 11.1 A non-verbal student can choose a story by eye pointing and can communicate his enjoyment of the story through body language. (Reproduced with permission of the family.)

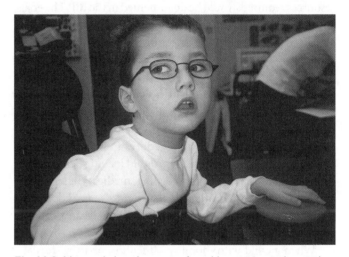

Fig. 11.2 Non-verbal students are often able to use a single switch to activate electronic devices or a computer program. (Reproduced with permission of the family.)

and effect and, with sufficient hand control, be able to use a single switch designed to activate a variety of electronic devices such as a tape deck, popcorn maker, blender, or toy. Others may be able to activate devices with prerecorded messages. Some non-verbal children recognize pictures or symbols and are able to use a simple communication board to make choices. Some children may be learning to scan while others might be using a more elaborate communication device or a programme on a computer (Figure 11.2). Once a device is chosen, intensive time and structured individual work with a speech language pathologist is required. After skills are introduced to a student, they can be practiced and used in the classroom in real life situations. Peers can be wonderful motivators, giving the child a purpose for using the new skills they are acquiring.

Some children have sufficient hand coordination and dexterity to use standard or a modified form of sign language. A teacher might arrange for someone fluent in sign language to come into the classroom to teach other children basic sign language skills. Sometimes a parent of a child who uses sign language is able and willing to do this.

Some children have sufficient coordination to use laser pointers enabling them to point to an appropriate response on a page, to a printed word that they do not understand, or to communicate a choice they have made. Other children are able, through intensive practice with a trained professional, to learn complicated language systems such as 'minspeak', which enables them to use more sophisticated modes of communication. A head mouse, which looks like a small dot attached to a child's forehead, can be used to point to letters and symbols on the screen of a computer which then produces a written message with voice output. This device can give a child independence and power. Not only can ideas and thoughts be shared but the child is able to plan, store, and present oral presentations. Questions can be asked in class discussions and the child can even interject with amusing comments. The child can move from a world of isolation to a world of new possibilities.

Some children have had normal functioning before the onset of a degenerative illness which either has taken or is taking communication and motor functioning away. These children often experience tremendous frustration and isolation. They previously have been able to communicate with their friends and have been able to participate in academic endeavours as well as activities such as swimming, gymnastics, and playing the piano. Now they are confined to wheelchairs, either losing or already having lost speech and motor function, and often needing to relearn skills to adapt to their current capabilities. Most of these children want desperately to participate with their peers whether by going to a textiles or foods class, choosing the colors of a T shirt, or deciding what to cook. Most are able to enjoy art and music activities with their peers and the social times at breaks and lunch hour.

Regular class and resource room

Many educational jurisdictions have resource teachers or special education resource teachers who give support to children with special needs either in the classroom or as a pull-out programme in a resource room. The classroom teacher is still responsible for the child's overall educational programme but the resource teacher has an opportunity to meet individual needs in a small group setting. The child might receive instruction in reading and writing, or math skills. He might receive assistance with projects or work that he has missed as a result of absences due to his illness. The resource room offers a

setting which can be less distracting and less competitive. It is often a place children can use if the classroom becomes too overwhelming [10]. Here, the resource teacher can listen to individual children and can help them problem solve and develop skills to cope with everyday school life. Resource teachers are sometimes able to offer support to children before and after school and resource rooms are often places where children feel comfortable hanging out during breaks. At the secondary level, structured peer tutoring programmes are often provided to give children an opportunity to receive further assistance as well as the opportunity to interact with their peers in a supportive, structured environment.

Alternative settings

Special classes

Until the 1960s, the most common way of serving children with special needs was through placement in a special class [10]. Some parents of children who are not able to follow a regular curriculum as a result of a progressive life-limiting illness prefer that their child be accommodated in a special class. These classes usually have teachers with special education training. Typically they have a smaller than usual class size and additional support such as special education assistants. The educational programme offered can be geared to meet specific needs such as life or communication skills. When choosing a placement for children, the educational and parent teams involved often find these classes to be more appropriate for secondary-aged children than a regular placement. In these classes it is possible for children to spend more time working on their individual goals than might be the case in an integrated setting. Additional services such as speech language therapy, communication support, physiotherapy, and nursing support may be more readily available than in a regular setting. Some parents believe that their child benefits from being with and making friends with children at a similar developmental level.

Some children who have been in an integrated setting for elementary school will have a special class placement for secondary school. At the secondary level it becomes increasingly difficult to modify material. A child in secondary school might have up to eight different teachers, each of whom might be responsible for part of the educational programme for more than two hundred students. The strong teacher–student relationship which is so important to successful inclusion can be lacking at the secondary level. Also, a child's previous peer group may have scattered. Some special classes provide for reverse integration by having students from regular classes come into the special class as peer tutors or for social interaction.

Part-time special class

Some children will be in a special class for core subjects and will join a regular class for other subjects such as music, art, physical education, foods, or textiles. Sometimes a child is also able to join a regular class for subjects such as computer technology or an alternate English or math class. Children in special classes at the secondary level usually appreciate the opportunity to be in regular classes with peers whom they may know from their elementary school.

Special day school

Some parents choose to have their child attend a special school, which can offer small classes, specialized services, and opportunities to progress with less pressure or stress than might be encountered in a regular school. These schools often cater to a particular population and offer nursing care and therapy. Some of these schools are privately operated and can be very expensive. One disadvantage of this type of school is that the children do not have the opportunity to socialize with children in a regular school environment.

Special residential school

Residential schools were once common. They were frequently provided for children who were hearing or visually impaired or who were cognitively lower functioning. Residential schools still exist for specific populations such as hearing or visually impaired [10]. In Vancouver, Canada there are currently two short-term-stay residential schools designed for assessment and rehabilitation following brain injury, neurological damage, stroke, or trauma from, for example, traffic accidents. Because children who stay at residential school are separated from their families, some residential schools encourage the child to live at home and commute to the school each day if possible [10].

Home instruction

Many local education authorities provide home instruction teachers who collaborate with the child's regular school teacher and provide instruction for the child, usually once or twice a week, at their home. This service is frequently accessed by children who are absent from school for significant periods of time due to the progress of their illness. Such children may be undergoing cancer treatment or may not be able to attend school during an outbreak of a communicable disease such as the flu or chickenpox. The home instruction teacher will collaborate with a child's regular school teacher and with parents to develop a programme suitable for the child. Where possible, instruction will follow the curriculum that is being covered in class. Children who have not been able to attend school and are not expected to return due to the progress of their illness

might work on appropriate projects or novel studies which interest and motivate them. The teacher will select and structure activities at which the student can be successful, taking into consideration fatigue and other health issues.

Hospital instruction

Many hospitals have school programmes available for children while they are in hospital. These programmes vary widely but are generally for in-patients, although some hospitals also offer programs for well siblings. On occasion, children might commute to a hospital from home to attend the school programme [20]. The aim of these programmes is to promote continuity of educational programming for children, to give children a sense of normality, to offer developmentally appropriate educational activities with which each child can be successful, and to facilitate successful reentry to school after hospitalization. Hospital programme teachers communicate with medical staff, regular school teachers, and parents to coordinate a programme which meets the child's current needs. Many children with palliative care needs are not well enough to go to a classroom while in hospital but the teacher is often able to come to the child's bedside where they may complete assignments or be read to. Communication is frequently encouraged between the child's classmates and the child in hospital.

Hospice school programmes

A child's right to an education has been acknowledged in the ACT [5] charter and in the Joint Briefing of the National Council for Hospice and Specialist Palliative Care Services [6]. Some pediatric hospices have recognized the importance of continuity of education for a child while at a hospice and have established their own school programmes. Hospices frequently offer respite services to children on a palliative care programme. Children on hospice respite programmes may come to the hospice several times during a school year, often for a week at a time. Having a school programme means that children can continue with their schoolwork while they are at the hospice so that they will not be behind when they return to school. School programs also ensure that children can continue with the normal routines of going to school and can engage in activities at which they can be successful. Any school-aged siblings staying at the hospice with their families may be included in the school programme. Frequent consultation with the home school and review of the child's IEP are important to ensure that the child's programme while at the hospice is consistent with their programme at their home school. End-of-life children may also be included in the school programme either in the classroom or at their bedside. Teachers are part of the hospice interdisciplinary team which enables them to be a part of a holistic approach to the care provided by a hospice.

Communication with parents is an important part of the programme and can occur informally for parents staying at the hospice or through phone calls or family meetings.

Schooling in a children's hospice—the Canuck Place experience

Canuck Place Children's Hospice in Vancouver, Canada, was opened in November, 1995. The education programme is staffed by one teacher and one SEA. A team of dedicated volunteers provides additional support in the classroom. These volunteers are an integral and crucial part of the programme.

Because the composition of the classroom at Canuck Place is constantly changing, it is impossible to duplicate the social dynamics of a regular classroom. Frequently, children who have similar illnesses and are of similar ages are booked into the hospice at the same time and, as their families get to know each other through social events and support groups, friendships are formed. It is not unusual to see a sibling reading to a younger child or to a child who is unable to read. Older children look out for younger children and quietly offer help to someone who needs assistance.

The makeup and needs of the classroom are constantly changing requiring staff flexibility. On any given day there may be children from kindergarten to grade 12. Some will be non-verbal, listening to stories and music, participating in a variety of multisensory activities including hand over hand art activities, and working on basic communication skills using eye pointing, communication boards, or switches. Some will be working on a modified programme and may receive assistance in reading a book or completing a math assignment. Some will be working on regular curriculum with adaptations.

In addition to close contact between the hospice teacher and the child's regular teacher and other involved specialists, contact with the student's classmates, either by email or by visits is encouraged. Parents are encouraged to offer input into the school programme for their child. For parents staying at Canuck Place the proximity of family suites to the school room, art room, and Snoezelen or multisensory room, encourages informal communication. One outgrowth of this is that the hospice teacher, at the parent's request, frequently becomes an advocate for the child at his regular school.

Inconsistent provision of education

During May and June of 2003 questionnaires were sent out to pediatric hospices in the United States, England, Wales, Australia, and New Zealand to determine education services provided to children, especially in hospice settings. Responses indicated either a lack of or a very inconsistent education services for children in hospice settings.

There are presently no children's hospices in New Zealand. In Australia, Bear Cottage in South Wales has an informal school programme that operates for two hours a day, staffed by a play therapist, with no separate funding.

Canuck Place in British Columbia, Canada, until recently the only free standing children's hospice in North America, has had a school programme since opening in 1995. The school programme has one full-time certified teacher and one special education assistant. Their salaries are funded by the provincial government. In the United States, George Mark Children's Hospice in California, the first freestanding pediatric hospice in the United States, opened this year, and is planning a have a school programme.

In the United Kingdom, there are almost thirty pediatric hospices but few have formal education programmes. Some hospices have trained teachers on staff but they are not hired to run a school programme. Because of the proximity of schools to hospices some children are able to attend their home school while they are at the hospice. Sometimes hospice staff is able to support the children with their homework and liaise with schools regarding homework or the implications of terminal illness. Helen House in Oxfordshire has recently hired a part time teacher and Quidenham in Norfolk has a teacher who runs a school programme 3 days a week.

While hospices have recognized in their national charters the importance of education for children with life-limiting illnesses [5,6] most hospices have not yet provided consistent educational programmes.

School reentry

Returning to school after the diagnosis of a progressive life-limiting illness or after a prolonged absence can be a very difficult for a child. [22] The child may have suffered major losses and lifestyle changes. His appearance may have changed due to medical procedures or he may require new equipment such as a ventilator or a gastrostomy tube. [23] These changes may affect a child's emotional health, social interactions, and school performance. Initially it might be necessary for the child to remain at home and receive home instruction. It might seem easier to continue instruction at home but the child would miss much of the social and emotional development that comes from interacting with peers in a school setting. 'School is the work of childhood.' [24] School is crucial to the development of the child's full potential and offers opportunities to grow, learn, and to be successful and creative. In school a child is seen as a student rather than as a patient [22]. School offers the child a sense of hope and the promise of a future. It is important that medical personnel communicate the importance of school to both the family and the child [23,24].

Both a child and his parents may have concerns about a return to school. It is important that a child life specialist or social worker talk with them about these concerns. The child should be prepared for the reactions and comments of other children and should, if possible, be introduced to another child who has faced similar challenges [22,24].

Communication and cooperation between the home, medical team, and school is vital. While a child is hospitalized, a liaison person should be assigned to communicate medical and home information to the school. A school liaison person, with the parent's permission, should be appointed to receive information and ensure appropriate information is related to all of the child's teachers and any siblings' teachers [22,24]. The teacher will need information about the child's illness and the effects this illness might have on school performance as well as concerns the child may have. The teacher should be aware of limitations the child may have and special accommodations needed. Social and emotional issues should also be discussed with the teacher. With this information the teacher can plan and develop appropriate educational strategies for the child and any necessary medical or educational resources or support can be put in place [22,24]. Some children may attend school for only part of the day or for only two or three days a week. At the secondary level children might attend certain subjects only. Each child's reentry will be unique and will require creativity on the part of teachers and other students.

It can be helpful for a class to retain regular contact with a hospitalized child. This can be done through letters, cards, emails or visits. This contact enables the child to feel that he is still a member of the class and that the class is expecting him back [22]. Before a child returns to school it may be appropriate for a child life specialist or a liaison nurse to make a presentation to the class. Some ill children choose to be present for this presentation and some would rather not. Written information on the illness might also be provided [22,24]. Classmates can be told what they can do to assist the child and to help make the adjustment easier.

It is important that there be ongoing follow-up and communication between the home, the medical team, and the school. For a student with an IEP this communication can occur naturally at designated times throughout the school year. Communication and follow-up should continue throughout the school years, including any transition from secondary school to post-secondary education.

Teachers in school settings

A teacher is an important person in any child's life and can be especially important in the life of a child with a progressive life-limiting illness. It is perhaps the teacher who has the greatest opportunity and responsibility to enhance the quality of life for that child [7]. The teacher, with support from special education resource teachers, has the responsibility of ensuring that appropriate learning resources are available and that any necessary adaptations or modifications are made to curriculum and to the physical environment. Perhaps even more crucial is the responsibility of the teacher to create a caring, supportive atmosphere in the classroom where each child is viewed as special and unique. In this setting a child with a progressive life-limiting illness would know that he is an important member of the class. The teacher might need to work with the class, giving children guidance on how to best make the child feel included. Support would be subtle and unobtrusive, not making the child feel as if he were being singled out. The teacher would also be able to assist with social interactions. He or she could ensure that the child is viewed as an important member of the class even when absent, by mentioning him, and by encouraging classmates to maintain contact with the child. Special events for which the child is absent might be videotaped and replayed for the child.

The teacher might also ensure that a child who is absent from school has access to assignments. For extended absences, a home instruction teacher could be arranged for. Assignments could be emailed to the child and the appropriate teacher contacted. When given updated information regarding the child's changing condition, the teacher would be able to make appropriate decisions about work expectations.

Case Michael is a keen, academically able grade five student who enjoys challenging math problems, reading books like *Lord of the Rings*, playing strategy games such as Mancala, and playing a wide variety of computer and video games.

Michael has spinal muscular atrophy. He uses a power wheelchair and follows the regular grade five curriculum. As he tires easily, assignments are often adapted in amount. For instance he might not do all the math questions assigned to other students, he might complete an assignment in class that others are assigned for homework, and he might be given additional time to complete a project in science or social studies. Michael frequently misses school either because of his illness or because of illness in the class to which he should not be exposed, and when he visits a local hospice for respite care. When Michael is unable to attend school his teacher emails assignments to him which, when completed, his mother emails back to the school. When he is at the hospice, all assignments are faxed to the hospice teacher with notes or telephone calls to update Michael on class activities. Michael's teacher emails Michael and encourages him to email her and the class. One task that the teacher asked Michael to complete while he was away was to design a new class seating plan. The design was faxed to his teacher. When Michael returned to school he felt some ownership of the new seating arrangement.

When Michael is absent his teacher mentions him frequently: 'I wonder what Michael would think about this?' or 'Which group shall we put Michael in?' This keeps Michael in the students' thoughts, as is evident by one boy's comment when the classroom floor was resurfaced. 'Too bad Michael isn't here. Think of the wheelies he could do around the room!' When Michael missed the Valentine's Day Party, his special education assistant, who helps him with physical tasks such as scribing for him and getting out his laptop, arranged to visit the hospice with two of his classmates, bringing all the valentine cards for Michael. His teacher has also visited the hospice several times, bringing different classmates each time. The students were able to play a game with Michael, see the hospice school room, and play with him on the new adapted outdoor merry-go-round. His teacher has reported that this contact has helped the other students, as they now know where Michael goes when he visits the hospice and can talk about what he might be doing. For next year the school staff has arranged for Michael to have the same teacher and most of the same students will be in his class.

Special education assistants

Assistants who work in a school, hospital, or hospice setting with children with progressive life-limiting illnesses are referred to in this chapter as special education assistants or SEAs. These people play an important role and are an integral part of the team that provides support for children with progressive life-limiting illnesses. Without their services it would be almost impossible for many children with palliative care needs to attend regular school.

The role of an SEA is to unobtrusively provide personal care such as feeding and toileting for children with palliative care needs. Children who are on a ventilator require frequent suctioning, and those who have other medical needs must be attended to by medically qualified staff. In these instances the SEA may have medical training as well as training to work in an educational setting. Sometimes there will be a nurse as well as an SEA to provide support for the child.

SEAs work under the direction of the classroom and resource teachers to adapt and modify curriculum and provide individual support to the child as needed. An SEA is trained to know when individual support is needed, and when it is better to remain in the background to foster independence, intervening before the child becomes too frustrated, thus preventing inappropriate behaviour. An SEA should move discreetly to the background in social situations, giving the child ample opportunity to socialize with his or her peers without adult intervention.

Often the child will feel comfortable confiding in the SEA who will then have an opportunity to help the child work through problems. The SEA also has the opportunity to make observations about social interactions of which the teacher may not be aware. Working together, the teacher and the SEA can often enhance social interactions. Sometimes a buddy system is put in place for recess and lunch, but often an SEA is able to foster inclusion in an even more natural way. An SEA has the opportunity to provide the child with the support he needs to be successful physically, academically, emotionally, and socially, enabling him to develop the confidence needed to take more risks in the school setting. As part of this an SEA should be aware of the importance of having the child feel that he or she is a part of, not separate from, the class. To foster normality the SEA will often direct parents to talk with the teacher about academic or social updates. The child will be encouraged to direct pertinent questions to the teacher and hand work in to the teacher rather than to the SEA.

Parents

Discovering that their child has a disability can be devastating for parents. Discovering that their child has a progressive life-limiting illness brings a new dimension to that devastation as it threatens one of the strongest of human bonds [25]. The degree to which parents are able to come to terms with and accept these conditions varies from parent to parent. For many parents, life following such a diagnosis is a series of crises. Parents find it difficult when their child first enters the school system and often are in the position of having to lobby for needed support for their child. At some point there may be a teacher or a special education assistant who they feel is not a good match for their child, which causes additional stress. As one parent said, 'I just feel that everything is under control and then I need to solve another problem.'

When children move from elementary school to secondary school there can be a great deal of parental anxiety especially when a change in the type of placement is being considered. It is crucial for parents to have the opportunity to be involved in the choice of placement and to know that their views are being taken into consideration. At times the pressure of the school day may seem overwhelming but most parents do want their child to have this normal experience.

Parents with children who have progressive life-limiting illnesses can be under tremendous physical and emotional strain. Their child often has complicated physical care needs including lifting and physiotherapy. Specialized equipment may be required and there are often numerous appointments related to the child's illness. It may not be possible for both parents to maintain full time employment, thus creating financial strains for the family. Parents often feel guilty that they are not able to spend enough time with their spouse or their other children. Although the time and energy of these parents is stretched, regular communication with them is still very important. Parents need to be involved in placement decisions, in school reentry plans, and in regular IEP meetings.

Parents can be kept informed about their child's programme and performance by telephone, meetings, or a communication book. Parents know their child better than anyone. They hold key information and knowledge [20] and should be full collaborative partners with the educational team.

There may be times in their child's school life when parents feel that, even after having gone through the process of IEP meetings and collaboration, the needs of their child are not being met. Many parents of special needs students have advocated publicly for what they believed their child needed. In some educational jurisdictions it is now possible to arrange for another person (a Parent Facilitator or an Independent Parental Supporter) to guide and support the parents to ensure that their voice is being heard. There may also be parent partnership groups that provide information, advice and guidance on issues and who are able to help guide a parent through an unfamiliar system [20, 26].

Siblings

Siblings have a special relationship that no other can duplicate. Although they may not always get along, may be jealous of each other, and even sometimes say they hate each other, there is always a great potential for support, companionship, and love. Siblings share a common history and common bonds [27].

The care of a child with a progressive life-limiting illness often totally consumes parents leaving little time for other children in the family. These children may feel overwhelmed and neglected and have been referred to as 'living in houses of chronic sorrow' [28].

During the progress of a terminal illness, a sibling may display a wide variety of behaviours at school. Some siblings may display no outward signs of emotional upset or disturbance. They may have a close relationship with their brother or sister and may find opportunities at recess or lunch to play with their brother or sister or give assistance with books or papers. Some siblings display amazing empathy and patience with classmates or other children in the school who have special needs (Figure 11.3).

Many siblings display behaviours that suggest they may be having difficulties adjusting to the illness of their brother or sister. Frequently they have attention-seeking behaviours and short attention spans. Many have difficulty sustaining effort on schoolwork and in learning new concepts. Others may have an overly strong desire to do everything perfectly and may become upset when they make mistakes. Some may seem to be overly anxious about the well being of other brothers and sisters in the family to the extent of taking on the role of a parent.

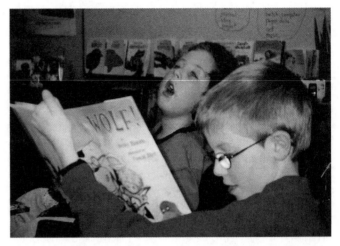

Fig. 11.3 Siblings often enjoy reading stories to children who are not able to read. (Reproduced with permission of the families.)

During this period, school can be a safe haven for some siblings. School may be the one place where siblings can be acknowledged for themselves rather than as the brother or sister of their ill sibling. At school, unlike at home, life tends to remain the same, including predictable routines [8]. School also provides opportunities to socialize with friends, whom they may no longer be able to see after school. Siblings can confide in their friends, socialize and enjoy the normal activities of childhood. During school hours it may be possible to forget what is going on at home.

It is important for teachers of siblings to have information about how the sibling is reacting to the progress of the illness outside the school setting. The teacher will be aware of any changes in school performance. The teacher should also look for any persistent signs of depression, social withdrawal, anxiety, aggression, or low self-esteem [27] which would indicate the possible necessity of intervention. The teacher may schedule times for the sibling to meet with a school counsellor.

The impact of the death of a brother or sister can last a lifetime but siblings who are 'comforted, taught, included, and validated' [27] can grow and develop into emotionally healthy adults. Teachers can play an important role in supporting siblings. Teachers can listen to them and provide opportunities for them to express their feelings through writing, art, physical education, music, and drama. They can ensure that siblings are included and important members of their class. Teachers have an important role in creating a supportive learning environment where caring classmates can also be part of the healing process. As well as arranging for counselling through the school, the teacher can assist in ensuring that the family is aware of outside resources that are available for siblings, including bereavement groups, play therapy, and private counselling.

Dealing with death

In some cultures death is an accepted part of life, but in many cultures it is a subject adults find very difficult to talk about [29]. The knowledge that death is irreversible, inevitable, and universal is usually assimilated by children around 7 or 8 years of age. Because children have a limited capacity to tolerate emotional pain and a limited ability to verbalize their feelings, they may avoid talking about their grief [29]. Children are interested in death as evidenced in their games and stories, and some educators feel that death education should be an integral part of the curriculum [30]. It is helpful for students to have had the opportunity to think about and discuss death before a death occurs in their lives, thus giving them opportunities to receive support and have questions answered [30].

The death of a classmate can be a very traumatic experience for the entire class resulting in changes which children may find difficult to deal with [31]. Many schools have protocols for informing children about the death of another child. Critical incident or response teams, which include an administrator, teachers, counsellors, and district specialists, give support to teachers and children [31,32]. The type of response made by this team at the time of death will depend on the ages and levels of emotional maturity of the children and the cause of death [31].

An anticipated death allows time to plan and prepare, making it important that the school personnel understand both the child's condition and prognosis [31]. Some research has shown that children fare best when honest discussions about a terminal illness occur from the time of diagnosis and when open communication appropriate to the child's developmental stage and emotional needs is maintained [33]. Teachers frequently use literature and discussion to help prepare children for the death of a classmate and to help deal with questions and emotions before and after the death. Some teachers will have attended professional development sessions on supporting children around death. In senior grades death can be touched on in literature, history, and biology [30]. Models of grief suggest that bereaved children need to understand, grieve, commemorate, and move on [34]. This means that is important for children to understand that death is universal and irreversible, they must be able to experience and express their feelings, they should be involved in some sort of remembrance or commemoration service, and then they must move on to other relationships. [34] It is usually the critical incident or response team that will initiate this response with follow up by counsellors and teachers.

The death of a child can have a great impact on teachers and other staff members who have worked closely with that child. Each teacher will react differently depending upon their own personal attitudes and beliefs about death, their personal experiences with death, and what is happening in their own life at that particular time. Some teachers may be able to cope effectively with little or no support while others may need to access school support groups or counselling provided by their educational jurisdiction. It is important that support be provided for staff by trained professionals not only for the teachers' own emotional and physical well being but also so that these teachers can effectively give support to the children with whom they are working. A school counsellor may be asked to come into the classroom to talk with the children or to provide resources and suggest strategies.

Some teachers may need support in dealing not only with their own attitudes and feelings about death and dying but also those of their students. Within present day Greek culture the death of a child is perceived as unnatural, unfair, and tragic. In 1997, a group of Greek educators were involved in a multidisciplinary year long training programme on supporting seriously ill and bereaved children. These educators have offered seminars and workshops in schools but many teachers have reported that they still feel unprepared to deal with the death of one of their students [35].

In France, death education was removed from the curriculum because of religious pressures [30]. In the United Kingdom, direct classroom instruction around death is part of the normal curriculum [36]. In 1999, a reflection time on matters of death and grieving was added to the curriculum. Training for some teachers was introduced and in September 2002, death and grieving education became a component of the school curriculum under the Personal, Social, and Health Education programme [30]. Hospice programmes in the United Kingdom sometimes act as resources to schools before and after the death of a child, as an extension to patient care [36].

The child with a progressive life-limiting illness

It is difficult to make generalizations about children with a progressive life-limiting illness. No two children with the same diagnosis will present identically. Working with these children only reinforces the belief that all children are unique and, as such, have very unique needs. There are, however, observations that can be made about these children. Many children with physical limitations are creative and resourceful. They are creative in the ways they have discovered they can do things. For instance, some children know which pens work best for art projects, which books will best support the mouse on the computer, and which type of calculator is easiest to use. They may not be able to run with a kite but they can fly a kite when the line is attached to their power chair and they will tell you where and how they want the line attached. They may not be able to cut with scissors but they can plan an entire model town complete with a tower to launch a rocket and will tell you exactly what they need you to do to help the project come to fruition.

There is a Tibetan saying that begins: 'Children are our real teachers. Listen carefully.' Perhaps because children with progressive life-limiting illnesses lose control in so many areas of their lives, it is even more important that they be given choices. Non verbal children may be able to tell you with their eyes which book they want and their body language can tell you that you have not interpreted their choice correctly. Other children may be very decisive about what they feel is important and what goals they want to work towards. Often activities of choice that adults might feel are important are not those that the child feels are important at all. When choices can be accommodated the child gains some control over his environment.

These children understand what it means to need help and how it feels to be vulnerable. Perhaps this is why so many are supportive of each other. It is not uncommon in a hospice setting to see one child asking for help on behalf of another child. Older children will consider younger children when planning outings and will offer to help younger or non-verbal children or read them a story.

As with all children, children living with progressive life-limiting illnesses are proud of their accomplishments. They feel good about their accomplishments, whether it be the good mark they received on a math test or the goal they scored in a power hockey or soccer game. They are able to take pride in attaining goals, whether the goal is to complete a math assignment, read a novel, or graduate from secondary school.

One of the most amazing attributes of many of these children is the ability to accept their illness in their stride. Yes, there are times when a teacher hears, 'It's just not fair!' but many of these children are strong, brave and courageous. Without flinching they can ask an adult to position their arms or legs, push their hair back, or blow their nose and then proceed with whatever it was that they were doing. These children are like any children. They want to learn, grow, play, laugh, and have fun. They have the same hopes and dreams as other children, the only difference being that they may not have as long to realize these hopes and dreams. Like a butterfly they need to stretch their wings and fly because they have much quality living to do in a limited period of time.

Case Greg is a 17-year-old boy who spends a significant amount of time at his computer, staying in contact with friends by email. He enjoys recreational activities, including indoor rock climbing with

the recreational therapist at Canuck Place. He would love to try sky diving some day.

Greg has been on an adapted programme at school. He often needs help scribing his work as he has Friedrich's ataxia which has made his hands weak and requires that he use a wheelchair. Greg tires easily and requires additional time to complete assignments. Over the past years, his teachers have often commented that he is a capable student but has difficulty keeping up with the workload of the regular secondary school curriculum. His teachers and counsellor recommended that Greg take 4 years to complete grades 11 and 12, his final years of school, before attending college.

Greg, however, set himself the goal of completing grades 11 and 12 in 2 years and graduating with his peers with whom he had attended school since kindergarten. Whenever he made respite visits to Canuck Place he was always keen to complete his assignments and keep up to date in his senior English course. Recently his case manager informed us that Greg had been on the Honour Roll at his school this past term, received a citizenship award, and a most inspiring person award. Greg requested that he be permitted to say a few words at the Awards Assembly. In his speech Greg told the audience that people thought he should take 4 years instead of 2 to graduate but that the most important thing for him was to graduate with his friends. He went on to say that after making this decision he decided what he had to do to make his dream come true. He concluded by saying, 'If I can do it, so can you!'

Conclusion

School is an important part of life for all children. For the child with a progressive life-limiting illness, the school is a place where children are able to develop their skills and abilities to their fullest potential and develop and maintain connections with peers. Schools also provide children with normal connections to the wider world, thus giving them a sense of hope. Many of these children require IEPs that necessitate additional planning, resources and support. There are challenges in meeting the individual needs of each child and ensuring they progress academically, socially, and emotionally. There is no road map, guidebook, or set of rules for this journey. Flexibility, creativity, good judgment, sensitivity, and love are required as each child's needs are assessed, the best possible placement is made, and all available resources and supports are put in place. With resources and services constantly in a state of flux, teachers, parents, and society must constantly be prepared to advocate for the best possible education for these children.

Having a child with a progressive life-limiting illness as a member of a class can be a very enriching experience for the teacher and the entire class. Together the children can learn and grow. Peers are able to offer friendship, understanding, and support. In return they will often develop empathy and a deeper appreciation for human worth and dignity. Children with progressive life-limiting illnesses often gain insights and wisdom beyond their years. Given opportunities and a willingness to share these thoughts and feelings, classmates may gain significant understandings and be challenged to think about issues beyond the prescribed curriculum.

Together, all members of the class, whether in a regular, special, hospital or hospice setting can learn the importance of taking time to listen and to learn. They can learn to truly listen to each other. They can learn how important it is to care for each other, to be a true friend, and to grow together. They can learn the importance of living in the moment and being present for each other. These children will be able to fully appreciate the words translated from Sanskrit:

> Look to this day for it is life, the very life of life,
> ....
> For yesterday is but a dream and tomorrow is only a vision,
> But today well spent makes every yesterday a dream
>   of happiness
>   and every tomorrow a vision of hope.
> Look well therefore to this day! [37]

Glossary

Adapted programme	student is following the regular curriculum for his or her grade level and will meet the learning outcomes with adaptations such as using a computer, having a scribe, having more time for assignments and tests
Augmentative technology	devices designed to support, augment, or assist communication using whatever skills an individual possesses
Case manager	the individual in the school designated to manage the 'case' of a student with special needs; this individual will arrange IEP meetings, coordinate services in the school and coordinate services from outside professionals such as doctors, nurses, occupational and physiotherapists, speech language therapists, social workers, etc.; see Special Education Resource Teacher/Special Needs Coordinator
Child	individuals of school age (5–18 years old)
Dependent	a child who is completely dependent on others for meeting all major daily living needs; assistance will be necessary for the child to attend school
Designation	the process by which a child is assessed for special needs and then assigned a government category for the purpose of funding and service
Elementary School	kindergarten to grade seven (usually 5–12)
Inclusion	unified systems of education with provision of appropriate education for all; all children are included, participating, valued members of the class
Individual Education Plan (IEP)	written plan developed by an educational team which includes parents and other appropriate professionals who are working with the child; plan consists of long and short term goals for the child and includes modifications or adaptations for the child and support which will be provided
Integration	sometimes referred to as mainstreaming; the provision of an appropriate education for children with special needs in a regular education setting
Modified Programme	child is following a parallel programme with learning activities which will enable the child to develop academic, social, and emotional skills; child will not meet the learning outcomes for his grade level
Regular	when referring to a regular school, class, setting, or placement this implies a setting where all children regardless of abilities, special needs, or health status are educated in the same environment. In this setting children with special needs learn side by side with their normally developing peers
Regular Programme	child's educational programme falls within the widely held expectations for his grade level
Secondary School	grades 8–12 (13–17 years old]
Special Education Assistants (SEA)	referred to as aides, teaching assistants, school and student support workers, child care workers; these paraprofessionals work in the classroom under the direction of the teacher supporting children with special needs physically, academically, and socially
Special Education Resource Teacher/Special Needs Coordinator	professional with training in special education; manages cases of children with special needs and often works with them individually, in small groups, or in the classroom
Statement	legal documentation, drawn up after assessment by the education authority, which outlines special education needs of a child and service required (In the United Kingdom)
Transition	the process of moving from one programme or environment to another

References

1. Desai, I. Inclusion: Disability and educational provision in Australia. *Proceedings of Pre-Conference Symposium; Disability and Policy in 21st Century: Refocus on and Old Issue*, Melbourne, Australia, 9 September 2001.

2. United Nations. Universal Declaration of Human Rights. Resolution 217 A (III). *Proceedings of the General Assembly of the United Nations.* Geneva, Switzerland, 10 December 1948.

3. United Nations. Convention on the Rights of the Child. Resolution 44/25. *Proceedings of General Assembly of the United Nations.* Geneva, Switzerland, 20 November 1989.

4. United Nations Educational, Scientific and Cultural Organization. The Salamanca statement and framework for action on special needs education. *Proceedings of World Conference on Special Needs Education: Access and Quality.* Salamanca, Spain, June 7–10, 1994.

5. Association for Children with Life-threatening or Terminal Conditions and their Families. ACT Charter for children with Life-Threatening or Terminal Conditions and their Families. (3rd edition. [pamphlet]). ACT, Bristol, 1998.

6. Elston, S. and Goldman, A. Joint briefing with ACT and ACH; palliative care for children [briefing bulletin]. National Council for Hospice and Specialist Palliative Care Services, London, 2001.

7. Jeffrey, P. Enhancing their lives: A challenge for education. In J.D. Baum, F. Dominica, R. Woodward, eds. *Listen My child has a Lot of Living to do*. London: Oxford University Press, 1990, pp. 133–7.

8. Trapp, A. Support for the family. In A. Goldman, eds. *Care of the Dying Child*. Oxford: Oxford University Press, 1994, pp. 76–92.

9. Lavelle, J. Education and the sick child. In L. Hill, ed. *Caring for Dying Children and Their Families*. London: Chapman and Hall 1994, pp. 87–105.

10. Winzer, M. Children with exceptionalities in Canadian classrooms (6th edition). Toronto: Prentice Hall, 2002.

11. Winzer, M. and Mazurek, K. (ed). From tolerance to acceptance to celebration: including students with severe disabilities. In *Special Education in the 21st Century: Issues of inclusion and reform*. Gallaudets University Press, Washington DC: 2000, pp. 175–97.

12. Winzer, M. and Mazurek, K. ed. The inclusion movement: a goal for restructuring special education. In: *Special education in the 21st Century: Issues of inclusion and reform.* pp. 27–40. Washington DC, Gallaudet University Press, 2000, 175–197.

13. Spalding, B. Special educational needs in the mainstream school. Liverpool: University of Liverpool, Department of Education, Liverpool, 1999. Available from: http://www.liv.ac.uk/education/inced/sen/index.html. Accessed 2003 June 5.

14. Smith, D. Introduction of progress report. Special committee on the disabled and handicapped. *Proceedings of the first session, 30 sec parliament*, June 1982, Ottawa, Canada.

15. Lindsay, G. Inclusive education: A critical perspective. *Br J Special Educat* 2003;30(1):3–12.

16. Ainscow, M., Haile-Giorgis, M. Educational arrangements for children categorized as having special needs. *Eur J Special Needs Educ* 1999;14(2):103–21.

17. Pierce, N. Editorial on Thailand. *Rehab Review* 2002;24(5):13–15.

18. Andrews, J. and Lupart, J. Historical foundations of inclusive education. *The Inclusive Classroom*. Scarborough, Nelson Thompson Learning, pp. 25–48.

19. Farrell, P. Special education in the last twenty years: Have things really got better? *Br J Special Edu* 28(1): 3–9.

20. Farrell, P. and Harris, K. Access to education for children with medical needs-a map of best practice. [pamphlet]. Sherwood Park: DfES Publications, 2001.

21. Canuck Place Children's Hospice. The Story of Canuck Place. Available at: http://www.canuckplace.com/about/story.html. Accessed: 2003 May 9.

22. Sexson, S.B. and Madan-Swain, A. School reentry for the child with chronic illness. *J Learn Disabil* 1993;26(2):115–37.

23. Hochu, J. The role of the child life specialist assisting the pediatric palliative patient return to school. *Hospice News* Spring 2003;7:16.

24. Leigh, L. and Miles, M.A. Education Issues for children with cancer. In P.A. Pizzo, and D.G. Poplack, eds. *Principles and Practice of Pediatric Oncology* 4th edition. Lippincott Williams and Wilkins, Philadelphia 2002, pp. 1463–76.

25. Overton, J. Development of children's hospices in the UK. *Eur J Palliat Care* 2001;8(1):30–3.

26. Vancouver School Board. Parent Advocacy Program. Available at: http://www.vsb.bc.ca/parents/parentadv.htm. Accessed: 2003 July 4.

27. Davies, B. The grief of siblings. In M.B. Webb, ed. *Helping Bereaved Children*. New York: Guilford Press, 2002, pp. 94–127.

28. Bluebond Langner, M. Worlds of dying children and their well siblings. In K. Doka, ed. *Children Mourning Mourning Children*. Washington: Hospice Association of America.

29. Webb, N.B. The child and death. In Webb N.B., editor. *Helping Bereaved Children*. New York: Guilford Press; 2002, pp. 3–18.

30. Abras, M. Teaching children to understand death and grieving. *Eur J Palliat Care* 2002;9(6):256–7.

31. Stevenson, R.G. Sudden death in schools. In N.B. Webb, ed. *Helping Bereaved Children*. New York: Guilford Press, pp. 194–213.

32. Vancouver School Board. School emergency and crisis response flipbook. Vancouver School Board, Vancouver, (revised 2003).

33. Weiner, L. and Septimus, A. Psychosocial support and ethical issues for the child and the family. In P. A. Pizzo and C. M. Wilfert, eds. *Pediatric AIDS: The Challenge of HIV Infection in Infants, Children, and Adolescents* (3rd edition). Baltimore MD: Williams and Wilkins, 1998, pp.703–27.

34. Fox, S. S. Tasks for bereaved children. In *Good grief: Helping Groups of Children When a Friend Dies*. 1998, Boston, MA: New England Association for the Education of Young Children, pp. 21–27.

35. Papadatou, D. The evolution of palliative care for children in Greece. *Eur J Palliat Care* 2001;8(1):35–8.

36. Gortler, E. Lessons in grief: A practical look at school programs. In A. Armstrong-Dailey and S. Z. Goltzer, eds. *Hospice Care for Children*. 1993, pp. 154–71. New York: Oxford University Press.

37. The Sanskrit. Salutation to the dawn translated from Sanskrit. In E. Roberts and E. Amidon, eds. *Earth Prayers from Around the World*. San Francisco, CA: 1991, Harper San Francisco.

12 The power of their voices: Child and family assessment in pediatric palliative care

Nancy Contro and Sarah Scofield

We are in need of medicine with a heart… The endless physical, emotional, and financial burdens that a family carries when their child dies… makes you totally incapable of dealing with incompetence and insensitivity…

Salvador Avila, parent 2001[1]

Importance of the family assessment

In the child's world, the family is the most central and enduring influence. The child's well-being is intrinsically linked to their parents' or caretakers' physical, emotional and social health, social circumstances, and child rearing practices [2].

Working with children in a medical setting inevitably entails working with their families and/or caretakers. Pediatric literature underscores the premise that physical and emotional outcomes for children are strongly linked to how well their families function, and that pediatricians are in a prime position to help nurture and support families, thus promoting optimal family functioning [2]. This is a unique quality of pediatric medicine, both challenging and compelling: the need to provide services within the confines and complexities of the family.

Understanding the relationship between the patient and family, and the needs of both, is critical to providing excellent care. This is recognized by the American Academy of Pediatrics (AAP) Task Force on the family, which includes screening, assessment and referral of parents for physical, emotional, social or health risk behaviors that can adversely affect the health and emotional/social well being of the child, in the role and responsibilities of the pediatrician.

To date there is very little in the literature that provides a comprehensive picture of the needs of families with a child facing incurable illness and death [1–3, 8]. This dearth of literature makes the task of a comprehensive family assessment in the context of pediatric palliative care even more critical. Careful interviewing of families not only provides invaluable information for the clinician but in the long run also contributes to our ongoing knowledge base regarding the needs of families in pediatric palliative care.

We, as care providers, must be able and willing to elicit and respond to this information. This responsibility may seem daunting, especially when coupled with the myriad of demands involved in providing medical care to a child with an incurable illness; but with training and practice, the tasks related to family assessment become not only manageable but well worth the effort.

In this chapter we examine the assessment of the child and family using a two-tiered approach. First we examine the necessary fundamentals of assessment and identify how various concepts apply through case discussion. Next we review a large-scale needs assessment research project conducted with bereaved families who identified critical components of quality care.

Defining assessment

What is assessment in pediatric palliative care? At an abstract level, it is the union of structure and flexibility, of science and art. When done well it can provide the foundation from which a caring professional may guide and accompany a family on the unimaginable journey through childhood illness, death, and bereavement.

On a practical level, assessment is a tool that will improve the quality of the patient's care and therefore the quality of both the child's remaining life and the child's death. It will provide the information that the caregiver requires to address the family's, and therefore the child's needs; to engage the family in a productive relationship; and to partner with the family in attaining the best care that state of the art palliation can offer.

Assessment is a semi-structured interview process that ideally acquires a fluid give-and-take dynamic. The more experienced and practiced the caregiver becomes, the more the caregiver will modify the assessment interview as needed during the process. On the simplest level, assessment means to ask, not to assume. Always ask what the family needs: just as a physician would ask a patient to describe his symptoms; just as you cannot provide proper treatment without proper diagnosis, you cannot provide proper services to children and families in palliative care without proper assessment.

Family concept

In modern times the concept of the family has expanded and changed to encompass many diverse situations. As we will see, one of the first tasks in assessing child and family needs is understanding the family composition. For the purposes of this chapter families may include parents, grandparents, extended family members, related or unrelated caretakers, full or half siblings or any combination of individuals who form the unit who cares for the patient. Not only is there tremendous variety in the composition of families, "there is also great variation in ethnic and racial heritage, religious practices, communication and life styles." [2] All of these factors must be taken under consideration in the family assessment because each individual and each family system comes to the situation with a unique background and perspective.

When first meeting a family, we must allow them to define of whom their family consists. It is not for the care provider to determine or judge the family composition but rather to ask the family for this information. This approach can set the tone for the ongoing caregiver relationship, and it sets up a critical foundation of quality care early on: always ask, never assume.

Individual child and family assessment

The assessment of the patient and family entering palliative care frequently occurs during treatment that is already in progress. In pediatric palliative care the patient and family have often been in ongoing treatment and are making a care transition rather than an initial entry into the system. The backdrop to this transition is the reality that the family is facing the most difficult situation imaginable: the incurable illness and impending death of their child. The death of a child is widely considered by the mental health profession to be one of the most psychologically catastrophic events a person can experience [4]. This fact makes the assessment of the family all the more critical and challenging. It requires the ability to sensitively approach a family experiencing overwhelming stress. The ability to perform the assessment competently and compassionately will shape the formation of the future caregiver/patient relationship.

It is well established in mental health/social work literature that the assessment process provides a critical opportunity for establishing a therapeutic relationship [5]. The term therapeutic relationship is not reserved only for psychotherapy settings; it applies as well to any caregiver/patient relationship and refers to the qualities of trust, mutual understanding, and respect that characterize a productive and collaborative relationship. Thus the family assessment not only provides essential information about the family's needs, it sets the stage for meeting those needs by beginning an open, thoughtful and attentive dialogue guided by the care provider.

How does this therapeutic bond develop during the assessment? It happens when the family experiences the caregiver as interested and attentive to their situation; to their thoughts, feelings, fears, questions, needs, ideas and experiences. As the caregiver asks questions to elicit this information, listens attentively and carefully, and responds compassionately and appropriately, the family is able to develop trust, a sense of safety, and a perception that their needs are being heard and addressed.

The assessment should involve the entire family if at all possible. All family members should be invited to participate as much as possible. This may mean contacting certain family members by phone or splitting the assessment into parts. Studies show that in "instances of anticipated grief, when death follows an incurable childhood illness, parental grief is diminished if the parents feel satisfied that they did all they could to contribute to their child's care and well being" [6]. The concept of involvement includes the participation of siblings as well. Evidence suggests that siblings welcome the opportunity to be a part of care and benefit from being incorporated whenever appropriate and possible [7].

What follows is a three-layered discussion regarding the basics of performing child- and family-assessments. First we will consider some key fundamentals that the caregiver will ideally incorporate. Then we will outline in detail the areas that any complete assessment should address. Finally we will utilize case histories to illustrate some focal areas of assessment that are almost universally relevant to families with an incurably ill child.

Basic fundamentals of child and family assessment

1. Provide protected time without interruption. Although often difficult to come by, this is necessary and will save resources in the future.

2. Provide a comfortable and confidential physical setting. This will help relax the family and lead to a more open discussion. For a child, make sure the room is stocked with age appropriate supplies such as art equipment and games.

3. Approach the child and family in a nonjudgmental, honest fashion. This helps families feel less intimidated and allows the care provider to better elicit information.

4. Let the child and family express their own opinions, whether or not you agree with them. This promotes accurate assessment through honest disclosure.

5. Watch and listen; show interest and respect for the child and family.

6. Monitor your own responses to the situation. Just as all families are different, each care provider comes with a unique background and trigger points.

7. Pace the assessment, making sure to check in with families in order to avoid overwhelming them. Break the assessment up into additional visits if necessary. Don't try to plow through the information. It will not be nearly as rich or useful and the interviewer and the family may become exhausted.

8. Ask questions in a way that reflects the participant's cognitive and educational levels and in an age-appropriate manner for children. Use techniques other than direct questioning with children such as drawing or engaging in activity while talking.

9. Families are usually very generous and forgiving. If you make a mistake, apologize and continue.

10. Be sure to verify your impressions with the child and family. Ask them if your impressions are accurate.

Child and family assessment outline

There is substantial overlap between various assessment areas; this is deliberate and is the nature of assessment. The awareness that information in one area may reveal important information in another will produce a more thorough and useful assessment. For example, an assessment of possible depression may be inherent when discussing coping, or an assessment of financial burdens may be inherent when discussing logistics. Likewise, much of what is revealed through the family assessment will be helpful in gaining a fuller understanding of the child.

Essential areas

Family composition/constellation

This area should explore the following: Who are the child's parents? Who are the primary caretakers—are they the parents or someone else? Who do the child and caretakers/parents identify as the immediate family unit? Who has legal and physical custody of the child? Who provides consent? Is the family system/unit intact? Are there disruptions in this unit, such as divorce or separation? Are there multiple primary family units?

Medical history of child

This area should explore the following: Is the information the medical team has about the child's medical history complete? Fill in any gaps, past or current. Include questions in this section about pain- and symptom-management. What has worked or not worked in the past? How has the child handled treatment? What are the family beliefs about pain and symptoms? Do they have fears or concerns about use of certain medications? What about care that has gone well so far and what does the family hope will be different in the future?

Medical history of family members

This area should explore whether there are any medical issues other family members have that may impact the family's ability to cope.

Emotional/psychiatric history

This area should explore any past history of emotional/psychiatric problems within the family members. For instance, a parent who has experienced prolonged bouts of depression prior to the palliative phases of treatment will have to be monitored closely and provided with additional supports. Questions might address reactions to difficult situations in the past; use of psychiatric medications; any current symptoms; a basic mental status exam; and any concerns the individual or family has about their emotional state. For children questions must be worded age/appropriately and the use of nonverbal communication, such as drawing, is encouraged.

Current coping

This area should explore the following: How is the child coping overall? How are family members coping overall? Are there any areas that are seriously problematic, and if so what are they? Is there anything that is impairing coping or functioning to the point that it interferes with the family's ability to be present for the child; to participate in care; to receive and process information; and to participate in decision making? Are additional resources needed to support the child and or family?

Immediate needs (logistics, concrete needs, forming a plan)

This area should explore the following: What does the family identify as their immediate needs? How are they managing their transportation, housing, finances, parking, travel, food, laundry, clothing, basic necessities, etc? Do they need to take turns coming to the hospital? How are the family members getting to the hospital? Are they able to be there as much as they would like and as needed by the patient? How are they managing needs at home, such as childcare and household responsibilities? How are they handling work and any needed time off? If the child is being cared for at home, are all the appropriate resources in place? Is there a need for respite care?

Informational needs

This area is critical and is often overlooked because assumptions are made that the family understands what the medical team understands about the child and his/her condition. This area should explore the following: What is the family's understanding of the child's condition, treatment and prognosis? What have they been told? Have they received conflicting information? Do they understand what they have been told and the implications? Do they have any questions? What do they feel they do not understand? How do they best receive, absorb, process and interpret information? Are there areas they are not asking about which the medical team believes they need to hear more? Do they have inaccurate information or misperceptions about anything? Do they understand the gray areas, where certainty and definite answers are not possible, and how do they absorb, process and handle uncertainty? Do they draw erroneous conclusions or focus unrealistically on one possible outcome when various outcomes are possible? Has the need for information been addressed with all family members or have key individuals been left out? How much does the child know about his or her medical situation? Does the child like to be a part of care discussions or would he or she prefer to hear information from parents or another support person? Is the family comfortable discussing difficult areas with the child and vice-versa or would they like help in this area? What style of communication works best for this child?

Religious/spiritual orientation

This area should explore: What is the family's religious/spiritual background and current orientation? Are family members consistent with one another or are there significant differences? If so, how to resolve these? For example, does one family member want prayers and/or blessings daily at the bedside while another does not? How do their religious beliefs impact their understanding of the medical situation, coping, and planning? Are there religious/spiritual support systems or beliefs that are helping the family cope? Is there conflict between religious needs and medical needs? Is there a crisis of faith? Are there any special accommodations that the family needs for religious practices in the medical setting?

Ethnic/cultural background

This area should explore: What is the family's ethnic, national or cultural background and how does that impact their experience at the hospital or with caregivers? Are they members of the dominant group that comprises the medical environment or are they members of a minority group? Special attention needs to be given to immigrant and minority families to check in if their experience is being impacted by their status. Are there any barriers, cultural or language-related, overt or subtle, that are affecting the family's experience? Is the family encountering any prejudice related to their background? What are their beliefs and values related to childhood illness, death, medical care and family involvement? For example in some cultures the father is considered the head of the household and the decision maker, and it would be offensive to provide major news or make major decisions without the father present.

Prior experience with trauma illness, death, bereavement

This area should explore the family's history with illness, death and loss. Knowing what the family has experienced or is currently experiencing will help the caregiver understand how the family is reacting to the current situation. For instance, has the family experienced the recent loss of an extended family member such as a grandparent? Has the family experienced any other significant deaths? If so, how have they coped? What resources have they relied on in the past? Even the death of a beloved pet may impact a family and be an important part of the assessment. The current situation may trigger strong memories or reactions to past losses, often to the surprise and distress of family members. Symptoms of post-traumatic stress and anxiety should be assessed if there is a history of trauma. Recognizing successful coping strategies from the past may provide hope and reassurance in the present.

Supports available

This area should explore the practical and emotional supports that the child and family has available to them and those that may need to be called to action. This discussion can help the family identify possible supports and it can give them opportunity or the incentive to ask for help from sources they were too timid or reluctant to approach. These may include extended family, friends, neighbors, the child's school, coworkers, church community groups or associations. Supports can be available on various levels, including individuals (professional helpers such as social workers, child-life workers or counselors as well as friends or the parent of another child who has undergone a similar illness); small informal groups such as family, friends and neighborhood; larger structured groups such as hospital support groups, work and school; and very large organizations such as the National Cancer Society.

Family roles, rules, and relationships

This area should explore what the communication patterns are within the family. This is often an area that can be understood through astute observations of the family. For instance, who does most of the talking? Do children have a voice in the family? Are grandparents or other family members important or primary communicators? Is there someone in the family who takes on the primary role of communicating or is it shared? Understanding these patterns will help guide the caregiver especially when there is difficult information to address. It is also important to understand the roles individuals play and how these roles impact the family caring for an ill child. For example, do grandparents perform a childcare role? Who is responsible for making sure the family is financially solvent? Are the older children in the family expected to take on additional responsibilities when the ill child has extended hospital stays? What are the family rules? Is certain information kept from children? Is there unspoken pressure that prevents anyone from expressing their needs or asking questions? What are the family relationships like? Is the marriage stressed? Does the family find ways to support one another?

Substance use/abuse

What are the family members' routine drinking and drug use patterns? Were these problematic before the child's illness? If so, what is happening currently? If not, has substance use become problematic since the illness? Are there differences of opinion in the family about whether alcohol and drug use is an issue? Are there dynamics of codependency and/or denial occurring in cases of problematic substance use? How does the substance use impact functioning related to the child's illness and participation in the child's care? Are referrals needed? Alcohol and drug use, while important to understand, are not necessarily problematic. If problems are suspected, the appropriate professional should complete a more specialized substance-abuse assessment.

Additional areas for assessment of the child

Child development

This area should focus on understanding the child's level of development. What is the developmental history of the child? Have developmental milestones typically been reached within an appropriate time frame? What is the child's developmental stage at this time especially with regard to understanding serious illness, death and spirituality? Has the child regressed during the course of the illness? What is the child's current cognitive functioning and level of understanding?

Play and leisure activities

This area should explore the following: What are the child's likes and dislikes? How does the child spend free time? How much have these activities been altered over the course of the illness? Does the child enjoy art, sports, music etc? Understanding these issues will not only inform the caregiver but will also provide an avenue of communication that the child can relate to. For instance, asking about a child's favorite activity or sports team during the assessment and then remembering to bring this information up in the future helps normalize the child's world and demonstrates care and concern on the part of the caregiver.

Social functioning and peer relationships

This area focuses on relationships with people outside of the family typically in the child's own age range. Who are the child's friends? What are the child's peer relationships like? Have they changed over the course of the illness? Have peers been involved with the child since he or she became ill? To the extent possible, is the child able to engage in age-appropriate social activities? Is there a way peers can be included or encouraged to participate in the treatment? Depending on the developmental stage of the child, these relationships will be more or less important. For instance, peer relationships for adolescents are very important and, if they are fostered during the illness, add a sense of normalcy most adolescents find helpful.

School

This area focuses on understanding the child's school history and current educational needs and desires. What is the child's educational history? Does he or she like school? Are there favorite subjects or activities that can be continued even when the child has lost functioning? Does the child enjoy reading or being read to? How much does the school community understand about what is happening to the child? Is there a way for the child to continue to have contact with the school if desired?

Further areas—that can help guide the team's efforts at interventions

What do you place a high value on as a family?

– Meals together?

– Taking trips?

– Quiet time?

– Other favorite activities?

The above list of topics is not meant to be exhaustive but rather a guide to help focus the assessment. One important area that the caregiver must always be willing to explore is the assessment of risk. Because of the critical nature of this area, we have chosen to provide a more in-depth exploration of the topic.

Risk assessment

In assessing family functioning when a child is dying, expect to find disturbances and disruptions in any or all aspects of functioning. For many such disruptions, the only intervention may be to educate the family and normalize the experience, or perhaps to offer some practical assistance. For example, the experience of a parent calling in sick frequently to work due to poor sleep and stress may be normalized by reassuring the parent that others in their situation also have difficulty coping with work. It is important to point out that a major purpose of assessment is to determine when a disturbance has gone beyond normal or safe limits and has become a risk to the family's or individual's health, safety or welfare.

Risk assessment involves identifying and evaluating areas or behaviors that endanger the family. Typically these may include substance-abuse, suicidal impulses, and family violence. Other examples include conduct resulting in job loss, which plunges the family into deep financial crisis; sleep or eating disturbances that have serious health consequences; or intense emotional reactivity that threatens the stability of a primary relationship, such as a marriage.

How to conduct a good risk assessment:

1. Get assistance if needed: if there is concern that some aspect of behavior or functioning is troubled enough to compromise individual or family safety or integrity, and that area is beyond your scope to assess, request a consultation from an appropriate professional.

2. Let the family or individual know that you are concerned about them and that you want to speak with them, or you want to ask someone else to speak with them, in order to determine if there is something that they need help with.

3. Create a non-judgmental, direct, comfortable and open atmosphere.

4. Ask the more difficult questions in a calm, non-threatening, straightforward manner. Be comfortable with the issues; your comfort level will dictate the interviewee's comfort level.

5. Be prepared for the answers; do not show shock or distress. Expressing empathy and concern is fine. Be prepared with the referrals and resources necessary for whatever you may discover. Offer hope and conviction that there is help for these problems and that the family can get through this crisis.

6. Finally, if you find that you are having difficulty addressing critical issues yourself, ask for consultation and help.

Assessment, and especially risk assessment, may come at unpredictable and inopportune times. Remember that assessment is structure wedded to flexibility. Some people will be ready and able to disclose issues only at their own pace, not at the appointment designated for such disclosure. For example, if you are a physician with whom a father feels particularly comfortable, and one day you casually ask the father at the bedside how he is doing, and he breaks down in tears and says, "Not so good, doctor. I'm at the point that I think my family might be better off without me", you need to be prepared to recognize the request for help and further assess the situation. Such a statement may indicate a suicide assessment is in order, and needs to be further explored without delay.

Practical considerations

Covering the above list may seem like an overwhelming task; however, keep in mind that not every question needs to be asked. Follow-up questions suggested in the outline of assessment areas are only to be used when indicated. For example, if the substance-use questions reveal casual alcohol use that has not changed with the current crisis, then further detail in this area is probably not necessary. Or, if a family reports that their religious practices have minor impact or interaction with the medical situation, then extensive detail is neither required nor appropriate.

Often a multidisciplinary team will share the components of an assessment. Ideally, the team will include a physician, a nurse, a chaplain, a social worker, a psychologist, a child-life specialist and other specialists as needed. The social worker or psychologist may take the lead role in the child and family-assessment and then collect information from other team members.

Depending on the situation family members might be interviewed individually or in subgroups. However, if at all possible, it is important to convene the family unit at some point during the assessment in order to observe the family functioning and to ensure that all members have appropriate input. Patterns of communication can be observed when the family meets together. Often one person will dominate the discussion. Care should be taken to ensure that each family member is addressed and has time to participate. Family members often carry private feelings or fears that they are reluctant to talk about in a group. Let the family know that individual follow-up meetings may be needed and may occur in the future. Notifying the family of the routine nature of an additional interview can prevent members from feeling singled out or frightened.

Family assessments are not finite as assessment is an ongoing fluid component of treatment. Many factors can stimulate the need for reassessment of the family. Changes in medical status or psychosocial functioning are probably the most common stimulants of reassessment although there are a myriad of possibilities that might call for reevaluating the needs of the family.

Case: **Marissa's family**

Marissa was born at 24 weeks to Juan and Claudia ages 31 and 27. She had two siblings, Miguel age 4 and Luis age 8. Claudia cleaned houses and Juan cleaned office buildings. They lived in a 1-bedroom apartment about 1½ h drive from the hospital. Claudia's mother came from Mexico when Marissa was born to help care for the other children. Claudia spent almost all of her time at the hospital where Marissa was in the Neonatal Intensive Care Unit. Juan occasionally came on weekends, as did grandma and the two older siblings. English was the primary language spoken in the hospital where the baby was hospitalized. Although Juan and Claudia spoke some English, they were much more comfortable speaking Spanish. Claudia was often seen crying but was agreeable and compliant with staff. Marissa was not expected to live long due to complications of extreme prematurity.

Because Juan was often absent from the hospital, staff formed judgments about his lack of involvement and often voiced them amongst themselves. They had initially tried contacting him by phone to pass on critical information but due to the difficulty of reaching him, they held the majority of the care conferences with only Claudia present. There was a scarcity of interpreters in the hospital so contacts with Claudia were less frequent and often more hurried than with English speaking families. When Marissa died after spending eight weeks in the NICU, many relatives came to the hospital to support the family. The family left and there was no additional contact with the hospital. Nine months after Marissa's death, the family was interviewed and asked to provide feedback about the care they had received.

***

Case Two interviewers met with the family in their home. The family was anxious to participate and immediately expressed their gratitude for being invited. The interview was conducted in Spanish. The small apartment was full of remembrances of Marissa. Pictures, articles of clothing, baby blankets and toys neatly filled up a bookcase in the corner. Initially Juan and Claudia praised the care their daughter had received. However, with probing, Claudia revealed the loneliness and insecurity she felt during her stay at the hospital. She expressed feelings of disappointment about not having her husband and mother present. She feared that she had at times made the wrong decisions about the care of her daughter and felt that her husband might blame her for the death of their baby. She expressed concern for her two other children and pointed out that her oldest boy had not yet cried for the loss of his sister.

Juan immediately stated that although he was grateful for the care his baby received, he did not feel respected by the staff. During Marissa's illness, he had worked additional hours to make up for the missing income from his wife. He felt pressure to keep the family going financially and to help care for the children at home. His dilapidated truck was unreliable for long-distance driving and had broken down twice while en route to the hospital. He felt his role as head of the household had been ignored and undue burden had been placed on his wife who was already over-wrought from the early delivery. Tearfully, he explained that he had not helped with his baby's care like he would have wanted to. On the occasions he was able to come to the hospital, he felt ignored by staff and stated that information was given mainly to his wife. He was surprised and unprepared when his baby died because his wife had assured him that Marissa was doing well just the night before.

In this case an initial family assessment was performed with Juan and Claudia shortly after the birth of Marissa. At that time, Claudia was exhausted and the NICU was extremely busy. The Spanish speaking social worker completed the assessment but due to the burden of a heavy caseload, failed to do so in a thorough fashion. Others on the care team were equally busy and also encountered the language barrier, which made it even more difficult to fully understand the family's situation. Although the social worker kept a close check on Claudia's emotional functioning, she too failed to gather critical information from the father, grandmother and children. A closer look at the financial resources of the family would have helped illuminate the difficulties the family had visiting the hospital. Also an exploration of who should be included in the discussion of critical information and a plan to incorporate father would have eased some of the grief felt by this family during the hospitalization and through bereavement. The father's role in the family was traditionally to have the final say in serious decisions. Regarding the care of his baby, he often felt this role was ignored. Although Marissa's siblings had visited the hospital a few times they had been left out of the assessment process. Claudia was asked by the medical team how her other children were doing but she usually gave simple, nondescript answers. Understandably, the children were in the care of grandmother and Claudia's attention was focused almost exclusively on the baby. Even if the siblings weren't able to visit regularly, an initial assessment might very well have laid the groundwork of a relationship that could be tapped into later if the need arose. Also, resources for the younger children such as books, supports at school and community resources could have been put into place. Claudia's compliance with the medical regime and lack of questions was misinterpreted and led the staff to assume that she was all right. In fact she was overwhelmed and intimidated by the University Hospital setting and without consistent use of her primary language she felt ill at ease. It is understandable that some of these issues would be missed on the initial assessment; however, a reassessment along the way should have helped to capture some of the missing elements. The meeting during bereavement helped the family to express some of their concerns, gather reassurances about the care they provided their daughter, and include the siblings in the process.

Case: **Dani's story**

Dani, an 8-year-old precocious girl with blonde hair and a face full of freckles was discharged home after unsuccessful treatment for rabdomyasarcoma. A family assessment was done as Dani transitioned to the palliative phases of treatment. Along with Dani, her parents, John and Linda, ages 46 and 54 were present for the assessment. John was a disabled war veteran still traumatized by his war experiences. During his military experience he had engaged in hand-to-hand combat and had witnessed many atrocities. He was a big man with a volatile disposition whose world centred on his daughter. Linda worked in a candy factory and was the main financial support for the family. Dani had no siblings nor did Linda or John have any other family. Before the conference began, John approached the medical team and indicated that he did not want his daughter told that she was going to die. He agreed to let the team tell her that she would be getting a different kind of treatment which would focus on making her feel comfortable. Linda strongly agreed with her husband and stated that they would leave the meeting if anyone failed to honor their wishes. The attending physician said he would abide by their wishes unless Dani asked the medical team directly whether or not she was going to live. The conference went fairly smoothly although several issues were not discussed due to John and Linda's request. The plan was to wait and reassess the family in the near future. The meeting ended and Dani's family prepared to go home. The social worker who had worked with the family for some time said goodbye to them and indicated that she would make a home visit in the next couple of days. At that point, Dani chased down the hallway after her, and tugging at her sleeve, announced with urgency, "I have to tell you a secret!" The social worker leaned over toward her and Dani whispered, "I am going to die, but don't tell my parents because they won't be able to take it. It has to be our secret." The social worker gave her a hug and assured her she wouldn't tell anyone but then added that they would talk about what to do when she came to the house to visit.

Case With regard to the assessment of this family there are several noteworthy areas.

Much of their energy and communication patterns focused on keeping from each other the secret of Dani's coming death. Keeping this secret is one way for families to maintain a sense of control when they have lost control over the most basic of functions: the parents' function to protect their child and the child's function to please their parents.

A family like this may experience substantial relief from the endless, overwhelming and ultimately impossible demands of maintaining a façade and letting go of the secrecy. But to reach such a family requires gentle, thorough, non-judgmental exploration. Time taken to meet with the parents both together and separately over several sessions to discuss their needs, fears, hopes and goals could open them to considering alternate ways of managing the situation. On the other hand, the assessment might reveal that while maintaining secrets is not ideal, this remains the best coping alternative, and to disrupt it may plunge the family into a destructive dynamic, harming the positive aspects of their remaining time with their child. If such were the case, the care team could formulate a clear and consistent plan on how to protect the fragile family from devastating disruption by allowing them to maintain their own coping strategies which include a long-standing pattern of maintaining secrets.

There is a clear need to assess the father's level of previous loss and trauma. His volatility, lack of close family connections and supports would warrant performing a thorough risk assessment. In a family which tries so hard to control information, the pace of assessment is critical. Pushing such a family too hard will almost surely alienate them from the care team. However, developing a relationship during the assessment process with frequent reassessments will help give the family an opportunity to form a trusting relationship with members of the care team and pave the way for future interventions.

There is much to be learned about the needs of families by listening to the power of their voices. When asked, they can provide the most enlightening reflection caregivers can find regarding what works well and what doesn't. The individual family assessment lays the foundation upon which to build a treatment plan and partnership for the future. As we have seen with our case examples, the well-done assessment can alleviate future suffering and pain. There are many who say that the initial interview with a family in crises is an art, something difficult to teach. However, the caring practitioner who takes the time to ask important questions and truly listen to the answers will find rich rewards in the relationship with the family.

Systemic assessment of the needs of families in pediatric palliative care

While the assessment with individual families is critical to providing optimal care, the systemic exploration of the families' needs on a broad scale can produce insights regarding the components necessary for high quality care and programmatic enhancements. In the remainder of this chapter we will review a selected portion of the results from one such needs assessment performed at Lucile Packard Children's Hospital at Stanford, an academic teaching hospital at the Stanford University Medical Center. Portions of this assessment have been reported earlier [8].

In order to assess the needs of families pediatric palliative care and to obtain receiving input regarding the desirability of initiating a palliative care service, we conducted extensive interviews with families. We asked about their needs, experiences and suggestions for improving the quality of end-of-life care. Participants were English- or Spanish-speaking family members of deceased pediatric patients who received care at Lucile Packard Children's Hospital at Stanford. Sixty-eight family members representing 44 deceased children were interviewed regarding treatment, transition to palliative care and bereavement follow-up. In addition, fourteen siblings participated in discussion groups about their experiences and offered suggestions about better meeting their needs.

Privacy and time for discussion

Although participants were understanding about the demands on staff, they stressed the importance of sufficient time for discussion and the need for privacy particularly when discussing sensitive issues. This need, although seemingly obvious, was at times ignored in an effort to "get the job done."

> Everyone was in too much of a hurry; they could not wait for me to formulate my questions. Sometimes we were in the hallway or a crowded spot on the unit (non-English speaking mother whose 5-year-old daughter died from leukemia).

Qualities of a good care provider

With striking consistency, families described the qualities of honesty, clinical accuracy, compassion and availability as the most highly valued in a care provider. Families also believed that their needs were best met when one care provider acted as their primary advocate throughout the course of treatment.

Communication of difficult news

The ability to deliver difficult news in a sensitive, compassionate yet accurate fashion was seen as highly desirable by families. Families stated that a familiar person should convey difficult news especially when it involved an impending death. Language should be easy to understand and non-technical. A straightforward, simple and honest approach most effectively allowed families to absorb difficult information. The ability to convey difficult news while still allowing for hope was essential even if the hope was only for a miracle.

Family involvement in care

Families expressed a strong desire to be involved in care and to feel that they were participating as much as possible. They conveyed deep appreciation for those staff who embraced their contribution and expertise regarding the needs of their child. Conversely, families who felt their opinions were disregarded were deeply offended and wrestled with lasting ill feelings about care.

Relationship with the child

The staff's ability to form a relationship with the ill child was seen as imperative to good care. Staff who took the time to form a personal relationship with the child were highly praised while those who treated the child's sick body without recognizing the person inside were seen as less desirable.

> M. liked the staff best who were honest with him and who acknowledged him as a person, not just someone to be

poked and prodded. He was more than just a body...he liked chocolate ice cream and video games, his favorite color was blue...those who took the time to learn those things were the people he liked best. (Mother of a 7-year-old boy who died of osteosarcoma)

Unintentional hurtful remarks

A surprising number of families described incidents of unintentional hurtful remarks. In the worst cases these remarks haunted their thoughts long after the death and impeded the healing process. The prevalence and impact of these mistakes underscore the need for careful, compassionate communication. Interestingly, many family members stated that a simple apology or recognition of the error would have been enough to rebuild trust. However, apologies in these instances were rare.

*I think M said something to the second nurse like, "I had to wait a long time for the pain medication." The next thing I know, the nurse laid into him very badly. She said, "Don't you ever again tell anybody that I don't do my job. I do the best I can." Here's this poor little boy, he's in pain, he's in a burn bed, and I can remember her leaning over the bed, and her tone of voice, and then him looking up at her and it broke my heart. I'll never forget that. (Mother whose 16-year-old son died of graft vs. host disease)

Preparation for death

When confronted with end-of-life realities, most parents said they would have benefited from more preparatory information. Particularly in the case of home deaths, many parents were required to perform care-giving tasks that they had not anticipated. Not only did they feel inadequately prepared for these demands, they said this also prevented them from "just being" with their dying child.

The whole night before she died was the time I felt completely unprepared for. She really went through so much suffering. Even knowing that word, suffocating, I didn't get it. (Father of an 18-year-old daughter who died of CF)

Sibling needs

The participants' responses revealed the need for further outreach to the healthy siblings. In most instances siblings were deprived of attention because their parents were preoccupied with the ill child. In addition, siblings expressed a desire to be more included in the care of their brother or sister. Of note is that siblings reported that home deaths also compounded the emotional toll, as they could not count on home as a safe haven during the time their brother or sister was very ill or dying.

Several children believed that their parents' intense grief would only be exacerbated if they shared their own feelings of sadness, fear, shock and anger. Consequently, many children were left to wrestle with their own emotions without intervention until long after the death.

It's scary. I didn't want to be there when my sister died. My mom woke me up sobbing...Imagine; I was only 8 years old! (10-year-old boy)

Non-English speaking families

The problems arising from the language barrier between non-English speaking parents and hospital staff permeated virtually every aspect of the parents' hospital experience. Adult non-English participants reported feeling isolated, unsupported, and distrustful of the hospital system. It was the primary caregivers who took the time to show genuine concern who earned the trust of these families.

When I went to the hospital, I was very reserved, very quiet. I couldn't talk about my feelings. I felt ignored at the hospital because of the language barrier. (Non-English-speaking father whose 4-year-old son died of a brain tumor)

Home deaths

In recent years we have come to believe that dying at home is desirable and somehow better than death in other settings. For many this may be true but there are several points to keep in mind. Several of the families who experienced home deaths reported problems with accessing services, lack of knowledge/experience with pediatric care, and difficulty with pain management. In addition, siblings reported feeling frightened and disturbed by the loss of home as a 'safe haven'. Families expressed the need for stronger supports from the hospital and from the community when taking a child home to die.

Pain management

Observing children in pain was cited over and over as one of the most anguishing experiences that families endured. The need for pain- and symptom-management in all settings was given the utmost importance. Pediatric literature calls for improvement in pain and symptom management and underscores the fact that children still experience pain and other debilitating symptoms unnecessarily [9,10,11].

Bereavement follow-up

Many families stated that they had neither accessed bereavement services nor had contact with staff after the death occurred. Most families felt ongoing contact with staff would be helpful to ease the transition away from the connection to the care facility. The enthusiastic gratitude for the needs assessment interview expressed by families may well indicate that there is an unmet need for opportunities to discuss such tragic events as the death of a child.

> As soon as she died, there was no more help. (Father whose 1-year-old daughter died from leukemia)

Conclusion

Information gathered from this assessment illuminated difficulties caused by a lack of quality communication. The need for comprehensive information from a familiar, trusted and empathic staff person was a powerful and predominant theme. The quality of the relationship between staff and the children and their families was regarded as crucial to a positive appraisal of the overall experience.

There is a substantial body of knowledge available regarding the impact of a child's illness and death on siblings [7,12,13]. Even so, siblings continue to be a low priority on the care continuum. Both the family interviews and sibling groups revealed that a comprehensive program that includes attention to siblings is a necessary and lacking component in quality care.

Summary

The purpose of this chapter was to illuminate the value of assessment on several levels. The large-scale needs assessment performed with the assistance of scores of bereaved family members taught us invaluable lessons about not only how to improve our health care systems, but about what to look for when we sit down with individual families to ask how they are doing. We must never assume what they need; we must always ask. We must ask from the position of knowledge, openness and caring, using what we know about basic assessment practices.

It is difficult if not impossible to provide families what they need when we don't know what that is. Educated guesses and assumptions will most likely fail both our families and the care team. The most abundant resource for this information is at our fingertips: the families themselves. For the most part families will respond if we provide the time, setting, atmosphere, and guidance to engage them in a compassionate and truthful dialogue. Wasted time, miscommunication and negative feelings can be avoided if we make this effort. Best of all, with a thorough and systematic ongoing family assessment a child's life can be improved and death can be eased.

References

1. Institute of Medicine of the National Academies. Summary. In Marilyn Field and Richard Behrman, eds. *When Children Die*. Washington DC: The National Academies Press, 2001, pp. 1.

2. American Academy of Pediatrics Task Force on the Family. Family pediatrics. *Pediatrics,* 2003 lll (Suppl.):1541–68.

3. Rosen, E.J. Loss and the Life Cycle. *Families Facing Death*. San Francisco, CA: Jossey-Bass Publishers,1998, pp. 47–67.

4. Rosof, B. *The Worst Loss*. New York: Henry Holt and Company Inc, 1994, pp. 3–20.

5. Kadushin, A. *The Social Work Interview*. New York: Columbia University Press, 1972, pp. 25–60.

6. Shapiro, E.R. *The Death of a Child. Grief as a Family Process*. New York: The Guilford Press,1994, pp. 185–*213.

7. Sourkes, B. Siblings of the pediatric cancer patient. In: J. Kellerman, ed. *Psychological Aspects of Childhood Cancer*. Springfield Ill: Charles C Thomas Publishers, 1980, pp. 47–69.

8. Contro, N., Larson, J., Scofield, S., Sourkes, B., and Cohen, H. Family Perspectives on Pediatric Palliative Care. *Arch Pediatr Adolesc Med* 2001; 155:14–19.

9. Wolfe, J., Grier, H., Klar, N., *et al.* Symptoms and suffering at the end of life in children with cancer. *N Engl J Med*. 2000; 342:326–33.

10. Eland, J. and Anderson, J. The experience of pain in children. *In A. Jacox, ed. Pain: A Sourcebook for Nurses and Other Health Professionals*. Boston, MA: Little Brown and Company Inc,1997, pp. 453–78.

11. Schechter N., Allen, D., and Hanson, K. Status of pediatric pain control: A comparison of hospital analgesic use in children and adults. *Pediatrics*, 1986; 77:11–15.

12. Stahlman, S. Children and the death of a sibling. In: C. Corr, and D. Corr, eds. *Handbook of Childhood Death and Bereavement*. pp. 149–64. New York: Springer Publishing Co. Inc., 1996, pp. 149–64.

13. Hogan, N. and DeSantis, L. Basic constructs of a theory of adolescent sibling bereavement. In D. Klass, R. Silverman, and S. Nickman eds. *Continuing Bonds: New Understanding* Washington DC: Taylor and Francis, 1996, pp. 235–54.

13 Impact of life-limiting illness on the family

Mary Lewis and Helen Prescott

Introduction

When a child is diagnosed with a life-threatening condition, a family is cast into a world it probably did not even know existed. A world full of confusion, disbelief and anguish unfurls, where difficult decisions regarding care and treatment and the desperate need for hope will have to be balanced with the realism of diagnosis.

'Being a parent of a child like Kim is like going to another planet; there isn't a guide book'. (Julia, Kimberley's Mum)

This chapter introduces the reader to some information about the family living with a child with a life-threatening or life-limiting illness, and the impact on individual members within the family. In the first section, the notion of family is defined, and family functioning and roles are discussed. In the second section, the effects of long-term illness, dying and death of a child on individuals within a family are introduced. In the final section, the reader is acquainted with some strategies and suggestions on how professionals and services can work with families to offer effective and timely support and help.

It is our argument that a long-term family care model which incorporates an understanding of individuals' and systems' roles, their needs and their beliefs to ensure optimum quality of life, is required. This approach is in accord with the values and philosophy required for care within the context of contemporary society. It has been noted in the literature on families [1] that some authors focus upon individuals, and regard other members as the social context of the person, whilst others look at the family unit as a whole, with individual family members making up parts of the whole. In this chapter we hope to develop readers' thinking and practice beyond the current tendency towards individual focus [2], to caring for the family as a unit, although not at the expense of individuals.

We have also included parents' narratives with the aim of adding depth and lending coherence to the discussion [3]. This approach is in keeping with the contemporary health care policy in the United Kingdom of 'user involvement' [4–6]. Our acknowledgement and thanks go to all the families who have contributed so unreservedly with this endeavour.

The experience of conditions and long-term illnesses that are palliative encompasses two emerging concepts: a life span developmental perspective and quality of life. We believe these are keys to an understanding of the experiences of families, and of how to help them.

Life span perspective

A family, when a child member has a life-threatening or life-limiting illness, faces a series of biographical disruptions [7] and transitions to differing levels of adversity [8,9]. In an exploration of the meaning of health for adults with Cystic Fibrosis [7], health is suggested as a dynamic concept [9].

Laurence's narrative illustrates this.

Case 'We are on a long journey that is constantly changing; our journey has changed and our needs have changed, and we see now will continue to change. We have therefore needed services and people to adapt and change as time goes by in a non-prescriptive way. In the beginning we needed daily visits, both to help with Alice's care and to support and keep us going. Two years on and we need regular contact, not so regular visits and support to organise a family trip to EuroDisney, including a care plan in French.' (Laurence: Katy, Oliver, Alice and Isobel's dad)

A life-span perspective reflects health as a dynamic concept, and incorporates the formation of health beliefs and habits during the developmental years of childhood and adolescence, [10, p. 476] alongside a family unit's evolving experience of caring for a child with a life-threatening or life-limiting illness. This allows periods of both change and stability to be viewed in a social context [7,10].

Quality of life

Quality of life is an emerging and central concept [3,11–15] relevant to this group of families. Meaningful measures of quality of life should be used to evaluate health and social care interventions [16]: 'symptom response and survival rates are no longer enough'. Definitions and measurements of the notion of quality of life, however, are inconsistent, making meaningful comparisons difficult [17]. The validity of health professionals' specific attempts to influence quality of life has been questioned [18]. It is rather suggested that health is one of many constituents, and its relative importance changes at different levels over a life span [18,19]. An alternative approach may be the use of lay definitions [17] to understand quality of life from an individual's perspective, [3] and place an emphasis on listening very carefully to personal perceptions of family members about quality-of-life issues.

Definitions of the family

A review of the literature on family theories and methods suggests that researchers from a variety of disciplines have struggled to define the term 'family' [20]. Baggaley [2] points out that when 'family' is used in the course of social interaction, it is readily understood by others. However, if we take time to consider what might be a definition of a family, the potential for different interpretations becomes apparent. Families do not exist in a social vacuum, but are partly determined by the surrounding culture. Skynner [2, p. 27] considered the family to be both inward- and outward looking and emphasised that society both reflects change in families and that society effects change upon families over time. 'This mutuality means there are as many forms of families as there are societies' [2, p. 27].

The Oxford dictionary's definition of family is 'a household'; although household fits with the census definition of family, it does not take account of the notion of family relationships. In the context of family nursing, Wright and Leahey [21, p. 40] use the following definition: 'the family is who they say they are'. This appears to accord with Frude's [1] notion of selection criteria, that involves an individual stating who he/she regards as being a member of the family, involving feelings of 'affinity, obligation, intimacy and emotional attachment' [1, p. 4].

The advantage of this approach is the recognition of non-traditional family groupings that are a feature of contemporary society [22]. Examples include single parent households, cohabiting couples, homosexual couples and 'any variation that may be encountered when working with families from cultures other than that of the host country' [23, p. 7].

The approach suggested, therefore, is an acceptance of the family's own definition of itself that provides a way of recognising the importance of affectional bonds [22] which do not precisely fit with the conventional view of the family, but equally, do not devalue the strength of the traditional family.

Family systems

The traditional view of family involvement in health care has been uni-dimensional, with family either helping or hindering patient health [24,25]. A family system approach moves the focus away from individuals to their primary social context, the family system [10,24], and the notion of family-centred care in the direction of family health. In the reality of practice, it is recognised that the shift in focus from family as context to family as unit of care may vary in relation to episodes in the family's experience [23]. However, we believe that this change of focus is timely and relevant to contemporary health and social care. This approach has its roots within the *systems theory*, and a brief discussion follows to put this into context.

The systems theory provides a basis for models of adaptation, for example, of families, and supports both empirical and theoretical perspectives [26]. In systems theory, all levels are linked within a hierarchical continuum, linking larger subordinate units to less complex ones. This provides a focus on accommodation, through the life span, between the individual and his/her changing environment. In the context of life-threatening and life-limiting illness, this approach suggests a need to explore the multiple factors that affect outcomes, as well as a need to assess the impact on individuals, families and communities of these diagnoses. It also suggests the notion of continuous interaction of both constitutional and environmental factors over time [26]. A systems developmental perspective offers a framework for interdependence between the 'properties of the person and of the environment, the structures of the environmental settings and the processes taking place within and between them' [27].

Four levels of systems in society are described, which relate to individuals with long-term illnesses, and to family systems [10,26–28] (Table 13.1 and Figure 13.1).

Within this model reciprocity, interconnections and relations between settings, transitions and role shifts are central

Table 13.1 Four levels relating to family systems

1. **Microsystem** of the child and family in their immediate environment

2. **Mesosystem** with which the family interacts on a daily basis; health and social care workers, extended family, community

3. **Exosystem** in which the mesosystem is seated; media, voluntary agencies, health and social care systems

4. **Macrosystem** that makes up the broad values and beliefs of the culture within which the individual lives. This includes ethnic, cultural, socio-economic and political factors

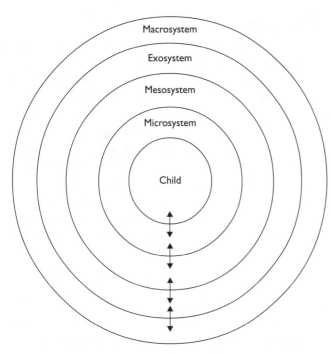

Fig. 13.1 Diagram representing the family systems framework. (Adapted from Thompson and Gustafson [26]; Bronfenbrenner [29]; Wright and Leabey [30].)

across the life span of a child and his illness journey [26]. There is much evidence now of the impact of parents' child-rearing behaviour on children's development. The systems theory identifies the crucial role of parenting as one of the adaptations that occur through the life span between a child and his or her environment. Life-threatening and life-limiting illnesses present a substantial challenge to the adaptation process, representing a major stressor to which the child and family systems endeavour to adapt.

The family is a system in which the sum is more than the total of its parts. Anything that affects the system as a whole will affect the individual members, while anything that affects the individual members will necessarily affect the system as a

whole. Like all systems, the family system struggles to maintain its balance and equilibrium. Bluebond-Langner's [31] ethnography of well siblings of children with cystic fibrosis illustrates how chronic illness sets the family and its members apart from others, and creates challenges for individuals and relationships within families.

'Plans, roles, duties, obligations and priorities change as family life is interrupted by the burdens of care and treatment' [12, p. 200].

It is suggested that this way of conceptualising the effects on family functioning takes account of the dynamic processes involved, and incorporates social and psychological elements [10,26]. Although strategies are adopted that enable family members to live with some sense of normalcy and control, it is not suggested that these strategies remove the conflicts or pain of the illness [31]. 'No more than all physical illnesses can be cured, can all social and psychological problems be prevented or remedied...' [31]. This is an important concept when assessing the outcomes and potentiality of the notion of professional support for families and family members.

Families develop specific roles, rules, communication patterns, expectations and patterns of behaviour that reflect their beliefs, values, norms, coping strategies, system alliances and coalitions to keep the system as consistent and stable as possible. A life-threatening or life-limiting condition is a diagnosis that affects the whole family, and the responses of the child, parents and siblings are highly interdependent. Laurence's narrative illustrates this.

'When our first child, Isobel, died at 9 months of age and when two days later we knew her twin, Alice, had the same unknown but life-threatening illness, our journey began and has affected our whole family. We were lost, totally confused; had lost control over everything we were doing. We have all adapted to accommodate Alice's needs. It has been very traumatic; there is no consolable or reasonable explanation for this happening to us. But we would like to think we are better people for it. As a family we are very close, we share a common experience and all know that Alice is special. She is a child who brings drama and extreme emotions to our lives.' (Laurence: Katy, Oliver, Alice and Isobel's dad)

Although the focus of this chapter is the family, it is recognised that a balance must be found in acknowledgement of Friedemann's [32, p. 15] suggestion that 'if the whole family system is viewed as the person who receives the care, the focus on each individual in the family is lost'. In order for the family as a whole to be balanced, the health and well-being of the individuals needs to be both understood and maintained as far as is possible. This concords with Mackenzie's [33] view that to provide support, (nurses) 'need to be able to "see" into the heart of each family and understand the experience from its perspective' [33, p. 82]. This needs to be balanced with the requirement to consider the welfare of the child, child protection [34] and the rights of the child.

The next section provides a brief overview of roles within a family before reviewing the impact on individual family members of life-threatening and life-limiting illness.

Roles within the family

Family members occupy a specific position, or status, within the family—that of mother, father, brother or sister. The conceptualisation of these roles in families has evolved and changed with the evolution of the family and contemporary society. For example, in Western society, fathers have tended to become more involved in the care of children, and mothers may continue with their careers. For each role within a family's culture, there is a prescription of appropriate relationships and behaviour that influences daily life. Role theory espouses that family roles are reciprocal and directly relate to other roles in the family [35]. Existing family relationships and dynamics are well established, and need to be 'discovered' [36] in order to enable successful work with families (Box 13.1).

Box 13.1 Roles and patterns within families

Examples of patterns a family may have adopted

- One parent may be less able to face stress than the other and choose to avoid situations or accept responsibility (for example, avoiding helping with caring for ill child).

- Parental relationship may be based on one partner being treated as a child by the other partner, and so, unused to being a supportive person within the relationship.

- Parents may be over-protective of their children.

- One child in the family may have a very close relationship with another family member, causing feelings of exclusion in the others.

- Parents may have an existing poor or difficult relationship with the child who becomes ill.

- One parent may seek support from his or her own parents or friends, rather than his or her partner.

- The marital relationship may be unsatisfactory, with poor communication and low levels of mutual support.

(Adapted from [Trapp 36, p. 78])

When a child as a family member becomes unwell, the role pattern changes, and the family members have to work out differing role patterns [35]. During this process of reallocation and reorganization of family roles, siblings' and parents' personal and social development may be affected. Families are dealing with a number of concurrent stressors at this time, some linked to the illness and others independent of it, for example, existing financial pressures. The diagnosis has far reaching implications for daily routines, hopes and ambitions [37].

When faced with a diagnosis of a life-threatening condition, family members, particularly mothers, become carers in addition to their existing roles. Innovations in medical practice, advances in technology, and government policy emphasising the community and primary care sectors as the arenas for long-term care [4,34,38–42] have led to children with long-term care needs being cared for in the community, rather than in institutional settings. This is evident in the growth of hospital-at-home schemes, palliative care services and other domiciliary services, including the role of education and social services [43–46]. Together, these factors have resulted in growing numbers of children being able to live at home, while dependent on their families and medical technology [47–50]. The family, and more specifically the parents, take on the burden and responsibility of the care of the child, [51] and in many cases, provide highly technical and intensive care that previously has been the domain of professionals [52].

'The responsibility of being a parent to two well children is huge; the responsibility of caring for an ill child has been unnerving and we have needed time and space to come to terms with everything.' (Laurence, father)

Parents can often take on the dual roles of co-ordinating care: finding the appropriate professional support whilst at the same time, caring for their child and being parents. In addition, they may also have to provide emotional support for the rest of the family system.

The loss of existing relationships within a family unit can be very difficult, and places a burden on individuals. A sibling, for example, not only experiences the loss of his or her relationship with the ill child, but also is in an environment where the parents' role is changing to one of caring for an ill child. Families need to be enabled and supported in making the right decisions and choices for themselves that they can be comfortable with in the future [36]. Before trying to bring about change when working with families, it is necessary to gain an understanding of how they work and communicate, and to assess whether any change is actually necessary.

Cultural and ethnic variables

The impact of culture and ethnicity on individual and family coping and functioning, and the various role expectations of individual family members and the extended family [53] cannot be underestimated. An understanding of the impact of culture and cultural diversity is essential in order to establish and develop effective and safe practice within health and social care. Many health care practices in the United Kingdom, for example, reflect the traditions of British society and its underpinnings of Christianity. Alongside unfamiliar organisational and health care practices, this can cause distress for families from ethnic minorities when they are most in need of support [54]. There is a requirement to elicit families' models of beliefs about the illness, its meaning for them, their expectations and their needs [55]. As with birth, death and dying are perceived as bio-social events, impacting spiritually as well as being physiological processes.

Pickett [55] defines culture as 'the values, norms, beliefs and practices of a particular group that are learned from generation, to generation, and share and guide thinking, decisions and actions in a patterned way'. A second variant, suggested by Kuper [56], is that the teaching of how to behave and act distinguishes different populations from one another. This may relate to, for example, religion, marriage practices, language and the care of sick and disabled people. Anthropological studies indicate that the key concepts listed in Table 13.2 are not necessarily held in the same way by all cultures [56]. However, there are few studies that focus on the impact of culture on the care of children with palliative care needs and their families.

This area is challenging and complex on a number of levels. While it is recognised that all societies have culture, and belonging to a culture can give a sense of identity and belonging, the juxtaposition is that culture can also be excluding, marking out differences amongst individuals [56]. It cannot be assumed that families from a particular cultural background share the same values, norms and beliefs. Within one family unit, principles affecting decision-making may differ, particularly if members have been influenced by exposure to other cultural traditions. Additionally, just as a life span is dynamic and changing, it cannot be assumed that a cultural perspective is static or unchanging.

Hall *et al.* [55] acknowledges that ethnic groups and different cultures may have varying perspectives about ill children and their care. These views may differ from that of the professional care provider, and make the processes of assessment, intervention and evaluation complex. Professionals will need to compare their own framework with that of the family, and develop a shared model that ensures that what is important for the child and the family is central.

We will now introduce a number of examples of the dilemmas that arise when trying to work in a culturally competent way with families that can be challenging.

Challenges for practice

Some illnesses may already hold a cultural context, due, for example, to the high incidence of a condition in one population. The Human Immuno Deficiency virus (HIV) in the African population is an example of this. Individual differences that may be apparent include the personal and social meaning of the illness, expectations of the illness and treatment and expectations of the role of health workers.

Case A family of Bangaladeshi origin that had recently moved to the United Kingdom was perceived by the hospital care team to be unco-operative and disinterested in learning about their child's care needs prior to the child being discharged. With the aid of an independent translator, it became apparent that the family members were not aware of the expectation that they would participate and take on their child's care, within their own tradition, this would not have been a parental role.

Once this understanding had been achieved, the family was both able and willing to fully learn about the child's care, and could take her home with appropriate support.

The way a family reacts to a diagnosis of life-threatening illness in a child member and the way meaning and value to such an event is accorded varies widely across cultures, and it is important to accommodate the wishes of the child and his or her family at all stages of the child's illness by understanding this.

'Each culture attributes a unique significance to the death of a child. Each holds various beliefs about where children come from before they are born, and where they will go to after they die'. [57, p. 92].

The following are a few examples of the differing values and needs, of families during the course of a child's illness, that significantly impact on the care and support they will want and need.

- In Western society, a child is a source of meaning and purpose in the parents' lives. The death of a child, consequently,

Table 13.2 Key concepts that reflect cultural diversity [56]
1. How childhood is viewed
2. The home environment of care
3. Communication patterns
4. Health beliefs

is particularly threatening to a parent's identity as a protector and provider, and can lead to a sense of failure.

- Egyptian mothers are expected to be withdrawn, mute and inactive for seven years after the death of a child; this behaviour is normal by their cultural standards. In contrast, a Western mother is expected to grieve in private, and return to normal activities soon.

- In some cultures, gender differences affect reactions. For example, if a male child is diagnosed, this will be more traumatic than a female child being diagnosed for a family whose expectation culturally is that he will perpetuate the family name, and be a provider as an adult.

- A variety of traditions relating to preparation for death and for arrangements afterwards exist, and it may be that the rituals that are followed for adults differ from those for children. For example, the Greeks dress a child who has died in wedding attire, as death before marriage is perceived to be especially traumatic. In the Chinese tradition, the death of a child is seen as 'bad' and family members do not attend the funeral or discuss the death, as it is considered shameful to the family [57].

- Infant deaths (and illnesses) may be afforded a special status, with abbreviated rites of bereavement, probably linked with low expectation of survival in some populations. For example, in West Africa, the death of a child under one year of age is seen as a minor loss, and is disregarded by society, and sometimes, the parents themselves. Hindu infants are buried, not cremated, as they are expected to return to earthly life.

- In societies influenced by Western medicine, hospitals have become the focus of care, with professionals delivering this care [57] and attempting to prolong life through a series of interventions. In other societies, care of the dying is still seen as the responsibility of the family and community, and the focus will be on the home.

Within any society, the needs of a cultural minority are generally inadequately met by health and social care services. There is a low uptake of palliative care services by ethnic minority groups in the United Kingdom, for example [55]. This is a matter of concern, as it may lead to culturally diverse perspectives being ignored, and to culturally insensitive decisions and health policies, especially where systems are located within a Western tradition. The difficulties lie beyond barriers relating to language differences, in barriers created by ethnocentric beliefs professionals may hold, that need to be overcome.

In a study of a South Asian population living in the United Kingdom, Randhawa *et al.* [58] found that among the reasons for poor uptake of services were lack of knowledge about service availability and communication difficulties between families and service providers. This would suggest the need for services, and professionals working in them, to develop what Randhawa *et al.* [58] call 'cultural competence'. To take the example of communication differences, however, the problem is not easily resolved using translators, due to the inavailability of personnel with the appropriate knowledge or skills. Family members, notably child members, are relied on, and this can cause difficulties, particularly when sensitive, distressing, and at times, personal information needs to be conveyed. The use of children as interpreters has been said to be 'unprofessional, unethical, uncivilised and totally unacceptable' [58]), but may be the only option available in some circumstances. We would suggest that it is important, in establishing communication to understand the significance of gender and language, for example, and to develop an understanding of the perceptions, knowledge and attitude of the family. This is worth striving for, as good communication lies at the heart of a culturally competent model of palliative care [59].

In concluding this section, we would reinforce the importance of developing an understanding of the interpretation of life-threatening illnesses with culturally diverse families, and their approaches to the care of ill children. We would suggest that this is imperative to reduce stigma and social distancing between providers and recipients of palliative care.

Effects of illness, dying and death of a child on the family

We will now focus on a consideration of the impact of illness, dying and death on family members. As has been noted, the reactions of individuals affect the family system as a whole, and maintaining equilibrium requires both understanding and finding ways of supporting both individuals and the family unit as a whole.

Parents

The course and treatment for a child with a life-threatening illness varies under different conditions, and with different children. Many aspects of the experience of the illness, however, are determined not so much by the particular illness as by developmental, family and social issues. Continuous adaptation occurs at all points on the illness trajectory, the timescale of which varies greatly according to the child's underlying disease process. The families' adaptation will be influenced by both internal and external factors that are influencing the family systems at any one point in time. Parents move through a series of changing biographical disruptions, moving from diagnosis, to coming to terms with, and living with, the illness, to when death is imminent, to when the child dies. At each of these phases, parents and other family members experience a series of losses. Loss can be actual, potential or anticipated. However, since each individual has a unique relationship with the ill child, different things will constitute loss to him or her. This needs to be recognised on an ongoing basis, as the nature and effect of the loss for individuals in the family will directly affect their emotional well-being and ability to adapt and cope with each phase of the child's life.

Diagnosis

There is no easy way for parents to learn that their child is seriously ill. Their sense of shock, numbness and disbelief is much like the experience of bereavement, of mourning for the loss of the healthy child they had known or hoped for. Denial, anger, guilt and despair in varying degrees may all play a part in this initial period. A sense of isolation and loneliness may also be experienced. For some parents, diagnosis may come as confirmation of fears they have harboured for some time, and for some of these parents, the certainty of diagnosis can be a relief. Families have been found to employ a number of different coping strategies at this time [54]. Some enter a period of mourning, while others adopt a proactive caring role [54] and yet others begin a quest for information [60].

It is well recognised that the manner in which news of a life-threatening diagnosis is given to a family is very important. There is some acceptance that in reality, this is often done in a less than satisfactory way [40], with recipients perceiving an uncaring and insensitive response from the professional involved. This can have a major and long-term adverse impact on recipients, affecting adaptation and coping (Fallowfield 1993 in [61]) and trust in the care team [54]. Parents have difficulty absorbing information, and incorrect assumptions can be made relating to parental understanding. If presented poorly, parents will recall the distress and remain angry for many years, as the following narrative illustrates . . . .

> 'The appointment at which we were told about our son, Edward's devastating diagnosis and prognosis was in itself a traumatic experience which because of the way it was conducted by the Consultant Neurologist, has continued to haunt and scare us over seven years on.
>
> We feel it was handled badly for the following reasons:
>
> • The consultant never once said he was sorry or saddened by the news he was giving us.
>
> • His 'triumphalism' at correctly diagnosing Edward's rare diagnosis (Adrenoleukodystrophy) was all too evident.

> • When we asked for information he suggested we go away and find out about it and suggested we watched the film 'Lorenzo's Oil'.
>
> • When we asked about support available he did not offer to find out on our behalf, even though we now know there was a local service for children with life-threatening and life-limiting illnesses.
>
> This experience left us traumatised, very frightened, bewildered and with an overwhelming feeling of being abandoned.' (Helen and Keith, Edward's parents)

In the United Kingdom, there has been a focus on educating and supporting physicians to improve their skills in breaking bad news. However, handling information-giving and early contact with family members need to be done well by all professionals [61], and education in this area should have a multi-professional and collaborative focus.

A key concept for those involved is the recognition of the uniqueness of the event for the individual family receiving the news. Even though the professional may have delivered similar news to a number of families, each individual situation must convey and reflect an essence of caring that is unique [61]. Good interpersonal skills are a central requirement, and a number of attributes are reported to be important in the person delivering the news. Examples include honesty, frankness, gentleness, sympathy and empathy. Box 13.2 suggests other strategies that may be helpful in supporting effective practice in difficult conversations (see also Chapter 3, Communication). A central concept is to remember the significance of this time for the family, as the following narrative illustrates:

> 'Every word said is in my mind, I can remember the smell of the room; I won't ever forget' (mother of child with a cardiac condition).

It is recognized that this is very challenging, especially if a diagnosis, and therefore, prognosis, remains in doubt. In this situation, we would suggest that there is a need to acknowledge what is unknown. However, even this should be communicated sensitively, and as much information as possible should be given. Ongoing management and support of the child and family should not be affected.

Living with the illness

Mastroyannopoulou *et al.* [62], in a study of 93 mothers and 73 fathers of children with life-limiting conditions, found that overall, mothers and fathers coped very differently. Mothers were more likely to cope through emotional release, whereas fathers coped through withdrawal and by being practical. However, these styles of coping were not always perceived to be as effective by the parents themselves.

Box 13.2 Strategies for difficult conversations

Planning

- Respectful and clear communication
- Time, place and a way of delivering the news agreed upon
- Availability of professional or friend for afterwards
- Significant family members present
- Translator available
- Private, quiet, and comfortable setting
- All have enough available time

The conversation

- Tape the conversation, and give a copy to family
- Indicate initially that the news is not good
- Listen very carefully
- Ascertain existing family knowledge and concerns
- Use non-jargonistic language
- Provide diagrams, notes, and information for family to keep
- Avoid evasions while realizing the family will have a need to maintain hope
- Make short-term follow up arrangements

Lengthy treatment, frequent hospitalization, relapse and progression of the underlying disease and the burden of care increase the risks of parental distress, which can result in detrimental effects on employment and in financial difficulties, in addition to impacting on family functioning.

> 'When she first came home she was ill all the time. She was re-admitted and when she goes back in it is really bad and you think she is going to die . . . It is very, very, frightening.' (Mother of a child requiring home-ventilation).

The grief reactions associated with the initial diagnosis can re-surface with heightened intensity when a child relapses or deteriorates. Parents may, at this time, experience feelings of hopelessness and helplessness, in addition to grief, fear, depression, anger and denial. For a child who has experienced a period of being very well, a change in his or her condition can have the same effects, with uncertainty about the next steps in the child's illness. This period needs to be handled as sensitively as the discussions at the time of the initial diagnosis.

Case Kimberley had been diagnosed with a complex cardiac condition at birth that her parents were told would be life-limiting.

As an infant, she survived a number of life-threatening surgical procedures that were palliative. She then had a number of years of being very well, with minimal contact with health care services, although her underlying prognosis had not altered. When she was 7 years old, she developed severe problems with secondary pulmonary hypertension. Her parents were given a very poor prognosis, with no clear plans about future care, except that she didn't have long to live.

More sensitive handling of information at this time, as well as planning and availability of ongoing support, would have been extremely beneficial to the family's coping and adaptation to what, to them, felt like a new diagnosis.

The family of a child with an inherited condition has additional difficulties. Family members may have feelings of guilt and blame, and they will need genetic counselling and information about prenatal diagnosis in the future. An added loss that may be experienced is the loss of future children, if parents decide to follow genetic counselling advice that might advocate this. The extent of this will be dependent on existing and future plans and ambitions that the parents had.

Mothers are usually the main care-givers for their children and therefore, are often primarily responsible for the daily medication, treatment routines and often complex nursing care. A life-limiting disease can create some very practical demands at a domestic level. Mothers, more than fathers, may feel that the child's illness limits their opportunities to work outside the family home, and that their career choices are compromised, adding to their sense of isolation, and potentially increasing the likelihood of them experiencing emotional problems [63].

The literature which exists to address the mental health of parents with a child with a life-threatening illness, points consistently to the fact that mothers have poorer mental health than mothers of healthy children, for example, in relation to suffering from anxiety and depression [64].

Bailey *et al.* [65] (1999) compared the needs of mothers and fathers of children with learning difficulties, and found that mothers expressed significantly more need for family and social support. This group of children are likely to be suffering from degenerative conditions, meaning their illness is characterized by a slow and gradual decline over a number of years. Mothers were reported to need support to manage their stress, conflict and aggressiveness when compared to fathers, who needed more practical information. The longevity of this situation indicates an ongoing and increasing burden, which is compounded by a series of losses as the child's physical and/or cognitive abilities gradually decline.

Studies investigating differences in mothers' and fathers' responses to their child's illness, although limited, have found that women generally respond more 'emotionally' (with anxiety, depression, concern), when compared to men [66]. In comparing the impact of childhood non-malignant life-threatening illness on parents, Mastroyann *et al.* [62], found that low cohesion (characterised by commitment, help and support), length of time since diagnosis of less than two years, and being female were significantly more predictive of higher mental health adjustment difficulties.

The child's illness and care needs can have a profound effect on family social activities, either due to the burden of caring and access difficulties, if the condition is disabling, or due to a need to adhere to strict medication routines and hospital admissions, if the child has cancer, for example. Families describe having to lead a 'divided life', with one parent staying with the ill child, and the other one going to work, or being with the siblings. This places a strain on existing relationships. A family's private world can be difficult to maintain due to the need to have professional involvement, and in some cases, carers in their home to help them with their child's care. This can place further strain on family relationships.

> 'We know we need them (carers) there, but we would much rather we didn't, so sometimes we get angry with them— but it's not them actually, it's the reminder that we can't manage without them because of our child's illness' (Mother of a child with complex needs).

Additional burdens for the family come in the form of practical difficulties with, for example, obtaining equipment when it is required, or in having adaptations done to the home to accommodate a child who becomes immobile; a young man with muscular dystrophy would be an example. These difficulties and frustrations that families may experience leave them with unmet needs and compromise their ability to care and feel in control of their situation. Another frequently reported source of frustration in our experience is lack of access to adequate or appropriate respite care to enable parents to take a break form caring, and provide them with time for their own personal and social needs.

When death is imminent

At the pre-terminal stage of illness, the inevitability of death dominates family life. However, recognising this stage of a child's life is problematic for a number of reasons. For those children who are undergoing treatment with a hope of cure, such as children with cancer who have relapsed, or a child with a cardiac condition who is in intensive care following a surgical procedure, the transition is more clearly defined. For this group the following description of this phase of their lives may be used: 'Terminal care begins at the point in an illness trajectory where nothing can be done to arrest the disease process, and the fundamental goal for the patient shifts from recovery to comfort' [54].

This contrasts with the children who have conditions where cure has never been a possibility, such as those with a neurological condition, or a neuromuscular one such as Duchenne Dystrophy, where the focus of care has always been essentially palliative.

For the first group of children, it can be hard to know when to stop intensive treatment. Physicians following Western traditions tend to focus on cure, and can therefore see dying as failure [67]. Families may have an expectation of treatment continuing. Advances in medicine and technology have created increasing expectations in Western society that death does not have to be inevitable, and that a 'cure' will be found eventually. In following this pathway, the care team and family may collude, and the child may not receive the appropriate treatment and palliative support he or she requires [54]. It is not uncommon for family members to have differing opinions on how long to continue with treatment, and there may be differing cultural expectations. A further complicating factor is if the view of the family does not concord with that of the care team. Within this the child's spoken and unspoken preferences can often be unheard.

Case The family of an Afghanistani child, who as an infant was found to have multiple neurological complications that were not felt by the medical team to be compatible with good quality for her ongoing life, was reluctant to agree to a 'do not resuscitate' policy, as the family members felt that her life and future would be decided by God. They therefore wanted the care team to do everything possible to keep the child alive, as their belief was that if she was not meant to live, it would be God's decision, and not theirs, in agreeing to a DNR policy. The infant's physician's experience was that to try and resuscitate the child would not be in her best interests, and so, he felt unable to agree unreservedly with the father's wishes.

Seeking a resolution in this sort of situation requires sensitive handling and mutual respect, and understanding through good communication.

For the second group of children, the family will have been living with the possibility of death for the whole of the child's life, or since the diagnosis was made. Families report being given a prognosis about when the child is likely to die, for example, before the age of three years. Leading up to this time, the family may go through a period of preparation and anticipation of imminent death. However, if the child lives past this age, as is often the case there is a tendency to view the child's potential for living more positively. Conversely, if the child dies prior to this time, the family may feel that they have missed out on expected time with the child, and that they were not ready for the child's death. Some children in this group may appear to be very stable, but then die unexpectedly. For others, the possibility of technological interventions, such as ventilation, introduces another dimension to the dilemmas they face.

Many children in both groups live lives that are characterised by multiple relapses, but they may confound both parents and professionals by recovering. Each relapse or serious deterioration can then be viewed as survival, and it can be hard for family members to reconcile this with the actual prognosis, and eventual death. It can also mean prolonged periods where the family members are, as one mother described it, 'living on a knife edge', with great uncertainty over long periods of time.

Case The parents of a boy with complex and multiple problems understood from the paediatric team that he had only a year at the most to live. During the following months, his parents made preparations for his death, including planning his funeral, informing people at school and arranging special trips and outings for him. During the year, he experienced a number of acute life-threatening episodes, but survived them all.

A year later, he has now reached a plateau, is not experiencing so many acute episodes, and is back at school full-time. His parents have now reversed their previous decision that he not be resuscitated, their rationale being that the prognosis they were previously given was wrong and they need to give their son every chance of survival.

A review of the literature [68] indicated that the quality of care offered during the terminal or last phase of a child's life may have a profound effect on the bereaved. Furthermore, Dominica [69] asserts that family involvement is never more important than in the terminal phase. Recognizing this phase and providing appropriate and timely support is vital; however, there is some evidence to suggest that health care staff underestimate the magnitude of the emotional problems that families experience [68]. Additionally, professionals tend to overestimate opportunities that are available for parents and other family members to express their concerns. For example, when there has not been a definable period relating to the end stage, parents report a lack of information about the prognosis, and at times, inappropriate communication from professionals [68]. The concept of 'professional distancing' has been noted, as death is imminent and must be guarded against.

The amount of time available to a family is significant for them. If the child's illness means he or she will die as an infant, or in a short time following diagnosis, there is much less time for the family to adjust, and there are less opportunities for choices about the care to be made. Parents need clarity and support through the difficult decisions they are facing. Parents may be unwilling or unsure about making preparations for death if they do not yet accept the inevitable, or if they feel that

doing this will be 'wishing the child away'. Alternatively, they may view their child's needs from the perspective of living rather than dying, and not be able, or willing, to adjust to an alternative stance.

However, it is our experience that in the time leading up to the child's death, and the death itself, planning care arrangements, with attention to the smallest details, can make a big difference to families, minimising the potential for regret that they may experience in bereavement. This extends the notion of end-of-life planning, it is suggested, beyond resuscitation plans to planning for pre- and post-death activities by all family members [70].

Another key task for the family when death is imminent is planning where the preferred place of death is for the child. It is worth noting that these may differ; for example, an adolescent may prefer to be in hospital, recognizing the burden being at home places on his or her parents, and needing to be slightly independent of his or her family, but the family may want him or her to be at the family home. There is general acceptance that a hospital environment requires the parents to alter their usual parenting roles [71]. Many studies over a number of years have emphasised both the feasibility and the desirability of home as the preferred place for children with cancer [72,73]. There is increasing evidence of similar advantages for other children and their families, too [38,45,74,75]. However, for parents, siblings, and the ill child, the availability of a choice of place is the key and ideally their options would include home, hospice or the hospital, with appropriate levels of support being available to them in all of these settings. Each family situation will be unique, and a central principle needs to be that whatever decisions a family makes can be changed at any time.

When a child dies

When a child dies (see Chapter 15, Bereavement), the parents have lost their family as they have known it. Although the family will continue after the death, the family system will be changed by the loss of the presence of the deceased child. Given that a basic function of the parent is to preserve the family and protect the child, there is an implicit expectation that the parent will die before the child.

Where the death results from genetic factors, as indicated previously, parents can hold themselves responsible for not producing a healthy child that could survive longer, and may feel deficient and worthless as a result.

One of the most difficult aspects of parental bereavement is that the death of a child strikes both parents at the same time, and confronts each of them with overwhelming loss. Consequently, a parent's most valuable resource is unavailable, as the person to whom either would normally turn for support is also deeply involved in grief. The parents, therefore, may experience loss, upon loss and may have to deal with the grief of their partners as well as their own. Since each parent had a separate and individual relationship with the child, different things will constitute losses to each parent after the child has died. This will be specifically pertinent at anniversary points, or when they see their child's peers undertaking activities that their child is no longer part of, for example, taking their exams or leaving school.

Children

Age and developmental stage influence the impact of illness on children in at least two important ways: their understanding of their condition, and their overall development, including physical, emotional and cognitive development.

Young children tend to understand illness in terms that are concrete, global and magical. They often give explanations of illnesses that involve contagion. A significant number may believe illness is in some way a punishment for bad behaviour. Older children understand that illness means that some part of their body is not working properly. Adolescents are able to appreciate that illness results from an interaction of factors inside and outside the body. The developmental tasks appropriate to the age of the child can be most vulnerable to the disruption caused by the phases and progression of an illness, including the medications, treatment and hospitalisations. A pre-school child is busy gaining increasing mastery over his or her own body and environment. He or she becomes increasingly independent, and begins to socialise outside the family, while learning about roles within the family. Repeated admissions and increased dependency on parents and medical staff may pose a threat to these aspects of development.

For ten or more years of their lives, school is the major social and educational setting for children. Many children with a life-threatening condition can miss significant amounts of schooling. They can fall behind academically, and can be separated from their friends. They can find it hard to keep up with activities that require physical exertion, and they may stand out from their peers at a time when being just like everyone else is important.

Adolescence is a period of great change, and its developmental tasks are challenging, even for healthy young people. Serious illness can force adolescents to become emotionally and physically dependent on their parents and medical staff at a time when establishing independence and planning for the future are key tasks within this period of development. The demands of their illness may cut them off from their peers, and their activities may be restricted. Planning can also become difficult when facing an uncertain future.

Adjustment

Psychological adjustment is central in addressing the psychological functioning of children with a chronic disorder. Good adjustment can be defined as behaviour that is age-appropriate, normative, and healthy, and follows a trajectory toward positive adult functioning. Maladjustment is mainly evidenced in behaviour that is inappropriate for the particular age, especially when this behaviour is qualitatively pathological or clinical in nature [76].

Children with chronic disorders constitute a group vulnerable to maladjustment, but this is not the most common outcome [60]. The variability in their responses would indicate considerable individual differences. As a consequence of this, studies have addressed the risk and resistant factors that may explain these individual differences to chronic childhood disorders.

Wallander and Varni [77,78] proposed a generic model intended to be potentially applicable to a wide range of paediatric chronic physical disorders. Within a theoretical framework on stress and coping, a paediatric chronic physical disorder is conceptualised as an ongoing chronic strain for both the children and their parents. The model does not assume that a chronically ill child represents an adverse event for the family *per se*. Rather, the primary factor thought to increase the risk of adjustment problems is stress. Stress results from a combination of the medical condition and related functional limitations, as well as from more general causes that occur in everyday life. Adjustment is hypothesised to be influenced by personal, social and coping processes.

Within the Wallander and Varni model of adjustment, risk factors in adjustment include:

(1) Disease and disability parameters, including, for example, diagnosis, medical complications, and cognitive functioning;

(2) Functional dependence in the activities of daily living;

(3) Psycho-social stressors disability related problems, major life events, and daily hassles.

Resistance factors are defined as:

(1) Intrapersonal factors, such as competence, temperament and problem-solving ability;

(2) Social–ecological factors, such as family psychological environment, social support, and practical resources available to the family;

(3) Stress processing factors, such as cognitive appraisal and coping strategies.

Risk factors therefore elevate the likelihood of adjustment problems, and resistance factors moderate their influence. For example, a sibling's emotional ability to cope will depend crucially on the way the family as a whole manages. If a family has previously been dysfunctional (with poor communication, emotional involvement and problem solving), it is likely they will be less able to provide a supportive environment for a sibling to express his or her feelings in. An assessment of family functioning, however, can only be made in the context of family cultural practices.

Case A 7-year-old boy living with a complex neuromuscular problem since birth had been cared for by his family at home, with relatively minimal support from professionals. His parents and two elder siblings as well as extended family and the local village community provided the majority of the required practical, social and psychological support required.

As his siblings grew up, one was leaving home, and extended family members became unwell, and so, less able to help. The equilibrium of the family system became disrupted, and the family risk factors more significant, until adjustments and increased input from outside agencies could assist the family to address the imbalance and enable it to find new ways of coping very successfully.

Siblings

The devastating impact of a life-threatening/life-limiting condition and childhood death on parents is well recognized, but the effects on siblings are also significant.

> 'But I still get worried about Britt. I just know that with CF (cystic fibrosis) you could die from it. And you get all skinny. And your lungs fill up with mucus. And you can't breathe. And you die'. (Tyler Foster, age 9, talking about his sister, Chapter 12, [12]).

Sibling relationships are complex, extending beyond the traditional notions of rivalry and jealousy [68]. The emotional relationships that children and their families have are dynamic, encompassing rivalry, loyalty, affection and aggression in varying degrees [36,68]. Children may feel lonely, isolated, sad and displaced in their family. They are surrounded by fear and uncertainty when their established boundaries have changed and are no longer fixed. Children's age, gender, and cognitive and emotional development will differentiate and affect their experience of having an ill child in their family. For example, Wass [28] argues that adolescents, in a sense, are experiencing loss, anyway—loss of childhood and the protective support of their parents. The potential death of a sibling at this time, as well as their parents' inevitable distraction, will interfere at every level with their business of being young persons. There will inevitably be conflict and potentially irreconcilable needs.

In a study of 52 healthy siblings of children with life-limiting conditions, Stallard *et al.* [79] identified significant communication needs in younger children, particularly boys. Despite this, the majority of parents perceived them to be coping well with their sibling's illness. This finding is consistent with that found in other areas of research, including research of siblings children with cancer, and particularly those of post-traumatic stress disorder where adults have been found to repeatedly under estimate the effects of traumatic events on children [80]. The perception of the parents that the child is coping, may be one explanation as to why they are not talking with, or providing more information to their healthy children. Alternatively, parents may be preoccupied with the ill child, and are therefore unable to fully appreciate the needs of the healthy siblings. It is clear, however, that although children do not ask questions, this does not mean that they are not concerned or worried. The reported lack of information provided to younger children may be due to parental uncertainty about what to tell their children, and at what age to do so, or it may reflect a general anxiety about talking with children about painful and distressing events. Whatever the reason, it is clear that parental reports alone must not be relied on to assess the effects on siblings, or to assess what their needs are. Sibling self-reports are very important.

Siblings may have their own versions of the causation of their brother's/sister's illness, and may hold some misconceptions about the nature of the illness, hospital and treatment programmes. They may be fearful of developing the same illness, and alongside this fear, they may experience guilt and relief that they have not developed the illness. They may also experience shame at having a child in the family who is ill or dying. Other feelings about their sick brother or sister include resentment or envy as parents, grandparents and other members of the extended family may be preoccupied with the sick child, [81] which may in turn compromise academic and social functioning [82].

The sick child needs a tremendous amount of parental attention, time and activity, which limits the parents' capacity to attend to and support well siblings.

> 'There is an imbalance with attention and care to other siblings—this has an impact. Other siblings get left out.' (Mother of a child requiring home-ventilation).

The demands on the expected roles of parents, such as the mother staying with the sick child in hospital whilst the father cares for the well siblings, or the siblings' stay with other relatives, creates drastic changes in the family dynamics, allowing the well siblings to potentially feel psychologically and emotionally isolated. It is not uncommon, therefore, for siblings to demonstrate difficult and challenging behaviour.

> 'They went to their grandparents when our son was in hospital. It was hard for them.' (Father of a young boy requiring home-ventilation).

A disturbing feature in siblings that can result from family separation is the manifestation of a number of psychological problems, such as enuresis, separation anxiety, abdominal pain and constipation. A number of behaviours that siblings may display, such as aggression or anti-social behaviour, are assumed to be aimed at gaining parental attention. Murray [83] identifies siblings as: 'the most emotionally overlooked and sad of all family members during childhood cancer'.

Siblings may also adopt a parental role in responsibility for the other brothers and sisters, and may also participate in the care of their ill brother or sister, or in domestic chores [68].

Some studies, however, report more positive effects of life-threatening illness in siblings [84]. Some siblings appear to benefit emotionally and psychologically from the experience, and are apparently no more at risk of psychological impairment than other siblings. Siblings of disabled children have been found to be more compassionate, sensitive and appreciative of good health than their other peers [68]. Iles [68], in a study of siblings of children with cancer, found that although they experienced the illness as a loss and stressor, they also found it to be potentially a time of growth, with increased empathy for their parents' needs.

It is suggested that there are a number of variables mediating sibling adjustment, but this is an under-researched area Box 13.3.

The wider family: grandparents and others

In discussing the significance for the wider family, it is important to remember that the child and family determine who significant family members are [30,85] and this may, or may not, include grandparents. It is our experience that grandparents and extended family members can either be a source of support, practical help and strength, or, in contrast, an

Box 13.3 Mediating variables of sibling adjustment

- Type of disease
- Type of disability
- Disease severity
- Gender
- Age and age spacing between sibling and the ill child
- Marital and family relationships
- Social support
- Family communication (open or closed)

(Adapted form Drotar and Crawford 1983 in While et al. [68])

additional pressure on the nuclear family. A key determinant will be the nature of existing relationships between the grandparents and their adult children, and the grandchildren. These relationships and existing communication patterns will be further influenced by cultural values and beliefs.

The wider family members are involved in the child's life at two levels; firstly, in supporting their adult children through a very painful time, and secondly, in their own grief for the child. From the grandparents' perspective, they are not in a position to have any information, or control, over any aspect of what is taking place, including decisions that are made about the child's care and treatment [36]. There is a paucity of literature relating to the role of grandparents in, and influence on, the family system [86]. It is generally recognized that they can go through a number of emotions, in addition to providing practical help and advice, without necessarily receiving support, or acknowledgement of their own needs [36].

In a study of grandparents of disabled children, Katz and Kessel [86] found that their satisfaction with their roles related to their views of the illness or disability, their relationship with their adult children, and their own life experiences. For many grandparents, when a child is diagnosed with a life-threatening illness, there can be an overwhelming feeling of guilt that they are alive, while their grandchild is now likely to die before them [36]. In the order of family lifecycles this creates disorder and can be hard to accept, and lead to feelings of helplessness and loss of control. Grandparents can feel anxious, exhausted and powerless. They can also, in some instances, be perceived as domineering and over-protective, and may be resented by the parents if they are felt to be in competition for the rule of the primary carer. However, in working with families, there is some evidence that involving the extended family in a care culture can influence the possibilities of them becoming involved in a positive way [87], and that support from grandparents may be more important to family adaptation than professional help [86].

Families may identify other significant people from within their communities who will be important for professionals to work with, and who may fulfil a role as substitute extended family members in terms of offering support and practical help. However, families also report difficult interactions with the wider community, often feeling isolated and excluded from activities that had previously been important to them, but now no longer seem to hold the same value for them. Many report instances of misplaced sympathy, not welcoming intrusions into their private worlds, [36] and hearing inappropriate things being said. Some report interactions where the subject of their child's illness is ignored completely, some sense that people are avoiding contact with them. Another feature of this changed perception and interaction can be found in the example of parents in the school playground, who may hear other parents complaining about what they now perceive as a trivial matter.

In understanding the impact of the child's illness on the wider family, and the potential positive and negative effects on the equilibrium of the family unit of these members and individuals, efforts to support the family in adapting and coping with the situation can be set within the real context of the families' existing systems and processes.

Helping the family

In this final section, the intention is to discuss how families and individual members can be enabled, as far as possible, to cope and live with the reality of childhood life-threatening and life-limiting illness. The term 'professional' is used to encompass all those involved with supporting and caring for families as part of their work.

We propose that to re-focus using a conceptual framework based on partnership and quality of life across a life span requires system changes and innovation at micro and macro levels. The systems framework, described above, is used to locate the emerging themes relating to helping the family. This has been chosen for its simplicity and relevance to practice, allowing readers to identify the arena within which they may be able to influence the family experience, and enabling them to act appropriately and effectively.

Whyte ([23], p. 10) presents a statement of principles that relate to family systems thinking (Box 13.4); these seem fundamental to an understanding of family assessment, and of a model of care that is relevant for this group of families.

It has been suggested that three processes influence family systems [26; Figure 13.2]:

(1) Cognitive processes;

(2) Social support;

(3) Coping methods.

Box 13.4 Principles of family systems

[23, p. 10]

- Parts of the family are related to each other.
- One part of the family cannot be understood in isolation from the rest of the system.
- Family functioning is more than just the sum of the parts.
- A family's structure and organisation are important in determining the behaviour of family members.
- Communication and feedback mechanisms between family members are important in the functioning of the family system.

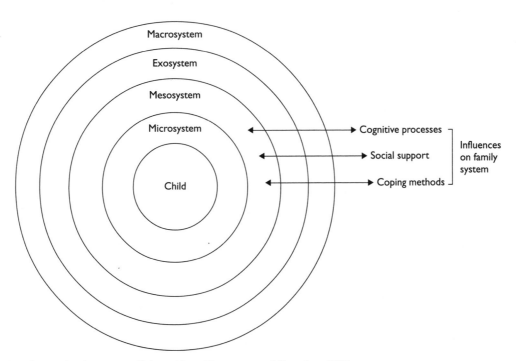

Fig. 13.2 Principles affecting family systems. (Adapted from Thompson and Gustafson [26].)

Our view is that social support and coping methods can realistically be the focus for inter-agency and inter-professional services to facilitate and support adaptation. The discussion presented should be viewed as our interpretation and suggestions based on experience of working with families, and on families' own stories, as they have been told to us.

Child and family (micro level)

The micro level relates to the child and family, and an exploration of ways of enabling, supporting and empowering individual family members and family units to cope and adapt to the threatening situation they are in, as well as possible.

Assessment (See also Chapter 12, Assessment)

Lewis [88] suggests that services for children with life-threatening conditions should be family-focused, in order to address the needs, including psychological needs of all family members. Early psychological, social and nursing assessment offers the opportunity to pre-empt problems and to facilitate more effective communication in the family. At a micro level, family disequilibrium occurs at critical times, such as exacerbation of illness [9]. By predicting these critical times, health and social care professionals can optimise the timing and effectiveness of their interventions [9,89].

Our experience has been that a systematic assessment [15, 40] process is essential to ensure that family health is fully appreciated, and that both individual and family needs are addressed in partnership. Getting the assessment right for families is the one of the most important factors in delivering an effective service that will meet individual and family needs. It is particularly relevant in the context of inter-professional and inter-agency working, to minimise duplication and ensure all aspects are assessed. The assessment framework triangle (Figure 13.3) has been adopted in the United Kingdom and building on this, a Common Assessment Framework is being developed [6] based on inter-professional and inter-agency work.

The assessment process can be viewed as the first stage in establishing an interactive working relationship with a family, and an opportunity to explore existing relationships within a family. Time spent at this stage of the professional–family relationship can be viewed as an essential and integral part of the caring process. Trusting relationships that can lead to acceptance by a family of a professional in their lives need to be developed sensitively and gradually [36]. A central aim of the assessment stage of establishing a relationship with a family is to ascertain what the family sees as important for professionals to work on with them and help them with. There will be unique needs, and a robust assessment, undertaken

sensitively, will ensure work can be targeted to areas families are able and willing to work on.

An example of this can be related to stress theories; the emphasis here is on family coping not only being related to the nature of the stress, but also to the perception of the meaning of that stress for an individual family [90]. In working with families, professionals need to avoid bracketing families together according to diagnostic groupings when assessing and planning interventions. It is important that value judgements are not made about families who are perceived as either coping or not, when they are in what appear to be similar circumstances.

Following the assessment framework introduced above, we suggest that utilising an assessment process in a systematic way enables families and those working with them to plan individualised care and support that will meet the needs of families and individual members at any given point in time. Our experience, for example, has been that a series of cue questions can have some utility in facilitating 'an exploratory and interactional experience in which the content and pace are mutually defined' [23, p. 15] (Table 13.3).

Trapp [36] also uses the notion of cue questions that can be used by professionals as they begin, through assessment, to establish an effective working relationship with a family, incorporating mutual understanding.

• Who are this family?

• Who do they consist of?

• What do they value, need, demand and fear?

• What are their dreams, now and for the future?

[36, p. 77]

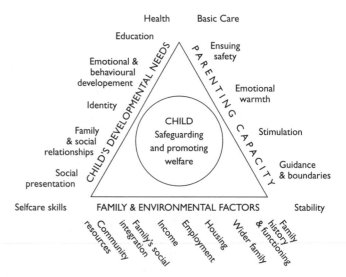

Fig. 13.3 Assessment framework triangle [40].

Table 13.3 The Lifetime Service Model [88]: cue questions for assessment

The Lifetime Service Model of Care, Assessment tool
What are the functional effects of having a life-threatening condition on this child's abilities?
How is this child's condition affecting other family members?
What are the social/ financial effects of the child's condition on the family's functioning?
To sibling: What do you know about your brother's/ sister's illness?
To parent: How much do your healthy children understand about the situation?
What information do other members of the multidisciplinary team require in order to enable them to improve the quality of life for this child and his/her family?

This approach offers the potential to guide the professional and family, to ensure that all families have an equal opportunity to review all aspects of their lives and make choices about the priorities for interventions and the nature of professional relationships they engage in at any one point in time. In the Lifetime assessment, for example, alongside the cue questions, standardised assessment measures are incorporated (relating to functional ability as well as psychological measures) to provide internal consistency and for evaluation purposes. An essential part of the assessment process is building in evaluation and reassessment with the family, to reflect the dynamic and changing nature of the family's life span.

Assessment of family structure, functioning and social networks is as necessary as identifying the ill child's symptoms and care needs. This approach directs professionals to take into account the systems within which the family is nested, and moves the focus from family pathology [23] to family health. Common themes arising from assessment relate to a need for information, practical help, emotional support and an understanding of normal family coping and adaptation, and parenting capacity.

Coping and adaptation

It is important to recognise that not all parents of children with a life-threatening or life-limiting condition will experience difficulties with adjustment. Research to date has shown that although mothers have increased risk of adjustment problems, good adjustment is possible. The general outcome for parents, therefore, appears to be much like that for children, particularly when applying Wallander and Varni's model, in that they are at risk of maladjustment, but there is a considerable individual

variation in adjustment [91]. There will also be variations during the course of a child's illness trajectory that will affect coping and adjustment, and this means that ongoing support and assessment are needed to inform the appropriate interventions, preventing or reducing distress at specific points in time [91].

There have been few controlled evaluations of interventions to improve the adjustment of children with chronic physical disorders. Both stresses associated with the child's condition and influences within the family system appear to be important for longer-term adjustment [91]. It would seem helpful to identify risk factors in families early [92], along with looking at modifiable factors associated with increasing resistance to the distress being experienced. Relating this to a model of stress and coping [90], it is suggested that the individual's perception of factors [37], and not his or her objective characteristics are the most important determinant of outcome. For example, perceived support may be more important than social network characteristics. If a parent has a negative fatalistic attitude, he or she is less likely to adapt successfully.

Information about the condition and subsequent treatment will need to be given more than once, and over a period of time. It is highly unlikely that it will have been heard or absorbed during the early stages of shock. Quine and Rutter [93] report that a major component of parental satisfaction at diagnosis is the feeling that the paediatrician had communicated the information in a sympathetic manner.

Mothers and recently diagnosed families who experience a family environment of low commitment, limited help and support are going to be at more risk of poor adjustment. Identification of those families who are most at risk is crucial, and interventions must be tailored appropriately. It is important that services address the continual stress that families experience within the context of their environment and provide on-going support, rather than crisis intervention [62]. A proactive model of working is therefore espoused. One example of this is working with individuals and groups of parents to establish coping behaviours and offer specific psychological care. Susan discusses what this has meant for her.

'Sometime as a parent you get so immersed in the continuous care and support of the rest of the family that one's own needs and feelings are not recognised. Last year I very hesitantly agreed to attend a counselling course . . . which I found illuminating and extremely helpful. I found, for the first time, that I was able to explore my own anxieties and emotions in a totally secure environment. I know this course proved to be a success with the other parents for we felt the need to meet up again for lunch and a chat' (Susan, mother).

The types of support that are found to be useful by parents vary, but it is often the qualities of the professionals they choose to support them, rather their occupational roles, which are seen as important by families [68]. Other factors in the professional that are seen as important by parents are knowledge of their child's disorder, accessibility and approachability, willingness to seek support from others, a flexible approach to service delivery, and an ability to work them as a whole family. In reality, insufficiency in what is actually available, due to lack of provision or resources, can be problematic in many places.

Parents also report the benefits of meeting with parents of other children, either through disease-specific self-help groups, or through local networking. Parents may use other parents to help them to problem solve, for practical advice and for emotional support [94]. Providing families with information about the availability of groups and other networking opportunities can be valuable for them. Family members may have to seek support outside the family unit, and this can work well for them. However, differing coping styles may lead to individuals misunderstanding the reasons whereby differing forms of support are used by close family members.

Parents need information and practical details to enable them to maintain a sense of control and confidence in their own abilities. Their hopes and fears need to be normalised, and they need encouragement that they will be strong enough to manage what they are being faced with. By giving them details about what may or may not happen, for example, they can develop a full understanding, and also be assured that they are being given honest opinions and information.

Bereavement support should be available when a child dies, wherever he or she dies and at whatever age death occurs. A range of flexible, sensitive services is required to provide support through bereavement if needed. The support needs to extend to parents, carers, siblings and extended family, and to the dying children themselves. Preparation for bereavement is an essential element of this process, as Susan's narrative illustrates:

'No one can say how they will cope at the time of their child's death, but it feels important to us to have these arrangements agreed and put away so that when the time comes our attention can be focused on each other and our children' (Susan, mother).

Susan's narrative continues, illustrating the requirement for individualised, sensitive and responsive care at the time of a child's death. Her family had chosen for their child to die at home. However, when the time came, she was taken to hospital, but the family quickly realised they wanted to revert to their previously made plans:

'I'll never forget your care when Emily died, and 6 years on, one of my most treasured memories is of Brenda (the community children's nurse) coming into A&E and 'rescuing us' by taking us all, including Emmy, home' (Susan, Emily's mum).

The needs of the parents, siblings and other involved family members are special, and they require a unique network of services and support [68]. In whichever setting the family may have chosen, they require high-quality care that fully integrates family support. When death is imminent, the family requires space to be together as a family unit. This may be a physical space, such as a room in the house, as well as space without interruptions from professionals or well-meaning friends or neighbours. Professionals can enable and empower families to find ways of ensuring they have this protected and private time. Often, families will want to do special things that mean a lot to them and their ill child. It is a time of preparation and sharing, during which they need access to appropriate information and help when they feel they want it. A flexible team approach is as vital at this stage as it will have been throughout the child's life.

In the basic model of care for families with a dying child that has developed in the Western culture, parents become primary caregivers, with a team (usually led by a nurse and physician) available to them as a facilitator of care, assisting them in assessing, planning and delivering the required care [68]. Of particular concern for care at this stage is the maintenance of quality of life and symptom control [68] and parents need to feel well supported twenty-four hours a day. There are many concerns and fears that parents may experience at this stage, and professionals need to explore which ones are important for each family member so they can work to alleviate them. Some examples of such fears are given in Box 13.5.

Box 13.5 Concerns for parents when death is imminent

- Uncontrollable symptoms
- Addiction to pain medication
- Anxiety and being over-burdened with their caring role
- What will actually happen at the time of death
- Lack of community or family resources
- Financial difficulties
- Lack of communication with multiple caregivers

The processes necessary to enable family coping and adaptation need to continue into bereavement for as long as a family requires them, and the same principles applied.

Working with siblings

There has been little work about what are effective interventions to assist sibling adjustment and coping, and it is likely that it is influenced by a number of factors in combination. Nevertheless, it is important for professionals to both have an understanding of the siblings' experience and use the information that is available, to try and make a difference in a positive way to their experience.

> 'We tell the siblings what is going on. You have to be open with the children . . . They realise mortality is a greater threat for their sister than for them' (mother of a child needing home ventilation).

Supportive relationships are very important for siblings to, enable them to have an opportunity to express their feelings, gain information and to understand why their family life has been so disrupted. Susan's narrative illustrates the need to consider a variety of approaches to meet the needs of siblings:

> 'Our children have received counselling from special psychologists. This not only helped them to understand more about their sister's condition, but also has given them opportunities to ask questions and explore their own feelings, individually and in confidence. They also attended two sibling groups, where they have not only made friends with other brothers and sisters, but explored their feelings through art and play' (Susan, mother).

Relationships with peers and school are thought to be especially important and essential micro systems of the well child's life that can provide some sense of equilibrium for them. Peers can be a source of comfort, although the reverse can occur. Those in the siblings' extended community need to be made aware of the situation and given ideas about how they can help, for example, by recognising the stresses in the well child's life that existed anyway (exams, peer pressure) prior to the additional burden they now have, with changes in their family. School, can have a central role in identifying persons who the siblings can go to and share feelings with, feelings that they would want to protect their parents from. Equally, maintaining normal routines at school and in other activities can provide the one constant in the well child's life. A child will often need a close friend outside the family, and finding this person can be important for them to provide honesty and time to be listened to and heard.

Groups for siblings may also be of benefit by reducing the feelings of isolation. This may be achieved through a wide variety of activities, including art and play, which are age and developmentally appropriate. A number of sibling group programmes have been developed which provide a safe and structured environment for children and young people. These types of groups need to be facilitated by experienced professionals who are able to appropriately deal with the range of emotions and issues that may be raised for children, both during and following such a group. Box 13.6 describes some activities and strategies that have been found to work well in practice in running such a group.

The groups also aim to provide a peer group for these children and young people such as they may not have previously experienced, and a safe environment to discuss more sensitive issues associated with their siblings' mortality.

Siblings need to be told what is happening, why it is happening, and what is likely to happen in the future. If they are excluded, they will sense something is wrong, and in the absence of age-appropriate explanations, will be likely to fantasise [95]. When the death of their sibling is imminent for example, it is important that they are involved. Being

Box 13.6 Activities for sibling groups

Groups for siblings—examples of activities

- A session on how the body works, and on identifying how their own brothers and sisters are affected by their illnesses, in addition to being able to ask questions of the doctor relating to their siblings' illnesses.

- An opportunity to identify and discuss their feelings and emotions toward their siblings by identifying these emotions as leaves and placing them on a feelings tree, or representing them as coloured chalk placed in a jar to illustrate and normalise their own experiences of a wide range of emotions, and how these emotions at times can be quite mixed.

- Coping skills can be identified by encouraging the children to draw family portraits and to include all the important individuals in their lives, and to help them acknowledge that they are also a 'resource' to them when they are struggling to cope with different and difficult emotions.

- Children can make their own 'coping' boxes, which encourage them to think of additional mechanisms for coping with their emotions, and sharing strategies with each other. The contents of the boxes may include balloons or bubbles to help them to relax when they are feeling angry, or yo-yo's when they are feeling tense, gem stones as a representation of a really special time, for example, a birthday, which can be used to trigger a good memory when they are faced with difficult times in their lives.

there at the death and spending time with their dead brother or sister can be extremely beneficial, although painful, and they will require support. They need to be allowed to have their feelings acknowledged. This can be hard to achieve, as their parents may not recognise their needs and want to protect them form the pain they themselves are feeling. In traditional culture, children will observe and be active participants in family rituals of dying and death, and no arrangements will be made to shield or protect them [57]. By contrast, in Western culture, children's exposure to death is likely to have been through the media, and they will have limited opportunities to learn about death. Some helpful literature and material are now emerging for children, parents and professionals to use, but they need to be used with 'cultural competence'.

Working with the wider family

It is important to assess and recognise the significant influence of grandparents on family dynamics and adaptation [86], and to work in partnership with the family, to determine the extent of involvement of extended family members. There is some evidence in the literature of the benefits of involving and supporting the wider family in the care of a child and the nuclear family [86], although further studies relating specifically to this group of children and their families are required. Our experience also suggests that involving, including and educating grandparents and other significant people in a child's needs, and in supporting them emotionally to enable successful coping, is beneficial. For example, a professional can help educate grandparents by giving them information and ideas about ways in which they may be able to help a family and make a real difference.

However, while considering ways that grandparents and wider family may be involved, it is also important to recognise that sometimes they may not be a source of practical or emotional support. For example, in one family, a grandparent's reactions to the situation may be a source of increased stress for the parents. This is most likely if the grandparent denies or rejects the true meaning of the child's diagnosis, or becomes over-protective of the ill child or the siblings, or takes on a domineering role. Reasons for such situations include impaired existing relationships, unresolved conflicts, financial, educational and health-related factors, and geographical distance.

Professionals need to recognise the support needs of significant other people in the child and families system, and in doing so, can aid the process of adaptation and coping for the family unit. Some examples of the possibly helpful types of support that extended family members may provide are listed in Table 13.4.

Working as professionals with the family (meso level)

The meso level relates to the daily interaction of the family with the extended family, friends, the local community, and health and social care professionals. Key concepts relate to partnership, information sharing and the notion of social support. Service providers, while situated in an organisational culture, are a group who can contribute to making order out of chaos, and help provide families with a language or meaning to their experience with their ill child [28, p. 571]. Services are embedded in culture, but like families, they are also active in creating and influencing the world around them. For example, if a palliative care or hospice service is opened in any area, perceptions relating to children with life-threatening illnesses will gradually be altered in the professional and public arenas in that area. If no services develop, there will be no awareness, and the family's experience will be a very different one.

Partnership

It must be acknowledged that adapting to a life-threatening illness involves coping with a degree of uncertainty. Initially, this can be all-encompassing, but can be contained by familiarity with the illness and treatment routines .As far as possible, parents need to know what to expect, and short-term treatment plans can be helpful in bringing some order to their lives and enabling them to function. Helplessness and a sense of loss of the ability to care properly for their child are common experiences of parents. Taking control is the best antidote to helplessness, loss of hopes, and unpredictability. One of the best aspects of good practice is the extent to which parents are seen as partners in the care of their child. The information parents are given must be honest and consistent, as they will seek out information from all sources available to them.

Table 13.4 'Helpful' support from the wider family (Adapted from Katz & Kessel [86])

- Shopping
- Babysitting/ help with short breaks
- Help with household chores
- Emotional support—acceptance and involvement in the child's care
- Help with caring for siblings and giving them 'special time' too
- Financial help

Good palliative care is flexible, and involves a partnership between the child and family and professionals. Good communication, multi-professional and multi-agency team work and partnership are essential. An integrated approach by service providers, for example, health and social care, education providers and voluntary organizations, including hospices, will facilitate a less fragmented and more effective service for children and families.

The ideology of holism and active participation [96] assumes that negotiation and patient choice are central to high-quality care. A negotiated position of the contemporary professional–family relationship is proposed, arising from the transfer of responsibility for caring to families in the community [44,50,97,98]. This requires a move away from paternalistic models of care. A spirit of partnership based on agreement, rather than unconditional collaboration [99], is proposed as a pragmatic way forward. The concept of case management has been suggested in a number of studies as potentially reducing stress significantly for parents of children with complex needs [100]. It is our experience that this model is transferable to children's palliative care. A key need is for families to receive the right amount and type of support over what may be a long period of time.

The interfaces between formal and informal care have changed, as more children are being cared for at home, in a reflection of the contemporary policy theme of participation at macro level [5,101,102]. Participation is a pivotal concept in child health practice, however, there is lack of consensus on how far the concept should be extended [103]. One dilemma in defining the concept of informal caring is that its key features mirror those of parenting, drawing on feelings of love, obligation and duty. The problematic nature of this is reflected in reports of the confused relationship between professionals and parents [44, 104]. The extent of parental participation should be determined by personal choice and based on developing trust, retaining control, and being assured about the competency of professionals and carers. These are central issues for families, and need to be accounted for by professionals and services [44,96].

A father's narrative illustrates this:

'We need, as a family, to facilitate the most out of life. Enabling this is all part of the care process that we are engaged in with the team working with us.

We will continue to need whatever is appropriate for the phase we are in at any point in time. The knowledge that we have this relationship with a service (and preferably personnel) is invaluable to us. This sounds very simple, and you would only know the value of it if you were in our situation' (father of child with metabolic condition).

Relationships and involvement

The themes of relationships, involvement, knowing the family, holism, negotiation and participation are inter-linked, and central to contemporary notions of professional support. The centrality of relationships to the family's experience and to professional practice is illustrated in the following two narratives:

'At the beginning, we were introduced to a community nurse from our local children's service (the Lifetime service). She gradually helped to begin to move us out of this "confused phase". We needed at this time confident and knowledgeable people who had the ability and flexibility to act on our behalf, at a time when we were unable to and had entered a world we did not understand' (mother of child with unknown, life-threatening diagnosis).

'We have needed a caring and supportive professional alongside us, with the strength to carry us when we've needed it and perception to let us be when we've needed that' (Laurence, father).

An individual's notion of involvement and non-involvement underwrites these patient/parent–professional relationships [105, 106]. An individual's norms and values regarding the nature of 'helping' and being helped have, it is suggested, a direct influence on the approach of the professional, and consequently, on the families' experience. May [105], in an account of professional relations (nurses), recognises the necessity, in describing involvement, to disentangle involvement enhancing the quality of care from personal attachments to specific patients. Laurence's narrative continues and sums this up: 'Done wrongly, this involvement could have been intrusive and very wrong for us'.

It has emerged in a recent study [107] that knowing the child and family is an essential prerequisite for the provision of high quality care, from the perspective of Community Children's Nurses working in a community palliative care team. Early contact with the family, and ensuring continuity of care, are valued and highlighted by both professionals [105, 107,108] and families [44,50]. It is recognised that maintaining this level of practice at micro and meso levels is a potential source of tension in the context of antipathetic changes and agendas at the exo-and macro levels.

The impact of relationships and involvement in decision-making, for example, on a family's experience is not fully understood. However it involves notions of collaboration and partnership. Kirk [52] specifically identified caring and respect for family's views and needs, and recognition of the significant role of parents as carers, as especially important aspects of positive professional–family relationships.

Communication and information sharing

A parent's vulnerability can lead to misunderstandings, not hearing and misinterpretations. Professionals need to be attentive to this, and perceptive about timing and sensitivity of content, and account for variations in how a family—and its individual members—need to hear and receive information, and crucially, ensure they are listened to. Professionals have a responsibility to respond appropriately and honestly to requests for information, and provide time for discussions and building relationships that will enhance care.

Clinicians should encourage parents to communicate openly and honestly with their child about the illness. This means there is a need to work with parents in order to empower and facilitate their ability to communicate with their children effectively and appropriately. Information should be provided on an on-going basis, particularly following changes in the ill child's condition or treatment at an age-appropriate level, consistent with the child's level of understanding. These principles need to be extended to siblings.

Organizations and systems (exo level)

The exo level relates to the wider context of health and social care systems, and encompasses other agencies with both direct and indirect contact with the family unit. Organizations providing services for families engage in a variety of practices that impact directly and indirectly on a family's environment. These services are always part of the family's exo-system, and may or may not become part of their meso-system, if they choose to engage with or use that service or occupational group.

This level reflects the themes within contemporary health and social care of inter-agency and inter-professional working, care pathways and integrated systems of care [119]. Emancipatory practice by professionals and policy leaders to facilitate the notion of 'blurring boundaries' [109], rather than delineating differences, is suggested. Achieving this could offer a real opportunity to improve the quality of life of individual and family's experiences, and ensure they have the agency to achieve their quality of life.

A useful illustration of working at this level is the use of a palliative care plan. Such a plan necessitates the use of a multidisciplinary approach, including, health, education and social services, in partnership with parents, whereby decisions can be made with the parents having the most appropriate information available to them.

'Perhaps one of the most significant aspects of the provision of services to us as a family has been the creation of a palliative care plan for Emily and a resuscitation policy. These have been given to social services, various health authorities, the children's hospice Emily attends and, of course, her school. The community children's nurse spent many hours helping and guiding us through very difficult decisions regarding resuscitation procedures and now it is finalised we can relax in the knowledge that should anything happen to Emily whilst she is away from home our wishes will be adhered to' (Susan, mother of Emily).

We would suggest that it is at this level that organizations need to make some decisions relating to establishing or developing services for this group of children and their families (Box 13.7). The family systems model presented here provides a broad framework, and we suggest that these discussions and decisions can be made within this framework.

The overarching cultural and sub-cultural environment (macro level)

The macro level refers to the underpinning values and belief systems within which the other levels are seated. A comprehensive illumination and discussion of this level is outside the scope of this text, and so, only some brief examples of culture and ethnicity and policy will be used.

Culturally sensitive care

In order to deliver culturally sensitive, and therefore effective, care, there is a requirement for recognition and reflection by

Box 13.7 Service development

Service development: issues to consider, using a family systems framework.

- Where will the work of this organisation be situated in relation to the systems of the child and their family?

- List the activities and interventions your organisation can do, or plans to do, for family members. How will these influence the systems of the family?

- What sources of support will your organisation be providing to other levels and other systems?

- What else needs to be in place for this to be achieved?

- How can services be evaluated and modified to identify differing levels of intervention and their effectiveness?

- How can the respective systems of family members be made as favourable as possible to facilitate their adaptation and ongoing development as individuals and as a family unit?

(Adapted from Rolls [28, p. 572])

individuals at all levels on the implications of personal and professional cultural backgrounds. An additional requirement is for an increase in the knowledge of the cultural needs of individuals and family units through research, education and, at a micro level, through assessment. Hall *et al.* [51] proposes that for professionals to work in partnership with families, a model of their belief about the illness needs to be elicited that is meaningful for them, and encompasses their needs and expectations. Using a reflexive approach, a shared model of care can be negotiated when assessing a family's needs [51]. A number of studies have evaluated professional support services for children [110–112]. However, these are problematic when considering the cultural needs of families, as they regard the care both given and received as being culturally neutral [56]. Contemporary health and social care require that further investigation be undertaken to inform and guide culturally sensitive practice.

Policy

A child with palliative care needs and his or her family live in a society where illness and disability are stigmatised, and normalcy, control and order are valued [31]. Changes in policies within health, education and social services in the UK [5,39] reflect the influence of many factors [4,40,113]. The process of change required to address palliative care and family support is enormous but will require a broader policy environment, including children and their families, health care organisations and communities, and include legislation, leadership and policy integration. Smaller steps may offer opportunities to at least begin making a difference within a long-term strategy. There needs to be investment in long-term and palliative care from the perspective of the family at all levels, and it will require re-conceptualisation and attitude change among policy makers, professionals, communities and family members [114,115].

Summary

'Palliative care for children and young people with life-limiting conditions is an active and total approach to care, embracing physical, emotional, social and spiritual elements. It focuses on enhancement of quality of life for the child and support for the family, and includes the management of distressing symptoms, provision of respite, and care through death and bereavement' [14]. In order to put this well-accepted espoused definition of children's palliative care into practice, an understanding of the role of the family is required, and has been presented here.

A long-term family care paradigm, that concords with strategies for chronic care [42] and focuses on family members'

perspectives of quality of life [3,18], has been proposed as the appropriate direction for services and professionals. The challenge for practitioners is to ' design and implement intervention programmes that take into account the entire multifaceted and dynamic context in which any given response is situated' [31].

A family systems approach requires a high level of expertise and experiential understandings of families' cultures, which have been found in other areas (health visiting) to be as important as scientific knowledge about conditions [116, 117]. The challenges of this approach in practice are recognised, as professionals move away from a traditional conceptualisation of 'professional activities'. The focus of family systems is to restore or establish 'normalcy' in the balance of all systems, uncovering the more positive aspects of long-term and life-threatening illness [49,118]. This shift away from an illness-focus, it has been suggested, should be integral to contemporary health and social care.

It has been our argument that collaborative working at all levels, putting child and family health at the centre, is a central requirement to ensure the child's best interests are met. Juxtaposing ideology with the reality of contemporary health care and society, it is recognised that this may be an unrealistic aspiration. A pragmatic way forward may be for dialogue at all levels, that includes the child, young person and family members. To achieve at least this, it is necessary for all involved to listen and speak very carefully. Laurence concludes:

> 'As we have continued on our journey we live daily with the long-standing probability of loosing our child. We have needed to hang on to people—professionals—we have met along the way who we can confidently work with, and be with. What I mean by this is, someone who can "join your life" in a supportive capacity, but not over tread the boundaries' (Laurence, father).

Acknowledgements

We would like to acknowledge the valuable contribution made to this chapter in its early stages by Susan Hayward, Social Worker, and Linda Lee, Head of Care, Little Bridge House Hospice.

References

1. Frude, N. *Understanding Family Problems: A Psychological approach*; Chichester: J.Wiley & Sons,1990.
2. Baggaley, S.E. The family: Images, definitions and development In *Explorations in Family Nursing.* 1997; (Chapter 2, 27–39), London: Routledge,1997.

3. Brown, R.I. *Quality of Life for People with Disabilities*. Cheltenham: Stanley Thornes (Publishers) Ltd,1997.

4. Department of Health (DoH). *The NHS Plan. A Plan for Investment. A Plan for Reform*. London: The Stationery Office, 2000a.

5. Department of Health (DoH). *Getting the Right Start: The National Service Framework for Children and Young People and Maternity Services—Standards for Hospital Services*. London: Department of Health, 2003a.

6. Department of Health (DoH). *National Service Framework for Children, Young People and Maternity Services: Change for Children—Every Child Matters*. London: Department of Health, Department of Education and Skills, 2004.

7. Lowton, K. and Gabe, J. 'Life on a Slippery Slope'—Perceptions of Health in Adults with Cystic Fibrosis. *Sociology of Health and Illness* 2003;25(4):289–319.

8. Woolley, H., Stein, A., Forrest, G.C., and Baum, J.D. Life threatening illness and hospice care. *Arch Dis Childhood* 1989;64(5):697–702.

9. Gravelle, A.M. Caring for a child with a progressive illness during the complex phase: Parent's experience of facing adversity. *J Adv Nurs* 1997;25:738–745.

10. Sarafino, E.P. *Health Psychology* (4th edition). New York: John Wiley & Sons, 2002.

11. Walters, S. Doctor—patient relationship in cystic fibrosis—a patient's perspective. *Holistic Med* 1990;6:157–62.

12. Bluebond-Langner, M., Lask, B., and Angst, D.B., (eds.) *Psychosocial Aspects of Cystic Fibrosis*. London: Hodder Headline Group, 2001.

13. Association for Children with Life-Threatening or Terminal Conditions and their Families (ACT). *Palliative Care for Young People aged 13–24*, 2001. (A joint report by ACT, National Council for Hospice and Specialist Palliative Care and Scottish Partnership Agency for Palliative and Cancer Care), Bristol: ACT.

14. Association for Children with Life-Threatening or Terminal Conditions and their Families and Royal College of Paediatrics and Child Health (ACT) (2nd edition). *A Guide to the Development of Children's Palliative Care Services*. 2003a; Bristol: ACT

15. Association for Children with Life-Threatening or Terminal Conditions and their Families (ACT). *Assessment of Children with Life limiting Conditions and their Families: A Guide to Effective Care Planning*. 2003b; Bristol: ACT

16. Bowling, A. *Measuring Health: A Review of Quality of Life Measurement Scales*.(2nd Edition). Buckingham: Open University Press,1997.

17. Farquhar, M. Definitions of quality of life: a taxonomy. *J Adv Nurs* 1995;22(3):502–8.

18. Anderson, K.L. and Burckhardt, C. Conceptualisation and measurement of quality of life as an outcome variable for healthcare intervention and research. *J Adv Nurs* 1999;29(2):298–306.

19. Wilson, I. B. Linking clinical variables in health-related quality of life: a conceptual model of patient outcomes. *J Am Med Assoc.* 1995;273 (1):59–65.

20. McClement, S.E. and Woodgate, R.L. Research with families in palliative care: Conceptual and methodological challenges, *Eur J Cancer Care* 1998; 7: 247–54.

21. Wright, L. and Leahey, M. (1994) *Nurses and Families: A Guide to family assessment and intervention*. 2nd Edition, Philidelphia. Davis Company.

22. Adams, J. Caring for the 'new family' in palliative care, *Br J Nurs*1995;(21):1253–72.

23. Whyte, D.A. Family Nursing—a systematic approach to nursing work with families. In D.A. Whyte, (ed.) *Explorations in Family Nursing*. Chapter 1, London: Routledge, 1997.

24. Patterson, J.M. A family systems perspective for working with youth with disability. *Pediatrician* 1991;18:129–41.

25. Faux, S.A. Historical overview of responses of children and their families to chronic illness. In M.E. Broome, K. Knafl, K. Pridham, and S. Feetham, (eds.) *Children and Families in Health and Illness*. London: Sage Publications Ltd, 1998.

26. Thompson, R.J. and Gustafson, K.E. *Adaptation to Chronic Illness*. 1996; Washington: American Psychological Association,1996.

27. Mitchell, D. and Winslade, J. Developmental systems and narrative approaches to working with families of persons with disabilities. In R.I. Brown, *Quality of Life for People with Disabilities* (2nd edition), Chapter 8. Cheltenham: Stanley Thornes (Publishers) Ltd, 1997.

28. Rolls, L. Families and children facing loss and bereavement. In S. Payne, J. Seymour, and Ingleton (eds.) *Palliative Care Nursing: Principles and Evidence for Practice*. Maidenhead: Open University Press, 2004.

29. Bronfenbrenner, U. (1992) Ecological systems theory, in R. Vasta (ed) *Six Theories of Child Development*. London: Jessica Kingsley

30. Wright,L. and Leahey, M. *Nurses and Families: A guide to family assessment and intervention* 3rd edition. Philidelphia, PA: F.A. Davis Company, 2000.

31. Bluebond-Langner, M. *In the Shadow of Illness. Parents and Siblings of the Chronically Ill-Child*. Princeton, NJ: Princeton University Press, 1996.

32. Friedemann, M. The concept of family nursing. In G.D. Wegner and R.J. Alexander, (eds.) *Readings Family Nurs*. Philadelphia, PA: Lippincott, 1993.

33. MacKenzie, H. The terminally ill child: Supporting the family anticipating loss in Whyte, D.A. *Explorations in Family Nursing*. Chapter 5, London: Routledge, 1997.

34. Department of Health (DoH). *Childrens Act*. London: The Stationery Office, 1989b.

35. Williams, P.D. Siblings and pediatric chronic illness: A review of the literature, *Intl J Nurs Stud* 1997;34(4):312–23.

36. Trapp, A. Support for the family. In A. Goldman, (ed.) *Care of the Dying Child*. Chapter 4, Oxford: Oxford University Press, 2002.

37. Eiser, C. *Growing up with a chronic disease: The impact on children and families*. London: Jessica Kingsley Publishers, 1993.

38. Kirk, S. Caring for technology-dependent children at home, *Br J Commun Nurs* 1999;4(8):390–4.

39. Department of Health (DoH). *Caring for People: Community Care in the Next Decade and Beyond*. London: HMSO, 1989a.

40. Department of Health (DoH). *The NHS Cancer Plan. A Plan for Investment. A Plan for Reform*. London: HMSO, 2000b.

41. Department of Health (DoH). *Framework for the Assessment of Children in Need and their Families*. London: The Stationery Office, 2000c.

42. World Health Organization (WHO). *Innovative Care for Chronic Conditions. Building Blocks for Action*. Geneva: World Health Organization,2002.

43. Danvers, L., Freshwater, D., Cheater, F., and Wilson, A. Providing a seamless service for children with life-limiting illness: Experiences

and recommendations of professional staff at the Diana Princess of Wales Children's Community Service *J Clin Nurs* 2003;12:351–9.

44. Kirk, S. Negotiating lay and professional roles in the care of children with complex health care needs, *J Adv Nurs* 2001;34(5): 593–602.

45. Carter, B. Ways of working: CCNs and chronic illness, *J Child Health Care* 2000;4(2):66–72.

46. Eaton, N. Models of community children's nursing. *Paediatr Nurs* 2001;13(1):32–6.

47. Glendinning, C., Kirk, S., Guiffrida, A., Lawton, D. (2001) Technology-dependent children in the community. Definitions, numbers and costs. *Child: Care, Health and Development*, Vol. 27, No.4. 321–334.

48. Bradley, S. Better late then never? An evaluation of community nursing services for children in the UK. *J Clin Nurs* 1997;6(5): 411–18.

49. Cummings, J.M. Exploring family systems nursing and the community children's nurse's role in caring for children with cystic fibrosis. *J Child Health Care* 2002;6(2):120–32.

50. Kirk, S. and Glendinning, C. Supporting 'expert' parents—professional support and families caring for a child with complex healthcare needs in the community, *Int J Nurs Stud* 2002;39: 625–35.

51. Katz, S. When the child's illness is life threatening: impact on the parents. *Pediatr Nurs* 2002;28(5):453–63.

52. Kirk, S. Families' experiences of caring at home for a technology-dependent child: A review of the literature, *Child: Care, Health Dev* 1998;24(2):101–14.

53. Leavitt, M., Martinson, I.M., Liu, C.U., Armstrong, V., Hornberger, L., Zhang, J., and Han, X. Common themes and ethnic differences in family care giving in the first year after diagnosis of childhood cancer: Part II, *J Pediatr Nurs* 1999;14(2):110–121.

54. While, A.E., Citrone, C., and Cornish, J.C. *A Study of the Needs and Provisions for Families Caring for Children with Life-Limiting Incurable Disorders*. Unpublished report, London: Kings College, 1995.

55. Hall, P., Stone, G., and Fiset, V.J. Palliative care: How can we meet the needs of our multicultural communities? *J Palliat Care* 1998; 15(2):46.

56. Kelly, P. and Uddin, S. (2000) Cultural Issues in Community Children's Nursing, in Muir, J. and Sidey, A. (2000) *Textbook of Community Children's Nursing. Chapter 16*. 1st Edition, Bailliere Tindall.

57. Young, B. and Papadatou, D. Childhood death and bereavement across cultures. In C. Murray-Parkes, P. Laungani, and B. Young, (eds.) *Death and Bereavement Across Cultures*. London: Routledge, 1997.

58. Randhawa, G., Owens, A., Fitches, R., and Khan, Z. Communication in the development of culturally competent palliative care services in the UK: A case study. *Int J Palliat Nurs* 2003; 9(1):24–31.

59. Oliviere, D. Culture and ethnicity. *Eur J Palliat Care* 1999;6(2): 53–6.

60. Eiser, C. *Childhood Chronic Disease: An Introduction to Psychological Theory and Research*. Cambridge: Cambridge University Press, 1990.

61. Farrell, M., Ryan, S., and Langrick, B. 'Breaking bad news' within a paediatric setting: An evaluation report of a collaborative education workshop to support health professionals, *J Adv Nur* 2001; 36(6): 765–75.

62. Mastroyannopoulou, K., Stallard, P., Lewis, M., and Lenton, S. The impact of childhood non-malignant life-threatening illness on parents: gender differences and predictors of parental adjustment, *J Child Psychol Psychiatr* 1997;38(7):823–9.

63. Sloper, P. and Turner, S. (1992) Service needs of families of children with severe physical disability. *Child: Care, Health and Development*. Vol. 18, 259–282.

64. Wallander, J.L., Varni, J.W., Babani, L., Tweddle Banis, H., and Wilcox, T. Family resources as resistance factors for psychological maladjustment in chronically ill and handicapped children. *J Paediatr Psychol* 1989;14:157–73.

65. Bailey, D.B., Blasco, P.M. Simeonsson, R.J (1992) Needs Expressed by mothers and fathers of young children with disabilities, *American Journal on Mental Retardation*. Vol.97, No.!, 1–10.

66. Affleck, G., Tennen, H., and Rowe, J. Mothers, fathers and the crisis of newborn intensive care. *Infant Mental Health J* 1990;11:12–25.

67. Chapman, J.A. and Goodall, J. Helping the child to live whilst dying. *Lancet* 1980;5:753–6.

68. While, A.E., Citrone, C., Cornish, J.C. *Bereaved Parents' Views of Caring for a Child with a Life-Limiting Incurable Disorder*. Unpublished Report, London: Kings College, 1996.

69. Dominica, F. Caring for the dying child and the family in J. Robbins, (ed.) *Caring for the Dying Patient and Family*. London: Harpers & Row Publishers, 1989.

70. Poon,M., Finlay, F., Lewis, M., and Lenton, S. To develop a framework for end of life plans, *RCPCH Annual summer meeting University of York, 23 September*, 2003.

71. Webb, B. Trauma and tedium: An account of living on a children's ward In J. Walmsley, and J. Reynolds, P. Shakespeare, and R. Woolfe, (eds). *Health, Welfare and Practice*. London: Sage Publications, 1993.

72. Goldman, A., Beardsmore, S., and Hunt, J. Palliative care for children with cancer—home, hospital or hospice? *Arch Dis Childhood* 1990;68:423–25.

73. Martinson, I.M. An approach for studying the feasibility and desirability of home care for the child dying from cancer. In M.C. Cahoon, (ed.) *Cancer Nursing*. Edinburgh: Churchill Livingstone 1982.

74. Cohen, M.S. Families coping with childhood chronic illness: a research review, *Family, Systems and Health*. 1999;17(2): 149–64.

75. Jerrett, M.D. Parents' experience of coming to know the care of a chronically ill child. *J Adv Nurs* 1994;19:1050–6.

76. Wallander, J.L. and Thompson, R.J. Jr (1995) Psychosocial adjustment of children with chronic physical conditions, in M.C. Roberts (Ed) *Handbook of Paediatric Psychology*. (2nd Edition) p 124–141. New York: Guilford Press.

77. Wallander, J.L. and Varni, J.W. Adjustment in children with chronic physical disorders; Programmatic research on a disability-stress-coping model. In A.M. LaGreca, L.Siegal, J.L. Wallander, and C.E Walker, (eds.) *Stress and coping with paediatric conditions*. New York: Guilford Press, 1992;279–98.

78. Wallander, J.L. and Varni, J.W. Appraisal, coping and adjustment in adolescents with a physical disorder. In J.L. Wallander and L.J. Seigal, (eds.) *Adolescent health problems: Behavioural perspectives*. New York: Guilford Press, 1995.

79. Stallard, P., Mastroyannopoulou, K., Lewis, M., and Lenton, S. The Siblings of Children with Life-threatening Conditions. *Child Psychol Psychiatr Rev* 1997;1:26–33.

80. Yule, W. and Williams, R.M. Post-traumatic stress reactions in children. *J Traumat Stress* 1990;3:279–95.

81. Sloper, P. Experiences and support needs of siblings of children with cancer. *Health Soc Care Commun* 2000a;8(5):298–306.

82. Sourkes, B. *Armfuls of Time. The Psychological Experience of the Child with a Life-Threatening Illness.* London: Routledge, 1995.

83. Murray, J.S. Siblings of children with cancer: A review of the literature. *J Pediatr Oncol Nurs* 1999;16:25–34.

84. Ferrari, M. Chronic Illness: Psychosocial effects on siblings—I Chronically ill boy, *Child Psychol Psychiatry* 1983;25(3):459–76.

85. Wright, L.M. and Leahey, M. Families and Life-Threatening Illness: Assumptions, assessment and intervention. In M. Leahey, and L. Wrights, (eds.) *Families and Life-threatening illness.* Springhouse, PA: Springhouse Corp 1987;45–58.

86. Katz, S. and Kessel, L. Grandparents of children with developmental disabilities: Perceptions, beliefs and involvement in care, *Issues Comprehens Pediat Nurs* 2002;25:113–28

87. Andershed, B. and Ternestedt, B. Development of a theoretical framework describing relatives' involvement in palliative care. *J Adv Nurs* 2001;34(4):554–62.

88. Lewis, M. The Lifetime Service: A Model for children with Life-threatening illnesses and their families. *Paediatri Nurs* 1999; 11(7):21–33.

89. Sloper, P. Models of service support for parents of disabled children. What do we know? What do we need to know? *Child: Care. Health Dev* 1999;25(2):85–9.

90. Lazarus, R.S. and Folkman, S. *Stress, Appraisal and Coping.* New York: Springer, 1984.

91. Sloper, P. Predictors of distress in parents of children with cancer: A prospective study. *J Pediatr Psychol* 2000b;25(2):79–91.

92. Wallander, J.L. and Varni, J.W. Effects of paediatric chronic physical disorders on child and family adjustment. *J Child Psychol Psychiatr* 1998;39(1):29–46.

93. Quine, L. and Rutter, D.R. First diagnosis of severe mental and physical disability: A study of doctor–patient communication. *J Psychol Psychiatr* 1994;34:1273–87.

94. Parker, D., Maddocks, I., Stern, L.M. The role of palliative care in advanced muscular dystrophy and spinal muscular atrophy, *J Paediatr Child Health* 1999;35:245–50.

95. Lansdown, R. and Goldman, A. The psychological care of children with malignant disease. *J Child Psychol Psychiatr* 1988;29: 278–83.

96. Gastrell, P. and Edwards, J. *Community Health Nursing. Frameworks for Practice.* London: Bailliere Tindall, 1996.

97. Whyte, D.A., Barton, M.E., Lamb, A., Magennis, C., Mallinson, A., Marshall, L., Oliver, R., Reid, P., Richardson, H., and Walford, C. Clinical effectiveness in community children's nursing. *Clin Effect Nurs* 1998;2:139–44.

98. Ratliffe, C.E., Harrigan, R.C., Haley, J., Tse, A., and Olson, T., Stress in Families with Medically Fragile Children, *Issues Comprehen Pediatr Nurs* 2002;25:167–88.

99. Bywaters, P. Social work and the medical Profession—Arguments against unconditional collaboration, *Br J Soc Work* 1986;16: 661–77.

100. Glendinning, C., Kirk, S., Guiffrida, A., and Lawton, D. Technology-dependent children in the community: definitions, numbers and costs. *Child: Care Health Dev* 2001;27(4):321–34.

101. DoH (2003b).

102. Boatang, P. *Every Child Matters. Green Paper consultation document.* London: Stationery Office, 2003.

103. Kirk, S. and Glendinning, C. Trends in community care and patient participation: Implications for the roles of informal carers and community nurses in the United Kingdom, *J Adv Nurs* 1998;28(2):370–81.

104. Harrigan, R.C., Ratliffe, C., Patrinos, M., and Tse, A. Medically fragile children: an integrative review of the literature nad recommendations for future research, *Issues Comprehen Pediatr Nurs* 2002;25:1–20.

105. May, C. Affective neutrality and involvement in nurse-patient relationships: Perceptions of appropriate behaviour among nurses in acute medical and surgical wards. *J Adv Nurs* 1991;16: 552–8.

106. Luker, K.A., Austin, L., Caress, A., and Hallett, C.E. the importance of 'knowing the patient': community nurses' constructs of quality in providing palliative care. *J Adv Nurs* 2000;31(4):775–82.

107. Lewis, M. An Exploratory Qualitative Study of Community Children's Nurses' Decisions on how to manage their Caseloads, *MSc Dissertation Thesis, Bath Spa University, Bath.* Unpublished, 2004.

108. Kennedy, C. The work of district nurses: First assessment visits. *J Adv Nurs* 2002;40(6):710–20.

109. Todd, A. *Crossing boundaries—opportunities and challenges of NHS and academic partnerships.* Concurrent session: Royal College of Nursing International Research conference. Manchester 9th–12th April, 2003.

110. While, A.E. An evaluation of a paediatric home care scheme. *J Adv Nurs* 1991;16:1413–21.

111. Tatman, M. and Lessing, D. Paediatric Home Care , In Spencer, N. (ed.) *Progress in Community Child Health.* Churchill Livingston, 1997;103–19.

112. Coyne, I. Chronic illness: The importance of support for families caring for a child with cystic fibrosis. *J Clin Nurs* 1997;6(2): 121–29.

113. Sarafino, E.P. (2002) *Health Psychology.* (4th Edition) New York: John Wiley & Sons.

114. Tattersall, R. the expert patient: A new approach to chronic disease management for the twenty first century. *Clin Med* 2002; 2(3):227–9.

115. Tregaskis, C. Social model theory: the Story so Far. *Disabil Soc* 2002;17(4):457–70.

116. Cohen (2003).

117. Cowley, S. In health visiting, a routine visit is one that has passed. *J Adv Nurs* 1995;22(2):276–84.

118. Thorne, S. and Patterson, B. Shifting images of chronic illness. *J Nurs Scholarship* 1998;30(2):173–8.

119. A framework for the development of integrated multi-agency care pathways for children with life-threatening and life-limiting conditions. Ed Elston S on behalf of ACT (Association for the care of children with lefe-threatening and terminal illness). Published 2004, by ACT, Orchard Lane Bristol, BS1 5DT.

14 After the child's death: Family care

Sister Frances Dominica

To live through the death of your child is perhaps one of the most painful experiences known to humankind. It is instinctive in parents to nourish and protect their child. Death is to be fought, even to the point of sacrificing your own life. If the fight is lost, life is quite literally beyond control. The death of your child leaves you feeling helpless, guilty, powerless and broken.

Nothing can take away the pain you experience, but there are small ways in which it can be made a little less appalling. If you feel that you have some control, not over the fact of death itself—would that it could be so!—but over the events, encounters and exchanges surrounding death, then maybe you can find a little comfort in the midst of the hell of it all.

I have come to believe that there is in every human being the instinct to meet death with a nobility and a 'rightness' which we rarely know we possess ahead of time. It is an instinct at the gut level, far deeper than reason or rationale. The more developed and sophisticated and cerebral the society in which we live, the deeper that instinct tends to be buried. But it is there. Those of us who find ourselves alongside those who grieve the death of a child need to have an unfaltering belief in that inherent instinct. The families are the experts, but they need others to affirm them. Those others are not there to tell them how they should think or behave, but to stay with them while they discover the answers within themselves.

The circumstances of death

The death of a child in this country is rare, yet for approximately 10,000 families in England and Wales annual statistics are irrelevant. The thing every parent dreads most is happening; their child will die from a life-limiting illness.

Children die in very different circumstances. Many die in early infancy. At two extremes, some die instantaneously, others live for many years with a progressive illness. In the case of sudden death there is no opportunity for preparation or anticipatory grieving.

With illness or handicap which is compatible with life for a period of time the family will experience bereavement long before their child dies. They may want to make plans for the time of their child's death while the child is still alive, or they may feel unable or unwilling to do so. We need to remember that no two situations are ever the same.

Many families, given the choice and the necessary support, choose to care for their child at home. Every effort should be made to make this possible. In any case what matters most is that the child and the family feel 'at home' wherever they are.

Towards the time of death

The most important people in a child's life, usually the parents, brothers and sisters, should, where at all possible, be with the child when he or she is dying, whether at home, in hospital, hospice or elsewhere.

To be in bed with the child, sharing a sofa or a large enough, comfortable armchair, may be best, given the choice.

If the child is still conscious, he or she may still have questions to ask and hopes or fears to express. These need to be met with honesty and simplicity and the reassurance that they are being heard.

It is natural to cuddle a child, to stroke the child gently, to talk to him or her. It is important to remember that hearing is usually one of the last faculties to be lost and that just because the child is no longer able to respond, it does not mean that he or she cannot hear.

The professional person's task at this stage, or that of the caring friend, is to ensure that the child is as comfortable as possible and is suffering the minimum of distress (see also

Chapter 34, Symptom control at the end of life, Davies), all the while giving gentle reassurance.

Sisters and brothers at the time of death

It has been our experience that it is best for sisters and brothers to be closely involved at this stage, as at all other stages, whatever their age or understanding. To be excluded often leads to deep-seated distress and anger for years to come.

Including them means answering questions honestly, asking them their wishes and their views and explaining things in a simple, straightforward way.

We may instinctively try to protect children from such pain, but to exclude them from the death of their sister or brother may give rise to fantasies more terrible than reality. Reality can more often be contained and controlled in the memory. Fantasy readily runs out of control.

Ideally the room where the sick child is being cared for should be arranged to allow other children to come and go freely. Someone should have the job of taking care of their immediate needs and focusing attention on them. These needs may be very great in the hours following the death of their brother or sister. They may feel an urgent need to protect themselves or to be protected in their extreme vulnerability.

However strongly *we* may feel about the benefits of including well children at every stage, once we have offered the view and given support for their inclusion, the parents—and the children themselves—must feel free to make their own decision. They usually know better than anyone else.

Grandparents, relatives, and friends

The grandparents' position is very painful. Not only are they watching their grandchild die, but they are also having to stand by and see the extreme distress of their own child. Their presence and practical role at this stage can only be decided with the parents.

Other relatives and close friends may or may not be welcome when the child is dying.

A time like this often brings the best out of human relationships but it can also bring out the worst. It needs great skill to deal with arguments and dissension in such a setting. It is not for the friend or professional to take sides but to try to ensure the greatest comfort and well-being of the sick child.

The trusted friend or professional person may well need to protect the child's family when relatives or friends try to make decisions on behalf of the family. This attempt to take over is often made with the best motives and with a genuine desire to help the family but it may be unhelpful. Given time and support parents will make their own decisions. Meanwhile it may be that the friend or professional can offer the greatest

help by giving time to relatives and friends, thus taking some of the pressure away from the family.

When a child dies—the death having been expected

The parents will often ask if the child has died. Their next question will be, 'What do we have to do?' *There is no hurry to do anything.*

Those closest to the child may want time just to be there with the child. They may want to pray or they may ask someone else to pray with them for their child, either formally or informally. For some parents this may be the moment when they say 'Goodbye' to their child.

When the parents are ready they may choose, with or without help, to do the various things necessary for their child themselves, they may ask someone else to do these things for them or they may have specific needs related to their culture or religion (see below). All families need the opportunity to discuss the choices and their preference.

The child may be washed. Nails may need attention. Wounds may be re-dressed, using waterproof dressings. It may sometimes seem advisable to introduce cotton wool into the anus but other orifices do not normally need packing. If the child has a central intravenous line the funeral directors will usually remove it. However if the parents want it removed sooner it can be tied off firmly just below the skin level (by pulling it gently forward) and then cutting it distally, and the tied end will slip back below the skin.

The child is dressed in whatever clothes the parents choose (nightdress or pyjamas, favourite track suit, first Communion dress, Batman outfit, shroud—nothing is inappropriate if it is the choice of the family.) The child's hair is brushed or combed in the usual style, and the body gently straightened on the bed.

It may be helpful to place a small cushion or pillow under the child's chin for 2 or 3 h to ensure that the jaw does not fall open. Likewise the eyelids may be gently closed and pads of wet cotton wool may be placed on them for a time. If there is any problem with this the funeral director will be able to help.

When the death of a child is sudden and unexpected

When a child dies suddenly and unexpectedly the coroner is informed, normally by the doctor. A coroner's officer (who may be police or civilian) will follow up enquiries. If police visit the child's home they will normally be in an unmarked car and where possible in civilian clothes. The child's body will normally be taken with the minimum of delay to a hospital mortuary by a funeral director acting under instructions from the coroner's office. A post-mortem may follow.

The lack of time and opportunity for the family to say goodbye to their child or to do anything for their child at this stage can be extremely distressing.

Once the coroner is satisfied and the body is released it may continue to be cared for in the hospital mortuary, or may be taken home or to the chapel of rest belonging to a funeral director.

After the death

The place where the child's body will lie until the funeral

The choices listed below assume that the coroner is not involved or that he has been involved and has subsequently released the body.

When a child dies the parents may choose:

- To have their child's body taken to a chapel of rest in a hospital or at a funeral directors'.

- To care for their child's body at home for some or all of the days leading up to the funeral.

- To use the 'special room' of a children's hospice, if this is available. Such rooms are designed to be like an ordinary bedroom but will have a built-in cooling system, sufficient to allow the child's body to remain there for several days, regardless of outside temperatures.

When a child dies at school or in any other place, whether from illness or accident, after the initial necessary action is taken and legal requirements are met, the parents should still be given the choice of where their child's body will be cared for until the funeral.

Caring for the child's body at home

Many people do not realise that in the United Kingdom parents have the option to care for their child's body at home unless the death has been reported to the coroner, and even then it may be possible once the coroner has released the body.

A child who dies in hospital or anywhere else other than home and who is small enough can simply be wrapped in a blanket and carried to a car and so transported home. A funeral director will give the necessary help for a child who cannot be transported in this way.

Hospital staff and others should co-operate fully in implementing the parents' choice. Parents may like to wait until they reach home before washing and dressing their child. In preparing the bed which is to be used it may be helpful to place waterproof protection over the mattress. The bed may be in the child's bedroom or any other suitable room. Family members may want to arrange flowers, toys, photographs and candles, and to make the room special for the child. They may want to remove equipment which the child has needed and which is no longer necessary, but they may not yet be ready to do this.

The room needs to be kept as cool as possible, with fresh air circulating freely. This can be helped with the use of a portable air-conditioning unit. This will help to delay the changes in the body, which sometimes give off an unpleasant smell. Air fresheners may help.

Once relatives and friends have overcome their initial apprehension, usually due to unfamiliarity with death in their own homes, they may well find that some of their fears are overcome by seeing and even touching the body of the child, in the more natural environment of home as opposed to hospital or chapel of rest.

In hot weather or in circumstances where it is difficult to keep the room sufficiently cool it may be best for the child's body to be taken to a chapel of rest after 2 or 3 days, but this is not always necessary.

The child's family will often find themselves in the unexpected role of comforter to those who come to visit in the days following their child's death. If the family has been allowed to be in control of events surrounding the death and to grieve in their own particular way, supported by those around them, they will be more able to meet the shock and raw grief of others.

Sisters and brothers seeing the body of the child who has died

Children of all ages often have frightening and lurid ideas of what people look like when they have died, for example, lots of blood, the body decapitated or squashed, the flesh turned black. These ideas often originate from films, videos or comics.

Children may also wonder how you know for sure that someone is dead. Older children may be reluctant to admit that they do not know the answers to their own questions. It is almost always helpful for them to see their sister or brother after the death, whether they have been present at the time or not. They will need to know that when someone dies their body temperature gradually drops until eventually they feel very cold to touch.

They may ask many questions to which we do not have the answers but, if they see their sister or brother for themselves, at least some of their fears may be dispelled. Some may find the analogy of a butterfly emerging and leaving its chrysalis behind helpful. Others may like to think of the body as a shell.

If the child's body is badly mutilated it may still be possible for sisters or brothers to see some part of the body, for example, a hand or foot, or the face, while the rest of the body is covered. Children—and adults—find it harder to believe that someone has really died if they never see the body. However, the fact that part of the body remains covered may in itself give rise to uncontrolled fantasy and fear. Nothing is perfect in such traumatic situations and one can only do what one believes to be right at the time.

If the brother or sister does not see the body either through choice or circumstance, it may be important to encourage them to talk about it at a later stage. Drawing or playing may be useful ways of working out a way of living with the reality of what has happened.

Telling relatives and friends of the death of a child

Parents will often want to tell relatives and close friends of the death of their child themselves, either in person, or by telephone or letter. Word of such a tragedy spreads fast but one way in which friends may be able to help is to offer to inform specific people.

The family may welcome the offer of a friend to spend time with them in the early days of bereavement with the intention of protecting them when they do not feel able to answer the door to visitors or to cope with telephone calls. This is a very personal thing and can only be done with common sense and great sensitivity. The family may be overwhelmed by callers at this stage but would often welcome them in the loneliness of the weeks and months to come.

Telling children in school

Telling children in school that one of their number has died is a particularly difficult task, requiring great sensitivity on the part of the head-teacher, chaplain, or other members of staff. Honesty, directness and simplicity should be the mark of such an announcement. The same principles apply in telling youth groups and other organisations, to which the child may have belonged.

It will help the children in their shock and grief if they can see for themselves that the adults around them are experiencing the same emotions. To make brief reference to the death of someone who has been amongst them as one of them, and then to carry on as if nothing has happened, is at best, bewildering to the other children, however young.

It is helpful to be given permission to cry, however young or old you are, and to be assured that tears are, in themselves, healing in the outpouring of emotion. To be told that, 'Big boys don't cry' or that, 'Nice girls don't get angry' is unhelpful and blatantly untrue.

Children like to know that they can talk privately to a teacher or other adult if and when they need to, without having to display their ignorance or vulnerability to their peers.

Some sort of remembrance event at the school or other organisation, marking and celebrating the child's life and giving an opportunity to express sorrow and all the conflicting emotions that will arise, may be creative and healing.

Special sensitivity is needed in welcoming back the brothers or sisters of a child who has died. They may appreciate being asked if they mind their brother or sister being talked about and if anything can be done to make this time easier for them. The bereaved child will not 'get over' the death in days or weeks, or even months, and will need great patience and understanding on everyone's part. Grief may manifest itself in many ways, sometimes in behaviour which is difficult to accept.

Deaths which are reported to the coroner

The rules regulating which deaths should be reported vary from country to country. In the United Kingdom, they include:

- a child who has not been seen by a doctor in the 14 days prior to death;
- any sudden or unexpected death;
- death at operation or procedure before full recovery from anaesthetic;
- death occurring within a year and a day of an accident considered to be the direct cause of death;
- any suspicious circumstances, for example, violence, neglect, poisoning.

The coroner will decide whether a post-mortem is required.

Post-mortem examination

As well as in situations when a post mortem is required by law consent may also be sought from parents where a post-mortem is not obligatory but where it is thought that it would be useful in revealing the effects of the disease on the child, or for other reasons which the doctors concerned will explain to the parents. This decision may be exceedingly difficult to make. The parents may find it a little easier if they know that other children with a similar condition may be helped by the knowledge gained through a post-mortem examination on their child. In some cases, the findings of a post-mortem examination may affect decisions made by the parents about further pregnancies.

Where a choice must be made, those standing by the parents while they reach their decision must be sensitive and never coercive. The parents may feel that their child's body has already suffered enough trauma and they must not be made to feel guilty if they refuse permission.

Parents can be reassured that if they do decide to give permission for a post-mortem examination it will still be possible for them to see the body of their child afterwards and, possibly, to care for it. It is a surgical operation and is not mutilating; any necessary incisions will have been closed and dressed as in normal surgical procedures. In many cases examination is limited to a specific organ or organs and parents who agree to a post-mortem may ask that it should be limited in this way. They will also want to be reassured that the organs will be returned to the body unless they give permission otherwise. Nevertheless some parents may feel emotionally unable to see or touch their child's body after a post-mortem examination and they must be given plenty of time and, where possible, the right environment in which to say their goodbyes before the procedure.

Many parents find that meeting with their doctors to hear the result of the post-mortem, both what was found and what was not, and why the child died, is in the long term a comfort. At a later stage they may feel the need to discuss the findings again.

Donor organs

Some parents will find it comforting to think that, by allowing a part of their child's body to be used, another child may be given the gift of life and health. They can be assured that the recovery of organs and tissues is carried out with great care by qualified surgeons. The body of their child will not be disfigured.

The use of donor organs does of course depend on those organs being healthy and also, with the exception of the cornea and heart valves, on the donor dying in hospital. The donor must not have malignant disease (with the exception of some cerebral tumours), major sepsis, viral hepatitis, or be HIV positive.

Two doctors will carry out a series of tests independently in order to confirm that the child is 'brain stem dead' before any procedure to remove organs can take place. Brain stem death usually follows a severe brain injury which causes all brain stem activity to stop. This may be the result of a major accident or of a clot, haemorrhage or severe swelling causing interruption of blood supply to the brain. It can be very painful for parents to say goodbye to their child while the child is still being ventilated and therefore appears to be 'alive'. They need to know ahead of time that although they may be able to accompany them to theatre, they will not be with them when they are disconnected from the ventilator. To know that someone understands their distress in this respect will help a little.

If, for whatever reason, the parents' offer to donate organs from their child is refused, they may feel a sense of hurt and rejection. The reasons for the refusal need to be carefully explained and genuine gratitude expressed for the generosity of the parents.

The transplant co-ordinator will always be willing to spend time with the family if requested.

Embalming and the use of cosmetics

Embalming is sometimes useful if the child's body is to remain at home until the funeral, or if there is a longer than usual delay between the time of death and the funeral.

It is a process performed by the funeral director at his premises in which blood in the arteries is replaced by a preservative, normally a solution of formalin. This delays decomposition of the body and the resultant smell.

Cosmetics will not often need to be used for a child though, appropriately and discreetly used, they may sometimes help to lessen the appearance of bruising for example, or to give the lips a more natural appearance. Cosmetics should not normally be used without the express permission of the child's parents.

Preparing for the funeral

The funeral director

The choice of funeral director is very important. If it is possible to choose one who is sensitive to the particular needs of a family whose child has died, this is of immense help. The funeral director can do much to help or hinder the family in the initial days of their grief following the death of their child.

The funeral director's role is to inform the parents, in a straightforward and uncomplicated way, of the various choices available to them. Many parents will not know that they can shape the funeral service so that it is fitting for their child and family.

The funeral director's advice may be sought, but the family should never feel coerced into making decisions against their will or before they are ready.

The funeral director can make the difference between an appalling experience which does nothing to convey the love and respect felt for the child, and an event which, in all its unspeakable tragedy, can be looked back on as right for this special child.

The family may choose to make most of the arrangements or may ask the funeral director to do so on their behalf. Whatever is decided, the funeral director should give an itemised written estimate of the costs to the family before acting for them. This will include the fees paid on behalf of the family, for example, crematorium fees, burial fees, doctor's fees for cremation papers, minister's fees etc., as well as professional fees paid to the funeral directors. Occasionally some of these fees may be waived; therefore it is not always possible to give an exact estimate.

Many funeral directors make no charge for the funerals of babies or small children. They will in any case be able to give advice if there are financial difficulties, as will a social worker.

The minister of religion

The degree of involvement of a minister of religion at the time of a child's death will depend on many things, not the least of which are:

- any previous relationship with the child or family;
- requirements of the religion to which the family may belong;
- the character of the minister and whether the support he or she offers is perceived by the family to be relevant.

The majority of families living in the United Kingdom will ask for a minister of the appropriate religion to conduct the child's funeral, although this is not essential. (See section on 'The person who will officiate'.) If the family does not know whom to contact, the funeral director will offer to do this on their behalf.

The person who will officiate at the funeral

This may be:

- a minister of religion;
- a member of the family or close friend who is able to conduct a meeting;
- a representative of an appropriate organisation.

If the person officiating has not known the child it is essential for him or her to be told something about the child. Sometimes a person who has known the child but who is not the officiant may be invited to give the address or homily. Anyone may be invited to take a particular part in the service, for example to read a chosen passage, to sing, to play a musical instrument or to offer some of the prayers.

Announcement of the death

The funeral director will normally offer to arrange for an announcement of the death of a child to be placed in either national or local newspapers or both, but the family may prefer to do this themselves, or not to make such an announcement at all.

The announcement may be brief and factual with the name and date of death only, or it may include as many details as the parents choose—for example, date of birth, illness or accident, place of death, names of family members, funeral arrangements, 'in memoriam' requests, suitable quotations or messages. There are however restrictions in most national daily newspapers.

If this is to be the chief way of notifying those who wish to attend the funeral, it is helpful to place the notice with the newspaper as soon as conveniently possible. Many details of the arrangements may be omitted in the announcement by simply giving the name and telephone number of the funeral director.

Suggested forms for national and local papers

National

BROWN John Alan, beloved son of Mary and Paul, dear brother of Samantha and Joshua, died peacefully on November 1st at home, aged 11 years. Funeral enquiries: F. H. Bloggs and Son, 3, West Street, Markham, Oxon. Tel 01865 333812.

Local

BROWN John Alan, beloved son of Mary and Paul, dear brother of Samantha and Joshua and much loved grandson of Edith, Joe and Jane; died peacefully on November 1st at his home after a courageous and fun-filled life, aged 11 years. Funeral on Thursday November 6th at 3 p.m. at All Saints' Church, Littleham, Oxon., and afterwards at St Edmund's School, Markham. Family flowers only but donations welcomed for The Muscular Dystrophy Group to F. H. Bloggs and Son, Funeral Directors, 3, West Street, Markham, Oxon. 0X3 7EW.

'A bright light has gone out of our lives.'

Registering the death

In the United Kingdom the death of all children (including unborn babies over 24 weeks gestation) must be registered with the Registrar of Births, Deaths and Marriages within 5 days of death. Parents may choose to register their child's death themselves, but if they do not wish to do so, or are unable, the task can be delegated to a number of other people, including a person present at the death or a relative present at the death, attending in the last illness or residing in the district where the death occurred.

The doctor who has seen the child after death will provide a signed medical certificate of cause of death or stillbirth to the informant who will register the death. Legible writing on the part of the doctor may save unnecessary distress when presenting the certificate to the registrar. If the doctor is uncertain as to the cause of death, or has not seen the child in the past 14 days, or if death occurs within 24 h of surgery or as a result of suspicious circumstances, the doctor is not permitted to issue a death certificate but must inform the coroner. The coroner will then make the necessary arrangements to ascertain the cause of death.

The certificate is taken to the registrar's office in the sub-district in which the death took place. The doctor will probably be able to give the necessary information about the place and office hours of the registrar. Alternatively the telephone directory entry is headed Registration of Births, Deaths and Marriages. An appointment is sometimes required, and in any case it is wise to check office hours before setting out.

A simple question and answer interview will take place between the registrar and the person registering the death. Information needed is:

- certificate of the cause of death;
- date and place of death;
- the child's full name, home address, the date and place of birth;
- the parents' full names, home addresses and occupations.

The correct entry is made in the register and signed by the informant and the registrar. Copies of the entry can be obtained for a small fee.

The registrar will supply the certificate of burial or cremation which will be required by the funeral director.

Planning the funeral

Many people think that it is good to 'get the funeral over' as soon as possible. Some religions and cultures require that the funeral and disposal of the body happens within 1 or 2 days of death.

For others, however, it may feel better to allow sufficient time to plan all the details of the funeral without a feeling of hurry. For many families the optimum time for the funeral to take place is about 5 days after the death of their child. There is more likelihood that relatives and friends who wish to attend the funeral will be able to do so, given more notice.

The choice of the day and time will partly depend on the availability of the services and amenities needed.

Choosing the coffin

The funeral director will make the parents aware of the range of designs from which they can choose a coffin. White coffins are normally available for children as well as various types of wooden or wood veneer coffins. Parents may choose the lining for the coffin.

A family may make or supply a coffin themselves but it must be strong enough and adequate for the purpose. Some people may prefer to call the coffin a casket, the definition being 'a place for treasure'.

Flowers

In some cultures, the gift of flowers is one way of expressing love and respect for the person who has died and sympathy for the child's family. Flowers can be bought and then sent by the florist to the funeral director or the child's home, according to the family's wish with a message and the names of those sending them. Alternatively the person giving the flowers can bring them to the home or to the funeral. The funeral director will normally give the family a list of those who sent flowers and will collect the flower cards for the family if asked to do so.

The family may prefer that only garden or wild flowers are given. Sometimes those who come to the funeral may be invited to bring a single flower and to put it on the coffin or into the grave. On other occasions only the immediate family will give flowers asking that friends and relatives express their love and sympathy in other ways.

It is not uncommon to see the new grave of a child and the area surrounding it carpeted with gifts of flowers, some of them in the form of elaborate arrangements—a teddy bear, a football or the name of the child for example. If this is comforting to the family then it is entirely appropriate regardless of the cost.

Gifts to charity in memory of a child

Some families will decide to ask relatives and friends to make a gift in memory of the child rather than give flowers at the time of the funeral.

These gifts might be to a favourite charity; to research into the disease which has caused the death of the child; to the place where the child has been cared for; to an organisation or family support group which has meant a lot to the family concerned; or to any other good cause which they may choose.

The suggestion that such gifts may be made in memory of the child may be placed in newspaper announcements. The funeral director will also convey this wish to any who enquire. He will, if asked, receive cheques, forwarding the final sum to the appropriate charity.

The funeral director will list those who contribute so that the family may be fully informed.

Specific items in memory of a child

Parents may choose to collect money to buy furniture or equipment for a place or organisation which has special links with their child.

Gifts towards the planting of a tree or a shrub is another way in which parents may ask others to mark the life and death of their child, living, growing things being symbolic and bringing comfort as time goes by.

An award at school or a trust fund is another way of keeping the memory of their child alive. Occasionally a charity is set up in memory of the child, but the formalising of such a major project is not often completed at this very early stage of bereavement.

The choice between burial or cremation

For many parents this is an agonising decision to have to make: to consign the body of their beloved child either to the earth or to flames is too painful even to contemplate.

If burial is being considered, it is important to discover where a plot is available. This may be in ground belonging to a church or in a local authority burial ground or one which is privately owned.

It is possible to arrange for burial to take place on private land, for example in a garden or field, or in woodland, following discussion with local planning authorities. Permission cannot be denied but the exact position may have to be negotiated. Problems can arise if the family subsequently considers moving house.

If cremation is being considered the superintendent of a crematorium is usually willing to meet members of a newly bereaved family and to answer their questions openly and honestly, often allaying misplaced fears or misconceptions. Families can be assured that the ashes they will be given are the ashes of their child and that they are never mixed with those of anyone else.

Some crematoria do not make any charge in the case of a child under the age of sixteen.

Burial

Those who choose burial often do so because they want to be able to visit the child's grave and to tend it, like a small garden. Some find that the grave becomes a place where they feel particularly close to their son or daughter, and where they can talk to the child. It may be comforting to the family if it is possible for their child to be buried in a family grave, for example with grandparents.

If a child is to be buried the funeral service will normally take place in a church or other building belonging to the relevant faith or in a cemetery chapel, though it can take place in any other appropriate place of the parents' choosing. Parents may choose whether the burial itself (the interment) is attended by relatives and friends or whether only the immediate family is present, others being invited to remain inside the building until the burial ceremony is complete.

The coffin is usually lowered into the grave by the funeral director and his assistants, but this may be done by family members. According to some traditions handfuls of earth may be thrown on to the coffin by some or all present. The grave will not normally be filled in until family and friends have left but, if they so wish, they may fill in the grave themselves. The grave may be lined with flowers or with artificial grass ahead of time. Sometimes flowers are thrown on to the coffin after it has been lowered into the ground.

As at all stages, we have come to believe that it is better to include other children in all that is happening. There are many ways of involving them. For example, one imaginative idea is to invite them to set helium balloons free as they stand by the grave, the number of balloons according to the age of the child who has died.

Parents may like to consider reserving the plot next to their child, or buying a family plot.

The headstone

It will probably be some months before a headstone can be placed on the grave so there is plenty of time to choose this and the words which will be inscribed on it.

If the grave is in a churchyard the agreement of the ordained minister acting on behalf of the diocese is needed concerning the choice of material used and the words of the inscription. Similarly, if the grave is in a municipal cemetery the agreement of the appropriate authority must be obtained.

Cremation

If cremation is chosen, a certificate of examination corroborated by two doctors must be completed in addition to the medical certificate of the cause of death. The funeral director will supply a form applying for cremation, to be completed and signed by the next of kin.

The service preceding cremation may take place in the crematorium chapel. Before choosing this option however, the parents should know that the service cannot normally take longer than 30 min, including the time taken for the congregation to enter and leave the chapel. The coffin may be placed in the crematorium chapel before the congregation is invited to enter, or it may be carried in procession with the congregation, or be brought in after the congregation has assembled.

Another option is to hold the main part of the service in a church or other suitable place, using the crematorium chapel only for the brief words of committal. The family may choose for the committal to be private so that only those invited will attend. A further possibility is for the cremation to take place following a brief service of committal in the crematorium chapel attended by the family only or those they may invite; indeed it is possible for the cremation to be private, without family or friends being present. The ashes may then be placed in a casket and taken to a suitable place where a less hurried funeral service can follow. However, this may not be possible until the following day.

It would seem to be helpful in accepting the painful reality of what has happened for the coffin to disappear from sight before the conclusion of the service, but occasionally this is too traumatic for the parents. They may wish to leave the chapel while the coffin is still present and in this, as in all things, their wishes must be respected.

Next of kin, usually only two people, are allowed to be present when the coffin is placed in the cremator. While this is the norm for those who practice Hinduism it is unusual for others.

Small babies are often cremated at the end of the day, allowing the heat of the fire to become less intense.

Ashes

Ashes may be collected from the crematorium by the funeral director or the family, by arrangement, usually at least 24 h after the cremation. The parents may choose to scatter the ashes in the grounds of the crematorium or in a beautiful place, on the sea, in the hills, or in a place of particular significance for the child.

Another possibility is to bury the ashes. This can be done in the grounds of the crematorium, in a churchyard, or anywhere of the parents' choosing, perhaps in their own garden. It is also possible to bury the ashes in a casket which can be supplied for the purpose by the funeral director. Sometimes the place of burial may be marked by a stone or a plaque, or by a shrub or tree in memory of the child. Families are often invited to plant a rose in the grounds of the crematorium.

Decisions concerning ashes do not need to be made immediately. The crematorium or funeral director will normally agree to take care of them, as will some churches, sometimes for a considerable length of time, before a decision need be reached. Alternatively, the family may take the ashes home in a suitable container supplied by the crematorium or funeral director and make their decision at a later date.

Placing the child in the coffin

The child's body will be placed in the coffin at a time arranged between the parents and the funeral director. The mother and father may wish to lift the child into the coffin themselves, continuing their tending and caring to the very last, but they may prefer that this is done by someone else.

The coffin may be left open until immediately before the funeral or throughout the funeral, or the lid may be fitted at an earlier stage if it seems advisable and if the parents are in full agreement.

Some may like to keep a lock of the child's hair, or a handprint or foot-print of their child, before the coffin is closed.

If photographs have not already been taken, this is the last opportunity. It may not be the parents' wish to have photographs. Other parents may find it is a long time before they can look at the photographs, or they may choose never to look at them, but if they have been taken, then they have the choice.

Placing things with the child in the coffin

It may seem right to the family to place favourite toys or possessions treasured by the child in the coffin. A religious symbol, a flower, a photograph or a gift may also seem appropriate.

Thoughts and wishes, words which a mother or father, a brother or sister may have wanted to say but have not been able to until now, a prayer or a poem—these may be placed in the coffin with the child. Sometimes the child's 'best friends' will like to write a letter to place in the coffin.

Some families will not think it helpful or appropriate to do any of these things.

If the child's body is to be cremated there are restrictions as to objects which may remain in the coffin when the lid is fitted. These restrictions normally include metal and man-made fibres. The funeral director will offer advice if asked.

Dressing for the funeral

Culture, social custom or the practice of a particular religion may require that those attending a funeral, or at least the closest relatives, will wear distinctive clothing. In Western culture this had traditionally been black. In Eastern practice it is often white. Many young families will not be expected to conform to a particular way of dressing but have freedom of choice. Some may specifically ask that mourners do not wear black.

All that matters is that the family feels comfortable with their choice. One factor they may well feel is the most important is whether their child would have approved of their choice.

Non-Christian customs surrounding death

Families who practice a religion such as Judaism, Islam, Hinduism or Buddhism may be well-informed about the rituals surrounding death and the funeral rites approved by the particular faith to which they belong. For others, support in finding information will be welcomed and local faith leaders can be a valuable resource. Families will have differing needs within the spectrum of their faith and each family's personal views should be sought as they may differ from staff's expectations. The following information may also be helpful (please also see cross reference: Rituals and Religion, Chapter 16 Brown).

Judaism

Strictly Orthodox Jews may place a feather over the nostrils and the mouth of the dead person for about 8 min following death.

It is general practice in orthodox Judaism for the nearest relative of the same sex as the child to

- gently close the eyes and mouth and place the arms by the side of the body;
- bind the lower jaw;
- remove tubes and instruments;
- place the body on the floor with the feet towards the door;
- wrap the body in a plain white sheet;
- light a candle and place it by the head.

In the absence of a relative anyone may perform these rites but orthodox families may prefer them to wear gloves when handling the child's body. It may be impossible to contact relatives in an Orthodox Jewish family on the Sabbath (sun-down on Friday to sun-down on Saturday).

Ritual cleansing and preparation of the body will be done by the community. Embalming is not permitted. Mourners do not view the body.

The body is never left alone. A 'watcher' may stay with the body from the time of death until the burial. The dead are buried as soon as possible, often on the day of death or within 24 h after death. Orthodox Jews do not permit cremation but progressive Jews sometimes do, as do nonobservant Jews.

Post-mortem examination is forbidden for Orthodox Jews except where required by civil law.

Organ transplant is rarely agreed to, with the exception of the cornea.

Over the following year a formal pattern of mourning provides the bereaved with support in the community. The shivah, or 7-day period of formal mourning, follows the burial and the bereaved remain at home and receive visitors. Prayers are said in the home each evening. A central part of the prayers is the recitation of the Kaddish said or sung by the close male relatives. After the period of shivah, Kaddish is said at communal prayers by the male relatives for the period up to stone setting which is 11 months to a year after the funeral.

Islam

The word Islam means submission to the will of God. Its followers are Muslims. The attitude of Muslims towards death is strongly influenced by their belief that suffering and death are part of God's will for them.

The dying child should face Mecca (south-east in the United Kingdom). Members of the family may pray at the bedside, whispering into the ear of the child. The child should never be left unclothed as nakedness is deeply shocking to Muslims.

Non-Muslims should not touch the body after death. If it is essential that they do, they should wear disposable gloves. With the family's permission:

- the eyes are closed and the limbs straightened
- the head is turned towards the right shoulder
- the body remains unwashed and is wrapped in a plain white sheet.

At death the family will normally perform the necessary rites and recite the prayers. They will appreciate privacy and access to water during this time. They will:

- close the eyes and straighten the limbs
- tie the feet together at the big toes
- bandage the face to keep the mouth closed
- take the body home or to the mosque for ritual washing
- place camphor in the armpits and orifices
- dress the body in white garments.

Strictly speaking a woman is forbidden to touch a dead body for 40 days after the delivery of her baby. If her baby or older child dies within this period any encouragement to hold the dead child should be very tentative.

Post-mortem examinations are not generally accepted except where required by civil law. It is important to assure the family that all the organs removed will be returned to the body for burial.

Organ donation is not generally acceptable.

Burial takes place within 24 h.

UK law requires the use of a coffin, which is contrary to Islamic law, and for this and other reasons some families may decide to take their child's body to their country of origin.

Duty binds relatives and friends in a supportive programme of mourning. The family remains at home receiving visitors for the first 3 days. Formal mourning continues for 1 month and anniversary remembrances remain important.

Hinduism

Hinduism involves the worship of many gods, each one being a manifestation of the Supreme Being.

There are many different practices concerning the rites surrounding death within the Hindu religion.

There is a common belief in reincarnation. A dying child is often given holy water from the River Ganges. A thread is sometimes tied around the child's neck or wrist as a sign of blessing and it should not be removed. Non-Hindus may touch the body after death provided they wear gloves or the body is wrapped in a plain sheet. There is likely to be opposition to post-mortem examinations but they are permitted if required by civil law. Organ donation is permitted.

Hindus are normally cremated, but children under the age of 4 years are usually buried, as it is believed that they are without sin and will not corrupt the earth. Ideally the cremation or burial takes place on the day of death but this may prove impossible in the United Kingdom. It is important for close relatives to witness the body entering the cremator.

A mourning period is observed and a remembrance ceremony may be held on the anniversary of the death.

Sikhism

Sikhs believe in reincarnation. The family is normally responsible for the last offices. A non-Sikh may close the eyes, straighten the limbs and wrap the body in a plain white sheet. The family will wash and dress the body. There are usually no religious objections to post-mortem examination. Organ donation is allowed.

Cremation will take place as quickly as possible, the exception being for an infant dying within a few days of birth, where burial is the norm. The closest relatives may want to be present when the coffin is placed in the cremator, the nearest equivalent to lighting the funeral pyre. The ashes are scattered on a river or in the sea. The family remains at home receiving visitors for the period of mourning.

Buddhism

Buddhists do not worship a godhead. The Buddha is revered as an example to his followers. The teaching is based on non-violence and compassion for all forms of life, with great emphasis on spiritual growth.

There is a belief in rebirth, not reincarnation. In each life, learning from past experience, the Buddhist progresses towards the state of perfection known as nirvana. This is a state of mind within the individual rather than a place beyond to be reached. Because of the importance of the state of mind, medications which may make clear thinking difficult are sometimes unacceptable.

There are no special requirements in caring for the body of the child. It is wrapped in a sheet without emblems. Post-mortem examination is accepted where necessary.

Organ donation is permitted. When a child dies special prayers are said for between 3 and 7 days before burial or cremation. Cremation is more usual. The ceremony is conducted by a relative or by a Buddhist monk (bhikku) or nun (sister). Practices and ritual vary greatly within different Buddhist groups, but there is a universally calm acceptance of death.

The funeral service and afterwards

Suggested structure for a Christian funeral service

The bidding

Welcoming those present
Suggesting the reasons for the gathering

* remembering
* giving thanks
* praying for the child and the family
* saying goodbye
* grieving.

The word

From scripture
From non-scriptural sources—prose, poetry
An Address or Homily

Prayer

For the child
For those who grieve
In penitence
In thanksgiving
(This may take the form of a celebration of the Eucharist.)

The commendation

Praying for God's blessing on the child in the life beyond death
Saying goodbye

The committal

Lowering the coffin into the grave or moving it towards the cremator.

Psalms, hymns, songs may be chosen and used in any part of the service. Sometimes music is played, either taped or live. It is not wrong to include a child's favourite nursery rhymes or a piece of pop or classical music if this speaks to those present of the child they knew and continue to love.

An alternative style of funeral service

A much less structured form of service may be chosen. An example is the style usually adopted by the Society of Friends (Quakers) in which silence is shared, interspersed with words offered by anyone who feels drawn to speak, read or pray as a tribute or expression of love for the one who has died.

The committal is the only essential part of the funeral rite, anything else being added from choice.

Some families have found it very helpful to be invited by the officiant at the funeral to place things which remind them of their child on a table near the coffin, for example a photograph, a favourite item of clothing, a well-loved toy. Each member of the family may be invited to bring something for the occasion and to take it home with them afterwards.

If the funeral takes place in a church or other suitable place, everyone present may like to light a candle, either during the service or at the end of the service when the coffin has been taken out. This is not normally possible in a crematorium chapel.

The service sheet

The service sheet is not only of practical help to those taking part in the funeral service but is a personal memento for them. It can also be given or sent to those who are unable to be present. There may be a member of the family or a friend who will type the service sheet, which can then be photocopied or printed. If not, the funeral director can arrange this.

The cover may have a design, a drawing or photographs on it. As well as the full name of the child (and sometimes the pet name by which he or she has been known), the dates of birth and death are often printed. The family may choose a quotation to be included on the front cover. The words of the service will follow. An invitation to a reception or gathering of friends after the service is sometimes included at the end of the service sheet. The family may choose to include thanks to individuals or groups of people who have helped in the care of their child.

Transporting the coffin

The coffin may be carried in a hearse provided by the funeral director. However the family may choose to use their own car or to borrow one from a friend. An ordinary estate car may be more appropriate for a small coffin. The car does not have to be black; white or another colour may be more suitable.

In some places it is traditional to use a horse-drawn hearse. The funeral director may walk in front of the hearse for part of the journey. In a village the coffin may sometimes be carried without needing to use a hearse or car. The cortege may pause as a mark of respect at particular places, for example outside the child's home if the journey has begun somewhere else.

It may be important for the family to decide with the funeral director whether the coffin will be carried or wheeled into the place where the funeral service will take place and who will do this.

Carrying the coffin into church the night before the funeral

In some Christian traditions this has been common practice for centuries. To some parents it may be comforting—as if it symbolises that their child is a step closer on the journey to heaven.

It may provide an opportunity for the father, both parents or other members of the immediate family to carry the coffin into church themselves. For some the ordeal of doing this in front of the whole congregation at the funeral service may be too great.

Simple prayers may be offered as the child is brought into the church. The coffin, depending on the size, may be placed on a table or on a bier, in a suitable place in the church. Flowers may be placed on the coffin or around it. A candle, perhaps the Easter candle, may be left burning close to the coffin. Light in the darkness can be comforting on a practical as well as a symbolic level.

This occasion may be attended only by the parents and the minister of religion or by anyone the parents may invite. If the building is normally locked overnight, it may be kind to offer to lend the key to the family.

Recording the service

A tape recording of the funeral service may be a source of great consolation in the months and years which follow. There may well be times when members of the family find it too painful to listen to the tape, some may never want to do so, but if a recording has been made then they have the choice. This is something which a friend or relative may be asked to do, or the funeral director may be asked to arrange for the recording to be made.

Who comes to the funeral?

Some parents may choose to give an open invitation to anyone who would like to attend the funeral. Others may choose to keep some part of it private, for example:

- bringing the coffin into church the night before
- committal of the body at the crematorium
- burial at the grave side.

They may invite others to join them for the remainder of the service. Another possibility is to have a private funeral service followed, at a later date, by a memorial service or service of thanksgiving.

Many adults worry about whether it is right to bring children—brothers, sisters, cousins, friends—to the funeral service. This is a very personal decision but, where at all possible, it does seem sensible to ask the child himself or herself. To be included usually feels better than to be excluded, even in the presence of raw grief, but some will have their own reasons for not wanting to be there.

If, for whatever reason, children are not present at the funeral, it may be important for them to be doing something significant at the time of the funeral so that they do not feel left out, guilty or empty. This could be visiting a special place, listening to favourite music, drawing or painting with someone with whom they feel comfortable.

It may be difficult for the family to remember who was present at the funeral, so those who attend may be asked to sign a sheet of paper or a book, either when they arrive before the service begins or before they leave. The funeral director or a friend will be responsible for this if asked.

Reception after the funeral

Some families will want to invite those who attend the funeral to return to the family home or the house of a relative or friend for refreshments afterwards. Some may prefer to meet in a hotel, pub or restaurant. Preparing the food and drink may be one way in which relatives and friends can help. Alternatively a catering firm may be employed.

People often find it hard to know what to say on such an occasion. They should not be afraid of talking about the child who has died.

Some parents may prefer to be alone or with the immediate family only after the service and relatives and friends will understand and respect this.

What friends can do

Practical ways in which friends may help

These are many and varied. A basic list is given, to which many suggested ways of helping may be added.

- calling on the family
- cooking for them
- offering to wash clothes or bed linen
- doing some housework
- shopping
- driving
- being with other children in the family
- informing named relatives or friends of the death and the funeral arrangements
- preparing refreshments to be offered to relatives and friends after the funeral
- making a tape recording of the funeral service
- listening and not 'doing' anything.

As the weeks go by the needs of the bereaved family will often become greater rather than less (see also Bereavement, Chapter 15 Davies). The most urgent need will be for someone who will listen without giving advice or referring to any experience they themselves may have had, except in so far as it may serve to convince the grieving person that he or she is normal in grieving this way. Anger is an integral part of grief and the friend must be prepared to be a receptacle for that anger without necessarily colluding with it. One subject bereaved people often want to talk about is the person who has died, yet so often it is the last subject other people want to broach. It is helpful to give the bereaved person the opportunity of talking about the child who has died.

Grief is an exhausting process, exhausting physically, mentally, emotionally and spiritually. Remembering this, good friends will find many ways of helping through the months and years of acute bereavement. Grief following the death of a child may go on getting worse for 2 years or more. In a society which expects you to be 'back to normal' in six weeks, the reality can quickly leave the child's family believing they are either sick or abnormal—'Am I going mad?'

Loss of identity or role is very painful—realising that you are no longer a parent, or that you have become an 'only child'.

Friends who will stay alongside, recognising the right of the grieving person to grieve in his or her own way, knowing that no two people, however loving or close they may be, grieve in the same way, are invaluable. It is usually a help rather than a hindrance when a friend shows his or her own true feelings. Bereaved parents or brothers or sisters know that other people are embarrassed or frightened of saying the wrong thing. It is often enough to say, 'I am so very sorry', or, 'How are you?' and then wait long enough to hear the honest answer.

Many families welcome friends' recognition of the anniversaries of the child's birth and death and difficult times such as Christmas, Mothers' Day or Fathers' Day. Friends need not fear reminding the family; they will not have forgotten and may well feel comforted and supported that others have not forgotten either.

Unhelpful things to say or do

Euphemisms—'falling asleep', 'passed away', 'lost'—are normally unhelpful. 'He has died' is true and straightforward and not offensive.

In all the pain and confusion it is easy to resort to clichés when talking to newly bereaved families. For example:

'God took her because she was so special.'

'Jesus has called him to be a little sunbeam . . .'

'God needed another baby angel.'

'It's a mercy—with his handicap he could never have lived a full life.'

'Time will heal.'

'At least you have got the other children.'

'You're young enough to have more.'

'She's gone to sleep with Jesus.'

These examples could be multiplied. There may be elements of truth in some of the remarks, but those who grieve the death of their children are unlikely to find any help and comfort in them, unless they themselves introduce the idea.

The anguish of separation is overwhelming. It feels as if half of them has been amputated. Can they survive?

Belief in God may bring comfort and consolation but it may also bring confusion and anger. There are far more questions than answers. It is unhelpful to try to fill the yawning abyss of unknowing with easy answers.

The real friend will stay alongside, often silent, through the unknowing, the anger and accusations, the guilt, the if-onlys. Guilt is powerful and overwhelming—about surviving beyond the death of your child; about not preventing that death or even in some way causing it; guilt the first time you laugh or live through an hour without thinking about your child. Raw grief is neither reasonable nor rational all the time. It operates at a level much deeper than the intellect.

Do not tell people how they should be grieving

To stay alongside a grieving person means listening to the same part of the story again and again without trying to correct it. Each person has his or her own way of grieving. Even those who are very close to one another will grieve differently. In the state of exhaustion brought about by grief it may or may not be helpful to suggest a game of tennis or joining a drama group. Do not make people feel that they ought to do something because it would 'do you good'.

Do not avoid coming face to face with a bereaved person out of fear or embarrassment. If you cannot find the right words then a hug, a touch or even a smile will help.

Deciding what to do with clothes, toys and other things which have belonged to the child, and rearranging the bedroom should only be done when the parents are ready. There is no hurry. It may be years rather than days or months before they are ready. This is normal.

Conclusion

The early hours and days following the death of a child are crucial in affecting the unfolding grief that ensues in the months and years to come. Nothing can take away the searing anguish, so unpredictable in its course. The heartache and bleak misery are all-invasive. Nothing will ever be the same again even if, given time, it is possible to adjust to a different way of living. At least if there has been the opportunity and the encouragement to do things their way at the time of death and the days following the family will be able to look back in the knowledge that, in a horrendously imperfect world, they ensured that everything was as perfect as it could be for their beloved child, to the very last.

'Some material previously published in *Just My Reflection* by Sr Frances Dominica, published and copyright 1997 by Darton Longman and Todd Ltd, and used by permission from the publishers.'

Further reading

Frances Dominica. *Just my Reflection*. Darton Longman and Todd Ltd, 1977.

Walter, T. *Funerals and How to Improve Them*. Hodder and Stoughton, London, 1990.

The New Natural Death Book Alberrry, N. and Wienrich, S. ed. Rider, London, 2000.

Gill, S. and Fox, J. *The Dead Good Funerals Book*. Engineers of the Imagination, Welfare State International. The Ellers, Ulverston Cumbria, 1997.

Davies, B. *Shadows in the Sun: Experiences of Sibling Bereavement in Childhood*. Brunner Mazel, Philadelphia, PA, 1999.

Emmanuel, L. and Neuberger, J. *Caring for People of Different Faiths* Oxford: Radcliffe Medical, 2004.

Sheikh, A. and Gatrad, A. *Caring for Muslim patients* Oxford: Radcliffe Medical, 2000.

15 Bereavement

Betty Davies, Thomas Attig, and Michael Towne

Case A Chinese-American father sits in a pediatric Intensive care unit (ICU) outside his child's room. He grieves for both his 2-week-old son who will probably die over the weekend of a congenital heart defect and another son who died of sudden infant death syndrome (SIDS) 10 years previously. Chinese New Year is the approaching Saturday. Three previous attempts have failed to remove the son from life support. The medical team and parents have discussed whether one final attempt should be made. The parents, neither a practising Buddhist, request that any attempt should take place after the holiday. This is for the sake of the maternal grandmother, a practising Buddhist, and because their culture and community believe that how one spends the New Year predicts the family's fortune for the rest of the year.

Though medical science has contributed much to the treatment of children with life-threatening conditions, children still die. In modern medical culture we define the death of a child as a tragedy. A family is profoundly affected by this experience prior to an anticipated death, at the time of the death, and many years thereafter. The father from the story above is preparing himself for the death of his fourth son while actively grieving again the earlier death of his second son. While the parents exercise their legal rights to make decisions about their baby's health, they do not do so in a familial or cultural vacuum. The extended family, family friends, and the community within which this family lives are all affected. One can easily imagine the import of a baby dying on Chinese New Year discussed by the members of this family's Chinese-American community.

Among those affected are the staff of the ICU who witness and support the family's reactions and responses to what is happening. The experience of bearing witness to the dying of a child has its impact, even though many staff may purport to the contrary. The impact is reflected in the exacting and impassioned efforts to save a child's life when possible, in the dark humor outside of the earshot of families, and in the emotional aftermath when team efforts are unsuccessful. Identification with the situation in a personal way happens, and for some that process may not be at easily accessible conscious levels. The communities that feel the effects of a death are multiple, including the family, the family's community, and the family's and the child's caretakers during the dying process.

While this father and mother are at the deathbed of their fourth son, they are struggling to support their 15- and 8-year-old sons. These well children, guided by their parents, peers, extended family and teachers, will make a psycho-social transition through this second difficult time in their family's experience. The father describes lessons learned from the first death, even though it was not anticipated and therefore quite different. His family went through a significant restructuring 10 years ago and will do so again. From his words one can also hear, and the literature supports, that the child who died of SIDS 10 years earlier still has his place in the family. Though they may change over time, feelings and connections never go away.

The development of modern medical technology has resulted in a shift in expectations of infant and child mortality in countries where such technology is widely available. In a society that expects children to live beyond childhood, the expectations themselves become integrated into the grieving process. Grieving parents often speak of having joined a club of which they did not want to become a member, given that the entrée is their child's death.

From infancy, humans learn to cope with loss. It is factored into our existence from early days of separation anxiety through adolescent individuation and on to young adulthood when we leave childhood behind. With each successive stage of maturation, we experience loss and progress, and so we grieve and rejoice. Furthermore, since all of us are living, we must all face death. The hoped-for pattern is that we learn lessons through earlier experiences of death that will help us contend with difficult deaths in later life. The death of a child, though, sits outside of that hoped-for pattern.

Contextual variables in bereavement and grieving

Each person's experience of loss and grieving is dependent upon a variety of factors, including both situational factors, individual and environmental factors [1]. These variables provide the context within which each grieves in his or her own way.

Circumstances of the child's death

The most immediate context is the history of the child's dying and death. Often a dying child and family members have already experienced many secondary losses through a relatively long course of living with a terminal illness. Such losses include having a 'normal' child, dreams and expectations for their family and their future together, lifestyle due to the disruptions of caring for an ill child, financial setbacks and hardships, social relationships, their sense of comfort and security in the world, mobility and the capacity to do things that 'normal' families do. They may then come to the death of the child in an already vulnerable position.

Ideally, in an anticipated death, the location (home, hospital, or hospice) of a child's death will have been based upon the family's specific needs and requests. Sometimes, even though the family and the healthcare team know their ideal location, it may not be achieved, for a variety of reasons (insurance issues, nursing shortages, and transportation problems).

A parent may have had to face decisions around the time of death about such things as experimental treatment, resuscitation status, or removal from life support. Or the decision may have been dictated more by the child's disease. Some families must contend with suspicions that either negligence or iatrogenesis contributed to the death. Others may believe (rightly or wrongly) that they bear some responsibility for the death, for example, in cases of accident or genetic illness or when it may be easier to blame themselves than to face total loss of control. Families carry within them images, sounds, and smells from the healthcare setting, including memories of pain or other distressing symptoms.

A child's life may have ended after full resuscitation or a gradual, peaceful slipping into an unconscious state. He or she may have died after years of treatment or very suddenly and unexpectedly. Extended periods of caregiving may leave family members numbed and with little energy for grieving. In contrast a shorter dying trajectory often leaves families less time to prepare and to create support systems for the deep sorrow and disorientation of their bereavement.

Personal history with bereavement

Some of those who grieve have had little or no previous history with bereavement. For a grieving child, perhaps no one close to them has died till now, or perhaps parents have tried with some success to protect him or her from harsh realities. For some adults the death of a child may also be their first experience of a major loss and even a first exposure to medical institutions and technologies. Others will have experienced a major loss before and then often aspects of those earlier deaths, including the memories and feelings (distressing or pleasant) will replay themselves when the grievers confront their new losses. In some cases, grievers may still be actively engaged in intense grieving over a prior loss when this new loss looms or has occurred. Those with experience of grief may bring learned patterns of grieving from the past to bear in coming to terms with a current loss and such lessons may or may not serve them in their current situation; for example, the father at the beginning of this chapter whose "pessimism" about his child's surviving is a means of coping derived from the earlier death of another son.

History and relationship with the child

Each parent, sibling, or grandparent has had a unique history and relationship with the deceased child. The older the child, the more complex and varied will have been the interweaving of the life of the child into the pattern of the daily lives and the life histories of those who grieve for him or her. When newborns die, family members may struggle with never really having the opportunity to know their child well. Grievers will have found different places in the daily life and growth of the child when he or she was well, joined in diverse experiences and activities, achieved different levels of intimacy with him or her, taken different roles in caring for the ill child, and found different meanings in the life they shared. Some histories will have been predominantly untroubled and others filled with tension and conflict.

Personality of the griever

Temperaments vary widely. Some grievers have high tolerances for change, vulnerability, ambiguity, and uncertainty, and others are more daunted by them. Some more extroverted grievers may be receptive to or seek the benefits of companionship and discussion with others, while more introverted grievers may prefer solitude, meditation, or prayer. Some grievers may focus their attention on the details of present and profoundly changed realities, while others may focus their attention on the future and emerging possibilities. Grievers will differ in their ways of choosing how to reshape and redirect their lives in the aftermath of loss depending upon how they are disposed to value control or spontaneity, and whether they attend to the facts and evaluate options objectively or factor in personal values, assessing how deeply they or others care about the alternatives. Some grievers are action-oriented problem-solvers disposed to change the world around them and reshape their daily life patterns deliberately, while others are more inclined to pause to process feelings, make themselves receptive to unanticipated opportunities and allow themselves to be changed by their profound experience.

Social and cultural circumstances

No one grieves in isolation from others. An individual's response to the death of a child is shaped by distinct social and cultural circumstances, and, in turn, each griever plays many roles in shaping responses of the family and the community. Family functioning during bereavement varies widely depending upon how the family communicates, deals with feelings, defines roles, solves problems, utilizes resources, accommodates change, invokes beliefs, and considers others' viewpoints and needs [1–3]. Friends, extended family, and community support also influence how the family unit and individual family members function and come to terms with loss.

Individuals and families grieve within their broader cultural contexts. Some, like the Chinese-American father at the beginning of this chapter, strongly identify with cultural beliefs and mores. They turn to culture and tradition to find support and comfort in the answers, rituals and ceremonies, behavioral prescriptions, and spiritual practices they provide. Since modern medical care is based on its own culture of bioethics, practices, and language, caregivers need to take care to avoid a clash between a Cartesian belief in the schism between body and soul and cultural views where treating the spirit is to also treat the body [4]. Some grievers, however, do not identify strongly with the beliefs and mores of their cultures of origin, even when other members of their own families may do so. Some may even experience cultural expectations as impositions. While it is useful to know how grieving is typically expressed within a particular cultural group, caregivers must respect the uniqueness of an individual's experiences within this broader context, presuming nothing and exploring with them their personal approach.

Grieving the death of a child

It is not the purpose of this chapter to provide a detailed review of the rich history of theory about the grieving process but rather to acquaint the reader with the major trends that have occurred when responding to those who are grieving the death of a child. Changing theory about grieving finds its way into everyday understandings and expectations of family members and caregivers alike.

Table 15.1 summarizes the major theories and the two major trends in thinking about grieving, and the references to works by leading proponents of the theories provide access to

Table 15.1 History of thinking about grieving

Stage or phase models

Emphasis: the physical, emotional, behavioral, social, and intellectual consequences that befall us after bereavement in some expectable sequence.

Leading proponents: Erich Lindemann [5], John Bowlby [6], George Engel [7], Colin Murray Parkes [8], and Elisabeth Kubler-Ross [9].

Medical models

Emphasis: the ways in which grieving is a matter of recovering from symptoms, a view sometimes confined to 'complicated' or 'pathological' grief.

Leading proponents: Erich Lindemann [5], George Engel [10], Colin Murray Parkes [8], Therese Rando [11], and Beverly Raphael [12].

Problems with stage/phase and medical models

Descriptive inadequacy: oversimplifying complex experiences; implying a definitive end to grieving; mischaracterizing normal grieving as pathological.

Failure to respect the individuality of the bereaved: emphasizing how grievers are alike and predictable; misapplying statistical generalizations to individuals; even imposing inappropriate expectations on grievers.

Reinforcing helplessness: implying that grieving is something more that happens after loss; ignoring how grieving is active and choice-filled.

Providing little guidance for caregivers: implying that caregiving means either waiting with, comforting, and listening to grievers or treating symptoms.

Grief work theories

Emphasis: grieving takes both time and effort, defining the efforts involved in actively responding to challenges bereavement presents.

Leading proponents: Erich Lindemann [5], Colin Murray Parkes and Robert Weiss [13], William Worden [14], Therese Rando [11], and Thomas Attig [15].

Virtues of grief work theories

Descriptive adequacy: recognizing that grieving is an active response to emotional, psychological, behavioral, social, intellectual, and spiritual challenges in loss.

Encouraging respect for individuality: encouraging attunement to the unique challenges each griever is contending with.

Responding to helplessness: appreciating how grievers implicitly address their helplessness as they actively engage with the challenges of loss.

Providing guidance for caregivers: expanding caregiver roles beyond passively waiting with the bereaved to actively. supporting the efforts of addressing the 'tasks' of grieving.

Theories of the relationship with the deceased

Emphasis: grieving requires ending the relationship with the deceased *or* grieving involves transforming the relationship.

Leading theorists: Ending the relationship—Sigmund Freud [16] and John Bowlby [6].

Sustaining the relationship: Dennis Klass, Phyllis Silverman, and Steven Nickman [17], Margaret.

Stroebe and Henk Schut [18], and Thomas Attig [15].

Table 15.1 (*Continued*)

Virtues of theories of sustained connection
  Descriptive adequacy: recognizing that grievers both continue to miss those they mourn and find ways to sustain constructive connection with them.
  Encouraging respect for individuality: encouraging appreciation of the unique meanings grievers find in sustained connection.
  Responding to helplessness: recognizing both the futility of longing for a return of the deceased and the possibility of establishing connection in separation.
  Providing guidance for caregivers: expanding caregiver roles to include supporting remembering the deceased and embracing their positive legacies.

major works in the history of grief theory. One trend in that history has been a move away from stage/phase or medical models toward grief work models. The other trend is a move away from the view that grieving requires ending the relationship with the deceased to the view that grieving involves transforming that relationship. The currently preferred theories

- describe the phenomena of grieving more accurately and adequately
- encourage respect for the unique suffering and distinctive struggles of the individual griever
- respond to griever helplessness by underscoring how grieving is an active response to bereavement
- provide more appropriate guidance for caregivers.

Here, we have chosen to offer an understanding of grieving the death of a child that we believe reflects the best of theories of grief work and transforming the relationship with the child.

Grieving as relearning the world

Fundamentally, grieving is a normal, active, choice-filled, evolving response to a "choiceless" event—bereavement, a process that both takes time and requires considerable effort. As grievers address the challenges that bereavement brings into their lives, they implicitly address the passivity and helplessness of bereavement. In describing the work of grieving, Attig [15] urges that grieving is nothing less than a process of 'relearning the world'. Contending with the death of a child shakes the foundations of the survivors' ways of being in the world and will be unique to each person. 'Relearning the world' requires that grievers learn how to be and act in a world transformed by the death of the child. There is no right way or easy formula for relearning the world, only the ways that grievers choose for themselves. Grievers must contend with virtually all elements in their experience, including their

physical and social surroundings, aspects of themselves and their relationship with the deceased.

Relearning physical surroundings

Those who grieve the death of a child face physical surroundings that are permeated with reminders of the child who died, including painful reminders of the child's absence and, in some cases, of his or her suffering (a sick bed or room, medical items, etc.) as well as cherished memories. Parents and siblings return to their homes once filled with the child's history (their words, arguments, laughter, and tears) and their personal possessions (clothing, art works mounted on walls or refrigerator doors, photographs, the child's favorite foods and music). Some return to cherished items that the child gave to them while others face items that distress them on discovery, for example, drug paraphernalia. Grandparents and friends who did not share home life with the child may nevertheless find returning to their own home or visiting the child's home challenging because of the distinctive reminders they find there. Many grievers also find that things and places outside of the home that were touched by the life of the child are difficult for them; these may include such things as family automobiles and many features of the neighborhood (e.g. schools, playgrounds, hospitals, particular stores, and vacation spots). Some parents and siblings return to homes with nurseries that the child never occupied, where life with the child was only anticipated.

Relearning social surroundings

Grievers must relearn their social surroundings, life with family members, friends, and others who may or may not have known the child. These social contexts are also permeated with reminders of the child, both painful and positive (such as family resemblances, habits and shared histories). Experiences, activities, and patterns of interaction that comprised family life patterns when the child was an active participant in them cannot be as they were before the child's death. Special occasions and anniversaries, holidays, birthdays, anniversaries of the illness and death, parties, the beginning of the school year, graduations, and family traditions can be especially challenging.

Each parent or sibling is uniquely anguished and vulnerable, in need of comfort and support, challenged by expectations of others, uncertain of appropriate things to say or do or roles to play, caught up in relearning the unique world of his or her experience, and limited in his or her understanding or capacity to help others. Anguish can be compounded as family members witness one another's individual struggles with the child's death and realize the limits of their own abilities to reach out to and support one another. None can grieve in pristine isolation from the others. Desires and choices of one family member about how to live with things, within places, with one another, in daily routines, and on new paths into uncharted futures implicate all of the others profoundly and individually. Family members are challenged to find the sensitivity, compassion, tolerance for difference, and skills in cooperation, compromise, and negotiation necessary to recover and sustain smooth family functioning in new family life patterns. Often families struggle with issues of conceiving and welcoming a new child into the family. Grandparents, other members of the extended family, and friends who do not share home life with the immediate family must also contend with new concerns, issues, tensions, and patterns of interaction with members of the immediate family even as they come to terms with their own bereavement.

Parents, siblings, and other grievers may find other social interactions challenging, including encounters with health care professionals, funeral directors, clergy, insurance agents, friends, colleagues at work, schoolmates, persons who knew the child but had not learned of the death, people who innocently ask about the number of one's children or siblings, and anyone who resembles the child in some way. Grievers may feel isolated or alienated from cultural support. Members of immigrant families may have to contend with language or legal complications of their status or with being outside of familiar cultural norms and support systems. A society that is vastly different from that of their origins may not readily support rituals or ways of expressing grief that they learned as children. Others may have to contend with unwelcome cultural pressures and expectations that they do not find supportive or that actually inhibit or interfere with their grieving.

Relearning aspects of the self

Those who grieve the death of a child must relearn their very selves, including their characters, histories, roles in life, commitments, and the identities they find in them. Parents contend with concerns such as the extent to which they are identified with their roles and histories as parents; the quality of their characters as reflected in their parenting, especially at the end of the child's life; what it means to be the mother, father, or stepparent of a dead child; what is to become of them now that their child has died; and their motivations and capacities for parenting other surviving children or children yet to be conceived. Siblings contend with similar concerns about their roles and places in the family; the quality of their characters as reflected in interactions with their dead brother or sister; what it means to be the brother or sister of a dead sibling; what is to become of them; and how the death is likely to affect the ways their parents and siblings care for, value, and respect them as individuals. Some must contend with parents and others who look upon them as replacements for the dead

child or expect them to be or become like them in some way. Parents and siblings alike are challenged to relearn their self-confidence and self-esteem. Those who knew and loved the child struggle to change and to fit with the new reality; reassess their commitments to family, work, and other major life projects and commitments; grow in understanding and modify perspectives on the greater scheme of things and their places in it; adapt their faiths and recover a sense of daily purpose, hope, and meaning in life. Family members and friends wonder about how they are different for knowing and loving the dead child and about how, if at all, they can understand or meaningfully embody these aspects of themselves in separation from the child.

Relearning the relationship with the child

Grievers also struggle to relearn and reassess their relationships with the child who died. Parents often experience raising their children as the central business of their lives. No matter what the age of a child who dies, parents can feel as if their experiencing the world with their child and witnessing his or her growth and accomplishments have been cut short. Many of their fondest hopes and aspirations for their child have been dashed. Parents, siblings and others often struggle with words unspoken and deeds not done in interactions with the child, especially words of love and affection and goodbyes. Attig [15] urges that the heart of grieving is making the transition from loving someone when he or she is physically present to loving him or her in separation. "Closure" is simply a myth: parents, siblings, grandparents, members of the extended family, and friends will always carry some pain over missing the child they loved, and they will never stop loving them. They struggle to learn ways of expressing their abiding love for the child and of feeling that the child's love is still with them. They carry within them memories and stories of the child's life that do not die when the child dies. Remembering itself can be painful as it, too, reminds them of their separation from the child. But memories are also filled with meanings, which can be cherished for a lifetime, and are the principal means of sustaining connection with the child's life. Parents, siblings, and others can feel the child's love for them as through memory they come to recognize how much the child gave them when he or she was alive: influences on their practical lives, including interests and projects that have come to matter to them; influences on their souls, including their ways of caring deeply and loving one another; and influences on their spirits, including their ways of overcoming difficulty, striving to improve lifes, and finding hope, meaning, and joy in life. Parents, siblings, and others can express their love for the dead child through remembering privately, sharing memories, and appreciatively embracing their practical, soulful, and spiritual legacies.

Relearning their world

Much of the work of grieving is a matter of working towards completing tasks by taking incremental steps in all aspects of the grievers' lives. They relearn and reframe their worlds in piecemeal experiences, not all at once. In this process the work is best understood as a cluster of life-long, open-ended endeavors (again rendering the expectation of 'closure' inappropriate). Grieving families and individuals return to worlds filled with painful reminders of the absence of the dead child and of a life with him or her that is no longer possible. The work of grieving involves coming to terms with the great agony of missing the child and reaching through the pain to affirm the meaning of life in separation from him or her. Family and individual daily lives are in disarray, often following an extended period of illness where familiar routines were disrupted frequently or set aside entirely. The work of grieving involves reshaping tattered lives, weaving together still viable threads from life prior to the death with new threads of activity and caring into inevitably new daily patterns. Family and individual life histories have veered from their expected courses, often through unwelcome chapters of anguish and dislocation while the child suffered and died over an extended period. The work of grieving involves redirecting life stories, carrying forward meanings familiar from past chapters while struggling to find and make new meanings in unanticipated chapters of individual and family narratives [19].

Grievers often experience disconnection from something greater than themselves that gave meaning to their lives, including the vital caring connection with the child, connections within the family or with the wider community, and a sense of belonging and purpose within the greater scheme of things. The work of grieving involves reconnecting in meaningful ways with family and community and seeking meaning and purpose in the greater scheme of things. Grievers must also actively engage with some of the most profound 'mysteries' of life such as death, suffering, loss, the meaning of life, and love. Unlike everyday problems, mysteries are constants that cannot be overcome, managed, controlled, or solved definitively. The work of grieving here does not involve changing the mysteries, but rather changing in response to them.

Suggestions and strategies for helping grieving families

Caregivers in the pediatric palliative care setting can help grievers to understand the basic contours of the grieving process: the challenges before them in bereavement and what relearning how to be and act in a world transformed by the child's death requires.

They can help them to appreciate the value of putting in the effort that grief work requires: helping them to grasp that effectively relearning the world of their experience will ameliorate their distress and anguish (though not eliminate all residual pain of missing the child), return them home to aspects of their lives that still hold meanings familiar to them from life prior to the death, engage them in reshaping and redirecting their lives in meaningful ways, and enable them to continue loving the child in separation. Such understandings can foster self-understanding; allay self-doubts about what is 'normal' in grief; undermine unrealistic expectations of closure such as having to let go entirely of the dead child and elimination of the pain of missing the child; define direction and purpose for grieving; and motivate the griever.

Helping as mentoring

Just as no one can learn for others, caregivers cannot relearn the world for anyone grieving the death of a child. They cannot rescue them from the pain and suffering that loss and transition entail. However caregivers can model their helping on what effective parents, mentors, and teachers do when they acknowledge that they cannot learn for those they are helping and when they help them to become active and self-directed in their learning. Some approaches they can take are:

- To comfort grievers, offer their presence, listen to their stories sympathetically and nonjudgmentally, and provide them places of safety and security.

- To support them as they reshape their daily lives and redirect their life stories. Caregivers can express confidence in grievers' abilities to face and meet the many challenges before them; refrain from offering pat answers, simple formulas, recipes, and directions; concentrate on helping them to find their own paths; and serve as sounding-boards, active listeners, companions in exploration of options and possibilities and constructive critics.

- To reassure grievers that they need not address all of the most difficult challenges at once.

- To help them focus their attention selectively, prioritize tasks, and set their own pace in relearning their worlds.

- To help mourners recognize and draw upon their strengths in meeting emotional, psychological, behavioral, social, intellectual, and spiritual challenges; recognize and overcome their weaknesses; and learn, and recover from, mistakes.

Helping grievers in all dimensions of their being

Caregivers can support and encourage persons in any or all of the dimensions of their grieving, depending on where help is requested or needed.

Psychologically. Caregivers can help grievers to cope emotionally as they listen actively, normalize feelings, empathize and comfort, encourage satisfying or meaningful expression, tolerate the expressions, and help to dissipate or constructively redirect the most corrosive feelings, for example, guilt or anger. They can help them with changing personal identities, supporting them as they puzzle over who they are now, return to familiar roles and ways of doing things, and try new roles and unfamiliar ways of doing things. They can help them to recover self-confidence by reassuring them as they either test still viable life patterns or build new ones. They can support self-esteem by showing that their presence is welcome and their contributions are valued.

Behaviorally. Caregivers can encourage and support grievers as they test, and recover confidence in, familiar dispositions, motivations, habits, and behaviors. They can help them recognize when old dispositions, motivations, habits or behaviors lead to frustration or obstruct progress in grieving. Where new patterns of living must be learned, caregivers can help them to identify, gather information about, and evaluate options; choose from among them; enact their choices; and reflect on whether they have chosen well or want to try some other course.

Physically. Caregivers can help grievers to recognize and secure means to meet their physical needs for food, rest and shelter. If exhaustion threatens, professionals can prescribe sedatives when appropriate. Caregivers can also reinforce personal bonds necessary for physical health through presence, touch, comfort, and reassurance of personal worth. And they can encourage others to offer the same rather than making excessive demands, adding to stress, or compounding feelings of isolation or abandonment.

Socially. Caregivers can support grievers as they reconfigure patterns of interaction with and maintain relationships with others. They can help them to overcome excessive self-reliance or pride, and encourage them to ask for support from individuals, support groups, or professionals. Caregivers can help them to balance demands from others for support with their own needs. They can help them anticipate and rehearse difficult conversations or situations; offer to be with them in difficult social circumstances; avoid, deflect, or otherwise effectively deal with insensitive, disrespectful, or destructive actions of others; offer to intercede with others; help them to recognize needs to seek distance from or even to break off relations with others, either temporarily or permanently; and support them if they make such difficult choices. Caregivers can help members of families and communities to recognize how they together face challenges to reshape and redirect family and community life; learn the importance of tolerance of and respect for individual differences; and learn ways to cooperate, negotiate, and compromise effectively. Caregivers can help grievers as they establish new relationships.

Intellectually. Caregivers can help grievers to develop understandings and perspectives on the concrete realities of death and bereavement. They can help them gather, sort, and interpret information about events surrounding the death; learn more about expectable impacts of loss and the challenges grieving persons face; evaluate their own strengths and limits in coping; and identify their own desires and hopes about where coping will lead them.

Spiritually. Caregivers can encourage the bereaved to explore the potential of ritual and ceremony (traditional or otherwise) to help them to contend with sorrow or embrace memories and legacies of the child who died. They can support them as they struggle to recover old or discover new goals and purposes in daily life. They can support them as they redirect their life stories and struggle to find meaning and bases for hope. They can help them see that they will relearn the world in grieving again and again throughout their lives as they learn an acceptable way of going on for a time and then find that they must change course once again. Caregivers can help grievers modify their beliefs and faiths and support them as they seek security, peace, consolation and a return to feeling 'at home' in the world despite human limitation and vulnerability and the mystery that pervades the human condition.

Helping grievers to find lasting love

Caregivers can be especially effective when they understand how lasting love can motivate relearning, temper pain and anguish, and restore wholeness for individual grievers as well as their families and communities. They can listen to the stories about the dead child that grievers have to tell, share stories of their own, encourage grievers to remember, preserve their memories, and share them with others. They can join with grievers and encourage them to join with others in exploring meanings of the stories and memories. They can help them to identify legacies from the child's life, deep lessons in living and ways in which they are different for having known and loved the child and having been known and loved in return. They can encourage them to explore and discuss with them how they can preserve those legacies and embrace them in the daily lives and the unfolding of their life narratives. As they do these things, they can help grievers learn to love and continue to feel loved by the child who died.

Issues in establishing bereavement support services

Families develop relationships with staff members, sometimes over many years. Some want to maintain an ongoing relationship with those who cared for the child. They often worry that the child will be forgotten. During the transition after the child's death, when medical care is not needed any more, families and staff have to navigate a changing relationship [20]. Issues of professional boundaries come into question. Many families express anger and resentment when either the care providers or the institution itself do not acknowledge the death of the child. This is when a bereavement program within palliative care, or as part of another area within the institution, can be of great service to both families and staff. They are commonly found in the array of services offered by hospices, and in some hospital-based and community palliative care programs but less often in general hospital services.

A bereavement program allows professional caregivers to refer a family and transfer their care to those who are adequately trained and have the time and resources to support families through their grief process. Furthermore, they offer all families the same services, including support groups, memorial services, and grief education programs. Technology has provided innovative approaches such as grief-list-serves for families to connect over vast geography or to not have to enter the hospice or hospital again. Families no longer have to contend with not knowing whether the individual physician, nurse or mental health worker will be available to support them. Sensitive programs develop means for families to see those who actually cared for the child at events like memorial services when staff are welcomed as well. Most importantly, bereavement programs connect grieving families to each other, while providing them with support resources. A bereavement program reflects commitment to care of the family since typically these services are offered free of charge.

A bereavement program can be an important bridge between families and staff. *For families* the program can make professional end-of-life care more sensitive to the needs of families through provision of information and education that communicates to staff what families experience. Services like offering handprints of a child for the family to take home with them after the death signal the caring nature of the institution. Many palliative care services offer photographs of the child (either before or after the death), a lock of the child's hair, plaster handprints, or keepsakes (blankets, stuffed animals, signs from the bed, etc.) that were part of the child's life. Families consistently report that the moments immediately prior to and following the death are never forgotten. Staff and volunteers need to be well informed about how to be sensitive in all, even brief, exchanges with families at this time. Caregivers can influence families' experiences in either positive or negative ways with significantly long lasting impressions.

For professionals and volunteers who help children and families through these difficult times in their lives, witness some heart-wrenching scenes, and are constantly reminded of the frailty and preciousness of life, the program can offer help too. Often staff members and volunteers have their own grief issues and need support. A bereavement program can help in debriefing after a death, validating feelings, helping with retention, and avoiding burnout. Historically, medical professionals were taught to desensitize themselves to these experiences and to maintain an "emotional detachment". New thinking has tempered that approach. Rather than "desensitizing", professionals are encouraged to sensitize to this powerful human material. They too must find ways to incorporate grief, death, loss and mystery into their practice. This is challenging given the western medical approach of science "having the answers". Professionals can learn over time to move through the pain of providing this kind of care and come to a place where they can offer a deep compassion to families [21]. Self awareness of one's own personal history of loss and beliefs about death, dying and afterlife is crucial. Without it, caregiver beliefs and cultural/spiritual biases can interfere with the experience of the family. For caregivers, strong coping techniques, good self-care and ongoing education and support are necessary components not only to do the work, but also to avoid burnout.

Training bereavement professionals and volunteers need to receive includes understanding of models and theories of grief, how to facilitate support groups, and systems and resources in the community that are of support to families. Many hospitals offer a menu approach (support groups, memorial services, grief workshops, etc.) for families to choose which is useful. But the individual intervention should be tailored to the unique experience of the griever. Even within groups there is a delicate balance between supporting the needs of the group, while allowing for the individual's process. Interviews need to carefully assess the meaning of the experience as filtered through cultural and spiritual beliefs. Discussion should include the person's life story, and its current set of issues.

Working with children who are grieving brings all of the above with the extra challenge of knowing how development interfaces with grief and loss. Therefore, comfort with interventions that include play and art are necessary skills. Many activities can be used to elucidate feelings, expand understanding, and develop a sense of normalcy in an unusual situation. One type of play that has been of use is playing with a tray of dirt, toy coffins, flowers, rocks, material for headstones and little people. Children explore the material in whatever way makes sense for them. Often they will recreate the grave site of their sibling. Some siblings report that the only way they have "visited" their sibling since the death is in this manner. While adults often find this a morbid activity, children gravitate to it with relish.

Case One 10-year-old, who had attended grief support groups for the 2 years since her brother's death, normally did not speak much in group. It was believed by the facilitators to be due to a combination of preadolescence and personal temperament. When she heard that 'burial play' was the activity for the evening, she ran into the room stating, "I love this activity", and then proceeded to unfold her story and that of her brother's death with both innocence and wisdom.

Circumstances where special services are more likely to be needed

It is important to identify when grievers are at risk of unnecessary suffering and more likely to need specialized professional services. It would be a mistake to conclude that grievers will always benefit from specialized services; most are remarkably resilient using their own resources and drawing upon the support of family and friends. However, grievers sometimes meet with extraordinary complications in the challenges they face that compromise, inhibit, interfere with, undermine, or even block their effectiveness in grieving.

Often grievers recognize when they are becoming frustrated, preoccupied, mired, or stuck in their grieving. And they are often able to take some responsibility for reaching out for help. But sometimes caregiving professionals or volunteers have to recognize that some grievers are not doing well on their own or in a support group and are likely to benefit from specialized interventions. Professionals should learn as much as possible about grievers' vulnerability to extraordinary complications in grieving [11, 22]. They should learn to recognize when they are out of their depth and refer grievers when appropriate to others who are specially trained, including psychologists, psychiatrists, child life specialists, trauma specialists, family therapists, social workers, clergy, and other spiritual and cultural advisors. They should also take some responsibility for reaching out and making services available to developmentally-challenged populations and survivors of traumatizing deaths.

Here we discuss four major types of extraordinary complication where the need for specialized intervention increases.

Extraordinary challenges in the relationship between the child who died and the griever

Grievers are vulnerable to some extraordinary complications that relate to their relationships with the dead child. Wishing that the child were still alive is a common aspect of missing him or her. It is nearly inevitable since feelings, desires, motivations, habits, and dispositions that took root in the expectation that he or she would still be alive are not extinguished the instant the child dies. Such wishing is harmless and episodic

and the grievers do not seriously imagine that such wishes can or will come true. However preoccupying and fervent longing for the child's return, by contrast, is dangerous. It hinders or stalls grieving as it undermines the griever's motivation to reshape and redirect his or her life. The griever "knows" the child is gone. Yet, paradoxically, the griever desires the child's return with every fiber of his or her being. This desire can motivate no action and nothing can fulfill it since the return is impossible. Such longing frustrates the griever, induces helplessness, and can paralyze him or her. It persists as the griever stays in retreat from a new and frightening reality, dwells in a desire that once held close a beloved child, receives secondary rewards for his or her obvious distress, or fears that he or she will forget or stop loving the dead child.

In some situations the griever may have to contend with unfinished business with the child who died: words unsaid and deeds undone (especially when the death was sudden or unexpected) or, more profoundly, the very life of the child that may be experienced as unfinished. The griever may become preoccupied with such unfinished business with the dead child. In general, the greater the burden of unfinished business, as the griever experiences it, the more likely it will distract him or her from relearning the world effectively. Given the common perception that they have not finished, or have even failed in, raising and nurturing the child, parents are especially susceptible to having extraordinary difficulty here [23].

Some grievers must contend with hurtful or dysfunctional aspects of their relationships with the child who died. Loss of a less than fully loving relationship is not less difficult to deal with. Negative ties can bind more tightly than positive ones and often destructively. A griever may become caught up in extreme anger for what a child did or failed to do, for example being careless, saying or doing hurtful things, rebelling, abusing substances, getting in trouble with the law, or attempting suicide. Or a griever may become caught up in extreme guilt for what he or she did or failed to do in life with the child, for example, tension and conflict, being too controlling, saying or doing hurtful things, jealousy, abuse, failure to protect, neglect, having actually contributed to the death, or feeling relief when the child died. Grievers may fervently long for the child's return to address these issues. Resentment, frustration, and bitterness may prevail. Grievers struggle even to acknowledge or express such negative ties or feelings. Family and social pressures may reinforce their reluctance.

Extraordinary complications deriving from attributes of the bereaved

Grievers are also vulnerable to some extraordinary complications that have to do with their own limitations in ability to relearn. He or she may lack well-developed emotional, psychological, behavioral, social, intellectual, or spiritual capacities needed to relearn the world but have the potential to acquire them. Or the griever may be compromised because he or she is a child, adolescent, developmentally delayed, or because his or her coping capacities have been affected by injury, physical illness or dementia. The griever may suffer from any of a wide variety of diagnosable psychological disorders, which may have been present prior to bereavement or been acquired subsequently. In either case, they can block or interfere with effectively relearning the world.

Children may suffer from the myth that they do not grieve which can lead some to neglect them and exclude them from family or community responses to death; siblings, in particular, are indeed the forgotten grievers. Children's reality changes too, but without developed orientation to reality prior to the death, their disorientation is greater unless someone answers their questions honestly and helps them understand and experience what the realities of death and loss entail. What they overhear or misunderstand in adult conversation often confuses them. Some children lack linguistic abilities to explain what troubles them; express their thoughts, feelings and other reactions; or state what they need or hope for in response. Unprecedented feelings frighten some and leave them at a loss as to what to do or say. Some imagine wrongly that they are responsible for the death, for example, because they wished the child dead. Loss often disrupts or undermines development of self-confidence, self-esteem and self-identity. Some feel helpless and need to learn they have choices in response to choiceless events. Regressive behavior is common, as is reenactment in play. Children lack models for, and need guidance and support in finding, appropriate things to do in the mourning period and in putting together new life patterns. Dependence makes them more likely anxious about the basic necessities of life, including food, shelter and love. Death often breaks bonds just when children are testing and learning to value and trust them.

Siblings especially, must contend with the loss of one of the commonly longest lasting relationships of a lifetime the significance of which is too often underappreciated [1]. Their responses fall into four categories:

1. 'I hurt inside' including the range of feelings and behaviors that are part of grief.

2. 'I don't understand' relating both to their developmental level and how, without explanation, they are bewildered by the death and related events.

3. 'I don't belong' including both their desire to help but now knowing how to and also to their being excluded from decisions and events.

4. 'I am not enough' referring to siblings particular vulnerability to comparisons with the dead brother or sister [1].

Children typically lack mature beliefs about such things as the meanings of life, death, and suffering. When a sibling or peer dies, some realize for the first time that they too could die. Children may need specialized professional help when their disorientation, emotional distress, or dysfunctional behaviors at home or at school persist in ways that seem not to be subsiding, when they have been involved in the death in some way, or when support from family or peers is lacking.

Extraordinary complications deriving from characteristics of the death

Grievers are vulnerable to extraordinary complications that relate to difficult circumstances surrounding the death itself. A griever may suffer fixating trauma, typically from horrific circumstances of death or experiences where he or she has unexpectedly witnessed something appalling. Another may be traumatized by multiple deaths that occur all at once or so close together that he or she experiences the challenges of grieving as overwhelming. Such traumatic events hold the griever's attention and block him or her from dealing with the challenges of relearning the world. When a griever experiences the death of a child as preventable or caused by human action, he or she can become preoccupied with those responsible, mired in legal system and media distractions and interferences, or deeply fearful that he or she lives in a threatening, menacing and untrustworthy world [24]. Those grieving the death of a child in a car accident might imagine the horror and details of the circumstances and the child's damaged and disfigured body. A parent grieving their child's death by a violent act might imagine not only the images, but also the terror their child felt prior to death. The parent of a baby who has died from nonaccidental injury by a family member struggles with the loss, the complex family issues, and the challenge to his or her assumptions about whom he or she can trust.

Extraordinary complications in the social environment

The social circumstances of some grievers can seriously interfere with their relearning. Families and community members can hinder or undermine effective individual coping: They can visit unwelcome expectations or make excessive demands upon the griever. They can abuse power or authority, attempt to manipulate or control the griever, or interfere paternalistically in the name of "what is best" as they see it. Some families have been quite dysfunctional prior to the child's illness or death, and others may become so as a consequence of these pivotal events. For example, parents who are in a decomposing marriage may blame each other for the death of their child. Or a deeply troubled sibling may act out in ways that further threaten family equilibrium. Some grievers may experience themselves as "disenfranchised" in their grieving [25] Sometimes others fail to recognize their grief, for example when young children, a developmentally delayed relative or elderly grandparent is thought not to be affected by the child's death. Sometimes others dismiss the significance of the griever's relationship to the child, for example when a stillborn baby or neonate dies, or if the dead child was severely handicapped. Siblings or childhood friends may be forgotten or neglected, a noncustodial parent after a divorce may be excluded from rituals, or a gay man or lesbian who raised a child, but is not the birth parent faces legal or societal limitations on his or her rights to actively and visibly grieve. In still other instances grievers may be disenfranchised because something is repugnant about the death, for example, where suicide, homicide, violence, mutilation, or stigmatized diseases are involved. Unwillingness to acknowledge a griever's hurt and desire to remember and love the dead child, and lack of social support, or even sanction, compound challenges grievers face as they add secondary losses; intensify feelings of abandonment, alienation, guilt and shame, anger, depression, and meaninglessness; and exclude the griever from social responses to death such as funerals and other rituals.

Summary

In pediatric palliative care, we regularly face the death of children and we must extend our care to those who are bereaved. In doing so, it is helpful to remember that we each engage in life and death. We try to make meaning of our experiences. We learn to carry pain and sit with mystery. When faced with the death of a beloved child, we relearn a world that misses, honors and remembers that child. We do all of this whether we are a Chinese-American father who is anticipating the death of his son in a pediatric intensive care unit or a 10-year-old bereaved sister playing and telling stories about her brother who died.

References

1. Davies, B. *Shadows in the Sun: The Experience of Sibling Bereavement in Childhood*. Philadelphia, PA:Brunner/Mazell, 1999.

2. Davies, B., Chekryn Reimer, J., Brown, P., and Martens, N. *Fading Away: The Experience of Transition for Families with Terminal Illness*. Amityville, NY: Baywood Publishing Co, 1995.

3. Davies, B., Spinetta, J., Martinson, I., McClowry, S., and Kulenkamp, E. Manifestations of levels of functioning in grieving families. *J Fam Issues* 1986; 7(3):297–313.

4. Miller, S. *Finding Hope When A Child Dies: What Other Cultures Can Teach Us*. New York: Simon and Schuster, 1999.

5. Lindemann, E. Symptomatology and management of acute grief. *Am J Psychiatry* 1944;101:141–8.

6. Bowlby, J. *Attachment and Loss: Attachment*, Vol. 1. New York: Basic Books, 1969.

7. Engel, G. Grief and grieving. *Am J Nurs* 1964;64:93–8.

8. Parkes, C.M. *Bereavement: Studies of Grief in Adult Life*. New York: International Universities Press, 1972.

9. Kubler-Ross, E. *On Death and Dying*. New York: Macmillan, 1969.

10. Engel, G. Is grief a disease? A challenge for medical research. *Psychom Med* 1964; 23:18–22.

11. Rando, T. *Treatment of Complicated Mourning*. Champaign, IL: Research Press, 1993.

12. Raphael, B. *The Anatomy of Bereavement*. Champaign, IL: Research Press, 1983.

13. Parkes, C.M. and Weiss, R. *Recovery From Bereavement*. New York: Basic Books, 1983.

14. Worden, W. *Grief Counseling and Grief Therapy: A Handbook for the Mental Health Practitioner* (1st Edition; 2nd Edition (1991)). New York: Springer Publishing Co, 1982.

15. Attig, T.W. *How We Grieve: Relearning the World*. New York: Oxford University Press, 1996.

16. Freud, S. Mourning and melancholia. In *Sigmund Freud: Collected Papers*, Vol. 4. New York: Basic Books, 1917.

17. Klass, D., Silverman, P., and Nickman, S. *Continuing Bonds: New understandings of Grief*. Bristol, PA: Taylor & Francis, 1996.

18. Stroebe, M. and Schut, H. The dual process model of coping with bereavement: Rationale and description. *Death Stud* 1999:23: 197–224.

19. Neimeyer, R. The language of loss: Grief therapy as a process of meaning reconstruction. In R. Neimeyer, ed., *Meaning Reconstruction and the Experience of Loss*. Washington, DC: American Psychological Association, 2001, pp. 261–92.

20. McKlindon, D. and Barnsteiner, J. Therapeutic relationships: Evolution of the Children's Hospital of Philadelphia model. *Matern Child Nurs* 1999; 24(5):237–43.

21. Harper, B.C. *Death: The Coping Mechanism of the Health Professional*. Greenville, SC: Southeastern University Press, 1977.

22. Bendiksen, R.A., Cox, G.R., and Stevenson, R.G. *Complicated Grieving and Bereavement: Understanding and Treating People Experiencing Loss*. Amityville, NY: Baywood, 2002.

23. Rando, T. *Parental Loss of A Child*. Champaign, IL: Research Press, 1986.

24. Kauffman, J. *Loss of the Assumptive World: A Theory of Traumatic Loss*. New York: Brunner-Routledge, 2002.

25. Doka, K. *Disenfranchised Grief: New Directions, Challenges and Strategies for Practice*. Champaign, IL: Research Press, 2002.

26. Attig, T.W. *The Heart of Grief: Death and the Search for Everlasting Love*. New York: Oxford University Press, 2000.

16 Ritual and religion

Erica Brown

Introduction

In the body, a million births and deaths take place at every moment. The body is a miracle of re-birth in which our habits, our likes and dislikes, our hunger, and our states of mind are always driving the body towards change and development. Never for an instant does the body cease to die, cease to be born. We might say that we live through death at every moment.[1]

Birth and death are the two events experienced by all people and religions are concerned with them. Belief in survival beyond death is perhaps the oldest religious conviction of humankind. As long ago as prehistoric times bodies were buried together with tools and ornaments for use in the next life. Today there is a great variety of teaching in world religions about death and afterlife, ranging from belief in the resurrection taught by monotheistic faiths to belief in reincarnation held by the religions of India and beyond.

During the past decade parental bereavement has received considerable attention and a number of descriptive studies have brought to light the unique needs of life-limited children and their families [2,3,4]. However, while there is a growing amount of literature available on the psychological needs of families with a life-limited child, scant attention has been paid to cultural care [5].

There is sometimes an assumption that the needs of families from ethnic minority groups are met by resources within their own community [6], but evidence shows that, although they often do not come forward for help, their needs are often unmet, and they struggle with little support [7, 8]. Therefore the need to provide accessible and appropriate palliative care to ethnic minority groups has been recognised as a significant service development issue. A Report from the UK National Council for Hospice and Specialist Palliative Care Services [9] identified, amongst other needs, a need for the provision of culturally sensitive services in relation to the 'spiritual, language and dietary needs of black and ethnic minority service users.'

The chapter is divided into there parts. Part one discusses social, cultural, and ethnic aspects of death and the importance of equal access to care. Part two attempts to define religious needs and describes the findings of small-scale research at Acorns Children's Hospice in Birmingham, UK [10] concerning the experiences and expectations of Asian mothers with a life-limited child. Part three contains information that may act as a springboard for policy and practice in religious care with specific reference to Hindu, Sikh and Muslim families. See Chapter 14 (cross ref after the child's death Ch. 14, Francis Dominica) for additional information, including practices in some other faiths.

Effects of ethnicity/culture on bereavement

Many people have multiple ethnic and cultural identities, possessing mixed heritage with parents, grandparents and great-grandparents from different groups or communities. Ethnicity and culture profoundly affect the ways families experience death, dying, and bereavement. Furthermore, the ways in which a society deals with death, reveals a great deal about that society, especially about the ways in which people are valued.

In pre-industrial societies there were high rates of death at the beginning of life and often children did not enter the social world until a naming ceremony took place and the baby became recognized as a member of the community. Indeed babies who died before this time did not receive full funeral rites. Instead of birth and death being viewed as two separate events they were treated as though one cancelled out the other. Perinatal death rates were still high in the United Kingdom as recently as Victorian times. Parents saw about a quarter to a third of their children die before they reached ten years of age.

Today many societies see death as a transition for the person who dies. How people prepare for this transition and how survivors behave after a death has occurred varies a great deal. There are, however, some common themes. Most societies provide social sanction for the outward expression of this in the funeral rites and customs that follow death.

Ethnicity

The term 'ethnic' is often misunderstood and discussion about the meaning of ethnicity has been extensive [11,12,13]. For the purposes of this chapter, ethnicity is regarded as referring to a group of people, who share distinctive features, such as shared origin of descent, language, culture, physical appearance, religious affiliation, customs, and values.

Literature about death and ethnicity is limited in both its volume and its scope. Little is currently known about family roles in paediatric palliative care settings within different ethnic groups. There is, however, some literature available giving accounts of death beliefs and funeral rites, focussing on ways of dealing with the body, rather than the experience of death and dying within these groups [14,15,16]. A fundamental weakness of the literature has been its insensitivity to the processes of change, which occur as members of minority ethnic communities adapt to their new societies [17]. The view that families from minority ethnic groups 'look after their own' has rightly been criticised as a stereotyped over simplification. Traditional family structures are changing in Britain as elsewhere in the world, and often relatives may live too far away for them to be present at the time of death. Young Asians who have been brought up in Britain may not have experienced a death in their family until they themselves are adult.

Culture

Numerous definitions of culture abound. In general they tend to place emphasis on culture as a shared system of meaning, which derives from 'common rituals, values, rules and laws' [18]. For the purposes of this chapter culture is defined, as, *how people do and view things within the groups to which they belong.* Culture also includes a set of shared values, expectations, perceptions, and life-styles based on common history

and language, which enable members of a community to function together.

For many people it is important, that they are able to maintain their cultural values and practices, but cultures are not fixed and static. They change in response to new situations and pressures [19].

Some aspects of culture are visible and obvious [20]. These include dress, written and spoken language, rites of passage, architecture and art. The less obvious aspects of culture, consist of the shared norms and values of a group, community, or society. They are often invisible, but nevertheless they define standards of behaviour, how things are organised and ideas about the meaning of such things as illness, life, and death.

Most Western Europeans view physical illness as caused by some combination of bad luck, external factors, heredity and individual behaviour. In other societies, people may consider other possibilities including bad behaviour, divine punishment, jealousy, or another person's ill will.

It is often assumed that a child inherits the culture into which it is born, but cultural awareness is also nurtured through shared rituals, values, rules, and laws. In the words of Unger [21], *the word 'culture' is not a noun but a verb.*

The culture of the community in which people grow up has a predominant influence on their worldview, and on the way in which they behave. Each culture has its own approaches for dealing with loss although there may be differences concerning spiritual beliefs, rituals, expectations and etiquette. Research indicates that grief is experienced in similar ways across all cultures, but that within cultures there is a huge range of individual responses [22]. Furthermore micro cultures exist within cultures with individual differences.

Throughout the history of humankind, the deaths of babies and children have continued to be common events. Today in countries where the rates of infant mortality are still high, the death of a child may be considered inevitable with mourning lasting little longer than a few days.

In societies where medical and scientific advances have resulted in the decline in infant mortality, childhood death is likely to be perceived as tragic and unfair. Most societies designate the status of bereaved individuals referring to them for example as 'widows' or 'widowers' for those losing a spouse, or as 'orphans' for children losing parents. There are no culturally accepted terms to describe the state of the bereaved parent.

Each culture attributes unique significance to the death of a child. Individual cultures also hold a variety of beliefs about where children come from before they are born, and where they go after they die. Furthermore, the age, gender, family position, and cause of death, may affect the meaning attributed to the death, and determine the rites of passage for grieving behaviour within a given culture.

Religion

The word 'religion' probably derives from the Latin *religare,* which means 'to bind' [23]. Faith is the recognition on the part of humankind of an unseen power, worthy of obedience, reverence, and worship. In monotheistic faiths this power is referred to as 'God', and in polytheistic societies as, 'the Gods'. All religions agree that their deity or the deities have control over the destiny of a person's soul after earthly life is over.

The great world religions have evolved in diverse ways under the influence of the cultures into which they have spread. Some religions provide detailed codes of conduct covering aspects of daily life such as diet, modesty, worship, or personal hygiene. Others have looser frameworks within which people make their own decisions. There are also different groupings within most religions, each of which may have a variety of beliefs, requirements and traditions.

The influence of religion on people's lives varies a great deal. Religion may act as a form of social support, providing companionship, practical help and affirming a person's self esteem through shared values and beliefs. Many people find that their faith is a source of comfort, giving meaning to suffering, and providing hope for the future. However, people may also feel angry, and let down by their God or Gods, and lose their faith. People who do not aspire to belong to a faith may, nevertheless, have strong ethical and moral values and a sustaining spiritual dimension to their lives.

Different generations may hold different views within their own faith, particularly where the second generation has grown up in a different cultural milieu. Children absorb parental attitudes towards religion in the early years of their development without question or analysis. This can influence their thoughts and attitudes in later life.

Sometimes people turn to religion for an explanation of their personal tragedy. Most major faiths teach that physical death is not the end. However the precise form the continued existence takes varies within different religions and sometimes within different denominations. Major themes include:

• Belief in the cycle of birth, death and reincarnation;

• Judgement that results in reward or punishment for past behaviour and thoughts;

• Existing with God in an afterlife in heaven/paradise;

• Being reunited with loved ones who have died earlier;

• Sleeping or resting until spiritually or physically resurrected by God;

• Exclusion from God in purgatory or hell.

Ceremonies and rituals

Much of life is made up of rituals; but these are so much part of everyday activity that people do not necessarily think about their origins or their meanings. The ritual is acted out in such a way that there is instant recognition of the event. Indeed part of the importance of the 'acting out' is that there is little need to explain. Often a variety of non-verbal ways of expressing feelings come into play. Sometimes people create their own ways to give meaning and resonance to what has happened. Others find meaning and comfort in traditional ways of doing things, particularly if they are part of a cultural minority.

The coming together of family, friends at a funeral is a statement of ongoing love and respect even though a person has died. Those who watch what takes place are constantly made aware of the fact, that what is important is not so much what is said, as by what is implied by the coming together. The more ceremony and ritual that is present, the more opportunities there are for the expression of feelings.

Death rites

In virtually all religions there are clearly set out rules, religious laws and procedures about what is to be done during the dying process and after the death. Periods of mourning last for a clearly defined period in many cultures, allowing the bereaved a gradual time to come to terms with what has happened, and to adjust to changes in their lives both psychologically as well as adapt to their changed social status.

The value a culture holds for children and the significance of their death, is reflected in the care and disposal of the body and in funeral rites, which may be quite different from those performed, when an adult dies. In several cultures children are considered innocent and their premature death affords them heavenly status. Thus Puerto Ricans dress their child in white and paint the child's face like an angel. Some Orthodox Christians believe death to be particularly traumatic if it occurs before a young person is married since marriage is viewed as the consummation of earthly happiness. If a young person or a child dies, their body is dressed as if they were wearing wedding clothes and funeral laments are sung, that bear a striking resemblance to wedding songs. In other cultures, such as China, the death of a child is perceived as a 'bad' death and parents and grandparents are not expected to go to the funeral. People avoid talking about the child, because, the event is considered to be shameful. Hence the values, beliefs and practices held by families in Western cultures may clash with those held by families with a different cultural background.

The ways in which families commemorate their child's life demonstrate and reinforce their beliefs. Individual members may hold differing views about the role of children as participants in funerals and mourning rituals. Some parents may not feel able to discuss their own feelings with members of an older generation who may want to 'protect' children from the pain of death. Hence the attitudes and practices within families may clash.

Religious rituals can also have important spiritual, social, and emotional significance, strengthening bonds between members of a group, giving a shared sense of meaning and purpose. Ceremonies surrounding death often stress forgiveness, preparation for the life to come, transcendence, and hope. Sometimes religious rituals offer a person the chance to participate in religious behaviour without specifying the extent of their belief. They may provide comfort and reassurance to the mourners. The ritual dimension of religion encompasses actions and activities, which worshippers do in the practice of their religion. Activities may range from daily ablutions before prayer to taking part in a once-in-a-lifetime pilgrimage.

Signs and symbols

Symbols may have great significance for families. Religious symbols are inextricably associated with religious belief and observance. Sometimes these are large and displayed in the family home, or they may be small and private, such as pendant or a sacred thread worn by Hindu males, under clothing. Statues or pictures may be used decoratively or as a focal point for private worship.

Natural phenomena such as light and darkness also have powerful significance. The crescent moon and stars appears in Muslim countries, representative of light and guidance for persons on a spiritual journey. 'Guru', a word with particular significance for Sikhs may be translated as 'a teacher' or 'enlightener' and is derived from the word 'gu', meaning darkness and 'ru' meaning light. Thus a guru is a spiritual teacher who leads from the darkness of ignorance to enlightenment.

Worship

The basis of most religious observance is worship of a deity (or deities). The form which worship takes, and the expression and location of worship vary between religions, denominations, and individual worshippers.

Worship comprises components such as thanksgiving, praise, and repentance. Expression may be found through prayer, physical position, and movement, reading and reciting sacred scriptures and silence. In some faiths music is very important. For example in Hinduism the sound of a *mantra*

or sacred verse reflects deeper meaning and its repetition acts as a focus to concentrate the mind of the worshipper.

For some people, prayer is an essentially private matter, and it may be silent. For others it may be a corporate activity with family members. Worship at home is important in all faiths. Some religions prescribe set prayers at certain times. Others encourage silent prayer and meditation. In children's hospices where staff endeavours to create a homely environment, it is important that people have private space set aside for worship.

Most religions identify sites of historical and spiritual significance, particularly where the founder of the faith experienced a revelation. Sacred places may include cities such as Makka or Medina for Muslims or Jerusalem for Jews and Christians. Sometimes shrines commemorate miraculous events and appearances and they are the destination of pilgrimages. Muslims for example, aim at least once during their lifetime to complete the Hajj by visiting Makkah, the birthplace of Mohammad.

Children's experience of death

The context of many children's experience of death has changed. In the past, most deaths occurred at home. Death and illness were witnessed first-hand and children were often present at funerals. The ancient nursery rhyme 'Ring-a-ring o' Roses' describes a game played by children during the Great Plague and Black Death of the fourteenth century and seventeenth centuries in Britain. The 'rosie-ring' refers to swelling lymph nodes and 'a pocket-full of posie' to an amulet worn as a protection from the disease. 'Achoo' (which over the years has become 'ashes' in the United States) describes the flu like symptoms associated with the plague and 'all fall down' to the inevitable death of the victims. In the twenty-first century most people die in hospitals or other care settings and death will rarely be within most children's everyday experience.

However, in Great Britain approximately 15,000 children and young people under the age of twenty still die each year. Although Black [24] writes of the remoteness of childhood death in the twentieth century, for some children and their families it will remain a stark reality.

The religious and cultural development of children with life-limited conditions

A child's age, cognitive ability, anxiety level, and home background will all influence their understanding of what happens at the time of death and beyond. Each family is unique, and the culture or faith in which children are brought up, and the way in which they are taught at home, and at school will influence the way in which they perceive death. Therefore it is vitally important that life-limited children are given age and developmentally appropriate opportunities to share and explore their fears and concerns. Children often indicate their awareness of serious illness and communicate their beliefs about what happens after they die through drawing and painting. In order that carers are able to work effectively with children it is important that they are aware of what children have been taught by their families and communities.

In the early stages of their development, children are egocentric and their understanding of religion is based on their experience within their family. Some children will have engaged in religious practices; some will have had occasional experience of religion; others none at all. Many may have an awareness of symbolism in religion and they are likely to have heard stories about the lives of key figures and religious leaders. They may also understand that for some people, places, food, and occasions have special importance. At this stage it is important to provide a foundation on which to build children's increasing awareness of themselves as individuals and of their relationships with other people. Helping them to respond to different environments provides a framework for cultural, and religious experiences with which they may be familiar such as reflection or meditation.

In the middle years, children have a greater understanding of themselves and an awareness of the faiths, and cultures in which they grow up (See Figure 16.1). Some families may choose to talk about death and dying, and perhaps the concept of the soul moving on to another form of life. Children's relationships with members of the local and wider community will have an important influence on their sense of personal identity, and purpose. Many children will have an awareness of the contribution they make to the communities to which

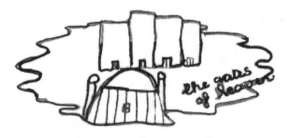

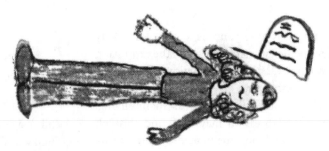

Fig. 16.1 A 10-year-old Muslim girl shows her understanding of burial and her hope for heaven in the next life. Interestingly, many Muslims would not depict the human body or heaven in pictorial form.

What happens when somebody dies ?

1. They go up to heaven.
2. Their body goes away.
3. They get a new body.
4. They go in a box and their body gets fired.

Fig. 16.2 An 8-year-old boy asked the question 'What happens when somebody dies?' He then attempted to give his own answers to his question.

they belong, and there should be opportunities to help them create memories for the people who will grieve after they have died.

Young adults are often fiercely independent and they seem to have an urgent need to get on with living their lives. This may conflict with having a life-limiting illness. There is often an impressive determination on the part of young people to deny the reality of the situation and carers need to respect this. Opportunities to explore the common ground between their own experiences and spiritual and religious questions of meaning and purpose may be helpful. Where young people are members of families with a religious belief their questions are likely to include a spiritual and religious context (See Figure 16. 2).

Bluebond-Langner [25] and Brown [26], describe how life-limited children with special educational needs may have a sophisticated understanding of death that includes a religious dimension. Turner and Graffam [27] have worked extensively with young people with learning disabilities and their research has included dreams about death. A consistent theme is the appearance in a dream of a person who has already died. Sometimes the deceased person invites the life-limited young person to join them.

Religious themes often appear in children's thoughts about death and an after–life. Heaven is nearly always regarded as a desirable place where life continues after earthly existence is over although mostly this life is in an altered form such as becoming an angel (See Figure 16.3). For some children hell appears as an alternative destination although young people rarely talk about it as a possibility for themselves.

For some children thinking about religion may be unhelpful (see Figure 16.4). The relationship between religion and death-anxiety has been studied by a number of researchers [28, 29]. Where young people are actively involved as worshipping members of a religious community, death-anxiety

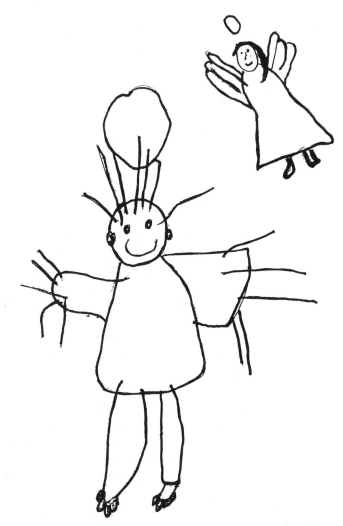

Fig. 16.3 A 5-year-old girl draws herself as a baby angel in heaven accompanied by her mummy, who will be there to look after her. Note the halos.

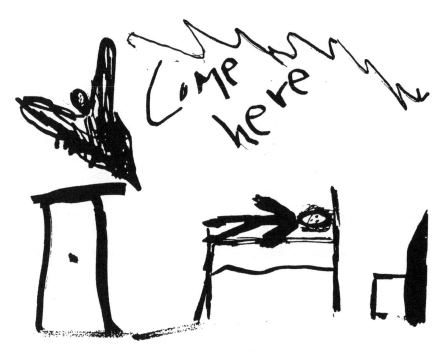

Fig. 16.4 An 8-year-old boy newly diagnosed with a life-limiting condition has night terrors about 'being taken' by the angel of death when he dies.

appears to be lower although personality, temperament and life experience all play their part.

Children's questions

Many children are curious about death and their questions about their illness may be accompanied by a fascination about what happens next. Religions seek to give responses to mysteries of human existence. Some children may question their faith, wondering how a just God can allow them to die. Others may turn to religion to find an explanation for what is happening to them. This may involve thoughts about sins they have committed, laws they have broken or faith they have lost. Thus, children's questions probe the world around them as they reflect on their past and present life and strive to make sense of the future.

As children grow through normal developmental stages their questions may change. Young children often ask questions based on their need for reassurance and they are very concerned with adult responses that give them a sense of security and safety. When they are older they are likely to need more detailed replies to questions as they try to satisfy their curiosity, uncertainty, and perplexity. By the time they are of secondary school age young people require more specific information, and their questions may include situations outside the belief and culture of their family. This may present a huge challenge for families and carers who feel ill-equipped to explore the complexity of young people's needs.

Fundamental to working with life-limited children is an ability of adults to understand what individual children really want to know. Some questions point to larger questions to which there may be no definitive answers. Comments such as 'there is nothing to be frightened about' may sell children short. A parent's own fear may also lead to denial of their child's inevitable death. Goodhall [31] emphasizes the importance of telling the truth, answering questions and using easily understood language instead of euphemisms and metaphors.

Children's attempts to answer questions such as, why do I suffer?, or why will I die?, may help them to make sense of what is happening in their own life story. Hitcham [32] writes, 'Inside every child there is a story waiting to be told but when that story involves difficult issues such as death and dying, it is neither easy to tell nor to listen to'.

Creating personal life-story books can help children to encapsulate their experiences. Some children may keep diaries that are important to them as private documents whilst they are alive. After their death these can provide their families with an insight into their child's journey. Other children may like to create a memory box in which they record their life story through writing, art and collections of symbolic objects.

Caring in practice

When people are ill or vulnerable they need care that is focussed on their needs, and what is important to them. Professionals require the skills, information, and confidence to find out what each family wants and organizational structures, which are sufficiently flexible to enable them to provide it. Practices, beliefs, and attitudes are continually emerging. Professional awareness of the range of such patterns can be a vital starting point in addressing the needs of ethnic minority families.

At a time when services are under great pressure and resources are stretched, the demand for holistic family-centred care that takes into account different cultural, religious, and personal needs may seem unrealistic. Holistic care for dying children and their families requires special skills, and sensitivity. Identifying and meeting individual, cultural, and religious needs are important parts of that care.

In order to be effective, members of the caring professions must be aware of their own social mores, prejudices, and worldview. People's attitudes and beliefs profoundly affect the way they respond to other people, particularly those whose lifestyles are different from their own. In 1995, Infield, Gordon, and Harper [33] concluded that 'while many people are individually knowledgeable and culturally sensitive, few hospices had systematically planned services to meet the needs of culturally diverse groups'. Therefore it is not surprising that generally, children's hospices are finding it difficult to attract referrals from minority ethnic groups [34].

Good service *can* be provided which *is* appropriate for families from a wide range of cultural and ethnic backgrounds, whether the child is being cared for at home, a children's hospital, or a hospice. Where service providers are committed to meeting the needs of different groups take-up has often been dramatic (Acorns Children's Hospice Trust, unpublished).

The experiences and expectations, of ethnic minorities with a child, with a life-limiting-condition, are under-researched areas of palliative care in children. Acorns Children's Hospice in the UK conducted one small-scale project [10] in 2002 examining the difficulties of Asian mothers. The study identified prejudice in their own faith or cultural communities, and common experiences of patronizing and dismissive approaches by professional groups when raising concerns about their child. This research has led to a number of changes in the way palliative care was delivered both at the hospice itself, and by other local health care providers. There is an Asian liaison officer who has worked with families to help them communicate their own needs actively, both within and outside the family unit. This has also helped families, particularly mothers, to understand options available to them, for example having a place set aside for worship or meditation or appropriate facilities to wash their child after they have died.

Religious and cultural artefacts are made available at Acorns hospices for families to use. Menus provide for a variety of dietary preferences and food is prepared and cooked in an appropriate way. Where possible, care for boys and girls, is given by staff and carers of the same sex.

At the heart of the philosophy of palliative care is holistic care for all families with a life-limited child, irrespective of religious, racial or cultural background. Education and training can raise staff and volunteer awareness of attitudes that can safeguard against stigmatisation and stereotyping of ethnic minority families. At the same time, their needs to be parallel research and development that can provide an evidence—base for a model of care that is matched to the individual needs of service users. Good practice in achieving accessible and appropriate palliative care services will only be experienced if the stated policies and practices are in harmony; the children and their families are made to feel welcomed; and their views are listened to and acted upon. Equal access means offering responsive, flexible services to families, in which individual needs are identified and accommodated so that each person benefits. This cannot be achieved by an ad hoc system or by individuals working in isolation. Equality must be supported by the ethos of the organization, be understood and implemented by all managers and employees, and backed up by training and practical support.

Caring for families

Over the last two decades there has been increasing awareness of the importance of listening to the views of parents of life-limited children and planning services which are sensitive to individual family needs. There has also been corresponding concern about the stereotypes which have been created concerning the level and nature of support which families would welcome.

The United Nations Convention on the Rights of the Child [35] makes several references to the importance of religious and cultural care. In the United Kingdom families embrace a wide diversity of religious beliefs, or none. Information for practitioners about different faiths and cultures is useful only if it is relevant to the people concerned, comes from reliable sources, is based on a commitment to the view that all faiths and cultures have intrinsic worth, and are equally worthy of respect, and acknowledges the complexity and variety of the real world. Therefore, it is essential that practitioners should have access to accurate information and advice [36].

Of course there is a danger that in attempting to describe and to classify beliefs and practices this leads to one-dimensional snapshots. Hence all guidelines are likely to contain some generalisations and crude stereotyping that ignores variation and idiosyncrasy.

The purpose of this part of the chapter is to introduce some examples of beliefs and observances of particular relevance to the everyday life, care, and well being of children and their families. Particular attention is given to caring for the dying child, and for the child's body after death. Space prohibits detailed or comprehensive information concerning all faiths. Therefore Asian traditions of Islam, Hinduism, and Sikhism have been chosen. In the course of writing, I have drawn on the advice and support of a great many people. Some are colleagues kind enough to share their knowledge; others are families who are practising members of a religion or leaders from faith communities.

Islam

The total size of the Muslim community living in the United Kingdom as recorded in the 2001 census is just over one and a half million. Muslims represent 3.1% of the total population of England and Islam is the second largest faith group in the United Kingdom. Although the largest concentration of Muslims is in the London Borough of Tower Hamlets, many people live in Birmingham and Bradford. Most of the Muslim community is very young with over half of all persons under the age of 25. There are more males than females.

Muslim families

Families are central to Muslim life and Muslim society. In the Qur'an, Allah gives specific guidance on the rights, responsibilities, and obligations of every Muslim within their own family, and stresses the family's value as a source of support, love and security. In Asian culture the family is traditionally a much larger unit often referred to as the extended family.

Marriage and the raising of children are fundamental to a good Muslim life and are religious duties.

Sons are considered responsible for the care and support of their parents, as they grow older. When a son marries, he and his wife often remain with his parents and bring up their children.

Sexual morality is strict. Sex is only permitted within the context of marriage, in which men have specific and clear responsibilities to protect and provide for women and children. Extra marital relations are forbidden and condemned in the Qur'an. In some communities it is considered responsible to segregate sexes after puberty.

Men and women

Within Muslim families, men and women generally share decisions, with women chiefly responsible for the comfort of the family, and the upbringing and moral education of the children. Outside the home, Muslim women are generally under the guardianship and protection of men: fathers, husbands, or sons if the woman is a widow.

A rigid code of public behaviour is often observed between the sexes. For example, on visits to Muslim families, men and women do not normally shake hands. It is considered courteous for the woman of the family to withdraw or remain silent when men or older people are talking to visitors. Outside the family, men and women usually socialize separately.

Religion

Muslims believe there is one God, Allah, and that Muhammad is his messenger. Allah is the Arabic word for God. God is the Eternal Creator, Compassionate and Merciful. He is All-Knowing and All-Powerful and His will must not be questioned in any way. He alone is to be worshipped.

Muslims believe that Muhammad was the last of a long line of Prophets. The Prophet Muhammad taught that he was a messenger, chosen to proclaim God's will. It is customary for Muslims, when they say the name of the Prophet Muhammad, to add the words 'Peace be upon him', immediately afterwards. Respect is paid in the same way to other Muslim Prophets.

Muslims have certain religious duties to perform. These include the 'five pillars' of Islam: faith in God, daily prayer, fasting during Ramadan, giving alms (if their means allows) and making a pilgrimage to Makkah.

Islam teaches about life after death and in resurrection from the dead at the Day of Judgement. Every individual should live on earth as perfectly as they can. When a person dies they will be judged by God and rewarded or punished for the life they have lived.

The duties of Islam

The five main duties which Muslim men and women perform are know as the 'Pillars' or Foundations of Islam. Not all Muslims practice every aspect of their faith strictly, but for those who do, the five pillars of Islam are extremely important.

The statement of faith (*Shahadah*)

All Muslims must make a statement of their faith in God, and in Muhammad as His Prophet.

'There is no God but God and Muhammad is the Prophet of God.'

Prayer (*Salah*)

Most adult Muslims will wish to say set prayers (*salah*) at five specified times every day. Children are encouraged to say prayers from about the age of seven years. The times of prayer are specified in the Qur'an:

- after dawn (*Fajr*)
- around noon (*Zuhr*)
- in the mid afternoon (*Asr*)
- early evening(after sunset) (*maghrib*)
- at night (*Isha*).

A certain amount of leeway is allowed so that people can pray at convenient times. Local times of prayer are published in the British Muslim newspapers, and by local mosques.

Before praying, Muslims should wash. When praying he or she should stand on clean ground (a prayer carpet is often used). This should face Makkah (south-east in Britain). Both men and women should remove their shoes and cover their heads before praying. During the prayers certain specified movements must be performed at different stages: standing, kneeling, bowing and touching the ground with the forehead.

Washing in preparation for prayer (*Wudu*)

For Muslims, physical and spiritual cleanliness are closely linked. It is stated in the Qur'an that every Muslim must always wash parts of the body thoroughly in running water three times before praying. Ritual washing follows a set routine: the face, ears, and forehead, the feet and the ankles, and the hands to the elbows. The nose should be cleaned by sniffing up water and the mouth should be rinsed out. Washing facilities are always provided in mosques.

Many Muslims will also wish to wash after using the toilet and most would not want to pray unless they have done this. People often take water for washing into the toilet with them if a washbasin is not provided in the lavatory cubicle. Women will wish to be particularly scrupulous about hygiene during menstruation.

Exemptions from the five daily prayers

Certain people are exempt from the set prayers although they may still want to say private prayers. This includes women for up to forty days after childbirth and during menstruation. Seriously ill people are exempted altogether but they may still wish to follow the requirements for prayer as far as they are able.

Friday prayers (*Jumu'ah*)

Friday is the Muslim holy day. Most male Muslims over the age of twelve will wish to go to the mosque for prayer. The precise time of Friday prayer varies depending on the committee of local mosques but it is usually at midday, or early afternoon. Some mosques provide a separate prayer room for women but many will wish to stay at home saying their normal noonday prayers.

Fasting (*Sawm*)

Healthy Muslims over the age of twelve will usually fast during Ramadan. Ramadan is the ninth month of the Muslim year, and the month in which the Qur'an was first revealed to the Prophet Muhammad.

Muslims consider that fasting enables them to reach a higher spiritual level, and therefore to come closer to God. During Ramadan Muslims will wish to abstain from all food, all liquids (including water), and tobacco between dawn and sunset. They also abstain from sexual relations at these times. The times of beginning and breaking the fast and of the five set daily prayer times during Ramadan are usually published and circulated by local mosques. Many Muslims will get up early during the month of Ramadan and eat a meal before the fast begins.

Exemptions from fasting

All Muslims except young children (under the age of 12 years) are required to fast, but there are certain exemptions:

- People who are ill may not fast but they will often make up for the number of days they have missed as soon as possible after Ramadan.

- Elderly people or children with special educational needs do not have to fast for the full month but some may abstain from eating if they are able to do so.

- Women who are menstruating are not allowed to fast, but they should make up the number of days of fasting they have missed at a later date.

- Women who are pregnant or who are breast-feeding are not bound to fast but they should also make up the days missed at a later date. However, some pregnant women may decide to fast, taking the opportunity of making a full and complete fast during Ramadan since they are not menstruating.

- People on a journey are not bound to fast but they should also make up the number of days they have missed as soon as possible after Ramadan.

Children are usually encouraged to fast for a few days from about the age of seven onwards. They often fast with their parents on Fridays and at weekends. From about twelve years young people will often fast during the entire month.

Alms giving (*Zakah*)

Alms giving is an integral part of Islam. The Qur'an requires every Muslim who can afford it to give approximately two and a half per cent of their disposable income every year to needy people or to the upkeep of the mosque.

Pilgrimage (*Hajj*)

The Qur'an teaches that every Muslim who is able, should make the *Hajj*, a pilgrimage to Makkah, at least once in their life. The *Hajj* is made during the second week of the twelfth month of the Islamic year (*Dhul-Hijjah*). Every pilgrim walks the same route and everyone joins in prayers. In the year 2002 over 3 million Muslims made the *Hajj*.

Muslims regard going on *Hajj* as a unique spiritual and emotional experience. The *Hajj* often has a profound and lasting effect on those who have made it. The pilgrimage takes 6 days.

The Qur'an

Muslims believe that the Qur'an is the word of Allah revealed through the Prophet Muhammad, and written down without alteration, in the words in which it was revealed. It is God's final statement on the whole meaning, purpose, and conduct of human existence.

Because the Qur'an consists of the actual words of Allah, it is treated with the utmost reverence. It must not be criticised or altered in any way, and its meaning cannot be changed, adapted or re-interpreted to suit people's wishes or values.

The Qur'an is written in Arabic. It is divided into 114 chapters (*surahs*) of varying lengths. It reveals the nature of God and His relationship with humankind and people's duties on earth. It also lays down detailed practical rules on many aspects of individual, family and community life, though it allows a good deal of leeway to take individual circumstances into account. For example, there is guidance on suitable food, proper dress, prayer, family duties, and responsibilities, borrowing and lending money, alms giving, gambling, alcohol, marriage, divorce, and inheritance. Devout Muslims turn to the Qur'an for guidance on most matters and problems. For areas that are not covered by the Qur'an, the Shari'ah, or Islamic law, gives guidance.

Care of the Qur'an

The Qur'an must be treated with great care. Nothing may be placed on top of it and it must not be touched by anyone who has not washed in the way which is required before prayer. The book is normally kept high on a shelf, wrapped in a cloth. It is placed on a stand when it is being read and should never be put on the floor. A small piece of cloth, leather or metal, containing words from the Qur'an may sometimes be worn as an amulet around a person's arm, the waist or neck. Unless it is unavoidable, other people should not remove this and it should be kept dry.

Learning to read the Qur'an

Most Muslim children go to a mosque school after school on weekdays or during the weekend for religious instruction. At the mosque school young people learn to read the text of the Qur'an in Arabic and memorise parts of it. Most children in the United Kingdom begin to attend mosque school at the age of five; girls attend till puberty, but many boys continue until they are fifteen years old. Most parents feel that it is essential that their children should be well grounded in the religion.

The mosque

In a Muslim country a mosque is primarily a place of worship for men and a centre for religious education for children. In the United Kingdom many mosques provide instruction for children in their mother tongue as well as in reading the Qur'an, and mosques still form an important focus in community life. In many communities women do not attend the mosque for prayer but pray at home. However, older, married women, well educated in the Qur'an and in Islam, may visit other women in the community in their homes to teach and pray with them. Women may attend the mosque for meetings and other functions

The organization of the mosque

Islam has no ordained priesthood. There is no central Islamic authority or hierarchy. Each community has its own religious leaders who are local men with status in the community (Imams).

The Imam

In the United Kingdom the Imam is the senior teacher or spiritual leader in the mosque. He performs all religious functions and teaches in the mosque school. Although it is not part of their traditional role, some Imams do fill pastoral functions.

The building

Each mosque usually contains a room for prayer, washing facilities, a schoolroom and a room for lectures or discussions. In the United Kingdom, some mosques are converted houses, though more and more communities are building new mosques with traditional Islamic architecture. The prayer room is usually very simple. The walls are normally bare but may have Qur'anic inscriptions on them. There are no seats. People stand, sit, or kneel on the carpeted floor. In the middle of the wall closest to Makkah (the south-east wall) there is a niche, (mihrab), towards which all the worshippers face while they pray. On the right of the Mihrab is a raised pulpit or chair (Minbar) from where sermons are delivered.

Before entering a prayer room all Muslims perform ablutions. Shoes must be removed and left outside, and heads must be covered. Both sexes must be modestly dressed.

Clothing

Muslim men and women are required to be modest about their bodies. Many Muslims find any exposure offensive and shocking. Muslims should traditionally be clothed from head to foot, except for the hands and faces, and their clothes should conceal the shape of their bodies. Women from Pakistan and Gujarat will usually wear shalwar kameez. A sari may also be worn on special occasions such as weddings. The kameez (shirt) is a loose tunic with long half sleeves. The shalwar (trousers) are usually cut very full to avoid immodesty. A long scarf (chuni or dupatta) is an integral part of the outfit. It is laid over the shoulders and across the chest to cover the breasts. A woman may cover her head with one end of the dupatta when she goes out, or as a sign of respect or modesty, in front of visiting strangers, older people and men. Muslim women from Bangladesh traditionally wear a sari with a waist length blouse and underskirt beneath. One end of the sari may be pulled over the head as a sign of respect or modesty. Muslim girls and women who wear western dress may wear trousers or long skirts to cover their legs. Jewellery may have important religious or cultural significance. For example, a woman may wear a taviz, a small cloth, or leather amulet containing words from the Qur'an. Some women may also wear a small medallion with words from the Qur'an engraved on it.

Traditional Pakistani male dress is a shirt (kameez) and loose trousers (pyjamas). The traditional dress of Bangladeshi men is a shirt and a lungi, a length of cloth wrapped around the waist, usually reaching down to the calfs. Muslim men cover their head, usually with a hat or cap (topi), while praying, and as a sign of respect at ceremonies such as marriages and funerals. Devout Muslim men may wear a hat or cap at all times.

Washing

Most Muslims prefer to take showers rather than baths, since they do not feel clean unless they have washed under running water. Where showers are not provided they may prefer to pour water over their heads. After using the toilet, Muslims wash themselves with water, using their left hand. Because the left hand is traditionally used for washing, the right hand is normally used for eating. Many people observe this custom.

Diet

Muslim food restrictions are clearly laid down in the Qur'an and are regarded as the direct command of God

- Muslims may not eat pork, or anything made from pork (sausages, bacon, and ham), or anything containing pork products (e.g. cakes, baked in tins greased with lard, eggs fried in bacon fat, suet puddings).

- Other meats or meat products are acceptable provided they are 'halal' or killed according to Islamic law. To be halal the name of Allah must be pronounced over the animal and its throat must be cut so that it bleeds to death. N.B. The opposite of halal is haram, meaning forbidden.

Many Muslims will refuse food if they are not certain of the ingredients. Muslim parents are likely to buy vegetarian baby food for children who are on a semi-liquid diet.

Fish is considered to have died naturally when it was taken out of the water and so the question of a special method of killing does not arise. Except for prawns, all fish, which does not have fins or scales, is forbidden.

Dairy products and eggs are permitted although cheese may be unsuitable if it contains non-halal animal rennet. Cottage, processed, curd and vegetarian cheese, which are not made from animal rennet, may be acceptable.

Alcohol is specifically forbidden in the Qur'an. It may only be used in medicines when there is no possible alternative.

Cooking and serving food

Muslims will not eat food, which has been in contact with prohibited foods. Families may refuse to allow their children to eat foods if it has not been prepared in separate pots and with separate utensils, on the grounds that if pots and utensils have been used for prohibited food they will contaminate all other food they come into contact with. Some Muslims may refuse any food prepared outside their own home, as they cannot be sure that the utensils have always been kept separate.

Birth and childhood ceremonies

Muslims babies are usually bathed immediately after their birth. This is done before the child is handed to the mother. The call to prayer (Adhan) is whispered as soon as possible into the child's right ear and a similar call into the left. This should be done by the father, a male relative or another male Muslim chosen by the family. The words are the first sounds that the child hears and they are important introduction to the Muslim faith.

Shaving the baby's head

The heads of babies are usually shaved as a symbol of removing the uncleanness of birth on the sixth or seventh day after a child is born. Oil and saffron may be rubbed into the child's head.

Naming the baby

The baby may be given its name on the day on which the hair is shaved. The names of siblings and other family members are often chosen.

Marriage

Marriage in Islam is a civil contract rather than a religious ceremony, regarded as a practical and social necessity, and as a landmark in life. Most Muslims would wish to marry. The ideal time for marriage is traditionally shortly after puberty but most countries now have national legislation, which defines the minimum age. Traditionally the families of the young people concerned arrange marriages. Today this practice is changing and young people often play an important part in the choice of a partner. Nevertheless, marriage is seen very much as a union between families, not just as a private union between two individuals.

Death and burial

Muslims believe in life after death. The death of a loved one is seen as a temporary separation. Muslims believe that the time of death is pre-determined by God and that suffering and death are part of God's plan. Therefore some people may feel that open expressions of grief and sorrow are sinful because these indicate a lack of acceptance of Allah's will. Some devout Muslims may discipline themselves to show no emotion at all after a death. Others, particularly women, will often express their grief openly.

Care of the dying child

Family members will often sit by a child's bedside and pray and recite verses from the Qur'an in order to give comfort. The family will also repeat the Muslim declaration of faith '*There is no God but God and Muhammad is His Prophet*'. If possible the dying child will sit up or lie with their face turned towards Makkah. A member of the family will usually whisper the call of prayer into the child's ear. If no family members are present any practising Muslim can be asked to give help and religious comfort.

Caring for the child's body after death

Many Muslims are very particular about who touches a dead body. The child's body should not be touched by non-Muslims. It should be treated with love, modesty and respect. Relatives may wish to close the child's eyes, straighten their limbs and turn the child's head towards the right shoulder. This is so that the body can be buried with the face towards Makkah. The body should then be wrapped in a plain sheet without religious emblems. It should not be washed; this is part of the funeral rites to be carried out later on. The child's body is generally taken home or to the mosque and washed three times, usually by the family. In the United Kingdom the family may wash the child's body at the undertakers or at the mortuary. Women will usually wash girls and men will wash boys. (Women are not allowed to do this for forty days after childbirth or during menstruation). Sometimes camphor is put into body orifices. The child's arms are usually placed across their chest. The body is then wrapped in clean white cotton either a seamless shirt, or a white covering sheet. Those who have washed the child's body will wish to carry out their own ablutions.

In Islam, the body is considered to belong to God and therefore, strictly speaking, no part of it should be cut, harmed or donated to anyone else. Post mortem examinations are

therefore forbidden unless absolutely necessary for legal reasons. If a post mortem is necessary, the reasons must be clearly explained to families.

Burial

According to Islamic law and practice, Muslims should be buried as soon as possible and generally within twenty-four hours. If this is not possible the child's body may be embalmed. After washing the body, passages from the Qur'an are recited and the family prays. Generally the funeral starts from the family home and the child's coffin may be left open so that relatives and members of the community can pay their last respects. Male members of the family will take the child's body to the mosque or the graveside for further prayers and Qur'anic readings before the burial. In the United Kingdom some Muslim communities allow flowers to be placed on the coffin. Women may go to the mosque or attend final prayers but Islamic law discourages them from going to the cemetery.

Graves should be aligned so that the child's face can be turned sideways towards Makkah. Generally flowers are not sent to Muslim funerals although this may in fact happen in Great Britain. Because it is not always possible to follow the rules for burial laid down in the Qur'an, some Muslim families will prefer to take their child's body back to their homeland. According to Islamic law the area above the grave must be slightly raised, the body must be buried facing Makkah and the grave must be unmarked.

Funerals are often very large.

Mourning

Mourning usually lasts for about a month. During this period relatives and close friends will come and keep the family company and given them comfort. They talk about the child who has died and grieve with the family, sharing the loss with them. The family usually stays indoors for the first three days after the funeral. Friends and relatives usually bring food to the house for them.

For 40 days after the funeral the grave may be visited every Friday and alms given to the poor. On certain days special prayers may be said.

Sikhism

The total size of the United Kingdom Sikh population as recorded in the 2001 census is just over three hundred and thirty thousand. Sikhs represent 0.7% of the population of England. Sikhism is the fourth largest faith group in the United Kingdom and this is believed to be one of the largest populations of Sikhs outside Punjab. The largest community in the United Kingdom is in Birmingham, closely followed by the London Borough of Ealing. There are approximately equal numbers of males and females.

Sikh families

Providing for the family and caring for all its members' emotional and spiritual well-being are religious duties for Sikhs. In Asian culture the family is traditionally an extended family, and in the United Kingdom obligations to family members in the Indian sub continent and in East Africa remain very strong.

Sons are considered responsible for the care, and support of their parents, as they grow older. Sikhs are expected to marry, and both men and women are expected to take an active part in bringing up children. There is generally a very strict code of sexual morality.

During his life Guru Nanak worked hard to raise the status of women. Thus men and women are considered equal in Sikh tradition. However, female virtues of modesty are important to Sikh women, and in Asian culture men and women may not mix socially outside the family. Boys and girls are generally segregated from puberty.

Religion

Sikhs believe in one God who is Eternal and the Creator of the Universe. Sikhs stress the need for each person to develop their own individual relationship with God, seeking truth and leading a virtuous life. Each individual must learn about God both from their life experience and through prayer and meditation.

Sikhs strive to become God-centred and less self-centred. Sikhism rejects ritual in the belief that this may prevent individuals from developing a direct and loving personal relationship with God.

Sikhism teaches that each soul may have to pass through many cycles of birth and re-birth through incarnation. The ultimate aim is to reach perfection and so, through God's grace, to become united with God and to avoid re-birth into the world. Re-incarnation is linked with belief in karma, the cycle of reward and punishment for thoughts and deeds. Every individual's present existence is directly determined by their behaviour in their past life, and how they live now will decide the manner in which they return in their next life. However, Sikhs also believe that a person's karma can be changed and improved through the grace of God.

The Sikh Gurus

The founder of Sikhism was Guru Nanak who lived in the fifteenth century. He was born into a Hindu family. Guru Nanak rejected the caste system and idolatry. He taught that one God should be worshipped; that all humankind are equal and that people should devote themselves to good actions and to God. When Guru Nanak died in 1539 his teaching was continued by a succession of nine Gurus, the last of whom was Guru Gobind Singh.

The Five signs of Sikhism and the turban

Guru Gobind Singh, the tenth and last Sikh Guru, gave five signs, known as the Five Ks, by which Sikh men and women could be identified and united. Each of the Five Ks has a symbolic meaning. The turban, traditionally worn by Sikh men, has also become an important symbol of Sikhism.

The Five Ks are:

1. *Kesh* or uncut body hair as a symbol of the sacred nature of a person's head.

2. *Kachera* or loose underwear (shorts) a symbol of self-discipline.

3. *Kangha,* a comb which fastens hair beneath the turban and is a symbol of cleanliness.

4. *Kara,* a steel bangle worn on the right wrist which symbolises the unbreakable link with the faith and a visual reminder of commitment.

5. Kirpan, the sword worn to symbolise the duty to fight against evil and to defend the faith.

Sikhs in the United Kingdom differ a great deal in how far they adhere to wearing the Five Ks.

Kesh: uncut hair and beard

In Asian tradition a person's head is regarded as sacred. Guru Gobind Singh forbade the cutting or shaving on any hair on the body or the head. The long hair (kesh) of the Sikhs is regarded as sacred and should be treated with respect. Most devout Sikh men and women never cut their hair, nor men shave their beards. A Sikh man with long hair wears it fixed in a bun (jura) on top of his head, usually concealed under a turban. His hair and beard will be washed regularly.

Most Sikh women never cut their hair. They usually wear it fixed in a bun or in a single plait. Young women (before marriage) may wear their hair in plaits, or sometimes lose. Older women may cover their hair with a scarf (called a dupatta or a chuni) as a sign of modesty. A few orthodox Sikh women may cover their hair with a tight black (or occasionally white) turban.

Sikh boys with uncut hair usually wear it plaited and tied in a bun (jura) on the top of their head. Very young boys may wear their hair in two coiled plaits pinned to the side of their heads. Young Sikh girls usually wear their hair loose or tied back in a plait or ponytail. Many Sikh parents in the United Kingdom decide to cut their children's hair. However, if a child's hair has been kept long it has the same significance as that of an adult and must be treated with the same respect.

Kangha: comb

A man or woman with uncut hair wears it in a bun (jura) kept in place by a kangha, a small wooden or plastic comb. Devout Sikhs who do not wear a turban may carry the kangha in a pocket, or they may wear a miniature kangha on a chain around their necks. A kangha should never be removed without permission.

Kara: steel bangle

Almost all Sikhs wear a steel bangle, or kara, on their right wrist. Left-handed people usually wear the kara on their left wrist. The circular shape is a symbol of unity with God, and of the community of Sikhs. The kara is also a constant and visible reminder to Sikhs that all their actions must be righteous. An adult Sikh should never remove his or her kara. Sikh children usually wear a kara from a very early age, and relatives may give a tiny kara, often gold or silver, to a new born baby.

Kirpan: symbolic sword

The kirpan symbolises a Sikh's readiness to defend their faith. It may vary in length from a small symbolic sword to one metre long. A kirpan is worn under clothes in a cloth sheath (gatra) slung over the right shoulder, and under the left arm at waist level. Left handed people usually wear their kirpan and sheath the other way round.

In the United Kingdom, most Sikhs wear only a small symbolic kirpan or wear a kirpan-shaped brooch or pendant. Some Sikhs may have a kirpan engraved on one side of their kangha (comb). People may wear a full sized kirpan in the gurdwara (temple) on formal religious occasions. Children of very devout Sikhs may wear a miniature kirpan from a very early age.

Kachera: special underwear

Kachera are underwear worn by Sikh men and women. They remind Sikhs of the duties of modesty and sexual morality. The legs of the kachera reached down to a person's knees. Nowadays some people wear ordinary underpants or boxer shorts instead of the traditional style but still regard them with the same importance.

When changing, many Sikhs are careful never to remove their kachera completely. One leg is put into the new pair before the old pair is removed. Kachera may be kept on while showering and the wet pair changed for a dry pair afterwards.

Sacred book

The Sikh Holy Book is called the *Guru Granth Sahib*. The word *'Granth'* means collection or anthology. Before he died, Guru Gobind Singh, the last living Guru, entrusted the Guru Granth Sahib to Sikhs as their Guru (teacher) and guide for the future in the place of human Gurus. The Guru Granth Sahib is now therefore the main religious authority for Sikhs. It is the focal point of the gurdwara and the basis of all Sikh ceremonies. Therefore it is treated with tremendous reverence and love and it is regarded as a unique and wonderful treasure of great beauty. The Guru Granth Sahib is usually consulted for advice at important times such as choosing a baby's name.

The Guru Granth Sahib is written in Punjabi in the Sikh alphabet, Gurmukhi. It is a collection of devotional hymns and poems by six of the Sikh Gurus and by other non-Sikh philosophers. Almost all the hymns and poems were set to music by Guru Arjan Dev who compiled it. Sikhs often learn the Gurumukhi script in order to be able to read and understand the Guru Granth Sahib. In Britain many gurdwaras run evening and weekend classes for Sikh children in their mother tongue to enable them to read the Guru Granth Sahib and to join in worship.

In the gurdwara the Guru Granth Sahib occupies the most important place and it is always the focal point for the congregation. It is placed on cushions on a decorated raised dais (*manji*) with a canopy over it. At night it is usually removed and kept in a safe place covered with a decorated cloth. A *'chauri'* is waved over the holy book by one of the congregation all the time it is open as a sign of respect. Any one entering the gurdwara bows in front of the Guru Granth Sahib before sitting down.

Physical and spiritual cleanliness are closely linked in Sikhism. Therefore everybody must wash before reading the Guru Granth Sahib. Washing facilities are always provided in a gurdwara.

Reciting hymns from the Guru Granth Sahib to music makes up the main part of Sikh congregational worship. Major festivals and events are often celebrated with an akhand path, a non-stop recitation of the Guru Granth Sahib, lasting about forty eight hours.

A few families may have a complete copy of the Guru Granth Sahib in their homes with a special room set aside where it can be treated with the same reverence as in the gurdwara. Many Sikhs also have their own prayer books (*'gutka'*) containing selections from the Guru Granth Sahib. Prayer books are kept carefully and may be wrapped in a small clean cloth, often of silk, or kept in a case for protection.

The Gurdwara

Sikhism is essentially a community-based religion. Congregational worship at the gurdwara (temple) is very important. Ceremonies such as engagements, weddings, name giving, and funerals also take place here.

Each gurdwara contains a prayer room (in which the Guru Granth Sahib is kept), facilities for washing, a kitchen, and a communal eating area for shared meals, and usually a small library. In the United Kingdom there are often rooms for children attending classes. The prayer room is generally bare with no seats. The congregation sits on the carpeted floor. There may be pictures of the Sikh Gurus on the walls. The focus of the room is a platform ('manji') on which the Guru Granth Sahib is placed during the day. Outside the gurdwara a yellow flag flies with the symbol of Sikhism printed on it. People arriving at the building may touch the flagstaff and bow as a sign of reverence.

Before going into the gurdwara people remove their shoes and cover their heads. Men or boys who do not wear a turban cover their heads with a hat or a handkerchief. Some people will wash their hands and feet. On entering the temple each person walks to the dais on which the Guru Granth Sahib is placed and bows low, touching the ground with his or her forehead. Some people give an offering of money or food for the kitchen (langar) and for poor people. By tradition men and women usually sit separately. When visiting a gurdwara, tobacco or cigarettes must be left outside.

Sikh families in the United Kingdom attend services at the gurdwara for several hours every Sunday and on special occasions. Some Sikhs, especially women go to the gurdwara on other days. There is no fixed day for Sikh worship but in the United Kingdom, Sikhs generally hold their main services on Sundays.

Congregational worship ('diwan') usually consists of reading and singing hymns from the Guru Granth Sahib accompanied by musicians ('ragi') playing drums and a harmonium. The singing of hymns is interspersed with sermons. The service always ends with set hymns and prayers. At the conclusion of worship the congregation are given a small portion of 'karah parshad', a specially prepared and blessed cooked sweet made of equal quantities of semolina or flour, sugar, and ghee, mixed while prayers are said. This is received with cupped hands. The sharing of 'karah parshad' emphasises the equality and fellowship of all Sikhs.

As part of the gurdwara there is also a communal kitchen ('langar') where food donated by worshippers is prepared by members of the congregation for everybody present to eat together. Hymns are sung and prayers are chanted while volunteers prepare the food. The meal is usually simple, and consists, for example, of a vegetable curry, yoghurt, chapatti and a dessert. It is always vegetarian. Visitors are welcome to share the food. Cooking and sharing a communal meal stresses the equality of all Sikhs and the rejection of the caste system.

There is no ordained priesthood or religious hierarchy in Sikhism. Any initiated Sikh can lead prayers and read the Guru Granth Sahib in the gurdwara. Most gurdwaras in the United Kingdom employ a granthi as a permanent caretaker and reader.

The gurdwara is supported by donations from the Sikh community. Money is also given to the gurdwara on special occasions such as weddings.

Prayer

Most Sikhs pray privately at home. Many devout Sikhs rise early to pray and recite hymns from the Guru Granth Sahib. A shower is taken beforehand. Short family prayers may also be said in the evening with readings from the Guru Granth Sahib. Further prayers may also be recited before going to bed.

A few Sikhs use a 'mala' or string of prayer beads to help as an aid to prayer. Devout Sikhs may carry a 'mala' or 'gutka' (prayer book) with them and these should be treated with respect.

Clothing

Many Sikh women will wish to cover their legs and upper arms. The most common form of dress is the salwar kameez. The kameez (shirt) is a long tunic with long sleeves. The salwar are trousers. The width of the salwar legs vary according to fashion, particularly among younger women. A long scarf called a chuni or dupatta may also be worn over the shoulders and across the breasts. Women may pull one end of the dupatta over their head as a sign of respect and modesty in front of strangers, older people or men.

Most Sikh men are very conservative in their dress. Nudity, even in the presence of other men, may be regarded as extremely offensive. Many men wear western style shirts and trousers but some may wear traditional dress to relax at home. Traditional dress is a shirt or kameez and loose trousers or pyjamas. Older men may wear their pyjamas and a shirt with a high collar with buttons down the front. This is called a kurta.

Personal hygiene

Most Asian meals are eaten with the fingers. People who eat with their fingers will wish to wash their hands before and after a meal. The left hand is traditionally restricted to washing private parts after using the lavatory. The right hand is therefore used for eating or handing things. When handing something to a Sikh it is considered courteous to do so using the right hand.

Some Sikh women, particularly older women, may consider that they are unclean during menstruation or for forty days after giving birth. At the end of the period of uncleanness they will normally take a ritual shower and clean themselves, their clothes and their surroundings thoroughly.

Diet

For Sikhs dietary restrictions are a matter of conscience and religious belief. Although, as a group, Sikhs are generally less strict than Hindus or Muslims in adhering to dietary restrictions, the dietary practices of each individual is still binding.

The only explicit Sikh prohibition regarding food is against eating meat. Many Sikhs are strict vegetarians, abstaining from eating anything considered as a source of life. Since a strict vegetarian Sikh cannot eat meat, fish, eggs or meat products, any dish containing non-vegetarian ingredients is prohibited, for example puddings containing suet, or cakes cooked in tins greased with lard or containing eggs. Many Sikhs would not wish to eat food that has been in contact with prohibited foods, for example, a salad from which a slice of ham has been removed since it has already been contaminated; or utensils that have not been washed since they last touched prohibited food, are not acceptable.

Non-vegetarian Sikhs generally abstain from eating beef, since the cow is regarded as sacred and is protected in India. Some people will not eat pork since the pig is a scavenging animal in most tropical countries.

In the United Kingdom, Sikhs have often become less strict about what they eat, and many men and children and young people eat chicken, lamb, fish and eggs. Sikh women tend to be more conservative about their food.

Alcohol is forbidden in Sikhism. However some less devout Sikh men drink, but this will be disapproved of by conservative and orthodox members of the faith.

Birth and childhood ceremonies

Ceremonies vary a great deal between different Sikh families and communities. At birth there is no religious ceremony for a Sikh baby. However, some Sikh parents may wish to know the exact time of their child's birth in order to prepare an astrological chart. This might be referred to in later life, for example, when a marriage is being arranged. About forty days after a child's birth, parents usually take the baby to the gurdwara with the family to pray, to give thanks and to perform a naming ceremony. The congregation says prayers.

To choose the baby's name the Guru Granth Sahib is opened at random and the first letter of the first word of the first complete paragraph on the left hand side of the page is read out. A name is then chosen for the baby to begin with that letter. The name is often selected by an older member of the family and is announced to the congregation. Some families may hold an 'akhand path', or non-stop reading of the Guru Granth Sahib, to celebrate the birth of their baby.

Marriage

Marriage is a sacrament as well as a highly valued social ceremony. The families of the young people concerned usually arrange marriages although this practice is being modified both in the Indian sub continent, and in the United Kingdom. Therefore, young people often play an increasingly important part in the choice of their partner. Nevertheless, marriage is seen very much as a union between two families.

Most Sikh communities give female dowries, although this is not strictly speaking part of Sikhism. In the United Kingdom, Sikh weddings usually take place in the gurdwara or occasionally in a hall or at home. During the short ceremony there are hymns and prayers and the bride and groom walk four times around the Guru Granth Sahib while the whole congregation sings a wedding hymn. At the end of the service the whole congregation receives 'karah parshad'. The bride traditionally wears a red and gold sari or salwar kameez and the groom's turban is usually yellow, orange or red. A wedding reception follows the ceremony. The bride's family usually pays for the wedding.

Marriage is regarded by Sikhs as an indissoluble sacrament. Although divorce has been permitted in Indian law since 1955 many Sikhs still regard divorce as shameful. There may be stigma attached to divorced people, particularly women. A woman who seeks a divorce may risk social disapproval and rejection by her community.

Death and cremation

In Sikhism references to death are often found associated with birth and the words 'janum' (birth) and 'maran' (death) generally occur together. According to Sikh belief humankind is not born sinful but in the grace of God.

Sikhism teaches that the Day of Judgement will come to every person immediately after his or her death. It also teaches that heaven and hell are not locations but that they are symbolically represented by joy or sorrow, bliss and agony, light and darkness. Hell is seen as a corrective experience, in which people suffer in continuous cycles of birth and death.

In Sikhism there are two distinct doctrines about re-birth. Firstly, the soul passes from one life to another in spiritual progress. 'Nadar', or grace, is eventually achieved through reincarnation. Secondly, re-birth in animal life is a punishment.

Care for the dying child

When a child is dying, friends and relatives usually read the 'sukhmani sahib' (Song of Peace) to console themselves. Some families will prefer people outside their community to refrain from comforting them. When death occurs, those present exclaim 'Waheguru!' (Wonderful Lord!), but loud lamentations are not appropriate.

Care for the child's body after death

The child's body is washed and dressed by members of the family or the religious community, and covered with a white sheet. Many parents would wish their child to wear the five Ks, including a turban for a young man. The body is usually taken home for friends and relatives to pay their last respects before the funeral. Gifts of dried fruit, clothes, or money may be put into the coffin. Often the coffin is kept open so that family and members of the community can pay their respects. In some communities flowers will be placed on the child's coffin for the journey to the crematorium.

Cremation

Cremation will take place as soon as possible after death but the child's body will normally be taken to the gurdwara first, although it is not taken into the presence of the Guru Granth Sahib. In India the body will be cremated on a funeral pyre but in the United Kingdom it will be taken to a crematorium. Some crematoria allow family members to press the button to start the coffin moving to the cremator, or to help push the coffin into the cremator. In either case, arrangements will be made for a close male relative to be present to press the button to light the fire. Prayers are recited as the fire is lit.

After the cremation, relatives and friends return to the gurdwara, to hear a sermon. A passage about death is read from the holy book and a hymn is offered. A prayer is recited and the Guru Granth Sahib is opened at random and a verse of guidance is read out. The service concludes with the distribution of food, which symbolises the continuity of social life and normal activities.

The child's ashes are usually scattered onto a river or the sea. In the United Kingdom some families may prefer to bury their child's ashes, or to have them taken to India to scatter them in the River Ganges.

Mourning

For about ten days after the funeral, relatives will gather, either at home or in the gurdwara for a complete reading of the Guru Granth Sahib. Donations to the temple or to a charity are normally given. Some families may wear white as a symbol of mourning.

Hinduism

The total size of the Hindu community living in the United Kingdom as recorded in the 2001 census is just over five hundred and fifty thousand. Hindus represent 1.1% of the total population of England, and Hinduism is the third largest faith group in the United Kingdom. The largest community in the United Kingdom is in the London Boroughs of Harrow and Brent, and in Leicester

The word 'Hinduism' is Persian in origin, meaning 'sindhu' or the river Sind, so 'Hindu' refers to people who live over the Sind. Today the river is called the Indus and over 80% of the population of India (about 900 million) are 'Hindu'. There is huge diversity of belief and practice, but in spite of this, there are a number of concepts, which are widely accepted by adherents.

Hindu families

The family is central to Hindu life and to Hindu communities. Hindus are encouraged to marry, and both men and women are expected to take an active part in bringing up children. Codes of morality are strict in order to protect the family, and the community. Parents remain responsible for their children all their lives. Children are considered to have a debt to their parents, which they should repay, by obedience, by caring for them in their old age, and by marrying and bringing up their family well.

In traditional Hindu society, the roles of men and women are clearly distinguished; men are responsible for all matters outside the home, and for supporting their families; women are responsible for rearing and educating children, looking after the family, and for running the home. These roles increasingly overlap. However, among a woman's most important duties is to teach her children and grandchildren about the religion, and to teach them moral and religious virtues. In many ways women are regarded as the custodians of family values and morals, including religious traditions and practices.

Sons are generally considered responsible for the care and support of their parents, as they grow older. In the Hindu tradition when a son marries he and his wife often remain with his parents and bring up their children there. The oldest son of a Hindu family also has the specific religious duty of lighting his father's funeral pyre. This is regarded as very important, and a Hindu father with no son to perform this crucial duty is considered extremely unlucky.

Within most families, men and women share decisions. However, one of the traditional religious duties of the Hindu woman is to honour and obey her husband. In turn Hinduism stresses that husbands must treat their wives with kindness and respect. Female virtues such as decorum and modesty remain important to most Hindu women, and in some communities men and women prefer not to mix socially and may be segregated from puberty onwards.

The Supreme Spirit

For Hindus there is one Ultimate Reality or Supreme Spirit, from which the whole universe emanates. This Supreme Spirit is without form or name; without gender, qualities or attributes. It is absolute and impersonal, infinite and all pervading. The Supreme Spirit resides in every human being in the form of a soul or life force—'atman'. This soul will ultimately be released to merge with the Supreme Spirit. The religious goal of all Hindus is to escape the illusory world through worship and devotion, and to be reunited with the Supreme Spirit.

Hindus believe that because human mental, emotional and intuitive powers are limited, they cannot begin to understand the Supreme Spirit, which is Ultimate Reality. Consequently, Hindus worship the Supreme Spirit by focusing on the different aspects of the created universe, in which the Supreme Spirit resides. Many of these aspects are personified and formalised as deities or gods.

Hindus recognise life events as creative, preserving or destructive. Everything in the universe is part of an eternal cycle; is growing or being created, is being maintained or preserved, or is decaying or dying. These three major aspects are personified or symbolised in the three main Hindu gods: Brahma, the Creator, who symbolises creative power; Vishnu the Preserver, who preserves and maintains all that has been created; and Shiva, the Destroyer, who brings all things to an end. Each of these major aspects and the qualities inherent in them, may be worshipped separately. They can also be personified and worshipped in other ways, for example, as a human incarnation of a deity, such as Rama or Krishna; or as a female deity who represents worthwhile areas of human endeavour, such as 'Saraswati' (or knowledge) or 'Lakshmi' (or prosperity).

Reincarnation and Karma

For Hindus, all living things in the world are subject to reincarnations; the cycle of birth, death and re-birth in a material world. This cycle is called 'samsara'. However, every living being also has an eternal soul or spirit, 'atma'. When any living thing dies, its immortal spirit does not die, it is reborn in another body.

The condition in which one's spirit is reborn depends entirely on what a person has done in previous lives including the ratio of good and evil deeds and attainments. In the same way each person's status, situation and good or ill fortune in this life is an investment in their future. This natural cycle of reward and punishment for all deeds and thoughts, is called 'karma'.

Belief in 'karma' leads to a clear sense of personal responsibility. Hindu belief stresses the importance of striving to do one's duty in any situation, and by so doing to ensure good 'karma' for the future. Good 'karma', or happiness and security in this life and in the next, can be actively ensured through doing one's duty.

Central to Hinduism is the belief, that all things in the world are inter-linked, and that everything affects everything else. 'Karmic, forces operate in everything. Therefore 'karma' affects groups and nations and families as well as individuals.

Hindus recognise that the cycle of birth, life and death in this world —samsara—and of punishment and reward—karma—inevitably involve pain and suffering. The ultimate aim of living things, is, therefore, to be released from the cycle of endless births and earthly existence and to be reunited with the Supreme Spirit. This final release is called moksha. All Hindus believe in 'moksha' or release as an ultimate goal. 'Moksha' is extremely difficult to achieve. Therefore, whilst recognising 'moksha' as the ultimate goal of all living things, Hindus concentrate on living a good life or doing their duty. Although they will not reach 'moksha' at the end of this life, they will be rewarded by good karma in the next, and so they will shorten the cycle of birth, life, and death.

Purity and impurity

The idea of purity and impurity is central to Hinduism. Purity and impurity have both physical and spiritual aspects. Decay is spiritually polluting and people who have been in contact with impurity must cleanse themselves before any act of worship or contact with sacred things. Many Hindu ceremonies concentrate on purification. Fire and water are regarded as symbols of cleansing and these are an important part of ceremonial worship. Bodily cleanliness is extremely important and most Hindus will wish to wash or shower frequently. Meat (dead flesh or dead bodies) are considered impure.

Hindu deities

Most Hindus worship the Supreme Spirit through a male or female deity. There are many different gods and goddesses, each with different qualities and characters. Vishnu, Shiva and Brahma are regarded as the three main gods. Most people worship Vishnu or Shiva, either directly or through another manifestation or an incarnation.

Some male gods also have a female counterpart, a goddess, the two complimenting each other to form a balanced whole.

Vishnu, Shiva and Brahma are usually depicted with Lakshmi, Parvati and Saraswati as their consorts.

Brahma

Brahma is often regarded as the Creator of the Universe and of other gods. He is usually shown having four heads and faces and four arms. He rides on a goose or a swan. He may carry objects such as a holy book, prayer beads, a water pot, or a bow. His wife is Saraswati, the goddess of music, arts, and literature.

Shiva

Shiva has many followers. He is a god with great power, representing creation and destruction, good and evil, simplicity and exuberance, kindliness and fear. He is often portrayed meditating in the Himalayan Mountains, seated on an animal skin, with his legs crossed in the lotus position. Shiva has four arms. One holds a drum, one a flame of destruction, a third gives a blessing, and a fourth points to his feet. It is at Shiva's feet that devotees find happiness and refuge. In his form as Nataraj or Lord of the Dance, Shiva dances in a circle of flames, representing the cycle of time, which has no beginning, and no end. He carries the moon on his forehead and beats out the rhythm of the universe on a small drum. His symbol is lingam—usually a stone pillar carved in a phallic form as a representation of his masculine creative energies. He has three eyes with which he is able to see the past, the present and the future.

Vishnu

Many Hindus in Great Britain worship Vishnu in the form of one of his avatars, usually Rama, or Krishna. The word avatar means 'one who descends' and avatars are forms which Vishnu took on earth when evil threatened. Vishnu is depicted as the observer of the universe and as the personification of goodness and mercy. He wears a jewelled crown and he is often shown seated on a throne or on a serpent. Sometimes he is seen riding Garuda, an eagle-like bird, together with his wife Lakshmi. He has four arms and he holds an object in each of them-a conch shell, a discus, a club and a lotus.

Sacred writings

There are many sacred writings. The oldest (the 'Vedas'), were compiled between four and five thousand years ago, and are regarded as immortal revelations. The Vedas are written in Sanskrit. They are concerned with the nature and purpose of human existence, and of the world. They also contain legends about the gods.

The Upanishads, also written in Sanskrit, date from between 500 and 200 BCE and are regarded as sacred revelations. They discuss the relationship of the human soul with the Supreme Spirit.

The two great Hindu epic poems, the Ramayana and the Mahabharata, were written between 300 BCE and 30 CE. Both poems describe human nature and moral values and their episodes cast light on human dilemmas and duties.

The Bhagavad-Gita

The most widely read of all Hindu sacred books is the Bhagavad-Gita, sometimes known as the Gita. It is an excerpt from the Mahabharata. In the Gita, Krishna, the human incarnation of Vishnu, teaches that humankind must love and worship the Supreme Spirit and must do their utmost to devote themselves selflessly to their sacred duties. Like all sacred Hindu texts the Gita must be kept clean and safe, and is usually wrapped in cotton or silk cloth for protection.

Hindu worship

Hindus worship both individually and with members of their community in the 'mandir' (temple). Most homes contain a small shrine. This may be in a separate room, or in a small glass fronted cabinet. The regularity of worship depends on family tradition, personal devotion, and opportunity. Very devout Hindus may pray several times a day; at sunrise, around noon, and at sunset. A devout Hindu should always take a shower and perform puja (devotion) before eating or drinking in the morning.

The exact details of each family shrine will differ, but there are usually statues of one or more gods particularly worshipped by the family and pictures and prints of others. Flowers may be placed on the shrine and also small symbolic offerings of food. Sometimes the shrine is in the kitchen, the purest and cleanest place in the house since it is a place where food is prepared.

In families where there is a separate shrine room this must be kept pure and should not be entered without an invitation. Anyone who enters must take off their shoes. Women may be asked to cover their heads. At special times Hindu families may organise a 'havan'. This is a special ceremony of purification in which fire is used to symbolise a purifying force. A 'havan' is performed, for example, at a marriage, after a birth, to celebrate or give thanks for a special event, or when someone has died. The ceremony itself is performed by a 'pandit' or priest, and may be held in the family home attended by relatives and close friends who are invited to the ceremony.

Private prayer

Private worship, and prayer are matters of individual decision. Some devout Hindus may wish to pray in the morning before they eat or drink. People may say prayers or repeat holy phrases, read a passage from a holy book, or meditate. Some Hindus use a '*mala*' or string of beads as an aid to prayer. A '*mala*' must be touched with clean hands and treated with reverence. It may be kept in a small cloth bag. Families may wish to perform special religious ceremonies for someone who is ill.

Worship at the temple

The '*mandir*' or temple may be an important place for Hindus to meet socially as well as for worship. Some people, who do not go to work, attend the '*mandir*' every day if they can. Others may go in the evenings after work. Many families attend on major festival days, and on Sundays.

No one should enter a '*mandir*' unless they are pure and physically clean. Everyone should remove their shoes, and women may be required to cover their heads.

In the '*mandir*' there are usually deities, and pictures of several gods with one in a central position, depending on the preferences of the congregation. The whole congregation sits on the floor, usually men and older boys on one side, women, girls, and very young children on the other. People pray individually before the deities, often bowing or kneeling as a sign of reverence. Sometimes there is congregational singing of hymns ('*bhajans*'), to a particular deity, whilst a priest performs rituals.

'*Mandirs*' have a resident priest ('*pandit*') appointed and paid for by the congregation to perform prescribed everyday ceremonies. They may also tend to shrines of the gods and officiate at special ceremonies and festivals.

Clothing

Hindu men and women are expected to be modest about their bodies. Some conservative Hindus find any exposure shocking and offensive.

Hindu women should traditionally cover their legs and upper arms. After puberty many females will not expect to undress fully except when they are alone. Some women wear a sari over a blouse and underskirt. The midriff may sometimes be left bare. Hindu women of Punjabi origin may wear shalwar kameez instead of a sari. The kameez (shirt) is a long tunic with long or half sleeves. The shalwar are loose trousers. The width of the shalwar legs varies according to fashion, particularly amongst young women. A long scarf known as a chuni or dupatta may also cover the head and breasts. Many married women will pull one end of the scarf or the end of their sari over their head as a sign of respect or modesty in front of strangers, older people or men.

Hindu women or girls who wear Western dress may prefer trousers or long skirts to ensure that their legs are covered.

Hindu widows traditionally wear white, with no jewellery or makeup.

Men often prefer to cover themselves from the waist downwards and nudity after adolescence is often considered offensive. In Great Britain men usually wear Western style shirt and trousers, but some may wear traditional dress at home. Traditional dress will usually be a kameez or a loose shirt with or without a collar and trousers with a draw–string (pyjama) or a '*dhoti*'. A dhoti is five or six meters in length wrapped around the waist and drawn between the legs. Older men may wear pyjamas and a shirt or coat with a high collar and buttons down the front. This is known as a '*kurta*'.

In some castes men and older boys may wear a sacred white thread or '*janeu*'. A janeu has three strands and it is worn over the right shoulder and around the body. It is given to a Hindu boy at a religious ceremony to mark his initiation to adulthood. A '*janeu*' should never be removed. Indeed a Hindu man is cremated still wearing his sacred thread.

Some males may wear a medallion with a picture of a personal god around their neck or arm or a ring containing a special gemstone. An amulet blessed by a priest may also be worn.

Ablutions

Much of traditional Hindu religious practice involves the removal, or avoidance of physical impurity, or pollution. Physical emanations from the body are considered polluting; for example urine, faeces, saliva, menstrual blood, mucous, sweat, and semen.

Most Hindus are extremely careful to wash or to shower frequently to rid themselves of physical impurities. Hindus often prefer to shower rather than to bath. Where showers are not provided, people may prefer to stand in a bath and use a small bowl to pour water over themselves.

Hindus may wish to wash themselves with running water after using the lavatory. The left hand is used for this purpose. Some people may clean out their nasal passages with water and spit out any phlegm. Material handkerchiefs may be considered distasteful after a person has blown their nose. Some people may wish to clean their tongue as well as their teeth. A metal or plastic tongue scraper is usually used. Some people will also wish to rinse out their mouth after a meal. Feet are regarded as the dirtiest part of the body and shoes may be considered polluting; therefore they should not be put with other possessions.

According to traditions of purity and pollution, Hindu women are considered unclean during menstruation, and for forty days after giving birth. They do not touch their family shrine, go to the temple, pray, or touch holy books. After child-birth, some women may stay in doors resting for forty days. At the end of the period of uncleanliness women usually take a special shower and cleanse themselves before returning to normal life.

Diet

Hinduism teaches that all forms of life are interdependent, and that all living things are sacred. Therefore most Hindus feel that they do not have the right to take the life of another living creature to sustain their own life. Consequently, most devout Hindus do not eat any food that has involved the taking of life. Meat may also be considered to be polluted, and therefore, many Hindus eat a vegetarian diet. However, Hinduism does not have dietary rules, so, within a general idea of vegetarianism, different communities, families, and individuals make their decisions about what they eat.

The cow is a sacred animal to Hindus. It is considered a symbol of gentleness and unselfish love and giving, and, as a mother, the antithesis of violence and greed. For these reasons the cow is protected and worshipped, and the eating of beef is strictly prohibited.

Eggs are potentially a source of life. Therefore in Asian tradition they are not generally eaten. Cheese is often unsuitable for vegetarians since it may be made with animal rennet. Cottage and curd cheese and vegetarian cheeses, which are not made with rennet, are acceptable in religious terms.

Many of the restrictions connected with the Hindu caste system relate to food. Cooked food may be considered to be polluted, and, in strict Hindu tradition, cannot be eaten if for example it has been touched by someone of a lower caste.

Fasting

Fasting is believed to bring both physical and spiritual benefits. In physical terms fasting is regarded as very important and healthy. Some Hindus fast on several days during each year and devout adherence may mean regular fasts, for example on special days of religious significance.

A Hindu fast does not necessarily involve abstaining from all food, although some people do make a complete fast. More usually, people who are fasting, have one meal a day, eating only foods that are considered pure, such as fruit or yoghurt, nuts or potatoes. They may refuse medication but circumstances will vary.

Alcohol is generally not permitted, and tobacco is regarded as a harmful narcotic.

Birth and childhood ceremonies

Customs connected with birth and childhood vary between communities, and between families. As soon as possible after a Hindu baby is born a member of the family may write the symbol 'OM' (representing the Supreme Spirit) on the baby's tongue with honey or with ghee. Most Hindu parents will wish to have their child's horoscope read by an astrologer, often a priest. Astrological influences are generally believed to have a strong influence on each individual's character, personality and future.

On the sixth day after a birth, the women of the family may gather to give thanks and to congratulate the mother and to bring presents for her, and for her child. The sixth day is also the day on which Hindus traditionally believe that a child's fate is written. Some parents may leave a symbolic blank sheet of paper and a pen near the baby's cot. They may also make an offering to Saraswati, the goddess of learning. Children are often given their chosen name by a priest at the 'mandir' (temple) on the tenth day after their birth. The first letter of the baby's name may be decided by the astrologer, who makes out the baby's horoscope. An older member of the family, a grandparent or an older aunt, then usually chooses a name beginning with that letter.

Marriage

For Hindus, marriage is a sacrament, as well as a contract, and a social ceremony. It is considered that every Hindu should marry and raise a family and that marriage is the beginning of a purposeful life. In Asian tradition the families of the young people concerned usually arrange marriages, though this practice is changing with the young people nowadays playing an increasingly important part in their choice of partners.

Hindu marriages are almost always arranged within the same caste and the couple's horoscopes are consulted to ensure that they will be compatible. Some Hindu communities give large dowries with their daughters. Other communities may give a dowry with a son. Traditionally wedding ceremonies and celebrations last several days. As many friends and relatives as possible are invited. The women of the family spend weeks before hand in preparation. The bride's family usually pays for the wedding, and is responsible for all the food and the hospitality.

Marriage is regarded by Hindus as a holy and an indissoluble sacrament. Divorce goes very much against this tradition. Although divorce has been permitted for Hindus under Indian law since 1955, it is extremely rare in conservative communities.

A woman who seeks a divorce may be risking social disapproval and rejection by her community.

Death and cremation

In life, the Hindu is said to pass through sixteen stages, or take sixteen steps each of which is dedicated to God through a ritual called 'Samskara'. The first of these takes place before birth and the last takes place after death. The sixteenth is the ceremony of cremation. The Hindu doctrine of 'karma' teaches that people who have performed good deeds in this life will be born into affluent families, but those whose behaviour has been evil will be born again as outcasts or animals.

In the last stages of life an adult Hindu would wish to spend time in prayer and contemplation of the next life.

Care of the dying child

Parents may wish to lay their child on the floor on a clean sheet or mattress before death occurs. Some families will moisten the child's lips with water from the holy river Ganges. Occasionally a sacred thread may be tied around the child's wrist. Comfort will be sought from reading holy books such as the Bhagavad-Gita.

Care for the child's body after death

After death, contact with the body is avoided as much as possible. After death a child's body is washed by the family or members of the religious community. It is then wrapped in a white shroud or white clothes. The child's body is usually placed in a coffin and a coin or a small piece of gold or a leaf from a sacred tulsi plant may be placed in their mouth. Family members will wish to keep the child's body close to them or close to the Hindu community until the funeral takes place. Large numbers of people may come to pay their last respects. Sometimes a lamp or an incense stick may be lit as a symbol of leading the child's soul to God.

Cremation usually takes place within twenty-four hours. Generally the family make the funeral arrangements themselves. Some families may fly the child's body back to the homeland for the funeral. In this case the body will be embalmed.

Cremation

In India, the coffin is tied to a funeral pyre, which is carried by six mourners to the cremation ground. The eldest member of the family leads the mourners. Ghee (clarified butter) is poured onto the pyre to help the fire catch alight, and the eldest son, or nearest male relation, lights the pyre. Sacred texts are recited by the priest throughout the cremation. The mourners process around the pyre in an anti-clockwise direction before either bathing in a river or taking a bath to wash away the spiritual pollution of death.

In the United Kingdom the child's body will generally be taken home for the first part of the funeral ceremony before the family accompany it to the crematorium. Mourners will walk anti-clockwise around the open coffin to symbolise unwinding the thread of life. The coffin is closed and taken to the crematorium.

The eldest male member of the family will play a key role in the funeral service and he will usually press the button to light the fire or help to push the coffin into the cremator. Prayers are said during the cremation. In some Hindu communities women do not attend the cremation.

N.B Babies and children under the age of three years may be buried.

Mourning

Family members traditionally wear white for the first ten days after a death. On the third day after the cremation the ashes are collected and, if possible, they are scattered onto a river. In the days following the child's death the whole family mourns. Women may not eat until after the funeral has taken place. A final ceremony is performed on the eleventh or thirteenth day after the funeral and this is known as the 'kriya' ceremony. All those who attended the cremation will be present. Offerings of food and milk may be made. After this ceremony the family will gradually return to normal living, although in the United Kingdom there may be rituals during the first year after the death, and the bereaved family may not partake in festivals and community events.

References

1. Prickett, J. Death. London: Lutterworth, 1980.
2. Brown, E. (ed.) The Death of a Child—Care for the Child, Support for the Family. Acorns Children's Hospice Trust, Birmingham, 2002.
3. Goldman, A. (ed.) Care of the Dying Child. Oxford: Oxford University Press, 2000.
4. Hill, L. Caring for Dying Children and their Families. London: Chapman and Hall, 1994.
5. Irish, D.P., Lundquist, K.S., and Nelson, V.J. Ethnic Variations in Dying, Death and Grief: Diversity in Universality. London: Taylor and Francis, 1999.
6. Atkins, K. and Rollings, J. Looking after their own? Family care-giving among Asian and Afro-Caribbean communities. In W. Ahmad and K. Atkin, (eds.) 'Race' and Community Care. Buckingham: Open University Press, 1998.
7. Firth, S. Wider Horizons—Care of the Dying in a Multicultural Society. National Council for Hospice and Specialist Palliative Care Services, 2001.
8. NHS Executive. The Vital Connection: An Equalities Framework for the NHS Department of Health. London: NHS, 2000.
9. Hill, D. and Penso, D. Opening Doors: Improving Access to Hospice and Specialist Care Services by Members of Black and Ethnic Minority Communities. National Council for Specialist and Palliative Care Services, Occasional paper 7, London, 1995.
10. Acorns Childrens Hospice. The experiences and expectations of Asian mothers with a life-limited child. Acorns Childrens Hospice, 2002.

11. Jenkins, K. On *What is History?* London: Routledge, 1995.

12. Smaje, C. *Health, 'Race' and Ethnicity: Making Sense of the Evidence.* London: King's Fund, 1995.

13. Hillier, S. The health and healthcare of ethnic minority groups. In G. Scambler (ed.) *Sociology as Applied to Medicine.* London: Bailliere Tindall, 1991.

14. Firth, S. Cross Cultural Perspectives on Bereavement. In D. Dickenson, M., Johnson, and J. Samson, eds. *Death, Dying and Bereavement.* London: SAGE and Open University, 2000.

15. Kalsi, S. Change and Continuity in the Funeral Rituals of Sikhs in Britain. In G. Howarth and P.C. Jupp, (eds.) *Contemporary Issues in the Sociology of Death, Dying and Disposal.* Basingstoke: Macmillan, 1996.

16. Jonker, G. The knife's edge: Muslim burial in the dispora. *Mortality* 1996;1(1):27–43.

17. Firth, S. The Good Death: Attitudes of British Hindus. In G., Howarth, and P.C. Jupp, (eds.) *Contemporary Issues in the Sociology of Death, Dying and Disposal.* Basingstoke: Macmillan, 1996.

18. Geertz, C. *The Interpretation of Cultures.* London: Fontana, 1993.

19. Ahmad, W. Family obligations and social change among Asian communities. In W. Ahmad and K. Atkin, (eds.) *'Race' and Community Care.* Buckingham: Open University Press, 1996.

20. Hofstede, G. Cultures and organisations—software of the mind. London: McGraw-Hill, 1991.

21. Unger, R. Some musings on paradigm shifts: feminist psychology and the psychology of women. *Psychol Women Sec Rev* 1999;21(2):58.

22. Cowles, K.V. Cultural perspectives of grief: an expanded concept analysis. *J Adv Nur* 1996;23:287–94.

23. Stoter, D. *Spiritual Aspects of Health Care.* London: Mosby, 1995.

24. Black, D. Life Threatening Illness, Children and Family Therapy. *J Family Ther* 1989;22:18–24.

25. Bluebond-Langner, M. Worlds of Dying Children and their Well Siblings. *Death Stud* 1989;13:1–16.

26. Brown, E. *Loss, Change and Grief—An Educational Perspective.* London: David Fulton, 1999.

27. Turner, J. and Graffam, J. Deceased loved ones in the dreams of mentally retarded young adults. *Am J Retard* 1987;92:282–9.

28. Kaczorowski, J.M. Spiritual well-being and anxiety. *Hospice J* 1989; 5:(4):105–15.

29. Peterson, S. and Greil, A. Death experience and religion. *Omega* 1990;21(1):75–82.

30. Templer, D. Death anxiety scales: A dialogue. *Omega* 1993;26(4): 239–53.

31. Goodhall. Thinking like a child about death and dying. In L. Hill, (ed.) *Caring for Dying Children and their Families.* London: Chapman and Hall, 1994.

32. Hitcham, M. *All About the Rainbow.* Newcastle: Royal Victoria Infirmary, 1993.

33. Infield, D.L., Gordon, A.K., and Harper, B.C. (eds.). *Hospice Care and Cultural Diversity.* New York: Haworth Press, 1995.

34. Association for children with life-threatening or terminal conditions and their families (ACT) and Royal College of Paediatrics and Child Health (RCPCH) A Guide to the Development of Children's Palliative Care Services, 1997.

35. UNICEF. The Convention on the Rights of the Child. London: UNICEF, 1995.

36. Kharbach, N. *Working Together in Westwood.* Liverpool: Barnardos, 1996.

Section 3

Symptom care

17 Symptoms in life-threatening illness: Overview and assessment

Gerri Frager and John J. Collins

Introduction

The aim of this chapter is to enhance and expand each reader's fund of knowledge with respect to the symptoms faced by children with life-limiting illnesses, particularly those with advanced and end-of-life illness. The chapter's components include the prevalence of symptoms in children with life-limiting illness, symptom assessment and measurement, the barriers to adequate symptom management, and practical resources for families and clinicians. This chapter will primarily be an overview of physical symptoms and their assessment, although it is well appreciated that physical symptoms do not exist in isolation, and that physical, psychological, and spiritual factors all impact on one another.

The prevalence of symptoms of children with life-limiting illnesses

The 1995 World Health Organization Report provided the dire statistics that 12.2 million children less than 5 years of age, die each year. Many of these children have life-limiting illnesses for whom palliative care could be beneficial [1]. A US-based study over a period of two decades examined the pattern of childhood and young adult deaths among 15,000 individuals, aged 0–24 years with complex chronic conditions. It was estimated that 5000 of these infants, children, adolescents, and young adults were within their last 6 months of life [2].

What children experience as a result of their life-limiting illness is largely dependent upon where they live in the world. The causes of mortality differ vastly if the child is born into a developing or a developed country, as evident from worldwide childhood mortality patterns. Even with the same illness, how children live and die with that illness may make it seem like an entirely different entity.

For example the treatment options available to children with HIV/AIDS varies according to geographical location. HIV/AIDS is known to cause pain and other systems from multiple causes, including the primary virus itself, opportunistic infections, and where treatment is provided, from the treatment of either the human immunodeficiency virus with anti-retroviral agents, or the treatment of the secondary infections [3]. Even in developed countries, where the knowledge, skills, and pharmaceutical agents are available for symptom relief, multi-factorial barriers continue to impede their access and implementation. Pain significant enough to be reported as having an impact on their life was reported by 59% of children with HIV infection in a US study [4]. The major symptom burden of HIV/AIDS in children is borne by the developing countries, where the numbers of children affected is tragically high, and where access to treatment of the HIV infection, attendant opportunistic infections, and analgesics may be poor (Table 17.1).

What frequently occurs in clinical practice is often not easily shared through the published literature. Parents and health care professionals develop ways of finding out how the child is feeling, tailored to the child. They may do this through trialing different language, facilitating their communication through the use of stuffed toys, through modeling, and non-verbal strategies and innovative verbal means. Comprehensive and consistent symptomatic relief can be a challenge because of the relatively small numbers of children within each diagnostic category.

The past decade has witnessed an exponential growth of interest in the field of pediatric palliative care. The interest and

Table 17.1 Estimates of life-limiting conditions of childhood (in developed countries, based on UK surveys)

Condition	Prevalence/10,000	Source
Cancer	1.1/10,000 children < 18 years of age	Draper, 1995
Duchenne Muscular Dystrophy	1.8/10,000 boys < 18 years of age	Green and Murton, 1993
Mucopolysaccharide diseases	0.2/10,000 children < 18 years of age	MPS Society, 1994
Overall: Life-limiting Conditions	13–18/10,000 children < 19 years of age	ACT and RCPCH, 1997
Annual Mortality	1/10,000 children with life-limiting conditions < 18 years of age	ACT and RCPCH, 1997

Draper, G. (1995). Cancer. In: Botting B, ed. *The Health of Our Children*. London: HMSO.

Green, J.M., Murton, F.E. (1993). Duchenne muscular dystrophy: The experience of 158 families. Centre for Family Research, University of Cambridge.

MPS Society (1994). *When a child dies*. Leaflet.

A Guide to the Development of Children's Palliative Care Services. Report of a Joint Working Party of the Association for Children with Life-threatening or Terminal Conditions and their Families (ACT) and the Royal College of Paediatrics and Child Health (RCPCH) (1997).

work has been primarily concentrated on pain in the oncology patient and pain assessment in the neonate. However, relative to the adult population, there remains a paucity of information about symptoms in the life-limiting illnesses of childhood. What is known comes largely from the oncology population, even though comprising only a third of childhood deaths. Where studies have been done, they tend to be focused on dying with an illness, inadequately addressing the child's experience of living with their illness.

Cancer-related symptomatology

The majority of studies have been based on caregiver report, whether that be a parent or health professional rather than from the perspective of the child experiencing the symptom. The pattern of symptoms, based on the self-report of US children aged 10–18 treated for cancer, was studied. Inpatients reported more symptoms than outpatients, with a mean of 12.7 ± 4.9 compared with 6.5 ± 5.7, respectively. Recent administration of chemotherapy was associated with significant symptomatology. Children with solid tumors were more symptomatic than children with a diagnosis of leukemia, lymphoma or cancer of a central nervous system. Lack of energy, pain, drowsiness, nausea, cough, anorexia, and psychological symptoms all had a prevalence rate greater than 35%. Review of the physically-based symptoms showed that pain, nausea, and anorexia were also associated with a high degree of reported distress [5].

A similar survey was conducted in children 7–12 years of age, also treated for cancer, who provided self-report of the symptoms they experienced over the 2 days preceding the survey. Although symptoms from the psychological realm were surveyed, the most prevalent physically based experiences were: pain, sleeping difficulty, itch, nausea, tiredness, lack of appetite, with the first 4 symptoms more often associated with high distress [6].

In a review of the records of 157 US children with cancer who were referred for a neurology opinion [7], the symptoms that prompted referral were analysed. Leukemias and lymphomas were the most common cancer (58%). The 42% of cancers represented by solid tumors included neuroblastoma, Ewing's sarcoma, and rhabdomyosarcoma. Headache and seizures were the most common symptoms for referral, in contrast with back pain and altered mental status which were the main symptoms in adults. This reinforces the notion that population-based studies specific to life-limiting conditions in children are both generally lacking and necessary.

More than a decade has passed since studies confirmed the clinical appreciation that procedure-related pain was a major focus of distress for children undergoing cancer treatment [8]. Despite significant advances in procedural pain management, a recent review from Sweden describes the persistent predominance of pain related to cancer-related procedure in the pediatric population [9]. This differs from the adult cancer population, where disease-related pain still predominates.

Pain relief for the vast majority of children with cancer should be achievable with what would be considered 'standard' or conventional doses of analgesics. It is unusual that 'extraordinary' doses or analgesia via unusual routes, such as the subarachnoid route or the provision of sedation to ensure comfort, are required [10]. However, this fact has unfortunately not directly translated into the action of providing 'standard' or 'conventional' opioid therapy. Barriers to appropriate analgesic therapy persist among patients, families and health professionals.

Symptoms at the end of a child's life

Relative to the adult population, few surveys of the symptoms of children with life-limiting illnesses have been performed. Of these, most have consisted of small numbers of participants, are often based at one site, and often have been carried

Table 17.2 Compilation of retrospective reviews of children's end-of-life symptomology

Study	Population/diagnosis	N	Country	Most prevalent symptoms	Author/Year
6 year chart review	Cancer	28 patients	Japan	Anorexia, dyspnea, pain, fatigue	Hongo, Watanabe et al 2003 [11]
30 mos. chart review	>1 day after admission, if chronically ill and >7 days from admission, if acutely ill	77 inpatients	Canada	Available for only 5% of patients	McCallum, Byrne et al 2000 [13]
2 year parent questionnaire	PICU patients	56 parents	US	Pain, non-pain symptoms not assessed	Meyer, Burns et al 2002 [14]
parent interview	Cancer	103 parents in/outpatients	US	Fatigue, pain, dyspnea	Wolfe, Grier, et al 2000 [12]
9 mos. chart review & nurse interview	Majority with cancer	30 inpatients	Australia	Lack of energy, drowsiness, pain, anorexia	Drake, Frost, et al 2003 [15]
5 year chart review & parent interview	Cancer	70 in and out patients	Finland	Pain, other symptoms inferred from medications	Sirkiä, Ahlgren et al, 1997 [16] Sirkiä K, Ahlgren B, et al, 1998 [17]
Chart review	Majority with cancer, others with neuro degenerative illnesses, HIV	28 patients of the Palliative Home Care Service (home & inpatient)	Canada	Pain, vomiting, respiratory problems, bedsores, seizures	St-Laurent-Gagnon 1998 [18]
4 year chart review	Majority with cancer	154 referrals to Supportive/ Palliative Care	US	Pain, disturbed sleep	Belasco, Danz et al 2000 [20]
9 year chart review	Cystic fibrosis	Deaths in 44 patients >5 years of age	US	Headache, chest pain, dyspnea	Robinson, Ravilly, et al 1997 [25]
5 year chart review	majority with neuro-degenerative illnesses	30 hospice inpatients	UK	Pain, dyspnea, oral symptoms	Hunt, 1990 [26]

out over several years. What is known about symptoms in dying children is frequently inferred from descriptive chart reviews that identify patients by age, diagnosis, and may include medication use. Symptom assessment has not often been part of the study, and where it has been, is frequently based on the report of someone other than the child, most commonly the parent or a health care professional (Table 17.2).

A chart review study based in Japan, over a 6-year period, examined the signs and symptoms occurring at the end-of-life in 28 children dying from cancer. The demographics of the children studied match the distribution of childhood cancers in the United Kingdom and North America with leukemia/lymphoma predominating at 39%, brain tumors making up 25%, and 35% of the group comprised of other solid tumors. All children experienced anorexia, 82.1% had dyspnea, and pain was documented in 75%. Fatigue was substantial at 71.4%,

nausea/vomiting in 57.1%, and other gastrointestinal symptoms notable for constipation at 46.4% and diarrhea at 21.4% [11]. This symptom profile closely matches that of a US-based study that reviewed symptoms in children in their last month of life. The predominant symptoms assessed by parental report, were fatigue, pain, and shortness of breath [12].

A retrospective chart review from Canada gathered information about 77 infants and children whose deaths occurred at least 7 days since admission to hospital. The majority (83%), who ranged in age from 8 days to 16.8 years, died in the intensive care unit with most (78%) intubated. Perhaps a surprising statistic, this is not unusual for many children who die in a tertiary care setting within a developed country. Documentation of non pain symptoms was sporadic. Even for children where pain had been noted to be a significant problem, complete pain assessments were lacking. Although a small number of children had symptoms evaluated, the pattern again reflects that of other pediatric end-of-life studies. Pain, anxiety/agitation, decreased level of consciousness, nausea/vomiting, dyspnea, constipation, and feeding difficulties were all featured [13].

Parents of children cared for at their end-of-life in several pediatric intensive care units retrospectively completed an anonymous questionnaire. Pain was only one component assessed and 55% of parents reported that their child was comfortable. Non-pain symptoms were not addressed [14].

The symptoms of children close to death were surveyed utilising the report of a proxy care-giver [15]. Respiratory failure and encephalopathy were noted as the most frequent physiologic disturbances, although they were not linked to how the child might feel as a consequence. The symptom profile in the last week of life demonstrated a significant constellation of 11.1 ± 5.6 symptoms per child with six symptoms occurring in at least 50% of the children. The most frequently occurring symptoms included lack of energy, drowsiness, skin changes, irritability, pain, and extremity swelling. Lack of energy was associated with the highest level of distress for 30.7% of the children. Although not notably prevalent, nervousness, worry, and numbness/tingling of distal extremities were the most distressing symptoms. The level of patient comfort as reflected by the health professionals' notes indicated that the majority of children were 'always comfortable' to 'usually comfortable' in the last week (64%), day (76.6%), and hour (93.4%) of life. The pattern of many pediatric deaths in the developed world was again reflected in this study with the majority (66.7%) of the hospitalized children dying in the intensive care unit [15].

Over a 5-year period, a Finnish study evaluated the pattern of end-of-life for children dying from cancer. Symptoms were largely inferred by the medications administered with the most detail for pain, as 89% of the children had received pain medication. Pain relief was reported by retrospective parental interview as inadequate in 19% of the children treated with analgesics [16,17].

Of the children cared for by a palliative home care program at a tertiary care hospital in Canada, a chart review documented that pain severe enough to require opioid therapy occurred in numbers approaching 90%. Parents reported that intractable pain, seizures, and dyspnea were the most distressing complications of their child's end-of-life phase [18].

A review of the deaths occurring over a 7-year period in the inpatient wards at an Australian children's hospital was carried out through chart review. Where the 18 charts did not document the symptoms experienced, inferences were made from the medication record. The diagnoses of cancer, cystic fibrosis, cerebral palsy, and neurodegenerative illnesses each

accounted for the deaths in nearly equal proportions other than for one child who died of herpetic encephalitis [19].

The palliative care service at a tertiary care pediatric hospital in the US described some of the characteristics of 154 infants, children, and young adults referred to the service over a 4-year period [20]. The majority of referrals were patients with cancer diagnoses with the balance being made up from a diverse array of childhood illnesses. Analgesic agents corresponding to Step-2 and 3 of the World Health Organization Ladder (WHO) [21] were provided for more than 80% of the patients. In addition to pain, another prominent symptom requiring intervention was sleep disturbance. 44% of the patients with cancer received chemotherapy concurrent with palliative care interventions. This dual model of care is representative of how palliative care in children is often best integrated with care directed to cure and/or to amelioration of the primary disease rather than either goal in isolation [22]. Of the 140 patients who died during the four years of the study period, 60% of them died at home.

The end-of-life care of patients more than 5 years of age and dying from cystic fibrosis was summarized through a chart review at a US tertiary care facility, where they had received their care [23]. Twenty-five percent of these patients had been receiving opioids for more than 3 months prior to their death for relief of chronic headache and/or chest pain. At end-of-life, the percentage of patients treated with opioids for dyspnea and/or chest pain increased to 86%.

Arthritis, headache, and chest pain are known sources of pain in patients living with cystic fibrosis. Osteoporosis may be a cause of pain, associated with protracted coughing with the risk of rib fractures. Headaches would be expected based on the physiology of hypercarbia and/or hypoxia, and/or sinus infection. The arthropathy seen in children with cystic fibrosis can be related to the hypertrophic pulmonary osteoarthropathy (HPOA), antibiotics, infections, or an associated kyphosis [24]. Of children dying of cystic fibrosis and reporting pain, 86% reported 'serious' pain with the most frequent locations being chest, headache, limb, abdomen, and back [25]. The increase in pain in their last three years of life may serve as a warning flag consistent with other signs of advanced, progressive disease [25].

Symptoms in children with neurodegenerative illnesses

While there have been missed opportunities to ask children how they feel in many life-limiting illnesses, many children with neurodegenerative illnesses have been even further marginalized. This population of children most often requires someone's assistance to observe and interpret how they feel. In a study at the first free-standing children's hospice in the United Kingdom, the demographics for 127 children was significant for 41% of children having neurodegenerative illness with virtually all children having no speech or impaired speech. The median age from their first admission to death was 2½ years [26].

Another study over an 11-year period, at the same hospice, reviewed the care of 30 children admitted in their last month of life. Half of the children were non-communicative, with half of that subgroup having neurodegenerative illnesses. Pain, breathlessness, and oral symptoms, such as difficulty with secretions, were the most common symptoms recorded by the children's caregivers in the last month of life and continued to be noted as frequent symptoms in the last week of life. The reports of excess secretions and cough increased in the last week of life [27].

Symptom assessment

The assessment, diagnosis, and measurement of symptoms is fundamental to the care of any child with a life-limiting illness. Palliative therapeutics should generally be implemented concurrently while investigating, as appropriate, the underlying causative mechanisms, since therapies directed at the primary cause may ultimately have a more effective outcome for symptom management. Symptom assessment is complemented by symptom measurement. Measurement refers to the application of some metric to a specific element of a symptom. There is an increasing interest in the measurement of other domains of symptom experience beyond intensity, frequency and distress, for example.

A historical approach to the assessment and management of symptoms

Consider the child with cystic fibrosis or primary cardiac disease presenting with shortness of breath. The traditional orientation to symptoms has been one focused on the symptom as an important indicator of the disease process, a 'signal' of the underlying pathophysiology and as a marker for the extent of disease. Clinical, research, and educational efforts relating to symptoms have been almost wholly directed to curing or ameliorating the condition responsible for the symptom. Exploring how the child interprets the symptom and addressing any accompanying distress have traditionally not carried as much importance as determining and documenting the symptom's presence, and treating its root cause. A standard of care to aspire to is one where clinical, research, and educational pursuits concurrently address the child's experience of the symptom and to provide relief

with the same enthusiasm and urgency as those efforts directed to the primary disease. Children have said or had their families, as witnesses to the child's distress, say that there "can be things worse than dying," or they didn't know "the cure could be worse than the disease." Symptom measurement may help facilitate an understanding of a child's subjective experience.

The rationale for a focus on symptoms

When faced with the diagnosis of a life-limiting and chronic illness, the parents, health professionals, and the child, as developmentally appropriate, want to know what to expect [28–30]. What does the future hold? How will the child feel throughout the course of the illness? How can they best prepare for what is to come? A proactive approach, discussing, and planning for what symptoms may occur, confers some measure of control for all involved in the child's care, at a time of tremendous vulnerability. Being able to plan for the 'what-ifs,' to discuss the likelihood of seizures or breathlessness provides reassurance through a discussion and plan. This helps the parent to continue to parent, to support the child through the difficult times, which can be a substantial comfort for both the child and for the parent. Although pain, breathlessness, or nausea may be a feature of the illness, it is reassuring to know that these and other symptoms, are able to be controlled with a variety of agents.

Several end-of-life studies have involved parents monitoring their child's symptoms [31,32] Parents reported a greater willingness to consider end-of-life care decisions when physical changes were observed. Symptoms have also been the basis for parents' choice of where their child receives end-of-life care [33–36]. In a feasibility study, parents of children who had died within the previous 2 years, were asked to identify the most troubling symptoms that their child had during the final week of life, final 24 hours of life, and what actions helped or did not help to manage the symptoms (Personal Communication Hinds, P.S. St Jude's Children's Research Hospital, Tennessee) [37]. A total of 34 symptoms were identified by all of the parents; with all parents reporting 2 to 6 symptoms. The most commonly reported were pain, changes in breathing, changes in responsiveness, and urinary output. All families indicated a worsening of the troubling symptoms in the final 24 h of their child's life. Helpful behaviors of professionals included being available to the family, providing information about the symptoms and features of dying, and assuring the parents that they had been good parents (Personal Communication Hinds, P.S. St Jude's Children's Research Hospital, Tennessee) [37]. In addition, a retrospective study examined the perspectives of 25 families of 26 ill children who had been cared for at the first children's hospice in the United Kingdom. While families reported feeling well supported for symptom management, they worried about breathlessness, seizures, and pain [38].

Understanding the link between symptoms and specific clinical conditions benefits the child through efforts directed to preventing the symptoms, lessening them, or helping a child and his/her family deal with them. Knowledge about these symptoms can also help health care professionals teach children how to identify and describe a symptom. Such information can further contribute to the prevention, amelioration, or resolution of symptoms.

Knowing the pattern of symptoms for a given life-limiting condition serves to drive interventions directed to relief of the symptom. Where existing therapies are either inadequate or absent, documentation of the symptom prevalence and associated distress can help advance research initiatives. For children who eventually die of their illness, the knowledge that their discomfort was proactively assessed and compassionately managed can, at best, ensure comfort for the bereaved survivors, or otherwise, at least not compound their distress.

Knowing what symptoms are likely to occur at the end-of-life and their time-course, may guide what supportive interventions might be recommended to pursue or help select those best not pursued. For example, a child very ill with end-stage cystic fibrosis has a massive gastrointestinal bleed and a decreased level of consciousness. Actively investigating the bleed and providing multiple transfusions may not necessarily be in this child's best interest, to subsequently have the child rally long enough to become significantly dyspneic as the lung function worsens. Such considerations are generally based on clinical judgement, best managed by discussions with colleagues, the family and child.

Symptoms and quality of life

It does not necessarily hold true that a child's quality of life is directly related to the degree of symptom burden. Quality of Life (QOL) is a complex, multifactorial, and a dynamic process. The words, meaning, and concepts used by quality of life assessment tools for adults require modifications unique to the illness, age and development of the child. In addition, the assessment is frequently delegated by default to someone other than the person whose QOL is being measured. This difficult task often falls to the parent, health professional or other proxy, although studies have demonstrated lack of concordance between self-assessment and proxy-assessments [39,40].

Despite the difficulties, there is a growing interest to supplement traditional outcomes in pediatric cancer clinical trials such as survival, relapse-free survival, event-free survival, disease-free survival or organ toxicity with those that reflect the impact of treatment on patients and families [41–43].

Despite this interest, quality of life, as an endpoint, has yet to make a significant impact on the design and the reporting of Phase III chemotherapeutic trials in pediatric oncology [44]. This is due, in part, to lack of validated measures. Although the measurement of symptoms is one aspect of QOL assessment [45], two of the three validated QOL measures developed for children with cancer, the *Play Performance Scale for Children* [46] and the *Pediatric Quality of Life Scale* [47] do not assess symptoms. *The Pediatric Cancer Quality of Life Inventory-32 (PCQL-32)* is a standardized patient self-report and parent proxy-report assessment instrument designed to systematically assess pediatric cancer patients' health-related quality of life outcomes [48,49]. It assesses five domains: disease and treatment-related symptoms/problems, and physical, psychological, social, and cognitive functioning. It focuses on pain and nausea in its assessment of physical symptoms.

There is, therefore, a need for the development and use of a comprehensive tool for the measurement of symptoms in the context of quality of life assessment of children with cancer and non-cancer diagnoses.

Other than the child: A bigger view on distress

There may be instances when the parent, family member, friend, or health professional may be the ones most distressed by what they perceive as the child's experience in the course of care. The child's perceptions should be the priority for the symptoms addressed but this is not to the exclusion of other's concern and distress. For example, the noisy pattern of breathing in a child who is unresponsive and unable to swallow or otherwise clear their oropharyngeal and bronchial secretions is a difficult sound to be present for. The distress of those present though this time can be significant despite repeated offered explanations that the child is not disturbed by this. The imperative to provide comfort extends to those accompanying the child at end-of-life as well as the child. Simple measures, including the use of an anti-cholinergic agent, confer a benefit beyond only the recipient of the medication.

When to assess symptoms and when to treat?

Ensuring comfort is a medical imperative throughout the child's entire illness, not one reserved for the period of time identified as solely 'palliative' or 'end-of-life'. Symptoms are not sequestered into a block of time identified as the palliative or end-of-life phase of a life-limiting illness. Rather, symptoms may predominate at diagnosis and any time throughout the entire course of the illness. A US-based study of pediatric oncology patients noted the greatest suffering in children who died of treatment-related complications [12]. Ensuring the relief of pain and other symptoms is the 'right' thing to do regardless of when the symptom presents in the course of the illness.

Clinicians are poor predictors of when a child may be approaching end-of-life. One study of clinicians and parents caring for children living with and dying from cancer reported that the understanding that the child had no realistic chance for cure was acquired at vastly different times along the illness trajectory. This ranged from a mean of 206 days before the child's death for physicians to roughly half that for parents [50]. The important message for clinicians is not to wait until the child is clearly deteriorating and has no realistic chance for cure, or until all involved come to such an understanding, before having discussions relating to decision-making and initiating appropriate interventions directed to comfort. Instead, such discussions and incorporation of the principles of palliative care, including the provision of comfort, need to occur throughout the child's entire illness course.

Physical symptoms may be related to different and multiple factors, including the underlying illness, varied treatment-related side-effects, or to causes unrelated to either the primary disease or its treatment. Symptoms, such as fatigue, anorexia, and agitation, tend to cross disease groupings and may have multi-factorial causation.

Symptoms may make a significant contribution to morbidity. Despite a high prevalence, many symptoms may be relatively easily treated with conventional management. This is important information, as there may be an assumption that one must "live with" certain common aspects of the illness. This misperception may prevent care-givers from initiating relatively simple measures to ensure that the child can feel well and be as active as they can while living with the illness. Even uncommon symptoms can have import because of the degree of associated distress. Breathlessness, pain, or fatigue confer a profound impact on the child's activities and overall QOL. The meaning and value linked with the symptom may carry broader implications, as in the familial anxiety engendered by anorexia and asthenia.

General principles of symptom assessment

A clinical history, detailing the associated aspects of a symptom, including temporal factors, exacerbating features, relieving measures, concurrent sensations etc. serves to clarify information leading to the best strategies for symptom relief. An assessment of the symptom's severity, and how bothersome it is to the child is measured either through self-report and/or observation. Knowing the child's usual intensity and pattern of activity, play, and reported or inferred enjoyment, is crucial to understanding the impact of the symptom on the child's quality of life, even when ill. Physical examination and investigations tailored as appropriate to the child's condition, illness trajectory, and goals of care, complete the picture.

Common symptoms of children with life-limiting illness

Pain

The adequate, proficient and timely assessment, measurement and management of pain in the dying child is of critical importance. Pain is one of the most feared symptoms in the context of life-limiting illness. Not only is it important from an humanitarian viewpoint, but also because the memory of unrelieved pain and other symptoms in dying children may be retained in the memory of parents many years later. It will be impossible for children and their families to negotiate the domains of psychological and spiritual care if pain and other physical symptomatology has not been adequately treated. As few controlled studies of symptom management have been performed in childhood, many of the analgesic and other therapeutic approaches used in children have been developed through experience based on best practice in adults.

Dyspnea

Dyspnea is the subjective sensation of shortness of breath and is a highly distressing symptom for children. The treatment for dyspneic relief is distinct from pain, where for the latter, quality of life is generally improved and function maximized with conventional doses of conventional analgesics. Relief of the sensation of breathlessness in advanced illness may be dependent on providing comfort through sedation.

Nausea

Nausea and vomiting are not uncommon in children receiving palliative care. Nausea and vomiting occur when the vomiting centre in the brain is activated by any of the following: cerebral cortex (e.g. anxiety), vestibular apparatus, chemoreceptor trigger zone (CTZ), vagus nerve, or by direct action on the vomiting centre. Identifying the clear etiologic mechanism can be helpful as the list of potential causes is great and therapies differ, depending on the putative mechanism. One of the most common disease-related cancer treatment effects is nausea and/or vomiting. Vomiting is easily quantified by frequency measurements and is obviously not reliant on self-report. Nausea is very difficult to assess in children, particularly those unable to self-report.

Fatigue

Fatigue is a noteworthy symptom because of its prevalence, impacting on what the child feels able to do, and the paucity of therapeutic interventions that provide relief. Parents ($n = 103$) of children who died of cancer reported fatigue to be the most common and troubling symptom during the final month of their child's life [12]. The etiology of fatigue in children dying of cancer may be due to a combination of factors including: anaemia, poor nutrition, insomnia, metabolic derangement, the increased work of breathing in patients with dyspnoea, side effects of medication, and a range of psychological factors.

In the assessment of fatigue in a child, and the matrix of its potential causes, it is important to establish if this symptom is distressing to the child and/or his family. If so, potential remediable causes should be considered. Therapies directed at the primary cause should be instituted only if these therapies are not a substantial burden to the patient and/or his family.

Seizures

Seizures in children with life-limiting illnesses may be anticipated and managed expectantly, as a component of a particular condition, such as in many of the neurodegenerative illnesses. Seizures may also newly present in a child with a known seizure history who previously had achieved control, as the child becomes more ill. They can also present denovo in an ill child related to biochemical abnormalities without other risk factors. Seizures may be distressing to the child or more evidently distressing for those who witness the child having a seizure.

Case Mitchell was an 11 year old with a brain tumor whose pattern of seizure would start in the fingers of one hand and then 'march in Jacksonian fashion' up the motor strip represented anatomically by the homunculus. His arm, shoulder, then upper torso would sequentially become involved. When the seizure activity reached his abdomen, he was able to be reassured first by his parents and then calm himself, knowing that the seizure would soon be over. He was distressed by seeing his arm shake and his parents learned to comfort him by covering his arm as soon as Mitchell voiced awareness of the impending seizure. These measures were used in combination with titration of his anticonvulsants until better pharmacologic control was achieved.

Hematologic symptoms/signs

Several of the signs manifested by many of the pediatric cancers relate to the effect on the bone marrow either because of direct marrow involvement by the cancer or the treatment's suppression of the marrow's production of white cells, red cells, and platelets. The potential for associated symptoms of infection, fatigue, breathlessness, or bleeding may be problematic for the child and/or the family and those who care for them. Interventions to address the neutropenia, anemia, or thrombocytopenia require discussion, decision-making, and periodic review.

The use of platelet transfusions at home for children with end-stage cancer was reviewed over a 5-year period by a UK children's hospital. 35 transfusions were provided to 12 children for the following indications: platelet counts less than 25×10^9 per mm^3 and bleeding for longer than an hour, or severe, painful bruising unresponsive to tranexamic acid. The average time between repeat transfusions was 4 days with the majority of transfusions noted to be successful for hemostasis [51].

Repeated transfusions, particularly in areas without the capacity for transfusions at home, requiring the child to be in hospital or 'hooked-up' for intermittent and extended periods, may not be how the child and/or family want to spend the remainder of the child's life. Even in the setting of platelet transfusions continuing to be provided at the end-of-life, it is prudent to have a contingency plan to provide rapid sedation for the child, to minimize the distress in the uncommon event that a massive bleed occurs.

Confusion or delirium

Although lacking the prevalence data, clinicians' impressions are that this is an uncommon but significantly troubling symptom. To have the child as they are known and loved, essentially 'lost' before being 'lost through death', compounds the distress of the child's family, friends, and care givers. There may be treatable causes of the confusion, such as hypoglycemia or medication influences, both of which can be resolved by a relatively simple intervention. The decision to change medications, such as opioid rotation, in the setting of confusion, is dependent to a large extent, upon the child's proximity to death. It may be reasonable to provide sedation until death rather than making changes in the child's regimen when death is proximate.

The assessment of symptoms at different stages of child development

An infant's symptoms—an infant's story

Proactive management of potential symptoms at end-of-life

Case Emily was a newborn with a congenital muscular disorder (Figure 17.1). She had severe hypotonia, ineffective respiratory effort, some facial and spontaneous eye movements, right clubfoot, and bilaterally dislocated hips. Emily had no spontaneous movement of her limbs, which had flexion contractures and markedly decreased muscle bulk.

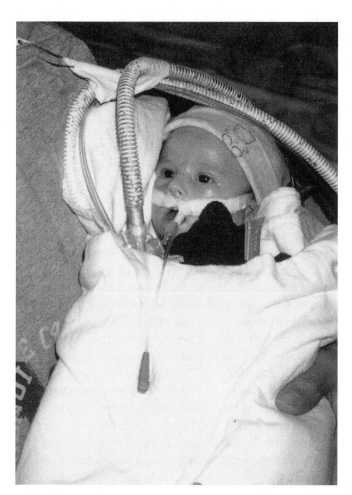

Fig. 17.1 Emily, a new born with a congenital muscular disorder.

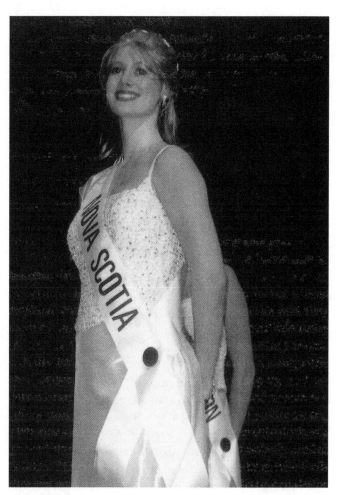

Fig. 17.2 Gina a 16-year-old who experienced many difficulties during treatment of Ewing's sarcoma.

At 15 days of age, in preparation for withdrawal of ventilatory support, Emily was pre-medicated with an anti-cholinergic as she was unable to manage her secretions. Emily also received an opioid and anxiolytic to ensure she did not experience distress related to not being able to adequately ventilate.

Emily was unable to express how she felt. Being unable to adequately ventilate is recognized as a likely distressing entity and knowing that she would be unable to cough or swallow her secretions, she was medicated prior to extubation. This approach is sometimes necessary in infants where what is known to be a potentially painful or distressing entity should be preemptively and proactively managed rather than waiting for care givers to observe, interpret, and act upon signs of distress [52].

An adolescent's symptoms—an adolescent's story

Whose symptom and whose associated distress?

Case Gina was a savvy, independent 16-year-old, who enjoyed cheerleading and a wide circle of friends (Figure 17.2). She experienced

many difficulties during treatment of Ewing's sarcoma. A feisty individual, she toughed it out through an extensive limb salvage procedure, chemotherapy, and radiotherapy, staying hopeful and celebrating the positive aspects of her life.

Gina's course was complicated by obstructive uropathy, necessitating a nephrostomy tube and external bag. Metastases to her lower spine resulted in urinary retention for which she self-catheterized for the the kidney not drained by the nephrostomy tube. Gina had significant neuropathic pain managed with a combination of opioids and multiple adjuvants, from which she had significant adverse reactions, requiring many changes to her analgesic regimen.

Despite achieving good analgesia and managing her nephrostomy and self-catheterizations, Gina became despondent because of fecal incontinence secondary to involvement of the cauda equina from spinal cord metastases. She expressed that she felt life was not worth living because of the incontinence.

With various techniques, Gina was able to achieve fecal continence, enabling her to relax in a hot tub, a goal Gina had for her trip to California with her boyfriend, father, and stepmother [52].

The importance of Gina's story is that it is the patient's distress with any given symptom that is the priority. The assumption might have been that having her pain well controlled was the priority of care. Such interventions had no import for Gina's quality of life if she could not also achieve fecal continence.

Symptom measurement in children

Pain (See also Chapter 20, Pain: Assessment)

Self-report scales

In the view of field experts, the best instruments for measuring the severity of pain are visual analogue scales using one of the preferred facial expression scales [53]. In the very young child (aged 3 to 4), the self-report should be simple, with a maximum of three to five options. In persistent, recurrent, or chronic pain, it is appropriate to consider multidimensional assessment, and because few self-report scales of this nature exist, semi structured interviews may be required.

Cognitively intact children aged 7 years and older can rate the severity of their pain or other symptoms with a modified Likert scale scored from 0 to 10, as used in the adult population. Self-report measures for the cognitively intact, younger verbal child of approximately 4 years of age generally use some form of pictorial or photographic representation of faces in various degrees of distress, as detailed in the chapter on pain assessment [54]. To use such a scale, the child needs to understand the concepts of proportionality, that pain or the symptom for which the scale is adapted, is experienced along a continuum, and be able to apply these concepts to visual representation, as in the Faces Pain Scale [55]. Modifications to the scales have been validated for use in pediatric pain assessment, through testing the strength of the tool's ability to measure what is intended. As the experience of pain is a subjective one, the process of validating a measurement tool, such as the visual analogue scale, is a complex one requiring input from multiple, often indirect sources, including behavioral observation. Of interest, is the description of Piaget's and Inhelder's early research from the 70's. This reference described that young children, yet unable to count, were able to understand the concept of quantity along a linear continuum by relating which pile of beads would result in the longer necklace [56,57]. Measuring other dimensions associated or causally related to having pain have been explored to a less extent in children, as described in a later section on multidimensional symptom assessment scales. Naming the affective state or emotional quality of pain and its severity, such as 'feeling sad' or the pain being 'unpleasant', is a more abstract task than the rating of pain's severity and is linked to a more advanced developmental understanding, proving difficult for children less than 8 years of age. [56] For clinical purposes, it is less critical what pain intensity scale is chosen. The guiding principle is that pain, especially persistent pain, should be assessed and monitored.

Modifications to these scales for non pain symptoms, although having clinical utility, have not generally been validated for this context.

Behavioral observation measures

The measurement of symptoms in children who are unable to self-report, because of their age, impaired cognition, or difficulty communicating with voice or by pointing requires methods reliant on behavioural observations. Unobtrusive observation of the child and/or a caregiver's description of their observations are incorporated in the assessment. Watching how the infant moves, appears with diaper changes, or positions itself in sleep and interacts while playing are all opportunities for assessing how the way they are feeling may be impacting on their behavior. Measurement tools to assist in gathering this information have been developed for children experiencing or likely to experience pain in certain circumstances, such as the post operative period, in the care of premature and other ill neonates, and in the context of procedures, such as veni punctures and bone marrow aspirates.

There is a paucity of measurement tools for pain that may be chronic or other non pain symptoms. The Gauvain-Piquard rating scale is designed for the assessment of chronic pain in oncology patients 2–6 years-of-age. The modified scale consists of 15 observed items, 9 of which are specific to pain assessment, 6 are related to what is referred to as 'psychomotor retardation', and 4 assess anxiety. There is a maximum possible score of 60 as each item is rated from 0 to 4, with a score greater than 12 indicative of pain [58].

The child with cognitive impairment

The reliance on functional measures as indicators of pain or other distressing symptoms, such as observing the child's behavior when sleeping or playing assumes greater relevance in the child unable to self-report. Biologic markers, such as heart rate and blood pressure or diaphoresis attenuate with time, may be influenced by medications or the child's illness, and are therefore unreliable indicators of pain, particularly when pain may be more longstanding.

The non-verbal child whose medical condition causes them to have facial grimacing, dystonic posturing, and/or spasticity accompanied by increased tone makes observational assessment of distress even more difficult. There have been efforts to assess pain in this patient population, many of whom have life-limiting illnesses in whom death in childhood would be anticipated. The input of a primary caregiver, someone who knows the child well, and who can help interpret their behavior is extremely helpful. The kind of items indicative of distress are fairly intuitive but it is helpful to have a checklist against which to compare and rate one's observations. The reader is referred to the chapter on pain assessment in this volume and primary references for additional detail [56,59,60].

Nausea and vomiting

Instruments for the assessment of nausea and vomiting have been studied in the context of childhood cancer. A rating scale for nausea and vomiting utilising verbal descriptors was used in a series of assessment studies in children with cancer aged 5–18 [61–64]. Children younger than 10 years had faces included above numbers on the scale. There was 80% agreement between parent and child rating when they were assessed independently.

A comparison of child and parental ratings of children's nausea and emesis symptoms was assessed among 33 children (aged 1.7–17.5 years, median 4.7 years) with acute lymphoblastic leukemia receiving identical chemotherapy [65]. The measures utilised nausea and vomiting vignettes designed to assess the frequency and severity of nausea and emesis symptoms as reported by children and their parents based on the previous chemotherapy experience of the child. The vignettes, based on the work of Zeltzer [66], consisted of 12 questions separately assessing nausea and emesis at three time intervals: prior to, during, and after chemotherapy. A 5-point Likert-type rating scale ranging from 'not at all' to 'all the time' for the frequency items and from 'not bad' to 'real bad' on the severity items were employed. A composite nausea/vomiting score was determined by calculating the mean of the 12 frequency and severity items. Children younger than 5 years were not asked to complete this measure because of their difficulty in understanding the instructions. This study demonstrated a significant correlation between child and parent ratings of nausea. Significant inter-rater correlations for nausea frequency and severity but not for emesis frequency or severity was found.

Fatigue

Recent work developing valid measures of child or adolescent cancer-related fatigue should help establish prevalence and incidence data about fatigue in children with varied life-limiting illnesses [67]. A new Children's Fatigue Scale (CFS), was tested in 7–12-year-old oncology patients ($n = 149$),

just over half of whom were within 6 months of diagnosis. The most frequently endorsed items included not being able to play, being tired in the morning, sleeping more at night, not being able to run, and laying around. Children and adolescents have noted distressing fatigue at the time of their cancer diagnosis, throughout treatment, and for several years following successful treatment [6,68,69]. Associated factors in cancer-related fatigue include altered sleep, sadness or depression, anemia, hospitalization, inadequate nutrition, and lack of enjoyment for social encounters [6,67,70].

Dyspnea

The many tools assessing apparent breathlessness have not been found to correlate with the patient's report of dyspnea, which is based on the self-report of a subjective sensation. Rather, these tools, such as the physiologic measures of respiratory rate, carbon dioxide or oxygen saturation or their functional counterparts of spirometry, or inspiratory nasal pressure, the walk, step or shuttle test which evaluate exercise capacity, do not correlate with the patient's sensory experience of breathing or their difficulty with it. There have been several tools developed and modified for subjective report by adults, such as the Borg Scale, also referred to as an RPE Scale (Report of Perceived Exertion). The original scale was used to calculate heart rate in athletes and had numbers ranging from 6 to 20 accompanied by verbal descriptors, such as 'maximal exertion' [71]. Such language is poorly understood by most children and has little clinical utility for this patient population. Even the ten descriptors arranged along a vertical line in the 'modified Borg' include 'moderate' or 'slight' and would similarly challenge the comprehension of many children. These scales need to be markedly modified by asking qualitative questions oriented to the sensation of ease or discomfort in breathing by asking modifiers like: "How much is your breathing bothering you, do you find breathing is hard for you?," or from the functional perspective, "Are there things you would like to do but can't because you have trouble catching your breath; is your breathing keeping you from running or playing?," etc.

For quantitative self-report, pictorial scales were developed for self-rating the sensation of dyspnea, based on focus groups of children living with asthma and cystic fibrosis. These four, 7-item scales were subsequently trialed in children with respiratory illnesses. Also evaluated were ratings of pain, fear, and sleep. Referred to as the 'Dalhousie Dyspnea Scale', this visual analogue scale has been shown to have reliability for self-rating the intensity of one's breathlessness for children 6 years of age and older [72].

Multidimensional symptom assessment tools for children

The Memorial Symptom Assessment Scale (MSAS) 10–18 is a 30-item patient-rated instrument adapted from a previously validated adult version to provide multidimensional information about the symptoms experienced by children with cancer aged 10–18 [5]. The scale was created to enable children to rate their own symptoms in terms of severity, frequency and distress. The analyses supported the reliability and validity of the MSAS 10–18 subscale scores as measures of physical, psychological, and global symptom distress, respectively. The majority of patients could easily complete the scale in a mean of 11 min.

A revised MSAS was created as an instrument for the self-assessment of symptoms by children with cancer aged 7–12 years [6]. Validity was evaluated by comparison with the medical record, parental report, and concurrent assessment on visual analogue scales for selected symptoms. The data provide evidence of the reliability and validity of MSAS (7–12) and demonstrated that children as young as 7 years with cancer could report clinically relevant and consistent information about their symptom experience. The completion rate for MSAS 7–12 was high and the majority of children completed the instrument in a short period of time and with little difficulty. The instrument appeared to be age appropriate and may be helpful to older children unable to independently complete MSAS 10–18.

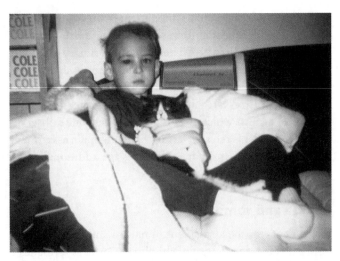

Fig. 17.3 Daniel a 5½-year-old with metastatic neuroblastoma.

A child's symptoms—a child's story

Breathlessness by whose assessment?

Case Daniel was a 5½-year-old with metastatic neuroblastoma, having relapsed following treatment with chemotherapy, radiation, surgery, and a bone marrow transplant (Figure 17.3). He had been able to describe his pain as an 'owie' and tell his parents when he was hurting ever since his diagnosis, when he was 3½ years old. With modifications by Daniel's mother, he was able to use the 'Faces Pain Scale' to self-report pain.

Daniel would describe his nausea as feeling 'like I have to spew' and 'tummy cramps'. His nausea and vomiting were managed with regular antiemetics including a pro-kinetic agent. Following occasional emesis, Daniel would continue to want small amounts of food and his family would have the foods he enjoyed readily available.

When Daniel developed a pleural effusion compounded by anemia with a hemoglobin of 62, he was reported as looking distressed with apparent breathlessness. However, he was unable to identify if he was 'breathless' or had 'trouble with his breathing', nor could he say if his 'breathing was bothering him' (Figure 17.4). His parents noted that he was self-restricting his activity and

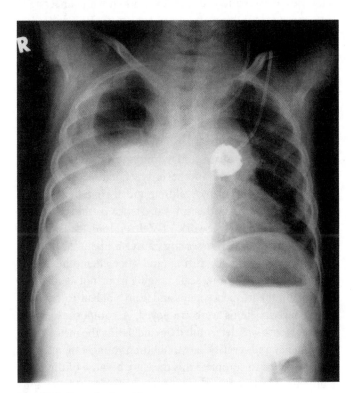

Fig. 17.4 Daniel's chest X-ray.

arranging himself on the couch to achieve a position of comfort. He would lie with the pleural effusion side dependent eventhough he had previously always preferred to lie in the opposite direction to watch the activities in the family room.

Daniel did not find supplemental oxygen help him feel better. His apparent breathlessness was managed with a blood transfusion, opioids, anxiolytics, and physical measures, such as positioning, and cool air to his face. His parents rearranged the family room, so that Daniel could continue to enjoy watching the family activity in comfort.

Daniel required modifications to the developmentally appropriate pain scale. His mother tailored the visual analogue scale so that it was both acceptable to him and able to provide useful information about his pain. Fastidious observers of their children, parents are reliable sources of information about how their child may be behaving differently. They can help interpret for the health professional what behaviors may be indicative of physical distress.

Barriers to symptom assessment

General barriers

Children and their families need to be provided with the rationale for the questions detailing the assessment. They may tire of the questions, particularly if they do not see an outcome that seems to be of benefit. Children may believe, 'If I tell them how I feel they're only going to poke at me and do more tests.'

There may be an assumption that symptoms are an expected part of the child's illness, and therefore, symptoms may not be reported. Congruent with this perception may be the child's or family's assumption that because the health professionals have a diagnosis, these clinicians would also know what the child would be experiencing. Children and families may have a view that the clinician would be addressing their symptoms if there was something that could be done about them [72].

Barriers specific to childhood development

The tools developed for use in the adult population are generally not applicable to pediatrics because of several factors. The items typically scored in adult symptom and QOL assessments would not be applicable to a child's life nor understood by a child because of developmental constraints.

Where assessment tools exist for children' symptoms and QOL, they are from the frequently narrow focus of a particular illness not easily generalizable or extrapolated to other illnesses. Life-limiting conditions of childhood are frequently unusual, uncommon, with an unclear prognosis. Both the diversity and the small number of life-limiting childhood conditions relative to the adult population compound the difficulty in acquiring knowledge about the patterns of the accompanying symptoms. The main contribution to the understanding of symptoms in childhood conditions to date has been in cancer and generally focused on pain. In general, the focus on physical symptoms has been on the acute pain measurement typical of the post operative period.

Whether and how children understand what is happening to their bodies and whether they perceive that they have any control over the situation can influence their degree of distress [72]. On occasion, illness can cause regression in the child's 'usual' capacity to understand and interact.

It is essential to the child's care that symptoms are anticipated and expectantly managed. Generally, compared with adults, children have little patience with medications that may make them feel some way they don't like, even if they are benefiting in some other way. Children are not known as masters of delayed gratification. This may be partially related to a relative lack of understanding about the relationship between cause and effect. A child who experiences nausea or itching as an unwanted opioid-related side effect, will be reluctant to continue with the opioid, despite excellent analgesia [73].

Care of the pediatric population includes those who are non verbal by virtue of their age and others with cognitive impairment, both unable to use even those scales specifically tailored for children. A substantial proportion of children living with or dying from a life-limiting illness are represented by these individuals, among them children less than one year of age who comprise the single largest age-related group of pediatric deaths.

Clinicians' obstacles to optimal symptom assessment

Despite the knowledge that medications exist to safely and adequately manage pain and other symptoms, clinicians do not necessarily use them appropriately or in a timely fashion. Despite the fact that opioids can be used safely and long-term, misperceptions and fears persist about their use [74].

Some clinicians continue to inappropriately choose to keep such agents 'in reserve', when the child 'really needs them' or restrict their use to a time that is clearly end-of-life. Perhaps physicians may find that bearing witness to the child's distress more tolerable if they do not ask about it and the patient and family inadvertently maintain an interaction of 'they don't ask and we don't tell'. This may also be related to clinicians feeling less than wholly competent in aspects related to symptom management. Despite its importance, this particular aspect of care has been poorly addressed in health care professionals' training.

If clinicians feel they are unable to conduct an accurate assessment of a child's pain or other symptom, they may be reluctant to trial an intervention, such as an opioid or an adjuvant for pain relief. The concern for potential adverse effects is generally greatly disproportionate to the reality. Unfortunately, such lack of understanding continues to be a formidable foe of excellent and appropriate care, being notably resilient, obstinate in the face of comprehensive evidence to the contrary.

Resources for symptoms in the life-limiting conditions of childhood

In addition to various references in the expanding literature relating to pediatric palliative care [75–79], some of the best current resources about symptoms in life-limiting conditions are through disease-specific internet-based organizations, often parent driven, such as the mucopolysaccharidoses (MPS) group. There may be parallel venues tailored for the child (as appropriate), family, or health professional frequently with national or regional links, support groups, and ask the 'expert' sections.

To help with the symptom profile of various illnesses

www.rarediseases.org	National Organization of Rare Disorders US-based (NORD)
www.eurordis.net	European Organization of Rare Diseases

To help with the assessment and management of symptoms

A listserv accessible worldwide through e-mail/internet for issues relating to pediatric palliative care is accessible by sending an e-mail to paedpalcare@act.org.uk with subscribe as the subject line.

A listserv accessible worldwide through e-mail/internet for issues relating to pediatric pain is accessible by sending an e-mail to LISTSERV@is.dal.ca with the message SUB PEDIATRIC-PAIN and your first then last name.

www.act.org.uk and www.cnpcc.ca   are two comprehensive web sites with excellent resources, including policies and educational materials and links for palliative care for children.

www.childendoflifecare.org   A web-based resource with information, including audio clips for health care professionals, and families.

www.ich.ucl.ac.uk/cpap   An initiative of the Institute of Child's Health and based at Great Ormond Street Hospital for Children, has developed The Children's Pain Assessment Project. Has links to other internet and paper-based resources.

www.ippcweb.org   The Initiative for Pediatric Palliative Care—A comprehensive website with curricula and resources.

UNIPAC Eight   A Hospice/Palliative Medicine Approach to caring for Pediatric Patients. A paper-based, self-study curriculum from the American Academy of Hospice and Palliative Medicine.

ChIPPS   Curriculum, from a collaboration between the Children's International Project on Palliative/Hospice Services and the National Hospice and Palliative Care Organization, www.nhpco.org.

To help with support for patients and their families (Information, Resources)

In addition to those listed above

www.Bravekids.org

www.faculty.fairfield.edu/fleitas/contents.html (also known as 'Bandaids and Blackboards').

www.virtualhospice.ca
Canadian Virtual Hospice is an interactive network for people dealing with life-threatening illness and loss.

Final thoughts and future directions

A recent study reported that 76% of the parents interviewed had noted that pain or discomfort was very important in guiding their decision to forgo life support for their children being cared for in several US-based pediatric intensive care units [28]. It should be contested that symptoms or the lack of their adequate management not be the driving force behind the decision-making in end-of-life care. The solace imagined to be offered by suggesting that, 'at least their child is no longer suffering' provides a shallow refuge and a hollow victory that clinicians must continually strive to reach beyond.

The numbers of children facing life-limiting illnesses will hopefully always be small, and so the barriers to research in this area will likely persist. What would improve research and positively influence care would be more collaborative initiatives, where several centers collectively pool their resources and experience. Potential research initiatives in this content area are vast, as there is much room for new initiatives and enhancement of existing work. Some thoughts include further exploration into the assessment of nonacute pain and non pain symptoms in children with cognitive impairment or non verbal expressive abilities. Commitment to greater integration into practice and clinical utility should be required of researchers developing pain and symptom measurement tools and those who fund them. Linking measurement development to the outcome assessment of therapeutic interventions, such as pharmacologic trials for the relief of dyspnea, is one strategy. Aligned efforts are needed to test the best ways for education and dissemination of the acquired knowledge, and evaluation of the impact on care and comfort of children with life-limiting conditions.

To improve this aspect of care, at least five things must happen

1. If what is already known about what can help relieve pain and other symptoms is applied in every location where children experience distressing symptoms, from tertiary care in patient units, intensive care units, at home and in small rural community hospitals, the collective symptom burden could be profoundly reduced.

2. The focus needs to be grounded first with the child. Efforts put into finding the right words and methods understandable and acceptable to the child should drive research initiatives on pain- and symptom-assessment in pediatrics. Systematic research directed to finding out how the children feel, from the children themselves, will lead to addressing what most bothers them, and helping them to feel better.

3. The enthusiasm with which health professionals face the challenge of curing the child's illness needs to be shared with addressing how the child's feels living with and dying from their illness.

4. Granting for any clinical research should be incumbent on ensuring the study has clinical utility and the investigators describe a feasible strategy for how the results of the proposed study will be disseminated and implemented to enhance care.

5. Research granting agencies need to develop and strengthen their commitment to funding beyond the research, to ensure the study results advance care.

The human and monetary resources currently designated for pediatric palliative care are inadequate to support the work that needs to be done, the work that would ultimately improve the lives of these children, and those who care for them. All who are involved in the health of children, whether from a personal, clinical, educational, or research focus, can be important activists for the advancement of pediatric palliative care.

Acknowledgements

Grateful thanks are extended to the families of Emily, Mitchell Fraser, Daniel Penman, and Gina Smith, who very generously allowed their children's stories and pictures to be shared.

The kind contribution of Pamela S. Hinds PhD, RN, CS, Director of Nursing Research at St Jude Children's Research Hospital, Tennessee, is very much appreciated through the generous sharing of her work and review of the draft manuscript.

References

1. WHO. The World Health Report 1995: Bridging the gap. Report of the Director General. Geneva: WHO, 1995.

2. Feudtner, C., Hays, R.M., Haynes, G., Geyer, J.R., Neff, J.M., and Koepsell, T.D. Deaths attributed to pediatric complex chronic conditions: National trends and implications for supportive services. *Pediatrics* 2001;107:99.

3. Oleske, J.M. and Czarniecki, L. Continuum of palliative care: Lessons from caring for children infected with HIV-1. *Lancet* 1999; 354:1287–90.

4. Hirschfeld, S., Moss, H., Dragisic, K., Smith, W., and Pizzo, P.A. Pain in pediatric immunodeficiency virus infection: Incidence and characteristics in a single-institution pilot study. *Pediatrics* 1996; 98:449–52.

5. Collins, J.J., Byrnes, M.E., Dunkel, I. *et al*. The Memorial Symptom Assessment Scale (MSAS): Validation study in children aged 10–18. *Pain Symptom Manage* 2000;23:363–77.

6. Collins, J.J., Devine, T.B., Dick, G. *et al*. The measurement of symptoms in young children with cancer: The validation of the Memorial Symptom Assessment Scale in children aged 7–12. *J Pain Symptom Manage* 2002;23:10–6.

7. Antunes, N.L. and De Angelis, L.M. Neurologic consultations in children with systemic cancer. *Pediatr Neurol* 1999;20:121–4.

8. McGrath, P.J., Hsu, E., Capelli, M., Luke, B., Goodman, J.T., and Dunn-Geir, J. Pain from paediatric cancer: A survey of an outpatient oncology clinic. *J Psychosocial Oncol* 1990;8:109–24.

9. Ljungman, G., Gordh, T., Sorensen, S., and Kreuger, A. Pain Variations during cancer treatment in children: A descriptive survey. *Pediatr Hematol Oncol* 2000;17(3):211–21.

10. Collins, J., Grier, H., Kinney, H., and Berde, C.B. Control of severe pain in children with terminal malignancy. *Pediatrics* 1995; 126:653–7.

11. Hongo, T., Watanabe, C., and Okada, S. Analysis of the circumstances at the end of life in children with cancer: symptoms, suffering and acceptance. *Pediatr Int* 2003;45:60–4.

12. Wolfe, J., Grier, H.E., Klar, N. *et al*. Symptoms and suffering at the end of life in children with cancer. *NEJM* 2000;342:326–33.

13. McCallum, D.E., Byrne, P., and Bruera, E. How children die in hospital. *JPSM* 2000;20:417–23.

14. Meyer, E.C., Burns, J.P., Griffith, J.L., and Truog, R.D. Parental perspectives on EOL care in the PICU. *Critical Care Med* 2002;2:226–231.

15. Drake, R., Frost, J., and Collins, J.J. The symptoms of dying children. *J Pain Symptom Manage* 2003;226:594–603.

16. Sirkiä, K., Ahlgren, B., and Hovi, L. Terminal care of the child with cancer at home. *Acta Paediatr* 1997;86:125–30.

17. Sirkiä, K., Ahlgren, B., Pouttu, J., and Saarinen-Pihkala, U.M. Pain medication during terminal care of children with cancer. *J Pain Symptom Manage* 1998;15:220–6.

18. St-Laurent-Gagnon, T. Paediatric palliative care in the home. *Paediatr Child Health* 1998;3:165–8.

19. Mallinson, J. and Jones, P.D. A 7-year review of deaths on the general paediatric wards at John Hunter Children's Hospital, 1991–97. *Child Health* 2000;36:252–5.

20. Belasco, J.B., Danz, P., Drill, A., Schmid, W., and Burkey, E. Supportive care: Palliative care in children, adolescents, and young adults—Model of care, interventions, and cost of care: A Retrospective review. *Care* 2000;16:39–46.

21. WHO. The World Health Organization. Cancer Pain Relief and Palliative Care in Children. In Geneva: (ed.) *World Health Organization*, 1998.

22. Frager, G. Pediatric Palliative Care: Building the Model, Bridging the Gaps. *J Palliat Care* 1996;12(3):9–12.

23. Robinson, W.M., Ravilly, S., Berde, C., and Wohl, M.E. End-of-life care in cystic fibrosis. *Pediatrics* 1997;100:205–9.

24. Massie, R.J., Towns, S.J., Bernard, E., Chaitow, J., Howman-Giles, R., and Van Asperen, P.P. The musculoskeletal complications of cystic fibrosis. *Paediatr Child Health* 1998;34:467–70.

25. Ravilly, S., Robinson, W.M., Suresh, S., Wohl, M.E., and Berde, C. Chronic pain in cystic fibrosis. *Pediatrics* 1996;98:741–7.

26. Hunt, A. and Burne, R. Medical and nursing problems of children with neurodegenerative disease. 1995;9:19–26.

27. Hunt, A.M. A survey of signs, symptoms and symptom control in 30 terminally ill children. *Dev Med Child Neurol* 1990;32: 341–6.

28. Angst, D.B. and Deatrick, J.A. Involvement in health care decisions: parents and children with chronic illness. *J Family Nurs* 1996;2(2):174–94.

29. James, L. and Johnson, B. The needs of parents of pediatric oncology patients during the palliative care phase. *J Pediatr Oncol Nurs* 1997;14:83–95.

30. Lewis, C., Knopf, D., Chastain-Lorber, K. *et al.* Patient, parent, and physician perspectives on pediatric oncology rounds. J *Pediatr* 1988;112:378–84.

31. Hinds, P., Bradshaw, G., Oakes, L., and Pritchard, M. Children and their rights in life and death situations. In R. Kastenbaum, (ed.) *Macmillan Encyclopedia of Death and Dying*. New York: Macmillan, 2003, pp. 139–47.

32. Kirschbaum, M.S. Life support decisions for children: What do parents value? *Adv Nurs Sci* 1996;19(1):51–71.

33. Martinson, I.M. Why don't we let them die at home? RN 1976; 39(1):58–64.

34. Martinson, I.M. and Henry, W.F. Home care for dying children. *Hastings Center Report* 1980;10(2):5–7.

35. Martinson, I.M., Moldow, D.G., Armstrong, G.D., Henry, W.R., and Nesbit, M.E. Home care for children dying of cancer. *Res Nurs Health* 1986;9(1):11–16.

36. Davies, B., Deveau, E., deVeber, B. *et al.* Experiences of mothers in five countries whose child died of cancer. *Cancer Nurs* 1998;21(5): 301–11.

37. Hinds, P.S. Personal communication.

38. Stein, A., Forrest, G.C., Woolley, H., and Baum, J.D. Life limiting illness and hospice care. *Arch Dis Child* 1989;64:697–702.

39. Gerharz, E.W., Eiser, C., and Woodhouse, C.R. Current approaches to assessing the quality of life in children and adolescents. *BJU Int* 2003;91(2):150–4.

40. Eiser, C. and Morse, R. Can parents rate their child's health-related quality of life? Results of a systematic review. *Qual Life Res* 2001;10(4):347–67.

41. Reaman, G.H. and Haase, G.M. Quality of life research in childhood cancer. *Cancer* 1996;78(6):1330–2.

42. Spieth, L.E. and Harris, C.V. Assessment of health-related quality of life in children and adolescents: An integrative review. *J Pediatr Psychol* 1996;21(2):175–93.

43. Bradlyn, A.S., Ritchey, A.K., Harris, C.V. *et al.* Quality of life research in pediatric oncology. *Cancer* 1996;78(6):1333–9.

44. Bradlyn, A.S., Harris, C.V., and Speith, L.E. Quality of life assessment in pediatric oncology: A retrospective review of Phase III reports. *Soc Sci Med* 1995;41(10):1463–5.

45. Moinpour, C.M., Feigl, P., Metch, B. *et al.* Quality of life end points in cancer clinical trials: review and recommendations. *J National Cancer Ins* 1989;81(7):485–95.

46. Lansky, S.B., List, M.A., Lansky, L.L., Ritter-Sterr, C., and Miller, D.R. The measurement of performance in childhood cancer patients. *Cancer* 1987;60:1651–6.

47. Goodwin, D.A., Boggs, S.R., and Graham-Pole, J. Development and validation of the Pediatric Quality of Life Scale. *Psychol Assess* 1994;6:321–8.

48. Varni, J.W., Katz, E.R., Seid, M. *et al.* The Pediatric Cancer Quality of Life Inventory-32 (PCQL-32). Reliability and validity. *Cancer*, 1998;82(11):84–96.

49. Varni, J.W., Seid, M., Knight, T.S., Uzark, K., and Szer, I.S. The PedsQL 4.0 Generic Core Scales: sensitivity, responsiveness, and impact on clinical decision-making. *J Behav Med* 2002;25(2):175–93.

50. Wolfe, J., Klar Neil, Grier, H. *et al.* Understanding of prognosis among parents of children who died of cancer: impact on treatment goals and integration of palliative care. *JAMA* 2000; 284:2469–75.

51. Brook, L., Vickers, J., and Pizer, B. Home platelet transfusion in pediatric oncology terminal care. *Med Pediatr Oncol* 2003;40:249–251.

52. McConnell, Y. and Frager, G. (internet) Decision-making in pediatric palliative care. An Educational Module. In The Ian Anderson Continuing Education Program in End-of-Life Care, University of Toronto and The Temmy Latner Centre For Palliative Care, Mount Sinai Hospital, 2003, with permission.

53. Champion, G.D., Goodenough, B., von Baeyer, C.L., and Thomas, W. Measurement of Pain by Self-Report. In G.A. Finley, P.J. McGrath, (ed.) *Progress in Pain Research and Management*, 1998; Vol. 10: Seattle: IASP Press.

54. Hicks, C.L., von Baeyer, C.L., Spafford, P., van Korlaar, I., and Goodenough, B. The Faces Pain Scale-Revised: Toward a common metric in pediatric pain measurement. *Pain* 2001;93:173–83.

55. Collins, J.J. Symptom control in life-limiting illness. In D. Doyle, G.W.C., Hanks, N. Cherny, K.C., Calman, (eds.) *Oxford Textbook of Palliative Medicine* (3rd Edition) Oxford: Oxford University Press, 2004; pp.789–798.

56. Gaffney, A., McGrath, P.J., and Dick B. Measuring pain in children: Developmental and instrument issues. In N. L. Schechter, C. B. Berde, M. Yaster, (ed.) *Pain in Infants, Children and Adolescents* Vol. 2: Williams & Wilkins, PA: Lippincott, 2003; pp. 128–41.

57. Piaget, J. and Inhelder B. *The Child's Construction of Quantities*. London: Routledge and Kegan Paul, 1977.

58. Gauvain-Piquard, A., Rodary, C., Rezvani, A., and Serbouti, S. The development of the DEGRR: A scale to assess pain in young children. *European J Pain*. 1999;3:165–76.

59. Breau, L.M., McGrath, P.J., Camfield, C.S., and Finley, G.A. Psychometric properties of the non-communicating children's pain checklist-revised. *Pain* 2002;99:349–57.

60. Stallard, P., Williams, L., Velleman, R., Lenton, S., and McGrath, P.J. Brief report: Behaviors identified by caregivers to detect pain in noncommunicating children. *J Pediatr Psychology* 2002;27: 209–14.

61. Zeltzer, L., Kellerman, J., Ellenberg, L., and Dash J. Hypnosis for reduction of vomiting associated with chemotherapy and disease in adolescents with cancer. *J Adolesc Health Care* 1983;4:77–84.

62. Zeltzer, L., LeBaron, S., and Zeltzer, P.M. The effectiveness of behavioral intervention for reducing nausea and vomiting in children and adolescents receiving chemotherapy. *J Clin Oncol* 1984;2:683–90.

63. Zeltzer, L.K., LeBaron, S., and Zeltzer. P.M. A prospective assessment of chemotherapy related nausea and vomiting in children with cancer. *Am J Pediatr Hematol/Oncol* 1984;6:5–16.

64. LeBaron, S. and Zeltzer L. Behavioral intervention for reducing chemotherapy-related nausea and vomiting in adolescents with cancer. *J Adoles Health Care* 1984;5:178–82.

65. Tyc, V.L., Mulhearn, R.K., Fairclough, D. *et al.* Chemotherapy induced nausea and emesis in pediatric cancer patients: External validity of child and parent ratings. *Dev Behav Pediatr* 1993;14(4): 236–41.

66. Zeltzer, L.K., LeBaron, S., Richie, D.M., and Reed, D. Can children understand and use a rating scale to quantify somatic symptoms? Assessment of nausea and vomiting as a model. *J Consult Clin Psychol* 1988;56(4):567–72.

67. Hockenberry, M.J., Hinds, P.S., Barrera, P. *et al.* Three instruments to assess fatigue in children with cancer: The child, parent and staff perspectives. *Pain Symptom Manage*, 2003;25: 319–28.

68. Hinds, P., Scholes, S., Gattuso, J., Riggins, M., and Heffner B. Adaptation to illness in adolescents with cancer. *J Pediatr Oncol Nurs* 1990;7:64–5.

69. Hinds, P.S., Quargnenti, A., Bush, A.J. *et al.* An evaluation of the impact of a self-care coping intervention on psychological and clinical outcomes in adolescents with newly diagnosed cancer. *Eur J Oncol Nurs* 2000;4:6–17.

70. Hinds, P.S., Hockenberry-Eaton, M., Gilger, E. *et al.* Comparing patient, parent, and staff descriptions of fatigue in pediatric oncology patients. *Cancer Nurs* 1999;22:277–89.

71. Borg, G. *Borg's Perceived Exertion and Pain Scales.* Stockholm: Human Kinetics, 1998.

72. Pianosi, P., McGrath, P.J., and Smith, C. Four pictorial scales to evaluate dyspnea in children. *Am J Resp Crit Care Med* 157 (Suppl), A782.

73. McGrath, P.J. and Frager, G. Psychological barriers to optimal pain management in infants and children. *Clin J Pain*, 1996;12:135–41.

74. Frager, G. Pediatric palliative care. In S.K. Joishy, (ed.) *Palliative Medicine Secrets*, Hanley & Belfus, 1999; pp. 158–73.

75. Liben, S. Pediatric palliative medicine: obstacles to overcome. *J Palliat Care* 1996;12:24–28.

76. Goldman, A., Frager, G., and Pomietto, M. Pain and Palliative Care. In N.L., Schechter, C.B. Berde, M. Yaster, (ed.) *Pain in Infants, Children and Adolescents*, Vol. 2: Williams & Wilkins, PA: Lippincott 2003, pp. 539–62.

77. Goldman, A. Life-limiting illnesses and symptom control in children. In D. Doyle, G.W.C. Hanks, and N. MacDonald, (ed.) *Oxford Textbook of Palliative Medicine*, Oxford: Oxford University Press, 1998; Vol.2:pp. 1033–43.

78. Levetown, M. Treatment of Symptoms Other than Pain in Pediatric Palliative Care. In R.K. Portenoy, E. Bruera, (eds.) *Topics in Palliative Care.* New York: Oxford University Press, 1998; pp. 51–72.

79. Goldman, A., Burne, Rees, P., and Duggan, C. Different Illnesses and Problems they Cause. In A. Goldman, (ed.) *Care of the Dying Child.* Oxford: Oxford University Press, 1999; pp. 14–51.

80. Miser, J.S. and Miser, A.W. Pain and symptom control. In A. Armstrong-Dailey, S.Z. Goltzer, (ed.) *Hospice Care for Children*, New York: Oxford University Press, 1993; pp. 22–59.

18   Using medications

Nigel Ballantine and Nicki Fitzmaurice

The term 'therapeutic orphans' was coined by Shirkey in 1968, when referring to the lack of a sound scientific base for the delivery of drug treatment to children and neonates [1]. More than three decades later, whilst our understanding of the maturation of physiological processes has undoubtedly grown, enabling drug treatment to be delivered to children from a more informed position, children, and particularly, certain groups of children, remain therapeutic orphans. This is particularly true of those receiving palliative care, where the complexities of the interaction between maturing physiological function, underlying disease, terminal illness, and ethical considerations result in a paucity of research and data. These difficulties are addressed in the following sections through an examination of the maturation of pharmacokinetic and pharmacodynamic functions, the effect of disease using the example of cystic fibrosis, and the effect of acute illness as a proxy for some of the changes that are likely to occur during palliative care.

Pharmacokinetics

Variability in drug response may be due to differences in:

- patient age
- organ maturation
- pharmacokinetics
- pharmacodynamics
- efficacy
- toxicity
- concomitant disease and drugs
- race or genetic status
- method of drug administration
- dosage forms
- stability and compatibility
- compliance with therapy [2].

Pharmacokinetics uses mathematical models to describe the ways in which the body handles administered drug, through the processes of absorption, distribution, metabolism, and excretion. Age-related changes in drug distribution and handling are not well understood, and yet, are crucial to appropriate dosing of children. In palliative care, the complexities of such changes in the well child must be taken into account, as also changes in drug handling associated with the patient's underlying disease, and also any changes specific to the palliative phase. This section aims to provide an overview, but data is often hard to find. Changes occurring within a particular age range may proceed at varying rates in individual subjects, and developing physiological functions vary in their rate of change over time [3]. Marked variations in the rate of change are seen around landmarks such as adolescence and transitions between growth phases. But younger age does not necessarily mean that drug handling mechanisms are less well-developed. Amongst children aged between 3 months to 17 years who were receiving chlorpromazine, Furlanut *et al* (1990) found a high correlation between age and half-life, with the mean half-life amongst the group shorter than that reported for adults [4]. The association between age and maturation of drug handling is dependent on interaction between anatomic, physiologic and chemical factors that are, in turn, age-dependent.

Research into drug handling mechanisms in children has largely focussed on the functional development that follows birth, and these have been reviewed in published papers and in textbooks [5,6].

Factors affecting GI absorption

The gastric mucosa is able to secrete gastric acid within minutes of birth at full term, with output increasing over several hours, but gastric pH may initially be alkaline, due to the presence of amniotic fluid. Subsequently, little is known about the secretion of gastric acid; such studies that have been carried out are difficult to compare, due to methodological differences.

Evidence suggests that in full-term neonates, basal and stimulated gastric acid secretions, expressed as mEq/kg/h, are similar in the first few days of life. A trough in both occurs at around 1 month, but by 1 year, stimulated acid secretion exceeds basal secretion, and by 2 years of age, acid output (kg^{-1}) is similar to that of adults [7], although essentially adult levels of function may be achieved considerably earlier [8].

Gastric emptying time (GET) is significantly influenced by gestational and postnatal age [8]. It is delayed in the first 24 hours of life for both full-term and premature neonates. Thereafter, a healthy neonate has a GET similar to an adult's (25–87 min vs 22–53 min), although significant differences have been reported, with others reporting adult GET by 6–8 months [7,8].

Intestinal transit time is less well studied than GET. Transit times of 3 to 13 hours have been reported in full-term neonates three to five days old. Longer transit times are found in breast-fed babies 45 days old, compared to those of the same age fed on formula milks. In the neonate and young infant, factors such as immaturity of the intestinal mucosa and biliary function, high intestinal β-glucuronidase activity, and variable intestinal colonisation may all influence drug absorption [7].

Amylase and other pancreatic enzymes show low activity in the duodenum up to the age of 4 months. α-amylase cannot be detected in the duodenum during the first month of life in premature neonates born at 32–34 weeks, and remains at low levels throughout the first year of life [8]. Lipase activity is present before birth, and increases 20-fold in the first 8 months of life [8]. Similarly, trypsin secretion, stimulated by pancreozymin and secretin, develops through the first year of life. Drugs requiring hydrolysis by pancreatic enzymes are unreliably absorbed in the first few months of life.

The bile acid pool in neonates is 50% of adult values in newborns, and 33–50% in premature neonates. The reduced pool is due to ineffective ileal reabsorption and increased jejunal permeability. The absorption of lipid soluble drugs and those that undergo enterohepatic re-circulation may be adversely affected.

Such differences suggest explanations for different drug bio-availability in neonates, and young children compared to adults, but many studies that seek to investigate these differences fail to consider all possible variables. In neonates, higher plasma concentrations and area under the concentration-time curve for several penicillins, compared with those found in older children and adults, are commonly explained by enhanced absorption due to achlorhydria. But it has been suggested that these differences may be due to decreased renal function.

Mucosal enterocytes in the small intestine possess cytochrome P450 drug metabolism enzymes [9]. Grapefruit juice markedly inhibits cytochrome enzymes in the intestinal mucosa, and may increase the absorption of drugs such as midazolam, ciclosporin and terfenadine by up to 50%, if taken in sufficient quantities an hour before drug ingestion. The flavenoids naringenin and quercetin are thought to be involved, and are also present in health food supplements available over-the-counter.

Drug absorption across other mucosal membranes

Percutaneous drug absorption depends on the effect of maturational changes in the skin, including vascularisation and development of exocrine and apocrine glands and the corneal strata. Little is known of how these changes affect percutaneous drug absorption, but the higher ratio of body surface area to body weight in the neonate, compared to an adult, is important. Drug absorption across the same area of skin will result in higher absorption, corrected for body weight, in the neonate. Such differences are responsible for the developmental problems associated with the use of hexachlorophene-containing products in neonates. The poorly developed epidermal barrier in pre-term infants has been exploited through the use of theophylline presented as a topical gel. However, absorption declined steadily after the first 24 h of life.

In the newborn and infant, the rectal route of drug administration can also be effectively utilized, using suitably formulated drug preparations [7].

Drug distribution

Factors affecting drug distribution include vascular perfusion, body composition, tissue binding, and binding to plasma protein. All are subject to maturational changes.

Whereas drug administered parenterally is distributed directly to the heart and lungs, drug administered orally is delivered primarily to the liver. First-pass metabolism, the metabolism which occurs during the drug's, transit through the liver, following absorption, and before it reaches the systemic circulation, may result in very little parent drug reaching its site of action, although for prodrugs it may be essential to producing physiologically active drug.

Vascular perfusion may have a significant effect on drug distribution. Persistent fetal circulation produces a shift in blood flow from the lungs to other organs and tissues. In such cases tolazoline may produce peripheral rather than pulmonary vasodilation when used to treat pulmonary hypertension.

Body composition differs considerably between the neonate and adult. Total body water, as a percentage of body weight, falls from 87% in the pre-term neonate, to 77% at full

Table 18.1 Effect of age on organ weight as percentage of body weight [5]

| | Organ weight as % of body weight | | |
	Fetus	Full term neonate (%)	Adult (%)
Skeletal muscle	25	25	40
Skin	13	4	6
Heart	0.6	0.5	0.4
Liver	4	5	2
Kidneys	0.7	1	0.5
Brain	13	12	2

Source: Originally published in 'Effect of maturation on drug disposition in pediatric patients,' © 1987, American Society of Health-system Pharmacists, Inc. All rights reserved. Reprinted with permission. (R 0516).

term, 73% at 3 months of age, 59% at 1 year and 55% in adulthood. Extracellular water falls from 45% of total body weight at full term to 33% at 3 months, 28% at 1 year and 20% in the adult. Adipose tissue changes both qualitatively and quantitatively through gestation and after birth. Quantity increases rapidly in the first year of life, and neonatal adipose tissue contains 57% water, compared to 26.3% in the adult [7]. At puberty, gender differences in percentage of adipose tissue become apparent. Males lose 50% of their body fat between the ages of 10 and 20 years, whilst females lose only 3% [7].

Tissue binding is predominantly determined by the physicochemical properties of the drug substance, as also by variables identified previously. In addition, the mass of organ tissue varies considerably with age (see Table 18.1).

Blood provides many sites for drug binding which may show age-related changes. Neonatal erythrocytes have 2.5 times more binding sites for digoxin than adults, with the erythrocyte: serum ratio for neonates stabilised on digoxin being 3.6, compared to 1.3 in adults. Such differences help to explain differences in neonatal and adult dosing requirements.

Plasma protein binding

Changes in plasma protein binding are due to changes in both the amount and quality of plasma protein, as well as the affinity of drug for binding sites. Albumin is the major drug binding protein in plasma for acidic drugs and other molecules, including fatty acids and bilirubin. Basic drugs favour α_1-acid glycoprotein and lipoproteins over albumin, whilst other drugs bind to transcortin, fibrinogen and thyroid-binding globulin. Serum levels of albumin in neonates are similar to those in adults, but α_1-acid glycoprotein levels are lower. Other age-related differences in plasma protein include the

persistence of fetal serum proteins, hypoproteinaemia and the presence of ligands, including endogenous plasma globulins and bilirubin, which compete for binding sites. Altered bound: free drug ratios in neonates may result with consequences for the pharmacologic profile of a drug. Many drugs are less bound to serum protein in neonates as compared to adults, although the opposite is true of dexamethasone, which is more highly bound to neonatal than maternal protein. Phenytoin, which is 94–98% bound to albumin in adults, but only 80–85% in neonates, illustrates this point [7]. Since bound and free drugs are in equilibrium, the total blood drug level for a given concentration of free (active) drug will be lower in the neonate than the adult. The therapeutic range, which is based on drug concentration in whole blood, will be lower in consequence. It is essential, when monitoring drug levels, to understand whether it is free or total drug concentrations that are being measured.

Many pathological conditions, including acidosis, malnutrition (hypoproteinaemia), hepatic and renal disease, cystic fibrosis, burns and trauma, and malignancy and surgery, have been shown to alter the protein binding of drugs. Typically, these increase the percentage of unbound drug, leading to increased pharmacological responses and toxicity. Following displacement, a greater amount of unbound drug is available for clearance, however, which explains why altered binding in disease, demonstrated *in vitro*, is not necessarily clinically significant.

Changes in drug–protein binding chiefly affect drugs with capacity-limited extraction and high protein binding (>85%). The best-known example of toxicity attributed to altered protein binding is probably the kernicterus, which may occur when highly protein-bound drugs such as sulphonamides are administered to neonates [10]. This explanation has been, disputed, however, since the affinity of bilirubin for protein-binding sites is greater than that of drugs, and the toxicity observed may be due to other mechanisms.

Age-related changes tend to increase the volume of distribution of water-soluble drugs, and decrease that of lipid-soluble drugs. Increased volume of distribution results in a greater amount of drug in the body, for a given serum concentration. Many age-related differences in drug distribution are relevant only in the first year of life. Thereafter, distribution is similar to that in adults.

Drug metabolism

Many organs in the body, including the blood, lung, GI tract, liver, and kidney are capable of metabolising drugs. Different metabolic pathways develop at different rates, both within and between individuals, and drug exposure *in utero* may induce such pathways. Such factors make prediction of the extent and efficiency of bio-transformation processes based on post-natal age extremely difficult. Normalization of volume of distribution and clearance to body weight, ideal or lean body weight, or body surface area is commonly carried out to correct for differences in parameters that are solely related to body size [11]. Which of these is most appropriate for individual drugs may depend on the particular pathways of bio-transformation and elimination.

Phase 1 reactions are principally non-synthetic, and are directed at detoxifying the drug molecule, although drug metabolites may be therapeutically active or toxic. The mixed function oxidase (MFO) system, which includes cytochrome (CYP) P-450, cytochrome b5 and NADPH cytochrome c reductase, is central to drug metabolism, and many factors control the rate of bio-transformation. These include the concentration of the metabolic enzyme, the proportion of the various forms, rates of reaction, and the affinity for the drug substrate. Furthermore, the presence of competing substrates, both exogenous and endogenous, affects the rate of bio-transformation.

The major components of the MFO system are present in preparations of human microsomes from both fetal and full-term samples. Cytochrome P-450 activity in the fetus and full-term neonate is between 50% and 75% of adult values. NADPH cytochrome c reductase activity is lower in the premature, compared to the full-term, neonate, and both are significantly lower than an adult. With both enzymes, there appears to be a relationship between activity and gestational and post-natal age.

The development of drug metabolising enzyme activity is well illustrated by the example of theophylline, a substrate for CYP1A2. In term infants at 6–12 weeks of age, the half-life is 8–18 h [7]. A linear relationship between age and half-life follows, with the latter falling to 3–4 h by 48 weeks of age. Adult levels of function of this iso-enzyme are reached by 3 months of postnatal age. Similarly, studies of CYP3A4, using carbamazepine and midazolam as substrates, demonstrate low levels of activity in the foetus, increasing rapidly in postnatal life to adult levels by 3–12 months of age. Development continues until adolescence, when activity declines to adult levels [7]. Substrates for this iso-enzyme include nifedipine, lidocaine, ciclosporin and tacrolimus, illustrating its importance to paediatric practice.

Studies of drugs commonly administered to infants, including diazepam, caffeine, phenobarbital and phenytoin, demonstrate a low capacity for oxidative transformation in full-term infants, and almost none in pre-term neonates. The biological half-life of drugs metabolised by the cytochrome P-450-dependent mono-oxygenase system, including phenytoin and amobarbital, is generally longer in infants, compared to adults. The metabolism of phenytoin, a substrate for CYP2C9, indicates that, like ibuprofen, this iso-enzyme is more active in young children than adolescents and adults. Increased oxidative metabolism in the liver in patients with head injuries explains the higher dose requirements for lorazepam and phenytoin [2].

Studies in older children demonstrate marked inter-subject variation. Metabolic clearance in this age group is considered to be greater than that in adults, as demonstrated by the elimination of theophylline (CYP1A2), phenytoin (CYP2C9), carbamazepine (CYP3A4), quinidine and pro-cainamide. This may be due in part to a greater liver weight, relative to body weight, in newborns and children, compared to adults [3]. When normalised for body weight or surface area, however, such differences were not seen with lorazepam, antipyrine and indocyanine green, respectively model substrates for glucuronidation, MFO bio-transformation and flow dependent metabolism [7]. Growth hormone activity at different stages of development may influence specific drug metabolising enzymes.

The cytochrome P450 system is subject to polymorphism, such that 3 variants of CYP2C9 associated with point mutations are recognised. The clearance of phenytoin and ibuprofen is influenced by the CYP2C9 genotype. Similarly, extensive metabolisers (93% of white and black patients) of tramodol, a substrate for CYP2D6, show significantly greater analgesic effects and frequency of adverse events, due to the increased formation of O-Desmethyl-tramodol, a metabolite with potency 6 times greater than the parent compound [7]. Some iso-enzymes of the cytochrome P450 system are male-specific, or regulated by male-specific factors, such as steroid hormones [12]. Establishment of the menstrual cycle may also be an important source of hormone related changes in hepatic metabolism. Menstrual-cycle-related changes in methaqualone metabolism result in clearance mid-cycle, twice that on day 1. C-oxidation (a cytochrome P450 function) was also greater on day 15, compared to day 1 [12]. Sexual maturation has also been shown to influence the activity of the CYP1A2 and CYP2C9 iso-enzymes, but not that of CYP3A4 [7]. Oral contraceptive use by post-pubertal women represents a special case of gender difference in drug handling. The mid-cycle increase in methaqualone metabolism is abolished by concurrent oral contraceptives, which inhibit the metabolism of a number of drugs subject to phase I oxidation, including aminopyrine, some benzodiazepines, caffeine and imipramine. This is believed to be due to a reduction of cytochrome P450 content, caused by the oestrogen component. In contrast, increased clearance of drugs eliminated by glucuronidation has been shown for paracetamol, clofibrate, diflunisal, lorazepam, oxazepam and temazepam.

Phase 2 reactions consist principally of conjugation of drug and/or metabolites with endogenous molecules to produce a compound with greater water solubility than the parent. Hepatic microsomal enzymes also catalyse these reactions, with the most common being glucuronidation, sulfation, acetylation and amino acid conjugation.

Thiopurine methyltransferase activity is 50% higher in newborn infants than in adults [7]. Women show 70% higher peak plasma concentrations of propranolol, compared to men, due to reduced side-chain oxidation and glucuronidation reactions, and subsequently clearance [12]. The case of methylprednisolone illustrates the complexity of competing processes. Women show greater sensitivity to methylprednisolone-induced cortisol suppression than men. But they also metabolise methylprednisolone more rapidly, possibly due to greater activity of CYP3A-mediated hydroxylation, resulting in similar net cortisol suppression in both sexes.

Sulfation is well developed in term newborns [13], and is an essential alternative conjugation pathway for acetaminophen in the neonate, since glucuronidation in this age group is less well-developed. Evidence exists that sulfation capacity decreases with age [13], with formation rate constants in patients aged 7 to 10 years exceeding adult values. Adolescent and adult handling of paracetamol by sulfation are not considered to differ. Premature neonates acetylate drugs such as sulphonamides more slowly than full-term neonates, while both do so more slowly than adults. In the case of this reaction, genetically determined fast or slow acetylator status may also be important, as it is in adults, although it is less well characterised in children. Amino acid conjugation is present at birth, and reaches adult values at around 6 months of age.

It is known that the ability to acetylate a number of drugs including isoniazid, sulfonamide antibiotics, hydralazine and procainamide shows a genetically determined bimodal distribution. Different ethnic groups demonstrate different proportions of fast acetylators; for example, 88% of Japanese–Americans compared to 56% of Caucasian Americans. Some evidence suggests that the proportion of fast acetylators increases with age [13]. Keruegis et al. showed that 62.5% of adolescents less than 15 years old demonstrated the fast acetylator phenotype, compared to 38% in older subjects, although this difference was not statistically significant. Singh found weight-adjusted clearance and elimination rate constants in children aged 7–12 to be twice those reported in adult studies, although the study could not exclude other explanations for the observed difference. The half-life of sulfamethoxazole correlates with age, showing a two-fold difference between children <10 years old and adults, when corrected for differences in volume of distribution [13].

Similarly, debrisoquine hydroxylase deficiency may be important both because of its relative rarity in Caucasians (5%), and because more than 30 drugs are known substrates for the enzyme [11].

Glucuronidation occurs mainly in the liver and kidney, and occurs through the donation of glucuronide groups by uridine diphosphate-glucuronic acid in reactions catalysed by the family of microsomal uridine diphosphate-glucuronyl transferases (UDPGT's). These reactions are important to the metabolism of a number of drugs administered to children, including morphine, paracetamol, zidovudine, lorazepam, naloxone, diclofenac and chloramphenicol, as well as endogenous substrates including steroids and bilirubin [7]. The inability of some neonates to conjugate bilirubin results in high levels of unconjugated bilirubin that can diffuse across the blood–brain barrier to cause kernicterus. The 'grey-baby' syndrome caused by chloramphenicol is also due to decreased capacity for glucuronidation, as well as increased bio-availability [2]. Glucuronidation formation reaches adult values between 2 months and 3 years of age [7].

Evidence existing shows for differences in glucuronidation between older children and adults. Crom et al. reported a trend towards increased clearance and shorter half-lives for lorazepam in three subject groups: less than 13 year old, 13–18 years olds and adults [13]. Differences between the patient groups (for example, the adults were healthy subjects, whilst the children had acute lymphoblastic leukaemia in remission, suggesting the possibility that the changes were due to differences in body composition) make interpretation of the data difficult, however. Similarly, evidence for increased clearance and shorter half-life for lorazepam in young women taking an oral contraceptive is contradictory [13].

Zidovudine is believed to be metabolised by a UDPGT, and some evidence exists for a correlation between age and weight-adjusted clearance [13]. Whilst no differences in apparent clearance, apparent volume of distribution or half-life were seen during the menstrual cycle, the overall half-life in post-pubertal women is 3–4 h longer than in studies which have used predominantly male subjects [13].

In general, the plasma kinetics of morphine in children over 1 year old are reported as being similar to those found in adults [14]. Differences are seen in plasma clearance between premature and full-term infants, whilst children and adolescents show similar or higher clearance values compared with adults (13–15). Clearance in infants less than 1 month old is only 25% of that of 6-month-old infants (half-life of 7.3 h compared to 2.3 h).

Ethnicity may influence morphine pharmacokinetics. It has been reported [16] that despite higher levels of morphine-6-glucuronide, Caucasians are less susceptible to morphine-induced depression of the ventilatory response to carbon dioxide re-breathing than native (South American) Indians or Latinos.

Similarly, paracetamol half-life shows no difference between young children, 12-year-olds and adults, although glucuronidation rates increase until they level off around the age of 12 years.

Nevertheless, there is a trend to higher oral clearance of paracetamol during the follicular and luteal phases of the menstrual cycle, compared to clearance in the menstrual phase and in males [13].

In general, bio-transformation of most drugs is decreased in the neonates, increasing from the ages of 1–5 years and then declining to adult values following puberty. An exception is amphotericin B, where the clearance is markedly decreased in patients between the ages of 1 and 10 years [2].

A further complication of many studies of drug metabolism in children is the co-administration of enzyme inducing drugs. These may induce the metabolism of other drugs or themselves. The mechanism is believed to be an increase in synthesis of enzyme protein. In the non-induced infant in the first 2 weeks of life, drug bio-transformation is reduced. For most drugs, this is not a major problem, since deficiency of the primary metabolic pathways is often compensated for by the presence of alternatives pathways, as with acetaminophen and salicylates. Problems may occur, as with chloramphenicol, when alternative pathways do not exist unless there is strict observance of dosage, and serum level monitoring is performed.

Such interactions can have significant effects. The area under the plasma concentration—time curve (AUC) for midazolam is reduced by 96% when rifampin is administered concurrently, making sedation using midazolam difficult, if not impossible [9].

There remains no proxy of liver metabolic function, such as serum creatinine provides in respect of renal function. Studies in older children have demonstrated a correlation between liver volume (standardised by unit of body weight) and age, whilst in adults, a correlation has been shown between antipyrine clearance and liver volume. Such data does not as yet, however, permit this approach to predict drug metabolic function in general.

Renal elimination

Whilst the liver is the primary organ of drug metabolism, the kidney is the major route of elimination of water-soluble drugs and metabolites. The three mechanisms involved are glomerular filtration, tubular secretion, and tubular reabsorption. Renal blood flow is an important determinant of glomerular filtration, and therefore, drug elimination.

The neonatal kidney is inefficient at drug elimination, which results in prolonged elimination half-lives for drugs such as aminoglycosides, digoxin and furosemide. Maturation of the processes of filtration, secretion and reabsorption occurs at different rates, and may be influenced by a number of factors, including maternal drug use.

The premature neonate is born with a reduced number of functioning nephrons, compared to its full-term counterpart [7]. The latter's kidneys, whilst having a similar number of nephrons to an adult, has greatly reduced renal function, compared to older children and adults, even when standardised for body weight, body surface area, extracellular fluid volume and kidney weight. Functional development of the kidney during the neonatal period, particularly between the 34th and 36th weeks of gestation, is the result of a balance between filtration and secretory mechanisms on the one hand, and reabsorption on the other. Glomerular filtration rates increase significantly in the first 2 weeks of life, and do so more quickly than tubular function. This imbalance persists until 6–10 months of age [7]. Clearance of drugs may be greater in infants than in older children, due to slower development of reabsorption processes. The underlying disease state may also be significant, with hypoxia causing impairment of tubular function in the neonate and changes to normal kidney development. Thereafter, renal function remains essentially constant through to adulthood, although there is substantial variability in renal function in the general population [11].

The renal handling of digoxin illustrates the differential maturation of the processes of renal function. In full term neonates, digoxin clearance exceeds creatinine clearance indicating the present of mechanisms other than filtration: a phenomenon not seen in other age groups [10]. The increase in digoxin clearance in the first few months of life indicates the initial immaturity of these mechanisms. Thus mean renal clearance of digoxin at 1 week of age is 32.9 ± 7.4 ml/min^{-1}·1.73 m^{-2}, increasing to 88.9 ± 23.8 ml min^{-1}·1.73 m^{-2} and 144.4 ± 38.4 ml min^{-1}·1.73 m^{-2} at 3 months and 1.5 years respectively. Premature neonates demonstrate longer half-lives than their full-term counterparts, with mean renal clearance of 10.4 ml min^{-1}·1.73 m^{-2} being determined from seven premature neonates studied. The half-life mirrors clearance, falling from 20 to 76 h in full-term neonates less than 2 months of age to 12–42 h at 16 months of age.

Passive filtration of drug is determined by the unbound fraction, renal blood flow and the area and nature of the glomerular membrane, and each of these is influenced by maturational changes. In the full term neonate, glomerular filtration is around 40% of the adult, reaching a maximal value at around 3 years or earlier [3], when corrected for body size. Glomerular filtration rate (GFR) is lower in premature neonates than in their full-term counterparts. Much has been published on the dosing of aminoglycoside antibiotics, including amikacin, gentamicin, and tobramycin, in neonates, since these drugs are primarily excreted by glomerular filtration. Most dosing recommendations suggest a starting dose, and subsequent serum level monitoring as a basis for dosing, since GFR and aminoglycoside clearance is reduced during the first week of life and subsequent maturation depends on birth weight, concurrent disease, and drug therapy.

Tubular function requires both energy and carrier molecules, and consists of separate systems for organic acids and bases. The capacity of the kidney to secrete weak acids, such as penicillins and cefalosporins, is markedly reduced in the neonate, although there is evidence that the secretory mechanism may be stimulated by repeated exposure to drug.

Tubular reabsorption of drug may involve both passive diffusion and active transport. The former is more common and depends on the degree of ionisation of the substance, urinary pH, urine flow and tubular surface area. Passive reabsorption in neonates is decreased, with the ability to reabsorb glucose, sodium and phosphate increasing with age. With their different sleep pattern, decrease in urinary pH during sleep does not occur in neonates as it does in adults. The elimination of acidic drugs is enhanced by the more alkaline environment, in which more drug is ionized, and therefore, less reabsorbed.

Renal function also matures due to changes in renal blood flow (arising from increased cardiac output or decrease in vascular resistance, or both) and redistribution of blood flow between the intrarenal regions and the cortex.

Gender differences can be found in respect of renal function, as with liver function. The renal clearance of amantadine has been reported as 14 L/h[1] in men and 9 L/h[1] in women. Concurrent administration of quinine or quinidine reduces the renal clearance of amantadine in men, but not in women [12].

Circadian rhythms

Drug absorption, distribution, metabolism, and renal elimination display significant daily variations in common with nearly all functions of the body [17]. Asthma attacks occur most commonly around 4 AM. Children show the same pattern of highest blood pressure and heart rate during the daytime, followed by a nightly drop and an early morning rise, as do normotensive adults and those with primary hypertension. Cardiovascular drugs, anti-asthmatics, anti-cancer drugs, psychotropics, analgesics, local anaesthetics and antibiotics demonstrate pharmacokinetics which are not constant throughout the day. Circadian rhythms undergo maturation with development, and the scheduling of doses has the potential to alter drug response. It is now inappropriate to consider that pharmacokinetic parameters are independent of the time of day.

Theophylline was one of the first drugs for which daily variations in pharmacokinetics were identified. Peak drug concentrations are lower, and time to peak drug concentration longer, after dosing in the evening, compared to the morning, possibly due to slower absorption. In consequence, theophylline should be given as a single evening dose, or the evening dose should be weighted, compared with doses given earlier in the day. The same picture is seen with terbutaline. In contrast, anticholinergics and inhaled beclomethasone (beclometasone) have a more pronounced effect at night. These results suggest that a plasma level: time relationship which is a flat line may not be the most appropriate to match drug exposure to clinical symptoms. Similarly, the assumption that a continuous infusion of drug produces a constant serum concentration is no longer valid. Continuous infusion of ranitidine produces greater increases in gastric pH during the daytime than at night. The proton pump inhibitors omeprazole and lansoprazole are also more effective if administered in the morning, although, at least for lansoprazole, this may be due to decreased absorption if dosed in the evening. The higher peak plasma levels and shorter time to peak levels for propranolol and calcium channel blockers when dosed in the morning are assumed to be due to faster gastric emptying time and higher gastro-intestinal perfusion at this time of day, compared to the evening.

Elimination, as well as absorption, is influenced by these rhythms. In children less than 1 year old, sulfisomidine elimination rate was 20% lower at night than during the day, indicating variation in non-ionic tubular reabsorption.

In children acute lymphoblastic leukaemia with (ALL), the elimination half-life of 6-mercaptopurine is significantly longer in the evening, compared to the morning, (7.1 v 2.9 h) during maintenance therapy. This difference is such that in 188 children studied, evening dosing, compared to morning dosing, resulted in a significant increase in disease-free survival.

Pharmacodynamics

Pharmacodynamics describes the biochemical and physiological effects of drugs, providing a correlation between action and chemical structure. Whilst the amount of information available on drug pharmacokinetics in children is relatively small, the situation is even less clear in respect to pharmacodynamics. This is partly due to the relatively recent appreciation of the importance of these phenomena, and partly due to the difficulty in separating the influence of pharmacokinetic variables from pharmacodynamic ones, unless the study is specifically designed to do so.

Some pharmacodynamic issues have been addressed in previous discussions, including differences in drug response apparently influenced by gender. Gender differences in response to a number of drugs have been reported, including general and local anaesthetics, salicylates, hypoglycaemics, imipramine, diazepam and phenothiazines [12]. Post pubertal women may respond differently to anti-psychotic drugs, possibly due to higher hormonal concentrations or hormonal effects on receptors. Responses and adverse reactions to anti-depressants may vary by gender [12]. Differences in insulin sensitivity have also been seen between male and female adolescents with insulin-dependent diabetes mellitus. The female subjects demonstrated reduced sensitivity to insulin compared to the males, an effect postulated to result from differences in levels of growth hormone between the sexes during the early phase of hypoglycaemia.

The maximum tolerated dose (MTD) for a number of anti-cancer drugs has been shown to be greater in children than in adults [11]. The MTD for etoposide in children is 1.2 times that for adults; for amsacrine and daunorubicin, 1.25 times, and for doxorubicin and teniposide, 1.33 times. These differences may be due to pharmacokinetic differences, such as more rapid clearance, or pharmacodynamic differences in, for example, end organ sensitivity. Children are known to clear methotrexate more quickly than adults, although significant variability exists at all ages.

The IC_{50} for IL-2 expression in peripheral blood monocytes exposed *in vitro* to ciclosporin has been shown in infants less than 12 months of age to be 50% of the value found in older children. This difference appears to be based on a true difference in drug: receptor interaction.

Cystic fibrosis

It is well established that in children and adults, underlying disease may affect the distribution of drugs, although this is much more widely studied in adults. In children, the disease most investigated in terms of altered drug distribution is cystic fibrosis (CF) [11]. CF may be the only disease in which certain parameters of drug metabolism are increased [9]. In 1975, Jusko *et al.* first demonstrated increased creatinine clearance and atypical drug distribution of dicloxacillin in patients with CF [18]. Since then, much work has elucidated the mechanisms by which drug handling is altered in CF. 85–90% of patients with CF have symptoms of GI dysfunction, including hypersecretion of gastric acid and duodenal aspirates which are small in volume, viscous, and containing low concentrations of bicarbonate and pancreatic enzymes [8]. In consequence, a number of drugs, including cloxacillin, ciprofloxacin, clindamycin and cefalexin have significantly

delayed absorption in patients with CF. The lower peak plasma/serum levels of cefalexin, dicloxacillin, epicillin and theophylline may in part be a consequence of impaired absorption, but may also result from increased volume of distribution and/or drug elimination.

Steatorrhoea in CF has been associated with malabsorption of fat-soluble vitamins, with clinical features of Vitamin A deficiency being seen even when pancreatic enzyme supplements are given. Vitamin K deficiency tends to occur in older patients, and correlates with the severity of liver and pulmonary disease, whilst deficiency of Vitamins A and D is common unless supplemented. Absorption of Vitamin B_{12} is impaired due to lack of a pancreatic factor and gastric hyperacidity.

Hypoalbuminaemia is common in patients with CF. It is most commonly due to increased plasma volume, secondary to pulmonary hypertension and cor pulmonale, but may also occur in infancy. As pulmonary disease progresses, serum immunoglobulins A and G concentrations may rise, and this hypergammaglobulinaemia may be important for the protein binding of basic drugs such as propranolol, methadone, tricyclic antidepressants and some local anaesthetics, which may counter-balance increased elimination. Only theophylline has been shown to have significantly decreased plasma protein binding, compared with controls.

It is proposed that the clearance of drugs should be normalised to lean body mass, in order to account for the significant differences in volume of distribution found for amikacin and ceftazidime. But this approach has been criticised for the difficulty it presents in comparing data from emaciated patients, in whom total body weight equals lean body mass, with that from better-nourished counterparts.

Typically the mean weight of the kidney in CF is 150% of that expected, and glomerulopathy has been demonstrated in patients as young as 4 months. Increases of 13.4% in glomerular filtration rate measured by insulin clearance have been demonstrated in patients with CF, with decreased tubular reabsorptive capacity for sodium. Other studies are contradictory, and comparisons are complicated by the different methodologies used. The expansion of plasma volume of 30–45% in patients with moderately severe CF may be another confounding factor.

In CF, increases in night time urine flow rate of 9.4–65.3% and 77% compared to controls have been demonstrated, consistent with an elevation of the filtration fraction. Dilution and a reduced time available for tubular reabsorption, resulting from increased urine volume and flow rate, may account for the 200% increase in the clearance of dicloxacillin in CF patients. The renal excretion of gentamicin and theophylline are also reported to be dependent on urine flow, and the increased elimination of trace elements may also be due to this effect.

Mechanisms that may account for increased non-renal clearance of drugs include elimination in bile and bronchial secretions. The elimination of lipid-soluble drugs such as cloxacillin and furosemide in bile is increased in patients with CF, and, in the case of furosemide, is accompanied by a fall in urinary excretion.

Tobramycin has been found in markedly higher levels than normal in the bronchial secretions of CF patients. Correlation between clearance and disease severity suggests leakage of drug from inflamed lung tissue. Clearance is decreased following treatment of acute exacerbations, and similar phenomena are seen in non-CF patients with severe chronic bronchiectasis [19]. That such mechanisms, or others, may be saturable is suggested by the reduction of trimethoprim clearance seen on repeated dosing.

The total body clearance of theophylline in CF patients is approximately twice that of healthy controls. This difference cannot be accounted for by changes in bio-availability or protein binding. Increased formation of theophylline metabolites suggests that it may be due to induction of hepatic microsomal enzyme activity [7]. Similarly, the clearance of lorazepam and indocyanine green, model substrates for glucuronidation and hepatic blood flow, was increased in CF, compared to patients with cancer whose surgical or radiotherapy treatment had not involved the liver [11]. Theophylline clearance increases with disease severity, a picture also seen with gentamicin.

Palliative care

It is not surprising that there is little information available as to the pharmacokinetics of drug treatments in the palliative phase, principally for ethical reasons that are immediately apparent. This is particularly true in the case of children. However, some insight may be gained from changes identified during periods of acute illness [20].

The lung is increasingly recognized as important in the clearance of a number of drugs and chemicals [19], since it receives the entire cardiac output. Acute and chronic pulmonary disease can significantly affect drug disposition, but these changes have been poorly studied in children. The mechanisms are most commonly indirect, rather than direct. Respiratory decompensation results in altered blood flow to major organs, reduced tissue perfusion, hypoxaemia, hypercapnia, acid-base imbalance, and multiple organ failure. Acute and chronic hypoxia decreases the hepatic clearance of drugs, a phenomenon illustrated by the significantly decreased clearance of theophylline in patients with acute asthma. Hepatic oxidation is decreased in acute pneumonia and chronic obstructive pulmonary disease. Chronic respiratory disease has also been reported to decrease the protein binding of

acidic drugs, thereby increasing the volume of distribution [19]. Acidosis, hypoxaemia and hypercarbia have been shown to enhance the penetration of theophylline into the CNS, with the possibility of enhanced toxicity.

Severe acute illness is often accompanied by organ dysfunction, resulting from sepsis, shock, trauma and severe burns, as well as primary diseases of the liver, kidneys, heart or lungs. Pharmacokinetic variables in such situations should not be considered separately from pharmacodynamic ones. It is recognised that in critical illness, the relationship between drug levels and tissue responsiveness is altered for digoxin, ranitidine and cimetidine, and that certain sub-groups of patients may not respond. In palliative care, acute illness may occur in the presence of chronic disease and organ failure.

Acute cardiovascular disease is likely to reduce hepatic and renal blood flow that, together with disturbances of fluid, electrolyte and acid–base balance and protein binding, will lead to an altered pharmacokinetic profile. As discussed previously, the therapeutic range of total drug concentration may be altered. Wide inter-patient variations are also seen, such as the marked variability in plasma clearance of theophylline in patients with pulmonary oedema.

Acute renal failure may be superimposed on physiological immaturity in the young, and chronic renal failure at any age. Changes in drug disposition may be due to compartmental fluid shifts, acid–base imbalance, altered metabolism and decreased plasma protein binding. As renal function declines, the half-life of morphine and its metabolites increases.

As with renal disease, acute liver disease may be superimposed on chronic. Biological tests of liver function correlate poorly with the liver's ability to metabolise drugs, as previously noted. Issues which need to be considered include the 'first-pass' extraction of drugs such as lidocaine, propranolol, labetalol and calcium antagonists, whose hepatic metabolism is flow-dependent, and may be significantly affected by reduced hepatic blood flow due to portosystemic shunts. Significant increases in bio-availability can result.

Malnutrition can decrease the clearance of drugs [2]. Lorazepam clearance in moderately malnourished children with ALL was significantly greater, corrected for body weight, than that in well-nourished controls with ALL [11]. A variety of studies have demonstrated that when children are less than 60% of the standard weight for their age, processes including absorption, disposition, bio-transformation (particularly, oxidative metabolism) and excretion of drugs are affected [21]. In general, chronic malnutrition results in steady-state drug levels that are higher than normal, and the available evidence suggests that the changes in drug handling are reversible when the malnutrition is corrected [22]. As might be expected, toxicity associated with drugs with a narrow therapeutic index may be more likely [21]. For example, cardiomyopathy due to anthracyclines may be more common in malnourished children, compared to those who are well-nourished [22]. However, most studies have been carried out in chronic severe malnutrition, and the effect of less severe malnutrition that is of shorter duration is less clear. Similarly, available studies have concentrated on the effect of protein–calorie malnutrition, and have not addressed the effects of micronutrient deficiency.

Drug administration

A stepwise approach to symptom management is essential, to avoid the use of sophisticated but invasive techniques, without exhausting the possibilities offered by conventional treatment strategies [23]. Over-prescribing should be avoided in order to encourage compliance and ensure that new drugs are not added simply to address problems caused by those the patient is already receiving. Constant review is the key to successful management.

Oral administration

As in other therapeutic contexts, the oral route is preferred [24]. Most children are able to take medicines orally. While liquid medicines are increasingly preferred over tablets and capsules, young children are able to take quite large solid dosage forms with appropriate explanation and encouragement.

Nevertheless, by the time palliative care is considered, preferences with respect to oral medication are likely to have become established, and it is an inappropriate time to introduce dosage forms with which the child is not familiar or actively dislikes, unless there is a therapeutic imperative.

A significant proportion of children can be managed with oral medication throughout the palliative period. Successful management of pain will be a priority for family [23] and professionals alike, and the optimal route of administration of morphine is oral [25]. However, while oral absorption during palliative care will often be normal, this is not necessarily so. The patient's state of hydration, bowel motility, and the area available for drug absorption will all have implications for the rate and extent of drug absorption. The formulation of the medicine administered may also be important, since significant amounts of propylene glycol, or sugars such as glucose, mannitol or sucrose may cause diarrhoea and other adverse GI events [24]. Similarly, many licensed and unlicensed liquid formulations of medicines contain significant amounts of alcohol [24]. Whilst the effect of this may not be apparent in the child who is relatively well, it may become significant as the child's condition deteriorates.

During palliative, care patients may have naso-gastric tubes, gastrostomy buttons or other devices through which drug therapy may given. Ileostomies and duodenostomies may also be used, when these offer the easiest methods by which to administer drugs into the GI tract. All of these, however, while offering convenience, have inherent problems. Reluctance on the part of the patient to have such routes accessed can result in a number of medicines being administered at the same time, with the possibility of interactions occurring. There are many documented interactions within the GI tract that reduce the absorption of one or more co-administered drugs. Nor are such interactions limited to those between drug entities. A recent meta-analysis of the published studies has concluded that the evidence favours an interaction between oral phenytoin and continuous naso-gastric feeding [28].

The use of stomas for drug administration is unlikely to be a preferred route, but may become one of few alternatives. The crucial question here is whether the drug will be available to its normal sites of absorption, and if not, whether alternative sites are available lower down the GI tract. Issues of retention and abnormal secretion, and flow of bowel contents, will also need to be assessed, in order to make a judgement as to whether such routes of administration are appropriate.

The most common reasons for medicines not being given orally are vomiting, difficulty in swallowing and decreased level of consciousness [29]. Difficulty or inability to swallow will have a significant effect on both the acceptability of the oral route and its efficacy and safety. Vomiting is unpleasant, and often poorly tolerated. If it occurs soon after drug administration, it can be assumed to have expelled most of the dose administered, but the same cannot be said if it occurs 30–60 min after administration. During that time, significant amounts of the dose may have been absorbed. In the former case, the whole dose may safely be repeated, but in the latter case, the extent to which the patient has been under-dosed is unknown, and any replacement dose becomes a matter of guesswork.

An inability to take medicines orally will often preclude the use of sustained-release preparations that are most commonly, but not exclusively, available as tablets and capsules. Splitting the dose form or crushing or chewing it will often destroy the sustained-release properties of the formulation [25]. However, this is not always the case, and an understanding of the formulation is necessary in order to maximise the benefit the patient obtains. MST® granules provide a liquid medicine with sustained-release properties [25], and also offer the possibility of dose titration in increments smaller than is possible by moving between sachets of different strengths.

Parenteral administration

When one or more of these problems occur, injectable therapy is the most usual alternative considered in palliative care. Some patients may still have an indwelling central venous access device (CVAD) that, provided it has not become blocked, can be used. When using such devices after a period of non-use, it is essential to exercise care to ensure that clots or vegetations on the end of the line are not thrown off by drug delivery. Once in use, standard aseptic precautions are vital, if the patient is not to be exposed to the risk of infection at a time when he or she is particularly vulnerable.

The use of CVAD's means that drugs can often be given as boluses in small volumes over short periods of time, because the tip of the line lies within a major blood vessel. This has the advantage that it is unnecessary for the patient to be connected to extended infusions, giving them greater mobility if they desire it.

By the time palliative care is started, such devices will often have been removed, and the subcutaneous route becomes the most convenient (Table 18.2). Subcutaneous administration has many advantages, including being seen as less invasive than intravenous therapy, not requiring venous access where such access may be difficult or impossible, being easily monitored for local irritation, and being easily re-located if such problems occur. It is also widely acceptable in the community setting, making it possible to manage patients at home when more invasive devices would preclude this. This route is not suitable for all drugs, and can be limited by concentration. Higher concentrations increase the likelihood of local irritation, and also compromise the stability of the infusion, whilst the mixing of up to four drugs in a single syringe increases the risk of physical and chemical incompatibility.

Drug compatibility

The issue of drug compatibility is complex, and in order to avoid problems, the manufacturer's recommendation should be followed, not least because to do otherwise renders the administration unlicensed. To follow such recommendations is, however, commonly impractical or impossible in paediatric practice, and palliative care in particular.

In palliative care, the use of subcutaneous infusions has become common practice in recent years, but raises a number of difficulties if treatment is to be given both safely and effectively. Palliative care aims to provide a continuous exposure to the therapeutic agent over a prolonged period, and in order to ensure this, the solubility of the drug, in a restricted volume suitable for subcutaneous infusion, and its stability in solution over an extended period, must be addressed. Factors that affect the stability of a drug in solution include pH, concentration, temperature, time, the presence of other drugs, and the material from which the syringe or infusion system is made.

It is important that drugs are prepared and diluted in solutions with which they are compatible, and one of the key determinants of compatibility is pH. A drug that is most stable in an acidic solution will be more stable in Dextrose 5% (ph 4–5) than in Sodium chloride 0.9% (pH 7). Further, drugs are less stable as their concentration in solution, the ambient temperature and the available time for reaction, the infusion time, increase. Thus, whilst diamorphine is the preferred opiate analgesic for subcutaneous infusion because of its greater solubility as compared to morphine [25], it should not be forgotten that exploiting this property to the full tends to compromise the stability of the solution. The use of continuous infusions at ambient temperature raises further problems. A drug that is sufficiently stable at room temperature for an intravenous bolus injection may not be stable enough to permit an infusion over several days (Table 18.3).

There is some literature on the stability of drugs in solution [26, 27], but it should be interpreted with caution. New data is continually reported (www.palliativedrugs.com; www.pallmed.net). Many published reports rely on visual inspection of the solution and the assumption that a lack of evidence of incompatibility, such as precipitation or crystallisation, colour change or effervescence, indicates compatibility. This is an oversimplification, since a lack of visual clues to incompatibility indicates only that whatever substances the solution contains are soluble in the volume of fluid available. The original substances in the solution may have decomposed,

Table 18.2 Drugs that are commonly given subcutaneously
Morphine
Diamorphine (heroin)
Hydromorphone
Misazoloam
Levomepromazine (methotrimeprazine)
Haloperidol
Prochlorperazine
Metoclopramide
Cyclizine
Octreotide
Hyoscine butylbromide
Hyoscine hydrobromide
Furosemide
Phenobarbital
Dexamethasone

Table 18.3 Stability of commonly used drugs in simple solution [26]

	Diluent	pH	Solubility	Stability in plastic syringe
Diamorphine	Dextrose 5% (preferred); Sodium chloride 0.9%.	2.5–6.0. Most stable between pH 3.8–4.5. Precipitates from sodium chloride 0.9% if pH > 6.0.	1 g in 1.6 ml	Solutions of 1 g/l and 20 g/l show negligible loss in 15 days in sodium chloride 0.9% at 4 and 24°C
Cyclizine	Dextrose 5% Less stable in sodium chloride 0.9%	3.3–3.7 Incompatible with any solution if pH > 6.8.	Supplied as 50 mg in 1 ml	
Dexamethasone	Dextrose 5%, Sodium chloride 0.9%.	7–8.5	Supplied as 4 mg in 1 ml	Solutions of 94 mg/L and 658 mg/l are stable for 14 days in Dextrose 5% at 24°C protected from light Solutions of 92 mg/l and 660 mg/l are stable for 14 days in Sodium chloride 0.9% at 24°C protected from light Solutions of 200 mg/l and 400 mg/l are stable for 30 days at 4°C, followed by 2 days at 23°C in sodium chloride 0.9%.
Haloperidol	Dextrose 5%	3.0–3.6	Supplied as 5 mg in 1 ml	Solutions of 100 mg/l are stable for 38 days in Dextrose 5% at 24°C Stability in sodium chloride 0.9% is concentration dependant
Hyoscine hydrobromide		3.5–6.5	Supplied as 0.4 mg in 1 ml	
Levomepromazine		3.0–5.0	Supplied as 25 mg in 1 ml	
Midazolam	Dextrose 5%, Sodium chloride 0.9%	≈3.5	Supplied as 5 mg in 1 ml	Solutions of 30 mg/l are stable for 3 days in Dextrose 5% at 20°C Solutions of 500 mg/l are stable for 36 days in Dextrose 5% or sodium chloride 0.9% at 4, 25 and 40°C protected from light Solutions of 100 mg/l 500 mg/l and 1g/l show 3–5% loss in 24 h in Dextrose 5% at ambient temperature Solutions of 100 mg/l, 500 mg/l, and 1 g/l show 8–10% loss in 24 h in sodium chloride 0.9% at ambient temperature
Diazepam				Unstable

or reacted to form other inactive or toxic compounds. Studies which report chemical analyses of the solutions tested can provide greater reassurance, but are fewer in number due to the greater technical resources required.

A further difficulty in relating this literature to the clinical situation is the fact that the stability of a drug in solution will be defined by the several variables listed previously. One is very fortunate to find a published study which reports the stability of a solution that matches all these variables. If the patient's circumstance or condition prevents the use of a solution that has been tested, to what extent can data be extrapolated? Can it be assumed that a concentration of 200 mg in 1 ml is stable if a study reports that 20 mg in 1 ml is stable, even if all other variables are matched?

But the greatest difficulty is created by the practice of infusing more than one drug from a single syringe. Whilst the clinical situation may justify such mixing, it is only appropriate if the combination can be shown to retain both efficacy and safety. The majority of the literature on combinations of two, three or four drugs in a single syringe is based on visual rather than analytical assessment, and the use of efficacy as a proxy for stability. Yet such mixtures create increasing potential for interaction by bringing together more chemical entities which may react with each other, and increasing the pressure on the system by, for example, increasing the concentration of drug(s) within the available fluid volume. Nor can efficacy be a true proxy for stability, since there is no comparative data of the efficacy of the same drugs and doses given as concurrent but separate infusions.

Notwithstanding the above, the mixing of two or more drugs in the same syringe is an accepted part of palliative care practice, and the number of textbooks [26,27] and internet sites (www.palliativedrugs.com; www.pallmed.net) which collate reports, varying from the anecdotal to formal studies, provide some reassurance to the practitioner who is faced with no alternative but to infuse a multi-drug mixture (Table 18.4).

Table 18.4 Compatibility of common mixtures in syringe (confirmed by chemical analysis) [26]

Concentration (mg/ml)	<=5% decomposition in 24 h	=10% decomposition in 7 days
Diamorphine		
0.67		Midazolam 0.67 mg in 1 ml Midazolam 5 mg in 1 ml
2		Cyclizine 6.7 mg in 1 ml Haloperidol 0.75 mg in 1 ml
6		Cyclizine 51 mg in 1 ml
9		Cyclizine 32 mg in 1 ml
10	Haloperidol 1.5 mg in 1 ml Hyoscine hydrobromide 0.06 mg in 1 ml	Cyclizine 28 mg in 1 ml Cyclizine 37 mg in 1 ml Cyclizine 39 mg in 1 ml
11		Cyclizine 16 mg/Haloperidol 2.2 mg in 1 ml
12		Cyclizine 51 mg in 1 ml
12.5		Haloperidol 0.3125 mg in 1 ml
15	Cyclizine 15 mg in 1 ml	
16		Cyclizine 25 mg/Haloperidol 2.2 mg in 1 ml Cyclizine 27 mg/Haloperidol 2.4 mg in 1 ml
17		Cyclizine 26 mg in 1 ml
20	Cyclizine 5 mg in 1 ml	Cyclizine 6.7 mg in 1 ml Cyclizine 10 mg in 1 ml Haloperidol 0.75 mg in 1 ml Haloperidol 2 mg in 1 ml Haloperidol 3 mg in 1 ml Haloperidol 4 mg in 1 ml
23		Cyclizine 18 mg in 1 ml
25	Haloperidol 1.5 mg in 1 ml Hyoscine hydrobromide 0.06 mg in 1 ml	
33.3		Midazolam 0.67 mg in 1 ml Midazolam 5 mg in 1 ml
40		Cyclizine 11 mg/Haloperidol 2.2 mg in 1 ml
42		Cyclizine 13 mg/Haloperidol 2.1 mg in 1 ml
48		Cyclizine 10 mg in 1 ml
49		Cyclizine 10 mg in 1 ml
50	Cyclizine 5 mg in 1 ml Haloperidol 1.5 mg in 1 ml Haloperidol 1.5 mg in 1 ml/Levomepromazine 2.5 mg in 1 ml Hyoscine hydrobromide 0.06 mg in 1 ml	Haloperidol 2 mg in 1 ml Haloperidol 3 mg in 1 ml Haloperidol 4 mg in 1 ml Hyoscine hydrobromide 0.4 mg in 1 ml
51		Cyclizine 4 mg in 1 ml

Table 18.4 (*Continued*)

Concentration (mg/ml)	<=5% decomposition in 24 h	=10% decomposition in 7 days
55		Cyclizine 9 mg/Haloperidol 2.1 mg in 1 ml
56		Cyclizine 13 mg/Haloperidol 2.1 mg in 1 ml
61		Cyclizine 8 mg in 1 ml
92		Cyclizine 10 mg in 1 ml
99		Cyclizine 4 mg in 1 ml
100	Cyclizine 5 mg in 1 ml Cyclizine 6.7 mg in 1 ml	Haloperidol 2 mg in 1 ml Haloperidol 3 mg in 1 ml
150		Hyoscine hydrobromide 0.4 mg in 1 ml
Cyclizine		
4		Diamorphine 51 mg in 1 ml Diamorphine 99 mg in 1 ml
5	Diamorphine 20 mg in 1ml Diamorphine 50 mg in 1 ml Diamorphine 100 mg in 1 ml	
6.7	Diamorphine 100 mg in 1 ml	Diamorphine 2 mg in 1 ml Diamorphine 20 mg in 1 ml
8		Diamorphine 61 mg in 1 ml
9		Diamorphine 55 mg/Haloperidol 2.1 mg in 1 ml
10		Diamorphine 20 mg in 1 ml Diamorphine 48 mg in 1 ml Diamorphine 49 mg in 1ml Diamorphine 92 mg in 1 ml
11		Diamorphine 40 mg/Haloperidol 2.2 mg in 1 ml
13		Diamorphine 42 mg/Haloperidol 2.1 mg in 1 ml Diamorphine 56 mg/Haloperidol 2.1 mg in 1 ml
15	Diamorphine 15 mg in 1 ml	
16		Diamorphine 11 mg/Haloperidol 2.2 mg in 1 ml
18		Diamorphine 23 mg in 1 ml
25		Diamorphine 16 mg/Haloperidol 2.2 mg in 1 ml
26		Diamorphine 17 mg in 1 ml
27		Diamorphine 16 mg/Haloperidol 2.4 mg in 1 ml
28		Diamorphine 10 mg in 1 ml
32		Diamorphine 9 mg in 1 ml
37		Diamorphine 10 mg in 1 ml
39		Diamorphine 10 mg in 1 ml
51		Diamorphine 6 mg in 1 ml Diamorphine 12 mg in 1 ml
Haloperidol		
0.3125		Diamorphine 12.5 mg in 1 ml
0.75		Diamorphine 2 mg in 1 ml Diamorphine 20 mg in 1 ml

Table 18.4 (*Continued*)

Concentration (mg/ml)	<=5% decomposition in 24 h	=10% decomposition in 7 days
1.5	Diamorphine 10 mg in 1 ml Diamorphine 25 mg in 1 ml Diamorphine 50 mg in 1 ml Diamorphine 50 mg in 1 ml / Levomepromazine 2.5 mg in 1 ml	
2		Diamorphine 20 mg in 1 ml Diamorphine 50 mg in 1 ml Diamorphine 100 mg in 1 ml
2.1		Diamorphine 42 mg in 1 ml / Cyclizine 13 mg in 1 ml Diamorphine 55 mg in 1 ml / Cyclizine 9 mg in 1 ml Diamorphine 56 mg in 1 ml / Cyclizine 13 mg in 1 ml Diamorphine 40 mg in 1 ml / Cyclizine 11 mg in 1 ml Diamorphine 16 mg in 1 ml / Cyclizine 25 mg in 1 ml Diamorphine 11 mg in 1 ml / Cyclizine 16 mg in 1 ml
2.4		Diamorphine 16 mg in 1 ml / Cyclizine 27 mg in 1 ml
3		Diamorphine 20 mg in 1 ml Diamorphine 50 mg in 1 ml Diamorphine 100 mg in 1 ml
4		Diamorphine 20 mg in 1 ml Diamorphine 50 mg in 1 ml
Hyoscine hydrobromide		
0.06	Diamorphine 10 mg in 1 ml Diamorphine 25 mg in 1 ml Diamorphine 50 mg in 1 ml	
0.4		Diamorphine 50 mg in 1 ml Diamorphine 150 mg in 1 ml
Levomepromazine		
2.5	Diamorphine 50 mg in 1 ml / Haloperidol 1.5 mg in 1 ml	
Midazolam c		
0.67 mg in 1 ml		Diamorphine 0.67 mg Diamorphine 33.3 mg
5 mg in 1 ml		Diamorphine 0.67 mg Diamorphine 33.3 mg

Transdermal/transmucosal administration

The oral and subcutaneous routes are appropriate to many clinical situations, but patient preference and the clinical situation may require consideration of other possibilities. The transdermal and transmucosal routes have been used for many years, but have remained within narrowly defined therapeutic situations. Examples include the administration of glyceryl trinitrate by both the transmucosal and transdermal routes, and transmucosal administration of β_2 sympathomimetic and corticosteroid in the treatment of asthma and other respiratory conditions [30]. Proliferation of 'off-label' uses of drugs has commonly resulted, as practitioners seek to exploit these routes of administration in a wider range of therapeutic situations.

Drug administration using such routes is not straightforward. Defining safe and effective doses requires an understanding of the mechanism, rate and extent of drug absorption across the membrane and, crucially in the context of palliative care, how such parameters are influenced by the patient's state of hydration, skin thickness and so on. These variables can only be defined through clinical studies, but this will never be easy in this patient group.

Many children will be familiar with transdermal drug administration through the use of EMLA cream. The rate and extent of transdermal drug absorption depends on a number of factors, including site of application; thickness and integrity of the stratum corneum epidermidis; size of the molecule; permeability of the membrane of the drug delivery system; state of skin hydration; pH of the drug; drug metabolism by skin flora; lipid solubility; depot effect of drug in skin and variability of blood flow in the skin.

Because skin thickness and blood flow vary with age, controlling the extent of drug uptake is a particular difficulty. Children have a relatively rich blood supply in the skin and thinner skin than adults, so that transdermal absorption defined from adult studies is not necessarily applicable to children. The route may have obvious attractions to children, but experience with drugs such as hexachlorophene, which produced damage to the CNS when used to bath babies with their relatively large body surface area and thin skin, highlights the difficulties.

Examples of transdermal drug delivery familiar to practitioners in palliative care include hyoscine patches for the control of secretions and nausea; fentanyl and buprenorphine patches for pain and topical corticosteroids.

Nevertheless, the potential for toxicity should not be minimised. Excessive absorption through the skin may occur, commonly the result of application to damaged skin. It should not be forgotten that transdermal drug delivery results in systemic drug levels, which may interact with concurrent therapy administered by other routes. Methaemoglobinaemia has been reported in infants treated with EMLA cream. Concurrent administration of drugs such as phenobarbital, phenytoin, paracetamol and sulphonamides, which may also elevate methaemoglobin levels, should be avoided.

The fentanyl patch (Durogesic®) illustrates some of the difficulties associated with this method of drug delivery. In adults, transdermal absorption of fentanyl commences one hour after application of the patch, achieves initial therapeutic levels after 6–8 h peaks at 24 h, and thereafter, slowly declines. Drug accumulates in the skin and produces a depot effect. These characteristics make it difficult to predict the dosage of another opiate analgesic which will be required during the time to peak plasma levels, and also the dosage and schedule for any narcotic prescribed to replace the patch, if this becomes necessary.

Transmucosal administration

Transmucosal drug delivery will also be familiar through the used of local therapy for respiratory diseases [30]. Other uses include inhalation anaesthesia and the delivery of vasoactive drugs such as epinephrine, lidocaine and atropine in resuscitation, sedatives and hypnotics. Mucosal surfaces usually have a rich blood supply, providing the potential for rapid drug absorption and delivery to the systemic circulation. In most cases, first-pass metabolism by the liver will be bypassed.

The amount of drug absorbed will depend on factors including drug concentration; vehicle for drug delivery; mucosal contact time; venous drainage of mucosal tissue; drug ionisation and pH of the site of absorption; size of the drug molecule and lipid solubility.

Licensed drug delivery systems include metered dose aerosols, powder inhalers, nebulisers and vapourisers. Direct instillation of solutions is usually unlicensed. Inhaled drugs are typically deposited in the upper airway, due to their relatively large particle size ($>4 \mu m$), but very small particles ($0.5-1 \mu m$) are also deposited here. To reach the lower airway, a particle size between these limits is required. Water-soluble drugs also tend to remain in the upper airway, while hydrophobic drugs are more likely to reach distal airways. Since drug delivery is by passive diffusion, absorption of fat-soluble drugs will be more rapid than water-soluble ones. Absorption of nebulized morphine is unpredictable, and is best avoided [25].

Potential problems associated with this route of administration include drug metabolism in the respiratory tract; possible conversion to carcinogens; protein binding; mucociliary transport altering drug contact time; local toxic effects such as oedema, and local toxicity due to propellants, carriers or preservatives.

Although the respiratory tract is a common route of drug administration, the nasal mucosa is less often used. Drug applied to the nasal mucosa may be absorbed by olfactory neurons, supporting cells and the capillary bed, and directly into the cerebrospinal fluid (CSF). Transneuronal absorption is slow, whereas absorption by supporting cells and the capillary bed is more rapid. For some drugs administered as a nasal spray, the CSF: plasma concentration is greater than when the drug is administered intravenously or orally. This suggests absorption through the perineural space around the olfactory nerves, which connects directly with the subarachnoid space.

Vasopressin and corticosteroids were amongst the first drugs given by this route. The ability to achieve a rapid response makes it useful for the administration of sedatives and opiates, although the exact route of absorption remains unclear. However, many children object to this method of administration, because of the sensation associated with the volume of solution delivered, and an unpleasant taste in the posterior pharynx.

There is little chance of delayed absorption by the intranasal route, but the possibility of continued absorption of swallowed drug needs to be considered. Further, neurotoxicity has been demonstrated following the direct application of ketamine and midazolam to neural tissues. Much remains to be done to identify all the possible risks associated with drug delivery by this route.

Oral transmucosal drug absorption is efficient for reasons similar to those associated with absorption across other mucosal surfaces. Typically, drug appears in the blood within 1 minute, and peak blood levels occur within 10–15 min. Buccal administration of midazolam has been shown to be as effective as rectal diazepam for the control of continuous seizures in children and adolescents [31]. Similarly, a bio-adhesive buccal morphine tablet has been shown to have the same bio-availability as a controlled-release oral tablet [32]. Oral transmucosal absorption has the potential benefit of avoiding drug degradation by gastric acid and first-pass metabolism in the liver. However, a prolonged contact time with the mucosal surface is necessary for significant drug absorption, and the palatability of the formulation will have a significant impact in this respect.

In order to achieve prolonged contact time, drug may either be administered as multiple small aliquots in suitably cooperative patients, or as sustained-release lozenges. Currently licensed for breakthrough pain, although not in children, the Actiq® formulation presents fentanyl as a lozenge in which a matrix of drug is fixed to a plastic applicator, providing a formulation which may be sucked, or wiped around the inside of the mouth. The formulation permits simple dose titration, although absorption will be dependent on factors, such as mucosal hydration, that vary significantly over time. It also offers the possibility of reducing the incidence and severity of side effects, such as respiratory depression and glottic and chest wall rigidity, which are commonly seen in patients receiving intravenous fentanyl. Any drug that is swallowed will be destroyed by gastric acid, precluding the possibility of uptake from other potential sites of absorption.

Rectal administration

The rectal route offers a further possibility for transmucosal drug delivery. Suppository and enema formulations of a limited range of drugs have been available for many years, particularly when a local effect is required. Benzodiazepines may be administered by this route for epileptic seizures [30], and antiemetics suppositories are valuable for treating vomiting patients. This route has also been used on paediatric hospital in-patients for whom the oral or intravenous routes were not available, commonly using formulations such as oral liquids or injection solutions not intended for this route. Such use was based largely on anecdotal evidence of efficacy, but there is increasing evidence of the suitability of this route of administration in suitable, compliant patients [33–35].

The rate of rectal absorption depends on formulation; volume of liquid; drug concentration; site of drug delivery; presence of stool; local pH; period over which drug is retained and differences in venous drainage across the rectosigmoid region. In consequence of these, and the loss of some drug through leakage or expulsion, significant inter-patient variability of drug absorption is seen in practice. Whilst drug absorption may be equivalent to administration of an intravenous bolus, it may conversely be delayed and/or prolonged. In addition, this route may not be appropriate for patients, such as the immuno-compromised, in whom even minor trauma to the rectum can result in abscess formation and prolonged bleeding.

As noted above, drug levels following rectal absorption will be influenced by the delivery of the drug. Drug delivered high into the rectum is subject to hepatic first-pass metabolism, since the superior rectal veins drain this area. Drugs administered lower in the rectum are delivered to the systemic circulation by the inferior and middle rectal veins and bypass such metabolism. The patient's posture and the method of drug delivery will influence drug availability, although the clinical implications of such variability are not well-defined. MST tablets have been successfully administered by the rectal route, although drug absorption is highly dependent on the height of insertion of the tablet. The use of such sustained-release formulations is likely to carry a significant risk of over-dosage, if absorption from one dose form is not complete before another is administered.

However, the concentration of the drug solution is also a key determinant of response. It has been shown that equivalent sedation was achieved with 25 mg/kg of a 10% solution and 15 mg/kg of a 2% solution. Such findings illustrate the need for consistency in the method of delivery, if predictable clinical effects are to be achieved. In general, the rectal dose required for similar clinical effect is higher than the oral or intravenous dose, with slow onset of duration and prolonged duration of effect. Initiation of such treatment, other than single doses, should ideally be managed in an in-patient setting, due to the unpredictability of drug absorption. However in the palliative situation, this will rarely be appropriate.

Unlicensed medicines

The issue of unlicensed medicines has its origins in the thalidomide disaster, and the public demand for stricter controls and safeguards around the pre-clinical testing of drugs.

The Medicines Act, 1968, addresses all aspects of the marketing, sale and supply of drugs. In the United kingdom, the Medicines Control Agency (MCA), advised by the Committee on the Safety of Medicines (CSM), administers the process by which drugs are licensed and granted a Marketing Authorisation (MA)—formerly known as a Product License [36].

A pharmaceutical company wishing to market a medicine must satisfy the MCA that there is sufficient evidence, gained through laboratory testing and clinical studies, that the substance as formulated is both safe and efficacious.

Historically, medicines have been licensed on a national basis, but it is becoming increasingly common for licensing approval to be granted on a Europe-wide basis by the European Medicines Evaluation Agency (EMEA), advised by the Committee on Proprietary Medicinal Products (CPMP).

The MA specifies the indications, patient population, dose, method of administration, contraindications and other precautions in use, as well as other information, and all of this defines the uses for which the manufacturer is permitted to promote the product. This information, central to the original philosophy of the Medicines Act and the licensing process, is seen as crucial to the safe prescribing and administration of medicines. It is made widely available as the Summary of Product Characteristics (SPC), formerly known as the data sheet, in both printed and electronic formats.

Following publication of the Marketing Authorisation Regulations on 1 January 1999, it is now a legal requirement that patient information leaflets (PIL), which must accurately reflect the SPC, be supplied with dispensed medicines [37]. Pharmacists commit an offence under the regulations if a leaflet is not supplied to all hospital out-patients and in the community.

As commercial enterprises, pharmaceutical companies are unlikely to research and develop products for markets that will not provide a return on the considerable financial investment required to obtain an MA. The paediatric market for most drugs is small, and it is widely believed that it is the issue of return in investment which results in many medicines not having an MA for use children, even though such a use might have been anticipated at the time the original MA was sought, or subsequently become apparent.

Because there is no incentive to research and license the use of medicines in this age group, children, in common with some adults, (particularly the elderly), do not have access to modern medicines that are licensed for use in their age group, or for indications for which they are regularly used.

In 1996, only 30% of 103 newly introduced drugs were licensed for use on children [38]. A further 20% clearly had the potential for use in this age group, but were not appropriately licensed, and of these, 50% had already been used in a large children's hospital in the United Kingdom. A similar study from Europe, in 1999, showed that of 45 new drugs, only 20% were licensed for children, even though 45% had such potential [39].

Some attempts have been made to address these issues, but none have made a significant impact to date. The Best Pharmaceuticals for Children Act, 2001, (USA), provides patent exclusivity to drug companies that conduct paediatric studies on new drugs, or those already marketed [40]. Twelve drugs, including baclofen, furosemide, heparin, lorazepam, and spironolactone have been identified for testing in accordance with this legislation, in 2003 [41]. However, the paediatric drug rule, a previous measure introduced by the FDA in 1988, which required all drugs to be studied in children at the same time as they come to market for adults, has recently been declared unlawful by a US District Court [42], despite wide acceptance by the industry, and despite some success in increasing the testing of drugs in children and in increasing the availability of licensed uses in this population.

The possibility that not all medicines would be licensed for all patient groups or therapeutic indications was envisaged, or at least catered for, by the Medicines Act. It permits the prescribing, supply and administration of unlicensed medicines, but this in no way diminishes the responsibility of medical, nursing and pharmacist practitioners to perform their role in an informed and conscientious manner that safeguards the interests and safety of the patient. In fact, that responsibility is increased, because the manufacturer will not be held accountable if a medicine has been used outside the terms of its MA. Recognising two separate issues, the term 'unlicensed' has come to be applied to a situation where the medicinal product is not available as a product with an MA, while 'off-label' is used to describe the use of a licensed product where treatment of the particular patient group, the indication, or the means of administration are not in line with the MA.

There are concerns that unlicensed medicines have not been subject to independent peer review in respect of their quality, efficacy and safety. These concerns are understandable, but in assessing the relative risks of licensed versus unlicensed medicines, it is important to recognise the limitations of the licensing process. When new medicines come to the market, they will have been evaluated in clinical studies involving a relatively small number of patients, who have been rigorously selected on the basis of the inclusion/exclusion criteria set out in the study protocol. Post-licensing use will be in a much wider and less rigorously selected population, and there are many examples of drugs that have been withdrawn soon after marketing, as a consequence of concern about their safety.

Similarly, the increasing requirement of regulatory bodies for randomised controlled studies against placebo preclude the comparison, at the pre-marketing stage, of a new substance against established treatments, if they exist.

Press comments that in using unlicensed medicines, doctors have to 'guess the dose' in the absence of available information from an MA, ignore the fact that such information in an MA may not be based on experience from a wide patient base, espcially when the drug is new to the market. Similarly, these comments ignore the possibility that the use of unlicensed medicines over a prolonged period may result in the accumulation of both clinical experience and published data that permit the drug to be used both safely and efficaciously.

An MA refers to both the drug and the formulation in which it is supplied. In predominantly aiming their products at the adult market, pharmaceutical manufacturers present their products in formulations, particularly tablets and capsules, which are often inappropriate for children, because of the dose contained within them, their physical size, or their palatability. Pharmacists have historically provided extemporaneously prepared liquid preparations from such formulations, and injections, although such products may increasingly be obtained from commercial sources, when they are known as 'Specials'. However, good quality data on the stability and shelf-life of such products, whatever their source, is often lacking. This is particularly true in the case of those products for which pharmaceutical ingredients are not available, such as treatments for certain metabolic diseases. Neither must it be forgotten that in preparing such presentations, the use of the drug becomes 'unlicensed', even though the original preparation used may be licensed in respect of both the age group and therapeutic indication.

This creates a tension, amongst all those involved in the case of the patient, between the desire to treat a condition with a medicine or a chemical for which there may be good evidence of efficacy of treatment, and the awareness that they will be held accountable for any harm that befalls the patient in consequence of that treatment. The accountability of health care professionals will inevitably be at a higher level if an unlicensed product, rather than a licensed one, is used.

A number of recent studies, in both the United Kingdom and Europe, have sought to identify the extent of unlicensed and off-label prescribing in both hospital and community settings [43—51]. In respect of children in hospitals, the extent of unlicensed and off-label use of medicines has been shown to be 25% in a general paediatric ward, 40% in a paediatric ICU and 80% in a neonatal ICU. In the community, 11% of prescribing in the United Kingdom is unlicensed or off-label, while 33% of prescribing is unlicensed or off-label in France.

Such figures raise two questions: is this a problem and, if it is, what should be done about it? Where unlicensed or off-label medicines are prescribed and supplied, and harm results, both the clinical staff involved and their employers may be held liable, unless they can demonstrate that they acted responsibly and in the patient's best interest. It is, therefore, most important that such prescribing is in accordance with the knowledge base available at the time, even though this may be extremely limited where rare conditions or new treatments are concerned. Disclaimers, signed by either the clinician or the patient or carers, almost certainly do nothing to diminish the responsibility of clinical staff to act in the best interests of the patient, whatever their roles in the delivery of care.

Whether the prescribing of unlicensed and off-label medicines does put children at greater risk is unproven, but a non-significant trend towards more adverse reactions occurring amongst hospital in-patients prescribed such treatment has been identified [43]. It is likely that at least one factor in any such trend will be the need to calculate and measure the required dose from the original adult dose form.

A further difficulty is the requirement to provide a PIL with each supply to hospital outpatients and patients treated in the community. In the case of 'off-label' prescribing this will result in the patient and family being given incorrect, confusing and misleading information. In the case of unlicensed medicines, PIL's may simply not be available or, if the medicine is imported, may be in a foreign language. To try to explain this situation, a joint committee of the Royal College of Paediatrics and Child Health (RCPCH) and the Neonatal and Paediatric Pharmacists Group (NPPG) have produced a policy statement and information leaflets for both patients/carers and older children, that can be supplied with dispensed medicines, or downloaded from their websites [52].

References

1. Shirkey, H. Editorial comment: Therapeutic orphans. *J Pediatr* 1968; 72:119–20.
2. Nahata, M.C. Variability in clinical pharmacology of drugs in children. *J Clin Pharm Therap* 1992;17:365–8.
3. O'Flaherty, E.J. Physiologic changes during growth and development. *Environ Health Perspect* 1994;102(Suppl. 11):103–6.
4. Geller, B. Psychopharmacology of children and adolescents: Pharmacokinetic relationships of plasma/serum levels to response. *Psychopharmaol Bull* 1991;27(4):401–9.
5. Stewart, C.F., and Hampton, E.M. Effect of maturation on drug disposition in pediatric patients. *Clin Pharm* 1987;6:548–64.
6. Walson, P.D. Paediatric clinical pharmacology and therapeutics. In T.M. Speight, N.H.G. Holford, ed. *Avery's Drug Treatment* (4th edition). Auckland, NZ: Adis International Limited 1997, pp. 127–71.
7. Kerans, G.L. Impact of developmental pharmacology on pediatric study design. Overcoming the challenges. *J Allergy Clin Immunol* 2000;106:S128–38.
8. Kearns, G.L. and Reed, M.D. Clinical pharmacokinetics in infants and children a reappraisal *Clin Pharma* 1989;17(Suppl 1):29–67.

9. Berlin C.M. Advances in pediatric pharmacology and toxicology. *Adv pediatr* 1997;44:545–74.

10. Skaer, T.L. Dosing considerations in the pediatric patient. *Clini Therap* 1991;13(5):526–44.

11. Crom, W.R. Pharmacokinetics in the child. *Environ Health Perspect* 1994;102(Suppl 11):111–8.

12. Letcher, C.V., Acosta, E.P., and Strykowski J.M. Gender differences in human pharmacokinetics and pharmacodynamics. *J Adolesc Health* 1994;15:619–29.

13. Capparelli, E. Pharmacokinetic considerations in the adolescent: Non-cytochrome P450 metabolic pathways. *J Adolesc Health* 1994;15:641–7.

14. Hain, R.D.W., Hardcastle, A., Pinkerton, C.R. and, Aherne G.W. Morphine and morphine-6-glucuronide in the plasma and cerebrospinal fluid of children. *Br J Clin Pharmacol* 1999;48:37–42.

15. Berlin, C.M. Advances in pediatric pharmacology and toxicology. *Adv Pediatr* 1997;42:593–629.

16. Cepeda, M.S. Farrar, J.T., Boston R, *et al.* Ethnicity influences morphine pharmacokinetics and pharmacodynamics. *Clin Pharmacol Ther* 2001;70(4):351–61.

17. Lemmer, B. Relevance for chronopharmacology on practical medicine. *Semin Perinatol* 2000;24(4):280–90.

18. Prandota, J. Drug disposition in cystic fibrosis: Progress in understanding pathophysiology and pharmacokinetics. *Pediatr Infect Dis J* 1987;6:1111–26.

19. Kelly, H.W. Pharmacotherapy of pediatric lung disease: Differences between children and adults. *Clin Chest Med* 1987;8(4):681–94.

20. Jellett, L.B. and Heazlewood V.J. Pharmacokinetics in acute illness 1990;153:534–41.

21. Krishnaswamy, K. Drug metabolism and pharmacokinetics in malnourished children. *Clin Pharma* 1989;17(Suppl 1):68–88.

22. Anderson, K.E . Influences of diet and nutrition on clinical pharmacokinetics. *Clin Pharma* 1988;14:325–46.

23. Beardsmore, S. and, Fitzmaurice, N. Palliative care in paediatric oncology. *Eur J Cancer* 2002;38:1900–7.

24. Sagraves, R. Pediatric dosing information for health care providers. *J Pediatr Health Care* 1995;9:272–7.

25. Expert Working Group of the European Association for Palliative Care Morphine in cancer pain. *BMJ* 1996;312:823–6.

26. Trissel L.A. Handbook on Injectable Drugs (12th edition). American Society of Health-System Pharmacists, 2003.

27. Dickman, A., Littlewood, C., and Varga, J. *The Syringe Driver*. Oxford: Oxford University Press, 2002.

28. Au Yeung, S.C.S. and Ensom, M.H.H. Phenytoin and enteral feedings: Does evidence support an interaction? *Ann Pharmacother* 2000;34:896–905.

29. Goldman, A. and Byrne, R. Symptom management. In A. Goldman, ed. *Care of the Dying Child*. Oxford, UK: Oxford University Press, 1994, pp.52–75.

30. Committee on Drugs, American Academy of Paediatrics (1997). Alternative routes of drug administration—advantages and disadvantages (Subject review)(RE9723). *Pediatrics* 1997;200(1).

31. Scott, R.C., Besag, F.M., and Neville, B.G. Buccal midazolam and rectal diazepam for treatment of prolonged seizures in childhood and adolescence: A randomised trial. *Lancet* 1999;353:623–6.

32. Beyssac, E., Touraref, F., Meyer, M., Jacob, L., Sandouk, P., and Aiache, J.M. Bioavailability of morphine after administration of a new bioadhesive buccal tablet. *Biopharm Drug Dispos* 1998;19(6):401–5.

33. Smith, S., Sharkey, I., and Campbell, D. Guidelines for rectal administration of anticonvulsant medication in children. *Paediatr Perinat Drug Ther* 2001;4(4):140–7.

34. Warren, D.E. Practical use of rectal medications in palliative care. *Journal of Pain Symptom Manage* 1996;11(6):378–87.

35. Motwani, J.G. and Lipworth B.J. Clinical pharmacokinetics of drugs administered bucally and sublingually. 1991;21(2):83–94.

36. Nunn, T. Using unlicensed and off-label medicines. *Pharma Manage* 2002;18(4):64–7.

37. *Pharma J* 2000;264(7087):401.

38. Nunn, A.J. and Turner, S. Paediatric therapeutics—need for appropriate information (letter). *Pharm J* 1999;262:322–3.

39. Impicciatore, P., and Choonara, I. Status of new medicines approved by the European Medicines Evaluation Agency regarding paediatric use. *Pharmacol* 1999;48:15–8.

40. Silverman, J. (2002). FDA decides to retain, update pediatric drug rule. *Pediat News* 2002;36(5).

41. Mechcatie, E. (2003) Twelve drugs picked for imminent pediatric study. *Pediatric News* 2003;37(3).

42. Silverman, J (2002). Federal judge says pediatric drug rule is invalid. *Pediat News* 2002;36(11).

43. Turner, S., Nunn, A.J., Fielding, K., and Choonara, I. Adverse drug reactions to unlicensed and off-label drugs on paediatric wards: A prospective study. *Acta Paediatr* 1999;88:965–8.

44. Turner, S., Longworth, A., Nunn, A.J., and Choonara, I. Unlicensed and off label drug use in paediatric wards: Prospective study. *Br Med J* 1998;316:343–5.

45. Turner, S., Gill, A., Nunn, A.J., Hewitt, B., and Choonara I. Use of 'off label' and unlicensed drugs in a paediatric intensive care unit. *Lancet* 1996;347:549–50.

46. Conroy, S., McIntyre, J., and Choonara I. Unlicensed and off label drug use in neonates. *Arch Dis Child* 1999;80(2):F142–4.

47. Conroy, S., Choonara, I., Impicciatore, P. *et al.* Survey of unlicensed and off label drug use in paediatric wards in European countries. *Br Med J* 2000;320:79–82.

48. 't Jong, G.W. *et al.* A survey of the use of off-label and unlicensed drugs in a Dutch children's hospital. *Paediatrics* 2001;108:1089–93.

49. Seyberth, H.W. (1984). Aktuelle probleme der klinischen pharmacologie im kindesalter. *Kinderarzt* 1984;15:309–14.

50. McIntyre, J., Conroy, S., Avery, A., Corns, H., and Choonara I Unlicensed and off label prescribing of drugs in general practice. *Arch Dis Child* 1999;83:498–501.

51. Chalumeau, M., Treluyer, J.M., and Salanave, B. Off label and unlicensed drug use among French office based paediatricians. *Arch Dis Child* 1999;83:502–5.

52. Joint Royal College of Paediatrics and Child Health/Neonatal and Paediatric Pharmacists Group Standing Committee on Medicines Text available from www.nppg.demon.co.uk and www.rcpch.ac.uk, 2000.

19 Pain: An introduction

John J. Collins and Suellen Walker

Introduction

The International Association for the Study of Pain (IASP) defines pain as "an unpleasant sensory and emotional experience associated with actual or potential tissue damage, or described in terms of such damage" [1]. Implicit in this definition is that pain is a subjective experience and is based on self-report of the experience. Anand and Craig [2] have critically examined the definition of pain in the context of the infant or child who cannot give self—report. In its present form, the definition of pain does not apply to living organisms incapable of self-report. They propose a broader definition of pain that applies also to those diverse, special populations, that communicate in a unique and effective manner through their biobehavioural responses [2]. These populations include infants and the cognitively impaired.

Clinicians and researchers have long observed the lack of co-relation between the extent of tissue injury and the intensity of pain or suffering. The experience of pain is subjective, and, as such is modulated not only by biological factors, but also by previously painful experiences, the meaning and context of the pain, fear, anxiety, depression, and a range of other factors. It is essential to assess the extent to which one or more of these modulating factors require specific interventions.

Pain is one of the most common symptoms experienced in children receiving palliative care, and one of the most feared. The severity of this symptom may increase with time, especially when the terminal phase is reached. Palliative therapeutics should generally only be implemented once the underlying causative mechanisms have been established, since therapies directed at the primary cause may ultimately have a more effective outcome for symptom management.

The following Chapter outlines the historical concepts of pain, the myths and misperceptions about pain in children, the epidemiology of pain in dying children, the mechanism of pain perception in humans, the changes in nociceptive processing during development, the long term consequences of early pain and injury, and the mode of action of opioids and adjuvant analgesics.

Historical concepts of pain

It is an integral component of the survival process to recognise a relationship between pain and physical experiences that are harmful to the body. However, there has been much debate about the concept of pain over the centuries. The main controversy has surrounded the relative components of the response to external injury, and the contribution of inner emotions and psychological factors. Homer thought pain was due to arrows shot by Gods, and thus an external physical insult was seen as the determinant of pain. Aristotle, who was the first to distinguish the five senses of sight, hearing, smell, taste, and touch, did not regard pain as a sensation, but rather an emotion. He classed it as one of the 'passions of the soul', and felt that pain may result from unduly violent forms of wave motion due to the other sensations. Plato argued that pain and pleasure were perceived in the heart and liver, and resulted from violent impacts of the four elements earth, air, fire and, water on the soul. In Roman times, Galen (131–200 AD) investigated sensory physiology and concluded that the brain was the centre of sensation [3–5].

Over the centuries the relative contributions of injury and emotion, continued to be debated. During the seventeeth century, Descartes developed a mechanistic concept of a neural connection from the periphery to the brain. According to this 'Cartesian model', one unit of pain stimulus, secondary to a peripheral insult would pass to the brain and result in one unit of pain being perceived centrally [5]. The ninteenth century saw great advances in physiology and anatomy. Specific end–organs, peripheral nerve fibres and nerve tracts were identified, and the electrical activity of sensory nerves was studied. As in the Cartesian model, pain was seen as a physiological process within a fairly hard-wired system, which did not allow for modulation of transmission by peripheral, spinal cord or cortical mechanisms. If there was no clearly identifiable physical source of pain, pain was presumed to be due to emotional causes and was seen as imaginary [3], as distinct from pain due to observable physical causes.

The Gate Control theory of Melzack and Wall [6], published in 1965, suggested that activity generated by large myelinated primary afferent fibres (A-beta fibres) would act via inhibitory circuits in the superficial laminae of the dorsal horn, to inhibit the transmission of activity in the small unmyelinated primary afferent C fibres thus closing a 'gate' on pain transmission. Although aspects of the original Gate Control theory have been disputed [7], it provided the framework for directing attention to the active modulation of pain transmission. Thus, the intensity and quality of pain perceived does not bear a push-button, straight-through, one-to-one relationship to the intensity of the stimulus, but is influenced by a multiplicity of physiological, psychological and environmental variables [5].

The epidemiology of pain in dying children

The symptom prevalence, characteristics and distress of 30 children (mean age 8.9 years) dying in hospital have been described [8]. Data from the last week of life were obtained from the medical records and symptoms and their characteristics during the last day of life were determined by nurse interview. The dominant disease process was cancer ($n = 18$), most likely location of death intensive care ($n = 20$) and the major physiological disturbances at the time of death were respiratory failure ($n = 9$) and encephalopathy ($n = 9$).

The mean ($\pm$SD) number of symptoms per patient in the last week of life was 11.1 ± 5.6 and six symptoms, including pain, irritability and fatigue, occurred with a prevalence of 50% or more. The location of death had a significant ($p < 0.02$) impact on the mean number of symptoms; ward (14.3 ± 6.1) vs. intensive care (9.5 ± 4.7). The prevalence of pain in intensive care was half that of those patients located in the ward (40% vs. 80%). Only fatigue and dry mouth were more prevalent and more distressing to those who experienced these symptoms [8].

These data indicate that pain is both prevalent and highly distressing to many dying children. This raises the importance of paediatric palliative care physicians to be soundly trained in comprehensive pain management strategies. Otherwise, the memory of poorly controlled symptoms in their dying child may be retained for many years in the memory of their parents (Table 19.1).

Myths and misperceptions about pain in children

The myths

The myth that children either do not experience pain, or do not experience pain as much as adults, have inhibited progress in pain management for children until recent times (Table 19.2). Since the 1980s there has been a growing movement towards improved pain control for infants, children, and adolescents. This movement was partly a response to the weight of evidence indicating that poor pain control negatively influenced outcome in post-operative neonates [9]. It was also partly due to improved measures of pain severity in infants and children and a critical mass of clinicians with developing expertise in this area. This latter has seen the development of multidisciplinary pain services in many paediatric centres around the world.

The misperceptions

Although there is an increasing consciousness towards improved pain control for children in general, there are some particular issues pertaining to children receiving palliative care. For example, the meaning of increasing pain severity for some families is that this is a marker of disease progression. Some children and families defer opioid dose increases because of the meaning associated with increasing pain. The names of the opioids have certain meanings for some families. Methadone, for example, can sometimes be an appropriate analgesic for children in certain circumstances. The mere mention of methadone can cause anxiety for some care-givers because of its association with the treatment of opioid drug addiction.

There is confusion about the terms tolerance, dependence, and drug addiction.

- Analgesic *tolerance* refers to the progressive decline in potency of an opioid with chronic use, so that increasingly higher doses are required to achieve the same analgesic effect. Parents are sometimes reluctant to increase opioid doses in their child because of a fear that tolerance will make opioids ineffective later. Reassurance should be given that tolerance, in the majority of cases, can be managed by simple dose escalation, use of adjuvant medications, or perhaps by an opioid switch in the setting of dose-limiting side-effects.

Table 19.1 Symptom prevalence (*n* = 29) and characteristics (*n* = 27) of dying children on the last day of life

Symptom	Overall prevalence (%)	Degree when symptom was present Frequency A lot-AA (%)[a]	Intensity mod-VSev (%)[b]	Distress QB-VM (%)[c]
Skin changes	51.7	NE	60.0	21.4
Lack of energy	48.3	92.8	78.6	30.7
Dry mouth	41.4	66.7	25.0	27.3
Swelling of arms/legs	41.4	NE	50.0	9.1
Feeling drowsy	31.0	88.9	66.7	0.0
Pain	31.0	33.3	11.1	25.0
Problems with urination	27.6	87.5	87.5	0.0
Difficulty swallowing	27.6	75.0	62.5	12.5
Lack of concentration	27.6	62.5	50.0	0.0
Cough	27.6	25.0	12.5	12.5
Lack of appetite	24.1	85.7	85.7	0.0
Diarrhoea	24.1	42.9	28.6	33.3
Dyspnoea	20.7	66.7	33.3	16.7
Feeling irritable	20.7	16.7	16.7	16.7
Weight loss	20.7	NE	50.0	0.0
Mouth sores	20.7	NE	33.3	20.0
Vomiting	20.7	0.0	0.0	16.7
Feeling nervous	13.8	50.0	25.0	75.0
Feeling sad	13.8	50.0	25.0	25.0
Sweating	13.8	50.0	25.0	0.0
Worrying	10.3	100.0	33.3	100.0
Insomnia	10.3	33.3	33.3	0.0
Itching	10.3	33.3	0.0	0.0
Numbness/tingling in hands/feet	6.9	50.0	100.0	100.0
Headache	6.9	50.0	50.0	50.0
Nausea	6.9	50.0	0.0	0.0
Dizziness	6.9	50.0	0.0	0.0
Constipation	6.9	NE	50.0	0.0
Hair loss	6.9	NE	0.0	0.0
Change in the way food tastes	3.4	NE	0.0	0.0
'I don't look like myself'	0.0	NE	0.0	0.0

Note: NE = not evaluated
[a] Percentage a lot to almost always.
[b] Percentage moderate to very severe.
[c] Percentage quite a bit to very much.

Source: Drake, R., Frost, J., and Collins, J.J. The symptoms of dying children. *Pain Symptom Management* 2003;27(7):6–10.

- Physical *dependence* is a physiologic state characterized by withdrawal (abstinence syndrome) after dose reduction or discontinuation of the opioid, or administration of an opioid antagonist. Initial manifestations of withdrawal include yawning, diaphoresis, lacrimation, coryza and tachycardia.

- *Addiction* is a psychological and behavioural syndrome characterized by drug craving and aberrant drug use. Some parents fear that an exposure to an opioid will result in their child subsequently becoming a drug addict. The incidence of opioid addiction was examined prospectively in 12,000 hospitalized adult patients, who received at least one dose of a strong opioid [10]. There were only four documented cases of subsequent addiction in patients without a prior history of drug abuse. These data suggest that iatrogenic opioid addiction is an uncommon problem in adults. This observation is also consistent with a large worldwide experience with opioid treatment of cancer pain in childhood.

Long-term consequences of early pain and injury

Pain and injury in early life are occurring on the background of a developing nervous system. This not only leads to changes in baseline nociceptive processing, but also changes pharmacodynamic responses to analgesic agents. In addition, structural and functional reorganisation of synaptic connections occurs in the postnatal period, and is dependent on activity within developing sensory pathways. As a result, abnormal or excessive activity related to pain and injury may alter normal development, and has the potential to produce behavioural and structural changes that are not seen when similar injuries occur in the adult. Although the laminar distribution of 'A' fibres changes during development, the segmental distribution of the terminal fields of peripheral nerves is somatotopically precise from early in development and allows localisation of a stimulus. However, nerve injury in the first postnatal week in rat pups produces sprouting of remaining terminal afferents into the denervated area [11], while early inflammation can produce an

expansion of terminal fields [12,13]. Clinical studies suggest that early pain related to surgical and procedural interventions during intensive care management of premature neonates can have long term consequences upon pain behaviour, and perception in later life [14,15]. Further investigation of the plasticity of developing pain pathways is required to evaluate potential long-term effects of pain and injury experienced in early life.

How do humans experience pain?

The somatosensory system has the ability to detect noxious stimuli that are potential sources of tissue injury, and then to process this information to elicit the perception of pain and appropriate behavioural responses. Lack of protective sensation can lead to a variety of medical complications, including compartment syndromes or decubitus ulcers. Conversely, there is often no protective significance to some types of pain, such as that of metastatic cancer, or migraine. Neuropathic pain refers to pain associated with abnormal excitability in peripheral or central neurons. Neuropathic pain may persist even after tissue injury or inflammation have subsided. Neuropathic pain often is described as burning, shooting, or stabbing in character, and it is often associated with paraesthesiae. The term 'allodynia' refers to a condition in which pain can be elicited by normally nonpainful stimuli, such as light stroking of the skin. In the absence of acute inflammation of the skin, allodynia generally implies the existence of an underlying neuropathic condition.

Peripheral mechanisms

The detection of noxious stimuli requires activation of peripheral sensory organs (nociceptors), and transduction of the energy into electrical signals for conduction to the central nervous system. Nociceptive afferents are widely distributed throughout the body (skin, muscle, joints, viscera, meninges), and encode stimulus modality, intensity, location and duration. The most numerous subclass of nociceptor is the C-fibre polymodal nociceptor (PMN), which responds to a variety of stimuli, including:

Chemical stimuli A large range of chemical stimuli and inflammatory mediators activate and/or sensitise PMNs [16,17]. These may act either directly via ligand–gated ion channels (e.g. capsaicin and the vanilloid receptor 1, (VR1), or via metabotropic receptors linked to second messenger systems (e.g. bradykinin at the B2 receptor activates intracellular protein kinase C, (PKC). ATP acts via a number of ligand–gated cation channels (P2X receptors) to excite nociceptors, and the $P2X_3$ subtype is expressed selectively in small diameter

Table 19.2 Myths and misperceptions about pain in children

Myths
Infants and children do not experience pain

Misperceptions
Opioid dose escalation should be avoided because:
   tolerance will develop and there will not be drugs available when pain progresses;
   increasing pain relief signifies worsening disease.
Methadone is used only in the drug addicted population
Exposure to opioids will result in drug addiction

non-peptidergic, dorsal root ganglion (DRG) neuron [18]. The pH of injured and inflamed tissue is often low, and protons enhance the responsiveness of VR1 [19,20] and P2X receptors, and also excite nociceptors directly [21]. In addition, a number of acid-sensing ion channels (ASIC1, ASIC2b, and ASIC3) which are selective ligand-gated cation channels, are activated by extracellular acidification [22].

Thermal stimuli The transition from a sensation of warmth, to that of heat pain occurs at approximately 45°C in mammals. This correlates with the threshold for action potential generation in PMNs and a steep increase in firing frequency is seen with further increases in temperature [23]. The transduction mechanism is not dependent on a signal molecule and is not gated by diffusible messengers, and it is likely that heat is signalled through a number of channels [24–26]. The VR1 capsaicin sensitive receptor responds to thermal stimuli in the noxious heat range (>43°C) [27]. The capsaicin-insensitive vanilloid receptor-like protein subtype 1 (VRL1) is activated by temperatures higher than about 52°C, but is most prominently expressed by medium to large-diameter rather than small diameter DRG neurons [27].

Mechanical stimuli With brief noxious mechanical stimuli, the discharge rate of PMNs increases with the force and pressure applied. With repetitive stimulation, temporal or spatial summations of the nociceptive discharge signal the magnitude of sensation [16]. A different subpopulation (mechano-insensitive nociceptors) may also become active with tonic sustained pressure [28]. The transduction mechanism for mechanical stimuli may involve a stretch-activated channel [29].

Once transduced into electrical stimuli, conduction of neuronal action potentials is dependent on voltage gated sodium channels (VGSCs). However, the sodium current from nociceptive afferents reflects activation of a number of distinct ion channels. A rapidly inactivating, fast sodium current which is sensitive to block by tetrodotoxin is present in all sensory neurons. In addition, PMN neurons express TTX-R currents. The channels responsible for TTX-R currents vary in their subtype, distribution and number in different pain states, and represent an endogenous mechanism to modulate excitability [25].

The cell body of C-fibre PMNs resides in the dorsal root ganglion (DRG), and the axon bifurcates into both the peripheral branch that innervates the skin, and a central branch that enters the spinal cord. Two subtypes of DRG cell have been identified: one group synthesizes peptides [substance P (SP); calcitonin gene related peptide (CGRP)], and expresses the high affinity nerve growth factor (NGF) receptor tyrosine kinase A (trkA); while the second group express the purinergic

P2X$_3$ receptor, an IB4-lectin binding site, and receptors for glial derived neurotrophic factor (GDNF) [30,31]. Both groups respond to similar types of noxious stimulation, and synapse within lamina I and II of the dorsal horn.

Following the synapse of the primary afferent neuron with the second order cell body in the dorsal horn, multiple ascending pathways relay pain transmission. Nocispecific fibres from lamina I neurons that express NK$_1$ receptor ascend to the parabrachial area of brainstem, and a large number of fibres (with connections via lamina V) project in the spinothalamic tract [30]. Small diameter afferents have an orderly somatotopic arrangement in which each portion of the skin surface is innervated by afferent fibres that terminate in preferred localities within the dorsal horn [29]. This somatotopic map is maintained by second order neurones within the ascending tracts in the spinal cord, and is finally represented in the somatosensory cortex, thus allowing localisation of the painful stimulus.

Peripheral sensitization

An increase in peripheral noxious stimulus intensity is encoded in PMNs by an increase in action potential firing. Nociceptors must reach a certain discharge frequency (about 0.5 impulses/sec) for pain to be perceived [16]. A progressive increase in primary afferent firing correlates with the level of pain experienced until tissue damage is produced. A subgroup of C fibres (silent nociceptors) that are chemically sensitive, but initially insensitive to mechanical and thermal stimuli, can be recruited following injury [32], and once activated have features of PMNs.

In the presence of inflammation, nociceptors acquire new characteristics and are said to be sensitized [33,34]; that is:

(1) they spontaneously discharge and therefore contribute to the continuing pain following tissue injury;

(2) their threshold for activation is decreased, such that innocuous stimuli may cause pain (*allodynia*) and contribute to the tenderness experienced in an injured region;

(3) their stimulus–response curves are shifted to the left, such that a noxious stimulus causes more pain than normal (*hyperalgesia*). Primary *hyperalgesia* is characterised by a decrease in pain threshold and increased response to supra–threshold stimuli within an area of injury [23].

A number of inflammatory mediators induce peripheral sensitisation in PMNs with a resultant increase in C fibre afferent discharge. Prostaglandins, serotonin and adenosine activate adenylate cyclase and increase cyclic AMP, leading to activation of protein kinase A (PKA). One target for PKA is the TTX-R sodium channel [35]. Phosphorylation of the channel decreases the action potential threshold, increases the activation rate and increases the current magnitude, thus resulting in more rapid depolarisation. In addition, the inactivation rate of the channel is increased, allowing a decrease in inter-spike interval and the potential for increased discharge frequency [36].

Spinal cord mechanisms

The spinal cord is an important site for modulation of pain transmission. The central terminals of C-fibre nociceptors project predominantly to lamina I and II in the superficial dorsal horn of the spinal cord. However, dorsal horn neurones not only receive information via synaptic transfer from primary afferent neurones, but also from interneurons and descending neural pathways. These multiple inputs have both excitatory and inhibitory influences on the subsequent output from the dorsal horn neuron. The nature and amount of transmitter released, the density and identity of pre- and post-synaptic receptors, the kinetics of receptor activation and ion-channel opening and closing, and the rate of removal or breakdown of transmitter can all modify sensory processing in the spinal cord.

Depolarization of the primary afferent terminal results in glutamate release. If the stimulus intensity is high enough, substance P is also released from dense core vesicles [37]. Glutamate receptors are widely distributed throughout the spinal cord dorsal horn [38], and are of three types: the kainate/AMPA (L-amino-3-hydroxy-5-methylsoxasole-propionoc acid) receptor; the ionotropic n-methyl-D-aspartate (NMDA) receptor; and the metabotropic (mGluR) receptor. Fast synaptic currents (tens of milliseconds) mediated by glutamate acting on ionotropic AMPA receptors signal information relating to the location, intensity, and duration of afferent fibre input. In this 'normal mode' where a high intensity stimulus elicits brief localized pain, the sensory processing, and the stimulus–response relationship between afferent input and dorsal horn neuron output is predictable and reproducible [39].

Central sensitization

Ionotropic NMDA receptors are blocked by magnesium under resting conditions. Repeated C-fibre input results in a progressively more depolarised postsynaptic membrane and removal of the magnesium block. Slow currents mediated by glutamate acting on ionotropic NMDA receptors and mGluR, and by substance P acting on neurokinin1 (NK1) receptors, allow temporal and spatial summation of C fibre input [39]. As a result, there is in an amplified response to each subsequent stimulus, and this rapid progressive increase in

dorsal horn neuron responsiveness, during the course of a train of inputs has been termed 'wind-up' [40]. Tissue damage, and persistent primary afferent input also induce more generalized, and long-term changes in the sensitivity of the dorsal horn neuron, termed central sensitisation. Central sensitisation manifests as a reduction in threshold, increase in the responsiveness of dorsal horn neurons, and expansion of the receptive field. This is the result of a number of changes at the primary afferent synapse and within the dorsal horn neuron, which include:

1. Enhanced transmitter release from the pre-synaptic terminal. Glutamate acts on pre-synaptic NMDA and kainate GluR5 receptors, resulting in a positive feedback loop [41,42]. Nitric oxide is synthesised following activation of nitric oxide synthase in the dorsal horn cell, and diffuses back to influence pre-synaptic release [43]. A reduction in pre-synaptic inhibition (via adenosine, serotonin, opioid and GABA) will also increase transmitter release.

2. Increased post-synaptic depolarisation and activation of intracellular cascades. Ongoing activation of ionotropic NMDA receptors, voltage gated calcium channels, and metabotropic mGluR and NK_1 receptors results in an increase in intracellular calcium, both via calcium inflow, and release from intracellular stores. A number of enzyme cascades are subsequently activated via PKC, PKA and mitogen–activated kinase (MAPK) [17,39]. Phosphorylation of the NMDA receptor further reduces the voltage-dependent Mg block and enhances the channel kinetics [38]. These post-translational changes increase the basal sensitivity of dorsal horn neurons, and result in hyperalgesia that extends beyond the site of the initiating stimulus [17]. This surrounding zone of secondary mechanical hyperalgesia occurs in uninjured tissue, and is dependent on both spinal and supraspinal mechanisms.

3. Activation of transcription factors, with resultant changes in gene and protein expression. Increased PKC is associated with increased expression and insertion of AMPA receptors into the post-synaptic membrane of DH neurons [44]. Changes occurring in DRG and DH neurons often act together. For example, production of substance P increases in DRG neurons and is matched by an increased expression of NK_1 receptors in dorsal horn cells [39]. NGF is upregulated in peripheral inflamed tissues, and increases the firing rate of nociceptors. NGF is also retrogradely transported to the DRG of trkA expressing C fibre nociceptors, and contributes to upregulation of TTX-R channels and VR1 receptors, which further increases excitability [31]. Brain-derived neurotrophic

factor (BDNF) is also upregulated in DRG neurones in the presence of NGF and inflammation [45]. BDNF transport to the dorsal horn increases [46], leading to increased phosphorylation of the NMDA receptor and potentiation of C-fibre mediated spinal reflexes [45,47]. These changes contribute to longer-term alterations in the relationship between the peripheral stimulus and the dorsal horn neuron response.

The area of tissue that responds to an applied stimulus and generates a neural response within a nerve fibre is described as its receptive field. Each primary afferent, branches on to many central cells (divergence), and dorsal horn neurons receive inputs from many primary afferents (convergence). Therefore, the receptive field of dorsal horn neurones is relatively large and complex, but each central neuron has its own unique temporal and spatial input of activity. Receptive fields can be altered by persistent afferent input [48], with increases in the spatial extent of the receptive field and recruitment of previously subthreshold components. In the presence of inflammation and increased central excitability, cells in the superficial dorsal horn of the rat spinal cord that are normally nociceptive specific respond to low threshold primary afferent mechanoreceptors [49]. This effect is mediated via increased N-methyl-D-aspartate (NMDA) receptor activity as the increase in dorsal horn neuron receptive field size induced by C-fibre stimulation can be blocked by NMDA antagonist [50]. NMDA-receptor antagonists depress central sensitisation in both laboratory and clinical studies [51–54]. Dextromethorphan, dextrorphan, ketamine, memantine and amantadine, among others have been shown to have NMDA-receptor antagonist activities. The clinical usefulness of some of these medications is compromised by an adverse effect to side effect ratio.

Inhibitory mechanisms

As a result of inhibitory modulation, dorsal horn neurones can also reduce their output with time. Inhibitory effects within the dorsal horn can be activated by a large number of mechanisms that include: non-nociceptive peripheral inputs; local interneuronal fibres with inhibitory transmitters glycine and GABA; descending bulbospinal noradrenergic, serotonergic, and opioid projections; and higher order brain function (distraction, cognitive input etc.). Descending pathways from the brainstem modulate pain transmission in the spinal cord [55,56]. Activation of presynaptic inhibitory receptors (e.g. mu and delta opioid, alpha-2 adrenergic) reduces transmitter release. Post-synaptic inhibitory receptors on the dorsal horn neuron (e.g. mu, delta and kappa opioid, adenosine, GABA) reduce the excitation evoked by

Table 19.3 How do humans experience pain?

Peripheral mechanisms vary according to input from:
     Chemical stimuli
     Thermal stimuli
     Mechanical stimuli

In the presence of inflammation, nociceptors acquire new characteristics and are said to be *sensitized*
The spinal cord is an important site for pain transmission and modulation
The rapid, progressive increase in dorsal horn neuron responsiveness during the course of a train of inputs is termed *wind-up*
Dorsal horn neurons can reduce their output with time as a result of inhibitory modulation

glutamate via a G-protein coupled increase in potassium conductance that hyperpolarizes the membrane [57]. Opioids reduce the slope of the intensity-response curve, and diminish the magnitude of the response evoked in the dorsal horn by C-fibre activity [58]. These inhibitory mechanisms are activated endogenously to reduce the excitatory responses to persistent C-fibre activity [59], and are also targets for exogenous analgesic agents [60].

A unique and different set of neurochemical changes occurs in the spinal cord and the DRGs as a result of inflammatory, neuropathic, and cancer pain states and many of these changes might be involved in generating or maintaining each pain state and might potentially influence therapeutics. For example, it is known clinically that chronic inflammatory pain, cancer pain, and neuropathic pain are best treated with different types of analgesia. While there is a significant upregulation of substance P and CGRP in the dorsal horn in inflammation, these same neurotransmitters are downregulated in neuropathic pain states. In metastatic bone pain there is no changes in these neurotransmitters [61]. The greatest change observed in the spinal cord in response to metastatic bone cancer pain is the upregulation of glial fibrillary acidic protein (GFAP) which is significantly greater than that induced by neuropathic pain (Table 19.3).

Development and changes in nociceptive processing

The reader is referred to previous reviews of the impact of the developing nervous system on nociceptive processing and response to tissue injury [62,63].

Peripheral mechanisms of nociception

C-fibre polymodal nociceptors are mature in their pattern of firing at birth, and are capable of being activated by exogenous stimuli [64]. Although peripheral C fibres are initially less able to produce neurogenic oedema, primary hyperalgesia has been demonstrated in a number of early developmental models [65,66]. Cutaneous withdrawal reflexes can be elicited by low intensity stimuli (that is have lower mechanical and thermal thresholds) early in development as receptive fields are large and inhibitory mechanisms are immature [63]. Developmental changes in the pattern of withdrawal reflexes in rat pups have been correlated with changes in human neonates [67], and the threshold and magnitude of the reflex EMG response correlate with the intensity of the cutaneous stimulus [68]. Similarly, both laboratory and clinical studies have established changes in reflex withdrawal thresholds and the development of hyperalgesia following tissue injury. In neonates, repeated heel prick blood sampling produces primary hyperalgesia in the area of injury with a reduction in the mechanical threshold for limb withdrawal [67] and these changes can be abolished by topical analgesia [69].

Spinal cord nociceptive processing

In the adult, C-fibre polymodal nociceptors project to the superficial dorsal horn (lamina I and II), while larger myelinated A-beta fibres which subserve light touch and pressure project to deeper layers of the dorsal horn (lamina III and IV). Developmentally regulated changes in the functional and anatomical relationships between C and A fibres have significant effects on nociceptive processing. C fibre afferents enter the spinal cord late relative to A fibre innervation [70], and the density of substance P containing fibres in the dorsal horn is initially low. Early in development, A-beta fibres extend up into laminae I and II and only withdraw to the deeper laminae as C fibres mature [71,72]. This initial overlap of terminals contributes to the large receptive fields of dorsal horn neurones in early development. Electrical stimulation of the hindpaw at C fibre strength does not evoke post-synaptic activity in dorsal horn cells in the first postnatal week [73], although this does not exclude the presence of subthreshold responses.

Recordings from spinal cord slices confirm that capsaicin increases glutamate release at synapses in the superficial dorsal horn during the first postnatal week, although the frequency of miniature excitatory postsynaptic currents is less at postnatal day (P) 1–5 than at P9–10 [74]. From P10, repetitive C fibre stimulation at three times the C fibre threshold produces 'wind-up', but is observed in an increased proportion of cells with further increases in age. Sensitisation can be observed early in development, but is produced by repeated A fibre (rather than C fibre) stimulation which evokes activity in both superficial and deep laminae at P3 [73].

Mechanisms of central sensitisation and secondary hyperalgesia differ according to age, as there are developmental changes in the dorsal horn responses evoked by C or A fibre stimulation, alterations in NMDA receptor distribution and function, and variable maturation of post-synaptic intracellular cascades. NMDA receptor activation is an important component of central sensitisation, and this receptor is present throughout the gray matter of the dorsal horn in a higher concentration and more generalised distribution early in development [75]. In addition, the receptor has a higher binding affinity for NMDA, and activation results in a greater influx of calcium ions [76] during the first postnatal week. This may relate to changes in the sub-unit composition of the receptor, as increased NR2A subunit expression increases channel open time and ion flow in developing neocortex [77]. A proportion of NMDA receptors in the developing spinal cord have been considered to be "silent" as they are not co-localised with AMPA receptors, but repetitive stimulation can drive action potential firing and affect neuron excitability in the absence of AMPA [78]. The influx of calcium ions following NMDA receptor channel opening activates a number of intracellular enzyme cascades, which further modulate activity. Nitric oxide synthase expression does not reach adult levels in lamina II until P20, and this parallels a delay in the development of c-fos expression in response to peripheral mustard oil application [79].

Descending inhibitory pathways and diffuse noxious inhibitory controls are not functional in the first two postnatal weeks in rat pups [80,81]. Descending fibres are present in the dorsolateral funiculus, but initially do not extend collateral branches into the dorsal horn. Inhibition of dorsal horn cell responses by stimulation of the dorsolateral funiculus is not present until P10–12, and until P22–24 is only activated by high-intensity stimulation [80]. Stimulus-produced analgesia from the peri–acqueductal gray is also not effective until P21 [82]. In addition, local interneuronal inhibitory mechanisms are initially immature, and GABA has excitatory rather than

Table 19.4 Development and changes in nociceptive processing
C-fibre polymodal nociceptors are mature in their pattern of firing at birth
Mechanisms of central sensitization and secondary hyperalgesia differ according to age
In early development there is/are: A relative excess of excitatory pain mechanisms Large receptive fields Immaturity of the inhibitory pain mechanisms A more generalized response to lower intensity pain stimuli

inhibitory actions early in development [83]. Therefore in early development, there is a relative excess of excitatory mechanisms, immature inhibitory mechanisms, and large receptive fields, which contribute to more generalized responses to lower intensity pain stimuli (Table 19.4).

From laboratory to bedside: the mode of action of opioids, NMDA antagonists, antidepressants, and anticonvulsants

Opioids

It is now recognized that opioid actions are subject to changes within the nervous system ('plasticity'), and also modulation by a number of other transmitters, which may enhance or decrease the action of exogenous opioids. Opioid analgesia may be decreased by anti-opioid peptides such as CCK and F8a, or by activity of excitatory amino acids on the NMDA receptor [84]. Degeneration and loss of pre-synaptic opioid receptors following nerve damage will reduce opioid responsiveness, but this should be overcome by titration of opioid and dose escalation [85] as supraspinal sites of action will not be affected by primary afferent damage.

Hyperalgesia and morphine tolerance are interrelated at the level of NMDA receptor activation in the dorsal horn of the spinal cord. Post-synaptic mu opioid receptor activation by an exogenous ligand such as morphine may mediate protein kinase C activation, leading to removal of the magnesium blockade and allowing activation of the NMDA receptor. It has been proposed that exogenous opioid administration may result not only in tolerance, but also lead to hyperalgesia by increasing the efficacy of NMDA-receptor activated calcium channels [86]. Clinically, hyperalgesia has developed following high doses of morphine administered orally, parenterally [87] and intrathecally [88]. Therefore, escalation to massive doses of opioids in patients with pain may not always be appropriate, and alternative routes of administration, or alternative drugs may be preferable. Similar excitatory amino acid receptor-mediated cellular and intracellular mechanisms have also been implicated in the development of morphine tolerance [86].

Early research suggested that a subtype of mu receptor agonist may improve analgesia without associated respiratory depression, but this has not been supported by subsequent studies. Endorphins, enkephalins, and dynorphins are endogenous opioid peptides which bind with only low to moderate specificity to the mu, delta and kappa opioid receptors. Recently, two peptides (endomorphin-1 and endomorphin-2)

have been identified in mammalian brain and have the highest specificity and affinity for the mu receptor of any endogenous substance so far described [89]. Cloning of opioid receptors led to the recognition of a novel G-protein coupled opioid-like receptor. Nociceptin/orphinan FQ, a 17 amino acid peptide resembling dynorphin, acts as a potent endogenous ligand of the opioid receptor-like 1 (ORL$_1$) receptor. The ORL$_1$ receptor is expressed widely in the nervous system [90]. The actions of nociceptin/orphinan FQ are site specific and in animal studies hyperalgesia and opioid antagonism was demonstrated at supraspinal sites, while analgesia was shown at spinal sites [91]. Its efficacy varies in neuropathic and inflammatory models [92]. The clinical application of these findings is yet unclear, but they may provide tools for further elucidation of nociceptive pathways [93], and the development of more specific opioid agonists.

NMDA antagonists

NMDA receptor antagonists have been shown to prevent and reverse opioid tolerance, reduce opioid withdrawal effects, and may have a role in patients whose pain is inadequately controlled with high dose opioids [94]. Therefore, clinically useful NMDA antagonists with a reduced side-effect profile would have potential advantages in combination with opioids for the management of chronic pain [95].

The NMDA receptor clearly has an important role in pain transmission, and NMDA receptor antagonists reduce the effects of wind-up and central sensitisation. Ketamine, a non-competitive NMDA antagonist, has analgesic effects at subanaesthetic doses, but its use remains limited by psychomimetic side-effects. Preoperative administration of small doses of ketamine has been shown to improve postoperative analgesia [96], reduce opioid requirements [97], and reduce postoperative wound hyperalgesia [97,98]. Ketamine has also been shown to benefit patients with chronic neuropathic pain [99,100], and cancer pain. Currently available oral agents with NMDA antagonist activity, such as dextromethorphan and memantine, appear to have limited efficacy [101,102], but further studies are required to determine dose ranges. More specific NMDA receptor antagonists with improved side-effect profiles are required.

Antidepressants

Antidepressants potentiate the effect of biogenic amines in endogenous analgesic systems. The efficacy in neuropathic pain may rely on both noradrenergic and serotonergic effects, as the specific serotonin reuptake blocker fluoxetine was no more effective than placebo [103]; and paroxetine and mianserin were less effective than imipramine in adult studies

[104]. Controlled trials supports a moderate effect for tricyclic antidepressant drugs in neuropathic pain which is not selective for the nature or quality of the pain. Pain relief is independent of their action on mood as the analgesic effect occurs at a lower dose and with more rapid onset than mood effects, and the analgesic efficacy is similar in depressed and non-depressed patients [105].

Anticonvulsants

The mode of action of the anticonvulsants is sodium channel blockade which suppresses ectopic neural firing and may offer relief from neuropathic pain. Anticonvulsants such as carbamazepine and sodium valproate have a long history of use for trigeminal neuralgia and other neuropathic pain states. Newer anticonvulsant drugs such as gabapentin [106,107] and lamotrigine [108], may have improved side-effect profiles but this remains to be confirmed by controlled trials in a larger number of patients.

Conclusion

Pain is a common symptom in dying children. Fears and concerns surrounding its management are often based on myths and misperceptions. The mechanisms by which pain is perceived in infants, children, and adolescents and the consequences of improperly managed pain is increasingly being understood. The changes in pharmacokinetic *and* pharmacodynamic parameters with development suggest that clinical analgesic administration should take into consideration the type of pain, weight and clinical status of the child, and also his/her developmental stage. In addition, genetic factors contribute to responses to opioid agonists. This variability emphasises the importance of ongoing assessment of pain, and adjustment of analgesic regimes according to individual needs. This developing body of knowledge combined with a greater understanding of the developmental aspects of analgesia may lead to improved palliative analgesic therapeutics in the future.

References

1. Merskey, H. and Bogduk, N., (ed.) Classification of Chronic Pain: Description of Chronic Pain Syndromes and Definitions of Pain Terms. Seattle: IASP Press; 1994.
2. Anand, K.J.S., Craig, K.D. New perspectives in the definition of pain. *Pain* 1996;67:3–6.
3. Merskey, H. Some features of the history of the idea of pain. *Pain* 1980; 9:3–8.
4. Bonica, J.J. *The Management of Pain*. Washington: Lea and Febiger, 1990.
5. Brown, D.L., Fink, R.B. In M.J. Counsins, P.O. Bridenbaugh, eds. *Neural Blockade in Clinical Anesthesia and Management of Pain* (3rd ed), Philadelphia PA: Lippincott-Raven *The History of Neural Blockade and Pain Management*, 1998; pp. 3–27.
6. Melzack, R.A. and Wall, P.D. Pain mechanisms: A new theory. *Science* 1965;150:971–9.
7. Nathan, P.W. The gate control theory of pain: A critical review. *Brain* 1976;99:123–58.
8. Drake, R., Frost, J., Collins, J.J. The symptoms of dying children. *J Pain and Symptom Manage* 2003;27(7):6–10.
9. Anand, K.J., Hansen, D.D., Hickey, P.R. Hormonal metabolic stress response in neonates undergoing surgery. *Anesthesiology* 1990;73:661–70.
10. Porter, J. and Lick, J. Addiction is rare in patients treated with narcotics [letter]. *N Eng J Med* 1980;302:123.
11. Shortland, P. and Fitzgerald, M. Neonatal sciatic nerve section results in a rearrangement of the central terminals of saphenous and axotomized sciatic nerve afferents in the dorsal horn of the spinal cord of the adult rat. *Eur J Neurosci* 1994;6:75–86.
12. Ruda, M.A., Ling, Q.D., Hohmann, A.G. *et al*. Altered nociceptive neuronal circuits after neonatal peripheral inflammation. *Science* 2000;289:628–30.
13. Walker, S., Meredith-Middleton, J., Cooke-Yarborough, C., Fitzgerald, M. Neonatal inflammation and primary afferent terminal plasticity in the rat dorsal horn. *Pain* 2003, (in press)
14. Grunau, R.E. Anand, K.J., Stevens, B.J., and McGrath, P.J. eds. Pain Research and Clinical Management. Amsterdam: Elsevier; 2000; Long-term consequences of pain in human neonates, p. 55–76.
15. Dostrovsky, J.O., Carr, D. B., and Koltzenburg, M. eds. *The Role of Activity in Developing Pain Pathways*. Seattle: IASP Press; 2003; 185 p. Progress in Pain Research and Management.
16. Raja, S.N., Meyer, R.A., Ringkamp, M. *et al*. Peripheral neural mechanisms of nociception In P.D. Wall and R.Melzack (eds). *Textbook of Pain* (4th edition) Churchill Livingstone, pp. 11–57.
17. Woolf, C.J., and Costigan, M. Transcriptional and post-translational plasticity and the generation of inflammatory pain. *Proc Natl Acad Sci USA* 1999;(96):7723–30.
18. Burnstock, G. P2X receptors in sensory neurones. *Br J Anaesthesia* 2000;84:476–88.
19. Caterina, M.J., Leffler, A., Malmberg, A.B. *et al*. Impaired nociception and pain sensation in mice lacking the capsaicin receptor. *Science* 2000;288:306–13.
20. Davis, J.B., Gray, J., Gunthorpe, M.J. *et al*. Vanilloid receptor-1 is essential for inflammatory thermal hyperalgesia. *Nature* 2000;405:183–7.
21. Carpenter, K.J., Nandi, M., and Dickenson, A.H. Peripheral administration of low pH solutions causes activation and sensitisation of convergent dorsal horn neurones in the anaesthetised rat. *Neurosci Lett* 2001;298:179–82.
22. Waldmann, R., and Lazdunski, M. H(+)-gated cation channels: neuronal acid sensors in the NaC/DEG family of ion channels. *Curr Opin Neurobiol* 1998 8:418–24.
23. Treede, R.D., Meyer, R.A., Raja, S.N., Campbell, J.N. Peripheral and central mechanisms of cutaneous hyperalgesia. *Prog Neurobiol* 1992;38:397–421.
24. Cesare, P., Moriondo, A., Vellani, V., McNaughton, P.A. Ion channels gated by heat. *Proc Natl Acad Sci USA* 1999;96:7658–63.
25. McCleskey, E.W., and Gold, M.S. Ion channels of nociception. *Annu Rec Physiol* 1999;61:835–56.

26. Reichling, D.B., and Levine, J.D. In hot pursuit of the elusive heat transducers. *Neuron* 2000;26:555–8.

27. Caterina, M.J., Rosen, T.A., Tominaga, M. *et al.* A capsaicin-receptor homologue with a high threshold for noxious heat. *Nature* 1999;398:436–41.

28. Schmidt, R., Schmelz, M., Torebjork, H.E., and Handwerker, H.O. Mechano-insensitive nociceptors encode pain evoked by tonic pressure to human skin. *Neuroscience* 2000;98:793–800.

29. Swett, J.E. and Woolf C.J. The somatotopic organization of primary afferent terminals in the superficial laminae of the dorsal horn of the rat spinal cord. *J Comp Neurol* 1985;231:66–77.

30. Hunt, S.P., and Mantyh, P.W. The molecular dynamics of pain control. *Nature Reviews (neuroscience)* 2001;2:83–91.

31. McMahon, S.B. and Bennett, D.L.H. Trophic factors and pain. In P.D., Wall, R. Melzack (eds). *Textbook of Pain.* (4th edition). Churchill Livingstone; 1999; pp. 105–27.

32. Xu, G.Y., Huang, L.Y., and Zhao, Z.Q. Activation of silent mechanoreceptive cat C and A sensory neurons and their substance P expression following peripheral inflammation. *J Physiol* 2000;528:339–48.

33. Bennett, G.J. Update on the neurophysiology of oain transmission and modulation: focus on the NMDA-receptor. *Journal of Pain and Symptom Management* 2000;19 (Suppl.):S2–S6.

34. Andrew, D. and Greenspan, J.D. Mechanical and heat sensitization of cutaneous nociceptors after peripheral inflammation in the rat. *J Neurophysiol* 1999;82:2649–56.

35. Akopian, A.N, Souslova, V., England, S. *et al.* The tetrodotoxin-resistant sodium channel SNS has a specialized function in pain pathways. *Nat Neurosci* 1994;2:541–8.

36. Gold, M.S. Tetrodotoxin-resistant Na+ currents and inflammatory hyperalgesia. *Proc Natl Acad Sci USA* 1999;96:7645–9.

37. Cao, Y., Mantyh, P.W., Carlson, E.J. *et al.* Primary afferent tachykinins are required to experience moderate to intense pain. *Nature,* 1998;392(390):394.

38. Yung, K.K. Localization of glutamate receptors in dorsal horn of rat spinal cord. *Neuroreport* 1998;9:1639–44.

39. Woolf, C.J. and Salter, M.W. Neuronal plasticity: Increasing the gain in pain. *Science* 2000;288:1765–9.

40. Herrero, J.F., Laird, J.M.A., and Lopez-Garcia, J.A. Wind-up of spinal cord neurones and pain sensation: much ado about something? *Progress in Neurobiology* 2000;61:169–203.

41. Stanfa, L.C. and Dickenson, A.H. The role of non-N-methyl-D-aspartate ionotropic glutamate receptors in the spinal transmission of nociception in normal animals and animals with carrageenan inflammation. *Neuroscience* 1999;93:1391–8.

42. Liu, H., Mantyh, P.W., and Basbaum, and AI. NMDA-receptor regulation of substance P release from primary afferent nociceptors. *Nature* 1997;386:721–4.

43. Meller, S.T., and Gebhart, G.F. Nitric oxide (NO) and nociceptive processing in the spinal cord. *Pain* 1993;52:127–36.

44. Li, P., Kerchner, G.A., Sala, C. *et al.* AMPA receptor–PDZ interactions in facilitation of spinal sensory synapses. *Nature Neurosci* 1999;2(972):977.

45. Kerr, B.J., Bradbury, E.J., Bennett, D.L. *et al.* Brain-derived neurotrophic factor modulates nociceptive sensory inputs and NMDA-evoked responses in the rat spinal cord. *J Neurosci* 1999;19:5138–48.

46. Cho, H.J., Kim, J.K., Zhou, X.F., and Rush, R.A. Increased brain-derived neurotrophic factor immunoreactivity in rat dorsal root ganglia and spinal cord following peripheral inflammation. *Brain Res* 1997;764:269–72.

47. Mannion, R.J., Costigan, M., Decosterd, I. *et al.* Neurotrophins: Peripherally and centrally acting modulators of tactile stimulus-induced inflammatory pain hypersensitivity. Proc *Natl Acad Sci USA* 1999;96:9385–90.

48. Woolf, C.J., and King, A.E. Dynamic alterations in the cutaneous mechanoreceptive fields of dorsal horn neurons in the rat spinal cord. *J Neurosci* 1990;10:2717–26.

49. Woolf, C.J., Shortland, P., and Sivilotti, L.G. Sensitization of high mechanothreshold superficial dorsal horn and flexor motor neurones following chemosensitive primary afferent activation. *Pain* 1994;58:141–55.

50. Dickenson, A.H., and Sullivan, A.F. Evidence for a role of the NMDA receptor in the frequency dependent potentiation of deep rat dorsal horn nociceptive neurones following C fibre stimulation. *Neuropharmacology* 1987;26:1235–8.

51. Eide, P.K., Jorum, E., Stubhaug, A., *et al.* Relief of post-herpetic neuralgia with the N-methyl-D-aspartic acid receptor antagonist ketamine: A double-blind cross-over comparison with morphine an dplacebo. *Pain* 1994;58:347–54.

52. Persson, J., Axelsson, G., Hallin, R.G., *et al.* Beneficial effects of ketamine in a chronic pain state with allodynia. *Pain* 1995;60:217–22.

53. Nelson, K.A., Park, K.M., Robinovitz, E., *et al.* High dose dextromethorphan versus placebo in painful diabetic neuropathy and postherpetic neuralgia. *Neurology* 1997;48:1212–8.

54. Eisenberg, E. and Pud, D. Can patients with chronic neuropathic pain be cured by acute administration of the NMDA-receptor antagonist amantadine? *Pain* 1994;74:37–9.

55. Millan, M.J. Descending control of pain. *Prog Neurobiol* 2002 66:355–474.

56. Ren. K., and Dubner. R. Descending modulation in persistent *pain* An update. *Pain* 2002;100:1–6.

57. Yaksh. T.L. Cental Pharmalcology of nocieptive transmission In P.D. Wall, and R., Melzack eds. *Textbook of Pain*, London: Churchill Livingstone, 1999; pp. 253–308.

58. Jones, S.L. and Gebhart, G.F. Inhibition of spinal nociceptive transmission from the midbrain, pons and medulla in the rat: Activation of descending inhibition by morphine, glutamate and electrical stimulation. *Brain* 1998;460:281–96.

59. Chapman, V., Diaz, A., and Dickenson, A.H. Distinct inhibitory effects of spinal endomorphin-1 and endomorphin-2 on evoked dorsal horn neuronal responses in the rat. *Br J Pharmacol* 1997;122:1537–9.

60. Reeve, A.J. and Dickenson, A.H. Electrophysiological study on spinal antinociceptive interactions between adenosine and morphine in the dorsal horn of the rat 1995;194:81–4.

61. Giamberardino, M.A. ed. *Understanding the Neurobiology of Chronic Pain: Molecular and Cellular.* Seattle: IASP Press 2002; p. 237

62. Fitzgerald, M., and Howard, R.F. The neuroiological basis of pediatric pain. In N.L. Schechter, C.B. Berde, M. Yaster eds. *Pain in Infants, Children, and Adolescents* (2nd edition), Philadelphia, PA: Lippincott Williams and Wilkins 2003; Vol.2 pp. 19–42.

63. Fitzgerald, M. K.J., Anand. B.J., Stevens. P.J., McGrath. eds. Pain in Neonates (2nd edition). Amsterdam: Elsevier; Development of the peripheral and spinal pain system 2000;pp. 9–22.

64. Fitzgerald, M. Cutaneous primary afferent properties in the hindlimb of the neonatal rat. *J Physiol* 1987;383:79–92.

65. Koltzenburg, M., and Lewin, G.R. Receptive properties of embryonic chick sensory neurons innervating skin. *J Neurophysiol* 1997; 78:2560–8.

66. Walker, S., Howard, R.F., and Fitzgerald, M. Effect of developmental age on mustard oil-induced primary and secondary hyperalgesia. [Abstract] 6th International Symposium on Paediatric Pain 2003;156:91.

67. Fitzgerald, M., Shaw, A., and MacIntosh, N. The postnatal development of the cutaneous flexor reflex: A comparative study in premature infants and newborn rat pups. Dev Med Child *Neurol* 1988; 30:520–6.

68. Andrews, K.A., and Fitzgerald, M. The cutaneous flexion reflex in human neonates: A quantitative study of threshold and stimulus/response characteristics, following single and repeated stimuli. *Dev Med Child Neurol* 1999;41:696–703.

69. Fitzgerald, M., Millard, C., and McIntosh, N. Cutaneous hypersensitivity following peripheral tissue damage in newborn infants and its reversal with topical anaesthesia. *Pain* 1989;39:31–6.

70. Jackman, A., and Fitzgerald, M. Development of peripheral hindlimb and central spinal cord innervation by subpopulations of dorsal root ganglion cells in the embryonic rat. *J Comp Neurol* 2000;418:281–98.

71. Beggs, S., Torsney, C., Drew L.J., and Fitzgerald, M. The postnatal reorganization of primary afferent input and dorsal horn cell receptive fields in the rat spinal cord is an activity-dependent process. *Nueroscience* 2002;16:1249–58.

72. Fitzgerald, M., Butcher T., and Shortland, P. Developmental changes in the laminar termination of A-fibre cutaneous sensory afferents in the rat spinal cord dorsal horn. 1994;348:225–33.

73. Jennings, E. and Fitzgerald, M. Postnatal changes in responses of rat dorsal horn cells to afferent stimulation: a fibre-induced sensitization. *J Physiol* 2003;509(3):859–68.

74. Baccei, M.L., Bardoni, R., and Fitzgerald, M. Development of nociceptive synaptic inputs to the neonatal rat dorsal horn: Glutamate release by capsaicin and menthol. *J Physiol* 2003;549:231–42.

75. Gonzalez, D.L., Fuchs. J.L, and Droge, M.H. Distribution of NMDA receptor binding in developing mouse spinal cord. *Neurosci Lett* 1993;151:134–7.

76. Hori, Y., and Kanda, K. Developmental alterations in NMDA receptor-mediated [Ca2+]i elevation in substantia gelatinosa neurons of neonatal rat spinal cord. *Dev Brain Res* 1994;80:141–8.

77. Flint, A.C., Maisch, U.S., Weishaupt, J.H., Kriegstein, A.R., and Monyer, H. NR2A subunit expression shortens NMDA receptor synaptic currents in developing neocortex. *Neuroscience* 1997;17:2469–76.

78. Bardoni, R., Magherini, P.C., and MacDermott, A.B. Activation of NMDA receptors drives action potentials in superficial dorsal horn from neonatal rats. *Neuroreport* 2000;11:1721–7.

79. Soyguder, Z., Schmidt, H.H., and Morris, R. Postnatal development of nitric oxide synthase type 1 expression in the lumbar spinal cord of the rat: A comparison with the induction of c-fos in response to peripheral application of mustard oil. 1994;180:188–92.

80. Fitzgerald, M, and Koltzenburg, M. The functional development of descending inhibitory pathways in the dorsolateral funiculus of the newborn rat spinal cord. *Brain* 1986;389:261–70.

81. Boucher, T., Jennings, E., and Fitzgerald, M. The onset of diffuse noxious inhibitory controls in postnatal rat pups: A C-Fos study. 1998;257:9–12.

82. van Praag, H., and Frenk, H. The development of stimulation-produced analgesia (SPA) in the rat. *Brain Research* 1991;64:71–6.

83. Ben-Ari, Y. Excitatory actions of GABA during development: the nature of the nurture. *Nat Rev Neurosci* 2002;3:728–39.

84. Dickenson, A.H. Where and how do opioids act? In G.F., Gebhart. D.L., Hammond. and T.S., Jensen eds. *Proceedings of the 7th World Congress on Pain.* Seattle: IASP Press 1994, pp. 525–52.

85. Portenoy, R.K., Foley, K.M., and Inturrisi, C.E. The nature of opioid responsiveness and its implications for neuropathic pain: New hypotheses derived from studies of opioid infusions. *Pain* 1990; 43:273–86.

86. Mao, J, Price, D.D., and Mayer, D.J. Mechanisms of hyperalgesia and morphine tolerance: a current view of their possible interactions. *Pain* 1995;62:259–74.

87. Sjorgen, P, Jensen, N.H., and Jensen, T.S. Disappearance of morphine-induced hyperalgesia after discontinuing or substituting morphine with other opioid agonists. *Pain* 1994;59:313–6.

88. De Conno, F., Caraceni, A., Martini, C., Spoldi. E., Salvetti M., and myoclonus with intathecal infusion of high-dose morphine. *Pain* 1991;47:129–33.

89. Zadina, J.E., Hackler, L., Ge L.J., and Kastin, A.J. A potent and selective endogenous agonist for the mu-opiate receptor. *Nature* 1997; 386:499–501.

90. Darland, T., Heinricher, M.M., and Grandy, D.K. Prphinan FQ/nociceptin: A role in pain and analgesia, but so much more. *Trends Neurosci* 1998;21:215–21.

91. Yamamoto, T., Nozaki-Taguchi, N., Kimura, S. Effects of intrathecally administered nociception, an opioid receptor-like 1 (ORL 1) agonist on the thermal hyperalgesia induced by unilateral constriction injury to the sciatic nerve in the rat. 1997;224:107–10.

92. Hao, J.X., Xu, I.S., Wiesenfeld-Hallin, Z, and Xu, X.J. Anti-hyperalgesic and anti-allodynic effects of intrathecal nociceptin/orphinan FQ in rats after spinal cord injury, peripheral nerve injury and inflammation. *Pain* 1998;76:385–93.

93. King, M.A., Rossi, G.C., Chang, A.H., Williams, L., and Pasternak, G.W. Spinal analgesic activity of orphinan FQ/nociceptin and its fragments. 1997;223:113–6.

94. Walker, S. and Cousins, M.J. Reduction in hyperalgesia and intrathecal morphine requirements by low-dose ketamine infusion. *Journal of Pain and Symptom Management* 1997;14:129–33.

95. Wiesenfeld-Hallin, Z. Combined opioid-NMDA antagonist therapies. What advantages do they offer for the control of pain syndromes? *Drugs* 1998;55:1–4.

96. Barbieri, M., Colnaghi, E., Tommasino, C., *et al.* In T.S. Jensen, J.A. Turner, Z.Wiesenfeld-Hallin, eds. *Progress in Pain Research and Management.* Seattle: IASP Press; Efficacy of the NMDA antagonist ketamine in preemptive analgesia. 1997, pp. 343–9.

97. Tverskoy, M., Oz, Y., Isakson A., Finger, J., Bradley, E.L., and Kissin, I. (1994) Preemptive effect of fentanyl and ketamine on postoperative pain and wound hyperalgesia. *Anaesth Analg* 78:205–9.

98. Stubhaug, A., Breivik, H., Eide, P.K., *et al.* (1997). Ketamine reduces postoperative hyperalgesia. In T.S. Jensen, J.A. Turner, Wiesenfeld-Hallin Z., eds. *Progress in Pain Research.* Seattle: IASP Press pp. 333–42.

99. Rabben, T., Skjelbred, P., and Oye, I. Prolonged analgesic effect of ketamine, and N-methyl-D-aspartate receptor inhibitor in pateinst with chronic pain. *J Pharmacol Exp Ther* 289:1060–6.

100. Nikolajsen, L., Hansen, C.L., *et al*. The effect of ketamine on phantom pain: a central neuropathic disorder maintained by peripheral input. *Pain* 1996;67:69–77.

101. Mercadante, S., Casuccio, A., and Genovese, G. Ineffectiveness of dextromethorphan in cancer pain. *Journal of Pain and Symptom Management* 1998;16:317–22.

102. Grace, R.F., Power, I., Umedaly. H., *et al*. Preoperative dextromethorphan reduces intraoperative but not postoperative morphine requirements after laparotomy. *Anesth Analg* 1998;87:1135–8.

103. Max, M., Lynch, S.A., Muir, J., Shoaf, S.E., Smoller, B., and Dubner, R. Effects of desipramine, amitriptyline, and fluoxetine on pain in diabetic neuropathy. *N Eng J Med* 326:1250–6.

104. McQuay, H.J, Tramer, M, Nye, B.A., *et al*. A systematic review of antidepressants in neuropathic pain. *Pain* 68:217–27.

105. Max, M.B. Anhelepresants as analgesics. In H.L, Fields J.C. Liebeskind eds. Progress in Pain Research and Pain Management. Seattle: IASP Press; pp. 229–46.

106. Rosenberg, J.M., Harrell, C., and Ristic, H. The effect of gabapentin on neuropathic pain. *Clin J Pain* 1997;13:251–5.

107. Rowbotham, M., Harden, N., Stacey, B., Bernstein, P., and Magnus-Miller, L., Gabapentin for the treatment of postherpetic neuralgia: a randomized controlled trial. *JAMA* 1998;280:1837–42.

108. Canavero, S, and Bonicalzi, V. Lamotrigine control of central pain. *Pain* 1996;68:179–81.

20 Pain: Assessment

Anne Hunt

If we are concerned to discover and ameliorate unacknowledged instances of suffering in the world, we must study creatures' lives, not their brains. What happens in their brains is of course highly relevant as a rich source of evidence about what they are doing and how they do it, but what they are doing is in the end just as visible—to a trained observer—as the activities of plants, mountain streams, or internal combustion engines. If we fail to find suffering in the lives we can see (studying them diligently, using all the methods of science), we can rest assured that there is no invisible suffering somewhere in their brains. If we find suffering, we will recognise it without difficulty. It is all too familiar.[1]

This chapter examines pain assessment within a philosophical and social context. Models of pain are introduced that impact on our understanding of pain as perceived by both the pain sufferer and the observer of the other's pain. A social model of pain is identified whereby pain is not viewed as purely subjective but as an experience that has subjective, objective and inter-subjective criteria. Viewed from an intersubjective or social perspective, observers can come to know another's pain. This intersubjective perspective is in turn supported by the idea of 'pain assessment'. Whilst communication of pain from one individual to another is not necessarily straightforward, it can be assisted by the use of pain assessment tools. Several such tools are introduced that may assist in the assessment of pain in children with life-limiting conditions. Their use is discussed in relation to the developmental and disease status of children with potentially life-limiting conditions.

In 1986, Neil Schecter wrote about the under-treatment of pain in children and about the incorrect assumptions that can be held or inappropriate myths that may be believed [2]. He wrote of the inadequacies in training and research and of the complexities of pain assessment in children. Nearly 20 years on, we have seen improvements, particularly in relation to the attention given to pain in the infant, and the assessment and management of acute pain, but we still have some way to go, especially in developing our approaches to pain assessment for children with chronic life-limiting diseases.

In comparison with the attention given to assessment and treatment of acute pain, pain assessment in children with life-limiting and chronic conditions has received relatively little consideration. Of the many chronic conditions suffered by children, pain assessment and management have been matters of primary concern in only a few. These conditions include, for example, pain related to cancer [3–5], rheumatoid arthritis [6,7], and sickle-cell anaemia [8,9]. However, neither pain nor pain assessment has been a primary focus for many of the diagnostic groups for which palliative care approaches are provided or needed. Little is known for instance, or at least little is described in the literature, of the pain experiences of children and young adults with neuromuscular conditions, cystic fibrosis, HIV aids, organ failure, and until recently, progressive and static encephalopathies [10–16]. In many of these conditions, if recognized at all, pain has been seen more as a diagnostic tool or a measure of disease progression than as something worthy of attention and relief in its own right. Kane writes, 'Medical interventions based solely on the diagnosis and treatment of disease, limit the medical care of the severely ill child. Such an approach is particularly detrimental when caring for the terminally ill'.[17]. The relief of pain and suffering is pivotal to achieving the best quality of life for patients and family.

Pains experienced by children with chronic and life-limiting conditions may be related to investigative procedures or treatment, the disease, to disability secondary to the disease process, or it may be coincidental to the disease. Even in conditions that are chronic and life-limiting, pain itself may be both acute and chronic. Whereas acute pain may serve as a warning of injury and tissue damage, this pain may not necessarily be associated with major or persistent changes in lifestyle or relationships. However, chronic pain, which may be persistent or recurrent, is often associated with substantial alterations in behaviour and in relationships. Pain associated with life-limiting disease may have substantial effects on child, family, and professional caregivers [11,14,18,19]. Pain has an effect on both the child and the perceivers of the child's pain. It has a social context, meaning, and impact.

Models of pain

What is pain? Each of us has experienced something that we might call 'pain' [20] and yet we have difficulty in providing a satisfactory definition of what the phenonemon is. Strawson says that whatever pain is, it is what the word 'pain' means [21, p. 215]. For him, and he claims for virtually every human being, it 'is simply a term for a certain class of unpleasant physical sensations, considered entirely independently of any of its behavioural or other publicly observable causes and effects'. Pain can disrupt activities and in some cases can indicate serious disease [22]. Few people desire pain, though some might be less careful to avoid it than others. As defined by the International Association for the Study of Pain (IASP), it is a subjective experience [23–25]. It can claim to be private, for no one else can know my pain [26].

Turk and Okifuji describe three conceptual models of the pain experience [27]. First, a traditional biomedical perspective that assumes a one-to-one relationship between pain and the nociceptive input. This model, however, fails to explain changes in the person's pain perception when, for instance, he or she reassured that the pain does not indicate a serious or malignant condition. Similarly, a one to one relationship between the pain experienced and the nociceptive input is not supported when, as sometimes can occur for instance in low back pain, individuals with no *apparent* tissue damage may report severe pain, whereas others with pathology can be free of pain.

The second model is one that views pain as either physical or mental. The risk of this view is that it creates a 'dualist perspective' of pain, that is it must be one or the other [27]. Wall describes this as the standard response of most doctors to the problem of pain when there is no obvious peripheral pathology [28]. Wall does not argue with the basic premise of a dualist perspective. He suggests, however, that it is arrogant to believe that we currently have the techniques of diagnosis capable of detecting all relevant forms of peripheral pathology. Research in the last 10–15 years has demonstrated that pathology at the periphery is capable of initiating a cascade of changes that may persist in the central nervous system long after the peripheral pathology itself has disappeared. In addition, sensory systems are not dedicated and hard wired but plastic. Whilst they are normally held in a stable state by elaborate dynamic control mechanisms, under certain conditions they can be pushed outside their normal working range into a state in which they oscillate or fire continuously, a state described as 'wind-up' [29]. The hyperalgesia associated with wind-up is accompanied by persisting genetic changes of the spinal cord cells which contribute to the chronification of pain [30,31].

The third model suggested by Turk and Okifuji [27], and the one that they propose, is a model that integrates organic, psychosocial, and functional processes. When a patient presents with a complaint of chronic pain, the clinician needs to address each element that comprises the model.

Alternative though related ways of viewing pain and pain treatment have been described, specifically the 'behavioural'

and the 'cognitive-behavioural' models. The behavioural model is associated largely with the work of Fordyce [32]. Fordyce used the term 'pain behaviour' to refer to behaviours that communicate the experience of pain to the surrounding environment [33]. The concept of pain behaviour as described by Fordyce, represents a wide variety of verbal and non-verbal behaviours that correlate with the pain experience and communicate to others that an individual is experiencing pain. Such behaviours may include, for instance, going to lie down, limping, bracing and grimacing. A basic postulate of the model is that behaviours are identifiable and readily observed [34]. Whilst the behavioural responses to pain can serve protective functions which promote healing [35], eventually, if pain persists into a chronic state, the behaviour can become detrimental, for example, lack of movement may ultimately impair function [33,36]. According to Fordyce's concept, pain behaviour is open to operant reinforcement and the responses of others to patients in pain may help or hinder patients' coping strategies and can be maladaptive. Fordyce [33] suggests that patients and significant others can be encouraged to promote and reinforce those behaviours that reduce pain and extinguish those that have potential to increase it.

However, pain is influenced not only by behaviour but also by emotions [20]. The behavioural model was, therefore, considered too simplistic because it concentrated purely on pain behaviour, ignoring the thoughts that could maintain or reduce the pain experience. The cognitive-behavioural model is concerned particularly with enhancing coping skills by reducing negative thoughts that can reinforce pain or overt pain behaviours. This model sees patients as active processors of information in which sensory data is not just transmitted from the periphery to the brain but transformed in and by the process. Sullivan [22] describes the cognitive-behavioural model as the psychological counterpoint of the physiological account offered by gate-control theory [26,37].

The intersubjective or social model of pain

Behaviourist and dualist approaches tend to see pain as not only subjective, that is accessible from the patient's first-person perspective, but also as private, that is *only* accessible from the patient's perspective. Sullivan [22] describes a further model of pain, an *intersubjective* model and draws upon the philosophical writings of Wittgenstein in doing so. *Intersubjectivity* also has roots in the writings of the phenomenologist, Schutz and in the child development literature of Newson [38], Kaye [39], Stern [40], Trevarthen [41], and Schaffer [42]. Intersubjectivity refers to the fact that much of daily life is taken-for-granted and assumes that other people think, perceive and otherwise understand things in pretty much the same terms as we do ourselves. It is this mutuality of knowledge that allows us to interact with others [43]. 'Although the individual defines his world from his own perspective, he is nevertheless a social being, rooted in an intersubjective reality. The world of daily life into which we are born is from the outset an intersubjective world' [44, Foreword].

How can we know that other persons or we have pain? Wittgenstein's writings suggest that we need to appeal to something independent of us and of the sensation itself, to establish that we are identifying the same sensation each time. We must have some imagined standard or criteria, else remembering and speaking, have no content [45]. Without criteria for pain and a public pain language, our memory of pain would lack any specificity or distinction. Hence, we apply metaphors [37]. In the McGill Pain Questionnaire for instance, pain has descriptors which 'feel like' something else, for example 'throbbing', 'tugging', or 'drilling' [46]. Thus, we can differentiate types of pain by their criteria, associating different sensations with different sources. Pain associated with a myocardial infarction presents differently and is described differently from neuropathic pain for instance. In turn, we can observe behaviour which 'looks like' something else; this behaviour of grimacing and crying, for example, can 'look like pain'. Harré writes 'to be in pain is a complex but integrated and unitary state, including the having of an unpleasant feeling and a tendency to groan. The groan is not a description of a feeling but an expression of it. So, when we have discursively transformed the groan into a verbal avowal, the same grammar applies. To be in pain is to experience an unpleasant feeling and to be disposed to say such things as 'I'm in pain' [47, p. 42]. Pain is not simply manifested and learned in terms of outward circumstances and expressions, these outward expressions help to define the experiences as pain. Pain, as with other sensations and emotions is differentiated by a characteristic expression [45].

Within a social system pain language is both learnt and taught. According to McGinn [48] in her guide to Wittgenstein, contexts in which the child has hurt himself are used to teach him, first of all, exclamations, and later words with which to express his pain. We train the child to use a technique which enables him to express what he feels, not merely in cries and exclamations, but in articulate language. Wittgenstein writes 'Here is one possibility: words are connected with the primitive, the natural, expressions of the sensation, and used in their place. A child has hurt himself and he cries; and then adults talk to him and teach him exclamations and later sentences. They teach the child new pain-behaviour. 'So you are saying the word "pain" really means crying?' On the contrary: the verbal expression replaces crying and does not describe it' [45, p. 89e, 244].

In the wider social system, rules of grammar or as referred to by Wittgenstein, 'language games', are created that govern the practices, activities, actions and reactions in characteristic contexts in which the use of a word is integrated [45]. The lessons that the child learns can vary across cultures, within families, or even in the case of the same parent with different children. The child, in Kaye's terms becomes an apprentice in a social system [39], and within this system, the meaning of words is negotiated [49]. Within a family, parents can, for instance, be more or less tolerant of the child's everyday falls or more or less critical of the language the child uses, or more or less critical of the behaviour the child displays. The mother may say 'It's not as bad as that'. As the child matures, the school, the child's peers, and later the physician or society in general may place limits on the appropriateness of the expression or the behaviour, even of the feeling itself. In operant conditioning terms, the pain display, whether in words or behaviour may be reinforced or punished by social pressures.

Pain before language

Sullivan suggests that, whilst it is very real, infant pain is a simple and undifferentiated experience. Research on infant pain has shown this in many ways to be the case. Neonates from as early as 26 weeks gestation, respond with reflexive behaviour not only to stimuli normally considered painful but in certain situations to stimuli which in the older infant would not provoke this behavioural response [50–53]. In comparison with adults, these cutaneous reflexes are exaggerated with lower thresholds and more synchronized and longer lasting reflex muscle contractions. Whereas the reflex tends in adults to habituate with repeated stimulation, in the neonate, the reflex becomes sensitized. In addition, the receptive field for the reflex in the neonate is considerably larger and decreases with postnatal age [54,55]. However, even in neonates as early as 28 weeks gestation, behavioural and physiological responses of increasing magnitude are observed in line with increasingly invasive procedures, and in line with the perceptions of observing adults [56]. So, just as pain becomes differentiated through social interactions, codified in language, the sensory pathways of the infant also mature and become biologically more differentiated. Hence, development of pain as a concept can be described in parallel languages, the languages of psychology, sociology and physiology at the very least [57,58]. Whilst pain may be described through each of these areas of study or languages, it is sometimes necessary to translate between them, and this is not always easy, particularly as certain forms of data come to be more highly valued than others [57].

Recently, a tendency to discount or under-value nonverbal behaviour as an expression of pain, particularly in nonverbal individuals, has become evident with a consequent debate [57,59–67]. Anand and Craig (1996) argued that the definition of pain framed by Merskey and Spear and taken up by the IASP [23,25], excluded certain groups of individuals who could not verbally report their pain. Whilst the IASP definition suggested that verbal reports, whether accompanied by evidence of tissue damage or not, are to be accepted as pain, it suggested that pain indicated by non-verbal behaviour be classified as only 'probable' or 'inferred'. Thus, it assumed a certainty for verbally reported pain that it did not give to non-verbal behaviour [62]. As any one of us, in verbally reporting our pain, can and often do vary our verbal report according to whom we are telling and in what circumstances [68,69], this certainty, given to verbal reports, as against non-verbal reports, seems questionable. Recently, a note has been added to the IASP definition of pain which at least allows for the possibility that an individual unable to communicate verbally may be experiencing pain and be in need of pain-relieving treatment. In relation to the IASP definition, Popper's assertion that 'By and large, definitions do not contribute to making oneself understood or making things clear' [70, p. 18–19], seems to be substantiated. Our intellectual efforts to define pain are in danger of making us less, rather than more, inclined to respond naturally and appropriately to it.

How, therefore, do we come to agreement on what can and cannot be taken as evidence of pain? As Cunningham notes, not only is pain a subjective experience, witnessing another in pain is also a subjective experience [61, p. 96]. As part of the debate described above, Derbyshire argued that infants less than 12 months of age do not feel pain [66,67]. His argument was that the ability to verbalize or to perform any other 'meaningful act of communication' is in principle a key marker of consciousness, and that without consciousness the individual does not feel pain. He argued that infants have no subjective awareness until about 12 months of age (presumably when they start to use speech) [66]. One might wish to determine what was meant by a 'meaningful act of communication' because this would raise the question 'meaningful to whom?' Even if not meaningful to the infant the behaviour takes on meaning for the observer. In contrast to Derbyshire's position, theorists and practitioners of child development view placing meaning on (or finding meaning in) the non-verbal behaviour of infants as both a natural process and one that is essential to the development of infants and children. Whilst some child development theorists take the view that human infants have the basic equipment needed to engage in face-to-face interpersonal communication right from birth [41,71], others believe that the tendency of parents and others to treat them *as if* they do, is vital to the development and survival of the infant [38, 39,42,49]. Dennett refers to this tendency to interpret the other's actions *as if*, as adopting the 'intentional stance', an attitude or perspective which we routinely adopt towards one

another. The intentional stance, according to Dennett is 'the strategy of interpreting the behaviour of an entity (person, animal, artefact, whatever) by treating it *as if* it were a rational agent who governed its choice or action by a consideration of its beliefs and desires' [1, p. 35]. He goes on to argue that 'the point of the intentional stance is to treat an entity as an agent in order to predict its actions. We have to suppose that it is a smart agent, since a stupid agent might do any dumb thing at all' [1, p. 45].

Newson argues that the interactions between mother and baby should be viewed as an attempt by the mother to 'enter into a *meaningful* set of exchanges with her infant' (italics in original) even though she herself is often very aware that the meaning of the communication lies more in her imagination than in the mental experience of the baby [38]. He stresses that to view this social interest in the infant's behaviour by parents or others as a 'kind of whimsical aberration' is a serious mistake. 'It is in practice almost impossible (or one might say pathological)', Newson claims, 'for a mother to react to her baby as if it were merely an inanimate thing' [38, p. 49]. Fridlund, a behavioural ecologist, has argued that parenthood and childhood co-evolve such that behavioural displays of the infant have co-evolved with vigilance of the adult for them. 'That human beings so readily recognize and respond to such actions as discrete, implies in turn that our human attentional capacities are similarly organized into acts of looking, listening etc., which resonate in harmony with the actions of other members of our own species'[72]. In support of this argument, recent work by Deyo *et al.* suggests that by the age of 5 years, children are able to discriminate the facial expressions of pain in others in a linear fashion [73]. Bateson describes how these interactions between parent and child have evolutionary significance [74]. 'Human infants, unlike ducklings, cannot walk away, are, in fact, extraordinarily helpless. Therefore, the immediate biological task is not to teach the infant to recognize the mother but to teach the mother to recognize, acknowledge, and care for the infant—to mobilize a set of maternal behaviours or, alternatively to set the stage so that she will learn these very fast. She must meet both the infant's physical needs and his or her emotional and communicative needs.'

Certainly the capacity of the mother (or alternative caregiver) to infer from the infant's behaviour that he or she is, for example, hungry or in pain would have immense survival advantage and the failure to do so could have dire consequences for the infant, a family and the human species. The capacity to differentiate between sources of distress also facilitates survival and this capacity is enhanced by parents' access to the context of the situation and their knowledge of the biography of the child [75].

The early communications of the child are often situation dependent and the gestures used only have specific reference in the context of that moment. Stern [49] emphasizes that no one set of behaviours has in itself a knowable signal value, but only an approximate one with built-in ambiguity. The more precise signal value is determined by what went before and what direction the negotiation is taking. 'The timing of the gesture and its contextual significance will often be much more important than the precise movements of which it is made up' [38]. The meaning of signals can never be assumed from their physical forms alone. They can often only be understood by the partners themselves by virtue of sharing a particular history of previous communication with each other [38]. There may be particular difficulties for parents of children who are sick or disabled. Unlike healthy infants in normal circumstances, infants and children with disabilities may be limited in their abilities to give signals and to respond reciprocally to the signals of others [76]. Likewise, parents may have difficulties in interpreting what may be the atypical cues of sick and disabled children. In healthy infants and mothers the reciprocal interaction that occurs is positive in nature and encourages both participants to persist in the interaction. In contrast, if the infant is impaired in some way, unclear cues of the infant can lead eventually to unclear cues being sent from the mother, setting up an interaction that may not be reciprocal (or positive) in nature [77].

Pain behaviour

The argument described here is that although primarily a subjective experience, pain is made evident to others through behaviour (both verbal and nonverbal). It is argued that careful observation of behaviour is extremely important because it is one of the few means we have for understanding another's pain experience [59, 78]. Pain behaviour has been widely studied, both in adults and children.

Behaviours that signal pain

Facial expression is widely discussed in the literature on neonatal and infant pain but its importance as an indicator of pain appears thereafter to decrease with age. This downward trend is associated with the development, in older children and adults, of a wider repertoire of behaviour which includes language and which makes the individual, in normal circumstances, less dependent on the response of caregivers [79]. Consequently the older child and the adult are less likely to emit behaviours with high 'signal value' such as crying and grimacing [72]. In addition, as children mature they learn to moderate their behaviour in line with the expectations of the culture within which they live [72,79].

Ethologists argue that the criteria for forms of behaviour with signal value are that they are conspicuous, restricted to particular social contexts, have little non-signal function, and possibly show typical intensity [80]. To have signal value they must be signals of *something to somebody*. Russell argues that there are two contexts—that of the displayer and that of the perceiver or judge [81]. In relation to pain, the urgency of the 'signal' is useless unless perceived as such by the observer. From an evolutionary perspective, Schiefenhovel [82] describes pain as a social signal and a releaser of empathy. In perceiving a child's pain, parents and other adults normally experience an empathetic distress which, in most circumstances moves them to take measures to relieve the child's pain. Craig suggests that sometimes the communication process fails because of a lack of precision in the cues. Too often there is a lack of correspondence between children's experience of pain and the adult's perception of it [83]. Craig et al. [84] introduce a Communication Model for understanding children's pain. The model describes four domains relating to pain: the child's 'experience' and 'expression' together with the adult's 'assessment' and 'action' taken (Figure 20.1).

Each of the domains is relevant to successfully understanding and responding to a child's pain experience. The successful management of the child's pain relies on the sensitivity of the adult to the child's cues, the interpretation they give, and their disposition to act upon their interpretation. Interpretation is particularly important for pain assessment. Philosophically, the Communication Model resonates with the symbolic interactionist approach of Mead and Blumer. Two types of interaction are described [85]. The first type is described as a 'conversation of gestures' through 'non-symbolic interaction', whereby direct response occurs without interpretation, a response that might be described in behavioural terms as reflexive or instinctual. The second system is the use of 'symbolic interaction' which involves an interpretation of the meaning of the other's action before one responds. According to Mead, human beings engage plentifully in non-symbolic interaction, responding immediately and reflexively to each other's bodily movements, expressions and tones of voice, but the characteristic mode is the second, where interaction occurs at the symbolic level, as they seek to understand the meaning of each other's action. The main tenants of Symbolic Interactions identified by Blumer [86] are that:

— Human beings act toward things on the basis of the meanings these things have for them.

— The meaning of these things is derived from, or arises out of the social interaction that one has with one's fellows.

— These meanings are handled in and modified through an interpretative process used by the person in dealing with the things he encounters.

	Child		Adult	
	(1) Experience	(2) Expression (Encoding)	(3) Assessment (Decoding)	(4) Action
Tissue Damage, Stress, and Other Physiological Events	Perception	Motor Program	Observation and Interpretation	Dispositions
	Intrinsic – Generic program – Maturation – Psychological capabilities – Affective mechanisms Formative – Family – Culture Situational – Transient states – Setting	Vocal – cry – scream Non-vocal – facial expression – limb movement – posture Verbal – emergent language	Sensitivity – attention – perceptivity Meaning – interpretation – acumen	Intervention – pharmacological – behavioural Withdrawal – withhold care Imposition – inflict for humane or brutal purposes

Fig. 20.1 A communication model for understanding children's pain. Figure reproduced with permission from publishers and author. Copyright © 2003, Lippincott Williams & Wilkins. All rights reserved.

Facial expression

Pain, at least in infancy, appears to have a unique facial expression [79]. Five facial movements have consistently been found to be associated with pain in healthy, full-term newborns subjected to heel lancing and to hypodermic injections. The facial actions most commonly described comprised brow lowering (brow bulge), eyes squeezed shut, deepening of the nasolabial furrow, open lips and mouth, and a taut cupped tongue. These five actions, along with five other variables, horizontal and vertical stretch mouth, lip purse, chin quiver, and tongue protrusion, made up Grunau and Craig's Neonatal Facial Coding Scheme (NFCS) [87,88]. Facial expression in adults has been found to be similar. Prkachin [89] described a set of four facial actions consistently shown and which carried the bulk of the information about pain. These four actions were brow lowering, tightening and closing of the eyelids, nose wrinkling and upper lip raising The tongue cupping described by Grunau and Craig [88] appears to be behaviour more associated with, or more visible in, young infants than the older child or adult.

Few studies have looked in detail at the facial actions that occur with pain in children after infancy. Changes in facial anatomy occur during the transition from infancy to the toddler years and the Child Facial Coding System (CFCS) was developed to incorporate those changes. This system focuses on 13 discrete facial actions which include both the gross and more subtle movements observed in the young child's facial pain display [90]. The facial actions are very similar to those observed in neonates and appear to occur consistently in response to brief pain events such as immunization, venepuncture and finger lance. However, the simultaneous display of all actions is uncommon and individual differences

are observed [91]. In a study of pain reaction in 8 adolescents with profound neurological impairments, video-raters' coding on CFCS failed to differentiate between occasions when a flu vaccination was administered and a dummy injection. Interestingly, global pain assessments made by observers were significantly higher in the vaccination group.

Although individuals do appear to show very similar facial, gestural, postural and physiological signs of pain even in different cultures [89,92], Izard, Ekman, and Fridlund [93] all agree that facial expressions cannot be understood independently of the context in which they occur. Context depends not only on the structural features of the situation but also has historical and biographical features as it depends also on the succession of interactants' displays and the responses made to them.

Vocal (non-verbal) expression of pain

Whilst facial expression appears to be the most salient pain cue in infants, cry, or other vocal cues are often taken as the most reliable indicators of pain in older children [94]. Experimental studies have shown that adults (including parents) can sometimes distinguish the causes of infant's crying. However, this was only *if* the range of eliciting conditions is sufficiently limited, *if* the cry exemplars are carefully preselected, and *if* the range of possible interpretations is narrowly constrained [95]. Early studies by Sherman of global response (rather than cry alone) showed that there was a considerable lack of agreement when adults had no information regarding the eliciting stimulus [95]. The stimulus that appeared to immediately precede the response (whether it was the actual initiating stimulus or not) was the best predictor of the adults, judgement as to cause of the infant's cry.

Just as observers have difficulty in discriminating between facial expressions of distress, Galati and Levene [96] demonstrated that parents had difficulty differentiating between cries and tended to attribute most of them to hunger, even those that were precipitated by painful stimuli. Within the normal home setting, it appears that cry alerts the parent, whereas any suppositions about the cause of crying are based on the individual's knowledge of the context [95,96].

Crying in the infant and young child is therefore not very specific. It can be difficult to distinguish cries of pain from those of hunger, anger or protest [97,98]. This is particularly so in the absence of contextual cues. It may be easier to differentiate between the cries of a specific infant with whom one has on going contact than to determine the differences between cries across a number of infants with their inevitable individual differences. As well as being accustomed to the intra-individual variation in their child's cries, parents have knowledge of such factors as the child's behavioural dispositions, health status, and time since feeding for instance which help them in distinguishing one cry from another [75].

Johnson and Strada suggest that it may be differences in pitch, frequency and latency of the cry rather than the cry itself that alerts the parent to a cry of pain [99]. 'Cry type' appears to be less specific and meaningful than 'cry gradation' with the early part of the cry appearing to impart more meaning than the later part [95]. Whereas, in the case of an acute pain stimulus, cry may start loud and then reduce, cries associated with hunger tend to start more softly and then become more intense with time. The sudden loud cry associated with an acute pain stimulus or startle of any kind is more likely to draw an immediate response from the parent [95].

When facial and cry variables were considered together, Hadjistavropoulos et al. [100] found cry variables added little to the prediction of ratings in comparison to facial variables. The authors concluded that whilst cry would seem to command attention, facial activity, rather than cry, accounts for the major variations in adults' judgements of neonatal pain.

Whilst crying may be a generalized distress signal in the infant, as the child matures, the nature of the vocal expression of pain is likely to widen in range, for example groaning, moaning [101,102] and sighing [103,104] become part of the repertoire. In relation to older children, Hamers et al. [94] found that vocal expression, especially crying, most influenced nurses' pain assessments and decisions to intervene with analgesic treatments. Other factors were the medical diagnosis, age, parent reports, and nurses' knowledge, experience, attitude and workload. Overall, the presence of a particular diagnosis appeared to legitimate the child's pain complaints. Here again, context, whether in this case truly related or not, appears to play as important a role in determining the cause attributed to the child's cries as does the nature of the cry itself.

Bodily movements and posture

Whilst facial expression and cry appear to have signal value and function to alert others to the sufferer's plight, bodily movements and changes in posture may have additional or alternative functions. Wall [35] has described the behaviour of animals in response to acute pain as agitation, aggressiveness, guarding, and splinting of the injured area. After those initial responses and when confronted with persistent pain, animals are quiet, solitary, antisocial with prolonged sleep and minimal movement. Humans, Wall states, respond to persistent pain by limiting movement of the injured part, restricting movement in general, sleeping for long periods, eating poorly, and restricting social contact.

In cancer, both acute and persistent pain can occur. In a study of pain behaviour in adults with lung cancer, patients reported that they used 42 different behaviours to control pain. Behaviours such as rotating or shrugging the shoulders served to alter ascending nociceptive input, whilst others, such as listening to music and reading diverted cortical attention and hence stimulated descending modulation. The number of behaviours reported correlated with pain intensity and predicted the length of time pain had been experienced. No behaviour was reported to be performed to express pain [105].

In line with the descriptions by Wall [35] and with the 'pain control' concept, Gauvin Piquard et al. [106] described an 'antalgic' group of behaviours through which a young child with cancer might take up a position which causes least pain. Another group of behaviours described was one of 'psycho-motor atonia' where the child takes on an attitude of helplessness and becomes still and withdrawn, avoiding eye contact or any participation with his surroundings.

Changes in posture and movements, therefore, can serve a variety of purposes and functions; to prevent pain, to control and relieve pain, and as behaviour associated with changes in mood, for instance through depression associated with persistent pain. Though the purpose may not be to communicate pain, whether intended to do so or not, these behaviours can signal pain to those around them [105].

Physiological changes

Pain evokes physiological changes that can be measured. These changes include changes in heart and respiratory rate, vagal tone, blood pressure, oxygen saturation, transcutaneous oxygen and carbon dioxide tension, and intracranial pressure. However, many of these changes will not be readily accessible to measurement in the clinical situation [107].

Heart rate

Several studies have reported that among the indicators used by professionals in their assessment of pain are increased heart and respiratory rate [108–110]. After an initial slowing of the heart rate following an acute pain stimulus, heart rate has been shown to increase [99,111]. In turn, this increase in heart rate has been shown to be responsive to analgesic treatments [112–114].

Respiratory rate

Changes in respiratory rate with pain are not consistent across studies [97]. In some studies, respiratory rate has tended to be reduced with a painful stimulus, in others, increased. In other studies, variability in rate has altered but not the rate itself [115]. Changes in rate or variability of respiration appear to be more important as indicators of pain than the direction of change.

Hormonal response to nociceptive events

Pain evokes a physiological stress response that includes outpouring of pituitary, adrenal and pancreatic hormones [116]. However, these responses are variable and not specific to pain. Although not specific to pain, a positive association has been demonstrated between plasma cortisol levels and nociceptive stimuli such as inoculation and circumcision [117]. Even the fetus has been shown to demonstrate a cortisol response to a noxious event [118]. Recognizing that drawing blood by heelstick or venepuncture is itself a stressful event [119], many of the more recent studies have used saliva cortisol in preference to plasma cortisol measurements. Positive relationships have been identified between saliva cortisol and acute noxious events such as inoculation [117,120–122], circumcision [123], and heelstick [119].

Few studies, have investigated physiological response to non-acute pain but there appears to be some relationship here too. Subacute pain and distress of neonates has been investigated. Compared to a control group, significantly higher concentrations of saliva cortisol were found in distressed infants being ventilated and in those with pain due to necrotising enterocolitis and meningits [124]. In a study of verbal children attending a hospital casualty department, positive correlations were noted between saliva cortisol and self-report (VAS $r = 0.35$, Faces score $r = 0.36$). Correlation was higher between saliva cortisol concentration and the extent of injury itself ($r = 0.63$) [125]. In the course of validating the Paediatric Pain Profile (PPP), a pain assessment scale for children with severe neurological impairment, saliva cortisol concentration correlated ($rs = 0.38–0.45$) with each of three observers' PPP scores of children filmed during everyday morning activities [13]. Generally, however, cortisol concentrations appeared low and may have been influenced by additional factors besides pain. Moore *et al.* [126] investigated the association between urinary cortisol excretion and chronic pain in a pain clinic population. Thirty percent of adult patients with chronic pain were shown to have urinary cortisol to creatinine ratios above the normal range. However, this response was higher in the patients with more recent onset of chronic pain suggesting that some habituation had occurred in the response.

Self-report of pain

The ability of children to describe and rate their own pain varies with their age, developmental stage, and health. Work has been ongoing over a number of years to develop assessment tools to facilitate the communication of the intensity of the child's pain to the child's caregivers. As children are less able than adults to quantify and qualify abstract phenomena, measuring techniques must be appropriate to the child's cognitive and developmental levels. The concepts of the psychologist, Piaget, are useful in understanding how the child's development affects his capacity to use pain assessment tools [127,128].

Piaget describes several stages through which the child's thought becomes more logically structured and increasingly free of the necessity for concrete situations [128]. Most pain assessment tools involve the concept of seriation, that is, placing or conceptualizing things in order of magnitude. After puberty, seriation problems can be solved abstractly, but prior to this the domain needs to be concretely present for the seriation to succeed. Piaget's stages 1, 11, and 111 in the development of seriation behaviour correspond respectively to the pre-conceptual, intuitive and concrete operational periods he describes [128]. Piaget's concepts of logic and order are supported by research on the ability of children at different ages to correctly order faces on faces pain scales [129–132].

Young children 3–11 years

• Preconceptual (Stage 1). Children from 3–4 years of age are at a 'pre-conceptual' level of development. At this age, children have limited sense of seriation and therefore difficulty in carrying out tasks which involve placing things in order, for instance they would be unable to reliably place in order of size ('to staircase') a series of 7 blocks [128].

• Intuitive (Stage 11). At the age of five or six, children have a sense of big and small and become more able to construct the perfect staircase, but only by means of trial and error. Once built, they may pick out extremes in it but would be unable to insert extra blocks once it is built. This suggests that pain assessment tools such as the poker chips [133], a small number of different size blocks [98], or faces scales with a minimum number of faces such as the Oucher [129] may be best suited for this age group. Younger children are unlikely to volunteer that they have pain and it is important to be vigilant for behavioural indications of pain. Use of a behaviour rating scale such as the DEGRr may be helpful [106].

- Concrete Operations (Stage 111). From 7 years to adolescence, children enter, in Piaget's terms, a period of concrete operations where they acquire the concept of conservation and reversibility. They can think in terms of longer, higher, bigger, and sort objects on the basis of col our, size, and shape. From 7 or 8 years, children can reliably build the 'staircase', starting with the longest or shortest and systematically adding the next in size and will now be able to add in an intermediate-sized block to the pre-existing staircase [128]. Children become capable now of elementary logic, but can still only apply it to concrete events. At this age they become more able to use tools to quantify pain. In addition to the earlier suggested tools, they can use other more schematic faces scales [130,132,134] (Figures 20.2–20.4), visual analogue scales (VAS) [135], or colour analogue scales [135] (Figure 20.5).

Adolescents 11–18 years

Adolescents are, in Piaget's terms, at a cognitive stage of formal operations and are able to abstract, quantify and qualify phenomena. At this stage they may be able to use scales as in adults and do not need any props to do so. For instance, adolescents

Faces Pain Scale—Revised (FPS-R).

The full-size version of the Faces Pain Scale (FPS-R), together with instructions for administration, are freely available for non-commercial clinical and research use from www.painsourcebook.ca.

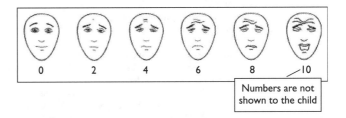

Instructions to the child are: 'These faces show how much something can hurt. This face [point to left-most face] shows no pain [or hurt]. The faces show more and more pain [point to each from left to right] up to this one [point to right-most face]-it shows very much pain. Point to the face that shows how much you hurt [right now]'.

Do not use words like 'happy or 'sad'. This scale is intended to measure how children feel inside, not how their face looks. Numbers are not shown to children; they are shown here only for reference.

The instructions for administration are currently available in 12 languages from www.painsourcebook.ca.

Fig. 20.4 Faces Pain Scale—Revised (FPS-R). Copyright ©2001 International Association for the Study of Pain (IASP).

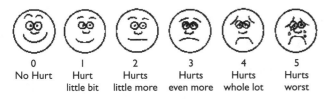

Fig. 20.2 The Wong baker faces scale. (From Wong, D.L., Hockenberry-Eaton M., Wilson, D., Winkelstein, M.L., and Schwartz, P. (eds). *Wong's Essentials of Pediatric Nursing*, St Louis, 2001, vol. 6: p. 1301. Copyrighted by Mosby, Inc. Reprinted by permission.)

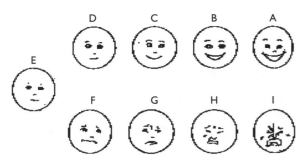

Fig. 20.3 Facial affective scale.

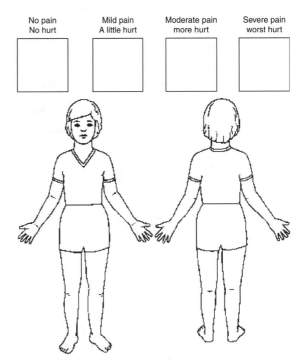

Fig. 20.5 Eland colour scale. (Reprinted with permission of J.M. Eland from McCaffery, M. and Beebe, A. *Pain: Clinical Manual for Nursing Practice*. St Louis: CV Mosby Co.; 1989.)

NAME:_____ MRN_____ DATE_____

Instructions:
We want to find out how you have been feeling the last 2 days.
Use a pencil or crayon to circle your answers.

EXAMPLE
Did you have any pain yesterday or today?
    Yes   or   No
If YES
* How much of the time did you have pain?
    1 – A very short time   2 – A medium amount   3 – Almost all the time
* How much pain did you feel?
    1 – A little   2 – A medium amount   3 – A lot
* How much did the pain bother you or trouble you?
    0 – Not at all   1 – A little   2 – A medium amount   3 – Very much

1. Did you feel more tired yesterday or today than you usually do?
    Yes   or   No
If YES
* How long did it last?
    1 – A very short time   2 – A medium amount   3 – Almost all the time
* How tired did you feel?
    1 – A little   2 – A medium amount   3 – Very tired
* How much did being tired bother you or trouble you?
    0 – Not at all   1 – A little   2 – A medium amount   3 – Very much

2. Did you feel sad yesterday or today?
    Yes   or   No
If YES
* How long did you feel sad?
    1 – A very short time   2 – A medium amount   3 – Almost all the time
* How sad did you feel?
    1 – A little   2 – A medium amount   3 – Very tired
* How much did feeling sad bother you or trouble you?
    0 – Not at all   1 – A little   2 – A medium amount   3 – Very much

3. Were you itchy yesterday or today?
    Yes   or   No
If YES
* How much of the time were you itchy?
    1 – A very short time   2 – A medium amount   3 – Almost all the time
* How itchy were you?
    1 – A little   2 – A medium amount   3 – Very tired
* How much did being itchy bother you or trouble you?
    0 – Not at all   1 – A little   2 – A medium amount   3 – Very much

4. Did you have any pain yesterday or today?
    Yes   or   No
If YES
* How much of the time did you have pain?
    1 – A very short time   2 – A medium amount   3 – Almost all the time
* How much pain did you feel?
    1 – A little   2 – A medium amount   3 – A lot
* How much did the paqin bother you or trouble you
    0 – Not at all   1 – A little   2 – A medium amount   3 – Very much

5. Did you feel worried yesterday or today?
    Yes   or   No
If YES
* How much of the time did you feel worried?
    1 – A very short time   2 – A medium amount   3 – Almost all the time

Fig. 20.6 Memorial Symptom Assessment Scale (7–12). (Reprinted from *J Pain Symptom Manage* 23(1), Collins, J.J., Devine, T.D., Dick, G.S., Johnson, E.A., Kiham, H.A., Pinkerton, C.R., Stevens, M.M., Thaler, H.T., and Portenoy, R.K. The measurement of symptoms in young children with cancer: The validation of the memorial symptom assesment scale in children aged 7–12. © 2002, with permission from U.S. Cancer Pain Relief Committt.)

* How worried did you feel?
   1 – A little   2 – A medium amount   3 – A lot
* How much did feeling worried bother you or trouble you
   0 – Not at all   1 – A little   2 – A medium amount   3 – Very much

6. Did you feel like eating yesterday or today like you normally do?
   Yes   or   No
If NO
* How long did it last?
   1 – A very short time   2 – A medium amount   3 – Almost all the time
* How much did this borther you or trouble you?
   0 – Not at all   1 – A little   2 – A medium amount   3 – Very much

7. Did you feel you were going to vomit (or going to throw up) yesterday or today?
   Yes   or   No
If YES
* How much of the time did you feel you could vomit (or could throw up)?
   1 – A very short time   2 – A medium amount   3 – Almost all the time
* How much did this feeling bother you or trouble you?
   0 – Not at all   1 – A little   2 – A medium amount   3 – Very much

8. Did you have trouble going to sleep the last two nights?
   Yes   or   No
If YES
* How much did not being able to sleep bother you or trouble you?
   0 – Not at all   1 – A little   2 – A medium amount   3 – Very much

Other:
If you had anything else which made you feel bad or sick yesterday or today, write it here*
*

* How much did not being able to sleep bother you or trouble you?
   0 – Not at all   1 – A little   2 – A medium amount   3 – Very much
*

* How much did not being able to sleep bother you or trouble you?
   0 – Not at all   1 – A little   2 – A medium amount   3 – Very much

Fig. 20.6 (*Continued*)

may use a numerical rating scale (0–10 scale) to scale their pain without any tool being present. They can be asked, for instance 'How would you rate your pain—on a scale of 0 to 10? 0 is no pain and 10 is the worst pain imaginable'. Verbal rating scales or VAS will also be appropriate. However, when ill, adolescents may regress to earlier stage of development and they may find it easier to use a more concrete tool. Faces scales appear popular at least in the short term.

At all ages, body maps may be useful in eliciting site, dimensions and intensity of pain [136] (Figure 20.6). The child's drawings can help the carer to gain an impression of the child's pain and provide an opportunity for conversation about the pain with the child and parents [137].

Pain is not alone in causing distress to children during chronic and life-limiting illness. Collins and colleagues have developed two scales based on the Memorial Symptom Assessment Scale to assess and monitor symptoms that can cause discomfort and distress for children with cancer [139, 140].

Assessing pain in children with severe to profound neurological disability

Children with severe neurological and cognitive impairments face significant barriers in both expressing pain and in obtaining appropriate and timely help [141]. Difficulties may lie on both sides, for the individual experiencing the pain, who can have difficulty encoding expressive behaviour, and for the caregiver, who may lack skills required to decode the behaviour. In the face of these difficulties, pain may go unrecognized and untreated [84] or be misinterpreted and treated inappropriately. In addition to difficulties in communicating the fact of pain itself, a multitude of potential pain sources in the child makes identifying the source and providing a useful treatment challenging [91]. There has been an increasing interest over the last 10 years in eliciting the types of behaviours which signal to caregivers that the child has pain [13,15,16,142–144]. These studies have resulted in a degree of consensus on the pain cues displayed (Table 20.1) and subsequently the development of behaviour rating scales which demonstrate satisfactory reliability and validity in this population of children [15,145]. The PPP is a behaviour rating scale developed to assess pain in children with severe motor and learning disabilities [13–15] (Figure 20.8). The tool is envisaged as a parent held document, and contains documentation of the child's pain history, baseline, and ongoing pain assessments.

Some children with neurological impairment, even those who are without speech, provided they have sufficient cognitive skills, may be able to use self-report tools when these are made

Name: Date:

SECTION 1:

INSTRUCTIONS: We have listed 22 symptoms below. Read each one carefully. If you have had the symptoms during this past week, circle *YES.* If *YES,* let us know how *OFTEN* you have had it, how *SEVERE* it was usually and how much it *BOTHERED OR DISTRESSED* you by circling the appropriate answer. If you *DID NOT HAVE* the symptom circle *NO.*

DURING THE PAST WEEK DID YOU HAVE ANY:

* DIFFICULTY CONCENTRATIING or PAYING ATTENTION?

1.   Yes   or   2.   NO
         If YES   How often did you have it?
                        1 — Almost never   2 — sometimes   3 — a lot   3 — Almost always
                        How severe was it usually?
                        1 — Slight   2 — Moderately   3 — Severe   4 — Very severe
                        How much did it bother you?
                        0 — Not at all   1 — A little bit 2 — Somewhat   3 — Quite a bit   4 — Very much

* PAIN?

1.   Yes   or   2.   NO
         If YES   How often did you have it?
                        1 — Almost never   2 — sometimes   3 — a lot   3 — Almost always
                        How severe was it usually?
                        1 — Slight   2 — Moderately   3 — Severe   4 — Very severe
                        How much did it bother you?
                        0 — Not at all   1 — A little bit 2 — Somewhat   3 — Quite a bit   4 — Very much

* COUGH?

1.   Yes   or   2.   NO
         If YES   How often did you have it?
                        1 — Almost never   2 — sometimes   3 — a lot   3 — Almost always
                        How severe was it usually?
                        1 — Slight   2 — Moderately   3 — Severe   4 — Very severe
                        How much did it bother you?
                        0 — Not at all   1 — A little bit 2 — Somewhat   3 — Quite a bit   4 — Very much

* FEELING OR BEING NERVOUS?

1.   Yes   or   2.   NO
         If YES   How often did you have it?
                        1 — Almost never   2 — sometime   3 — a lot   3 — Almost always
                        How severe was it usually?
                        1 — Slight   2 — Moderately   3 — Severe   4 — Very severe
                        How much did it bother you?
                        0 — Not at all   1 — A little bit 2 — Somewhat   3 — Quite a bit   4 — Very much

* DRY MOUTH?

1.   Yes   or   2.   NO
         If YES   How often did you have it?
                        1 — Almost never   2 — sometimes   3 — a lot   3 — Almost always
                        How severe was it usually?
                        1 — Slight   2 — Moderately   3 — Severe   4 — Very severe
                        How much did it bother you?
                        0 — Not at all   1 — A little bit 2 — Somewhat   3 — Quite a bit   4 — Very much

* NAUSEA or FEELING LIKE YOU COULD VOMIT?

1.   Yes   or   2.   NO
         If YES   How often did you have it?
                        1 — Almost never   2 — sometimes   3 — a lot   3 — Almost always
                        How severe was it usually?
                        1 — Slight   2 — Moderately   3 — Severe   4 — Very severe
                        How much did it bother you?
                        0 — Not at all   1 — A little bit 2 — Somewhat   3 — Quite a bit   4 — Very much

* A FEELING OF BEING DROWSY?

1.   Yes   or   2.   NO
         If YES   How often did you have it?
                        1 — Almost never   2 — sometimes   3 — a lot   3 — Almost always

Fig. 20.7 Memorial Symptom Assessment Scale (10–18). (Reprinted from *J of Pain Symptom Manage,* 19(5), Collins J.J., Byrnes M.E., Dunkel I.J., Laplin J., Nadel T., Thaler H.T., Polyak T., Rapkin B., and Portenoy R.K. The measurement of symptoms in children with cancer, pp. 363–77. © 2000 with permission from U.S. Cancer Pain Relief Committee.)

How severe was it usually?

| 1 — Slight | 2 — Moderately | 3 — Severe | 4 — Very severe |

How much did it bother or distress you?

| 0 — Not at all | 1 — A little bit | 2 — Somewhat | 3 — Quite a bit | 4 — Very much |

* NUMBNESS/TINGLING or PINS AND NEEDLES FEELING IN HANDS or FEET?

1.   Yes   or   2.   NO

If YES   How often did you have it?

| 1 — Almost never | 2 — sometimes | 3 — a lot | 3 — Almost always |

How severe was it usually?

| 1 — Slight | 2 — Moderately | 3 — Severe | 4 — Very severe |

How much did it bother or distress you?

| 0 — Not at all | 1 — A little bit | 2 — Somewhat | 3 — Quite a bit | 4 — Very much |

* DIFFICULTY SLEEPING?

1.   Yes   or   2.   NO

If YES   How often did you have it?

| 1 — Almost never | 2 — sometimes | 3 — a lot | 3 — Almost always |

How severe was it usually?

| 1 — Slight | 2 — Moderately | 3 — Severe | 4 — Very severe |

How much did it bother or distress you?

| 0 — Not at all | 1 — A little bit | 2 — Somewhat | 3 — Quite a bit | 4 — Very much |

* PROBLEMS WITH URINATION or PEEING?

1.   Yes   or   2.   NO

If YES   How often did you have it?

| 1 — Almost never | 2 — sometimes | 3 — a lot | 3 — Almost always |

How severe was it usually?

| 1 — Slight | 2 — Moderately | 3 — Severe | 4 — Very severe |

How much did it bother or distress you?

| 0 — Not at all | 1 — A little | 2 — Somewhat | 3 — Quite a bit | 4 — Very much |

* VOMITING or THROWING UP?

1.   Yes   or   2.   NO

If YES   How often did you have it?

| 1 — Almost never | 2 — sometimes | 3 — a lot | 3 — Almost always |

How severe was it usually?

| 1 — Slight | 2 — Moderately | 3 — Severe | 4 — Very severe |

How much did it bother or distress you?

| 0 — Not at all | 1 — A little bit | 2 — Somewhat | 3 — Quite a bit | 4 — Very much |

* SHORTNESS OF BREATH?

1.   Yes   or   2.   NO

If YES   How often did you have it?

| 1 — Almost never | 2 — sometimes | 3 — a lot | 3 — Almost always |

How severe was it usually?

| 1 — Slight | 2 — Moderately | 3 — Severe | 4 — Very severe |

How much did it bother or distress you?

| 0 — Not at all | 1 — A little bit | 2 — Somewhat | 3 — Quite a bit | 4 — Very much |

* DIARRHEA or LOOSE BOWEL MOVEMENT?

1.   Yes   or   2.   NO

If YES   How often did you have it?

| 1 — Almost never | 2 — sometimes | 3 — a lot | 3 — Almost always |

How severe was it usually?

| 1 — Slight | 2 — Moderately | 3 — Severe | 4 — Very severe |

How much did it bother or distress you?

| 0 — Not at all | 1 — A little bit | 2 — Somewhat | 3 — Quite a bit | 4 — Very much |

* FEELINGS OF BEING DROWSY?

1.   Yes   or   2.   NO

If YES   How often did you have it?

| 1 — Almost never | 2 — sometimes | 3 — a lot | 3 — Almost always |

How severe was it usually?

| 1 — Slight | 2 — Moderately | 3 — Severe | 4 — Very severe |

How much did it bother or distress you?

| 0 — Not at all | 1 — A little bit | 2 — Somewhat | 3 — Quite a bit | 4 — Very much |

* NUMBNESS/TINGLING or PINS AND NEEDLES FEELING IN HANDS or FEET?

1.   Yes   or   2.   NO

If YES   How often did you have it?

Fig. 20.7 (*Continued*)

	1— Almost never	2— sometimes	3— a lot	3— Almost always	

How severe was it usually?

1— Slight	2— Moderately	3— Severe	4— Very severe	

How much did it bother or distress you?

0— Not at all	1— A little bit	2— Somewhat	3— Quite a	4— Very much

* DIFFICULTY SEELPING?

1.   Yes   or   2.   NO

If YES   How often did you have it?

1— Almost never	2— sometimes	3— a lot	3— Almost always	

How severe was it usually?

1— Slight	2— Moderately	3— Severe	4— Very severe	

How much did it bother or distress you?

0— Not at all	1— A little bit	2— Somewhat	3— Quite a bit	4— Very much

* PROBLEMS WITH URINATION or PEEING?

1.   Yes   or   2.   NO

If YES   How often did you have it?

1— Almost never	2— sometimes	3— a lot	3— Almost always	

How severe was it usually?

1— Slight	2— Moderately	3— Severe	4— Very severe	

How much did it bother or distress you?

0— Not at all	1— A little bit	2— Somewhat	3— Quite a bit	4— Very much

* VOMITING or THROWING UP?

1.   Yes   or   2.   NO

If YES   How often did you have it?

1— Almost never	2— sometimes	3— a lot	3— Almost always	

How severe was it usually?

1— Slight	2— Moderately	3— Severe	4— Very severe	

How much did it bother or distress you?

0— Not at all	1— A little bit	2— Somewhat	3— Quite a bit	4— Very much

* SHORTNESS OF BREATH?

1.   Yes   or   2.   NO

If YES   How often did you have it?

1— Almost never	2— sometimes	3— a lot	3— Almost always	

How severe was it usually?

1— Slight	2— Moderately	3— Severe	4— Very severe	

How much did it bother or distress you?

0— Not at all	1— A little bit	2— Somewhat	3— Quite a bit	4— Very much

* DIARRHEA or LOOSE BOWEL MOVEMENT?

1.   Yes   or   2.   NO

If YES   How often did you have it?

1— Almost never	2— sometimes	3— a lot	3— Almost always	

How severe was it usually?

1— Slight	2— Moderately	3— Severe	4— Very severe	

How much did it bother or distress you?

0— Not at all	1— A little bit	2— Somewhat	3— Quite a bit	4— Very much

* FEELINGS OF SADNESS?

1.   Yes   or   2.   NO

If YES   How often did you have it?

1— Almost never	2— sometimes	3— a lot	3— Almost always	

How severe was it usually?

1— Slight	2— Moderately	3— Severe	4— Very severe	

How much did it bother or distress you?

0— Not at all	1— A little bit	2— Somewhat	3— Quite a bit	4— Very much

* SWEATS?

1.   Yes   or   2.   NO

If YES   How often did you have it?

1— Almost never	2— sometimes	3— a lot	3— Almost always	

How severe was it usually?

1— Slight	2— Moderately	3— Severe	4— Very severe	

How much did it bother or distress you?

0— Not at all	1— A little bit	2— Somewhat	3— Quite a bit	4— Very much

* WORRYING?

1.   Yes   or   2.   NO

Fig. 20.7 (Continued)

	If YES	How often did you have it?			
		1 — Almost never	2 — sometimes	3 — a lot	3 — Almost always
		How severe was it usually?			
		1 — Slight	2 — Moderately	3 — Severe	4 — Very severe
		How much did it bother or distress you?			
		0 — Not at all	1 — A little bit	2 — Somewhat	3 — Quite a bit	4 — Very much

* ITCHING?

1.	Yes	or	2.	NO	
	If YES	How often did you have it?			
		1 — Almost never	2 — sometimes	3 — a lot	3 — Almost always
		How severe was it usually?			
		1 — Slight	2 — Moderately	3 — Severe	4 — Very severe
		How much did it bother or distress you?			
		0 — Not at all	1 — A little bit	2 — Somewhat	3 — Quite a bit	4 — Very much

* LACK OF APPETITE OR NOT WANTING TO EAT?

1.	Yes	or	2.	NO	
	If YES	How often did you have it?			
		1 — Almost never	2 — sometimes	3 — a lot	3 — Almost always
		How severe was it usually?			
		1 — Slight	2 — Moderately	3 — Severe	4 — Very severe
		How much did it bother or distress you?			
		0 — Not at all	1 — A little bit	2 — Somewhat	3 — Quite a bit	4 — Very much

* DIZZINESS?

1.	Yes	or	2.	NO	
	If YES	How often did you have it?			
		1 — Almost never	2 — sometimes	3 — a lot	3 — Almost always
		How severe was it usually?			
		1 — Slight	2 — Moderately	3 — Severe	4 — Very severe
		How much did it bother or distress you?			
		0 — Not at all	1 — A little bit	2 — Somewhat	3 — Quite a bit	4 — Very much

* DIFFICULTY SWALLOWING?

1.	Yes	or	2.	NO	
	If YES	How often did you have it?			
		1 — Almost never	2 — sometimes	3 — a lot	3 — Almost always
		How severe was it usually?			
		1 — Slight	2 — Moderately	3 — Severe	4 — Very severe
		How much did it bother or distress you?			
		0 — Not at all	1 — A little bit	2 — Somewhat	3 — Quite a bit	4 — Very much

* FEELINGS OF BEING IRRITABLE?

1.	Yes	or	2.	NO	
	If YES	How often did you have it?			
		1 — Almost never	2 — sometimes	3 — a lot	3 — Almost always
		How severe was it usually?			
		1 — Slight	2 — Moderately	3 — Severe	4 — Very severe
		How much did it bother or distress			
		0 — Not at all	1 — A little bit	2 — Somewhat	3 — Quite a bit	4 — Very much

SECTION 2:

INSTRUCTIONS: We have listed 8 symptoms below. Read each one carefully. If you have had the symptom during this past week let us know how *SEVERE* it was usually and how much it *BOTHERED OR DISTRESSED* by circling the appropriate answer. If you *DID NOT HAVE* the symptom circle *NO*.

* MOUTH SORES?

1.	Yes	or	2.	NO	
	If YES	How severe was it usually?			
		1 — Slight	2 — Moderately	3 — Severe	4 — Very severe
		How much did it bother or distress you?			
		0 — Not at all	1 — A little bit	2 — Somewhat	3 — Quite a bit	4 — Very much

* CHANGE IN THE WAY FOOD TASTES?

1.	Yes	or	2.	NO	
	If YES	How severe was it usually?			
		1 — Slight	2 — Moderately	3 — Severe	4 — Very severe
		How much did it bother or distress you?			
		0 — Not at all	1 — A little bit	2 — Somewhat	3 — Quite a bit	4 — Very much

Fig. 20.7 (Continued)

* WEIGHT LOSS?
1.   Yes   or   2.   NO
          If YES   How severe was it usually?
                             1— Slight   2— Moderately   3— Severe   4— Very severe
                             How much did it bother or distress you?
                             0— Not at all   1— A little bit   2— Somewhat   3— Quite a bit   4— Very much

* HAIR LOSS?
1.   Yes   or   2.   NO
          If YES   How severe was it usually?
                             1— Slight   2— Moderately   3— Severe   4— Very severe
                             How much did it bother or distress you?
                             0— Not at all   1— A little bit   2— Somewhat   3— Quite a bit   4— Very much

* CONSTIPATION or UNCOMFORTABLE BECAUSE BOWEL MOVEMENTS ARE LESS OFTEN?
1.   Yes   or   2.   NO
          If YES   How severe was it usually?
                             1—Slight   2—Moderately   3—Severe   4—Very severe
                             How much did it bother or distress you?
                             0—Not at all   1—A little bit   2—Somewhat   3—Quite a bit   4—Very much

* SWELLING OF ARMS OR LEGS?
1.   Yes   or   2.   NO
          If YES   How severe was it usually?
                             1—Slight   2—Moderately   3—Severe   4—Very severe
                             How much did it bother or distress you?
                             0—Not at all   1—A little bit   2—Somewhat   3—Quite a bit   4—Very much

* "I DON'T LOOK LIKE MYSELF"?
1.   Yes   or   2.   NO
          If YES   How severe was it usually?
                             1—Slight   2—Moderately   3—Severe   4—Very severe
                             How much did it bother or distress you?
                             0—Not at all   1—A little bit   2—Somewhat   3—Quite a bit   4—Very much

* CHANGES IN SKIN?
1.   Yes   or   2.   NO
          If YES   How severe was it usually?
                             1—Slight   2—Moderately   3—Severe   4—Very severe
                             How much did it bother or distress you?
                             0—Not at all   1—A little bit   2—Somewhat   3—Quite a bit   4—Very much

Fig. 20.7 (Continued)

available to them [146]. This case history is presented as an example.

Case Kate was 16 years old and had a neurodegenerative disease. Her developmental level approximated that of a 7–8-year old. She had no speech and very limited voluntary movement. Most of her communication was by facial expression and by 'yes' and 'no' replies to questions. She signified 'yes' by glancing to the right and 'no' by glancing to the left, or alternatively 'yes' by raising her right arm. Whilst she was extremely expressive, it wasn't always easy to tell what she was expressing. Kate's pain was recorded using a pain diary in conjunction with the Facial Affective Scale [130]. The faces scale and a body map [137] were incorporated into her Bliss symbol communication book that went everywhere with her and from which she could chose subjects that she wanted to 'talk' about. It was possible to elicit from her on one occasion that she had toothache, which necessitated, rather to her dismay, a visit to the dentist for extraction of a decayed tooth, and later, on a more ongoing basis, pain in her back probably due

to increasing kypho-scoliosis. It was then possible to monitor relief from that pain with the administration of once daily sustained-release diclofenac.

The pain assessment process—measurement and meaning

The World Health Organization (WHO) provides guidelines on cancer pain relief in children [147], guidance which is equally relevant to children with other life-limiting conditions. In relation to pain assessment, they recommend the following 'ABC's':

- *Assess.* Always evaluate a child with cancer for potential pain. Children may experience pain, even though they may be unable to express the fact in words. Infants and toddlers can show their pain only by how they look and act; older children may deny their pain for fear of more painful treatment.

Table 20.1 Identification of pain cues of children with neurological and cognitive impairments

Author	San Salvador [144]	Non-communicating children's Pain checklist [142,145]	Paediatric Pain Profile [13,15]
Population	Patients attending institutions for multiply handicapped	Non-verbal individuals with learning disabilities	Children with severe to profound neurological and learning impairment
Cue generation	Elaborated by physicians and nurses based on clinical experience ($n =5$).	Interviews with primary caregivers of 22 children aged 6–29 years (mean 14.5 years).	Interviews (20) with parents of 21 children aged 2–18 (mean 11 years) Interviews with professionals (26). Questionnaires to parents (120) of children aged 1 to 25 (mean 11 yrs) (only 2/120 > 18 yrs)
Coding	22 items reduced to 10	Interviews reviewd and list of 31 items produced which was them used to code interviews.	56 behaviours identified through inductive coding of interviews and questionnaires. Each of 56 items, identified by > 5% of responders. 56 items subsequently reduced to 20 through process of combination and elimination.
Coding assessed		8 interviews coded by 2nd rater	12 interviews reviewed by 3 co-investigators
Study setting	31 patients likely to be suffering and 31 without reason to suffer. Age 2–33 years (mean 16.5). 22 items reduced to 10.	Daily life: Short sharp pain; Longer lasting pain	Daily life—any situation. Info re pain sources collected. Parents of 132 children +26 professionals from mixed disciplines
Vocal	Crying with or without tears Moaning or inaudible cries Shouting or crying	Moaning, whining, whimpering Crying Screaming / yelling Specific sound	Cried /moaned /groaned /screamed or whimpered

Facial expression	Painful expression
	    Anxious
	    Smirking
		Cringe/grimace
		Furrowed brow
		Change in eyes, including eyes tightly shut, eyes open wide; eyes as if frowning
		Turn down of mouth, not smiling
		Lips pucker up, tight, pout, or quiver
		Clenches teeth, grinds teeth, chews, thrusts tongue
			Grimaced/screwed up eyes or face
			Frowned/had furrowed brow/looked worried
			Looked frightened (eyes wide open)
			Ground teeth or made mouthing movements

Mood		Not co-operating, cranky, irritable, unhappy Less interaction, withdrawn Seeks comfort or physical closeness Difficult to distract, not able to satisfy or pacify	Less cheerful/sociable/responsive Appeared withdrawn or depressed Hard to console or comfort Bit self or banged head
Eating and sleeping		Eats less, not interested in food Increase in sleep Decrease in sleep	Was reluctant to eat/difficult to feed Had disturbed sleep
Protective (antalgic)	Co-ordinated defensive reaction Protection of painful areas	Flinches or moves body part away, sensitive to touch Gestures to or touches part of body that hurts Not moving, less active, quiet Protects, favours, or guards part of the body that hurts	Pulled away or flinched when touched Tended to touch or rub certain areas Resisted or was fearful of being moved
Movement and posture		Moves body in a specific way to show pain (e.g. head back, arms down, curls up)	Was restless/agitated or distressed Flexed inwards or drew legs up towards chest Tensed/stiffened or spasmed

Table 20.1 (*Continued*)

Author	San Salvador [144]	Non-communicating children's Pain checklist [142,145]	Paediatric Pain Profile [13,15]
		Stiff, spastic, tense, rigid Jumping around, agitated, fidgity Floppy	Twisted and turned/tossed head/writhed or arched back Had involuntary (or stereotypical) movements/ was jumpy/startled or had seizures
Physiologic		Shivering Change of colour, pallor Sweating, perspiring Tears Sharp intake of breath, gasping Breath-holding	In original 56 items were appeared hot, sweaty, altered breathing, pallor, redness

Pain Profile—ongoing assessments

1. For each item please circle the number that best describes your child's behaviour during the time you are assessing.
2. If you are unable to rate an item because the activity, for example 'feeding' or '. . . being touched' is not happening in the period being assessed, tick in the 'unable to assess' column and score the item as 0.

3. Copy the numbers you have circled in to the 'score' column.
4. Add up the numbers in the 'score' column to give the total score.
5. Then transfer the score to the Summary Pages.

In the last .... Name	Not at all	A little	Quite a lot	A great deal	Unable to assess	Score
Was cheerful	3	2	1	0		
Was sociable or responsive	3	2	1	0		
Appeared withdrawn or depressed	0	1	2	3		
Cried/moaned/groaned/screamed or whimpered	0	1	2	3		
Was hard to console or comfort	0	1	2	3		
Self-harmed e.g. bit self or banged head	0	1	2	3		
Was reluctant to eat/difficult to feed	0	1	2	3		
Had disturbed sleep	0	1	2	3		
Grimaced/screwed up face/screwed up eyes	0	1	2	3		
Frowned/had furrowed brow/looked worried	0	1	2	3		
Looked frightened (with eyes wide open)	0	1	2	3		
Ground teeth or made mouthing movements	0	1	2	3		
Was restless/agitated or distressed	0	1	2	3		
Tensed/stiffened or spasmed	0	1	2	3		
Flexed inwards or drew legs up towards chest	0	1	2	3		
Tended to touch or rub particular areas	0	1	2	3		
Resisted being moved	0	1	2	3		
Pulled away or flinched when touched	0	1	2	3		
Twisted and turned/tossed head/writhed or arched back	0	1	2	3		
Had involuntary or stereotypical movements/was jumpy/startled or had seizures	0	1	2	3		
Total						

Fig. 20.8 Paediatric pain profile.

- *Body.* Be careful to consider pain as an integral part of the physical examination. Physical examination should include a comprehensive check of all body areas for potential pain sites. The child's reactions during the examination — grimacing, contractures, rigidity, etc.—may indicate pain.

- *Context.* Consider the impact of family, health care and environmental factors on the child's pain.

- *Document.* Record the severity of the child's pain on a regular basis. Use a pain scale that is simple and appropriate both for the developmental level of the child and for the cultural context in which it is used.

- *Evaluate.* Assess the effectiveness of pain interventions regularly and modify the treatment plan as necessary, until the child's pain is alleviated or minimized.

Although validity and reliability of pain assessment instruments is important in both research and clinical settings, the provision of an aid to communication may be the most vital function of a pain measurement tool for children in the palliative care setting. When, for instance, a child lying rigid in bed is asked how bad his pain is on a 0–10 scale and he replies '11', the reply, though it might not be considered valid in psychometric terms, certainly conveys meaning.

The main purposes of pain measurement within the clinical setting are, therefore, to

- describe and quantify the experience,

- monitor the effects of treatment,

- provide the individual with a shared medium through which he or she can communicate the experience to others.

Pain measures may ultimately be most useful as a channel of communication between the clinician and the patient, not as an alternative to talking to the child and family, but as part of the conversation. Engaging with the child and family is necessary to understanding not only the nature and context of the child's pain, but also the family's fears, goals and aspirations, knowledge of which may help to determine the appropriate treatment.

References

1. Dennett, D.C. *Kinds of Minds. Towards an Understanding of Consciousness* (2nd edition). London: Phoenix, 1996.
2. Schecter, N.L., Allen, D.A., and Hanson, K. Status of pediatric pain control: A comparison of hospital anagesic usage in children and adults. *Pediatrics* 1986;77:11–15.
3. Beyer, J.E. and Wells, N. Assessment of cancer pain in children. In R.B. Patt, (ed.) *Cancer Pain*. Philadelphia, PA: J.B. Lippincott Company, 1993, pp. 57–84.
4. Berde, C., Ablin, A., Glazer, J., Miser, A., Shapiro, B., Weisman, S., et al. Report on the subcommittee on disease-related pain in children. *Pediatrics* 1990;86(5):818–33.
5. McGrath, P.J., Beyer, J., Cleeland, C., Eland J., McGrath, P.A., and Portenoy, R. Report of the subcommittee on assessment and methodological issues in the management of pain in childhood cancer. *Pediatrics* 1990;86(5):814–17.
6. Thompson, K.L. and Varni, J.W. A developmental cognitive-biobehavioral approach to pediatric pain assessment. *Pain* 1986; 25(3):283–96.
7. Varni, J.W., Walco, G.A., and Katz, E.R. Assessment and management of chronic and recurrent pain in children with chronic diseases. *Pediatrician* 1989;16(1–2):56–63.
8. Beyer, J.E., Platt, A.F., Kinney, T.R., and Treadwell, M. Practice guidelines for the assessment of children with sickle cell pain. *J Soc Pediatr Nurs* 1999;4(2):61–73.
9. Franck, L.S., Treadwell, M., Jacob, E., and Vichinsky, E. Assessment of sickle cell pain in children and young adults using the adolescent pediatric pain tool. *J Pain Symptom Manage* 2002;23(2):114–20.
10. Breau, L.M., Camfield, C.S., McGrath, P.J., and Finley, G.A. The incidence of pain in children with severe cognitive impairments. *Arch Pediatr Adolesc Med* 2003;157(12):1219–26.
11. Carter, B., McArthur, E., and Cunliffe, M. Dealing with uncertainty: Parental assessment of pain in their children with profound special needs. *J Adv Nurs* 2002;38(5):449–57.
12. Hunt, A. and Burne, R. Medical and nursing problems of children with neurodegenerative disease. *Palliat Med* 1995;9:19–26.
13. Hunt, A.M. Towards an understanding of pain in the child with severe neurological impairment. Development of a behaviour rating scale for assessing pain [PhD]. Manchester: University of Manchester, 2001.
14. Hunt, A., Mastroyannopoulou, K., Goldman, A., and Seers, K. Not knowing-the problem of pain in children with severe neurological impairment. *Int J Nurs Stud* 2003;40(2):171–83.
15. Hunt, A., Goldman A., Seers, K., Crichton, N., Mastroyannopoulou, K., Moffat, V., et al. Clinical validation of the Paediatric Pain Profile. *Dev Med Child Neurol* 2004;46(1):9–18.
16. Stallard, P., Williams, L., Lenton, S., and Velleman, R. Pain in cognitively impaired, non-communicating children. *Arch Dis Child* 2001;85(6):460–2.
17. Kane, J.R. and Primomo, M. Alleviating the suffering of seriously ill children. *Am J Hosp Palliat Care* 2001;18(3):161–9.
18. Ferrell, B.R., Rhiner, M., Shapiro, B., and Dierkes, M. The experience of pediatric cancer pain, Part I: Impact of pain on the family. *J Pediatr Nurs* 1994;9(6):368–79.
19. Treadwell, M.J., Franck, L.S., and Vichinsky, E. Using quality improvement strategies to enhance pediatric pain assessment. *Int J Qual Health Care* 2002;14(1):39–47.
20. Staats, P.S., Hekman, H., and Staats, A.W. The psychological behaviorism theory. *Pain forum* 1996;5(3):194–207.
21. Strawson, G. *Mental Reality*. Cambridge, MA: MIT Press, 1994.
22. Sullivan, M.D. Chronic pain: The need for a 'second-person' account. *Semin Clin Neuropsychiatr* 1999;4(3):195–202.
23. Merskey, H. and Bogduk, N. Classification of chronic pain: Description of chronic pain syndromes and definition of pain terms. Seattle: IASP Press, 1994.

24. Merskey, H. (ed). Descriptions of chronic pain syndromes and definitions of pain terms. New York: International Association for the Study of Pain. *Pain* 1986; (Suppl. 3).

25. IASP. International Association for the Study of Pain: Pain terms: a list of definitions and notes on usage recommended by the IASP Subcommittee on Taxonomy. *Pain* 1979;6:249–52.

26. Melzack, R. and Wall, P. *The Challenge of Pain*. Hammondsworth, Middlesex: Penguin Books, 1982.

27. Turk, D.C. and Okifuji, A. Assessment of patients' reporting of pain: An integrated perspective. *Lancet* 1999;353(9166):1784–8.

28. Wall, P.D. Introduction to the edition after this one. In R. Melzack (ed.) *Textbook of Pain*. New York: Churchill Livingstone, 1994; pp. 1–7.

29. Fitzgerald, M. The post-natal development of cutaneous afferent fibre input and receptive field organization in the rat dorsal horn. *J Physiol* 1985;364:1–18.

30. Dickenson, A.H., Chapman, V., and Green G.M. The pharmacology of excitatory and inhibitory amino acid—mediated events in the transmission and modulation of pain in the spinal cord. *Gen Pharmacol* 1997;28(5):633–8.

31. Herrero, J.F., Laird, J.M.A., and Lopez-Garcia, J.A. Wind-up of spinal cord neurones and pain sensation: Much ado about something? *Prog Neurobiol* 2000;61:169–203.

32. Fordyce, W.E. An operant conditioning method for managing chronic pain. *Postgrad Med* 1973;53(6):123–8.

33. Fordyce, W.E. *Behavioral Methods for Chronic Pain and Illness*. St Louis, MO: Mosby, 1976.

34. Keefe, F.J., Block, A.R., Williams, R.B., Jr., and Surwit, R.S. Behavioral treatment of chronic low back pain: Clinical outcome and individual differences in pain relief. *Pain* 1981;11(2):221–31.

35. Wall, P.D. Three phases of evil: The relation of injury to pain. *Ciba Foundation Symp* 1979;69:293–304.

36. Ahles, T.A., Blanchard, E.B., and Ruckdeschel, J.C. The multidimensional nature of cancer-related pain. *Pain* 1983;17(3):277–88.

37. Sullivan, M.D. Pain in language. From sentience to sapience. *Pain Forum* 1995;4(1):3

38. Newson, J. An intersubjective approach to the systematic description of mother-infant interaction. In H.R. Schaffer, (ed.) *Studies in Maternal-Infant interaction. Proceedings of the Loch Lomond Sympoium*; September 1975. Strathclyde: University of Stracthclyde, 1977, pp. 47–61.

39. Kaye, K. The Mental and Social Life of Babies. How Parents Create Persons. Chicago, IL: The University of Chicago Press, 1982.

40. Stern, D.N., Beebe, B., Jaffe, J., and Bennett S.L. The infant's stimulus world during social interaction: A study of caregiver behaviours with particular reference to repetition and timing. In H.R. Schaffer, (ed.) *Studies in Maternal-Infant interaction. Proceedings of the Loch Lomond Symposium.*; September 1975. Strathclyde: University of Strathclyde, 1977, pp. 177–200.

41. Trevarthen, C. Descriptive analyses of infant communicative behaviour. In H.R. Schaffer, (ed.) *Studies in Maternal-Infant interaction. Proceedings of the Loch Lomond Symposium.*, Septemper 1975. Strathclyde: University of Strathclyde, 1977, p. 227–70.

42. Schaffer H.R. Early interactive development. In H.R. Schaffer, (ed.) *Studies in Maternal-Infant interaction. Proceedings of the Loch Lomond Symposium*. Strathclyde: University of Strathclyde, 1977.

43. Layder, D. *Understanding Social Theory*. London: Sage Publications, 1994.

44. Schutz, A. *Collected papers. The Problem of Social Reality*. The Hague: Martinus Nijhoff, 1962.

45. Wittgenstein, L. *Philosophical Investigations* (3rd edition). Oxford: Blackwell Publishers, 1953.

46. Melzack, R. The McGill Pain Questionnaire: Major properties and scoring methods. *Pain* 1975;277–99.

47. Harré, R. *The Singular Self. An Introduction to the Psychology of Personhood*. London: Sage Publications, 1998.

48. McGinn, M. *Wittgenstein and the Philosophical Investigations*. London: Routledge, 1997.

49. Stern, D.N. *The Interpersonal World of the Infant*. London: Karnac Books, 1998.

50. Andrews, K. and Fitzgerald, M. Cutaneous flexion reflex in human neonates: A quantitative study of threshold and stimulus-response characteristics after single and repeated stimuli. *Dev Med Child Neurol* 1999;41(10):696–703.

51. Andrews K. and Fitzgerald, M. The cutaneous withdrawal reflex in human neonates: Sensitization, receptive fields, and the effects of contralateral stimulation. *Pain* 1994;56(1):95–101.

52. Anand, K.J., Coskun, V., Thrivikraman, K.V., Nemeroff, C.B., and Plotsky, P.M. Long-term behavioral effects of repetitive pain in neonatal rat pups. *Physiol Behav* 1999;66(4):627–37.

53. Anand, K.J. Effects of perinatal pain and stress. *Prog Brain Res* 2000; 122:117–29.

54. Fitzgerald, M. and Andrews, K. Flexion reflex properties in the human infant. In P.J. McGrath, (ed.) *Measurement of Pain in Infants and Children*. Seattle: IASP Press, 1998, pp. 47–58.

55. Lloyd-Thomas, A.R. and Fitzgerald, M. Do fetuses feel pain? Reflex responses do not necessarily signify pain. *BMJ* 1996;313(7060):797–8.

56. Porter, F.L., Wolf, C.M., and Miller, J.P. Procedural pain in newborn infants: the influence of intensity and development. *Pediatr* 1999; 104(1):e13.

57. Shapiro, B.S. Implications for our definition of pain. *Pain Forum* 1999;8(2):100–2.

58. Graham, D.T. Health, disease, and the mind-body problem: Linguistic parallelism. *Psychosom Med* 1967;29(1):52–71.

59. Anand, K.J.S. and Craig, K.D. New perspectives on the definition of pain. *Pain* 1996;67:3–6.

60. Anand, K.J.S, Rovnaghi, C., Walden, M., and Churchill, J. Consciousness, behavior, and clinical impact of the definition of pain. *Pain Forum* 1999;8(2):64–73.

61. Cunningham, N. Primary requirements for an ethical definition of pain. *Pain Forum* 1999;8(2):93–9.

62. Rollin, B.E. Some conceptual and ethical concerns about current views of pain. *Pain Forum* 1999;8(2):78–83.

63. McIntosh, N. Pain in the newborn, a possible new starting point. *Eur J Pediatr* 1997;156(3):173–7.

64. Kopelman, L.M. Acknowledging pain in others. *Pain Forum* 1999; 8(2):87–90.

65. Craig, K. and Badali, M. On knowing an infant's pain. *Pain Forum* 1999;8(2):74–7.

66. Derbyshire, S.W. Do fetuses feel pain? Analgesic and anaesthetic procedures are being introduced because of shoddy sentimental argument [letter; comment]. *BMJ* 1997;314(7088):1201.

67. Derbyshire, S.W.G. The IASP definition captures the essence of pain experience. *Pain Forum* 1999;8(2):106–9.

68. Williams, A.C., Davies, H.T., and Chadury, Y. Simple pain rating scales hide complex idiosyncratic meanings. *Pain* 2000;85(3):457–63.

69. Morley, S., Doyle, K., and Beese, A. Talking to others about pain: Suffering in silence. In Z. Wiesenfeld-Hallin, (ed.) Proceedings of the 9th World Congress on Pain, 1999; Vienna, Austria: IASP Press, 1999, pp. 1123–9.

70. Popper, K.R. Knowledge and the Body-Mind Problem. In *Defence of Interaction*. London: Routledge, 1994.

71. Trevarthen, C. and Aitken, K.J. Brain-Development, Infant Communication, and Empathy Disorders—Intrinsic-Factors in Child Mental-Health. *Dev Psychopathol* 1994;6(4):597–633.

72. Fridlund, A.J. The new ethology of human facial expression. In J.M. Fernandez-Dols, (ed.) *The Psychology of Facial Expression*. Cambridge: Cambridge University Press, 1997, pp. 103–129.

73. Deyo, K.S., Prkachin, K.M., and Mercer, S.R. Development of sensitivity to facail expression of pain. *Pain* 2004;107:16–21.

74. Bateson, M.C. 'The epigenesis of conversational interaction': A personal account of research development. In M. Bullowa, (ed.) *Before Speech: The Beginning of Interpersonal Communication*. Cambridge: Cambridge University Press, 1979.

75. Craig, K.D., Gilbert-MacLeod, C.A., and Lilley, C.M. Crying as an indicator of pain in infants. In J.A. Green, (ed.) *Crying as a Sign, a Symptom and a Signal. Clinical, emotional and Developmental Aspects of Infant and Toddler Crying*. Cambridge: Mac Keith Press. Cambridge University Press, 2000, pp. 23–40.

76. Calhoun, M.L., Rose, T.L., Hanft, B., and Sturkey, C. Social reciprocity interventions: Implications for developmental therapists. *Phys Occup Ther Pediatr* 1991;11(3):45–56.

77. Lobo, M.L. Parent-infant interaction during feeding when the infant has congenital heart disease. *J Pediatr Nurs* 1992;7(2):97–105.

78. Keefe, F.J. and Dunsmore, J. Pain behavior. Concepts and controversies. *APS Journal* 1992;1(2):92–100.

79. Izard, C.E., Hembree, E.A., and Huebner, R.R. Infants' emotion expressions to acute pain: Developmental change and stability of individual differences. *Dev Psychol* 1987;23(1):105–13.

80. Brannigan, C.R., and Humphries, D.A. Human non-verbal behaviour, a means of communication. In N. Blurton Jones, (ed.) *Ethological Studies of Child Behaviour*. Cambridge: Cambridge University Press, 1972, pp. 37–65.

81. Russell, J.A. Reading emotions from and into faces: Resurrecting a dimensional-contextual perspective. In J.M. Fernandez-Dols, (ed.) *The Psychology of Facial Expression*. Cambridge: Cambridge University Press, 1997, pp. 295–320.

82. Schiefenhovel, W. Perception, Expression, and Social Function of Pain—a Human Ethological View. *Sci Context* 1995;8(1):31–46.

83. Craig, K. The facial display of pain. In McGrath, P.J, (ed.) Measurement of Pain in Infants and Children. Seattle: IASP Press, 1998, pp. 103–121.

84. Craig, K.D., Lilley, C.M., and Gilbert, C.A. Social barriers to optimal pain management in infants and children. *Clin J Pain* 1996; 12(3):232–42.

85. Mead, G.H. *Mind, Self, and Society. From the Standpoint of a Social Behaviorist*. Paperback Edition 1967 ed. Chicago, IL: The University of Chicago Press, 1962.

86. Blumer, H. *Symbolic Interactionism. Perspecive and Method*. Berkeley, CA: University of California Press, 1969.

87. Grunau, R.V.E., Johnston, C.C., and Craig, K.D. Neonatal facial and cry responses to invasive and non-invasive procedures. *Pain* 1990; 42:293–305.

88. Grunau, R.V.E. and Craig, K.D. Pain expression in neonates: Facial action and cry. *Pain* 1987;28(3):395–410.

89. Prkachin, K.M. The consistency of facial expressions of pain: A comparison across modalities. In E. Rosenberg, (ed.) *What the Face Reveals. Basic and Applied Studies of Spontaneous Expression using the Facial Action Coding System (FACS)*. Oxford: Oxford University Press, 1997, pp. 181–200.

90. Gilbert, C.A., Lilley, C.M., Craig, K.D., McGrath, P.J., Court, C.A., Bennett S.M., *et al*. Postoperative pain expression in preschool children: Validation of the child facial coding system. *Clin J Pain* 1999;15(3):192–200.

91. Oberlander, T.F., Gilbert, C.A., Chambers, C.T., O'Donnell, M.E., and Craig, K.D. Biobehavioral responses to acute pain in adolescents with a significant neurologic impairment. *Clin J Pain* 1999;15:201–9.

92. Craig, K.D. On knowing another's pain. In E. Rosenberg (ed.) *What the Face Reveals. Basic and Applied Studies of Spontaneous Expression using the Facial Action Coding System* (FACS). Oxford: Oxford University Press, 1997, pp. 187–180.

93. Ginsburg, G.P. Faces: An epilogue and reconceptualization. In J.M. Fernandez-Dols, (ed.) *The Psychology of Facial Expression*. Cambridge: Cambridge University Press, 1997, pp. 349—82.

94. Hamers, J.P.H., Abu-Saad, H.H., Halfens, R., and Schumacher, J. Factors influencing nurses' pain assessment and interventions in children. *J Adv Nurs* 1994;20(5):853–60.

95. Gustafson, G.E., Wood, R.M., and Green, J.A. Can we hear the causes of infant's crying. In J.A. Green, (ed.) *Crying as a Sign, a Symptom and a Signal. Clinical, emotional amd Developmental Aspects of Infant and Toddler Crying*. Cambridge: Mac Keith Press, Cambridge University Press, 2000.

96. Muller, E., Hollien, H., and Murry, T. Infant crying as an elicitor of parental behaviour: An examination of two models. *J Child Lang* 1974;1:89–95.

97. McGrath, P.J. Behavioral measures of pain. In P.J. McGrath (ed.) *Measurement of Pain in Infants and Children Seattle*: IASP Press, 1998, p. 83–102.

98. Poulain, P.A., Pichard-Leandri, E.M., and Gauvin-Piquard, A.P. Assessment and treatment of pain in children in palliative care. *Eur J Palliat Care* 1994;1(1):31–5.

99. Johnston, C.C. and Strada, M.E. Acute pain response in infants: A multidimensional description. *Pain* 1986;24(3):373–82.

100. Hadjistavropoulos, H.D., Craig, K.D., Grunau, R.V., and Johnston, C.C. Judging pain in newborns: Facial and cry determinants. *J Pediatr Psychol* 1994;19(4):485–91.

101. Lichter, I. and Hunt, E. The last 48 hours of life. *J Palliat Care* 1990;6(4):7–15.

102. Elander, G., Hellstrom, G., and Qvarnstrom, B. Care of infants after major surgery: Observation of behavior and analgesic administration. *Pediatr Nurs* 1993;19(3):221–6.

103. McDaniel, L.K., Anderson, K.O., Bradley, L.A., Young, L.D., Turner, R.A., Agudelo, C.A. *et al*. Development of an observational

method for assessing pain behavior in rheumatoid arthritis patients. *Pain* 1986;24:165–84.

104. Jaworski, T.M., Bradley, L.A., Heck, L.W., Roca, A., and Alarcon, G.S. Development of an observation method for assessing pain behaviors in children with juvenile rheumatoid arthritis. *Arthritis Rheum* 1995;38:1142–51.

105. Wilkie, D.J., Keefe, F.J., Dodd, M.J., and Copp, L.A. Behavior of patients with lung cancer: Description and associations with oncologic and pain variables. *Pain* 1992;51(2):231–40.

106. Gauvin-Piquard A., Rodary G., Rezvani A., Serbouti S. The development of the DEGR^R: A scale to assess pain in young children with cancer. *Eur J Pain* 1999;3:165–76.

107. Sweet, S.D. and McGrath, P.J. Physiological measures of pain. In P.J. McGrath, (ed.) *Measurement of Pain in Infants and Children.* Seattle: IASP Press, 1998; pp. 59–81.

108. Osgood, P.F. and Szyfelbein, S.K. Management of burn pain in children. *Pediatr Clin North Am* 1989;36(4):1001–13.

109. Coffman, S., Alvarez, Y., Pyngolil, M., Petit, R., Hall, C., and Smyth, M. Nursing assessment and management of pain in critically ill children. *Heart Lung* 1997;26(3):221–8.

110. Howard, V.A. and Thurber, F.W. The interpretation of infant pain: physiological and behavioral indicators used by NICU nurses. *J Pediatr Nurs* 1998;13(3):164–74.

111. Owens, M.E. Pain in Infancy: Conceptual and methodological issues. *Pain* 1984;20:213–30.

112. Mudge, D. and Younger, J.B. The effects of topical lidocaine on infant response to circumcision. *J Nurs Midwifery* 1989;34(6): 335–40.

113. Lander, J., Brady-Fryer, B., Metcalfe, J.B., Nazarali, S., and Muttitt, S. Comparison of ring block, dorsal penile nerve block, and topical anesthesia for neonatal circumcision: A randomized controlled trial. *J Am Med Assoc* 1997;278(24):2157–62.

114. Guinsburg, R., Kopelman, B.I., Anand, K.J., de Almeida, M.F., Peres, C.d.A., and Miyoshi, M.H. Physiological, hormonal, and behavioral responses to a single fentanyl dose in intubated and ventilated preterm neonates. *J Pediatr* 1998;132(6):954–9.

115. McIntosh, N., van Veen, L., and Brameyer, H. Alleviation of the pain of heel prick in preterm infants. *Arch Dis Child Fetal Neonatal Ed* 1994;70(3):F177–81.

116. Anand, K.J.S. and Carr, D.B. The neuroanatomy, neurophysiology, and neurochemistry of pain, stress, and analgesia in newborns and children. *Pediatr Clin North Am* 1989;36(4):795–822.

117. Lewis, M. and Thomas, D. Cortisol release in infants in response to inoculation. *Child Dev* 1990;61(1):50–9.

118. Giannakoulopoulos, X., Sepulveda, W., Kourtis, P., Glover, V., and Fisk, N.M. Fetal plasma cortisol and beta-endorphin response to intrauterine needling. *Lancet* 1994;344(8915):77–81.

119. Gunnar, M.R., Porter, F.L., Wolf, C.M., Rigatuso, J., and Larson, M.C. Neonatal stress reactivity: Predictions to later emotional temperament. *Child Dev* 1995;66(1):1–13.

120. Gunnar, M.R., Brodersen, L., Krueger, K., and Rigatuso, J. Dampening of adrenocortical responses, during infancy: Normative changes and individual differences. *Child Dev* 1996; 67(3): 877–89.

121. Ramsay, D.S., and Lewis, M. The effects of birth condition on infants' cortisol response to stress. *Pediatrics* 1995;95(4):546–9.

122. Lewis, M., Ramsay, D.S., and Kawakami, K. Differences between Japanese infants and Caucasian American infants in behavioral and cortisol response to inoculation. *Child Dev* 1993;64(6):1722–31.

123. Kurtis, P.S., DeSilva, H.N., Bernstein, B.A., Malakh, L., and Schechter, N.L. A comparison of the Mogen and Gomco clamps in combination with dorsal penile nerve block in minimizing the pain of neonatal circumcision. *Pediatrics* 1999;103(2):E23.

124. Kidd, S., Reiss, J., McIntosh, N., Stephens, R., and Smith, J. Measuring subacute pain in the newborn. In Abstracts 5th International Symposium on Paediatric Pain. London, 2000.

125. Kidd, S., Lone, N., Midgley, P., McIntosh, N., Stephens, R., Smith, J. *et al.* Salivary hormones as markers of pain in children. In Abstracts 5th International Symposium on Paediatric Pain, 2000; London, 2000.

126. Moore, R.A., Evans, P.J., Smith, R.F., and Lloyd, J.W. Increased cortisol excretion in chronic pain. *Anaesthesia* 1983;38(8):788–91.

127. Piaget, J. and Inhelder, B. *The Psychology of the Child.* London: Routledge & Keegan Paul, 1969.

128. Boden, M.A. *Piaget.* London: Fontana Press, 1994.

129. Beyer, J.E., and Aradine, C.R. Content validity of an instrument to measure young children's perceptions of the intensity of their pain. *J Pediatr Nurs* 1986;1(6):386–95.

130. McGrath, P.A., deVeber, L.L., and Hearn, M.T. Multidimensional pain assessment in children. In F. Cervero, (ed.) *Advances in Pain Research and Therapy.* New York: Raven Press, 1985, pp. 387–393.

131. Shih, A.R. and von Baeyer, C.L. Preschool children's seriation of pain faces and happy faces in the Affective Facial Scale. *Psychol Rep* 1994;74(2):659–65.

132. Hicks, C.L., von Baeyer, C.L., Spafford, P., van Korlaar, I., and Goodenough, B. The Faces Pain Scale—Revised: Toward a common metric in pediatric pain measurement. *Pain* 2001; 93:173–83. Scale adapted from: Bieri, D., Reeve, R., Champion, G., Addicoat, L., and Ziegler, J. The Faces Pain Scale for the self-assessment of the severity of pain experienced by children: Development, initial validation and preliminary investigation for ratio scale properties. *Pain* 1990;41:139–50.

133. Hester, N.K. The preoperational child's reaction to immunization. *Nurs Res* 1979;28(4):250–5.

134. Wong, D.L. and Baker, C.M. Pain in children: Comparison of assessment scales. *Pediatr Nurs* 1988;14(1):9–17.

135. McGrath, P.A., Seifert, C.E., Speechley, K.N., Booth, J.C., Stitt, L., and Gibson, M.C. A new analogue scale for assessing children's pain: An initial validation study. *Pain* 1996;64(3):435–43.

136. McCaffery, M. and Beebe, A. Pain in Children. Special Considerations. In A. Beebe, (ed.) Pain. Clinical Manual of Nursing Practice. St Louis: The C.V. Mosby Company, 1989.

137. Unruh, A., McGrath, P., Cunningham, S.J., and Humphreys, P. Children's drawings of their pain. *Pain* 1983;17:385–492.

138. Collins, J.J., Byrnes, M.E., Dunkel, I.J., Lapin, J., Nadel, T., Thaler, H.T. *et al.* The measurement of symptoms in children with cancer. *J Pain Symptom Manage* 2000;19(5):363–77.

139. Collins, J.J., Devine, T.D., Dick, G.S., Johnson, E.A., Kilham, H.A., Pinkerton, C.R., *et al.* The measurement of symptoms in young children with cancer: The validation of the Memorial Symptom Assessment Scale in children aged 7–12. *J Pain Symptom Manage* 2002;23(1):10–16.

140. Oberlander, T.F., O'Donnell, M.E., and Montgomery, C.J. Pain in children with significant neurological impairment. *J Dev Behav Pediatr* 1999;20(4):235–43.

141. McGrath, P.J., Rosmus, C., Canfield, C., Campbell, M.A., and Hennigar, A. Behaviours caregivers use to determine pain in non-verbal, cognitively impaired individuals. *Dev Med Child Neurol* 1998;40(5):340–3.

142. Stallard, P., Williams, L., Velleman, R., Lenton, S., McGrath, P.J., and Taylor, G. The development and evaluation of the pain indicator for communicatively impaired children (PICIC). *Pain* 2002;98(1–2):145–9.

143. Collignon, P. and Giusiano, B. Validation of a pain evaluation scale for patients with severe cerebral palsy. *Eur J Pain* 2001;5(4): 433–42.

144. Breau, L.M., McGrath, P.J., Camfield, C.S., and Finley, G.A. Psychometric properties of the non-communicating children's pain checklist-revised. *Pain* 2002;99(1–2):349–57.

145. Fanuric, D., Koh, J.L., Harrison, R.D., Conard, T.M., and Tomerlin, C. Pain assessment in children with cognitive impairment. An exploration of self-report skills. *Clin Nurs Res* 1998;7(2):103–19; discussion 120–4.

146. World Health Organization. *Cancer Pain Relief and Palliative Care in Children.* Geneva: World Health Organization, 1998.

21 Pain—pharmacological management

Ross Drake and Richard Hain

Introduction

Children suffer from a wide range of malignant and non-malignant conditions that ultimately result in death in childhood or young adulthood. The disease trajectory may differ for individual illnesses, but in most, pain is both prevalent and distressing [1–3]. Control of pain, therefore, plays, a central role in maintaining a satisfactory quality of life, a primary aim of palliative care.

A multidisciplinary team of professionals, trained in paediatrics and with a family-centred care focus, should care for children. The team should be responsive to the requirements of individual children and their families, openly discuss treatment strategies, and anxieties and misconceptions (often particularly evident when opioids are being considered). Response to treatment needs to be monitored frequently and modified whenever appropriate. Pain management is not always straightforward and specialist advice should be sought if initial basic approaches are not effective.

The symptom of pain illustrates very well a number of fundamental precepts of good symptom management in palliative care. An approach to managing pain should flow from these basic principles.

The first is that pain is subjective; it is 'what the patient says it is'. The subjective nature of pain has been acknowledged in principle for many years. It means that in order to meet the needs of the individual patient, any pain management approach should be constantly subjected to review and modification in the light of its effectiveness. A continual cycle of prescription, review, and titration is necessary.

Pain, like all symptoms, occurs simultaneously in all domains of a child's experience. It is tempting to consider pain

to be a primarily physical phenomenon, but the reality is that it will have ramifications in emotional, psychosocial, and existential or spiritual domains. Furthermore, problems that occur in any of these other domains, will also influence pain. Any therapeutic approach that fails to take this into account is unlikely to succeed [4]. A combination of pharmacological and non-pharmacological approaches to pain is usually necessary.

A third guiding principle in palliative care is that its value to the patient should be carefully considered by weighing up its burden and its benefits. To do this clearly requires some knowledge of the pathophysiology of pain, and the pharmacology of drugs used to treat it. Ideally, this should be based on published evidence. This is not always available for those working in children's palliative care. Published evidence is generally rather sparse, and what there is usually comes from studies in adults who are either healthy or suffering from cancer. Extrapolation from these studies to children is often necessary, but should be undertaken with caution since children and adults differ in anatomy and physiology as well as their cognitive responses to pain and analgesia. This is particularly true in the neonatal period [5–8].

A rational approach to treatment is not, however, limited to deriving practice from published studies. It is intuitively reasonable to use medications for an individual that have been effective and well tolerated in the past. Where there is no evidence, an empirical approach based on an understanding of the drugs themselves and on observation of their effectiveness in patients is rational.

This chapter will consider the pharmacological management of pain in children with life-limiting conditions and, wherever possible, will draw on the pool of knowledge gained from studies in children themselves.

World Health Organization guidelines

Overview

In the 1980s, the World Health Organization identified a global problem in managing pain in adults with cancer [9]. It was recognized that underlying this were a number of uncertainties and misconceptions regarding pain and how it should be treated. Prominent among these was a widespread concern about the use of major opioids. At that time, major opioids were often seen primarily as drugs of addiction that should usually be avoided unless there was no alternative. Children were, by common consent, considered particularly vulnerable to the adverse effects of opioids and these were often withheld. This over-cautious approach was often justified by early studies that seemed to suggest that children experienced pain less intensely than adults [10].

In attempting to address some of the confusion and misunderstanding, the WHO drew up a simple and rational stepwise approach to the management of cancer pain in adults [9]. The guidelines were subsequently republished with little modification for children [4]. The WHO approach (Figure 21.1) is based on the assumption that, for most children, pain will gradually increase as their illness progresses, and that this increase in pain intensity should be matched by the stepwise introduction of progressively stronger analgesics.

On the first step are simple analgesics, essentially limited in children to paracetamol, on the second are minor or weak opioids, and on the third major or strong opioids. One aim of this model is to avoid cycling through alternative medications of the same potency as an alternative to selecting a stronger class of drug. If step 2 is no longer effective, a major opioid on step 3 is required.

Around this basic stepwise approach to analgesia, the WHO built a simple but rational set of guidelines. They were intended to be educational rather than definitive, but their

practical usefulness has been such that they remain more or less unchanged at the present time.

The WHO approach has been summarized in four phrases:

1. By the ladder—enabling a stepwise approach to treatment commencing with non-opioids and increasing to strong opioids (Figure 21.1). The level at which a child enters the ladder is determined by the child's needs, the intensity of pain and response to previous treatments.

2. By the clock—regular scheduling ensures a steady blood concentration, reducing the peaks and troughs of *pro re nata* (PRN) dosing.

3. By the appropriate route—use the least invasive route of administration. The oral route is convenient, non-invasive and cost effective.

4. By the child—individualize treatment according to the child's pain and response to treatment.

The extent to which these principles can be extended beyond management of cancer pain is not clear. There is little in the guidelines that is specific for a malignant cause and, in the absence of evidence to the contrary, it seems reasonable to assume that they can be usefully applied to the much wider range of conditions that characterizes palliative care in children. The following sections consider each of the steps in turn, as well as some of the more general principles of selecting a suitable drug, dose, and route as well as the use of appropriate adjuvants.

Caveats

Although the WHO approach remains the most widely accepted and standardized one, there is debate about some aspects. Perhaps the most important of these, are around the middle minor opioid step. With respect to their pharmacological effect, a minor opioid is little or no different from a small dose of a major opioid. The second step of the WHO ladder is, therefore, seen by some as effectively redundant and introducing an unnecessary complication [11].

Furthermore, some opioids traditionally classified as weak, such as tramadol, may in practice have a much higher analgesic potency through non-opioid mechanisms. These 'intermediate opioids' have no obvious place in the WHO ladder and yet can sometimes be of value in practice.

Debate has also surrounded the categorisation of non-steroidal anti-inflammatory drugs as adjuvants. By definition, an adjuvant has always been considered to be a drug that, while it can give relief from pain in certain situations, is not itself inherently analgesic. This definition is appropriate for carbamazepine, for example, which is of proven analgesic efficacy in many forms of neuropathic pain, but has no place in managing pain outside this indication. It is not equally suitable for non-steroidal anti-inflammatory drugs, which

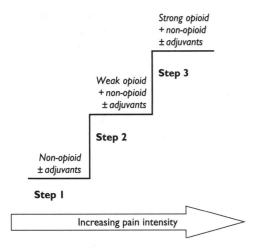

Fig. 21.1 World Health Organization Analgesic Ladder (adapted from (4)).

have considerable inherent analgesic activity [11] and this aspect is reflected in an update of the WHO guidelines in adults [12].

Despite these reservations, the WHO guidelines provide an uncomplicated and logical framework for managing pain, based on an understanding both of the nature of the pain and of the medications available to treat it.

Simple analgesia (Step 1)

The range of non-opioid analgesics available for use in children is very narrow. Aspirin (acetylsalicylic acid) is an effective analgesic with additional antipyretic and anti-inflammatory properties. It therefore has one of the properties of an ideal medication in palliative care, namely that the one drug can do several things.

The effectiveness of aspirin, however, is limited by the unfamiliarity of most paediatricians with the drug. In most countries, it was withdrawn from use in children under 12 following concerns in the 1980s regarding a possible association with Reye syndrome. Although this is not relevant for most indications in palliative care, aspirin is rarely used in practice.

Aspirin inhibits platelet aggregation, an irreversible effect whose duration is therefore the lifespan of the platelets, that is 2–3 weeks. This makes it unsuitable for use in most children with thrombocytopenia or dysfunctional platelets.

Paracetamol (Acetaminophen)

Paracetamol provides good relief for mild pain and alongside other analgesics plays an important role in the relief of moderate to severe pain. It is widely used and well tolerated in children, both for its analgesic and anti-pyretic properties. It has a central action through inhibition of prostaglandin synthesis in the hypothalamus and by blocking spinal hyperalgesia mediated by substance P and N-methyl D-aspartate (NMDA). It has no peripheral action or anti-inflammatory effect.

Oral doses are absorbed rapidly from the duodenum, but peak analgesic effects are not seen for 1–2 h. This is due to a lag between peak plasma and effect site concentrations in the CNS. The high oral absorption rate in conjunction with similar volumes of distribution at different ages means that loading doses vary little over age groups. Individual clearance values for paracetamol can be predicted from weight and age, with most of the age-related changes in clearance being completed by 1 year of age. After this age, increasing weight results in decreased clearance, although adult clearance is reportedly higher.

The anti-pyretic activity of paracetamol occurs at a plasma concentration of 10–20 mg/L [13]. This range correlates with analgesic activity and a target concentration of 10 mg/L produces 50% of the maximum pain relief in children [14].

In many countries the rectal route is no longer considered appropriate in children, for cultural and legal reasons. It is usually contraindicated anyway if there is a risk of neutro- or thrombocytopenia. Even when permissible, tolerated and safe, absorption of rectal paracetamol is slow and erratic [15,16]. It often fails to reach effective serum concentration and is not recommended in the palliative setting, except perhaps when short-term administration will allow analgesia to be maintained while a problem such as vomiting is controlled.

Metabolism of paracetamol occurs in the liver with around 5% excreted unchanged in the urine. The primary metabolites are a glucuronide (50–60%) and sulphate (25–35%). The majority of the remainder being metabolized by the cytochrome P450-catalyzed oxidative system forming N-acetyl-p-benzoquinone imine (NAPQI) and another catechol metabolite. NAPQI is hepatotoxic but is preferentially conjugated with intracellular tripeptide glutathione to a nontoxic metabolite. Hepatotoxicity, in the form of centrilobular necrosis of the liver, occurs when the hepatic synthesis of glutathione is overwhelmed. This is more likely to occur with doses greater than 150 mg/kg/day for 2–8 days [17], but has been reported at therapeutic doses [18,19]. Factors that may increase the risk of toxicity include chronic administration, concurrent viral infection, hepatic or renal disease, acute malnutrition, dehydration, and enzyme induction with medications like carbamazepine, phenobarbital, isoniazid, and rifampicin.

Non-steroidal anti-inflammatory drugs

Non-steroidal anti-inflammatory drugs other than aspirin, are considered in more detail under the adjuvants section (see below). Unlike other adjuvants, NSAIDs do have inherent analgesic activity [11] and some would consider them simple analgesics. However, this categorisation is not wholly satisfactory either. The potency of non-steroidals varies considerably and while some offer analgesia comparable with paracetamol, others can compare with the potency of major opioids [20]. For the purposes of this chapter, NSAIDs are considered to be adjuvants with a particular role in managing bone pain. It should be borne in mind that in practice, their application is much wider than this would suggest.

Opioids

Opioids are the mainstay of good analgesia for most children at some point in the palliative phase of their condition. They are divided somewhat arbitrarily into weak (or 'minor') opioids and strong ('major') opioids. The pharmacological distinction between them is unclear and indeed, at a receptor level, their actions are precisely the same. If there is a clear difference between the two groups, it is that the dose of a weak opioid cannot be escalated indefinitely if they are not adequately effective. This is not due to a true pharmacological ceiling effect (i.e. caused by full receptor occupancy so that further receptor-drug interaction is impossible). Rather, it seems to be a limit imposed in practice by the occurrence of adverse effects that make further increases simply intolerable.

There are, nevertheless, some practical advantages to distinguishing between weak and strong opioids. Many patients who could benefit from opioid therapy, particularly adolescents and young adults, are reluctant to start them. This can be for many reasons, many deriving from a culture disproportionately concerned about the risk of addiction. Other reasons for reluctance or poor compliance stem from the perception of morphine as a drug whose prescription marks the beginning of the road towards death.

Such fears and misconceptions should on the whole be explored rather than perpetuated by prescribing alternatives. For some patients, this is not enough and the choice for them is between a minor opioid and no analgesia at all. Irrespective of whether such fears are rational, they can powerfully compromise good pain control, and there is little point in prescribing the ideal drug regimen if it is clear that the child or young person will not comply. It is in this situation that the availability of effective alternatives that are perceived to be safer can be of real practical value.

The following section considers practical issues of prescribing opioids by addressing the following three questions:

- Which drug to select?
- How much, and how often?
- By what route?

Which drug to select?

Minor or weak opioids (Step 2)

Once simple analgesia is no longer effective to control pain, a weak opioid should be introduced. They should be added to, rather than substituted for, a non-opioid agent, and when they do not provide adequate pain relief, should be changed to a strong opioid. There is no rationale to substitute within the group.

Weak opioid analgesics are often described as having a 'ceiling effect', that is that above a certain concentration, further increases in dosage do not result in better effect. There is little to support this concept in therapeutic practice. Indeed, for codeine, it would be difficult to explain such a difference

from morphine, given the prominent role morphine itself plays in mediating analgesia after demethylation of codeine (see below). What is certainly true in practice, however, is that in higher doses, the analgesic effect of weak opioids is often out-weighed by adverse effects, imposing a *de facto* ceiling limit on the tolerability of this group of drugs. It is partly for this reason that this step of the ladder has been the subject of debate, with calls for it to be replaced by low dose morphine.

Codeine is the weak opioid agent recommended by WHO for children. There are few alternatives and, on the whole, little to separate them in terms of efficacy although tramadol has a more complex therapeutic and adverse effects profile than others in this group.

Codeine

Codeine is a derivative of morphine. It is about one tenth as potent as morphine, and 10% of it is converted to morphine by hepatic metabolism, making morphine the primary means through which codeine exerts its effect. Codeine has a similar half-life to morphine in adults, that is, 2.5–3.5 h. It has an oral bio-availability around 60% with an onset of analgesic action of 20 min, peaking at 1–2 h and lasting from 4 to 8 h. While there is some evidence that codeine itself has some direct analgesic capability [21], its analgesic action derives mainly from its metabolic by-products, and in particular from morphine and its active derivatives. The main metabolite is codeine-6-glucuronide, which has weak binding capacity. Other active metabolites include small amounts of norcodeine and morphine-6-glucuronide (M6G), as well as the inactive compound morphine-3-glucuronide (M3G), which has no affinity for opioid receptors.

Morphine is derived by demethylation via the cytochrome P450 system sub-type 2D6 (CYP2D6), for which over 50 different genetic variants have been identified. Some of these variations result in an enzyme which is unable to convert codeine to morphine. Individuals with enzyme variations of this type, derive limited analgesic effect from codeine and may account for, as much as, 30% of some populations [22].

Codeine has a side effect profile common to all opioids (Table 21.1). The most troublesome of these is constipation. The recommended oral dose is 0.5–1.0 mg/kg every 4 h for children 6 months of age and older, to a maximum of 60 mg/dose. It comes as a syrup, tablet and parenteral formulation. Parenteral administration confers no advantages over morphine and is associated with marked histamine release and hypotension.

Other minor opioids include dihydrocodeine and propoxyphene. Dihydrocodeine is a semi-synthetic analogue of codeine with a bioavailability of 20%. The onset of analgesic

Table 21.1 Adverse effects of opioids

Common	Occasional	Rare
Constipation	Dry mouth	Respiratory depression
Drowsiness	Sweating	Psychological dependence
Unsteadiness	Pruritus	
Confusion	Hallucinations	
Nausea and vomiting	Myoclonus	
	Urinary retention	

action is around 30 min and the duration of action ranges from 3 to 6 h. The low oral bioavailability means that it is equipotent to codeine when taken orally but has double the potency with parenteral administration. Propoxyphene is a congener of methadone, but only has an efficacy equivalent to that of paracetamol. It has an active metabolite, norpropoxyphene, which accumulates with repeated dosing and is toxic to the CNS.

Tramadol

Tramadol is a centrally acting synthetic derivative of codeine with weak affinity for the mu-opioid receptor, around 10 times weaker than codeine. There is also relatively weak non-opioid activity through inhibition of presynaptic serotonin and noradrenaline reuptake and stimulation of neuronal serotonin release. The active mono-O-de(s)methyl-tramadol (+) or M1 metabolite (via CYP2D6) has a mu-opioid affinity 200 times that of morphine. The combination is synergistic and gives tramadol, a potency of 1/5th to 1/10th that of morphine for oral and parenteral administration, respectively.

Oral bio-availability is around 70% but increases to 90–100% with multiple doses. Peak effect is achieved after 2 h and the duration of action is around 4–6 h. Tramadol is metabolized in the liver and around 90% excreted by the kidneys. The adverse effects are similar to those of other opioid agents and, in overdose, can result in severe respiratory depression and central nervous system symptoms such as convulsion [23].

Major or strong opioids (Step 3)—Morphine

The category of major opioids offers the greatest variety to professionals working in palliative care in children [24]. The wide range of products currently available in some countries reflects not only clinical need but also commercial expediency. The result has been a plethora of medications, all with very similar therapeutic and adverse-effects profiles. Most are little different from the archetype in this category, morphine itself, and none can boast the long history of safety and effectiveness that morphine offers.

Nevertheless, some new products do offer genuine advantages, either because of the drugs themselves or because of the formulations that are available. Additionally, there may be value for some patients in switching from one major opioid to another of a different class, even when the two are similar, since the patient may be less tolerant to some of the desirable effects of the new drug (see below).

There is, therefore, a role for many of the alternatives to morphine that have become available, providing they are used discriminatingly, and as a result of clinical decision making based on an understanding of the drugs themselves. Where there is no such advantage, morphine remains the drug of first choice for most children in whom the weak opioids of step 2 are no longer enough.

Opioid drugs are defined by their capacity to interact with mu-opioid receptors, of which there are a number of sub-types. Opiates are naturally occurring opioids such as morphine and diamorphine. Many opioids interact with other opioid receptors, notably kappa (e.g. oxycodone) and delta-opioid (e.g. methadone). Some also have activity at non-opioid receptors involved in analgesia (e.g. methadone, tramadol). In the following section, morphine will be considered first and other major opioids later, in so far as they differ from it.

Morphine acts in the CNS and with regular administration has an oral to parenteral (intravenous or subcutaneous) ratio between 1 : 2 and 1 : 3. After oral administration the onset of effect is seen after 20–30 min with peak activity reached at 60–90 min. The duration of action ranges from 3 to 6 h.

Thirty-five percent of the oral dose is made available, with the principal site of metabolism being the liver. The main metabolic process is glucuronidation with M3G and M6G, the main metabolites. M3G does not have analgesic activity, M6G does, and probably contributes significantly to the analgesic effect. M3G is the predominant metabolite in children, but the elimination clearance of M3G is greater than M6G. M3G:M6G ratios change with maturation of the hepatic and renal systems [5, 6, 8, 25]. M6G clearance is reduced in renal failure and a reduction in morphine dose is necessary to avoid toxicity.

The pharmacokinetics of morphine in neonates have been studied [5–8, 26]. Birth weight, gestational and postnatal age influence glucuronidation of morphine, and glucuronidation is present, albeit at a reduced level, in preterm and term neonates. The volume of distribution increases from 1.17 L/kg at birth to 1.94 L/kg in the first few months. Half-life decreases from around 10 hours in the preterm infant to 2 h in young children, while clearance increases from around 2 ml/kg/min to between 20 and 25 ml/kg/min, respectively. There is no evidence that morphine passes more easily into the cerebrospinal fluid of children than adults [26].

The oral, subcutaneous, intravenous, epidural, or intrathecal route can be used to administer morphine. Oral morphine comes as an immediate- and sustained-release preparation. Elixir and tablets provide the immediate-release options, while sustained-release preparations include tablets and capsules. The capsule contains granules that allow a controlled release of morphine. The capsule can be opened and the granules sprinkled in soft foods such as yoghurt or jam. If the granules are chewed, then the slow delivery effect is lost. In the opioid naïve child, the starting dose of morphine is equivalent to oral morphine 1.0–2.0 mg/kg every 24 h.

The increased half-life and reduced clearance in infants under 6 months of age warrants a more cautious approach when initiating therapy and the initial dose should be reduced by 25–30% of the dose recommended for older children. Treatment should then be adjusted according to analgesic effect and incidence of side effects.

Undue emphasis is often placed on the risk of inducing respiratory depression in children with the initiation of opioid analgesia. Children older than 3 months of age are probably at no greater risk of developing significant opioid-induced respiratory depression than adults [26,27], though vulnerability may be increased in younger infants as a result of metabolic and anatomical immaturity and consequent differences in pharmacokinetics [28,29].

This does not, of course, mean that pain in a neonate should remain untreated but that a more cautious approach should be taken to prescribing medication for younger infants. As in all age groups, the dose of opioids should then be carefully monitored and titrated as quickly as is necessary to provide symptom relief.

Major or strong opioids (Step 3)—Alternatives to morphine

Diamorphine (heroin)

Much of the important research in palliative medicine and symptom control has been in the use of diamorphine. In countries where it is available, it is usually used in effect as the parenteral form of morphine.

Diamorphine is a pro-drug that is quickly metabolized by deacetylation to an active metabolite, mono-acetylmorphine, and then more slowly to morphine through which its analgesic activity is largely mediated. In laboratory studies, however, both diamorphine and mono-acetyl morphine are also active in their own right at delta-opioid receptors [30, 31].

The characteristics of diamorphine are, as might be expected, similar to morphine except that it has increased solubility and is highly hydrophilic. This confers a significant clinical advantage that large doses can be given in small

volumes. Its potency is 1.5–2 times that of morphine when the two are given by the same route. It has gained a spurious reputation as a drug of addiction and because of this, is difficult to obtain in many countries. In reality, there is no evidence of any increased potential for addiction over morphine, and it is a useful and highly effective analgesic.

Fentanyl

Fentanyl is a highly lipophilic synthetic mu-agonist with around 100 times the potency of morphine. Many of its proven advantages over morphine, relate to the formulations in which it is available. It is, however, wholly synthetic and of a different class from morphine. It is, therefore, a suitable agent for opioid rotation (see below) where adverse effects of opiates have become dose-limiting. Like morphine/diamorphine, fentanyl has been studied reasonably extensively in children [32–36, 38–41, 43–45]. Perhaps for these reasons, it is usually considered the second-line major opioid in children after morphine/diamorphine.

It is not available as an oral formulation, but there are transdermal [32,38] and intranasal [39] delivery systems. Parenteral administration of fentanyl has an onset of action of less than a minute, but rapid redistribution to inactive tissues such as fat, rather than elimination, means a short duration of action, of around 30–45 min. However, large or multiple dosing increases the analgesic action as elimination becomes the determinant of effect duration. Elimination is hepatic with glucuronidation to inactive metabolites that are then excreted by the kidney. The pharmacokinetics of fentanyl are age-dependent with wider volumes of distribution and higher clearance values in neonates and infants [40,41], and adult values are reached around 2 months of age, when allometric scaling is used [42].

There are three fentanyl congeners. Alfentanil is about 5–10 times less potent and has an extremely short duration of action, usually less than 15–20 min. However, it can prove to be a useful alternative, especially when subcutaneous administration of fentanyl is compromised because of excess volume requirements and may cause less postoperative respiratory depression than either morphine or fentanyl. Sufentanil and Remifentanil are 10 times more potent than fentanyl. Application in palliative medicine is limited but intranasal Sufentanil can be helpful for rapid relief from incident pain. Remifentanil has unique pharmacokinetic properties characterized by small volumes, rapid clearance, and low variability compared with other intravenous anaesthetic agents.

Transdermal fentanyl

In a small, open label study in children with cancer pain [32], transdermal fentanyl was found to be well tolerated and have pharmacokinetic parameter estimates similar to those for adults but with less variability. Peak plasma concentrations of a 25 mcg/h fentanyl patch were reached around 24 h (18 to > 66 h) followed by a slow decline from the peak concentration, consistent with 72 h dosing, in most children.

The advantage of the transdermal formulation of fentanyl is that it is easy to use, requires no needles, and needs changing only every 48–72 hours, while usually providing a relatively consistent degree of analgesia. These make it an ideal major opioid formulation in the maintenance phase (see below). It is not usually suitable, however, in the initiating or titration phases. The smallest patch size, 25 mcg per hour, is equivalent to around 40 mg in 24 h of oral morphine. This is too large for most opioid naïve children. Furthermore, the patch sizes then go up in 25 mcg increments, making titration against an individual patient's pain very difficult. Attempts to divide the patch, either by cutting it or occluding part of it, are anecdotally successful but are not recommended by the manufacturer. This is because, until recently the nature of the transdermal delivery system was such that the drug could leak from a cut surface, and the rate of drug absorption is dependent on surface area so that covering half the patch does not necessarily mean the child receives half the dose of fentanyl in a given period. The manufacturers have recognized this potential weakness in an otherwise very valuable formulation, and are developing a new transdermal system which, like transdermal buprenorphine, can be cut down to allow fractions of a patch to be administered.

Oral transmucosal fentanyl citrate

OTFC is a flavoured, fentanyl impregnated sugar matrix presented as a lozenge. It has been found to be a safe and reliable pre-anaesthetic medication in healthy children prior to surgery [33–35, 43] and for analgesia during inpatient and outpatient burn-wound management [44,45]. It has a bioavailability of 33% in children [43], lower than the 50% quoted for adults probably because of either a higher first-pass extraction or increased swallowing in children. In adults, 25% is rapidly absorbed through the oral mucosa and 25% (i.e. one-third of 75%) is made available more slowly following gastrointestinal absorption and hepatic metabolism.

The lozenge is typically consumed within 20 min and analgesia first noted after 5–10 min with maximum effects at 25–45 min. The steady-state volume of distribution and clearance rates for children aged 2–10 years were comparable to adult's [43]. Effects can persist for several hours and, in adults, the plasma half-life is in the region of 7 hours. A randomized, placebo-controlled, double blind study in children [35] confirmed higher rates of pruritus and nausea compared with placebo. The incidence of nausea increases with higher OTFC doses.

The rescue dose for breakthrough pain is, as always, based on the regularly scheduled pain medication and can be given as fentanyl itself or as the equivalent dose of some other opioid such as morphine.

Hydromorphone

Hydromorphone is a hydrogenated ketone of morphine with very similar pharmacokinetic and pharmacodynamic properties to morphine [46]. It has an oral bioavailability of 40–60% with a rapid onset of action and duration of action of 4–6 h and is also effective when given by the subcutaneous, intravenous, epidural and intrathecal routes. The elimination half-life is 3 to 4 hours and, like morphine, shows wide intra-subject pharmacokinetic variability. It is between 5 and 7.5 times more potent [47], and 2–10 times more lipid soluble. Like morphine, it is metabolized in children to the 3- and the 6-glucuronide [46].

It is unclear whether hydromorphone has advantages over morphine in children [36,47]. In countries where diamorphine is not yet available, however, its greater potency than morphine can provide an alternative practical solution to the problem of dissolving high opioid doses for parenteral administration.

Methadone

Methadone has a very different chemical structure from morphine and is a racemic mixture. The analgesic efficacy is not only mediated through the mu-opioid receptor (L-enantiomer) but by desensitization of the d-opioid receptor and antagonism of the NMDA receptor (L- and D-enantiomers). This often makes it a useful agent in neuropathic pain syndromes. Activity of the d-receptor is critical for the development of morphine-induced tolerance and dependence and concomitant exposure to morphine and methadone suppresses the mechanisms leading to opioid tolerance.

Methadone is a basic and lipophilic drug that is known for its high oral bio-availability (80–90%), and very long duration of action (4–24 h). It is very slowly metabolized in the liver, does not rely on renal excretion and the elimination half-life averages 19 h in children aged 1–18 years, range 4–62 h [48]. There is also wide individual variation in plasma and elimination half-life in neonates [49,39]. Enzyme inducers such as carbamazepine, phenobarbitone (Phenobarbital), phenytoin, and rifampicin increase the metabolism of methadone while amitriptyline and cimetidine reduce metabolism. Methadone leads to higher plasma levels of zidovudine.

Outside some case reports [50–52], there is relatively little research on the use of methadone in children [24]. One direct comparison with morphine [53] showed that it was more effective for postoperative analgesia. A second study [54] suggests that methadone had a greater impact than morphine on respiratory depression, although this was of no clinical significance for either drug.

It is important that the safety and effectiveness of methadone should be established in children. Methadone potentially has a unique place among major opioids. It is of a very different chemical structure from morphine, making it a suitable opioid where opioid switching (see below) is considered. But the unique advantage of methadone is that in addition to analgesic efficacy mediated through the mu-opioid receptor, methadone also acts through antagonism of the N-methyl D-aspartate (NMDA) receptor [55]. The NMDA receptor is important in the pathophysiology of neuropathic pain. Methadone, therefore, combines in principle the pharmacological effects of both a major opioid such as morphine and those of an NMDA antagonist such as ketamine.

With this in mind, it is perhaps surprising that methadone is not more widely used in the management of pain in children. Certainly, in adults it has found a valuable role in the management of cancer pain [37,56,57]. Dextromethorphan, another combined opioid/NMDA antagonist [58] seems nevertheless to be a relatively poor analgesic [59].

Oxycodone

Oxycodone has similar properties to morphine but has additional kappa-receptor agonist activity and has been effective in providing analgesia for neuropathic pain syndromes in adults. Oral bio-availability is around 50–60% and potency equivalent to morphine. Parenteral potency is 75% of morphine. Onset of action is 20–30 min after oral administration, with duration of action of 4 h. The plasma half-life is around 3.5 h but increases during renal failure.

The pharmacokinetic profile was studied in 40 children, aged 6–93 months, undergoing surgery [60] . Patients received a single 0. 1 mg/kg dose of oxycodone under anaesthesia either by the intravenous, intramuscular, buccal, or nasogastric route with blood samples being evaluated over the next 12 h.

Peak drug concentrations were approximately twice as high after intravenous administration than after intramuscular dosing (mean 82 versus 34 mcg/L) and were considerably higher than buccal or gastric administration (9.8 and 0.2 mcg/L, respectively). Terminal elimination half-life was approximately 150 minutes in all groups. These parameters are similar to those observed in adults. On the other hand, the elimination half-life and clearance values have been found to be higher in adults and have been associated with greater ventilatory depression in children when given intravenously after surgery, at comparable analgesic doses of other opioids [61]. Anecdotally, vomiting, pruritus, and delirium appear to be less common in children than in adults.

Oxycodone is metabolized in the liver mediated by the CYP2D6 enzyme system. Metabolites are, generally, inactive except for oxymorphone. Oxymorphone has similar characteristics to morphine but has 10 times the potency and is manufactured in its own right as a parenteral formulation.

Buprenorphine

Buprenorphine also offers some potential advantages over morphine, related mainly to its formulation. It is available as, both a sublingual and a transdermal formulation, both of which have obvious advantages in paediatric practice.

Buprenorphine is a partial mu-agonist and has mixed agonist and antagonist properties at other receptors. In practice, its effects seem to be similar to those of morphine. Its onset of action is approximately 30 min and the peak around 3 h. Its half life is three hours, but the duration of action can be as long as 9 [62].

The sublingual formulation avoids first past metabolism without the need for an injection. 400 mcg of the sublingual preparation is approximately equivalent to 300 mcg parenterally.

Perhaps the biggest advantage of buprenorphine, however, is its availability in a transdermal patch that, unlike that of fentanyl, can be divided without apparently jeopardising its delivery. In the United Kingdom, there are three patch sizes releasing 35 mcg/h, 52.5 mcg/h, and 70 mcg/h, each for 72 h. The drug is held in a matrix [63]. It appears that this can be divided without compromising the drug delivery, although there remain few studies in children.

One theoretical problem with buprenorphine has been the fact that it is a partial agonist. This has two implications. The first is that there is a genuine pharmacological ceiling dose as receptor occupancy approaches 100%. However, it appears that this does not occur until 3–5 mg of buprenorphine daily in adults [62, 64]. The potency of buprenorphine is 60 times that of morphine, so this ceiling dose occurs at an oral morphine equivalent of 180–300 mg in 24 h. There are certainly some children who require these doses and this should be borne in mind when changing to buprenorphine.

The second consequence of the partial agonist nature of buprenorphine is, that it can block opioid receptors to the effect of morphine or other major opioids. Again, however, in practice this is probably only a problem in high doses when receptor occupancy becomes close to complete. Furthermore, since buprenorphine can be used for breakthrough pain, the solution is simply to avoid using other major opioids alongside buprenorphine at high doses [62].

Because buprenorphine has a very high affinity for opioid receptors, it is not easily displaced by the pure opioid antagonist naloxone, and considerable amounts of naloxone may be needed. Inadvertent overdoses, or idiosyncratic exaggerated responses to normal doses, should be treated additionally with respiratory stimulants such as doxapram.

Other opioids

Opioids such as pentazocine and butorphanol are less likely to cause respiratory depression than morphine but have an increased tendency toward sedation and other central nervous system toxicity including dysphoria, at therapeutic doses.

Pethidine (Meperidine) is a short half-life opioid which in the past was used for moderate to severe pain in children. It has little to recommend it, being both less potent, and more toxic than morphine. The enteral absorption of pethidine is erratic [54,65]. Furthermore, accumulation of its long-acting neurotoxic metabolite norpethidine causes convulsions [66–69]. They can also cause irritability, insomnia, myclonus and seizures. Toxicity is possible at any dose, but is more likely at high doses, with renal or hepatic insufficiency or with accumulation after repeated dosing for more than 2–3 days. With increasing evidence of the safety and efficacy of alternatives, pethidine now has little place in the management of pain in children.

Initiation phase

How much and how often?

The concept of a starting dose is central to good pain management, and is rather different from the way in which many other drugs are used. In most drug prescriptions, the expectation is that one standard dose per kilogram will be enough to achieve the desired effect. By contrast, the initial prescription for analgesics is a starting point from which it is expected that titration will occur until pain is under control. It is often helpful to make this clear to the child and the family, in order that they do not feel discouraged if the initial prescription is not quite enough to control the pain. In effect, there are three phases in the prescription of major opioids. The first is *initiation*. This is followed by a period of *titration* in which, the aim is to match the degree of pain with enough drug to provide analgesia but without exceeding this and incurring unnecessary adverse effects. The third phase is a *maintenance phase* in which a reasonably stable dose of medication has been reached. In reality, of course, this maintenance phase may simply represent a period of slower titration. A combination of disease progression and perhaps opioid tolerance means that a process of continual review is necessary even during the maintenance phase to ensure that adequate analgesia is achieved.

It may also be necessary to telescope the titration phase into a few hours or minutes by slow and careful infusion of parenteral opioid in cases where there is very severe pain that needs urgent intervention (see below). This is a relatively rare procedure in children, but has been described more often in adults [70–72].

The three phases (initiation, titration and maintenance) are characterized by specific approaches both to dosing and formulation.

Starting dose and frequency

Anxiety often surrounds the initial prescription of major opioids, particularly for those who are relatively inexperienced in their use in children. In practice, there are two ways to arrive at a safe and appropriate initial dose. If the child is not already receiving opioids, it should be calculated on the basis of the child's weight. For children who are already receiving opioids (minor or major), there is likely to be some tolerance and a dose-per-kilo approach will often underestimate the child's true requirements. Instead, the dose of opioids already required by the child should be used as a guide to the appropriate initial dose of the new drug. Typically, this occurs as a child moves from step 2 (minor opioids) to step 3 (major opioids). It is often useful to calculate the dose using both methods. The need to move to step 3 implies that the child's pain is not yet adequately controlled, so when the two calculations arrive at different doses, the higher figure is usually the more appropriate.

Calculating an initial dose using a 'dose per kilogram'

In countries where major opioids are available to children, most formularies will offer a suitable dose-per-kilogram of the child's weight. This is based on the assumption that the volume of distribution per kilogram is the same in children as for adults. In other words, that if 10 mg of morphine given to a 70 kilo adult results in a suitable and effective serum concentration, then half that dose given to a 35 kilo child will have the same result. Although this assumption may only be approximately correct [25, 26], in practice dosing guidelines based on it seem to work reasonably well.

Most formularies recommend as a starting dose an equivalent to oral morphine 1–2 mg/kg/24 h. There is relatively little direct evidence from paediatric studies, but one study [25] seems to suggest that this will usually result in adequate analgesia with little toxicity.

The importance of prescribing regular and breakthrough medication has already been emphasized (see above). Immediate release oral morphine is the preferred first line major opioid and a sixth of the total daily dose should be prescribed regularly 4 hourly. It is often undesirable and unnecessary to wake the child to receive the night time dose, and some clinicians will double the dose before bed-time to make up for this missing dose.

The breakthrough dose should be the same as the regular four hourly dose, that is one-sixth of the total daily dose. It is important to explain to families that although the breakthrough dose and the regular dose are the same, they perform two different functions. The regular dose is 'to try to keep the pain away' and the breakthrough dose is 'to treat pain if it happens despite that'. This is important because, without that understanding, parents may withhold a breakthrough dose if it is needed just before or just after a regular one, rather than giving the extra dose in addition.

The breakthrough dose achieves two things. It ensures that analgesia is available to the child should the regular analgesia be inadequate. It also provides some measure of the child's requirement for such additional analgesia, which allows a process of rational and safe titration (see below).

The frequency with which breakthrough medication should be made available is unclear, and practice varies from centre to centre. Traditional practice was to offer the break-through dose as needed four-hourly, but increasingly among adults, it is being offered as often as is necessary, even up to hourly. Once an oral breakthrough dose has been given, there is, perhaps, little to be gained by giving a further dose within an hour of a previous one, since it can take thirty to sixty min-utes for the effect of an oral dose to become apparent.

Opioids should usually be started enterally unless there is no alternative. Where it is thought necessary to commence them using a parenteral formulation, standard dosing proto-cols are usually available, or again, a dose can be calculated by conversion from any existing opioid requirements. Rarely, it may be necessary to intervene more urgently, and the appro-priate dose can be established on the basis of rapid titration to the child's requirements (see below).

Calculation of an initial dose by conversion from existing opioid requirements

An important and fundamental concept in the pharmacology of analgesia in palliative care is that of analgesic equivalence among opioids. Most major opioids work in the same way on the same receptors, but with differing potency. This means that the analgesic effectiveness of any opioid can be expressed in terms of how it compares with other opioids. Fentanyl, for example, is 75 times as potent as morphine when both are given parenterally.

The route should also be taken into consideration: mor-phine is twice as potent given by the parenteral route as it is when given orally, so that parenteral fentanyl is 150 times the potency of oral morphine.

The concept of analgesic equivalence can also be extended to minor opioids. For example, codeine is approximately one-tenth as potent as morphine, while pethidine is about one-sixth as potent. Equivalency can be made more complex if an opioid has more than one analgesic action. For example, oral tramadol is approximately one-fifth the opioid potency of

morphine, but has additional non-opioid analgesic properties that make its effects less predictable.

By convention, the potency of all opioids is expressed in terms of their equivalence to oral morphine (Table 21.2). This enables appropriate conversions to be made, not only between morphine and other opioids, but also among different non-morphine opioids. For example, since hydromorphone is approximately five oral morphine equivalents (OME), and oxycodone is approximately two OME, it is clear that hydro-morphone must be two and half times as potent as oxycodone. A patient on oxycodone wishing to convert to hydromorphone would therefore be expected to have the same pain relief if the dose were divided by two and a half (see Example 1).

In deciding on a starting dose of an opioid, it is important to consider what opioids, if any, a child is already receiving. A child whose pain is barely controlled on step 2 of the WHO ladder despite 30 mg of codeine six times a day, will need something in excess of 18 mg of oral morphine as an initial dose. Many standard texts in palliative care [62,73] include tables of opioid equivalence, and practitioners in palliative medicine in children should become familiar with these.

Table 21.2 Some oral morphine equivalents

Opioid	Potency relative to oral morphine	Notes
Morphine po	1	
Morphine sc or iv	2	
Diamorphine po	1.5	
Diamorphine sc or iv	3	
Fentanyl transdermal, OFTC sc or iv	150	Absorption from mouth is transmucosal, not enteral
Hydromorphone po	3.6–7.5	Variable (75, 132–134)
Hydromorphone sc	3.1–8.5	
Codeine po	0.1	
Tramadol po	0.2	Non-opioid analgesic effects may be more potent in practice
Buprenorphine transdermal	60	
Oxycodone po	2	
Oxycodone sc or iv	3	
Methadone	Variable	Complex, depends on dose (see text)

NB there is variability both in published evidence and in individual patients, and data are mainly from adults with cancer.

Example 1

Patient receiving 15 mg oral oxycodone in 24 h, needing to change to hydromorphone. Published tables suggest that relative potency of oral oxycodone is two OME (i.e. twice the potency of oral morphine) and relative potency of hydromorphone is 5 OME (i.e. five times the potency of oral morphine).

Oral morphine equivalent of oxycodone = 15 × 2 = 30 mg oral morphine

Oral hydromorphone equivalent = 30 ÷ 5 = 6 mg oral hydromorphone.

So, 15 mg oral oxycodone is equivalent to 6 mg oral hydromorphone. Total daily dose of hydromorphone should in principle, therefore, be 6 mg. In practice, the dose should be further reduced to take account of incomplete cross-tolerance, see below.

A further situation in which it may become necessary to select an initial dose, occurs in children already on strong opioids who need to change to a new one. This is termed 'opioid substitution' or, if repeated, 'rotation'. Although it is unusual for this to become necessary, in some children tolerance to strong analgesia probably occurs even in a therapeutic setting. The solution usually is simply to increase the dose of major opioid, but rarely such increases are constrained by dose-limiting toxicity, often by neuroexcitability. In this situation, it may be necessary to change to an alternative strong opioid of a different class [38,74]. A child who has become partially tolerant to the analgesic effects of morphine, may well be less tolerant to those of fentanyl, a phenomenon termed 'incomplete cross-tolerance'.

The effectiveness of opioid rotation or substitution in this way depends in part on the different adverse effects profiles of different opioids. It is mainly, however, because changing to a new opioid allows a reduction in the total opioid dose without any loss of analgesia. The dose reduction is conventionally twenty five per cent. In converting from one major opioid to another, therefore, there are two stages in the calculation (example 2). The first is calculation of an equianalgesic dose of the new opioid, based on oral morphine equivalency (see above). The second is a 25% reduction in that dosage to effect a reduction in toxicity.

Methadone, another potent opioid in a different class from morphine, would seem a useful alternative to fentanyl when considering substitution, particularly if there is an element of neuropathic pain. Its use is complicated by its unusual pharmacokinetics that mean the conversion factor is dependent on the dose of the previous opioid [75–77]. Furthermore, again because of its unpredictable pharmacokinetics, it is

Example 2 Opioid substitution

After titration, a child receiving a subcutaneous infusion of morphine receives 500 mg in 24 h but is becoming toxic, with neuroexcitability, sweating and myoclonus. The decision is made to switch to an alternative opioid. Parenteral fentanyl (150 times analgesic potency of oral morphine) is selected because it is a synthetic opioid with a structure very different from morphine.

Step 1: Calculating theoretical equianalgesic dose of fentanyl

Oral morphine equivalent of sc morphine = 500 × 2 = 1000 mg oral morphine

Parenteral fentanyl equivalent of 1000 mg oral morphine = 1000 mg ÷ 150 = 6.67 mg parenteral fentanyl in 24 h.

Step 2: Reducing dose by 25% to account for incomplete cross-tolerance

25% parenteral fentanyl dose = 0.25 × 6.67 = 1.67 mg parenteral fentanyl

Final dose of parenteral fentanyl, taking into account both equianalgesic potency in theory and incomplete cross-tolerance in practice, is:

6.67–1.67 = 5 mg in 24 h

(cross check: 5 × 150 = 750 mg oral morphine equivalent i.e. 75% of original 24 hrly opioid requirements).

usually recommended that methadone should be commenced in a hospital setting. This makes it unsuitable for use in children needing palliative care, in whom facilitating early discharge home is always a priority. The need for this caution is not, however, entirely clear in practice, as outpatient prescription has been reported to be safe [78] with careful monitoring.

Rarely, it is necessary to titrate rapidly against pain in order to establish an appropriate starting dose. The indication is for very severe pain for which, a more measured approach would condemn the child to prolonged suffering. In this situation, the parenteral route is the most appropriate. The opioid should be infused slowly over half and hour or so until analgesia is achieved. There are a number of methods used to calculate the total daily dose required, once this has been achieved; perhaps the simplest [72] is to assume that it represents the equivalent of a single four hourly dose, and accordingly give six times this dose in 24 h (Example 3). This can be given by any appropriate route, and as any opioid, providing appropriate conversions in doses are made.

Example 3 Rapid titration

A child with severe pain related to a sarcoma requires 6 mg intravenous morphine to achieve analgesia.

Oral morphine equivalent = 2×6 = 12 mg

Assume this represents four-hourly breakthrough requirement.

Total 24 hourly requirement = 6 × 6 = 36 mg oral morphine equivalent

Can give in several ways: 6 mg immediate release morphine 4 hrly

18 mg morphine via continuous sc infusion over 24 h

12 mg diamorphine via continuous sc infusion etc. over 24 h

Dose interval—how often should opioids be given ?

Another of the fundamental principles of the WHO pain ladder for children is that opioid medication should always be given 'by the clock' rather than simply being available when it is needed. There are numerous reasons for this.

It is comparatively unusual for pain that, at its worst, is intense enough to need a major opioid, to disappear completely at other times. There are exceptions to this, particularly in managing episodic pain (see below), but in general, if pain is severe enough to warrant major opioids, it is likely to require them to be given on a regular basis.

Perhaps more importantly, the aim of analgesia is to keep the patient free from pain. Any prescription that relies on the occurrence of pain to trigger an analgesic intervention is inherently unsatisfactory. To allow access to analgesia to be contingent on reporting the need for it, ensures that a child must inevitably experience pain and can never be free from it.

There are also sound theoretical reasons for always giving major opioids regularly. In the case of morphine, there is evidence [79, 80] that single doses are considerably less effective than repeated doses. In other words, the effectiveness of the first dose of morphine is less than that of the fifth or sixth regular dose. The explanation for this is thought to be accumulation of the active metabolite M6G, which has a longer-half life and therefore accumulates after repeated dosing. Regular repeated doses are, therefore, usually mandatory in the prescription of major opioids.

The exact dosage interval is governed largely by the half-life of the medication and its duration of action. The half-life of morphine in children is probably somewhat shorter than in adults [24–26]. But perhaps this difference is insignificant compared with the wide variability observed between individual patients [81,82]. Certainly, in practice a four-hourly dosing schedule for immediate-release oral morphine seems to work well in children as in adults.

It follows that where the half-life of a drug is increased, the dosage interval should also be lengthened to accommodate it. For children in the neonatal period, for example, renal clearance of morphine and its active metabolite M6G are less than in older children or adults. Dosage intervals of six, eight, or even twelve hours are therefore often suggested [83]. For children with poor renal function from other causes, such as those dying from renal failure, clearance of morphine may also be reduced and adjustments should be made to the dosing interval. One approach is to reduce the dosing interval of the immediate release morphine to 8 or 12 hourly. Where renal dysfunction is particularly severe, however, it may be preferable to give morphine one milligram per kilo as needed, with no regular dose at all. Although this appears to break one of the 'golden rules' of the WHO Pain Ladder, reduced clearance of morphine and M6G means that the child will maintain an acceptable serum level even with intermittent dosing.

In summary, when considering the appropriate frequency with which analgesia should be prescribed, the most important characteristics are those of the drug itself. However, it is also important to consider the characteristics of the patient, in particular as a result of coexistent disease, which may impact on clearance of the drug.

Management of episodic pain is considered elsewhere (see below).

Titration phase

The purpose of the titration phase is to match the dose of analgesia prescribed with the degree of pain experienced by the patient. If pain is counteracted by adequate analgesia, it is also true that some of the effects of analgesia are countered by pain. The risk of clinically significant respiratory depression, for example, is very small if the dose of opioid prescribed is not excessive in relation to the degree of pain experienced by the patient. Titration is the means by which the correct dose of analgesia is determined to keep the child comfortable without unnecessary toxicity.

The opioid of choice in the titration phase is oral morphine. Other oral medications with relatively short half-lives, such as hydromorphone, methadone or oxycodone could also be used. Formulations with long half-lives or slow release delivery systems, such as fentanyl patches or slow release preparations of morphine or oxycodone, would not be appropriate for titration.

The essence of titration is the ongoing review of the regular opioid dosage, based on the amount of breakthrough

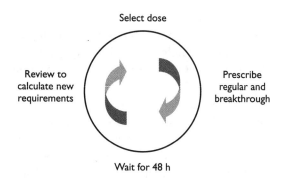

Fig. 21.2 Prescribe-review cycle in titration phase of opioid prescription.

medication the child has required (Figure 21.2). Once appropriate initial doses of regular and breakthrough opioid have been selected, the prescription should, if possible, be left for 48 h and then reviewed. If the child has needed only one or two breakthroughs in each 24-h period, then the dose of regular analgesia is probably about right and no alteration needs to be made. If, on the other hand, the child has needed more than this, the total daily dose of the regular opioid prescription should be increased by the amount of breakthrough that has been required (Example 4). It is imperative that each time the total daily dose of regular opioid is reviewed, the breakthrough dose should also be increased so that it remains approximately a sixth of the total daily dose. This is because, as tolerance develops, the breakthrough dose will become progressively less effective unless it is increased in proportion to the regular dose.

After a further 48 h, the process should be repeated and once again the total daily dose of regular opioid amended in line with the child's requirements for breakthrough opioid. In this way, it is usually possible to find a 24-h regular dose that allows the child to need only a small number of breakthrough doses.

This approach has a number of advantages. It allows the 24-h regular opioid dose to be very precisely titrated against the child's experience of pain. Furthermore, increases in regular opioid dose can be made with confidence since they only reflect what the child has already received over the previous 48 h, with no ill effect. This can be reassuring for parent and professional alike.

The reason for delaying changes to the regular opioid dosage for 48 h, is to allow the opioid to reach steady state at the new dose. Too frequent changes in dosage can result in increases being made disproportionately to the degree of pain, so that the child, in effect, receives too high a dose of opioids and is therefore at risk of some of the adverse effects. There are clearly situations however, in which more rapid titration is necessary, for example, where the pain is severe, or where there

Example 4 Prescription, titration and maintenance of opioids

Day 0: A child of 30 kg commences 1 mg/kg/24 h oral morphine that is 30 mg/24 h. This is prescribed as an immediate-release oral preparation of morphine. This **regular dose** is given as 5 mg every four hours. The additional **breakthrough** dose is one sixth of the total daily dose, that is 5mg, prescribed as needed (prn) orally 1–4 hourly.

Day 1: The child requires four breakthrough doses, each of 5 mg.

Day 2: The child requires two breakthrough doses, each of 5 mg.

Review after 48 h. Child has needed average of three breakthrough doses each day, implying that regular dose is not yet enough and needs to be increased.

- Regular dose: Increase in 24 hourly regular dose should be $3 \times 5 = 15$ mg, so new regular total daily dose is $30 + 15 = 45$ mg/24 h.

- Breakthrough dose: New breakthrough dose remains one sixth of total daily dose $45 \div 6 = 7.5$ mg prescribed as needed (prn) 1–4 hourly.

Day 3: The child requires two breakthrough doses, each of 7.5 mg.

Day 4: The child requires one breakthrough dose of 7.5 mg.

Review after 48 h. Child has needed average of 1.5 breakthrough doses each day, implying that regular dose is still not enough and needs to be increased further.

- Regular dose: Increase in 24 hourly regular dose should be $1.5 \times 7.5 = 10$ mg, so new regular total daily dose is $45 + 10 = 55$ mg/24 h.

- Breakthrough dose: New breakthrough dose remains one sixth of total daily dose $55 \div 6 = 9$ mg prescribed as needed (prn) 1–4 hourly.

Days 5–8. Child requires only occasional additional breakthrough doses.

Review every 48 h. Few additional breakthrough doses have been necessary, implying opioid prescription is now well matched against child's pain. This marks the end of the titration phase and the beginning of the maintenance phase:

- Regular dose: Change to more convenient formulation. Total daily morphine dose is 55 mg, approx = 30 mg twice daily of 12 hourly slow release morphine formulation.

- Breakthrough dose: Breakthrough dose remains one-sixth of total daily dose $60 \div 6 = 10$ mg prescribed as needed (prn) 1–4 hourly. Remains as immediate release preparation.

Continue regular review process, including changing needs for breakthrough, tolerability of the drug and formulation, and possibility of narcotisation.

is rapid disease progression such that the severity of pain is increasing faster than 48 hour titration would allow.

If titrating opioids in this way fails to impact adequately on the pain, it may be because the pain is inherently, wholly or partially, insensitive to opioids. The first of these is extremely unusual but the second is seen, not infrequently. Neuropathic pain (see below) is one cause; although opioids remain the most effective analgesic agent for neuropathic pain, additional approaches such as adjuvants or neurolytic procedures may improve the situation.

There are many other reasons for pain to be relatively resistant that are outside the scope of this chapter, but are considered elsewhere in the book. Among these, perhaps the most important to consider is that pharmacological management of pain tends to address mainly its physical aspects. Pain in which these physical elements are only a small contribution (often referred to, perhaps misleadingly, as 'total pain') will typically respond only poorly to the approaches to prescription and titration described above. 'Attempting to relieve pain without addressing the patient's non-physical concerns is likely to lead to frustration' [4].

Maintenance phase

For most children, the titration phase will come to an end when it is no longer necessary to keep adjusting the total daily dose of regular opioid. At this point, it is usually helpful to change to a long acting formulation if this has not already been done. In paediatric palliative medicine, slow release morphine preparations that can be given 12 or 24 hourly are first line, and in most countries fentanyl patch is second line. The relative potency of fentanyl means that the patches should really only be prescribed to a child receiving more than 30–40 mg of oral morphine equivalent in 24 h. In practice, however, fentanyl patches seem to be well tolerated even when they represent an increase in the dose of opioid.

It is not necessary for the breakthrough opioid to be the same as the regular one. There is, indeed, a theoretical advantage in combining some; for example, oral morphine (primarily a mu-1 receptor agonist) with fentanyl (primarily a mu-2 receptor agonist) may, in theory, give better overall blockade of receptors than either one alone.

The pharmacokinetics of some slow release preparations of morphine are not the same in children as in adults [25]. It appears that the absorption of slow release morphine formulations is erratic and their slow release nature may be less reliable. For this reason, slow-release-preparations of morphine in children are sometimes given 8 rather than 12 h. This rather reduces their usefulness and for children requiring 8-hourly slow release morphine; it may be better to consider an alternative.

Clinical experience is that some children find they need to change fentanyl patches every 48 rather than 72 h, in order to avoid increasing requirements for breakthrough towards the time of the next patch change.

Of course, even during the maintenance phase, the dose should be subject to review (Example 4). For most children, the maintenance phase is not a true plateau but a much more gradual gradient in the increase of their pain. Further increases will be needed as a result mainly of disease progression, but perhaps also due to the development of tolerance.

Sometimes, the dose may need to be revised downwards and reduced rather than increased. The need for such a decrease can be inferred from the sudden development of toxicity. A child, who is receiving an appropriate dose of opioid for the degree of pain, will typically experience very few of the side effects that are countered by pain, particularly drowsiness and respiratory depression.

Should adverse effects from opioids develop unexpectedly despite careful titration, the cause may be 'narcotisation'. There are three common reasons for narcotisation to occur.

1. The pain has become suddenly less severe. This is usually because some other therapeutic intervention has been effective. For example, radiotherapy to a malignant metastasis may reduce or even abolish pain at that point completely. Similarly, a nerve block or epidural anaesthetic may provide very effective analgesia, such that a previously appropriate dose of opioid is now too high. Less commonly progression of the disease itself can paradoxically provide symptom relief. For example, nerve damage that initially causes pain may, when it progresses, instead cause regional anaesthesia.

2. Clearance of the opioid may be acutely impaired. The commonest cause is a sudden deterioration in renal function, resulting in accumulation of morphine and its metabolites. The cause may not be immediately obvious; renal function may be impaired both by the underlying disease and by some of the interventions, palliative or otherwise, introduced in its management.

3. Interactions with other drugs. Polypharmacy is common in the palliative phase, even in the paediatric specialty. It is not always possible to predict how a certain combination of drugs will impact on a child's conscious level. The introduction of psychoactive drugs such as midazolam or phenothiazines may induce drowsiness that can masquerade as opioid toxicity.

Management of adverse effects

Opioids are the main pharmacological tools available and the majority of children will have a favourable outcome. However, excessive adverse effects will be suffered by a significant minority and when they occur, can jeopardize optimal management of pain. Children are likely to refuse medication that causes distressing side effects, even if it is effective. Adverse effects should be anticipated, specifically addressed with the patient and the family, and relieved as rapidly as possible.

Most evidence-based practice is derived from work in adults [74]. There is little evidence in children and it seems reasonable to apply these principles to paediatric patients, but, as always, extrapolating with caution.

The adverse effects (Table 21.1) can be dealt with in one of two ways:

- Substitution of a different opioid in order to reduce the total opioid dose
- Symptomatic management of the adverse effect

Dose reduction of systemic opioids

Unless there has been a reduction in pain, it is unlikely that a simple reduction in the dose of opioid will be possible without jeopardising good pain relief. Tolerance to the analgesic effects of one opioid does not necessarily mean it will have occurred equally to all of them, however. This gives the opportunity to reduce the total opioid dose (measured in oral morphine equivalents) by switching to an alternative opioid. This is more likely to be effective if the opioid is of a different class, since incomplete cross-tolerance is more probable. The technique of opioid 'substitution' or 'rotating' has been considered above.

Symptomatic management of the adverse effect

This involves the use of drugs to prevent or control adverse effects and adds to the child's medication burden. All children commencing a major opioid should, for example, also be prescribed stimulant and softening laxatives (see Chapter 23, Gastrointestinal symptoms). Generally speaking, additional medications should be avoided if possible, as children may be reluctant to take yet another medication and polypharmacy often increases the risk of further adverse effects or drug interactions.

The effects of underlying disease and of other drugs can mimic opioid toxicity, particularly in neuropsychiatric problems such as drowsiness, cognitive dysfunction, and myclonus [74]. As an initial step, it is important to ensure that opioids are indeed the cause. Substitution of a different opioid or (very rarely) replacement with an alternative, non-opioid approach may be required.

If these fail, it may be necessary to begin specific therapy. The agents recommended for symptomatic management of the adverse effects of opioids are often based on anecdotal experience and clinical observation. They lack support from prospective studies on efficacy or toxicity over the long-term or systematic evaluation of retrospective data.

Nausea and vomiting

This is relatively rare in children and antiemetics are not normally prescribed prophylactically. Alternative explanations should usually be sought if nausea or vomiting occurs on established treatment. Haloperidol is often recommended in adults for opioid induced symptoms [see Chapter 23, Gastrointestinal symptoms] but in children, other dopamine antagonists such as domperidone, ametoclopramide or broader-spectrum antiemetics such as levomepromazine may be more acceptable.

Constipation

Constipation is extremely common among children receiving opioids and should be anticipated and prophylactic laxatives prescribed as soon as the prescription is made. A combination stimulant and softener should be used. Lactulose, favoured by paediatricians in many countries for constipation in children, is not appropriate for opioid induced constipation.

Oral opioid antagonist naloxone may help reverse opioid induced constipation (see Chapter 23, Gastrointestinal symptoms). Transdermal fentanyl probably causes less constipation than morphine in adults [84–86].

Pruritus

The management of pruritus due to opioids is considered in more detail in Chapter 28, Skin symptoms. It is not uncommon in infants and young children [87], and seems to occur particularly around the nose and face. Substitution of an alternative opioid is usually effective.

Sedation

The patient and/or the family should be informed that there might be an initial period of drowsiness when opioid therapy is commenced or increased, but that this will generally subside within a few days. Unfortunately, on occasion, the sedative effect persists and contributing factors such as hepatic, renal or central nervous system disease should be considered. Reduced renal function can result in accumulation of morphine's centrally acting metabolite, M6G, and an opioid not reliant on renal excretion, may be better tolerated. Opioid rotation has had a positive effect on the prevalence and severity of drowsiness, as has a change from oral to subcutaneous morphine.

Psychostimulants such as methylphenidate (familiar to most paediatricians for its role in managing hyperactivity disorders) have had a demonstrable effect in a number of adult studies. They have also been effective in adolescents with cancer [88]. In all of the studies, however, the use of psychostimulants has been associated with adverse effects such as hallucinations, delirium, psychosis, decreased appetite and tremor. Psychostimulants are contraindicated when there is a history of psychiatric disorders, and relatively contraindicated in patients with substance abuse problems or paroxysmal tachyarrhythmia. There is little information about their use for this indication in younger children.

Cognitive impairment

Some patients, especially young children, receiving opioids become agitated rather than sedated. It may be appropriate to check their renal and/or hepatic function and adjust the dose of opioid accordingly. The adequacy of pain control dictates the approach taken. Good control allows a trial reduction in the dose of opioid or lengthening of the dosing interval but poor control indicates opioid rotation.

Myoclonus

Myoclonus is an involuntary muscle contraction while conscious and can occur with high opioid doses or in-patients on long-term opioid therapy due to the accumulation of neurotoxic metabolites such as morphine 3-glucuronide. It is an idiosyncratic reaction. Empirical approaches that have been used [74] are based on benzodiazepines, particularly midazolam or clonazepam, or muscle relaxants such as baclofen or dantrolene. Valproic acid has also been used with effect. Opioid rotation accompanied as always by a reduction in total opioid dose can also be helpful.

Urinary retention

Urinary retention can be caused by any opioid given by any route but, anecdotally, is more frequent when given epidurally or spinally, often after rapid dose escalation. Interventions to counter the effect include the application of external bladder pressure, starting a low dose infusion, or using intermittent catheterisation. Other options include substitution to an alternative opioid such as fentanyl, or trying a cholinomimetic agent, such as bethanecol, to stimulate effective bladder contractions.

Respiratory depression

Respiratory depression due to opioid administration in children is much feared but grossly overestimated. Pain is a very effective stimulant to respiratory drive and apnoea is highly unlikely if titration is carried out appropriately as above. An exception is if narcotisation occurs (see above), usually as a result of a sudden reduction in pain stimulus or in capacity to clear opioids. It is rarely necessary to administer opioid antagonist naloxone, and since doing so carries the certainty of simultaneously reversing analgesia, it should not be undertaken lightly.

Physiologic dependence, tolerance, and addiction

Many of the misconceptions around opioid use surround the issues of dependence, tolerance, and addiction. Such misconceptions are so common that they must be pro-actively addressed and reviewed with all health professionals, patients, and families. Dependence and tolerance are physiologic events and are not indicative of addiction, which is a psychological phenomenon.

Physiologic dependence may occur. Dependence is the occurrence of physical symptoms attributable to withdrawal, when the dose of opioids is reduced too quickly. If the dose of opioid needs to be reduced (for example, if there has been another analgesic intervention, and narcotisation is anticipated), it should be done slowly. One practical approach is to reduce the dose by 25% every two days, aiming to reduce the dose to zero over the course of one or two weeks.

Tolerance is defined as a requirement for increasing opioid doses to maintain the same degree of pain relief. There are many mechanisms underlying this phenomenon, including alterations in G-protein expression and opioid receptor regulation. The solution to increasing needs for opioids in the terminal phase is usually simply to increase the dose. The most common cause of increased opioid requirements is advancing disease; the contribution of tolerance, if any, is usually trivial.

Addiction, that is, an individual's craving for opioids for their psychological impact rather than for pain relief, is probably no more likely to occur in patients receiving opioids for pain than in the general population [89]. It is important that irrational fear of addiction does not interfere with proper prescribing as part of good palliative care, and similarly that useful therapeutic medications, such as diamorphine, do not remain unavailable to these vulnerable patients because of misunderstanding among lawmakers.

Which route ?

Oral or other enteral

An enteral route—usually oral but often gastrostomy—is always to be preferred if it is available. Oral medications can be administered without advanced skill and are relatively easy to titrate. They must be acceptable to children, so important considerations are palatability, tablet size, solution volume, and frequency of administration.

Palatability has been improved by the manufacture of better tasting flavoured vehicles; and a variety of syrups, ice creams, jam, and sauces can be used. Manufacturers have moved away from only providing medications in tablet form, which made it difficult for children who were unwilling or unable to swallow tablets, and have developed concentrated solutions for children requiring high doses of a medication. The frequency of administering a medication can be prohibitive to children. In general, analgesics that need to be taken every 4 h are impractical for anything but short-term administration. However, many analgesics are now available in sustained-release preparations. The preparation of some products means that even the contents of an opened capsule can be mixed with soft foods without losing their slow-release formulation. If they are actually chewed, however, these granules will, in effect, become immediate-release preparations, so this often remains an unpredictable approach.

The oral route is not appropriate when children:

- prefer a different route of administration;
- are actively vomiting;
- are unable to comply (e.g. if drowsy or unconscious);
- have a significant gastrointestinal or swallowing dysfunction with risk of aspirating, as might be seen in neurological impairment;
- are experiencing a severe pain crisis, when parenteral administration may become necessary for rapid titration.

Subcutaneous

Parenteral routes should be used when rapid titration is required or when a child is unable to tolerate the oral route. Several types of device are available to provide parenteral delivery of analgesics by continuous infusion, intermittent boluses or both. Opioids can be used alone or administered in combination with other medications such as anti-emetics, benzodiazepines and corticosteroids.

Patient controlled analgesia [PCA] permits even very young children to self-administer small doses of opioid analgesics parenterally at frequent intervals. Delivery systems have the versatility of being able to provide a continuous infusion, also known as a background infusion or basal rate, at the same time. A variation on the theme of PCA is 'parent/nurse controlled analgesia' (PNCA), which has been successfully and safely adopted for use in younger children or neurologically impaired children [90].

The pharmacokinetics and efficacy of subcutaneous delivery are equivalent to intravenous delivery (see below). The usual volume limit for a subcutaneous infusion is 3 ml/h. This does not normally pose a problem because of the availability of many highly potent and/or soluble opioid preparations, particularly diamorphine but also hydromorphone and oxymorphone.

A short gauge indwelling non-metallic needle system, most often placed over the upper arm or abdominal wall, provides intermittent and/or continuous delivery of medication. The chest can also be used as a site for needle placement but care must be taken, as a small risk of causing a pneumothorax exists. If irritation, erythema or induration occurs at the insertion site then the needle site should be changed. There are no firm rules on how long a needle should remain in situ. Anecdotally, non-metallic needles have been successfully used for periods up to 21 days. However, the site should be checked on a regular basis and carefully examined in the event of poor pain control, as inflammation of the area may be uncomfortable as well as impairing drug delivery.

Intravenous

The need for repeated and usually increasingly difficult re-siting of a peripheral cannula, combined with the challenge of safely maintaining it outside a hospital environment, means that this route is usually impractical for a child at home. A long-term percutaneous catheter or other central venous device is often used in children with difficult venous access or who need long-term therapy such as blood products or parenteral nutrition. It may also be available for palliative interventions, though this should be balanced against the risk of infections and their treatment.

Fortunately, the much simpler subcutaneous route is equally suitable for most medications in the palliative phase (see below). The intravenous route, whether central or peripheral, is rarely necessary.

Novel routes

One of the keys to delivering effective medication to children, is to find a route that they will find acceptable. The transdermal route has provided a valuable alternative to injections when oral dosing is not possible (see above).

A number of other routes have also been used in paediatric palliative medicine. The transmucosal route has been used, particularly for diamorphine and midazolam. It avoids first pass metabolism, and can provide rapid intervention for breakthrough pain, anxiety or dyspnoea. Buccal (transmucosal) midazolam can be of particular value in breaking the cycle of acute shortness of breath and anxiety.

A variation on the buccal transmucosal route is the nasal approach. The nasal approach has been used for many years to deliver some hormones and again has found a place in delivering midazolam either through a spray [91] or simply through a small dose in a syringe with no needle.

Opioids delivered through a nebulizer have been the subject of considerable study in the management of dyspnoea [92]. Although a consensus seems to be emerging that they are not generally effective, individual patients do seem to derive some benefit [93]. The effects of nebulised local anaesthetics on cough have been examined in adults [94].

Any facemask or nebulizer should be used with some caution. Many children find it claustrophobic and intolerable, and bronchospasm may, albeit rarely, complicate administration of any nebulized route.

Other routes

In many cultures, children dislike rectal administration, particularly on a chronic basis. The rectal route can, however, be useful as a means of avoiding parenteral administration over the short term, if children are unable to tolerate oral analgesics. The strength of analgesic suppositories is limited but oral sustained-release or immediate-release preparations can be given via the rectum at the usual intervals. The rectal route is usually contraindicated during episodes of neutropenia and thrombocytopenia because of the risk of infection and bleeding, respectively.

Intramuscular administration can rarely be justified in children, given the number of alternatives that are now available. Although the absorption profile of analgesia given by this route means that a single bolus can deliver sustained serum levels for longer than other parenteral routes, it is inevitably painful to administer. This forces the child in pain to have to consider whether the pain he/she is already in is severe enough to out-weigh the discomfort of the remedy. This is an invidious choice that a child should not have to make, and ensures that he/she will remain in pain.

Adjuvants

Identifying a patient's pain syndrome is important for both diagnosis and treatment. There are some general principles for adjuvant use [95].

1. Choose each medication based on the balance of intended effects and side effects. For example, the analgesic and sedating properties of amitriptyline can benefit a child with dysaesthesia who is also experiencing insomnia.

2. Be sure the child and/or family have a good understanding of what to expect, especially the slow onset of action, need for long-term use, and likely development of side effects and tolerance to these over time.

3. Start at low doses and increase the dose slowly to aid tolerance to side effects.

4. Increase the dose of each medication until analgesia is achieved, side effects are unmanageable, or high therapeutic drug levels are obtained.

5. Make sure that each drug is tried for long enough as many require several weeks to reach maximum efficacy.

For neuropathic pain

Neuropathic pain (Chapter 26, Neurological and neuromuscular symptoms) is characterized by altered sensation occurring in a recognisable nerve distribution which is usually dermatomal, but can also follow a vascular distribution in the case of sympathetic-mediated pain.

Alterations in sensation can range from simple hypoaesthesia or numbness to abnormal non-painful sensations such as tingling (paraesthesia) and abnormal noxious sensations such as burning (dysaesthesia). Clinically, simple touch becomes a painful stimulus (allodynia), painful responses become magnified (hyperalgesia), and responses to relatively innocuous stimuli are prolonged and exaggerated (hyperpathia). The patient's description, therefore, provides the best indication that the pain is neuropathic in origin. Historically, descriptions of two types of pain have been used to initiate treatment despite poor consistency in their predictive value. Epicritic pain is sharp, lancinating, and pricking pain that is likely to be associated with A-δ fibres and reported to respond to anti-convulsant therapy. Protopathic pain is dull, burning and poorly localized and postulated to be transmitted by the polymodal C-fibres and treated with an anti-depressant. Motor dysfunction is a late finding in neuropathic pain, implying considerable nerve damage.

The amino acid, glutamate, is a major neuroexcitatory transmitter in the CNS and plays a key role in the generation of neuropathic pain. The acute response to pain is mediated through glutamate activation of a-amino-3-hydroxy-5-methylisoxazole-4-proprioninc acid (AMPA) receptors. If the right conditions exist, including prolonged stimulation of the AMPA receptor, then released peptides and glutamate lead to activation of the N-methyl D-aspartate (NMDA) receptor and prolonged pain states are generated. This phenomenon is known as 'wind-up' and results in dramatic increases in the duration and magnitude of cell responses while the input into the spinal cord is unchanged.

The cause of neuropathic pain is very dependent on the disease process and is often related to compression, direct invasion, or infection of the peripheral nerves or spinal cord. Opioid therapy remains the central plank of pain management, [24] even where there is a neuropathic element. Although neuropathic pain is more likely than other types of pain to be partially opioid resistant [96], opioids are nevertheless more likely to be effective than other therapies. In other words, adjuvant therapies are more specific, but less potent.

Treatment of neuropathic pain involves the use of opioids and adjuvant analgesics. In adults with cancer, opioid responsiveness cannot be reliably predicted in individual patients solely on the basis of the type of pain [97]. In view of this, a trial of opioid therapy should not be withheld or limited, solely on the basis of inferred pathophysiology.

Once a diagnosis of neuropathic pain is made, an adjuvant should be added; this should not wait until other analgesic approaches have failed. Most adjuvants for neuropathic pain tend to be neuroactive; their primary site of action includes the central or peripheral nervous system. They are drawn from a wide range of medications that enhance pain relief and/or allow a reduction in the amount of opioid used. The dose of an adjuvant therapy required for analgesia is often less than that required for its primary indication.

Much of the data concerning management of neuropathic pain has been derived from studies on adults with painful diabetic neuropathy (PDN), post herpetic neuralgia (PHN), or trigeminal neuralgia (TN). There is discrepancy between the research findings and clinical experience in neuropathic pain syndromes other than TN [98]. There are many other medications in use, but information on efficacy is either very limited or contradictory. Agents in this group include systemic or topical administration of anaesthetic agents such as mexiletine and lidocaine, systemic administration of α-2 adrenergic receptor agonists like clonidine and the topical agent, capsaicin. This does not mean that such agents should be discarded as an option, but their application considered after failure of other options or for specific situations. For example, systemic lidocaine, either as a bolus or infusion, in anti-arrhythmic doses can be useful in gaining control of severe neuropathic pain exacerbation as an emergency measure.

The use of any benzodiazepine as an adjuvant agent for neuropathic pain should be actively discouraged, as a careful review of the literature reveals insufficient evidence to support any meaningful analgesic properties in most clinical circumstances [99].

Anticonvulsants

Many anti-convulsants have found a use in treating neuropathic pain. This may relate to the similar mechanisms that exist between seizures and pain propagation. The potential mechanisms of action include:

- Prolonged inactivation of the sodium channel—carbamazepine, phenytoin, lamotrigine, topirimate, valproic acid.

- Prolonged activation of the chloride channel through the γ-aminobutyric acid (GABA) receptor—vigabatrin, topirimate, valproate.

- Prolonged activation of the chloride channel as a direct effect on the channel—barbiturates, benzodiazepines.

- Calcium channel modulation—gabapentin.

Only carbamazepine, phenytoin, gabapentin, and lamotrigine have been studied in randomized clinical trials for relief of pain in neuropathic pain syndromes and of these agents, only carbamazepine and gabapentin have been shown to have a positive effect in all studies [98]. A systematic review of anti-convulsant drug management for neuropathic pain showed carbamazepine and phenytoin to be efficacious but there was not enough evidence for valproic acid [100].

Carbamazepine and its derivative oxcarbazepine [101] are effective in the treatment of neuropathic pain for patients with trigeminal neuralgia (TN). This class of drug has peripheral and central actions and has the ability to suppress spontaneous A∂ and C-fibre activity without affecting normal nerve conduction. The most common adverse effects are dizziness and light-headedness. Nystagmus, nausea and vomiting, gum hypertrophy and megaloblastic anaemia are other side effects.

Gabapentin seems to be well tolerated for this indication in children [102,103]. Other anti-convulsants have been associated with a variety of idiosyncratic adverse effects that include Stevens-Johnson syndrome, aplastic anaemia, hepatotoxicity, and systemic lupus-like syndromes. These are rare, but can be fatal.

Antidepressants

There is good evidence that tricyclic anti-depressants (TCA) have a beneficial effect in neuropathic pain [104, 105]. The mechanism is not fully elucidated but is likely to be due to their multi-modal activity, inhibition of presynaptic reuptake of norepinephrine and serotonin, NMDA receptor antagonism, and an inhibitory action on sodium channel activity. The more selective serotonin reuptake inhibitors do not seem to have as significant an effect on neuropathic pain independent of their anti-depressant activity.

The numbers needed to treat to get at least a 50% reduction in pain compared with placebo (NNT) for TCA, across different neuropathic pain conditions, is between 2 and 3. That is, every second or third patient will derive more than 50% pain relief. In a meta-analysis study of anti-depressants compared with placebo [104] of 100 patients treated for neuropathic pain, 30 would obtain more than 50% pain relief, 30 would have minor adverse reactions, and 4 would need to stop therapy because of a major adverse effect.

The most commonly used and most studied agent is the tertiary amine TCA, amitriptyline. Other tertiary agents in use include imipramine and doxepine while secondary amines include desipramine and nortryptiline. They are generally well absorbed from the gastrointestinal tract, peak in the plasma after 2–8 h, and have long half-lives ranging from 20 h for amitriptyline to 80 hours for protryptiline. This makes them ideal for once daily dosing, which is best given at night to either reduce or make use of their sedative side effect. They are lipophilic and strongly protein bound and widely distributed to the brain and other organs.

Adverse effects are common and may be dose-limiting although clinical experience suggests they may be better tolerated in children than in adults. Adverse effects are more likely with TCAs that include a tertiary amine group and include:

• Sedation

• Sympathomimetic—tremor, insomnia (use as morning dose)

• Anti-muscarinic—dry mouth, blurred vision, constipation, urinary hesitancy, confusion

• Cardiovascular—orthostatic hypotension, conduction defects (prolongation of QT interval), arrhythmia

• Neurologic—seizures

• Metabolic/endocrine—weight gain

• Psychiatric—withdrawal syndrome (avoid abrupt discontinuation of therapy).

Fortunately, the dose required for effectiveness against neuropathic pain is usually much less than that required for anti-depression and it is often possible to find a well-tolerated dose. Common practice for amitriptyline is to commence one tenth of the usual total daily dose for depression, given as a single nighttime dose. The dose is then escalated gradually until there is analgesia. If the total daily dose for depression is reached without analgesic effect, tricyclics should be considered ineffective and be discontinued.

NMDA antagonists

NMDA receptor antagonists have a potential use for any pain syndrome with the sensory abnormalities of neuropathic pain, inflammatory pain, phantom limb pain or peripheral vascular disease. Some opioids, particularly methadone (see above) combine opioid and NMDA antagonist properties, and are a good choice in principle for this indication.

Ketamine binds non-competitively with the NMDA receptor. It has been used most frequently as a dissociative anaesthetic agent by activating the limbic system, and depressing the cerebral cortex. The result is profound analgesia, slight respiratory depression, cardiovascular stimulation, and maintenance of protective reflexes and amnesia. At sub-anaesthetic doses, the analgesic effect continues but without impairment of consciousness. There are two enantiomers for ketamine and

the (+) isomer is 3× more potent as an analgesic, 1.5× more potent as an anaesthetic, and causes less excitation than the (−) isomer. Commercially available preparations contain equal concentrations of both enantiomers.

Parenteral bioavailability is around 93%, but a high hepatic first pass metabolism that means around 16%, is available after oral administration. Analgesic effects following oral administration are seen after 30 min and the half-life is around 1–3 h.

Ketamine is a homologue of phencyclidine (PCP, angel dust) and similarly has psychomimetic effects, such as vivid dreams, hallucinations, confusion, delirium and feelings of detachment from the body. This potential drawback typically occurs when emerging from an anaesthetic. They are less likely to be associated with the lower doses used for analgesia, in children under the age of 16 years and with slow administration, and can be managed in the same way as delirium using haloperidol and benzodiazepines. Additional adverse reactions involve skin reactions at the site of sub-cutaneous administration, cardiovascular excitability, excess salivation, and enhanced gastrointestinal transit. Ketamine is also a potent cerebral vasodilator and increases cerebral blood flow by about 60% and therefore, is not recommended for patients with increased intracranial pressure.

In the palliative setting, ketamine can improve analgesia in morphine tolerant patients with neuropathic pain [106] but 40% of patients had central adverse effects. In children receiving parenteral administration, a loading dose of 0.1 to 0.2 mg/kg, can be followed by an infusion rate of 0.1 to 0.3 mg/kg/h, and this can be increased to effect, intolerable side effects or a maximum infusion of 1.5 mg/kg/h.

For bone pain

In contrast with the nature of distribution of neuropathic pain, bone pain is typically well localized and may be indicated by a patient by pointing to a specific spot. It can be intense and very severe and is sometimes described as 'boring' or 'like a drill'. The timing of the pain depends on the underlying cause which can include marrow expansion from leukaemia or solid tumours, or metastatic spread to bone cortex (for example, with osteosarcoma or Ewing's sarcoma).

Non-malignant causes of bone pain can include:

• Primary defects and structural bone proteins (osteogenesis imperfecta)

• Bone abnormalities in the context of systemic disease (mucopolysaccharidosis)

• The effects of systemic treatment (especially steroids)

• The effects of immobilisation in neurodegenerative conditions and cerebral palsy.

Where it is due to a fracture, bone pain may be intermittently very severe or episodic in nature (see below) which can complicate its management since analgesia sufficient for pain, at its worst, may be too toxic for pain, at its least.

Procedures that immobilize the bone may be effective in reducing bone pain, particularly if associated with a fracture. Opioids are, as always, the most reliably effective analgesics. However, useful adjuvants include non-steroidal anti-inflammatory drugs, bisphosphonates, and radiotherapy.

Non-steroidal anti-inflammatory drugs

The NSAIDs are a heterogenous group of powerful anti-inflammatory agents that inhibit the activity of the cyclo-oxygenase (COX) enzyme, and thus the production of prostaglandin and thromboxane. The specific mechanism of analgesic action is not known, but blockade of prostaglandin production does not account for the total analgesic effect.

There is a wide array of essentially equi-analgesic agents [107]. The oldest NSAID (acetyl-salicylic acid or aspirin) is often considered an inferior analgesic and possesses two other undesirable features that make it less suitable for use as a primary analgesic in children. It has non-linear elimination kinetics (slower elimination at higher concentrations) that increases the risk of toxicity in the form of salicylate poisoning. Its use in children with febrile illness has been associated with the development of Reye's syndrome [108], though this is debated [109]. Depending on the stage of the child's disease, the latter concern may not be as relevant to children with palliative care needs.

NSAIDs are, broadly, grouped according to selectivity for the two isoforms of COX; constitutive COX-1 and inducible COX-2. COX-1 is present in all tissues and is involved in physiological functions, such as gastrointestinal mucosal protection, platelet function, and regulation of renal haemodynamics and electrolyte balance. COX-2, normally undetectable in tissue, is involved in inflammation, mitogenesis, and specialized signal transduction. There is considerable increase in COX-2 activity with inflammation. The non-selective NSAIDs inhibit both isoforms to varying degrees making them effective anti-inflammatory and analgesic agents, while the selective COX-2 inhibitors have poor analgesic activity outside of their anti-inflammatory action.

The mechanism of action in blocking the COX-1 pathway may not completely explain the analgesic efficacy, but does seem to account for their adverse effects. These are either predictable and dose-dependent or unpredictable and dose-independent.

Predictable effects include:

Haematological—decreased platelet adhesion. Decreased platelet aggregation and prolongation of bleeding time results from inhibition of platelet thromboxane A2 activity. Aspirin is the only agent to inhibit platelet aggregation irreversibly, and inhibition by other preparations depends on blood concentration and has not been a practical concern for children having surgery or dental extractions. It is generally held that children with pre-existing reduced platelet counts or bleeding disorders (such as those with relapsed leukaemias) should avoid NSAID where possible, though there is little published evidence to support this caution.

Gastrointestinal—dyspepsia, haemorrhage, peptic ulceration, perforation. Clinically significant gastropathies are unusual during chronic use in children with juvenile rheumatoid arthritis [110]. Taking these agents with food can minimize the gastrointestinal effects. Avoidance is advised in children with a history of peptic ulceration.

Renal—salt and water retention, interstitial nephritis. Renal toxicity is low in normal healthy children [111], but risk increases in those with pre-existing renal problems or hypovolaemia [112].

Pulmonary—bronchospasm. NSAID-induced bronchospasm occurs in 8–20% of asthmatic adults but seems to be uncommon in children [113, 114]. However, they should be avoided in children with previous reactions to NSAIDs and practitioners should remain alert to the possibility of idiosyncratic reactions.

Unpredictable events can include effects on the following systems:

- Central nervous system (CNS)—tinnitus, dizziness, headache, anxiety, aseptic meningitis, psychiatric-type reactions
- Gastrointestinal—diarrhoea
- Haematological—thrombocytopaenia, haemolytic anaemia, agranulocytosis, aplastic anaemia
- Immunological—anaphylaxis
- Hepatic—hepatitis, Reye's syndrome
- Skin—rash, pruritis, angioedema, severe skin reactions

COX-2 selectivity appears to correlate with a reduction in, but not elimination of, gastrointestinal adverse events and platelet aggregation problems. However, this has to be weighed against their relatively poor analgesic cover outside of their anti-inflammatory action and other potential adverse effects. This was highlighted in 2004 by the worldwide withdrawal of rofecoxib (Vioxx) after clinical trial data indicated an increased incidence of serious thrombotic events, myocardial infarction, and stroke among adult patients receiving long term rofecoxib compared with placebo.

Bisphosphonates

Bisphosphonates are analogues of pyrophosphate, a natural inhibitor for the formation of calcium phosphate crystals. Their effect is to decrease bone resorption by:

- Decreasing recruitment and function of osteoclasts—the mevalonate enzyme pathway is inhibited.

- Stimulating osteoblasts to produce an inhibitor of osteoclast formation.

- Direct binding to hydroxyapatite crystals in bone, making it inherently more resistant to resorption.

These actions do not impair bone architecture or mechanical strength and lead to an increased vertebral bone mass and bone density. They are available in intravenous and oral forms and biological action is dependent on the chemical side chain. First generation bisphosphonates such as etidronate and clodronate are the least potent; second generation aminobisphosponates like alendronate and pamidronate are 10–100 times as potent as first generation drugs, while third generation agents, such as risedronate and zoledronic acid, are 10,000 times more potent.

Bisphosphonates have been used in children for 25 years. The conditions for which they are used are very diverse. In contrast with adults, in whom there is considerable experience of their use for painful metastatic malignant disease [115], in children, most experience has been in congenital and acquired forms of osteoporosis [116]. There are only limited case reports of use for bone pain in children and none is related to malignancy.

Bisphosphonate therapy appears not only to be effective but also safe, even with prolonged use. The adverse effects described with pamidronate can be divided into short and long-term.

Immediate side effects include:

- Acute phase reaction—common influenza-like reaction that is fever, chills, myalgia, that occurs 24–48 h after the first treatment but usually not in subsequent infusions. The symptoms may be improved by prophylactic use of paracetamol or ibuprofen.

- Hypocalcaemia—uncommon problem that occurs within 72 h of infusion but can be prevented by a daily intake of 1 to 1.5 g calcium.

- Bone pain—only reported in adults with cystic fibrosis but diminishes with subsequent infusions.

- Iritis and/or uveitis—uncommon.

- Occasional long-term adverse effects have been reported. They include impaired bone mineralization, nephrocalcinosis and osteopetrosis [117]. There is a theoretical risk of altered bone re-modelling during periods of rapid growth, and in particular during adolescence, but this has not been demonstrated in practice [118].

Radiotherapy

Radiotherapy can be very effective if the cause of bone pain is localised metastatic malignant disease. This is true even for relatively radio-resistant tumours such as osteosarcoma, since a small reduction in the size of the lesion can have a significant effect on pain management. Some radiotherapy centres will offer a single fraction of palliative radiotherapy to sites of metastasis. This is well tolerated by children and young people, although they are often reluctant to undergo diagnostic interventions beforehand, such as plain x-ray or bone scan, that require attendance at hospital. Many radiotherapy centres will offer targeted radiation on clinical history alone in the palliative phase.

The effectiveness of radiotherapy is such that a degree of narcotisation (see above) should be anticipated among children on major opioids for metastatic bone pain.

Muscle spasm

Muscle spasm is a potent source of pain for many children with neurodegenerative conditions and particularly cerebral palsy. Benzodiazepines have been prescribed to patients in this group with good effect [119]. Baclofen and dantrolene may also be of benefit and should be offered alongside analgesic therapy.

More recently, botulinum toxin has been shown to have good efficacy in relieving the pain of muscle spasm in cerebral palsy [120–122]. The administration of botulinum toxin is a specialist skill requiring input from the local paediatric neurology or orthopaedic team. For children whose pain is significantly improved by botulinum toxin, it can often be inferred that an orthopaedic intervention to relieve muscle spasm will also be effective on a more permanent basis. The management of painful muscle spasm in cerebral palsy, therefore, requires a collaborative approach between paediatric palliative medicine, orthopaedics, and the paediatric teams mainly involved in the care of the child.

Opioids should not be withheld from children with non-malignant conditions. Given the expectation that they will survive for decades, however, it is often prudent to optimise management with non-opioid means first and proceed to opioids if these initial measures fail.

Cerebral irritation

The experience of pain is powerfully amplified by anxiety and incomprehension. Cerebral irritation, usually arising from acute hypoxic ischaemia or septic brain injury, can cause pain that is very difficult to treat using opioids and other analgesics alone. Benzodiazepines such as midazolam or lorazapam can be of benefit in reducing anxiety, but should be continued for only a few weeks, if possible. Phenobarbitone (Phenobarbital) is an effective sedative that has the additional advantage of being familiar to many neonatal paediatricians as an anticonvulsant. Again, it should be continued only for a few months in order to avoid the risk of unacceptable long-term side effects in these children who are likely to survive for some years. Once the acute brain injury has resolved, it is often possible to withdraw anxiolytic therapy over a period of some weeks.

Steroids

The use of corticosteroids as an analgesic adjuvant agent can be helpful in managing inflammatory-mediated pain or pain syndromes mediated by peri-tumour oedema, for example, headaches resulting from raised intracranial pressure [123], neuropathic pain secondary to spinal cord, nerve root or peripheral nerve compression, and pain resulting from capsular distension.

There are a variety of corticosteroids available, but those that have minimal or no salt-retaining properties, such as prednisolone, betamethasone and dexamethasone, are recommended. Dexamethasone is the most often used in most countries. It has a relative potency 25 times that of cortisone, and a biological half-life between 36–54 h despite a plasma half-life of 3.6 h. Betamethasone has similar characteristics to dexamethasone, while methyl-prednisone possesses 5 times the potency of cortisone, but a similar half-life.

The pharmacological actions of steroids are Protean, and this is equally true of therapeutic and adverse effects. Administration of any corticosteroid can result in a plethora of adverse events. All are more likely to occur with high doses and/or prolonged duration of treatment. They include:

- Cushingoid habitus—moon face, central adiposity
- Skin—striae, acne, skin fragility, increased bruising, poor wound healing
- Muscle—proximal myopathy, peripheral oedema
- Gastrointestinal—gastritis, bleeding, gastric ulceration and perforation
- Immunological—increased risk of infection, oral candidiasis
- Metabolic—osteoporosis, insatiable appetite, hyperglycaemia/ glucosuria
- Psychological—restlessness, agitation, sleep disturbance, anxiety, depression, frank psychosis. In children, behaviour and mood changes are common.

The progressive distortion of a child's physical appearance should not be underestimated for the effect it has on both the child and family, especially the body image conscious adolescent. As a result, the temporal relationship of steroid use

to projected life expectancy must be carefully considered and the lowest effective dose used. Options to prolonged use include maximizing opioids and other symptom-specific agents, prescribing corticosteroids as pulses. This is a brief, intense 3–5 day course repeated at set intervals or when symptoms dictate. Effective control of symptoms has been reported for up to 4 weeks [124]. In some situations, a large one-off dose can be helpful in a severe pain crisis.

A typical dose of corticosteroids for a child is 1–2 mg/kg/day of prednisolone, (maximum 60 mg/day) or 0.5 mg/kg/day (maximum 16 mg/day) of dexamethasone. The biological half-life data would suggest that once or, at most, twice daily dosing is required.

Palliative chemotherapy

The term 'palliative chemotherapy' has been used in many different ways [123]. In its most precise sense, chemotherapy can have a role in reducing symptoms due to advanced cancer. It should only be prescribed after carefully weighing up its potential benefit against the likely burden it will impose on the patient. This would include, for example, increased need for attendances to hospital for haemoglobin, platelet and white cell counts, the possibility of nausea and vomiting and also of hair loss. Oral etoposide [126–128] can relieve symptoms caused by tumour bulk, particularly in haematopoietic malignancies and brain tumours. Vincristine and steroids can be effective in managing the pain of medullary expansion due to leukaemic transformation of the marrow. The side effects of steroids have been considered (see above) and it should be remembered that vincristine needs to be given intravenously, requiring a cannula to be sited, and can cause painful neurotoxicity for some children. For most, however, it can offer a well-tolerated tumour reducing effect.

Not all chemotherapy given to children with cancer for whom there is no longer a chance of cure can be considered truly palliative. Chemotherapy given on phase I or II clinical trials, for example, is experimental and is not, therefore, prescribed with any likelihood that symptoms will be relieved. Nevertheless, trial chemotherapy can be very valuable for some children and particularly young people who will value the opportunity of taking part in a trial that may contribute to human understanding. Many will retain the hope that trial chemotherapy will work a miracle and it is important that patients and families realise that neither long term cure, nor even palliation of symptoms, is the expectation. Any impact on symptoms is incidental to the stated goal of the trial.

Many families request chemotherapy even when it is clear that it is futile. Again, this should not be confused with palliative chemotherapy, since the intention is not to palliate symptoms.

There may, occasionally, be a place for such futile chemotherapy but it is important to ensure that the needs of the family are carefully weighed against those of the child and that the child does not suffer simply in order to perpetuate false hope in the family.

Regional and neurolytic approaches

Neurolytic approaches include epidural, spinal and intrathecal anaesthesia as well as regional nerve blocks, or ablative therapy. They are the domain of specialist anaesthetic and neurosurgical services. Most require hospital attendance or even admission for invasive procedure, and are, therefore, relatively rarely used in children. They can be difficult for a family to manage at home.

Nevertheless, they should be considered in children for whom adequate pain relief cannot be obtained using the methods outlined elsewhere in this chapter [129]. Consultation with an appropriate colleague should be considered early when there is evidence of coeliac plexus pain or for the child with pelvic or lower limb pain, and particularly for the child who is in any case immobile.

Breakthrough and incident pain

The terms 'episodic' and 'breakthrough' are not precisely the same. Pain may be episodic for three rather distinct reasons. The dose of regular medication may simply be too small, resulting in intermittent breakthrough pain. Breakthrough pain itself has been defined as 'a transitory exacerbation of pain superimposed on a background of persistent, usually well controlled pain' [130]. The solution is to review the regular medication and adjust the dose as outlined above.

The cause of the pain may itself be episodic. For example, movement can provoke pain from a pathological fracture or from some bone metastases. This is often referred to as 'incident pain'. Identifying, anticipating, and where possible avoiding the provoking factors are the mainstays of treatment. Local radiation, chemotherapy or surgery can help, but even simple measures such as a sling to immobilise the affected part can be of value. Regional neurolytic approaches may also have a role.

Finally, the pain itself may simply be of an episodic nature, for example, intestinal colic or muscle spasm. This is a situation in which adjuvant therapy such as anticholinergics or muscle relaxants may be particularly helpful.

Because these causes for episodic or breakthrough pain are closely related, the definitions are often confused and the therefore incidence difficult to estimate [129]. Adult patients report a wide variety of types of pain that can break through their regular analgesia and similarly variable events that can precipitate it [132].

An ideal pharmacological intervention for breakthrough pain would be immediately accessible to the patient at the time the pain began, have a very rapid on- and off-set of action [133], and be highly potent. There is currently no such paragon. The peak effect of oral morphine, for example, may be up to an hour after its ingestion, meaning that it will often occur well after the episode of pain has subsided.

Though none is perfect, agents that approach the ideal include ketamine, inhaled nitrous oxide, parenteral opioids and oral fentanyl lozenges. More novel methods of administration include buccal diamorphine and intranasal sufentanil. Irrespective of what is chosen to treat the breakthrough pain itself, it is important to maintain the usual regular opioid schedule [133].

Summary

Managing analgesia is, of course, only one of the aspects of caring for a dying child. Palliative care means giving attention to physical, psychosocial, and spiritual issues simultaneously. It may seem that disproportionate emphasis has been placed on what is, after all, only one symptom among many.

The reality is that pain is the commonest symptom experienced by dying children, and that it overlaps with all dimensions of a child's existence. A child who is in severe pain cannot engage with carers in a way that allows meaningful exploration of other fears or concerns. Good pain management is, therefore, a necessary, though not sufficient, first step in addressing these wider issues.

Furthermore, pain itself is a symptom that is experienced in every existential dimension. Even where the primary painful stimulus is a physical one, its perception and experience by a child will be dictated by the spiritual and psychosocial context in which it occurs. The meaning of a painful ankle caused by a football injury is very different from that caused by recurrent cancer, even where the physical elements are identical. If we are to manage what has been described as 'total pain' effectively, we must recognise the need to address it in as broad a way as possible.

This chapter has dealt with pharmacological approaches and has focused largely on its physical aspects, but the reader is encouraged to refer to other chapters in the book that examine the wider experience of pain.

References

1. Drake, R., Frost, J., and Collins, J.J. The symptoms of dying children. *J Pain Symptom Manage* 2003;26(1):1–10.

2. Hunt, A.M. A survey of signs, symptoms and symptom control in 30 terminally ill children. *Dev Med Child Neurol* 1990;32(4):341–6.

3. Wolfe, J., Grier, H.E., Klar, N., Levin, S.B., Ellenbogen, J.M., Salem-Schatz, S. *et al*. Symptoms and suffering at the end of life in children with cancer. *N Eng J Med* 2000;342(5):326–33.

4. Organization WH. Cancer pain relief and palliative care in children. World Health Organization, 1998.

5. Choonara, Lawrence, Michalkiewicz, Bowhay, Ratcliffe. Morphine metabolism in neonates and infants. *Br J Clin Pharmac* 1994;437 (1994).

6. Choonara, I., McKay, P., Hain R.D.W., and Rane A. Morphine metabolism in children. *Br J Clin Pharmacol* 1989.

7. Kart, T., Christrup L.L., and Rasmussen, M. Recommended use of morphine in neonates, infants and children based on a literature review: Part 1—Pharmacokinetics. *Paediatr Anaesth* 1997;7(1): 5–11.

8. Bouwmeester, N., Anderson B.J., Tibboel, D., and Holford, N.H. Developmental pharmacokinetics of morphine and metabolites in neonates, infants and young children. *Br J Anaesthesia* 2004;92 (208–217).

9. Ventafridda, V., Tamburini, M., Caraceni C., De Conno, F., and Naldi, F. A validation study of the WHO method for cancer pain relief. *Cancer* 1987;59:850–6.

10. McGraw, M.B. Neural maturation as exemplified in the changing reactions of the infant to pin prick. *Child Dev* 1941;12(1):31–42.

11. McQuay, H.A.M. Acute pain: Conclusion. In H.A.M, McQuay ed. *An Evidence-Based Resource for Pain Relief*. Oxford, UK: Oxford University Press, 1998, pp. 187–92.

12. World Health Organization. Cancer Pain Relief with a guide to opioid availability (2nd edition). WHO, 1996.

13. Kelley, M.T., Walson, P.D., Edge, J.H., Cox, S., and Mortensen, M.E. Pharmacokinetics and pharmacodynamics of ibuprofen isomers and acetaminophen in febrile children. *Pharmacol Ther* 1992;52(2):181–9.

14. Anderson, B.J., Woollard G.A., and Holford, N.H. Acetaminophen analgesia in children: Placebo effet and pain resolution after tonsillectomy. *Eur J Clin Pharmacol* 2001;57(8):559–69.

15. Anderson, B.J. and Holford, N.H. Rectal paracetamol dosing regimens: Determination by computer simulation. *Paediatr Anaesth* 1997;7(6):451–5.

16. Montgomery, C.J., McCormack, J.P., Reichert, C.C., and Marsland, C.P. Plasma concentrations after high-dose (45 mg/kg) rectal acetaminophen in children. *Canad J Anaesth* 1995;42(11): 982–6.

17. Anderson B.J., Holford N.H., Armishaw J.C., and Aicken R. Predicting concentrations in children presenting with acetaminophen overdose. *J Pediatr* 1999;135(3):290–5.

18. Morton, N.S. and Arana, A. Paracetamol-induced fulminant hepatic failure in a child after 5 days of therapeutic doses. *Paediatr Anaesth* 1999;9(5):463–5.

19. Hynson J.L. and South, M. Childhood hepatotoxicity with paracetamol doses less than 150 mg/kg per day. *Med J Aus* 1999;171(9):487.

20. Forrest, J.B., Heitlinger E.L., and Revell, S. Ketorolac for postoperative pain management in children. *Drug Saf* 1997;16(5):309–29.

21. Quiding, H., Lundqvist, G., Boreus L.O., Bondesson, U., and Ohrvik, J. Analgesic effect and plasma concentrations of codeine and morphine after two dose levels of codeine following oral surgery. *Eur J Clin Pharmacol* 1993;44(4):319–23.

22. Mikus G., Somogyi A.A., Bochner F., and Chen Z.R. Polymorphic metabolism of opioid narcotic drugs: Possible clinical implications. *Ann Acad Med* Singapore 1991;20(1):9–12.

23. Riedel, F. and von Stockhausen, H.B. Severe cerebral depression after intoxication with tramadol in a 6-month-old infant. *Eur J Clin Pharmacol* 1984;26(5):631–2.

24. Hain, R.D.W., Miser, A., Devins M., and Wallace, W.H.B. Strong opioids in pediatric palliative medicine. *Pediatr Drugs* 2005;5(1):1–9.

25. Hunt, A.M., Joel, S., Dick, G., and Goldman, A. Population pharmacokinetics of oral morphine and its glucuronides in children receiving morphine as immediate—release liquid or sustained-release tablets for cancer pain. *J Pediatr* 1999;135(1):47–55.

26. Hain, R.D., Hardcastle, A., Pinkerton, C.R., and Aherne, G.W. Morphine and morphine-6-glucuronide in the plasma and cerebrospinal fluid of children. *Bri J Clin Pharmacol* 1999;48(1):37–42.

27. Gill, A.M., Cousins, A., Nunn, A.J., and Choonara, I.M. Opiate-induced respiratory depression in pediatric patients. *Ann Pharmacother* 1996;30:125–9.

28. Raddle, I.C. Pharmacology of the perinatal period. In I.C. Raddle, S.M. MacLeod, eds. *Pediatr Pharmacol Ther*. St Louis: Mosby, 1993, p. 423.

29. Koren, G. and Cohen, M.S. Special aspects of perinatal and pediatric pharmacology. In B.G. Katzung, ed. *Basic Clin Pharmacol*. East Norwalk: Appleton and Lange 1995, pp. 916–19.

30. Rady, J.J., Elmer, G.I., and Fujimoto, J.M. Opioid receptor selectivity of heroin given intracerebroventricularly differs in six strains of inbred mice. *J Pharmacol Exp Ther* 1999;288(2):438–45.

31. Rady, J.J., Takemori, A.E., Portoghese, P.S., and Fujimoto, J.M. Supraspinal delta receptor subtype activity of heroin and 6-monoacetylmorphine in Swiss Webster mice. *Life Sci* 1994; 55(8):603–9.

32. Collins, J.J., Dunkel, I.J., Gupta, S.K., Inturrisi, C.E., Lapin, J., and Palmer, L.N. Transdermal fentanyl in children with cancer pain: Feasibility, tolerability, and pharmacokinetic correlates. *J Pediatr* 1999;134(3):319–23.

33. Howell, T.K., Smith, S., Rushman, S.C., Walker, R.W., and Radivan, F. A comparison of oral transmucosal fentanyl and oral midazolam for premedication in children. *Anaesthesia* 2002;57(8):798–805.

34. Epstein, R.H., Mendel, H.G., Witkowski, T.A., Waters, R., Guarniari, K.M., Marr, A.T. *et al*. The safety and efficacy of oral transmucosal fentanyl citrate for preoperative sedation in young children. *Anesth Analg* 1996;83(6):1200–5.

35. Feld, L.H., Champeau, M.W., van Steennis, C.A., and Scott, J.C. Preanesthetic medication in children: A comparison of oral transmucosal fentanyl citrate versus placebo. *Anesthesiology* 1989;71(3): 374–7.

36. Goodarzi, M. Comparison of epidural morphine, hydromorphone and fentanyl for postoperative pain control in children undergoing orthopaedic surgery. *Paediatr Anaesth* 1999;9(5):419–22.

37. Ripamonti, C. and Bianchi, M. The use of methadone for cancer pain. *Hematol Oncol Clin North Am* 2002;16(3):543–55.

38. Noyes, M. and Irving, H. The use of transdermal fentanyl in pediatric oncology palliative care. *Am J Hosp Palliat Care* 2001;18(6): 411–6.

39. Borland, M.L., Jacobs, I., and Geelhoed, G. Intranasal fentanyl reduces acute pain in children in the emergency department: A safety and efficacy study. *Emerg Med* (Fremantle) 2002;14(3):275–80.

40. Johnson, K.L., Erickson, J.P., Holley, F.O., and Scott, J.C. Fentanyl pharmacokinetics in the pediatric population. *Anesthesiology* 1984;61(3A):A441.

41. Santeiro, M.L., Christie, J., Stromquist, C., Torres, B.A., and Markowsky, S.J. Pharmacokinetcis of continuous infusion fentanyl in newborns. *J Perinatol* 1997;17(2):135–9.

42. Anderson, B.J., McKee, A.D., and Holford, N.H. Size, myths and the clinical pharmacokinetics of analgesia in paediatric patients. *Clin Pharmacokinetics* 1997;33(5):313–27.

43. Dsida, R.M., Wheeler, M., Birmingham, P.K., Henthorn, T.K., Avram, M.J., Enders-Klein, C. *et al.* Premedication of pediatric tonsillectomy patients with oral transmucosal fentanyl citrate. *Anesth Analg* 1998;86(1):66–70.

44. Sharar, S.R., Bratton, S.L., Carrougher, G.J., Edwards, W.T., Summer, G., Levy F.H., *et al.* A comparison of oral transmucosal fentanyl citrate and oral hydromorphone for inpatient pediatric burn wound care analgesia. *J Burn Care Rehabil* 1998;19(6):516–21.

45. Sharar, S.R., Carrougher, G.J., Selzer, K., O'Donnell, F., Vavilala, M.S., and Lee, L.A. A comparison of oral transmucosal fentanyl citrate and oral oxycodone for pediatric outpatient wound care. *J Burn Care Rehabil* 2002;23(1):27–31.

46. Babul, N., Darke, A., and Hain, R.D.W. Hydromorphone and metabolite pharmacokinetics in children. *J Pain Symptom Manage* 1993;10(5):335–7.

47. Collins, J.J., Geake, J., Grier, H.E., Houck, C.S., Thaler, H.T., Weinstein, H.J., *et al.* Patient-controlled analgesia for mucositis pain in children: A three-period crossover study comparing morphine and hydromorphone. *J Pediatr* 1996;129(5):722–8.

48. Berde, C.B., Sethna, N.F., Holzman, R.S., Reidy, P., and Gondek, E.J. Pharmacokinetics of methadone in children and adolescents in the perioperative period. *Anesthesiology* 1987;67:A519.

49. Chana, S.K. and Anand, K.J. Can we use methadone for analgesia in neonates? *Arch Dis Childhood* (Fetal & Neonatal Edition) 2001;85(2):F79–81.

50. Shir, Y., Rosen, G., Zeldin, A., and Davidson, E.M. Methadone is safe for treating hospitalized patients with severe pain. *Canadi J Anaesth* 2001;48(11):1109–13.

51. Shir, Y., Shenkman, Z., Shavelson, V., Davidson, E.M., and Rosen, G. Oral methadone for the treatment of severe pain in hospitalized children: a report of five cases. *Clin J P* 1998;14(4):350–3.

52. Miser, A.W. and Miser, J.S. The Use of Oral Methadone to control moderate and severe pain in children and young adults with malignancy. *T Clin j Pain* 1986;1:243–8.

53. Berde, C.B., Beyer, J.E., Bournaki, M.C., Levin, C.R., and Sethna, N.F. Comparison of morphine and methadone for prevention of postoperative pain in 3- to 7-year-old children. *J Pediatr* 1991;119(1):136–41.

54. Hamunen, K. Ventilatory effects of morphine, pethidine and methadone in children. *Br J of Anaesth* 1993;70(4):414–18.

55. Callahan, R.J., Au, J.D., Paul, M., Liu, C., and Yost, C.S. Functional inhibition by methadone of N-methyl-D-aspartate receptors expressed in Xenopus oocytes: Stereospecific and subunit effects. *Anesth Analg* 2004;98(3):653–9, table of contents.

56. Hanks, G.W., Conno, F., Cherny N., Hanna, M., and Kalso, E., McQuay H.J. *et al.* Morphine and alternative opioids in cancer pain: The EAPC recommendations. *Br J Cancer* 2001;84(5):587–93.

57. Layson-Wolf, C., Goode, J.V., and Small, R.E. Clinical use of methadone. *J Pain Palliat Care Pharmacother* 2002;16(1):29–59.

58. Nelson, K.A., Park, K.M., Robinovitz, E., Tsigos, C., and Max, M.B. High-dose oral dextromethophan versus placebo in painful diabetic neuropathy and postherpetic neuralgia. *Neurology* 1997; 48(5):1212–18.

59. McQuay, H., Carroll, D., Jadad, A.R., Glynn, C.J., Jack, T., Moore, R.A., *et al.* Dextromethorphan for the treatment of neuropathic pain: A double-blind randomised controlled crossover trial with integral n-of-1 design. *Pain* 1994;59(1):127–33.

60. Kokki, H., Rasanen, I., Reinikainen, M., *et al.* Pharmacokinetics of oxycodone after intravenous, buccal, intramuscular and gastric administration in children. *Clin Pharma* 2004;43:613–22.

61. Olkkola, K.T., Hamunen, K., Seppala, T., and Maunuksela, E.L. Pharmacokinetics and ventilatory effects of intravenous oxycodone in postoperative children. *Br J Clin Pharmacol* 1994;38(1):71–6.

62. Twycross, R., Wilcock, A., Charlesworth, S., and Dickman, A. PCF2 Palliative Care Formulary (2 edition). Oxford: Radcliffe Medical Press, 2002.

63. Radbruch, L. and Vielvoye-Kerkmeer, A. Buprenorphine TDS: The clinical development rationale and results. *Int J Clin Pract Suppl* 2003(133):15–18; discussion 23–4.

64. Budd, K. Buprenorphine: A review. In: Evidence Based Medicine in Practice. Newmarket: Hayward Medical Communications, 2002.

65. Pokela, M.L., Olkkola, K.T., Koivisto, M., and Ryhanen, P. Pharmacokinetics and pharmacodynamics of intravenous meperidine in neonates and infants. *Clin Pharmacol Ther* 1992;52(4):342–9.

66. Kussman B.D. and Sethna N.F. Pethidine-associated seizure in a healthy adolescent receiving pethidine for postoperative pain control. *Paediatr Anaesth* 1998;8(4):349–52.

67. Pryle, B.J., Grech, H., Stoddart, P.A., Carson, R., O'Mahoney, T., and Reynolds, F. Toxicity of norpethidine in sickle cell crisis. *BMJ* 1992;304(6840):1478–9.

68. Kyff, J.V. and Rice, T.L. Meperidine-associated seizures in a child. *Clin Pharm* 1990;9(5):337–8.

69. Waterhouse, R.G. Epileptiform convulsions in children following premedication with Pamergan SP100. *Br J Anaesth* 1967;39(3): 268–70.

70. Soares, L.G., Martins, M., and Uchoa, R. Intravenous fentanyl for cancer pain: A 'fast titration' protocol for the emergency room. *J Pain Symptom Manage* 2003;26(3):876–81.

71. Harris, J.T., Suresh Kumar, K., and Rajagopal, M.R. Intravenous morphine for rapid control of severe cancer pain. *Palliat Med* 2003;17(3):248–56.

72. Mercadante, S., Villari, P., Ferrera, P., Casuccio, A., and Fulfaro, F. Rapid titration with intravenous morphine for severe cancer pain and immediate oral conversion. *Cancer* 2002;95(1):203–8.

73. Back IN. Palliative Medicine Handbook (3 edition.) Cardiff: BPM Books, 2001.

74. Cherny, N., Ripamonti, C., Pereira, J., Davis, C., Fallon, M., McQuay, H., *et al.* Strategies to manage the adverse effects of oral morphine: An evidence-based report. *J Clin Oncology* 2001;19(9):2542–54.

75. Bruera, E., Pereira, J., Watanabe, S., Belzile, M., Kuehn, N., and Hanson, J. Opioid rotation in patients with cancer pain. A retrospective comparison of dose ratios between methadone, hydromorphone, and morphine. *Cancer* 1996;78(4):852–7.

76. Mancini, I., Lossignol, D.A., and Body, J.J. Opioid switch to oral methadone in cancer pain. *Curr Opin Oncol* 2000;12(4):308–13.

77. Bruera, E. and Sweeney C. Methadone use in cancer patients with pain: A review. *J Palliat Med* 2002;5(1):127–38.

78. Hagen, N.A. and Wasylenko, E. Methadone: Outpatient titration and monitoring strategies in cancer patients. *J Pain Symptom Manage* 1999;18(5):369–75.

79. Hanks, G.W., Hoskin, P.J., Aherne, G.W., Turner, P., and Poulain, P. Explanation for potency of repeated oral doses of morphine? *Lancet* 1987;2:723–6.

80. Hoskin, P.J., Hanks, G.W., Heron, C.W., Aherne, G.W., and Chapman, D. M6G and its analgesic action in chronic use. *Clin J Pain* 1989;5(2):199–200.

81. Neumann, P.B., Henriksen, H., Grosman, N., and Christensen, C.B. Plasma morphine concentrations during chronic oral administration in patients with cancer pain. *Pain* 1982;13(3):247–52.

82. Nahata, M.C., Miser, A.W., Miser J.S., and Reuning, R.H. Variation in morphine pharmacokinetics in children with cancer. *Dev Pharmacol Ther* 1985;8(3):182–8.

83. Royal College of Paediatrics and Child Health, Group NaPP. Medicines for children (2 edition). London: Royal College of Paediatrics and Child Health, 2003.

84. Clark, A.J., Ahmedzai, S.H., Allan, L.G., Camacho, F., Horbay, G.L., Richarz, U. *et al*. Efficacy and safety of transdermal fentanyl and sustained-release oral morphine in patients with cancer and chronic non-cancer pain. *Curr Med Res Opin* 2004;20(9):1419–28.

85. Radbruch, L., Sabatowski, R., Loick, G., Kulbe, C., Kasper, M., Grond, S. *et al*. Constipation and the use of laxatives: A comparison between transdermal fentanyl and oral morphine. *Palliat Med* 2000;14(2):111–9.

86. Staats, P.S., Markowitz, J., and Schein, J. Incidence of constipation associated with long-acting opioid therapy: A comparative study. *South Med J* 2004;97(2):129–34.

87. Drake, R., Longworth J., and Collins, J.J. Opioid rotation in children with cancer. *J Palliat Med* 2004;7(3):419–22.

88. Yee, J.D. and Berde, C.B. Dextroamphetamine or methylphenidate as adjuvants to opioid analgesia for adolescents with cancer. *J Pain Symptom Manage* 1994;9(2):122–5.

89. Foley, K.M. Current issues in the management of cancer pain: Memorial Sloan-Kettering Cancer Center. *NIDA Res Monogr* 1981;36:169–81.

90. Grandinetti, C.A. and Buck, M.L. Patient-controlled analgesia: Guidelines for use in children. *Pediatr Pharmacother* 2000;6(11):1–4.

91. Knoester, P.D., Jonker, D.M., Van Der Hoeven, R.T., Vermeij, T.A., Edelbroek, P.M., Brekelmans, G.J., *et al*. Pharmacokinetics and pharmacodynamics of midazolam administered as a concentrated intranasal spray. A study in healthy volunteers. *Br J Clin Pharmacol* 2002;53(5):501–7.

92. Polosa, R., Simidchiev, A., and Walters, E.H. Nebulised morphine for severe interstitial lung disease. *Cochrane Database Syst Rev* 2002(3):CD002872.

93. Cohen, S.P. and Dawson, T.C. Nebulized morphine as a treatment for dyspnea in a child with cystic fibrosis. *Pediatrics* 2002;110(3):e38.

94. Hansson, L., Midgren, B., and Karlsson, J.A. Effects of inhaled lignocaine and adrenaline on capsaicin-induced cough in humans. *Thorax* 1994;49(11):1166–8.

95. Farrar, J.T. Neuropathic pain: Definition, diagnosis, and therapy. In M.C. Perry, ed. American Journal of Clinical Oncology Educational Book. Alexandria: *Am Soc Clin Oncol* 1999.

96. Collins, J.J., Grier, H.E., Kinnery, H.C., and Berde, C.B. Control of severe pain in children with terminal malignancy. *J Pediatr* 1995;126:653–57.

97. Cherny, N.I., Thaler, H.T., Friedlander-Klar, H., Lapin, J., Foley, K.M., Houde, R., *et al*. Opioid responsiveness of cancer pain syndromes caused by neuropathic or nociceptive mechanisms: A combined analysis of controlled, single-dose studies. *Neurology* 1994;44(5):857–61.

98. Backonja, M. Anticonvulsants and antiarrhythmics in the treatment of neuropathic pain syndromes. In P.T., Hansson, H.L., Fields R.G., Hill, P., Marchettini eds. *Neuropathic Pain: Pathophysiology and Treatment, Progress in Pain Research and Management*. Seattle: International Association for the Study of Pain, 2001, pp. 185–201.

99. Reddy, S. and Patt, R.B. The benzodiazepines as adjuvant analgesics. *J Pain Symptom Manage* 1994;9(8):510–14.

100. McQuary, H., Carroll, D., Jadad, A.R., Wiffen, P.J., and Moore, R.A. Anticonvulsant drugs for management of pain: A systematic review. *Br Med J* 1995;311(7012):1047–52.

101. Royal, M., Wienecke, G., Movva, V., Ward, S., Bhakta, B., and Jensen, M., *et al*. (225) open label trial of oxcarbazepine in neuropathic pain. *Pain Med* 2001;2(3):250–1.

102. Dougherty, J.A. and Rhoney, D.H. Gabapentin: A unique antiepileptic agent. *Neurol Res* 2001;23(8):821–9.

103. McGraw, T. and Stacey, B.R. Gabapentin for treatment of neuropathic pain in a 12-year-old girl. *Clin J Pain* 1998;14(4):354–6.

104. McQuay, H.J., Tramer, M., Nye, B.A., Carroll, D., Wiffen, P.J., and Moore, R.A. A systematic review of antidepressants in neuropathic pain. *Pain* 1996;68(2–3):217–27.

105. Sindrup, S.H. and Jensen, T.S. Efficacy of pharmacological treatments of neuropathic pain: An update and effect related to mechanism of drug action. *Pain* 1999;83(3):389–400.

106. Mercadante, S., Arcuri, E., Tirelli, W., and Casuccio, A. Analgesic effect of intravenous ketamine in cancer patients on morphine therapy: A randomized, controlled, double-blind, crossover, double-dose study. *J Pain Symptom Manage* 2000;20(4):246–52.

107. Munro, J.E. and Murray, K.J. Advances in paediatric rheumatology: Beyond NSAIDs and joint replacement. *J Paediatr Child Health* 2004;40:161–9.

108. Hurwitz, E.S., Barret, M.J., Bregman, D., Gumm, W.J., Schonberger, L.B., Fairweather, W.R., *et al*. Public Health Service study on Reye's syndrome and medications. Report on the main study. *JAMA* 1987;257(14):1905–11.

109. Orlowski J.P. Whatever happened to Reye's syndrome? Did it ever really exist? *Crit Care Med* 1999;27(8):1582–7.

110. Keenan, G.F., Giannini, E.H., and Athreya, B.H. Clinically significant gastropathy associated with nonsteroidal antiinflammatory drug use in children with juvenile rheumatoid arthritis. *J Rheumatol* 1995;22(6):1149–51.

111. Lesko, S.M. The safety of ibuprofen suspension in children. *Int J Clin Pract Suppl* 2003(135):50–3.

112. Ulinski, T., Guigonis, V., Dunan, O., and Bensman, A. Acute renal failure after treatment with non-steroidal anti-inflammatory drugs. *Eur J Pediatr* 2004;163(3):148–50.

113. Short, J.A., Barr, C.A., Palmer, C.D., Goddard, J.M., Stack, C.G., and Primhak, R.A. Use of diclofenac in children with asthma. *Anaesthesia* 2000;55(4):334–7.

114. Lesko, S.M., Louik, C., Vezina, R.M., and Mitchell, A.A. Asthma morbidity after the short-term use of ibuprofen in children with asthma. *Pediatrics* 2002;109(2):E20.

115. Fulfaro, F. and Casuccio, A. The role of bisphosphonates in the treatment of apinful metastitic bone disease: A review of phase III trials. *Pain* 1998;78(3):157–69.

116. Batch, J.A., Couper, J.J., Rodda, C., Cowell, C.T., and Zachaarin, M. Use of bisphosphonate therapy for osteoporosis in children and adolescence. *J Paediatr Child Health* 2003;39(88–92).

117. Whyte, M. P. *et al.* Bisphosphonate-induced osteopetrosis. *N Eng J Med* 2003;349:457–63.

118. Ward, K. *et al.* Quantification of metaphysical modelling in children treated with biphosphonates. *Bone* 2005;36:99–1002.

119. Geiduschek, J.M., Haberkern, C.M., McLaughlin, J.F., Jacobson, L.E., Hays R.M., and Roberts, T.S. Pain management for children following selective dorsal rhizotomy. *Can J Anaesth* 1994;41(6):492–6.

120. Bakheit, A.M. Botulinum toxin in the management of childhood muscle spasticity: Comparison of clinical practice of 17 treatment centres. *Eur J Neurol* 2003;10(4):415–9.

121. Barwood, S., Baillieu, C., Boyd, R., Brereton, K., Low, J., Nattrass, G., *et al.* Analgesic effects of botulinum toxin A: A randomized, placebo-controlled clinical trial. *Dev Med Child Neurol* 2000; 42(2):116–21.

122. Lee, L.R., Chuang, Y.C., Yang, B.J., Hsu, M.J., and Liu, Y.H. Botulinum toxin for lower limb spasticity in children with cerebral palsy: A single-blinded trial comparing dilution techniques. *Am J Phys Med Rehabil* 2004;83(10):766–73.

123. Waterson G., Goldman A., and Michalski A. Corticosteroids in the palliative phase of paediatric brain tumours. *Arch Dis in Childhood* 2002;86(Suppl 1):A76.

124. Glaser, A.W., Buxton, N., and Walker, D. Corticosterioids in the management of central nervouse system tumours. Kids Neuro-Oncology Workshop (KNOWS). *Arch Dis Childhood* 1997;76(1): 76–78.

125. Hain, R.D.W., Maisey, K., Cox, R., Kus T., Devins, M., and Davies, R.E. Ethical dimensions of palliative chemotherapy. *Arch Dis in Childhood* 2004;89(Supp 1):A35.

126. Schiavetti, A., Varrasso, G., Maurizi P., Cappelli, C., Clerico A., Properzi, E. *et al.* Ten-day schedule oral etoposide therapy in advanced childhood malignancies. *J Pediatr Hematol Oncol* 2000;22(2):119–24.

127. Haim, N., Ben-Shahar, M., and Epelbaum, R. Prolonged daily administration of oral etoposide in lymphoma following prior therapy with adriamycin, an ifosfamide-containing salvage combination, and intravenous etoposide. *Cancer Chemother Pharmacol* 1995; 36(4):352–5.

128. Davidson, A., Gowing, R., Lowis, S., Newell, D., Lewis, I., Dicks-Mireaux, C. *et al.* Phase II study of 21 day schedule oral etoposide in children. New Agents Group of the United Kingdom Children's Cancer Study Group (UKCCSG). *Eur J Cancer* 1997;33(11): 1816–22.

129. Collins, J.J., Grier, H.E., Sethna, N.F., Wilder, R.T., and Berde, C.B. Regional anesthesia for pain associated with terminal pediatric malignancy. *Pain* 1996;65(1):63–9.

130. Gomez-Batiste, X., Madrid, F., Moreno, F., Gracia, A., Trelis, J., Nabal, M. *et al.* Breakthrough cancer pain: Prevalence and characteristics in patients in Catalonia, Spain. *J Pain Symptom Manage* 2002;24(1):45–52.

131. Mercadante S., Radbruch, L., Caraceni, A., Cherny, N., Kaasa, S., Nauck, F. *et al.* Episodic (breakthrough) pain: Consensus conference of an expert working group of the European Association for Palliative Care. *Cancer* 2002;94(3):832–9.

132. Portenoy, R.K., Payne, D., and Jacobsen, P. Breakthrough pain: Characteristics and impact in patients with cancer pain. *Pain* 1999;81(1–2):129–34.

133. Farrar, J.T. Incident pain: Definition, diagnosis, and therapy. In M.C. Perry, ed. American Society of Clinical Oncology Educational Book. Alexandria: *Am Soc Clin Oncol*, 1999, pp. 402–4.

134. Dunbar, P.J., Chapman, C.R., Buckley, F.P., and Gavrin, J.R. Clinical analgesic equivalence for morphine and hydromorphone with prolonged PCA. *Pain* 1996;68(2–3):265–70.

135. Sarhill, N., Walsh, D., and Nelson, K.A. Hydromorphone: pharmacology and clinical applications in cancer patients. *Support Care Cancer* 2001;9(2):84–96.

136. Lawlor, P., Turner, K., Hanson, J., and Bruera, E. Dose ratio between morphine and hydromorphone in patients with cancer pain: A retrospective study. *Pain* 1997;72(1–2):79–85.

22 Pain—an integrative approach

Leora Kuttner

Introduction

Pharmacological methods—those that rely for their effect on the use of drugs—remain the standard approach for managing pain in most centres. They should no longer, however, be considered the only options [1–8]. Furthermore, there is a risk that because they are standard, pharmacotherapeutic strategies are assumed, sometimes without evidence, to be always the most effective.

Pain has been described as 'indivisibly a psychobiological unity' [9] and approaches to managing it must avoid inappropriately dichotomizing methods of pain management into those that are purely psychological and those that are purely physical. In searching for how to refer to the panoply of techniques that do not rely on medication, terms such as 'mind-body' are over-inclusive and 'cognitive-behavioural' are too narrow. The term 'Integrative' has emerged in recent years [3] to encompass methods that integrate physical and psychological approaches. Integrative approaches include, for example, biofeedback, hypnosis, imagery and relaxation as well as TENS (transcutaneous electrical stimulation), aromatherapy, massage and other physical therapies (Table 22.1).

Integration of all these methods, together with pharmacotherapy, is needed to achieve total pain management. Research has shown that children experience less distress and cope better with painful procedures and symptoms when they understand what is happening and are encouraged to participate fully in the process to relieve their pain [10–14]. This

Table 22.1: Integrative methods of pain management across developmental ages

Age	Physical comforts	Distraction	Cognitive behavioural
Infants: 0–1 years	Rocking, swaddling, kangaroo care, pacifier, sucrose, decrease light & noise, massage, Therapeutic Touch.	Music, singing, soothing & familiar voice, bubbles, pacifier, mobiles, lullabies & other rhyming patters.	Parent support & guided teaching on how to increase infant's comfort
Preschoolers: 2–5 years	Rocking & cuddling, pacifier, sucrose, decrease light & noise, massage. TENS, Therapeutic Touch, positioning for comfort, heat/cold packs, Acupressure, Physical Therapy	Familiar songs, music, pop-up books, puppets, videos, bubble-blowing, stories, stories-on-tape, clowning, pet visits.	Art & music therapy, imagery & hypnosis, therapeutic play, relaxation games (e.g. rag doll), participation in favourite stories, simple explanations. Parent support and guidance.
School-aged: 6–11 years	Comfort rocking, cuddling, decrease light & noise, massage, TENS, Therapeutic Touch, positioning for comfort, heat/cold packs, Acupressure & Acupuncture, Physical Therapy	Familiar songs, music, pop-up books, puppets, favourite toys & games, videos, bubble-blowing, stories, stories-on-tape, clowning, pet visits	Art & music therapy, imagery & hypnosis, relaxation games (e.g. rag doll, belly breathing), participation in favourite stories, information, biofeedback, psychotherapy. Parent support & guidance.
***Adolescents* 12–18 years**	Massage, TENS, Therapeutic Touch, positioning for comfort, heat/cold packs, Acupressure & Acupuncture, Physical Therapy, adjust environment to teen's preference.	Favourite music, games, stories-on-tape, videos, pet visits, books read aloud.	Imagery & hypnosis, art & music therapy, relaxation & deep breathing, information, biofeedback, psychotherapy. Parent support & guidance.

may mean that the child receives regular analgesic medication, with boluses for breakthrough pain, has therapeutic massages to release muscle tension and uses imagery as needed to increase comfort and control pain. Comprehensive pain control requires tailoring the interventions to the needs of the individual child and integrating a multimodality of pain management methods.

Children with chronic and life-limiting conditions have many losses. Knowing how to cope and deal with distressing symptoms has great value in enhancing the quality of remaining time [15]. This applies not only to children and teens, but to their parents and other care-givers. Methods that develop internal coping skills also empower children and teens and enhance their quality of life [16]. Being supported in learning to actively participate in pain relief and coping becomes even more important for children who will not have a lengthy lifetime in which to develop internal resources.

For children in palliative care who struggle with pain and other distressing symptoms such as fatigue, nausea, sleep and breathing difficulties integrative methods can become woven into the child's day with long-term benefits ameliorating these symptoms. Methods include cognitive behavioural techniques such as imagery, hypnosis, abdominal breathing, distraction, music massage, TENS, hydrotherapy, heat, cold, positioning and other techniques (see Chapter 31). Once learned, children and teens can use self-regulatory methods independently or with supportive guidance [17]. TENS, biofeedback and therapeutic touch require a trained professional [18]. In contrast, massage and music are part of contact comfort and everyday life, and can be most beneficial when the touch and sound is familiar, and when words are difficult or seem inadequate [19–21] Even when a child is severely ill or feeling depleted, the knowledge of what is available to help ease pain and suffering supports ego-strength allowing energy for end of life concerns (22, p.541).

Excellent pain and symptom management at end of life promotes control and frees the child, parent(s) and family members to deal with loss, grief, and changes in relationships and identity.

In this chapter, the integrated use of imagery, breathing, music and massage will be discussed, and illustrated with case examples. These techniques are naturally occuring phenomena that children and parents are familiar with and can comfortably use. The more specialized methods of TENS, hypnosis, and biofeedback where training or equipment is required will not be covered, although there is much evidence for their benefit in relieving children's pain [3,7,9,11–14,17,18,23]. The emphasis in this chapter will be on methods that parents and health care providers find relatively easy to use at home, in hospice, or in hospital to control pain, reduce distressing symptoms such as fear or fatigue, and to increase feeling of well-being and peace at the end of life.

Total pain management

Pain is a complex multidimensional phenomenon. It is a subjective, unpleasant, and often noxious mind-body experience. We have a long history of under-estimating children's pain—particularly that of neonates, babies, non-verbal or developmentally delayed children and children at end of life [4,5, 24]. This under-assessment led to a systematic under-treatment of children's pain and a lack of recognizing the long term negative effects of poorly treated or untreated pain on the lives of babies and children [25]. In the last 25 years a revolution in research, teaching, practice and protocol in managing the complex nature of children's pain has led to greater improvements in care. There are still significant strides to be made. A greater appreciation of the total picture, in which the interaction of cultural, social, familial, personal, as well as physiological factors remains to be better understood [8,10], is needed. This in turn will further improve pain management. Methods that are not pharmacological have a significant role in this process to achieve a comprehensive management of pain and suffering.

Integrative methods of pain management shift a child's attention from pain and suffering onto a more pleasant alternative. The measure of success tends to accord with the degree of imaginative absorption the child attains in this alternate experience [26,27]. Often the experience will be integrated with invitations to calm emotions, maintain hopeful beliefs and increasingly experience positive body sensations. The child's creative imagination is enlisted to enhance these beneficial effects. Research, clinical studies and cases have shown that involving the child's attention through an absorbing pleasant experience, image or focus will maintain an experience of comfort so that acute, recurrent, chronic and pain at the end of life pain is controlled [7,11,13,14, 28]. Staff don't need to choose between giving an analgesic or providing comfort care by doing imagery with a child. Thinking in an 'either/or' manner greatly limits the possibility of total pain relief. These various methods work hand in hand to provide total pain management.

One of the necessary steps in caring for children with life-limiting and life-threatening illness is to include them early as part of the team. This means sharing information and discussing care options. It also requires that the child be adequately prepared for painful procedures, or sudden turns in the status of their illness for which unexpected pain management interventions may occur. Even young children need to understand the role, impact and side effects of analgesics, such as constipation, and their options. The child's threshold of pain and tolerance even for minor procedures can be severely compromised when the child is ill, fatigued or experiencing other distressing symptoms. Even a finger stick or minor blood draw can become trying or distressing. It is at these times that the child who hasn't developed coping skills is at greater risk for developing anxiety responses. Having information, being supported to question, explore, be listened to and participate in the decision making, is a central part of total pain management. Children are less likely to feel helpless and more likely to draw on internal or interpersonal resources.

Research indicates that children report that painful treatments and interventions can be worse than the experience of the disease itself [13]. As a result, child's preferences for painful medical invasive procedures must be considered. They need to be respected and wherever possible accommodated, for example, how a procedure works best, in which position, and with which adjunctive support or therapy. Though important, the criterion should not be the clinician's level of comfort—as is often the practice—but the child's. If not too traumatised by previous procedures, and with well-supported experiences and encouragement, children develop a range of coping skills to sustain them during invasive treatment related procedures [27]. Throughout the terminal phase of life, children and teens are often aware of their diminishing options. This adds to the importance of heeding preferences and concerns in providing comprehensive pain management.

Parents are an important component of the pain management team and total pain management. They can be their child's best advocate. Often if the child's condition has been long-term, parents become skilled both at assessing pain and knowing what kind of intervention will have optimum impact. In some cases however, parents may also fall into the pattern of under-estimating the level of pain, particularly if the child is by nature stoical or protecting the parent. In general, the child's perspective is that parents are the key to feeling safe, supported and protected. When asked what helped the most during painful procedures, children answered, 'The presence of their parent' [28]. Consequently pain interventions with parental presence in the team have a greater likelihood of being effective.

Understanding the meaning of the pain

At end of life pain has increased significance. It can signify that the disease is progressing and/or that the child's death may be imminent. As a result, pain symptoms can carry added emotional distress and fears [22,15]. How the child describes the pain, what words are used, emotional intensity, and associated behavioural signs become part of pain assessment. The integration of all these, together with parents and staff observations, build the 'Gestalt', a more complete picture than each discrete variable.

Case For many years 16-year-old Jenny had used relaxation and imagery to help control the back pain she experienced with Ewing's sarcoma. She used pain coping techniques pre- and post-surgery to remove a cancerous rib, during chemotherapy, and through a harrowing bone marrow transplantation. She was highly skilled and practised at involving herself in her own pain management.

When she came to clinic walking more slowly than usual, her face drawn and pale, and reported in a tight tense voice that her back pain felt somehow different, in a way that was hard to describe, alarm bells went off for the oncology team. She was immediately scheduled for a bone scan, which sadly revealed progression of the tumour in her lumbar spine, well below the original surgery site. She understood ahead of everyone else that the pain signalled a turn for the worse. The quality of her voice was not one of fear, but of quiet dread, knowing that this time had arrived.

Assessment of pain quality

Children in palliative care often have more than one pain and many have concurrent pains and a number of distressing symptoms, including fatigue, nausea, difficulty going to and/or maintaining sleep [30]. Each pain and symptom needs to be assessed individually, noting its severity and character, and monitored over time. The characteristics of the pain—its quality (throbbing, burning, sharp, achy) its location, duration, whether intermittent or ongoing—help to determine the source of the pain, whether it is bone, nerve, soft tissue, or organ system. Knowing what precipitates and provides relief is part of pain assessment, and is crucial in determining optimum ongoing management.

Knowing the character of the pain can be used in a therapeutic integrative manner by providing a direct suggestion for comfort. Hope needs to be sustained and nourished during difficult painful times. For example, if the child reports a burning neuropathic pain:

'Now as the pain relieving medicine goes into your IV, close your eyes and breathe out and you'll probably already begin to notice that your pain is moving from that 'burny' sharp pain you felt earlier to be less bothersome...breathe and let go allowing the sense of comfort you know so well to become stronger...nod your head to let me know when you feel that happening...'

We don't know whether this type of intervention alters pain threshold, but clinical experience suggests that it does influence the child's pain tolerance. The supportive intervention allows the child to focus on how it bothers him less and to notice the other positive changes, instead of remaining tense, fearful and distressed until the medication takes full effect. The child's ability to create comfort through abdominal breathing and imaginal involvement is not an indication that the pain wasn't as severe as reported, but as per the Gate Control theory of pain, it is a natural function of the brain's ability for downward modulation of pain signals. Responsiveness to suggestion, images, physical positioning deserve to be noted and charted as part of total pain management.

The therapeutic relationship: A component of pain management

In the terminal phase of life there tends to be a diminishing of energy and a narrowing of the circle of people with whom the child wishes to spend time. An established relationship built on deep understanding and respect, will provide the foundation to choose the methods that best fits the child's current symptoms or pain problems [16]. Relationships with history and continuity are most often those with the greatest potential for therapeutic benefit. Children at end of life are particularly sensitive to issues of abandonment and loss, as they prepare and move towards their ultimate separation. Not heeding or being sensitive to this can damage a previously good therapeutic relationship.

Understandably, it is harder to begin a relationship as the child is nearing end of life than when the child first enters palliative care or is first diagnosed. It is furthermore important to note that:

In working with a child facing death, the therapist must be able to enter the threat with the child and accompany him or her down the road towards ultimate separation (Sourkes, p 266.)

With the hardships of living with a life-limiting illness and its many unpleasant treatments and procedures, children in palliative care form special attachments to favourite staff members. As a result, there are occasions a child will request to wait for the return of a preferred staff member before being willing to proceed with a painful procedure. These special attachments, like the parental attachment, are an important part of total pain management. The bonds are an important source of comfort, particularly during painful and uncertain times. The staff member has become attuned to the child and built a trusted and successful working alliance. Sometimes the child and staff member have worked out a system in which the child feels mastery and a greater feeling of safety. While special relationships can be supported by others, the pain relieving information 'system' must be charted and shared with other members of the team so that competent care and beneficial therapy for the child isn't interrupted, causing problems in the day to day pain management.

There are occasions where there isn't the luxury of forming long relationships, when an invasive medical procedure needs to be done when the preferred staff member is away. This should not be an impediment. Without knowing a child well, empathic health care professionals can engage with a child in a

sincere and professional manner and establish sufficient trust in a short time in order to proceed [6,8–11]. Asking the child or parent to provide some history of how the painful procedure was previously best managed, what interventions were most helpful and what were not, and given that, what would the child like in the upcoming procedure. This scenario applies not only in hospitals, but in home-care and hospice.

One of the benefits of having some history with a child is that the health care professional can, if time is on one's side, develop a 'bag of favourite tricks' with which the child has experienced pain and anxiety relief. These techniques then become a mainstay or reliable source of comfort at end of life. Methods and styles vary with developmental age (see Table 1), taking into account cultural and ethnic factors. Parents' input is often invaluable. As part of the care plan all professionals working with the child and family know these preferences.

Supporting parents to provide pain relief and contact comfort

With continuing illness and fatigue a dying child tends to draw into him/herself and reliance on parents changes, becoming either stronger or more distant [16]. This can take the form of the child preferring quiet and more privacy, or communicating non-verbally or using mere sounds, which some parents, attuned to their children, may more easily interpret. Staff need to empathically support parents to adjust to these changes. Parents find that providing a variety of comfort measures for mild, wearing types of pain, like using a hot or cold pack or gentle massage with or without familiar music can provide some easing of distress and maintain some connection. Symptoms of fatigue, or restlessness can be similarly addressed.

Parents unsure of what to do when their child is in pain can draw from this list of suggestions:

- familiar physical comfort-contact from earlier years, such as stroking or tickling back, arm or face
- a foot massage with peppermint oil
- favourite music or song
- story-telling, or stories on tape
- 'remember when . . .' experiences, recalling a special event or enjoyable holiday experience

The child is supported to experience a more pleasant alternative, such as the soothing sensation in a non-painful limb, when other body parts are feeling pain or discomfort. These shifts in attention and absorption for both parents and child provide a healing framework within which to decrease mutual feelings of helplessness. Providing and sharing memories can be part of creating memories. These are child-centred, intimate and life-affirming ways of relating to a child when energy is low and the child has little strength for talk or play.

Parents can be guided to do imagery and breathing, simply and directly with their sick child, as in this example:

Case Seven-year-old Sarah, dying of spinal muscular atrophy, chose to be cared for at home through her terminal illness. She became irritable and restless a few days before her death. Her mother Margaret thought she was in pain, indicating she didn't know how to make Sarah more comfortable. On a visit to the home the Hospice nurse suggested that Margaret increase Sarah's sustained release morphine. They then discussed times when Sarah had been especially happy. The nurse demonstrated, guiding Margaret to lead Sarah towards easier deeper breathing, and coached her on suggesting memories and images of a happy family camping trip. Margaret then directed Sarah's attention to the playful fun-filled experiences that they had shared, and added that she could leave the pain far far away. Sarah's anxiety began to lessen. Margaret felt relieved that she was still able to help her daughter. The imagery of that happy holiday provided a bridge for Mom to then say what she longed to say to her daughter: 'Just as we have remembered this wonderful camping trip, we will always remember you... We will always love you... You will always be a part of our family'.

Integrative methods

The methods of imagery, music and massage will be discussed in greater depth, with examples on how to integrate these into a healing experiences to better manage pain and other distressing symptoms that cause suffering.

Imagery

Therapeutic imagery is gentle, non-intrusive, child-centered, and energy conserving for children and teens in pain and distress [31–33]. A picture is worth a thousand words, and for those in palliative care without verbal facility, an image can convey a great deal when energy is diminished and time is precious. Furthermore, imagery can provide a meaningful alternate experience when the present reality is fraught with pain, fear, or physical tension or fatigue. Absorption in an imagery experience can sustain or develop greater inner strength and peace. It helps a child manage an intolerable situation, and aids in the process of letting go as death approaches.

Imagery has a power and a gentleness that are consistent with the psyche's best ability to heal itself. (35, p.165).

Images are an aspect of the expression of self, as much as words, feelings or thoughts. Over time children and teens learn to feel empowered by, and often to take delight in the creation and healing use of images.

When used for pain control, imagery works synergistically with analgesics to reduce pain and discomfort [31]. As the child's attention and absorption in the imagery increases, the capacity to increase comfort, dissociate from the pain, reduce anxiety, or alter the pain sensations and perceptions, becomes greater [6,9,11,13,14]. Imagery can be applied in many ways. Broadly there are two approaches: focus directly on the pain as an image to alter, or create an image that is disparate from the pain. It is unclear whether associating with the pain or dissociating from it is more effective [36,37]. Nor do we know how imagery through the 'neuromatrix' of the brain-pain system provides pain relief. Pediatrician Dr. Karen Olness writes:

In controlled studies our research has documented the abilities of children to control voluntarily certain physiological processes previously believed to be autonomic (such as, transcutaneous oxygen, peripheral temperature, and brainstem auditory evoked potential). As children succeed in accomplishing the desired control, they often describe spontaneous images which they used to effect the changes. Images vary from child to child; they are unique and unexpected. We are convinced that understanding the source and nature of the images that trigger the neuro-humoral cascade is more important than the machines to which the children are connected [38, p.173].

How to begin

Imagery is a natural process for all of us, but particularly for children aged 3 to 6 years whose cognitive boundaries between fantasy and reality are quite fluid [11]. Pre-school children move easily into 'Let's pretend...'. or 'Let's imagine...' as easily as they move into playing. These familiar and comfortable introductions make it easy to engage the younger child in therapeutic imagery. Developmental age and ability influence which approach is best suited (Table 1). The child's energy level, ability to focus, willingness to talk, and type of pain and symptom will also guide in the choice of technique.

Older children may need a little more formal invitation, such as, 'How about travelling into your inner world...',or 'Let's use your imagination to...', or 'Would you like to experience how you're able to change what is happening by using your imagination...'.

It's crucial to know which image experiences the child prefers, dislikes, or wishes to avoid. For example, if a child is afraid of heights, imagery such as 'going up in a helium balloon, or a flying carpet' would be counter-productive. Information from the parents or other members of the family help establish the therapeutic experiences and images that enhance comfort, create a sense of well-being and deal effectively with fatigue and fear.

Use all sensory modalities

With some skill and considerable sensitivity, imagery is rarely, if ever, frightening or disturbing. Children who are dying seem to be particularly receptive and responsive to imagery, perhaps even more so than adults. The child's experiences can be surprising, helpful, illuminating, and informative. For the dying child, discoveries can be transformative in shedding fears common to children who are profoundly ill. In order to pull the most out of the imagery experience, one can draw on all the senses, or support the child's primary sense with the other modalities.

Music

Music can be highly therapeutic [19,39,40] (see Chapter 10, Children expressing themselves), whether used in a systematic intervention as music therapy within a hospital setting or in an more informal way to provide another focus or to improve the emotional climate. There are numerous articles on the use of music in palliative care with adults, yet few on the use of music therapy with children during palliation [19,37]. Music therapy addresses a need for self-expression, provided through music-assisted creative play, or through song-writing dealing with issues of loss, pain, and separation.

Case A 12-year-old girl with cystic fibrosis referred herself for music therapy during one of her many hospitalizations. The therapist used techniques of song-writing and parody. The pre-teen wrote 'Hospital Blues'. As her condition deteriorated, she shared the process of music and song writing with her therapist to address her pain, fears and separation from friends, easing the process for both herself and her family. [38, p.37]

Music is a natural way to bring children's normal world more strongly to the fore, especially when in pain, severely ill and/or nearing end of life. In its many forms, such as listening to a walkman through headphones, or a personal stereo, playing an instrument or singing, music can change a tense or fearful atmosphere to one of greater ease when a child is tense suffering or in ongoing pain. Appropriately chosen music will promote relaxation especially if it is a familiar or favourite melody. Playing a favourite nursery rhyme is an easy addition to enhance comfort, for example, during a blood transfusion for a toddler or pre-schooler, or playing hip-hop music can do the same for a teen. Singing, creating new verses, or writing a song together can bring more meaning to times of greater restriction, such as being being bedridden. It creates interest, helps minimize restlessness, and can make long periods of time feel shorter.

In contrast to a hospice, parents in hospital report feeling worried that the child's music will be intrusive to the ward. They need to be reassured that this is generally not the case. Most staff members welcome the change of sound, and appreciate the therapeutic benefit of music.

Massage

Massage is used therapeutically when children are in pain to decrease muscular-skeletal pain, decrease muscle-tension, ease spasms and contractures, create sensations of comfort, increase children's capacity to achieve a deeper restful state or fall asleep. It can be initially guided or directed by the child. Children will tend to opt for massage on a part of their body that is unaffected by pain or disease, as this experience seems to create a 'white noise' effectively blocking continual low-level discomfort from various pain sources. Despite its obvious value, massage is not yet widely practised in pediatric palliative settings [20].

Massage is probably one of the most underused therapies in Pediatrics. It has few contraindications; common sense precludes the use of vigorous massage over a surgical wound, skin infections, abrasions or burns. Although time intensive, massage can be provided inexpensively if parents or other family members are trained to do it. We have found it one of the most helpful adjunctive treatments for patients with chronic pain, particularly because it empowers the family to take an active role in helping reduce a child's symptoms. [20, p.456]

There are informal and formal techniques of massage. Formal massage includes pressure point techniques such as shiatsu and acupressure, long gliding strokes of Swedish massage, and the deep tissue massage of Rolfing. In most cases pressure point techniques are reserved only for particular tension related pain and Rolfing is rarely used with children. Successful physical therapy management of children's pain 'ideally takes place in an environment of integrated care . . . to address the multifaceted issues involved in the treatment of pain' [18, p. 434].

The informal methods have great value in easing pain and discomfort for children in palliative care. Massage is often given with lighter gentler strokes and there is no assumption that the nurse or parent has specialized training in one of the many forms of massage. At end of life, a very gentle caring touch is preferred, avoiding painful areas where the child or teens experiences sensitivity or discomfort. Children may opt to have their favourite staff member give this more intimate therapy, often aided by nicely scented creams, such as lavender, peppermint or citrus.

Case When 15-year-old Jenny was in isolation struggling with graft versus host complications from a bone marrow transplantation, the only part of her body that was not tender and painful were her feet. She found it hurt to talk yet she did not want to be alone. When offered a number of suggestions, such as music, TV, a story or a foot massage, she chose the latter. She was given a gentle foot massage. She began to drift off as each toe was gently rubbed with peppermint cream, avoiding pressure in the soles of her feet. This remained a favourite pain-relieving technique for Jenny, which her Mom continued when she was discharged home.

Integrating imagery music and massage

Imagery can be initiated and integrated with other methods in a few ways.

A. Imagery can be spontaneous, generated freely by the child, or by asking:

'What would you like to do be doing now if you were not here?'

'I'd be playing baseball'

'Good. You know you could play baseball right now in your mind. You know the game so well. Would you like that? OK. Close your eyes and go off to the Baseball field…that's it…..So tell me what's happening?'

If needed, other methods such as massage or suggestions for greater energy resulting from the game can be added to amplify the therapeutic impact.

B. A specific image or scene that is known to have positive meaning can be proposed. The child is invited to go along to experience and in so doing distance or dissolve the pain, fear or nausea and become more comfortable. A CD or favourite music tape can be played simultaneously to enhance the effect so that the child is able to more easily shift or dissociate.

Case In her final hours of life, Tracy, a 7-year-old girl, was in a light coma. Although her pain appeared to be fairly well managed, Tracy's facial expression indicated pain, anxiety and possibly nausea, which had previously distressed her. Her brow was wrinkled, and her mouth was open and turned down. Knowing that 'taking her to the beach' was an image that had, in the past, evoked a strong relaxation response and reduction in her anxiety and pain, Tracy was invited to 'come to the beach and feel the easing warm sun all over her body and especially relaxing her tummy….' Her father on his own initiative put on a CD of the sounds of waves. As the familiar image unfolded, Tracy's facial expression relaxed. Her brow smoothed out, her mouth closed, and her lips turned up. She retained that peaceful expression, while the seascape sounds continued until her death, 5 hours later.

C. Imagery can be controlled by taking a spontaneous image and using it in a deliberate therapeutic way to release the child from pain or fear. This can easily be integrated with other techniques like using music or massage.

Case Thirteen-year-old David was a boy who couldn't talk. For eight years he battled with a rhabdomyosarcoma in the right maxillary sinus, and subsequently an osteosarcoma in the radiotherapy field. A quiet boy, David never revealed much of his inner self, thoughts or feelings. Building a trusting relationship with David took 8 months, answering the few questions he posed, giving information when necessary, and supporting him as his symptoms, especially pain, worsened.

Over the course of 8 months, David's tumor remained localized, expanding over his face, pushing his right eye outward and growing down through his hard, and later soft, palate. Towards the end of his life it was virtually impossible to understand him when he talked. David chose not to discuss any aspect of his impending death, until the day before he died. As his last hours approached, David's fear and anxiety overcame his natural reserve, in a display of tears. Drawing on her relationship with David, Clinical Nurse Specialist Cindy Stutzer reported the following:

CS: I heard you wanted to see me.

D: (nod, closes eyes).

CS: You look tired, David.

D: (nod)

CS: But it sounds like there's something else going on. Is there?

D: (nod; tears fall from his one eye)

CS: Do you want to talk to me about it?

D: (nod and says something that Cindy cannot understand)

CS: Are you afraid, David?

D: (nod)

CS: Are you afraid of dying?

D: (nod)

CS: Do you want to try some things to help you relax; to help make the fear go away?

D: (nod)

CS: I know you have some music you've been listening to. Shall we put that on?

D: (nod; Cindy puts on David's soft music)

CS: Close your eyes, David, and listen to the music.

D: (closes eye; his facial expressions are difficult to read, since the tumor has invaded most of his face. His brow is furrowed, one side of his mouth is turned down, his eye is closed. David is lying on his side, knees and arms drawn up)

CS: Are you feeling the fear now, David?

D: (nod)

CS: Sometimes when we feel fear, our bodies feel it too. Sometimes our stomachs feel like they're in a knot. Does yours?

D: (nod)

CS: Sometimes our muscles get tight, so tight they almost ache (nod), and our head hurts. Are you experiencing these things David?

D: (nod)

CS: Picture your fear as a big ball in the pit of your stomach, a black one.

D: (frowns)

CS: Is that how you imagine your fear to be?

D: (Shakes his head)

CS: Tell me how the fear looks to you, David.

D: Like a cloud, a dark storm cloud.

CS: So the fear is like a dark storm cloud. Does it fill up your body? (nod) And it makes all the muscles tense and puts knots in your stomach? (nod) Well, David, you know that clouds have no substance; they're not solid at all. They're just wisps of air, really. You are stronger than those wisps, David. And wisps can't hurt you. Now close your eyes and picture dark, ugly storm clouds in the sky. Picture a bright blue sky, with the storm clouds coming and coming. You know there are two ways to get rid of storm clouds. One way is for the wind to blow them away—one wisp at a time. You can break up those storm clouds, David... Let the music be carried on the wind.... Let it enter your body and blow those wisps away.... only Let the music surround your body and lift it up and carry your body. Can you feel it enter your body? (nod) Let it enter all the places where the fear is, David, and allow the music to blow the fear clouds away.

(Pause for almost a minute)

Can you feel the music enter your body and surround your body? (nod) Are some of the fear clouds gone? (nod) You know there's another way that clouds in the sky disappear. When the sun shines on them, they evaporate. Picture in your mind a soft, bright white light entering your body and evaporating the fear clouds. The light shines on you and in you. It feels warm, and soft, and good. And wisp by wisp, it evaporates the fear clouds while the music blows some more wisps away. Can you feel that? (nod)....

You are stronger than the wisps of clouds, David, and you are stronger than the fear. Fear and clouds cannot run your life. You are stronger than they are. What's happened to the fear now, David?

D: gone

CS: David, you are stronger than the fear. Listen to the music for a while and let it carry you... relax into the music and the light.

Indication and contraindications

When integrative methods of pain management are introduced and developed during the earlier stages of the illness they become an extra therapeutic aid and competency during tougher times in palliative care. Particularly for those children who need greater self-control, these methods meet that need.

Methods such as imagery are not appropriate for every child or adolescent. Imagery is more difficult to implement with non-verbal children and not suitable for those who are significantly developmentally delayed or mentally handicapped. However, music, contact comfort, and massage methods can be used with all children at most times, and can be introduced as part of total pain management.

Children who have developed their own coping techniques, relying on spontaneous imagery and relaxation to ease pain, often become remarkably creative: Ten year old Kyle told us that it works best for him when he makes his body 'like a wet noodle.' These resourceful children develop a strong 'inner sense' and great sensitivity to their body signals. For Gerard, relaxation and imagery became an 'internal scanner' that built self-reliance and a relationship with his failing body.

Case Diagnosed with leukemia 13-year-old Gerard had a rough course of medical treatment. Through the years, particularly while in isolation during transplantation, he developed his ability to relax and using sensory-based imagery. He would lie down, focus on his breath following it with all of his attention as it moved in, around his body and out. He would do this until the pain in his body become more distant. He started from the top of his head and systematically through his body, focusing on each part that needed easing and release from pain. He practised, perfecting this systematic technique which he called 'my scanner'. He insisted on a quiet room, no interruptions and the freedom to do it by himself. He loved the independence of this process and how it calmed and gave him self-control. One of the benefits of this self-regulatory technique was that he became very aware of how each part of his body felt, his typical body sensations, and what they meant. This enabled him to speak with greater authority to the staff about his status of health.

Gerard continued to use his relaxation and imagery in a quiet and personal way throughout the remaining 18 months of his life. It had become fully integrated into his way of coping with any pain and discomfort and helped him maintain an impressive composure and dignity to his last days.

Monitor the impact of the intervention

It is advisable to pay close attention to how the child responds to these integrative pain techniques, and to stop if the child's attention dissipates or fatigue sets in. If fatiguing is a consistent pattern, it could help to suggest ways that through the imagery experience the child could gather needed energy from the relaxation, or increase the depth of the sleep that follows.

Non-verbal behaviours are as important cues as verbal ones. These include facial expressions, position and movements of the body throughout the experience. For example, Tracy (above) provided only non-verbal clues to her inner experience. Monitoring these physical changes indicated her increasing involvement with the imagery and the relief that was provided. If there is the sense that something is amiss, check with the child: 'If anything disturbs you let me know' or 'You can change anything that you don't like'. When freed in this way to enter the experience more fully, children usually enhance the effectiveness of the imagery, music or massage for pain relief.

Integrative methods in hospital

In contrast to Hospices, Hospital can be non-restful place for children. Music, imagery, or the two in combination can be a means to creating a more restful and supportive environment for children in pain. Once learned these practices can easily be audio-taped and transferred for use at home.

Case Fifteen-year-old Jamie was wary of using imagery, but agreed to discuss its possibilities. She was having a difficult time sleeping in the hospital. Achy bone-pain, from osteogenic sarcoma, IV pumps with alarms, the lights and the interruptions at night, as well as her own active mind, contributed to insomnia. After exploring several options with her, she agreed to listen to relaxing music to calm and focus her mind and to see what images came to her. She saw her hip as a throbbing red fire-ball, hot and burning and emitting spurts of fire down her leg and through her pelvis (this is neuropathic pain). Together, using her imagery we made an audiotape with background music she had chosen from her CD collection.

'How about making snow balls and let's start throwing them on the fire one after the other....' The quenching of the pain began slowly. She was simultaneously receiving IV opioids, but control of this pain through opioids was proving difficult to achieve. Her comfort was partially increased by her older sister massaging her feet so that she could focus on the pleasant, non-painful sensations in her body. Adjunctive medication was added over the next hour. Despite her clear discomfort Jamie remained involved in the imagery, reporting that it gave her a sense of greater self-control.

Jamie used the tape at times throughout her hospitalization and at home. She told us that it took her away from the hospital, its noises, and her 'achiness'. She reported that sometimes she would fall asleep before she was aware of any images at all.

Conclusion

Palliative care is about living as well as possible despite the presence of a life-threatening condition. Part of our mandate is to bolster families' strength and ability to cope, maximizing the quality of time together for child and family. Fundamental to achieving this is the development and active practice of comprehensive pain management to address acute, procedural, recurring and chronic persistent pain. Pharmacological, psychological and physical methods can be integrated to achieve this. These methods can also be effectively used to address and control distressing symptoms such as fatigue, restlessness, fear and nausea and despair at end of life.

Biopsychosocial considerations are a cornerstone of good palliative care. Integrating pain-relieving methods such as, imagery, music and massage can be effective as part of the panoply of methods other than pharmacological, and can be synergistically and effectively used by children, their parents and health care professionals to control a child's distressing symptoms during palliation.

'Pain must be controlled if families are to say their good-byes and recover from their grief rather than dwell on memories of a loved one in agony.' [41, p.2].

Acknowledgements

Thanks to Cindy Stutzer MSN and Dr Stefan Friedrichsdorf for their helpful comments in preparing this chapter.

References

1. Franck, L.S. Relieving Pain: What's in a name? *Can J Nursing Research* 2000; 31:4, 9–16.
2. Liebeskind, J. Teaching about pain: Semantic and ethical issues *Am Pain Society Bulletin* 1991;1(2);2–4.
3. Culbert, T., Kajander. R., Rearney. J. Pediatric integrative medicine: Special issue. *Biofeedback* 2003; 31(1):4–29.
4. Schechter, N.L. The status of pediatric pain control. In S.J. Weisman ed. *Child & Adolescent Psychiatric Clinics of North America.* 6,4, Oct. 1997; pp. 687–702.
5. Schechter, N.L., Berde. C.B, and Yaster. M. Pain in infants, children and adolescents, an overview. In N.L. Schechter, C.B. Berde, and M. Yaster eds. *Pain in Infants, Children & Adolescents* (2nd edition) Lippincott Williams & Wilkins, 2003, pp. 3–18.
6. Kuttner, L. Mind-body methods of pain management. In S.J. Weiman, ed. *Child & Adolescent Psychiatric Clinics of North America* 6,4, Oct. 1997, pp. 783–95.
7. Conte, P.M, Walco, G.A, Sterling, C.M, Engel, R.G, and Kuppenheimer, M.A. Procedural pain management in pediatric oncology: A review of the literature. *Cancer Investig* 1999; 17(6):448–59.
8. McGrath, P.A. *Pain in children: Nature assessment and treatment.* New York: The Guilford Press, 1990.
9. Kuttner, L. and Solomon, R. Hypnotherapy and imagery for managing children's pain. In N.L. Schechter, C.B. Berde and M. Yaster eds. *Pain in Infants, Children & Adolescents* (2nd edition) Lippincott Williams & Wilkins, 2003, pp. 317–28.
10. McGrath, P.A. and Hillier, L. Modifying the psychologic factors that intensify children's pain and prolong disability. In N.L. Schechter, C.B. Berde. M. Yaster, eds. *Pain in Infants, Children & Adolescents.* (2nd edition) Lippincott Williams & Wilkins, 2003, pp. 85–104.
11. Kuttner, L. Favourite stories: A hypnotic pain-reduction technique for children in acute pain. *Am J Clin Hypn* 1998;30(4):289–95.
12. Chen, E., Zeltzer, L.K., Craske, M.G., and Katz, E.R. Children's memories for painful cancer treatment procedures: Implications for distress. *Child Dev* 2001;71:933–47.

13. Zeltzer. L.K. and LeBaron. S. Hypnosis and non-hypnotic techniques for reduction of pain and anxiety during painful procedures in children and adolescents with cancer. *J Peds* 1982;101: 1032–5.

14. LeBaron, S. and Zeltzer, L.K. (1984). Behavioral intervention for reducing chemotherapy-related nausea and vomiting in adolescents with cancer. *J Adol Health Care* 1984; 5:178–82.

15. Frager, G. Palliative care and terminal care of children In, S.J. Weisman ed. *Child &Adolescent Psychiatric Clinics of North America*. 6,4, Oct 1987, pp. 889–910.

16. Sourkes, B.M. Psychotherapy with the dying child In, H. Chochinov, and W. Breitbart, eds. *Psychiatric Dimensions of Palliative Medicine*. New York: Oxford University Press, 2000, pp. 265–72.

17. Culbert, T.P. and Banez, G.A. Pediatric applications other than headache. In *Biofeedback: A Practitioner's Guide* (3rd edition). M.S. Schwartz, and F. Andrasik, eds. pp. 696–724. New York: The Guilford Press, 2003, pp. 699–724.

18. McCarthy, C.F., Shea, A.M., and Sullivan, P. (2003) Physical therapy management of pain in children. In N.L. Schechter, C.B. Berde, M. Yaster, eds. *Pain in Infants, Children & Adolescents* (2nd edition). Lippincott Williams & Wilkins, 2003, pp. 434–48.

19. Aasgaard, T. (2001). An ecology of love: Aspects of music therapy in the pediatric oncology environment. *J of Pall Care* 2001;17;3: 177–81.

20. Kemper, K. and Gradiner, P. Complementary and alternative medical therapies in pediatric pain treatment. In N.L. Schechter, C.B. Berde, M. Yaster, eds. *Pain in Infants, Children & Adolescents* (2nd edition). Lippincott Williams & Wilkins, 2003, pp. 449–61.

21. Buckley, J. (2002). Message and aromatherapy massage: Nursing art and science. *Int J Pall Nursing* 2002; 8(6):276–80.

22. Goldman, A., Frager, G. and Pomietto, M. (2003) Pain and palliative care. In N.L. Schechter, C.B. Berde, M. Yaster, eds. *Pain in Infants, Children & Adolescents* (2nd edition). Lippincott Williams & Wilkins, 2003, pp. 539–62.

23. Merkel, S.I., Gutstein, H., and Malviya, S. Use of transcutaneous electrical nerve stimulation in a young child with pain from open perineal lesions. *J Pain Symptom Man*. 1999;18(5):376–81.

24. Oberlander, T.F. and Craig, K.D. (Pain and children with developmental disabilites) In N.L. Schechter, C.B. Berde, and M. Yaster. eds. *Pain in Infants, Children & Adolescents* (2nd edition). Lippincott Williams & Wilkins, 2003, pp. 599–619.

25. Anand, K.J., Grunau, R.E., and Oberlander, T.F. (1997). Developmental character and long-term consequnces of pain in infants and children. In S.J. Weisman ed. *Child & Adolescent Psychiatric Clinics of North America*. 6,4, Oct. 1997; pp. 703–24.

26. LeBaron, S., Zeltzer, L.K., and Fanurik, D. (1988). Imaginative involvement and hypnotizability in childhood. *Int J Clin Exp Hypnosis* 1988;36(4):284–95.

27. Zeltzer, L.K. and LeBaron, S. (1986) Fantasy in children and adolescents with chronic illness: Review article. *Dev & Behav Peds*, 1986; 7(3): 195–8.

28. Gardner, G.G. Childhood, death and human dignity: Hypnotherapy for David. *Int J Clin & Exp Hypnosis* 1976;24(2):122–9.

29. Ross, D.M. and Ross, S.A. *Childhood Pain: Current Issues, Research and Management*. Baltimore, MO: Urban and Schwarzenberg, 1988.

30. Management of pain and Other Symptoms, Section 3 In *Compendium of Pediatric Palliative Care*. Alexandria, Virginia: National Hospice and Palliative Care Organization, 2000. http://www.nhpo.org.

31. Kuttner. L. and Stutzer. C. Imagery for children in pain: Experiencing threat to life and the approach of death. In D.W. Adams and E.J. Deveau, eds. *Beyond the Innocence of Childhood*, Vol 2. D.W. Adams and E.J. Deveau, eds. New York: Baywood Publishing Co. Amityville, 1995, pp. 251–65.

32. Murdock, M. *Spinning Inwards*. Boston, MA: Shambhala Publications Inc, 1987.

33. Epstein, G. *Healing Visualizations. Creating Health through Imagery*. New York: Bantam Books, 1989.

34. LeBaron. S. and Zeltzer, L.K. The role of imagery in the treatment of dying children and adolescents. *J Dev & Behav Peds*, 1985;6:252–8.

35. Hyde, N.D. and Watson, C. Voices from the silence: Use of imagery with incest survivors. In T. Laidlaw and C. Malmo, eds. *Healing Voices: Feminist Approaches to Therapy with Women*. San Francisco, CA: Jossey-Bass,1990, pp. 163–93.

36. Fanurik D., Zeltzer L., and Roberts M., Blount R. The relationship between children's coping styles and psychological interventions for cold pressor pain *Pain* 1993;53(2):213–22.

37. Tsao J., FanurikD., and Zeltzer L. Long term effects of a brief distraction intervention on children's laboratory pain reactivity *Behav modif* 2003;27(2):212–32.

38. Olness, K.N. Little people, images and child health. *American Journal of Clinical Hypnosis* 1985;27(3):169–74.

39. Daveson, B.A. Music Therapy in Palliative Care for Hospitalized Children and Adolescents. *J Pall Care* 2000;16(1):135–38.

40. O'Callaghan, C. Bringing music to life: A study of music therapy and palliative care experiences in a cancer hospital. *J Pall Care* 2001;17(3):155–60.

41. Abrahm. J.L. Pain Control Near the End of Life. In *Pain. Clinical Updates* International Association for the Study of Pain 2003;10(1):1–6.

23 Gastrointestinal symptoms

Marek W. Karwacki

Introduction

Providing the best possible care for the child and the family is the first consideration for professionals working in paediatric palliative care. Dying children and their families generally prefer home care and even intense symptoms can usually be managed in this environment with appropriate planning, expertise and support [1–9]. Currently toddlers and adolescents with neurodegenerative life-threatening illnesses (NLTIs) account for a significant proportion of children requiring palliative care [1,7–9]. The high prevalence of neurological syndromes and genetic disorders in population of dying children is reflected in a spectrum of symptoms in which gastrointestinal (GI) problems are of great significance. Our experience at the Warsaw Hospice for Children (WHC[1]), is similar to that of other hospices worldwide in this respect. The most frequently documented GI symptoms are: Nausea and vomiting, constipation, sialorrhoea, hiccup, anorexia (Table 23.1), swallowing difficulties, precutaneous endoscopic gastrostomy, diarrhoea. This chapter will consider each of these common GI symptoms in turn.

The gastrointestinal tract is a sensitive and highly reactive system that not only monitors the material flowing through it, but also provides information about dysfunction and disintegration of the entire body. Symptoms arising from this system are among the most frequent complaints in childhood. Constipation is a particular problem, but nausea and vomiting

as well as diarrhoea are common symptoms even among healthy children. In the population of children suffering from chronic, intractable disorders, GI symptoms are common [10]. Specific medical conditions and developmental disabilities are often associated with certain feeding complications, among which gastro-oesophageal reflux is the most prevalent condition [11]. Feeding problems in children with neurological impairment are common and severe [12]. These issues may be of major concern to parents, and careful appraisal of the suffering child and of the parent-child interaction is always indicated. The occurrence (Table 23.1) and escalation of particular GI problems depend on the specific cause and rapidity of disease progression, any coexisting conditions and of course the child's general health.

This chapter covers the most common gastrointestinal problems encountered in a palliative practice setting. It is organised by symptoms and offers practical guidelines on pathogenesis and treatment. Aetiology and criteria for diagnosis are also highlighted. Emphasis is on the approach to the patient and palliative care practices. A rational strategy for symptom control, depending on the predicted survival of the child and the rate of disease progression, is the aim of the chapter.

Nausea and vomiting

Nausea and vomiting (N&V) are often considered as a single phenomenon when, in fact, they are distinct physiologic conditions and may occur independently.

Nausea ('*sickness of the stomach; feeling sick*') is defined as an unpleasant sensation, usually vaguely located in the epigastrium and abdomen and often accompanied by a tendency to vomit. The term comes via Latin (*meaning: seasickness*) from

---

[1] Warsaw Hospice for Children (a Non-Governmental Organization) is a home-based palliative care programme responsible for 24-h-a-day, and 7-days-a-week care for incurable children with progressive diseases inevitably leading to death. It closely cooperates with Department of Palliative Care, National Research Institute for Mother and Child, Warsaw, Poland. The latter is an institution responsible for scientific supervision on on-going clinical trials, which are financed by WHC, and training in paediatric palliative care.

Table 23.1 Prevalence of GI symptoms among 235 children treated in Warsaw hospice for children (9-years experience: September 1994–September 2003)

GI symptom	Prevalence (%)		
	In population of treated children	In children with malignancy	In children with non-oncological disorders
Constipation	67	62	73
Nausea and vomiting	62	70	52
Diarrhoea	13	11	14
Terminal dehydration	44	52	34
Swallowing difficulties	51	39	65
Nasogastric tube	31	19	44
PEG	15	2	30
Local complications	9	0	19
Severe complications	2	0	5

the Greek word 'naus' (ship) and has been used in English since 16th Century. This highly subjective symptom is objectively described by science as a 'conscious recognition of the need to vomit'.

Vomit (emesis) or the *act of vomiting* means a spasmodic, forceful ejection of gastric contents through the mouth as the result of involuntary muscular spasms of the stomach and oesophagus. The word comes from Latin 'vomere'. It starts with a sensation of nausea, then closing of the glottis, strong contraction of the abdominal muscles which forces the stomach contents to be ejected as the gastro-oesophageal sphincter relaxes. Repeated regurgitation of stomach contents is elicited by a variety of stimuli, including touching the region of the fauces of the tonsils. Nausea may occur independently of vomiting.

Regurgitation is distinct from vomiting. It is not preceded or accompanied by nausea. It seems to occur whenever the barriers that should prevent it, the oesophageal sphincters, do not hold against elevated pressures in the fluid-filled stomach or oesophagus.

Causes may not be physical. Emotionally children very often respond to stress with nausea or vomiting. *Anticipatory nausea and vomiting* is a classic conditioned response that can be activated by a number of triggers (such as memory of the hospital, sight of syringe or the presence of a nurse). The process is exaggerated by anxiety. Anticipatory nausea or vomiting significantly impacts on the quality of life of children undergoing treatment for malignancy. It may start well before they reach the oncology ward for chemotherapy. The sensation may be so deeply rooted that even at home, long after treatment has finished, memories of the ward can provoke nausea.

Pathophysiology of nausea and vomiting

Nausea and vomiting are different entities but may represent extremes of a continuum [13]. Emesis is a highly conserved evolutional mechanism designed to protect the organism from ingested substances that are interpreted as being poisonous or toxic.

Nausea, which is mediated by the autonomic nervous system, is usually accompanied by symptoms such as pallor, tachycardia, increased salivation and cold sweat. The vagal nerve and its neurotransmitter, acetylcholine, mediates this mechanism. Nausea corresponds to the first phase of emesis, called *pre-ejection*. The stomach relaxes and gastric acid secretion is inhibited. The next step of the vomiting reflex, *the ejection phase*, comprises a single retrograde giant contraction (RGC) of the small intestine. This alkalinises and confines ingested toxins to the stomach. Retching and vomiting do not occur until RGC reaches the stomach. During retching, intra-thoracic pressure decreases while intra-abdominal pressure increases. Contractions of the abdominal muscles and the diaphragm become coordinated and increasing pressures in thorax and abdomen compress the stomach, forcing its contents upward through the mouth and nose.

The period following a vomiting episode (*post-ejection phase*) is often characterized by relief of nausea. Retching may occur long after gastric contents have been expelled and has become an important indicator of effectiveness in the evaluation of new antiemetics. The number of retching episodes, as well as the number of emetic episodes and self-report of the severity of nausea, are currently considered the most appropriate outcome measures in antiemetic clinical trials.

Both nausea and vomiting are controlled by the central nervous system, but through different mechanisms [14–16]. Nausea is mainly mediated through the autonomic nervous system. Rapid enlargement of an encapsulated organ, or distension of a hollow viscus are important factors provoking nausea in many abdominal diseases. It accompanies, for example, sudden distension of the stomach, billiary tract, or intestine and rapid enlargement of the liver or pancreas, but not distension of oesophagus, and only weakly of the colon. Gastric mechanoreceptors are the main initiators. Less frequently, nausea may arise from direct excitation of receptors in the medulla by systemic toxins. This explains the sensation of nausea that accompanies many systemic infections and elevated intracranial pressure associated with brain tumours. It can also be elicited by vestibular stimulation.

Vomiting centre

Emesis, in contrast, requires stimulation of a complex reflex, coordinated by a putative true vomiting centre (VC). Rather than a discrete anatomical entity, the VC is better considered as a central integrating complex within the reticular formation of the brain stem. It comprises a network of neuroanatomical connections of several brain-stem nuclei, including the parvicellular reticular formation (PCRF), the nucleus tractus solitarus (NTS), and the somatic motor nuclei involved with the act of emesis. These include dorsal motor vagal nucleus innervating the abdominal viscera and the dorsal and ventral respiratory groups. The VC receives convergent afferent stimulation from several central neurologic pathways:

(1) a chemoreceptor trigger zone (CTZ);

(2) the cerebral cortex and the limbic system;

(3) the vestibular-labyrinthine apparatus of the inner ear;

(4) peripheral stimuli (Figure 23.1).

It is anatomically less well defined than the CTZ, and is separated from the blood by the blood-brain barrier.

The vomiting centre of the third ventricle is the central emetic generator. Interestingly, the opioid μ_2 receptors of the third ventricle are antiemetic (not emetogenic, as might be expected from the clinical side effect profile of opioids). Acetylcholine (ACh), dopamine (D_2), gamma amino butyric acid (GABA), histaminic (H_1), and serotonin ($5HT_2$) receptors are emetogenic.

Chemoreceptor trigger zone

The CTZ is located in the area postrema, one of the circumventricular regions of the brain, on the dorsal surface of the medulla oblongata at the caudal end of the fourth ventricle, in close proximity to the nucleus tractus solitarus. Unlike vasculature within the blood-brain barrier, the area postrema is highly vascularised with fenestrated blood vessels that lack tight junctions (zonae occludentes) between capillary endothelial cells. There is therefore free passage of solute between blood and CTZ. The CTZ is anatomically specialised to detect elements present in the circulating blood and cerebrospinal fluid, such as drugs, biochemical products and other toxins. The CTZ plays a general role as a chemoreceptor, and is also implicated in controlling food intake, conditioned taste aversion, and modulating GI tract motility. The CTZ contains emetogenic receptors for acetylcholine (muscarinic receptors—M_{ACh}), dopamine (D_2), opioids (μ_2) and serotonin ($5HT_3$). There are many other neurotransmitters in or around the CTZ, including noradrenaline, somatostatin, substance P(SP), histamine, enkephalins, and corresponding receptors.

Other regions of CNS

The cerebral cortex and the limbic system respond to sensory stimulation, particularly smell and taste, psychological distress, and pain. The vestibular-labyrinthine apparatus of the inner ear is sensitive to body motion. Motion sickness, labyrinthitis and ototoxic drugs are the most common stimuli. Tumour is a rare cause. Higher cortical centres can modulate vomiting and nausea reflexes and taste aversions, but the connections involved have not yet been clarified.

Peripheral stimuli

Input seems to come from several sources. Peripheral stimuli come from visceral organs and vasculature via vagal and spinal sympathetic nerves, as a result of excitation by exogenous chemicals and by endogenous substances that accumulate during inflammation, ischaemia, and irritation. The vagus nerve plays a key role in acute emesis associated with chemotherapy, radiation therapy to the epigastrium, and abdominal distension or obstruction. Different receptors are found in the stomach wall: D_2 receptors, which mediate gastroparesis; vagal $5HT_3$ emetogenic receptors; and enteric $5HT_4$ prokinetic receptors. The $5HT_4$ receptors require ACh as a mediator within the myenteric plexus. Prokinesis is therefore antagonised by anticholinergics, and the two should never be co-prescribed.

The gastrointestinal wall contains $5HT_3$ receptors for SP a neuropeptide also found in the central nervous system in the area postrema. SP induces nausea by binding neurokinin-1 receptors (NK_1). NK_1 receptor antagonists have broad-spectrum emetogenic activity and have shown promise in clinical trials.

Other neurochemicals found in the upper GI tract, including dopamine, neurotensin, vasoactive intestinal peptide (VIP) and polypeptide (PYY), may also play a role in emesis.

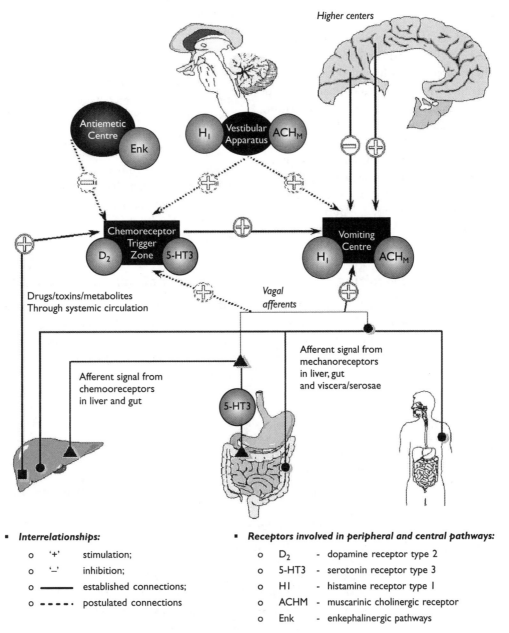

Fig. 23.1 Main receptors and pathways involved in emesis.

Mechanoreceptors within the gut wall respond to contraction and overdistension, and stimulate the vagal and splanchnic nerves.

Incidental causes of nausea and vomiting

Vomiting and nausea are often multifactorial in origin [14]. Even in children with life-limiting conditions, incidental age-related causes have to be considered. The most common is gastroenteritis. Congenital abnormalities and anatomic obstruction (e.g. pyloric stenosis), gastric chalasia, gastro-oesophageal reflux, overfeeding, and systemic as well local (e.g. otitis media) infection represent the most common cause for N&V in infants. Posseting ('innocent vomiting' and 'spitting-up'), are terms used to describe the repeated, effort-less regurgitation of small quantities of milk into the mouth after feeding. It occurs almost universally in the early months of life and, by definition, the child is well and thriving. Gastro-oesophageal reflux disease (GORD) may co-exist with posseting and in contrast can impact on growth. Both usually resolve over the first year of life. The underlying mechanism in the young infant is immaturity of the gastro-oesophageal sphincter mechanism.

Emotional causes

When N&V occur with no associated symptoms, an emotional origin should be considered. Emotional emeses are often seen in healthy children in stressful situations. Some may successfully conceal other symptoms of emotional illness, but it is hard to hide vomiting. Nausea is a common presenting complaint in depression and anxiety in children. The term 'nervous vomiting' has been used to describe a syndrome of infant stress [17]. Infant rumination syndrome, another functional vomiting disorder, has been associated with emotional distance of the main caregiver [17]. The baby learns to bring up gastric contents into the mouth for the purpose of self-stimulation. These illustrate that recurrent vomiting may indicate psychological issues, rather than organic disease.

Opioid-induced nausea and vomiting

Opioid-induced nausea frequently resolves spontaneously a few days after initiation of treatment [16]. It may persist in some patients, from the accumulation of toxic opioid metabolites. Combined with anaesthetics, opioids can trigger Ach-mediated nausea in the vestibular apparatus. Furthermore, opioids invariably produce constipation if prophylactic measures are not taken and constipation itself is a cause of nausea. Stimulation of visceral mechanoreceptors and chemoreceptors by distension of the gut, and retention of toxins from the bowel are the probable mechanism. Autonomic dysfunction often accompanies neurodegenerative conditions, and can result in decreased gastrointestinal motility, early satiety, and chronic nausea.

Patients who associate nausea with opioid analgesia may be reluctant to take more, creating a potential barrier to effective pain management. It has recently been proposed that δ and κ opioid receptors are emetogenic, while μ receptors are antiemetic, but it is unclear how important this distinction is in clinical practice [16].

Assessment of nausea and vomiting

A thorough knowledge of the aetiology and pathophysiology of N&V is crucial as different causes will require distinct interventions (Tables 23.2 and 23.3). The optimal management of N&V is based on ongoing assessment and historical documentation of the patient. Work in adult patients showed a significant

Table 23.2 Potentially reversible causes of vomiting

Cause of vomiting	Treatment
Hypercalcaemia	Rehydration and bisphosphonates
Systemic infection	Antibiotics, antivirals, antifungals, antiprotozoals, dopamine, and histamine antagonists
Raised intracranial pressure	Dexamethasone 　Cyclizine (if dexamethasone is contraindicated or ineffective)
Gastric irritation or ulceration	Discontinuation of non-steroidal anti-inflammatory drug 　Cytoprotective drugs or antacids 　Proton pump inhibitors or h2 receptor antagonist 　'Triple therapy' (2 antibiotics and proton pump inhibitor) for gastric ulcers
Opioid induced vomiting	Prophylaxis: metoclopramide or haloperidol and laxatives treatment: haloperidol, or methotrimeprazine (for intractable vomiting)
Cytotoxic chemotherapy	5-HT$_3$ receptor antagonists combined with dexamethasone. 　High dose metoclopramide and lorazepam (reduce anticipatory anxiety and nausea)
Constipation	Rectal measures and laxatives
Anxiety	Explanation and reassurance, possibly also anxiolytic drugs
Functional gastric stasis	Prokinetics (metoclopramide, domperidone, or cisapride)
Inoperable obstruction	Metoclopramide (partial obstruction) 　Dexamethasone (shrink inflammatory oedema around an obstructive lesion; reduce perineuronal oedema in a functional obstruction; direct antiemetic effect) 　Octreotide or high dose hyoscine
Vestibular disturbance	Cyclizine; sublingual or transdermal hyoscine
Congestive heart failure	Oxygen, opioids, dopamine, and histamine antagonists, anxiolytics
Renal or liver failure	Dopamine and histamine antagonists, anxiolytics, corticosteroids; serum electrolytes correction

Table 23.3 Antiemetic drugs: indications and dosage

Substance	Site of action	Indications	Dosage
Prokinetic drugs			
Metoclopramide	**D2** receptors in chemoreceptor trigger zone **D2 and 5-HT4** receptors in gastrointestinal tract *At high doses:* **5-HT3** receptors in chemoreceptor trigger zone and peripherally in gastrointestinal tract	Gastric stasis; Ileus chemotherapy	po, iv, sc: 0.033–0.1 mg/kg/dose q8h; postoperative po, iv, sc: 0.1–0.2 mg/kg/dose q6–8h; chemotherapy po, iv, sc: 1–2 mg/kg/dose q2–4h (with diphenhydramine to avoid extrapyramidal reactions).
Domperidon	**D2** receptors in chemoreceptor trigger zone **D2 and 5-HT4** receptors in gastrointestinal tract	Gastric stasis; Ileus	
Cisaprid	**5-HT4** receptors in gastrointestinal tract	Gastric stasis; Ileus	**Currently it is available on a limited basis to patients who fit strict criteria (no actual or previous heart disease and arrhythmias and not taking numerous additional medications as well)** Children: 0.15–0.3 mg/kg/dose q8h. Adults: 5–10 mg q6–8h.
Phenotiazides Prochlorperazine Chlorpromazine Thietylperazine Levopromzine	D_2 receptors in chemoreceptor trigger zone and peripherally in gastrointestinal tract; some acts on H_1, $Ach_M R$, $\alpha 1AD$ also centrally and peripherally	Various potency in all types of N&V	Chlorpromazine: *children:* po: 0.5–1 mg/kg/dose q4–6h; pr: 1 mg/kg/dose q6–8h; iv: 0.5–1 mg/kg/dose q6–8h.; *adults:* po, iv: 10–25 mg q4–6h; pr: 50–100 mg q 6–8h. Prochlorperazine: *children:* po, pr: 0.4 mg/kg/d tid/qid; adults: po, pr: 5–10 mg q6–8h.
Antihistamines Cyclizine Cinnarizine Diphenylhydram Prometazine	H_1 receptors in vomiting centre, vestibular afferents, brain substance **AchM** receptors in vomiting centre	Intestinal obstruction, peritonitis; vestibular stimulation, raised intracranial pressure	Prometazine: po: 0.5 mg/kg/dose; pr, iv, im: 0.25–1 mg/kg/dose q4–6h. Diphenylhydramine: po iv, im: 5 mg/kg/d qid; max. 300 mg/d. Cyclizine: *6–12y.* po: 25 mg q8h; *>12 y.* po, im: 50 mg q4–6h up to 200 mg/d
Butyrophenones Haloperidol Droperial	D_2 receptors in chemoreceptor trigger zone	N&V induced by opioids and/or metabolic and chemical irritation	Haloperidol: *3–12 y.* po: loading 0.25–0.5 mg/kg/d bid/tid; up to max. 0.15 mg/kg/d; *6–12 y.* im: 1–3 mg/dose q4-6h, up to max. 0.15 mg/kg/d; *adults:* po: 0.5–5 mg/dose q8–12h; im: 2-5mg q4–8h. A ceiling effect: at 30 mg/day. Droperidol: *2–12 y.* iv, im: 0.05–0.06 mg/kg/dose q4–6h; *12y.* iv, im: 2.5–5 mg/dose q6–8h.
Anticholinergics Hyoscine (scopolamine)	**AchM** receptors in vomiting centre and gastrointestinal tract	Intestinal obstruction peritonitis; vestibular stimulation raised intracranial pressure, excess secretion	Children: im, iv, sc: 6 mcg/kg/dose q6-8h, transdermal patch 0.25–1 patch q72h Adults: im, iv, sc: 0.3–0.65 mg/dose q6-8h.
5-HT₃ Antaginists Granisetron Ondansetron Tropisetron and others	**5-HT3** receptors in chemoreceptor trigger zone (possibly in vomiting centre) and peripherally in gastrointestinal tract	N&V induced by chemoirritation: chemotherapy, radiotherapy, surgery anaesthesia (postoperative)	Ondansetron: iv: 0.15 mg/kg/dose q8h; continous infusion: 0.45 mg/kg/d (max. 24–32 mg/d); po: 4–8 mg q8–12h. Graniseron: po: 1mg q12h; iv: 10–20 mcg/kg/dose q 8–12h.

mismatch between physicians', nurses' and patients' ratings of the severity of nausea and vomiting, and underline the need for simple symptom score scale [17].

Management of nausea and vomiting

The basis for pharmacological antiemetic therapy is neurochemical control of vomiting [14,15]. Peripheral neuroreceptors and the CTZ as well as VC express receptors for serotonin (5-HT$_3$ or 5-HT$_4$), histamine (H$_1$ and H$_2$), dopamine (D$_2$), acetylcholine (Ach$_M$), opioids and numerous other endogenous neurotransmitters (Figure 1). D$_2$-mediated nausea is probably the most frequently targeted for initial symptom management, even when the precise mechanism of nausea is not known. Refractory cases of N&V often require combinations of medications from different classes (Table 23.3).

Phenothiazines

Phenothiazines and butyrophenones are divided into three categories according to their receptor profiles: narrow (e.g. haloperidol); medium (e.g. prochlorperazine, promethazine, and chlorpromazine); and wide spectrum (e.g. levomepromazine and olanzapine). Chlorpromazine, thiethylperazine and perphenazine act both peripherally and centrally on dopaminergic receptors, but are also cholinergic and histamine receptor antagonists. Wide-spectrum phenothiazines are in effect 'broad spectrum antiemetics' which block D$_2$, ACh, 5HT$_2$, and 5HT$_4$ receptors. Hypotension may result if intravenous phenothiazines are administered rapidly at high doses.

This broad spectrum of action means that aliphatic phenothiazines can cause sedation and anticholinergic effects. Piperazines (e.g. prochlorperazine, thiethylperazine, perphenazine, and fluphenazine) are associated with less sedation but greater incidence of extrapyramidal reactions. These may include acute dystonias, akathisias, and rarely akinesias and dyskinesias, as well as neuroleptic malignant syndrome. Levomepromazine, though an aliphatic phenothiazine, is minimally sedating at low, but usually still powerfully antiemetic, doses.

Some reports on *olanzapine*, a new atypical antipsychotic wide-spectrum phenothiazine, have suggested a role as an adjuvant in opioid and chemotherapy induced N&V [18].

Butyrophenones

Another class of D$_2$ subtype receptor antagonist, structurally and pharmacologically similar to the phenothiazines, butrophenones, is represented by droperidol and haloperidol. Both have potent antiemetic activity. Both induce extrapyramidal reactions. Although these are usually self limiting and harmless, they can be frightening for patient and family.

Haloperidol is an ideal agent when delirium accompanies nausea, though this is rare in children. Its anticholinergic activity is negligible. It produces little drowsiness but has greater risk of extrapyramidal side effects than other phenothiazines.

D2 Antagonists

Metoclopramide is an antagonist at dopaminergic receptors and, at higher doses, 5HT$_{3+4}$ agonist. Beside its central (CTZ) and the peripheral activities, metoclopramide also increases lower oesophageal sphincter pressure and enhances the rate of gastric emptying. Prokinesis is mediated by the myenteric plexus system which relies on acetyl choline and is therefore antagonised by co-prescription of anticholinergic drugs. Dexamethasone adds to its antiemetic potential. Metoclopramide is associated with akathisia, particularly in patients over 30 years of age, and dystonic extrapyramidal effects, more commonly observed in persons under the age of 30. Diphenhydramine, benztropine (benzatropine) mesylate, and trihexyphenidyl can be used to counter the risk.

Anticholinergics

The vagus has a crucial role to play in mediating vomiting of all causes, and anticholinergics may be effective in most clinical situations. They include cyclizine and hyoscine. Cyclizine is also antihistamine and is often used in N&V associated with raised intracranial pressure, though its usefulness can be compromised by drowsiness and practical difficulties with administering it subcutaneously.

5-HT3 Antagonists

This group of very potent antiemetics, is particularly effective in N&V associated with chemotherapy and have also been used for treatment and prevention of perioperative N&V. Currently, this class includes *ondansetron*, *granisetron*, *tropisetron*, and *dolasetron*. They prevent serotonin, which is released from enterochromaffin cells in the gastrointestinal mucosa, from initiating afferent transmission to the CNS via vagal and spinal sympathetic nerves. 5-HT3 antagonists may also block serotonin stimulation at the CTZ and other CNS structures. The advantage of 5-HT3 antagonists over other entiemetics is a superior toxicity profile with equal or superior to high doses of metoclopramide antiemetic response. The major adverse effects include constipation, headache (which can be treated with mild analgesics), diarrhoea, fatigue and dry mouth. Recent data suggests no major differences in efficacy or toxicity between 5HT3 receptor antagonists in the treatment of chemotherapy-induced acute N&V [19]. Dolasetron differs from the others in its long half-life. These agents demonstrate greater antiemetic efficacy in combination with corticosteroids [18].

Other agents

Agents used as prophylaxis and treatment for chemotherapy-induced N&V, alone or in combination antiemetic regimens, include corticosteroids dexamethasone, and methylprednisolone, and a cannabinoid, dronabinol.

Corticosteroids possess intrinsic antiemetic properties and enhance the effect of some other antiemetics. The mechanism may involve changed permeability of blood-brain barrier to chemicals, reduced release of neurochemicals from damaged cells, changed GABA concentration in medullary antiemetic neurones and decreased release of leu-enkephalins in the brainstem.

Cannabinoids have been used in N&V associated with chemotherapy, human immunodeficiency virus therapy, and gastrointestinal malignant metastases [20]. They can be potent antiemetics in anticipatory N&V. Dronabinol (9-tetrahydro-cannabinol, one of the main ingredients in cannabis) and the synthetic cannabinoid compound nabilone are currently available by prescription in some countries. The mechanism is not clear. It is possible that cannabinoids act at specific cannabinoid receptors (e.g. CB-1) in the cortex, hippocampus, and hypothalamus to inhibit cyclic adenosine monophosphate (cAMP). They may even act at opioid receptors [21]. It has recently been suggested that 'endocannabinoids' constitute a novel neuroregulatory system involved in the control of emesis [22]. The class has yielded many potential areas of clinical application, including pain relief, antiemesis, appetite stimulation, relief of muscle spasticity, movement disorders, epilepsy, and glaucoma. The most promising clinical applications for cannabinoids are in stimulation of appetite, relief of nausea and vomiting, and analgesia [22,23].

Recently published studies concerning substance P antagonists and *neurokinin-1 receptor antagonists* have demonstrated an improvement of the control of chemotherapy induced acute N&V. NK$_1$ receptor antagonists have antiemetic activity against emetogenic chemotherapy, opioids, and radiation. One important advantage was control of delayed N&V compared with placebo [14].

Octreotide, synthetic analogue of somatostatin, reduces intestinal secretions. It can moderate nausea, vomiting, and abdominal cramps, particularly malignant bowel obstruction [24]. This is partly due to inhibition of motilin and vasoactive intestinal peptide hormone release [19]. Its main indication is N&V where the volume is high, where over-distension of the gastrointestinal tract is a probable factor.

Benzodiazepines are valuable adjuncts in combination with acute as well as chronic antiemetic regimens, especially in depressed or anxious children. They bind to type-2 GABA$_2$ receptors that are widely distributed throughout the CNS (cortex, reticular formation, and limbic region) [25].

Multiple antiemetic regimens have been proposed for the management of chronic nausea [1,26,14,15,16]. Metoclopramide or domperidone are generally recommended as first-line agents because they improve gastrointestinal motility and are anti-D$_2$ at the chemoreceptor trigger zone. A continuous parenteral infusion of metoclopramide may relieve intractable chronic nausea in children. Judicious use of corticosteroids such as dexamethasone, in selected patients, can also be useful in conjunction with other antiemetics. In complete bowel obstruction prokinetics are contraindicated as they simply induce painful colic.

Nausea and vomiting can be treated orally but this route may be ineffective. When vomiting persists, parenteral routes are preferable. Some antiemetics can be given rectally (in suppository or soluble tablet form).

Non-drug methods are important. These can include avoidance of food smells or unpleasant odours, diversion, and relaxation. Relaxation with guided imagery includes hypnosis, passive relaxation, active relaxation, and EMG biofeedback. Other relaxation techniques include systematic desensitization, and attentional distraction, and require a therapist with specific training, usually a psychologist. These techniques may well be useful adjuncts, but they have not been systematically tested [27].

Some patients report benefit from acupuncture or acupressure bands. A small but growing body of research suggests that acupressure (transcutaneous electrical and manual) is effective alone, or can enhance the antiemetic effects of ondansetron, metoclopramide, and phenothiazines following surgery or chemotherapy [28,29].

Dietary modifications are useful adjuncts to antiemetics and must be individualised for each patient.

Constipation

There is no single definition of *constipation*. It is often described as the slow movement of faeces through the large intestine that results in the passage of dry, hard stool. The longer the transit time of stool in the large intestine, the greater the fluid absorption and the drier and harder the stool becomes. For some children it may be normal to pass stools only every few days, but hard stools that are difficult to pass accompanied by pain or a sense of incomplete bowel evacuation should be considered constipation.

Prolonged constipation may be mistaken for diarrhoea by parents, as liquid faeces can leak around hard stool in the rectum and escape voluntary control.

Normal bowel habit

This changes markedly between birth and adolescence. Breast fed babies pass stool more frequently than those fed formula milk, up to ten daily. At 2–3 years of age, the mean is two bowel motions per day. From age three years to adulthood, normal variation is huge; between three times per day and three times per week. Concern for bowel habit should be reserved for recent change, or where there are symptoms.

Scope of the problem

Constipation occurs in up to 10% of a healthy paediatric population [30,31,32]. Chronic constipation with or without soiling is reported to make up 3% of referrals to out-patient general paediatric clinics, occurs in 1–3% of primary school children and is more prevalent in males than females.

The population of children needing palliative care is significantly at risk of constipation. Children with profound neurological deficit are particularly prone, such as cerebral palsy, neuromuscular and neurodegenerative disorders or spinal cord injury [33]. The major causes are:

- altered muscle tone
- prolonged time in one position
- reduced physical activity
- abnormal colon movement
- lack of muscle coordination
- reduced intake of fluid and dietary fibre [34].

In other groups, causes can include depression, coercive toilet training, attention deficit disorders, and sexual abuse. Over-the-counter cold medications and antacids as well as antidepressants, anticonvulsants or opioids can contribute to the problem (Table 23.4).

Table 23.4 Commonly used drugs exacerbating constipation

Opioids	Verapamil
Anticholinergics	Salts of: lithium
	Bismuth
	Iron
	Aluminium
	and Calcium
Tricyclic antidepressants	
Scopolomine	
Oxybutinin	
Promethazine	
Diphenhydramine	

Constipation is a common problem in people with intellectual disability (ID). Laxatives are frequently prescribed with disappointing results. In a population of 215 patients with severe intellectual disability [35], 69.3% suffered symptomatic constipation. It was significantly correlated with being non-ambulant, cerebral palsy, the use of anticonvulsive medication or benzodiazepines, H_2- receptor antagonists or proton pump inhibitors, food refusal, and IQ lower than 35. Faecal soiling was found in 15% of subjects, while manual evacuation of faeces was performed in nearly 7% of cases.

Physiology of normal defaecation reflex

Normal defaecation is a combination of autonomic and voluntary functions. It is voluntarily controlled in healthy people. It requires a concerted complex action, coordination and sequential activation of a large number of muscles in the anal canal and pelvic floor. Distension of the rectum is the stimulus that initiates reflex defaecation. There is voluntary contraction of the abdominal wall muscles and diaphragm, raising intra-abdominal pressure to force the rectal contents toward and into the anal canal. This intensifies the sensation of defaecation and marks the end of the voluntary phase. When the faecal bolus distends the rectum, sensory receptors in the rectal wall are stimulated, leading to conscious perception of rectal distension and involuntary relaxation of the internal anal sphincter. In the absence of voluntary contraction of the puborectalis muscle and the external anal sphincter, the faecal bolus is expelled.

The defaecation response is probably mediated in the distal spinal cord. The neural pathways involve parasympathetic, sympathetic, and somatic innervation to the colon, rectum, and anus. The intrinsic enteric nervous system, comprising submucosal Meissner and myenteric Auerbach plexuses, regulates segment-to-segment movement of the gastrointestinal tract. The vagus supplies the upper segments of the gastrointestinal tract up to the splenic flexure. The pelvic splanchnic nerves (*nervi erigentes*) carry parasympathetic fibres from the S2-S4 spinal cord levels to the descending colon and rectum. The hypogastric nerve sends out sympathetic innervation from the L1, L2, L3 spinal segments to the lower colon, rectum, and sphincters. The pudendal nerve (S2-S4) provides somatic innervation to the external anal sphincter and pelvic floor.

Spinal cord lesions above the *conus medullaris* are upper motor neuron lesions. They result in underactive propulsive peristalsis, overactive segmental peristalsis, and rectal distension. A lesion at the level of the *conus medullaris*, *cauda equina*, or inferior splanchnic nerve is a lower motor neuron lesion and leads to colonic slowing, resulting in constipation, faecal incontinence, and difficulty with emptying.

Intestinal transit time is closely related to defaecation frequency and decreases as childhood progresses. In the first month of life transit of stool takes 8 hours, whereas at age 2—16 h and between 3 and 13 years—26 h. Normal transit time in adults can be 48 hours or more; in all ages it is largely influenced by the amount of fibre in the diet. Fibre-rich diets favour the retention of water and result in increased stool weight and volume, shorter transit time and more frequent defaecation. The water content of normal stools is 60–85%. The desiccation of colonic contents in constipation is due to increased duration of mucosal contact rather than an alteration of mucosal absorptive function.

Pathophysiology of constipation

Constipation is frequently multifactorial in origin and can result from systemic or neurologic disorders as well as from medications. Causes of the symptom are usually classified into three broad categories:

- normal-transit constipation,
- slow-transit (functional) constipation, and
- disorders of defaecatory or rectal evacuation [36].

1. **Normal-transit constipation**   Stool traverses at a normal rate through the colon and the stool frequency is normal. Patients believe they are constipated, as they perceive difficulty with evacuation or the presence of hard stools. Factors responsible for the sense of constipation include bloating and abdominal pain or discomfort, increased psychosocial distress, increased rectal compliance and reduced rectal sensation.

2. **Slow-transit defaecation**   Infrequent urge to defaecate, bloating, and abdominal pain or discomfort are often symptoms associated with slow-transit constipation. Hirschsprung's disease represents an extreme form. Histopathological studies have shown alterations in the number of myenteric plexus neurons expressing the excitatory neurotransmitter SP, abnormalities in the inhibitory transmitters vasoactive intestinal peptide and nitric oxide, and a reduction in the number of interstitial cells of Cajal, which are thought to regulate GI motility [37–39]. In patients with a minimal delay in colonic transit, a high-fibre diet may increase stool weight, decrease colon-transit time, and relieve constipation. Patients with more severe problems, who have infrequent bowel movements (once a week or fewer), have a poor response to dietary fibre and laxatives. In such patients, there is often delayed emptying of the proximal colon and relatively few high-amplitude peristaltic contractions after meals that normally induce movement of content through the colon. Colonic inertia, a related condition, is characterised by slow colonic transit and the lack of an increase in motor activity after meals,

and after the administration of bisacodyl, cholinergic agents, or anticholinesterases [40].

3. **Defaecation disorder**   Anismus, pelvic-floor dyssynergia, paradoxical pelvic-floor contraction, obstructed constipation, functional rectosigmoid obstruction, the spastic pelvic-floor syndrome, and functional faecal retention in childhood are frequently used terms to describe defaecatory disorders. It results from dysfunction of the pelvic floor or anal sphincter. Failure of the rectum to empty effectively may be due to an inability to coordinate the abdominal, rectoanal, and pelvic-floor muscles during defaecation [41] and can be functional or organic. Functional defaecatory dysfunction can be provoked by prolonged avoidance of the pain, for example in association with anal fissure. There may be a history of sexual or physical abuse, or an eating disorder. Ignoring or suppressing the urge to defaecate is a widespread cause of chronic constipation in general population in both adults and children. Secondary encopresis often accompanies functional faecal retention in children. Extensive leakage of liquid stool around impacted stool may lead to an initial misdiagnosis of diarrhoea [42].

Signs, symptoms, and complications of chronic constipation

Symptoms and signs can include [32–34]:

- vague abdominal pain around the navel or even severe attacks of abdominal pain
- decreased appetite, nausea, or vomiting
- urinary incontinence, frequent urination, or bed-wetting
- recurrent urinary tract infections

Faecal impaction occurs in up to 80% of adult patients with chronic constipation. [27,43]. Impaction refers to the accumulation of dry, hardened faeces in the rectum or colon. Left untreated, impaction can result in bowel distension and megacolon. This in turn can be further complicated by chronic inflammation, infection, intestinal perforation and even death.

Management of constipation

The principle of treating constipation is to use the minimum intervention that will relieve the symptoms. Management plan includes attention to comfort and privacy, possible elimination of medical factors that may contribute to constipation, as well as therapeutic interventions. The type of medical procedure used depends on the child's age and exact problem [45–46].

Classes of laxative drugs

There are numerous types of laxatives, including bulk-forming agents and surfactants, lubricants, osmotic agents, contact cathartics, prokinetic drugs, and agents for colonic lavage.

Bulk laxatives

Fibre supplementation should be started at a low subtherapeutic dose and titrated upwards on a weekly basis until the desired effect is achieved. Combined with diet and liquids, bulk laxatives institute a 'natural', but also hardly effective long-term treatment for constipation. Their slow onset of action (between 12 and 72 h) limits their usefulness in acute management of constipation. Providing there is enough fluid intake and adequate gut motility, added fibre can helpful. However, many dying patients have neither of these, and additional fibre can worsen the situation, causing a 'soft impaction' and abdominal discomfort. Wheat bran is one of the best and least expensive of the bulk laxatives. Methylcellulose, psyllium (e.g. Metamucil), and polycarbophil are bulk laxatives that are safe, more refined, and more concentrated than wheat bran.

Osmotic laxatives

The osmotic agents cause retention of fluid, which distends the colon and increases peristaltic activity. Reduced absorption of water from stool and increased secretion into the gut lumen may be achieved by adding osmotically active particles such as magnesium and phosphorus salts, or non-absorbable sugars, such as lactulose or polyethylene glycol.

Magnesium citrate and magnesium hydroxide (Milk of Magnesia) decrease colonic transit time by stimulating cholecystokinin and drawing fluid into the colon by their osmotic effect. Their rapid onset of action (between 30 min and 3 h) makes them an excellent choice for acute management of constipation. These laxatives commonly cause abdominal cramping and, in patients with renal failure, may cause magnesium toxicity.

Polyethylene glycol is often considered the laxative of choice. The onset of action is between 24 and 48 h. It is equally effective, but better tolerated than the older osmotics, lactulose and sorbitol [47]. Because it is not fermented, gas and cramps are minimal. Sickly-sweet sorbitol and lactulose may not be palatable and may have the side effect of cramps, abdominal distension, and flatulence. Both are poorly absorbed sugars, likewise have rapid onset of action (8–12 h), but flatulence and abdominal distension may limit tolerance. Lactulose, whose breakdown products are mainly stimulant, is a particular culprit and is not usually recommended in paediatric palliative care.

Hyperosmolar solutions may worsen dehydration by drawing body water into the gut lumen and some are contraindicated in renal failure.

Stimulant laxatives

The stimulant laxatives include diphenylmethanes, the antraquinones, and castor oil. They are more potent than bulk or osmotic laxatives. Bisacodyl, a diphenylmethane, alters electrolyte transportation within intestinal mucosa and stimulates peristalsis. These actions may cause abdominal cramping and hypokalemia. Cascara, senna, and aloe (the strongest) are all anthraquinones. Colonic bacteria hydrolyse casanthranol and senna alkaloids into its active compounds. These stimulate peristalsis by excitement of the colonic myenteric plexuses and alter water and electrolyte secretion by the gut lining, resulting in net intestinal fluid accumulation. Aloe and *Cascara sagrada* directly irritate the intestinal mucosa, alter fluid and electrolyte secretion and increase colonic motility. All are available for both oral and rectal administration. Castor oil is reduced to ricinoleic acid that acts on the small intestine to decrease net absorption of fluid and electrolytes and stimulate peristalsis. As a general rule, the more potent the laxative substance, the more it is likely to cause unacceptable abdominal cramping. Spreading the dose out over the day, perhaps giving small doses with each meal and a slightly larger dose at bedtime, may diminish this effect. Constipated or impacted stool should be removed before introduction of drugs increasing gut motility to avoid exacerbating cramps.

Lubricants

Adequate lubrication of stool simply eases colonic passage and minimises pain that can interfere with excretion. Mineral oils lubricate by decreasing water absorption from intestine. Mineral oils can be used as an enema as well. Its long-term use is accompanied by concerns of lipid pneumonia, lymphoid hyperplasia, and foreign body reactions. Prolonged administration may also produce deficiency of fat-soluble vitamins. Docusate sodium causes increased systemic absorption of mineral oils, so the concomitant usage of both substances should be avoided. Glycerine suppositories can provide lubrication and draw-in water due to osmotically active particles. Instead of oils the most commonly used lubricants are dioctyl sodium sulfosuccinate (DSS), which decreases stool surface tension much like soap. DSS liquid is unpleasant to taste, so it may be given to tube-fed patients or use orally in other pharmaceutical formulation. DSS is commonly used in combination with senna in opioid-induced constipation, but is generally inadequate as a sole agent.

A selection of important medications and their modes of action is summarised in Table 23.5. In summary, stimulant laxatives combined with softeners should be considered first-line therapy for children undergoing palliative care. The effects of stimulants alone can attenuate over time [35,38]. In our practice, polyethylene glycol (PeGl) without electrolytes has become the first option for many patients and is well-tolerated [48]. Lubricant mineral oil and softening magnesium hydroxide can be used over long periods [27,49,50].

Table 23.5 Pharmacological treatment of constipation in children

Substance	Paediatric dose	Adolescent and adult dose
Osmotic laxatives—Produce osmotic effect in colon that results in distention and promotes peristalsis		
Lactulose *may cause cramps*	1–3 ml/kg/d PO divided qd/bid	10–30 ml PO qd
Sorbitol *may cause cramps*	1–3 ml/kg/d PO divided qd/bid	30–150 ml PO qd prn

Magnesium hydroxide
Contraindicated in patients
with renal failure
	1–3 ml/kg/d (as 400 mg/5 ml suspension) PO
	  qd or divided bid
		30–60 ml/d (as 400 mg/5 ml oral suspension)
		  PO qd or divided bid

Magnesium citrate *Contraindicated in patients* *with renal failure*	*<6 years:* 1–3 mL/kg/d PO qd *6–12 years:* 100–150 ml/d PO qd *>12 years:* Administer as in adults	150–300 ml/d PO qd
Polyethylene glycol	*For disimpaction:* 20 ml/kg/h q4–6h; not to exceed 1000 ml *Maintenance therapy in children >2 years:* 5–10 mL/kg/d	*Occasional constipation:* 17 g mixed in 240 ml of water PO qd prn
Sodium phosphate (Fleet enema) *Contraindicated in patients with* *renal failure*	*5–10 years:* 1 tsp PO *10–12 years:* 2 tsp PO *>12 years:* Administer as in adults	*Laxative:* 4 tsp PO *Purgative:* 3 tbsp PO
Colonic stimulants—Used to promote peristalsis		
Bisacodyl	*6–12 years:* 1 tab/d PO or 1 pediatric supp/d PR *>12 years:* 2–3 tab/d PO or 1 supp/d PR	2–3 tab/d PO or 1 supp/d PR
Cascara sagrada	*Infants:* 0.5–1.5 ml/d prn. *2–11 years:* 1–3 ml/d prn	5–6 ml or 1 tab PO hs

Senna	*2–6 years:* 1/2 tab/d to 1 tab bid PO or
	  1/4 tsp/d to 1/2 tsp bid PO
	6–12 years: 1 tab/d to 2 tab bid PO or 1 tsp/d to
	  2 tsp/d PO
		2 tab/d to 4 tab bid PO or 1 tsp/d to 2 tsp bid
		  PO

Castor oil *for use only when prompt catharsis is desired*	5–10 ml PO once	15–60 mL PO once
Casanthranol	*<6 years:* Not recommended	*>6 years:* 0.12–0.25 g PO qd
Lubricants—Soften stools and decrease water absorption from GI		
Mineral oil *Do not give mineral oil by mouth, as* *aspiration may cause pneumonitis;* *depletion of A, D, E, K vitamines*	*<1 year:* Not recommended *>1 year:* 1–3 mL/kg/d qd/bid	15–45 ml PO qd pr
Bulking agents—Absorb water in intestine to form viscous liquid that promotes peristalsis and reduces transit time		
Psyllium *should be mixed with water to prevent* *choking; low fluid intake may cause impaction*	*6–12 years:* 0.5 tsp/dose PO qd/bid	1 tsp/dose PO qd/bid;
Methylcellulose *low fluid intake may cause impaction*		Pediatric: Adults:
Emollient stool softeners—Help keep stools soft for easy natural passage		
Docusate sodium Docusate calcium *Inadequate alone to counteract* *opoid-induced constipation*	*<3 years:* 10–40 mg/d PO *3–6 years:* 20–60 mg/d PO *6–12 years:* 40–120 mg/d PO	50–200 mg/d PO
Emollient stool softeners in combination with stimulants		
Docusate sodium and casanthranol combination		

Experimental therapies

In recent years some specific and experimental therapies have been tried. It is believed that the laxative effect of prostaglandins may be due to changes in water and electrolyte absorption in the intestines and the motor effect. Researchers found that misoprostol increased the weight and frequency of stools and shortened colonic transit time in patients with severe chronic constipation[51]. Cisapride is an agent currently available in some countries that stimulates the upper GI tract and is useful in patients with spinal cord injury or Parkinson's disease as well as in chronic constipation with encopresis in children [36,52]. Colchicine, used to treat gouty arthritis, is useful in treatment of chronic constipation [53]. Erythromycin exerts its prokinetic effect by acting as a motilin agonist and has long been used in gastrointestinal motility disorders [54]. It under investigation in idiopathic and chronic constipation in children. One double-blind, placebo-controlled, crossover study [55] showed the efficacy of erythromycin in the treatment of refractory chronic constipation presenting with megarectum and faecal impaction. Another colonic prokinetic drug, tegaserod that is a selective 5-HT4 partial agonist improves stool consistency and frequency in children with chronic constipation [56].

Among recently introduced pharmaceuticals tested in multiple clinical trials, the selective antagonists of the muscarinic type-3 receptor (zamifenacin and darifenacin) and selective antagonists for neurokinin receptors type 1 and type 2 (ezlopitant and nepadudant) seem to be effective in reducing the symptoms of abdominal pain, bloating, and constipation [57]. Neurotrophin-3 (NT-3) in particular increased stool frequency, enhanced colon transit, and improved symptoms of chronic constipation. It seems to be a novel, safe, and effective agent for the treatment of functional constipation [58].

Children with internal anal sphincter achalasia have clinical characteristics that distinguish them from children with functional constipation. Intra-anal injection of botulinum toxin is a safe and effective medium-term treatment for these children. Injection of botulinum type A toxin into the puborectalis muscle may also be effective in the treatment of other defaecatory disorders involving spastic pelvic-floor muscles [59].

Alternative therapies

The options to laxatives capable to relieve symptoms accompanying chronic constipation in severely neurologically impaired children include *biofeedback and behavioural training* and a *pulse irrigation evacuation system*.

Biofeedback and *behavioural training* are of benefit to improve sensory and motor awareness in children with incomplete neurogenic bowel lesions. They can be used to train patients to relax their pelvic-floor muscles during straining and to coordinate this relaxation with abdominal manoeuvres to enhance the entry of stool into the rectum. It is usually performed with anorectal electromyography or a manometry catheter. Biofeedback is a simple, cost-effective technique with few adverse effects. It remains an attractive option, especially considering the complexity of the functional disorders of the colon, rectum, anus, and pelvic floor. The benefits of biofeedback appear to be long-lasting. However, it does require the presence of some degree of sphincter contraction and rectal sensitivity. Biofeedback may be less effective for patients with the descending perineum syndrome than for patients with other defaecatory disorders [60].

Pulse irrigations exploit intermittent rapid pulses of warm water to break up stool impactions and stimulate peristalsis. Some clinicians advocate use of a bowel management tube with attached balloon (e.g. Foley catheter) and subsequent administration of saline, phosphates or mannitol enema for faecal evacuation in children with neurogenic bowel dysfunction. The balloon helps to provide anal occlusion to retain the enema fluid in persons with weak or absent anal sphincter function. Enemas should be used sparingly. They tend to wash out the normal mucus in the colon that provides lubrication for stools.

Opioid-induced constipation

The pathophysiology of opioid-induced constipation has now been well characterised [61,62]. At least two types of opioid receptor, μ and δ, have been located in gut smooth muscle, with μ directly affecting the myenteric plexus [63]. Endogenous opioids modulate the resting tone of gut muscle [64]. Opioids delay gastric emptying by producing gastroparesis secondary to spasm in the antropyloric region. This action appears to stem from the central nervous system and is dopamine mediated [64]. Opioids also delay stool transit through the small bowel, an effect that is greatest in the jejunum and is related to an increase in nonpropulsive contractions. Colonic transit time as well as anal sphincter tone is also increased. Exogenous opioids inhibit detection of stool in the upper anal canal and therefore interfere with the defaecation reflex, and also inhibit relaxation of the internal anal sphincter. The result is impaired defaecation response, decreased peristalsis and increased stool transit time, which in turn lead to increased electrolyte and water absorption, drying of the stool and ultimately constipation. The constipating effect of opioids is immediate and dose related, and unlike most other side-effects, patients never become tolerant to it [64,65].

Opioid-induced constipation may also contribute to abdominal pain, distension, nausea and anorexia or gastroesophageal reflux, and constipation may even occasionally may progress to bowel obstruction. While opioids are prescribed, bowel habit should be monitored carefully on a daily basis, beginning with a thorough history of individual habits before commencing opioids. Factors that frequently aggravate and compound opioid-induced constipation during palliative care include dehydration, confusion, other drugs and immobility.

The most important way to manage opioid-induced constipation is prophylaxis against it. Anecdotally, children receiving opioids may not develop constipation quite as universally as adults. Nevertheless, the majority of children will, and it is more difficult to treat than to avoid. Laxatives should always be considered, and usually prescribed, prior to commencing opioid therapy. It has to be remembered that usual measures of constipation prophylaxis (e.g. fibre, fluids, exercise) may not be sufficient for patients receiving palliative care. Fibre-based laxatives may even be dangerous in children with faecal impaction, resulting in obstruction if fluid intake is inadequate, as is often the case in those with non-malignant LLC. Similarly, osmotic laxatives such as lactulose are not appropriate. Instead, a combination of stimulant laxatives such as senna or dantron, combined with stool softeners such as magnesium hydroxide or docusate, are the mainstay of prophylaxis. In some countries convenient formulations are available combining laxatives of both classes, such as codantramer or codantrusate in the United Kingdom.

Despite adequate prophylaxis, some children receiving opioids will go on to develop constipation. Management of the symptom once it occurs relies on an understanding of physiologic response to opioids [16,66,67,68].

Given the role of peripheral opioid receptors in developing constipation [69], blockade of receptors in the gut seems a logical therapeutic target for managing the problem. Given orally, naloxone and other opioid antagonists were the first among effective agents used to prevent opioid-induced constipation. Methylnaltrexone and alvimopan, newer opioid antagonists that are more selective for peripheral activity, have been introduced into clinical practice more recently [70]. Both have demonstrated the ability to reverse opioid-induced bowel dysfunction without reversing analgesia or precipitating central nervous system withdrawal signs. Interestingly, oral naloxone also been effective in other causes of constipation [71–76].

Patients who experience nausea or constipation while taking a particular opioid may benefit from opioid rotation [77] or switching to a different route. Opioids are not all equally constipating in relation to their analgesic activity; codeine, for example, is more likely to cause constipation than fentanyl or oxycodone [78]. Given the relatively weak analgesic potency of codeine, constipation may in effect impose a 'ceiling' on the dose of codeine that can be given.

Painful defaecation

Eliminating any pain associated with the passage of bowel movements is extremely important. Painful defaecation is the primary precipitant of constipation during early childhood [78]. Using large doses of laxatives to produce very soft stools may be necessary. Continuing laxative therapy for a number of months is often necessary. Reassuring caregivers of the safety of long-term laxative usage is of utmost important. There are many popular misconceptions about their use, and even abuse [45,46].

If the child has anal fissures, using Xylocaine ointment or hydrocortisone suppositories for a short period of time to provide symptomatic relief, may be appropriate. Rectal agents should be avoided in children who are at risk for thrombocytopenia, leukopenia, and/or mucositis from cancer and its treatment.

Excessive intestinal gas

The other, clinically important problem often complicated prolong constipation is gaseous distension. The most common symptoms associated with excessive intestinal gas are painful eructation, flatulence, and abdominal bloating and distention. Unfortunately, few therapies have been shown to be effective in treating these symptoms. Decreasing air swallowing can treat excessive eructation. Bloating and gaseous distension can improve in some patients by avoiding foods containing partially digested or absorbed polysaccharides, by taking replacement enzymes such as alpha-galactosidase or lactase, or occasionally, by taking antibiotics directed toward altering the colonic flora. For some children replacement of cow milk proteins with the substitutes (soy or peptide and amino acid formulas) may be beneficial [79].

Faecal impaction

For hard faecal impaction, a series of enemas or aggressive use of oral cathartics can avoid the need for digital disimpaction. Effective treatments include phosphates, mannitol, senna alkaloids and mineral oil or polyethylene glycol. Such interventions may need to be accompanied by a short-acting anxiolytic benzodiazepine, or an analgesic. After disimpaction, patients should be placed on a vigorous bowel regimen to avoid recurrence.

In extreme situations, caecostomy may permit decompression in megacolon, and antegrade enemas are of value in in colonic inertia. Antegrade enemas through a caecostomy are a safe option for children who are neurologically intact and who have severe constipation that does not respond to medical treatment. There seems to be no significant difference in the rate of continence or complication between caecostomy at ileal or appendiceal segment [49].

Intestinal obstruction

Intestinal obstruction is caused by an occlusion to the lumen or a lack of normal propulsion that prevents or delays intestinal contents from passing along the gastrointestinal tract. It is not restricted to children with malignant disorders, but can also occur and even cause death in children with non-malignant LLC [80,81,82]. Patients in the terminal phase are often unfit for surgery and require alternative management to relieve distressing symptoms [15] associated with obstruction. The distinction is often made between complete or partial, paralytic or mechanical obstructions. In patients with advanced disease the onset is usually insidious and takes even some weeks. Symptoms usually worsen gradually and intermittent obstructive episodes often resolve spontaneously, albeit sometimes only temporarily.

Difficult cases need medical, ethical and sometimes even legal considerations. The need for surgical intervention should always be decided on an individual basis. If palliative care is the only option, all symptoms should be adequately control. Appropriate conservative treatment can be effective in controlling nausea, vomiting and abdominal pain, secondary to bowel obstruction [26,83]. Currently octreotide seems to be very effective in symptoms control combination with traditional pharmacological treatment to ameliorate the symptoms of inoperable bowel obstruction in terminal patients [84,85].

Sialorrhoea

Sialorrhoea (drooling) is loss of control over one's own saliva [86]. Other terms, for example salivary incompetence, hypersalivation, ptyalism, are often (not always accurately) used synonymously.

Hypersalivation refers to the excessive production of saliva. Ptyalism is a term that includes both hypersalivation and sialorrhoea. Secretions that pool in the hypopharynx and contribute to aspiration can cause choking, dysphagia, and breathing difficulties. Sialorrhoea is a serious social handicap experienced by many neurologically impaired patients [87,88]. It carries considerable social stigma, can interfere with communication devices, and is a barrier to interpersonal relationships. Sialorrhoea may therefore have significant negative effects on the physical, social, and psychological well being of affected children as well as their families. It also

impacts on other caregivers, who may have to change the child's clothing or bib 10 to 20 times each day.

It is unlikely to cause physical harm, unless the body's normal reflex coughing mechanisms are also impaired in which case persistent micro-aspirations can result. Physical problems associated with excessive sialorrhoea include facial chapping, responsible for irritation, rash or chapping arising around the mouth and chin, chilling from facial wetness in cold weather, dental caries, lip cracking and fissures, and the possibility of transmission of infectious diseases.

Sialorrhoea is therefore a serious symptom at the terminal stage of many life-limiting diseases, but particularly non-malignant ones.

Scope of the problem

It is estimated that between as many as 58% of children with cerebral palsy, and 10% of children with other neurological disorders are faced with severe sialorrhoea that requires intervention [88,89]. Cerebral palsy (CP) alone affects approximately 1 in 200 to 300 newborns, so the absolute number of patients who should receive effective treatment is very significant.

Whilst neurological causes (Table 23.6) are the commonest in paediatric palliative care, other causes include structural abnormalities, of mouth, jaw and nasopharynx, emotional and psychological factors as well as side effects of some drugs, particularly neuroleptics and nitrazepam.

Pathophysiology of sialorrhea

Sialorrhoea may be caused by excess production of saliva, inability to retain saliva within the mouth, or problems with swallowing. Overproduction of saliva in the absence of swallowing impairment usually does not cause sialorrhoea.

Salivary flow rates in children with CP who drool are no different from normal children [89]. The predominant pathophysiologic mechanism is not overproduction of saliva, but

Table 23.6 Neurological conditions frequently associated with drooling

Cerebral palsy
Cranial nerve palsies: VII, IX, and XII
Global developmental disorder
Stroke
Amyotrophic lateral sclerosis
Down syndrome
Motor neurone diseases
Parkinsonism
Congenital suprabulbar palsy

disturbed coordination of the highly complex, sequential patterns of swallowing. It is the oral/voluntary phase of swallowing that is most severely affected. Inefficient swallow results from poor coordination of the lips, tongue, palate, jaws, pharynx, larynx, and respiratory muscles.

Nevertheless, although hypersalivation is rarely the cause of severe sialorrhoea, the pathophysiology of saliva excretion and oral cavity structure's innervation holds the key to rational therapy. Ninety per cent of saliva is normally secreted by three major pairs of salivary glands and numerous minor glands located on the palate, buccal mucosa, and tongue. Depending on demand and autonomic regulation, saliva consists of two phases—thin, watery secretions and thick, mucus-containing secretions. Daily production of saliva in adults usually reaches 1.5 l. The parotid glands are responsible for about 30% of the volume, producing mostly thin, serous secretions. The submandibular glands produce between 50 and 70% of the saliva. The quality of the secretions is more viscous because of a greater mucoid component. Sublingual glands account for about 5% of saliva and again produce predominantly mucoid secretions.

The secretory innervation of the salivary glands is primarily under the control of the parasympathetic nervous system. Stimulation of the parasympathetic nerves causes profuse secretion of watery saliva. Sympathetic stimulation may also occur but is thought to be a synergistic effect that results in an increase in the flow of saliva primarily through smooth muscle contraction at the duct level. Finally, some secretions come from the respiratory tree, as part of the physiological protective mechanisms.

Saliva serves many important physiological functions (Table 23.7). Any treatment plan that changes the amount, consistency, or flow of saliva in the oral cavity must consider the impact on these. The neuroanatomy is also important for both medical and surgical therapeutic considerations.

Management of sialorrhoea

Sialorrhoea becomes less of a problem once permanent dentition has appeared [90] and invasive techniques should be postponed until this time. Most treatments, which have been developed to date, are directed at reducing the volume of saliva produced. An appropriate therapeutic strategy for sialorrhoea should be based on the individual needs of the patient and family including the severity of the problem, previous interventions, and the level of neurological dysfunction. A major problem in treatment planning is that the magnitude of the problem varies considerably, so that control is a constantly changing need. Its impact may depend on factors other than simple saliva volume. A child who is less affected but more

Table 23.7 Physiological functions of saliva

Domain	Function
Digestive	Facilitates chewing
	Initializing enzymatic breakdown of food (proteins and carbohydrates)
	Facilitates swallowing
	Enhances taste
	Decreases breath odour
	Protects lower oesophageal sphincter from acid
Protective	Maintains oral health (contains gingival crevicular fluid)
	Prevents caries/periodontal disease
	Buffers as an antibacterial agent
Speech	Lubricates (facilitates articulation by moistening surface of tongue, lip, and palate)

cognitively aware of the problem may suffer a greater degree of social isolation and disability than one with a greater degree of sialorrhoea, but less awareness.

Management techniques can include behavioural, pharmacological, and surgical interventions (Table 23.8). The use of non-pharmaceutical modalities is often limited by cognitive ability and is usually unhelpful. Pharmacotherapy alone may have a useful role in many patients, especially those with only mild sialorrhoea and mild to moderate intellectual delay. Aggressive surgical interventions should be considered in many children with LLC but are not always appropriate.

Published literature and clinical observations suggest that pharmacotherapy offers only short-term solutions, often at the cost of considerable side effects [89,91,92,93]. Even surgical approaches seem to lose effectiveness with time [92]. Adverse side-effects are inevitable, irrespective of modality. Excessive dryness of mouth epithelium can exacerbate existing swallowing difficulties and aggravate rate of respiratory infections and breathing difficulties. Mucus producing respiratory glands are not regulated by any major nerve supply that can be blocked. The result is that saliva production is blocked, but not production of mucus. As saliva volumes diminished, mucus thickens and can accumulate in the back of the throat, with a tendency to block airways or make food stick in the throat. Coughing it up can be a tiring and arduous process, and take its toll on children and caregivers. In the presence of swallowing difficulties, especially in children with bulbar paralysis, successful treatment of sialorrhoea may therefore paradoxically worsen symptoms.

Adequate fluid intake is the first essential step in prevention of this problem. By reducing mucosal inflammation, antihistamines and NSAID may help [94,95]. Suction with appropriate catheters to clear phlegm and secretions from the throat and

Table 23.8 Treatment options for drooling

Reassurance
Elimination of a situational factors
　Posture control
　Dental caries, gingivitis, severe malocclusion
　Upper aerodigestive obstruction or inflammation

Alternative therapies
　Oral-motor therapy
　Behaviour modification
　Biofeedback
　Hypnotherapy

Pharmacologic treatment
　Anticholinergics
　Sympathomimetics
　Tricyclic antidepressants
　Other established or experimental therapies

Surgery
　Wharton's duct relocation, sublingual gland excision
　Submandibular gland excision, parotid duct ligation

Miscellaneous
　Botulin toxin A
　Dental prostheses
　Radiation

mouth is often helpful. In the experience of the Warsaw Hospital for Children, the 'Cough-Assist Mechanical Insufflation-Exsufflation device (MI-E)' has been of value in patients whose swallowing is impaired, especially those suffering from acute respiratory infections. It safely and effectively clears retained broncho-pulmonary secretions by gradually applying a positive pressure to the airway, and then rapidly shifting to negative pressure. The rapid shift in pressure produces a high expiratory flow from the lungs, simulating a cough.

Factors that exacerbate sialorrhoea include teething as well as sensitive and painful gums, mouth ulceration, lack of sleep and crying. Over-the-counter treatments are available which provide pain relief in the form of analgesic and anaesthetic gels, some of which also possess antiseptic or anti-inflammatory properties. There is also a wide range of home remedies, such as teething rings.

Pharmacotherapy

Medications that modify sialorrhoea do so by reducing saliva production and/or by altering its consistency. Anticholinergic drugs inhibit salivary secretion by reversible blockade of the acetylcholine-mediated activation of muscarinic receptors. They include atropine sulphate, prantheline bromide, benzhexal*,

benztropine (benzatropine), saltropine, glycopyrrolate, trihexyphenidyl and scopolamine. Scopolamine, glycopyrrolate, benztropine (benzatropine) and saltropine have received the most attention in children. They are not always effective; of patients treated, 45% can expect no change in their sialorrhoea, 30% minimal to modest improvement, and only 20% complete resolution. Some have maintained an excellent result for more than five years. Adverse effects of anticholinergics in children are largely attributable to other antimuscarinic effects and include:

- behavioral irritability
- restlessness
- sedation, and
- changes in cognition

Large doses may suppress intestinal motility, exacerbating constipation. Anticholinergics may also precipitate retention in children with neurogenic bladder. Reduced bronchial secretions can lead to formation of bronchial plugs. Inhibition of sweat glands can cause disturbances in temperature regulation. Other adverse effects include photophobia and facial flushing and anticholinergics are contraindicated for individuals with glaucoma.

Drug interactions with other medications must also be considered.

Scopolamine (hyosine)

Scopolamine can be inhaled [96] or used orally and in transdermal system as well [83,97,98]. The transdermal formulation has a significant advantage over enterally absorbed as it avoids the first passage hepatic deactivation and can be used effectively in lower doses. Unfortunately its effectiveness diminishes with time [99]. Dizziness, vomiting, nausea, headache, and vertigo may occur if the patch is discontinued too suddenly.

Atropine sulphate can also be used to reduce salivation and bronchial. Scopolamine and atropine, as well as glycopyrrolate (see below) have been used in nebulisers with no superior effect [100].

Glycopyrrolate

Glycopyrrolate may have fewer adverse effects [91] and better effectiveness [101,102] than other anticholinergics. Nevertheless, side effects require glycopyrrolate to be discontinued in approximately 20% of children [102].

Botulinum Toxin A

Clinical studies suggest that botulinum toxin A (BTX) injections into salivary glands are effective in decreasing sialorrhoea. It is reliable and well-tolerated [103–106]. The toxin originates from Clostridium botulinum and works by blocking acetylcholine release from nerve endings, at or near the place of injection. Typically BTX is injected into each parotid or submandibular gland only. The parotids are more important; as they are major glands producing the thin, watery part of the saliva. It takes a week to 10 days for the maximum effect of BTX injection to be seen. In patients who respond, blockade of salivary glands gradually diminished over 3–8 months. The injections can be repeated.

Of six patients treated in the Warsaw Hospice, there was no effect in two and good effect in another two. In the remaining two there was a therapeutic effect, but it was accompanied by a worsening of breathing difficulty, probably from thickening of bronchial plugs. If injected at the wrong site or if it spreads, BTX can paralyse muscles in the injection area and increase dysphagia and dysarthria, but if injections are given under ultrasound guidance, this is unlikely [107]. One study reports recurrent jaw dislocation as a side effect [108].

Others

Efficacy and side effects of trihexyphenidyl are similar to glycopyrrolate [109,110]. An additional potential benefit for children with rigid or dystonic cerebral palsy is reduction in muscle tone [110].

Dryness of the mouth, is a side effect of tricyclic antidepressants (amitriptyline, imipramine) which can be turned to advantage in sialorrhoea. Central effects on mood and psyche are of additional value of treatment of sialorrhoea with these drugs.

Experimental therapies include metoprolol and clonidine [111]. Drugs blocking beta adrenergic receptors also inhibit mucus producing glands located in epithelial layer of mouth cavity and respiratory tract.

In some patients, activity against sialorrhoea has been found with older and some newer antihistamine medications and sympathomimetic agents such as ephedrine and pseudoephredrine. Sympathomimetic agents produce constriction of the blood vessels within the mucous membranes. Sympathomimetics are only effective for a short period and and can induce ischaemia. Treatment should be limited to 4–6 days. Some antihistamines possess additional anticholinergic activity [95,96,112,113], and may be of value if secretions have an allergic component. Mucolytic agents alter not only mucus formation but also the consistency of saliva. Mucolytics are mainly used to reduce the thick, ropy secretions in throat and mouth that can interfere with swallowing and remain in respiratory tract.

Surgery

Surgery for severe sialorrhoea was first described in 1967 [114]. In general, surgery is reserved for children with non-progressive neurological disorders such as cerebral palsy, who do not respond adequately to non-surgical therapies.

Many surgical approaches have been reported. They are divided into two main categories: those that reduce the amount of saliva produced, and those that divert the saliva posteriorly so that spontaneous swallowing may occur more readily.

In patients who are at risk of aspiration, the former is preferable. There are 3 surgical approaches to decreasing salivary flow, including:

- removing salivary glands
- ligating salivary ducts
- sectioning the nerves involved in salivary production.

Unfortunately results of all three have been disappointing [115,116]. Nerve fibres regenerate and this limits long-term effectiveness. Children with severe impairment of volitional motor function and profuse sialorrhoea tended to have a poorer outcome compared with those with milder impairments [116,117].

One of the newest procedures is combined ligation of the submandibular and parotid ducts. Currently four-duct ligation should be considered when surgery is indicated to treat sialorrhoea [117].

Other therapies

Saliva can be also reduced by irradiating the submandibular and sublingual salivary gland [118]. [There is a risk of xerostomia and secondary malignancy which may limit its usefulness in children whose life expectancy is long enough for them to become likely.]

Hiccup

Hiccup comprises an involuntary contraction of the diaphragm and the auxiliary respiratory muscles, occurring mostly in irregular series, followed by an abrupt closure of the glottis. It is a physiological phenomenon, which already exists even *in utero*, but its function is unknown. It is a gastrointestinal rather than a respiratory phenomenon. It may result in part from neuronal dysfunction, at the level of nerve roots or the reflex arc between inspiratory and glottic closure complexes [119]. The reflex is probably mediated by phrenic and vagus nerves and a central (brainstem) reflex centre. Irritation of the diaphragm [120] is often the underlying pathophysiological mechanism. Brief episodes of hiccup are benign and usually self-limiting. If a single episode lasts longer than 48 h it is termed persistent; if longer than one month, it becomes intractable. Prolonged attacks have been responsible for patient's tiredness and significantly interfered with both: quality of life and quality of care. Usually, the cause remains unknown, but persistent and intractable hiccups may indicate an organic disorder. Detailed evaluation based on history and physical examination can be helpful. Selected laboratory tests are sometimes indicated.

Causes of hiccup

The causes of hiccup are many and varied [121]. The most common are gastrointestinal in origin. GORD is perhaps the most important [121]. Hiccup may be induced by some drugs (such as digoxin); the same agents that are used to treat hiccups may also induce them. According to one source (114), 23% drug-induced hiccups were related to corticosteroids; 15% to psychiatric drugs, mainly antidepressants, and 13% to neurologic drugs, mainly dopaminergic antiparkinsonians. Other culprits include antibiotics, digoxin and analgesics, including opioids themselves, and it has been suggested that corticosteroids may lower the threshold for synaptic transmission in the midbrain, and directly stimulate the hiccup reflex arc [122].

Idiopathic hiccup often accompanies stress and hiccup may accompany organic conditions including malignancy, myocardial infarction, gastric distension and liver dysfunction. Uraemia and other metabolic abnormalities (such as disturbances of serum glucose, calcium, and potassium) may cause hiccup. Hiccups that are psychogenic in origin commonly abate with sleep and may be temporally related to stressful circumstances.

Management of hiccup

An evidence-based approach to management of hiccup is hard to define [123]. Virtually all current data is anecdotal. Treatment should be if possible directed at the underlying cause where one is identified. The patient's prognosis, current level of function and potential adverse effects from any proposed treatment should all be considered [124,125].

Many drugs have been proposed to treat hiccup (Table 23.9). Baclofen, a centrally acting muscle relaxant, is the only one studied in a double blind randomised controlled study [126,127]. Its effectiveness may be increased by combination with gabapentin [128]. Among other well-established treatment modalities chlorpromazine is the most studied and appears to be the drug of choice. Its effectiveness reaches almost 80% [125].

Some older anticonvulsants include phenytoin, valproic acid and carbamazepine seem effective, especially in patients with hiccups of CNS origin. Metoclopramide has also been used successfully, especially if stomach distension is the

aetiology. Haloperidol has also been used. Ketamine has been effective at a dose of 0.4 mg/kg, that is, one fifth of the usual anaesthetic dose.

The efficacy of combination therapy with cisapride, omeprazole, and baclofen (*COB* regimen) for treatment of idiopathic chronic hiccup (ICH) has been shown [129,130]. Cisapride is no longer available for children in the United Kingdom following concerns regarding cardiac toxicity. Substituting gabapentin for baclofen in baclofen resistant ICH cases can occasionally be successful (*COG* regimen). COB and COG combination is considered by some to be 'therapy of choice' for hiccups [129].

Infusion of lidocaine has been effective when other agents were unsuccessful [131]. Even in subanaesthetic doses, lidocaine possesses membrane-stabilizing properties that diminish neuronal excitability and reduce ectopic discharges. It seems logical therefore that it might prove beneficial in the treatment of certain patients with hiccup, particularly those in whom a neurogenic aetiology is postulated.

Other approaches have included the muscle relaxant, orphenadrine, sedatives such as amitriptyline and chloral hydrate, analgesics such as morphine and inhaled lidocaine, and stimulants such as ephedrine, methylphenidate, amphetamine (amfetamine) and nikethamide. Rarely used drugs, including edrophonium, dexamethasone and amantadine, have also been tried with equivocal results [125,126]. Benzodiazepines may exacerbate or precipitate hiccups and should be avoided [132,133], but sublingual nifedipine is safe and may be tried if other interventions have failed.

Non-pharmacological approaches

Time-honoured home remedies for hiccups include: gargling with water, biting a lemon, swallowing sugar or producing a fright response, and many others. Most of these, if they work at all, do so through vagal stimulation. More sophisticated techniques include:

- interrupting the respiratory cycle through sneezing, coughing, breath holding, hyperventilation, or breathing into a paper bag.

- vagal stimulation through carotid massage or valsalva manoeuvre;

- interruption of phrenic nerve transmission via rubbing over the fifth cervical vertebrae;

In intractable hiccups, when other treatments fail, other approaches such as acupuncture, diaphragmatic pacing electrodes or surgical ablation of the reflex arc by cervical phrenic nerve block can also be considered [134].

Table 23.9 Pharmacological interventions in the treatment of patients with hiccup

Substance	Mode of action	Dosage
Chlorpromazine	Antidopaminergic drug; blocks postsynaptic mesolimbic dopamine receptors; has anticholinergic effect; can depress the reticular activating system (possibly all are responsible for relieving nausea and vomiting); blocks alpha-adrenergic receptors; depresses release of hypophyseal and hypothalamic hormones	*Children:* po: 0.5–1 mg/kg/dose q4–6h; pr: 1 mg/kg/dose q6–8h iv: 0.5–1 mg/kg/dose q6–8h *Adults:* 25–50 mg po tid/qid; slow iv infusion with patient lying flat when symptoms persist; 25–50 mg in addition to 500–1000 ml of saline (monitor blood pressure); 25–50 mg im if symptoms persist for 2–3 days
Metoclopramide	Blocks dopamine receptors in the chemoreceptor trigger zone of CNS.	*Children:* 1–2 mg/kg po tid/qid for 7 d till *Grownup:* 10–20 mg po tid/qid for 7 d
Phenytoin	Inhibits spread of motor activity by acting in motor cortex.	*Loading dose:* 15–20 mg/kg po/iv; *followed by* an initial dose of 5 mg/kg/d po/iv bid/tid *Maintenance dose in children:* 4–8 mg/kg po/iv bid/tid; *Maintenance dose in adults:* 2–3 mg/kg po bid;
Valproic acid	Increases brain levels of gamma-aminobutyric acid (GABA), or enhances GABA action; may potentate postsynaptic GABA responses, affects potassium channel, possesses directly membrane-stablizing effect	10–15 mg/kg/d po in 1–3 divided doses irrespective of the age
Carbamazepine	Blocks post-tetanic potentation by reducing summation of temporal stimulation	*<6 years:* 10–20 mg/kg/d po bid/tid (qid with suspension) *6–12 years:* 100 mg po bid (50 mg qid of suspension) *>12 years:* not to exceed 1000 mg/d in children 12–15 years or 1200 mg/d in >15 years
Ketamine	Acts on the cortex and limbic system, decreasing muscle spasms	*Children:* po: 6–10 mg/kg/dose *Adults:* po: 3–8 mg/kg; *Intravenously:* 0.4 mg/kg (one-fifth of the usual anesthetic dose) iv; supplemental dose of 1/3 to 1/2 initial dose may be given for maintenance
Lidocaine	Inhibits depolarisation of type C sensory neurons by blocking sodium channels	1–1.5 mg/kg loading dose (max. 3 mg/kg) followed by an infusion of 20–50 mcg/kg/min.; locally: up to 3 mg/kg/dose in 2-h interval
Orphenadrine	While exact mode of action not well understood, has shown clinical effectiveness in treating hiccups	*Children:* not established *Adults:* 100 mg po bid prn
Baclofen	Induces the hyperpolarization of afferent terminals and inhibit both monosynaptic and polysynaptic reflexes at the spinal level useful in patients for whom other agents are contraindicated (e.g., those with renal impairment)	*From the 2nd year of life:* 5 mg q8h titrated up to 40 mg/d in children and 80 mg/d in adults
Haloperidol	Useful in treatment of irregular spasmodic movements of muscles	0.05–0.15 mg/kg/d po in 2–3 divided doses (not to exceed 0.15 mg/kg/d)
Chloral hydrate	Central nervous system depressant effects (mechanism unknown)	50–75 mg/kg po/pr; not to exceed 2 g divided bid
Ephedrine	Stimulates release of epinephrine stores, producing alpha-adrenergic and beta-adrenergic effects	*Children:* 4 mg/kg/d po q6–12h *Adults:* 60 mg/dose, q6–8h; max. 240 mg/d
Amitriptyline	Inhibits reuptake of serotonin and/or norepinephrine at presynaptic neuronal membrane, which increases concentration in CNS; may have analgesic effects	*Children:* 0.1 mg/kg at bedtime; increase, as tolerated, to 0.5–2 mg/d. *Adolescents and adults:* 25–50 mg/d initially; increase gradually to 200 mg/d (adolescents) and 300 mg/d (adults)
Doxycycline		*Children:* 1–3 mg/kg/d *Adolescents:* 25–50 mg/d initially; increase gradually to 100 mg/d *Adults:* 30–150 mg/d initially; increase gradually to and 300 mg/d (maximal single dose 150 mg)
Methylphenidate	Stimulates cerebral cortex and subcortical structures	*Children:* 0.3–0.7 mg/kg/dose (max. 2mg/kg/d) divided bid/tid; *Adults:* 10 mg bid/tid, not to exceed 60 mg/d

Cachexia and anorexia syndrome

There has been considerable medical interest and remarkable progress in basic research in cachexia, despite there being no standard definition. Its Greek origins reveal that 'cachexia' means simply 'poor condition'. In adults with cancer, cachexia is considered to be present if there is involuntary weight loss within a 6-month period, representing more than 5% of premorbid weight. It is a complex syndrome that combines a dramatic decrease in appetite and an increase in metabolism of fat and lean body mass.

Anorexia, which frequently accompanies malignant LLC, is one contributor to the syndrome of cachexia. However, the pattern of weight loss in cachexia differs from that seen with pure nutrient deprivation.

The *'anorexia-cachexia syndrome'* is a multidimensional maladaptation, encompassing a variety of alterations that range from physiological to behavioural. It can be associated with poor quality of life as well as short prognosis, and is therefore a legitimate therapeutic target for specialists in paediatric palliative medicine.

Causes of cachexia/anorexia syndrome

The characteristic feature of cachexia is accelerated loss of skeletal muscle, occurring in the context of a chronic inflammatory response [135]. An enormous variety of chronic or end-stage diseases demonstrate some nutritional changes of cachexia [136,136]. In general, patients with solid tumours are more likely to suffer cachexia than those with haematological malignancies.

Pathophysiology of cachexia

Whilst the clinical features of cachexia are readily apparent, its pathogenesis is complex and poorly understood. In contrast with starvation, which is characterised by pure caloric deficiency, cachexia additionally evokes the body's acute phase response. Simply augmenting caloric intake does not reverse the process. Under normal circumstances, starvation leads to an increase in appetite, sparing of lean mass and a decrease in metabolic rate [137]. In cachectic malnutrition, on the other hand, appetite is diminished, lean body mass is reduced and there is an increase in metabolic rate [138]. Again, loss of skeletal muscle cannot be attributed simply to decreased food intake [139]. The damage to muscle is characteristic: pale muscle fibres are affected more than red ones, and damage predominantly involves myofibrillar proteins [140]. At the same time, there is an increase in visceral protein synthesis [141]. The adenosine triphosphate–dependent ubiquitin–proteasome pathway is probably the major mediator of protein degradation in cachexia [141]. Several proinflammatory cytokines stimulate production of ubiquitin messenger RNA.

Several factors may influence changes in body composition, including the patient's gender. Women lose more fat than lean mass (85% vs. 15%), while men lose similar amounts of both [142].

A milestone in the understanding and management of cachexia was the recognition that it represents an endogenous *response* to illness and injury. Rather than a simple increase in energy consumption by the tumour, and reduced caloric intake by the patient, cachexia is currently perceived as a metabolic abnormality resulting from a combination of host cytokine release and tumour products [139].

The key hormone responsible for coordination of the homeostatic loop regulating body weight is leptin [143]. Secreted by adipose tissue, leptin controls food intake and energy expenditure via neuropeptidergic effector molecules within the hypothalamus.

Many cytokines participate as mediators in the cachectic process [144], including tumour necrosis factor-α (TNF-α) and interleukins 1 and 6 (IL-1 & IL-6). In addition to their immunologic and physiologic functions these proinflammatory cytokines exert a variety of behavioural and nutritional effects. They can also affect the bowel, causing altered gastric emptying, decreased intestinal blood flow, changes small bowel motility and cellular proliferation of the villi, and alterations in ion fluxes. All of these can in their turn affect the patient's nutritional status [144].

Cytokines may also play a pivotal role in suppressing appetite, by mimicking the hypothalamic effect of excessive negative feedback signalling from leptin [144]. This may result either from the persistent stimulation of anorexigenic neuropeptides, such as corticotropin-releasing factor (CRF), or from the inhibition of neuropeptide Y (NPY) orexigenic network [144]. Lipid and protein mobilizing factors (such as lipid mobilizing factors [LMF] and proteolysis-inducing factor [PIF]) produced by a tumour itself can also directly mobilise fatty and amino acids from adipose tissue and skeletal muscles, respectively [139]. This argues a role for brain serotoninergic system in the aetiology of cancer anorexia-cachexia syndrome.

Recent studies have revealed new biochemical pathways in regulation of body mass. Such research will hopefully identify molecular targets that can help in developing effective pharmacological interventions. Most are currently directed at obesity treatment, but therapies for anorexia-cachexia syndromes may also become possible [139,143].

Clinical consequences of cachexia

Cachexia can significantly compromise quality of life. It may contribute both to morbidity and mortality [139,143]. As patients with lose muscle mass, they become profoundly weak and tired, finding even the most basic activities difficult. It can alter social interaction; affecting self-image and the individual's 'role' in the family and society. Patients with cardiac or pulmonary insufficiency may develop cachexia in association with severe dyspnoea, weakness and exhaustion [144]. Cachexia may even influence response to curative therapy in cancer [145,146].

Management of cachexia

Cachexia, like all symptoms, does not occur in isolation but in a complex multi-dimensional context. Whilst there are often physical dysfunctions underpinning it, they are only part of the experience the child and family have to go through.

Ensuring that one's child is adequately fed is a primal drive. Watching a child choose not to eat, to lose weight and change in appearance is very distressing for parents. For the child, on the other hand, losing appetite may be a relatively insignificant issue but the accompanying changes in body image can be profound and disturbing. Management needs to consider not only the underlying physical basis but the response of the child and the family to it.

In managing cachexia, therapies that are effective may incidentally, and sometimes inappropriately, extend life [139,143]. Strategies that are currently under investigation include anabolic steroid and human growth hormone therapy, some appetite stimulants, nutritional supplementation, and more recently cytokine antagonists (Table 23.10). Some have shown early promise.

Hypercaloric diets

The ineffectiveness of simply increasing caloric intake partly defines cachexia (see above). Increasing calorie intake will not increase muscle mass [139,143] because protein degradation exceeds synthesis. Poor food intake and cachexia may, however, co-exist. A first step in managing cachexia is therefore to optimise feeding. This can be done by encouraging flexibility in the type, quantity and timing of meals. Families may need encouragement and permission to offer the child favourite foods that they may have previously considered to be unhealthy, such as hamburgers, crisps, chips and other 'fast food'.

Presentation of meals in an attractive manner can stimulate appetite. It is often easier to eat a complete meal if it is small, particularly when served on a small plate. This offers positive reinforcement to the child, who is enabled to finish the whole meal. Often a child who finds a normal sized meal intolerable can manage many small meals through the day. Again, families who have always had the traditional three meals a day may need 'permission' to offer instead smaller meals five or six times a day.

Table 23.10 Existing and potential therapies for cachexia

Existing therapies	Experimental therapies
Hypercaloric feeding	Cytokine inhibition
Appetite stimulants	Antisense therapy directed at
Megestrol acetate	nuclear factor-κ B
medroxyprogesterone	Anti-IL 6 receptor monoclonal
dronabinol	antibody
	Anti-TNF monoclonal antibody
	Soluble TNF receptor
Anabolic agents	
human recombinant	
growth hormone	
testosterone	
anabolic steroids	
Anti-inflammatory agents	Metabolic regulators
Resistance exercise training	Insulin-sensitizing agents
Omega-3 fatty acids	β-Adrenergic agonists
Cytokine inhibition	(clenbuterol)
Pentoxifylline	Lipoprotein lipase activators
thalidomide	(benzfibrate)
antioxidants	Serotonin type 3 receptor
melatonin	antagonists (ondansetron)
medroxyprogesterone	
megestrol acetate	
Δ-9-tetrahydrocannabinol	
L-carntiine	
human recombinant erythropoietin	

Factors that potentially suppress appetite, such as nausea, vomiting, constipation, pain, fatigue and taste changes may be modifiable and should be treated where possible [136].

Anorexia/cachexia and depression often co-exist. Each can be a cause of the other. Recognition of depression in childhood is very important and appropriate intervention (cross ref psych symptoms chapter ch 25 Hammel), including antidepressant drugs, can lead to an elevation of mood and improved appetite. Weight gain is side-effect associated with some psychoactive drugs, including antidepressants, anxiolytics and antipsychotics [137]. This is probably through a combination of actions, relieving the underlying condition, directly stimulating appetite centrally, and perhaps through the suppression of pro-inflammatory cytokine secretions [137].

Appetite stimulants

Appetite stimulants may increase caloric intake of some cachectic patients, especially in an outpatient ambulatory setting. Megestrol acetate (MA) and medroxy-progesterone acetate (MPA) have been found to improve appetite, caloric intake, and nutritional status [147–149]. The mechanism of action of progestational drugs is complex, and might be related to stimulation of NPY in the hypothalamus, modulation of calcium channels in the satiety centre and inhibition of the activity of proinflammatory cytokines. There are reports of adrenal insufficiency during megestrol therapy [150,151,152,153].

Appetite stimulation and weight gain are well-recognised effects of the use of marijuana and its derivatives. They are often familiar to those treating chemotherapy-induced nausea and vomiting in children, and are often accompanied by improvement in mood. The mechanism by which cannabinoids exert their effect is still under debate. It is probable that they act via endorphin receptors, by inhibiting prostaglandin synthesis and by inhibiting IL-1 secretion [139]. Recent studies suggest that endogenous cannabinoids are present in the hypothalamus, and may activate CB-1 receptors to maintain food intake, forming part of the leptin regulatory system [154].

Serotonin suppresses appetite when injected into the VMH of animals [155]. Cyproheptadine, which inhibits serotonin, may stimulate appetite in patients with advanced carcinoid tumours [156] as do ondansetron and other 5HT3 antagonists [139]. Although corticosterioids can stimulate appetite, prolonged treatment may lead to weakness, delirium, osteoporosis, and immunosuppression as well as serious disruption of body image [157] and they should not usually be considered for this indication.

Anabolic drugs

Most effective treatments for cachexia either promote protein synthesis or inhibit protein breakdown. Although controversial, the use of growth hormone and its analogues have been reported in patients of cachexia [158]. Growth hormone (GH) diverts protein synthesis towards lean mass and away from acute phase response. There is evidence that mortality rates are increased by the use of GH [145,159] perhaps as a result of its effect on the immune system [143] or on promoting tumour growth.

Testosterone and anabolic steroids can cause increases in fat-free mass in adults with non-malignant life limiting conditions [157]. The efficacy of anabolic steroids in adults with malignancy is still unclear [160] and there is no evidence in children.

Anticytokine therapies

In vitro studies have shown that inhibition of proinflammatory cytokine activity can decrease protein breakdown [139,143,144]. Many drugs exert anticytokine properties in vitro, including appetite stimulants megestrol acetate, medroxyprogesterone, and 9-tetrahydrocannabinols. Pentoxiphylline and thalidomide reduce TNF activity. Many of these agents have been shown to promote weight gain [161,162] but few have been studied in children [144,163,164].

Fluorinated pyrimidine nucleoside (5';-deoxy-5-fluorouridine: 5'-dFUrd; 5-FU precursor) attenuates progression of cachexia in mice bearing murine or human cancer cell lines. The mechanisms include inhibition of IL-6 and PIF [165]. Another potentially active substance is melatonin, a circadian neurohormone secreted by the pineal gland that decreases the level of circulating TNF-α in experimental animals [139,166].

Anti-inflammatories

Anti-inflammatory therapies may provide an alternative to anticytokines, since signal transduction may involve arachidonic acid metabolites. Addition of NSAIDs or steroids to other anti-cachectic therapies results in improvements in quality of life, inutritional status and exercise capacity in some adult cancer patients [167,168,169]. NSAIDs may have a particular role in non-malignant cachectic conditions, such as rheumatologic diseases.

A novel approach is based on anti-inflammatory activity of omega-3 fatty acids, which inhibit the production of IL-1 and TNF, and may improve the efficacy of nutritional support [139]. Other therapy that has been tried with some success is the administration of branched-chain amino acids (BCAA: leucine, isoleucine, and valine). They may serve as a protein-sparing metabolic 'fuel', providing substrate both for muscle metabolism and gluconeogenesis. Total parenteral nutrition enriched in BCAA has resulted in improved protein synthesis [170]. Anti-oxidants may limit protein losses in experimental cachexia models [143].

Emerging drugs and other therapies

As in so many areas of palliative care in children, many unproven measures have been tried. Some alternative medicine practitioners promote hydrazine sulphate. Hydrazine inhibits phosphoenol-pyruvate carboxykinase, a key enzyme in gluconeogenesis [139]. Efficacy has not been shown and neurotoxicity is a risk.

On the other hand, beta 2 adrenoceptor agonists such as salbutamol may suppress muscle breakdown through its action on the ubiquitin-dependent proteolytic system [139,143]. Polyunsaturated omega-3 fatty acids inhibit cachexia model and counteract lipid mobilizing and proteolysis-inducing factors. Two substances have been studied to date: eicosapentanoic acid (EPA) and docosahexaenoic acid (DHA). Inclusion of EPA in nutritional supplements may increase weight gain and lean body mass and lead to an improvement in performance status [171].

Autonomic failure with decreased gastrointestinal motility is a recognised complication of cancer cachexia, associated with anorexia, chronic nausea, early satiety, and constipation, further compromising caloric intake [172]. Prokinetic agents, such as metoclopramide, domperidone and erythromycin have been used in cancer patients with some success [139].

Novel approaches to cytokine inhibition are currently being evaluated [143]. They include an antisense therapy which binds to the promoter region of DNA and slows transcription of cytokine mRNA [173]; anti–interleukin-6 receptor antibodies [174]; anti-TNF antibodies [175]; and soluble TNF receptors [176]. The place of these therapies in palliative management is unclear.

Among metabolic regulators tested in preclinical studies, promising results have been obtained with antagonists of TNF [177]; the hypolipidaemic agent benzfibrate [178]; and a novel activator of tissue lipoprotein lipase [179].

Ethical issues in disturbed swallowing and food intake

Anorexia and marked weight loss are common in dying patients [180,181]. Malignancy in children is only one cause; they are also a feature of many progressive and debilitating diseases.

Evidence suggests that artificial hydration and nutrition, whether parenteral or by tube, neither prolong life nor increase the comfort of imminently dying patients [1,7,182–186]. Assisted feeding may indeed compromise the quality of life for some, and palliative care physicians often see the complications of too aggressive interventions to maintain food intake. They include abdominal discomfort, nausea and vomiting, difficult breathing and increased pulmonary secretions. Parenteral fluids delivered either intravenously or subcutaneously may have adverse effects that are not always considered [184,187]. Intravenous lines can be cumbersome and particularly painful; many patients are difficult to cannulate.

Conversely, starvation and dehydration may exert analgesic effects and reduce discomfort at death [180,181,186,187,188]. The only common discomfort associated with dehydration near death is xerostomia, which can usually be relieved with oral swabs or ice chips [188,187]. Many children refuse to eat just before death, and they should not be forced.

The right to forgo food and water, whether by mouth or by artificial means, derives from the fundamental right of competent patients to refuse medical treatment and to be free of unwanted bodily intrusion [188,189]. Force-feeding a competent patient who clearly refuses food and water violates autonomy, liberty, and dignity. Many ethicists have sought to blur the ethical distinction between introducing an intervention that will kill, and refraining from starting one that may prolong life. The distinction is a fundamental one in palliative

medicine. One of the logical consequences is the 'principle of double effect'. The principle argues that an intervention (or the withholding of an intervention) may not be morally wrong, even if it results in an outcome that is not desired. This remains true, argues the principle, even if the unintended consequence is foreseen.

The principle of double effect was articulated by Roman Catholic moral theologians in the Middle Ages, but derives from the basic ethical principle of justice. The principle has an ethical validity that is independent of religious framework.

In considering the withdrawal of feeding, the issue is one of weighing up the balance of benefit and burden to the patient. To withdraw fluids or feeding simply in order to shorten life would not be ethically justifiable. However, if the intention is to reduce the severity of some symptoms such as secretions, bloating, or nausea and vomiting, it can usually be justified. It is unusual for withdrawal of hydration or feeding to be the primary cause of death. Even on those rare occasions when it occurs, however, the principle of double effect would argue that if the intention was primarily to relieve symptoms, the fact that death was a foreseen outcome does not mean it was the intended one.

Despite research, myths about eating and drinking at the end of life persist among patients, their families, and many healthcare professionals. Those working with dying children can come under considerable pressure to initiate or to continue inappropriate hydration and/or feeding. The need to nourish ones child is a very basic one. A child's refusal, or even inability, to eat and drink is often perceived by parents to be a failure on their part to fulfil this basic role [1,27].

It can therefore be very difficult for parents to accept, but families should usually be counselled that neither food nor hydration is necessary to maintain a patient's comfort. They need to be reassured that, near the end of life, food will not increase the patient's strength nor will it substantially delay death. At the same time, families should be given concrete recommendations such as advice on positioning the patient, use of favourite foods, small portions of simple meals and foods that are easy to swallow. Children who find it difficult to swallow may, for example, prefer milk puddings, fruit yoghurts or cottage cheese preparations and similar simple meals. Pieces of fruit frozen so that they can be sucked to moisten the mouth may help. Pineapple is a traditional recommendation for this, but individual patients may prefer apples, pears, oranges and bananas.

Xerostomia is one of the few adverse effects of not providing artificial hydration. It can be relieved using artificial saliva spray, petroleum jelly on the lips and careful oral hygiene. Once again, these interventions can involve the family and enable them to feel, rightly, that they are caring for the child even without needing artificial hydration or feeding.

For some families, the symbolic emotional meaning of artificial fluids or nutrition is so important to the family (or indeed the patient, or even health care professionals) that they become inescapable. It may then be necessary to modify the rates in order to avoid some of the adverse effects. For example, 50% or two-thirds maintenance will usually be enough hydration and may reduce the risk of excess secretions.

Inability to swallow

Inability to swallow can create a number of medical problems, among them the high risk of aspiration. Feeding may nevertheless be considered appropriate in children unable to swallow who are expected to survive more then 7–14 days, when there is a true hunger and thirst in the setting of a functional gut. Thus, nasogastric tubes or gastrostomies should be limited to patients who are able to benefit from nutrition as well as hydration. In general, enteral feeding is preferred to parenteral options [1,27,190,191].

In general nasogastric tubes (NGT) are useful only in the short term. Potential complications make them inadvisable for periods longer than 2–3 weeks. The useful life of some silicone NGTs can be extended beyond this [192]. Complications of NGT include aspiration pneumonia or mechanical difficulties (occluded or clogged tube, nasal irritation or erosion, sinusitis and epistaxis, tube displacement). Any tube which traverses the gastro-oesophageal junction promotes GORD.

Direct enteral access is preferred when feeding extends beyond 30 days [192,193]. Children may benefit from a gastrostomy for feeding or administering medications, to decompress the stomach, or both. The choice of access route—gastrostomy, gastrojejunostomy, or jejunostomy—and the choice of placement technique—surgical, endoscopic, or radiologic—depend on the needs of the individual patient [194].

Percutaneous endoscopic gastrostomy

Introduction of percutaneous endoscopic gastrostomy (PEG) into clinical practice has radically changed the approach to gastrostomy access. This minimally invasive procedure has largely replaced surgical gastrostomy [195]. Endoscopic gastrojejunostomy and direct endoscopic jejunostomy have also been used, [196]. Gastrostomy tubes may still predispose to gastro-oesophageal reflux and many patients are at risk of aspiration [196–199].

Uncorrectable coagulopathy and the absence of a safe access route are considered contraindications [195]. Nissen fundoplication or a similar procedure may be helpful if reflux is shown in preoperative studies and is often performed simultaneously to minimise the number of anaesthetics. Complications of PEG (Table 23.11) are infrequent [194–207] but can include wound infection, peritonitis, septicaemia, peristomal leakage, tube dislodgement, aspiration, bowel perforation, and gastrocolic fistula. Pneumoperitoneum after PEG is usually of no significance, unless of course accompanied by peritonitis. Dislodged tubes can often be replaced without imaging guidance. External rings or fasteners, and intraluminal balloons or special clips may be useful in preventing the exit of gastric contents, and development of cellulitis, erythema and tenderness around the catheter. Muscle atrophy, severe spasticity and obesity increase the risk of such problems. They often resolve rapidly with local antiseptic wound care.

Table 23.11 Complications of gastrostomy

Early	Later	
	Local	General
Haemorrhage	Site leakage and skin irritation	Overfeeding and obesity
Bowel perforation	Superficial skin infection	Vomiting
Peritonitis	Accidental device removal	Diarrhoea
Wound separation	Formation of granulomatous tissue	Gastrooesophageal reflux
Local or generalized infection	Discomfort	Aspiration
Adhesive bowel obstruction	Internal tube migration causing erosiohns or obstructions	Oral aversion
		Generalised infection or peritonitis

Diarrhoea

Persistent chronic diarrhoea is rare in children dying from most life-limiting diseases [27,45,208]. It commonly complicates *immunodeficiency*, particularly in HIV/AIDS (cross ref. HIV AIDs, chapter 32. Norval) [27]. Villous atrophy due to immune-mediated HIV enteropathy and necrotizing enterocolitis resulting from chronic intestinal infections is a common gastroenterological complication of late HIV infection. The treatment of HIV-related diarrhoea consists of specific antimicrobial, fungicidal and antiparasitic drug regimens. These are combined with cholestyramine (colestyramine) to absorb toxins. Antimotility agents are not indicated routinely for infectious diarrhoea, except for refractory cases of Cryptosporidium infection. Racecadotril, an oral enkephalinase inhibitor, is safe and has been successfully used in the treatment of acute diarrhoea of infectious origin, but especially in patients with HIV infection [209].

Pancreatic exocrine deficiency is another cause of chronic diarrhoea. Poor dietary control and inadequate supplementation of pancreatic enzymes during the course of cystic fibrosis and other rare hereditary disorders can result in diarrhoea in the terminal phase of disease.

In cancer patients severe polymucositis and diarrhoea often complicate high dose chemotherapy and occasionally radiotherapy.

The management of diarrhoea should usually be tailored to the underlying cause. It is often self-limiting. Opioids such as codeine and loperamide may be effective. For high output diarrhoea, octreotide may have a role. Ocreotide is a synthetic analogue of somatostatin which increases fluid resorption from the bowel. It is given subcutaneously, either as a bolus or as an infusion. The dosage range is usually between 60 and 1200 μg depending on the size of the child.

Closing remarks

Children deserve the best of care at all times, but perhaps especially at the end of life. The experience of palliative team members suggests that greater attention to symptom control and the overall well being of children with advanced disease can ease their suffering. The care of children at the end of life is gradually improving. Nevertheless, more than half suffer from intractable symptoms before dying.

Gastrointestinal symptoms are among the most common problems of terminal illness. The range of problems includes dysphagia, nausea, vomiting, anorexia, cachexia, constipation, diarrhoea and bowel obstruction. GI issues are a major chronic problem in 80 to 90% of with neurodevelopmental disabilities who represent the growing population among children required palliative care [35]. Many different malignancies and other intractable and/or chronic diseases can give rise to gastrointestinal dysfunction and specific symptoms needing appropriate pharmacological, surgical or complementary management. Beside the basic principles and pathophysiology of symptoms, some new drugs and innovative endoscopic and surgical techniques in the management of gastrointestinal symptoms have also been presented in the chapter.

It should be of some concern to the paediatric palliative care specialist that many currently available therapies have been introduced into every day practice without well-documented evidence concerning their efficacy and safety in children. Many—perhaps most—drugs are administered according to a regimen that is simply extrapolated from practice in adults. In reality, although the principles of palliative care apply equally to children and adult patients, a number of fundamental differences influence their application in the paediatric population. Palliative medicine has developed as a specialised field of practice in recent decades, but the focus has until recently been very much on adults with incurable malignancies. The issues in children are fundamentally different; they include a heterogeneous patient population, pathophysiological factors and developmental issues. Children are not little adults; their immaturity, developing cognition and dependence on caregivers all influence the diagnosis and multidimensional management of symptoms.

The paediatric palliative care team gives professional medical care, and provides sophisticated symptom relief. When evidence is lacking, an empirical approach is often necessary and appropriate. There is still a lack of specialised knowledge concerning the population of children dying from chronic, progressive diseases. Further research is needed to increase the evidence base for practice. Recent concerns over toxic effects of drugs in newborns, infants and children have stressed the need for better knowledge of drug kinetics during development. Children with life-limiting problems need a systematic and comprehensive approach if we are to ensure that their particular needs are met.

The management of gastrointestinal symptoms in dying children illustrates very well many of the principles that should underlie good symptom management. Treatment should be evidence-based where possible and empirical where necessary. The benefit to the patient of an intervention should always be expected to outweigh the burden before it is introduced. The ethical issues around withdrawing or withholding hydration or nutrition, for example, are often finely balanced. However, a clear understanding of the ethical principles involved, and in particular of the principle of double effect, will usually enable professionals to put the individual child's needs first, without putting themselves in ethical peril.

References

1. Goldman, A. *Care of the Dying Child* (Reprint with revisions), Oxford: Oxford University Press, 1998.

2. Goldman, A., Beardsmore, S., and Hunt, J. Palliative care for children with cancer—home, hospital, or hospice? *Arch Dis Child* 1990; 65(6):641–3.

3. Liben, S. and Goldman, A. Home care for children with life-threatening illness. *J Palliat Care* 1998;14(3):33–8.

4. Goldman, A. Home care of the dying child. *J Palliat Care* 1996; 12(3):16–9.

5. Goldman, A. Palliative care for children. *Palliat Med* 1995;9(3): 179–80.

6. Liben, S. Palliative care for children: is it really needed? *Am J Hosp Palliat Care* 2000;17(5):294–5.

7. Liben, S. Pediatric palliative medicine: Obstacles to overcome. *J Palliat Care* 1996;12(3):24–8.

8. Goldman, A. Recent advances in palliative care. Importance of palliative care for children is being increasingly recognised. *BMJ* 2001;322(7280):234.

9. Goldman, A. ABC of palliative care. Special problems of children. *BMJ* 1998;316(7124):49–52.

10. Afzal, N., Murch, S., Thirrupathy, K., Berger, L., Fagbemi A., and Heuschkel R. Constipation with acquired megarectum in children with autism. *Pediatrics* 2003;112(4):939–42.

11. Field, D., Garland, M., and Williams, K. Correlates of specific childhood feeding problems. *J Paediatr Child Health* 2003;39(4): 299–304.

12. Sullivan, P.B., Lambert, B., Rose, M., Ford-Adams, M., Johnson, A., and Griffiths P. Prevalence and severity of feeding and nutritional problems in children with neurological impairment: Oxford Feeding Study. *Dev Med Child Neurol* 2001;43(5):358.

13. Leslie, R.A. Reynolds, DJM Neurotransmitters and receptors in the emetic pathway. In P.L.R., Andrews and G.J. Sanger, eds. *Emesis in Anti-cancer Treatment: Mechanisms and Treatment* London: Chapman & Hall Medical 1993, pp. 91–112.

14. Mannix, K.A. Palliation of nausea and vomiting. In D. Doyle, G.W.C. Hanks, N., and MacDonald eds. *Oxford Textbook of Palliative Medicine* (2nd edition), Oxford: Oxford University Press, 1998.

15. Baines, M.J. ABC of palliative care: Nausea, vomiting, and intestinal obstruction. *BMJ* 1997;315:1148–50.

16. Herndon C.M., Jackson KCII, and Hallin P.A. Management of opioid-induced gastrointestinal effects in patients receiving palliative care *Pharmacotherapy* 2002;22(2):240–50.

17. Olver, I.N., Matthews, J.P., Bishop, J.F., and Smith, R.A. The roles of patient and observer assessments in anti-emetic trials. *Eur J Cancer* 1994;30A(9):1223–7.

18. Passik, S.D., Lundberg J., Kirsh, K.L., Theobald, D., Donaghy K., Holtsclaw, E., Cooper, M., and Dugan W. A pilot exploration of the antiemetic activity of olanzapine for the relief of nausea in patients with advanced cancer and pain. *J Pain Symptom Manage* 2002;23(6):526–32.

19. Walton, S.M., Advances in use of the 5-HT3 receptor antagonists. *Expert Opin Pharmacother* 2000;1(2):207–23.

20. Hubbard, J.R., Franco, S.E., and Onaivi, E.S. Marijuana: Medical implications. *Am Fam Physician* 1999;60: 2583–93.

21. Darmani, N.A., Sim-Selley, L.J., Martin B.R., Janoyan J.J., Crim, J.L., Parekh, B., and Breivogel, C.S. Antiemetic and motor-depressive actions of CP55,940: cannabinoid CB1 receptor characterization, distribution, and G-protein activation. *Eur J Pharmacol* 2003; 459(1):83–95.

22. Van Sickle M.D., Oland, L.D., Ho, W., Hillard C.J., Mackie, K., Davison, J.S., and Sharkey, K.A. Cannabinoids inhibit emesis through CB1 receptors in the brainstem of the ferret. *Gastroenterology* 2001; 121(4): 767–74.

23. Hall, W., Degenhardt L. Medical marijuana initiatives: are they justified? How successful are they likely to be? *CNS Drugs* 2003; 17(10):689–97.

24. Davis M.P. and Nouneh C. Modern management of cancer-related intestinal obstruction. *Curr Pain Headache Rep* 2001;5(3):257–64.

25. Mitchelson, F. Pharmacological agents affecting emesis: A review (part I). *Drugs* 1992;43:295–315.

26. Levetown, M. Treatment of symptoms other than pain in pediatric palliative care. In R.K. and Portenoy, E. Bruera eds: *Topics in Palliative Care*, Vol. 3, New York, Oxford University Press, 1998;51–69.

27. Redd, W.H. Behavioral intervention for cancer treatment side effects. *Acta Oncologica* 1994;33:113–6,

28. Vickers, A.J. Can acupuncture have specific effects on health? A systematic review of acupuncture antiemesis trials. *J R Soc Med* 1996;89:303–11.

29. Hogan, C.M. Nausea and vomiting. In J Yasko, ed: Nursing management of symptoms associated with chemotherapy (3rd edition) Philadelphia PA: Meniscus, 1993, pp. 89–108.

30. Baker, S.S., Liptak, G.S., Colletti, R.B., Croffie, J.M., Di Lorenzo, C., Ector, W., and Nurko S. Constipation in infants and children: Evaluation and treatment. A medical position statement of the North American Society for Pediatric Gastroenterology and Nutrition. *J Pediatr Gastroenterol Nutr* 1999;29(5):612–26.

31. Di Lorenzo, C. Childhood constipation: finally some hard data about hard stools! *J Pediatr* 2000;136(1):4–7.

32. Youssef, N.N. and Di Lorenzo C. Childhood constipation: evaluation and treatment. *J Clin Gastroenterol* 2001;33(3):199–205.

33. Chong, S.K. Gastrointestinal problems in the handicapped child. *Curr Opin Pediatr* 2001;13(5):441–6.

34. Goetz, L.L., Hurvitz E.A., and Nelson, V.S. Waring W III: Bowel management in children and adolescents with spinal cord injury. *J Spinal Cord* Med 1998;21(4):335–41.

35. Bohmer, C.J., Taminiau J.A., Klinkenberg-Knol E.C., and Meuwissen S.G. The prevalence of constipation in institutionalised people with intellectual disability. *J Intellect Disabil Res* 2001;45(Pt 3):212–8.

36. Lembo, A. and Camilleri, M. Chronic constipation. *N Engl J Med* 2003;349(14):1360–8.

37. Tzavella, K., Riepl, R.L., Klauser, A.G., Voderholzer W.A., Schindlbeck, N.E., and Muller-Lissner, S.A. Decreased substance P levels in rectal biopsies from patients with slow transit constipation. *Eur J Gastroenterol Hepatol* 1996;8:1207–11.

38. Cortesini, C., Cianchi, F., Infantino A., and Lise, M. Nitric oxide synthase and VIP distribution in enteric nervous system in idiopathic chronic constipation. *Dig Dis Sci* 1995;40:2450–55.

39. He, C.L., Soffer, E.E., Ferris, C.D., Walsh, R.M., and Szurszewski, J.H., Farrugia G. Loss of interstitial cells of cajal and inhibitory innervation in insulin-dependent diabetes. *Gastroenterology* 2001;121(2):427–34.

40. Bassotti, G., Chiarioni, G., Imbimbo, BP, Betti, C, Bonfante F, Vantini, I., Morelli, A., and Whitehead W.E. Impaired colonic motor response to cholinergic stimulation in patients with severe chronic idiopathic (slow transit type) constipation. *Dig Dis Sci* 1993;38(6):1040–5.

41. Doig, C.M. ABC of colorectal diseases: Paediatric problems. *BMJ* 1992;305:462–4.

42. Loening-Baucke, V. Encopresis and soiling. *Pediatr Clin North Am* 1996;43:279–98.

43. Sykes, N.P. Constipation and diarrhoea. In D. Doyle G.W.C., Hanks N. MacDonald ed. *Oxford Textbook of Palliative Medicine* (2nd edition), Oxford: Oxford University Press, 1998.

44. Schiller, L.R. Clinical pharmacology and use of laxatives and lavage solutions. *J Clin Gastroenterol* 1999;28(1):11–18.

45. Fallon, M. and O'Neill B. ABC of palliative care. Constipation and diarrhoea. *BMJ* 1997;315(7118):1293–6.

46. Pappagallo, M. Incidence, prevalence, and management of opioid bowel dysfunction. *Am J Surg* 2001;182(5A Suppl):11S–18S.

47. Tiongco, F., Tsang, T., and Pollack, J. Use of oral GoLytely solution in relief of refractory faecal impaction. *Dig Dis Sci* 1997; 42:1454–7.

48. Wald, A. Slow transit constipation. *Curr Treat Options Gastroenterol* 2002;5(4):279–83.

49. Weed H.G. Lactulose vs sorbitol for treatment of obstipation in hospice programs. *Mayo Clin Proc* 2000;75(5):541.

50. Agra, Y., Sacristan, A., Gonzalez, M., Ferrari, M., Portugues, A., and Calvo, M.J. Efficacy of senna versus lactulose in terminal cancer patients treated with opioids. *J Pain Symptom Manage* 1998;15(1):1–7.

51. Soffer, E.E., Metcalf, A., and Launspach J. Misoprostol is effective treatment for patients with severe chronic constipation. *Dig Dis Sci* 1994;39:929–33.

52. Nurko, S., Garcia-Aranda J.A., and Worona L.B., and Zlochisty O. Cisapride for the treatment of constipation in children: A double-blind study. *J Pediatr* 2000;136(1):35–40.

53. Verne, G.N., Eaker, E.Y., Davis, R.H., and Sninsky C.A. Colchicine is an effective treatment for patients with chronic constipation: An open-label trial. *Dig Dis Sci* 1997;42:1959–63.

54. Bassotti, G., Chiarioni, G., Vantini, I., Morelli, A., and Whitehead, W.E. Effect of different doses of erythromycin on colonic motility in patients with slow transit constipation. *Z Gastroenterol* 1998;36(3): 209–13.

55. Bellomo-Brand o M.A., Collares E.F., and Da-Costa-Pinto E.A. Use of erythromycin for the treatment of severe chronic constipation in children. *Braz J Med Biol Res* 2003;36(10):1391–6.

56. Rivkin, A. Tegaserod maleate in the treatment of irritable bowel syndrome: A clinical review. *Clin Ther* 2003;25(7):1952–74.

57. Davis, M.P., Nouneh C Modern management of cancer-related intestinal obstruction. *Curr Pain Headache Rep* 2001;5(3): 257–64.

58. Parkman, H.P., Rao, S.S., Reynolds, J.C., Schiller L.R., Wald, A., Miner, P.B., Lembo, A.J., Gordon, J.M., Drossman, D.A., Waltzman, L., Stambler, N., and Cedarbaum, J.M. Functional Constipation Study Investigators.: Neurotrophin-3 improves functional constipation. *Am J Gastroenterol* 2003;98(6):1338–47.

59. Ciamarra, P., Nurko, S., Barksdale, E., Fishman, S., and Di Lorenzo, C. Internal anal sphincter achalasia in children: clinical characteristics and treatment with Clostridium botulinum toxin. *J Pediatr Gastroenterol Nutr* 2003;37(3):315–9.

60. Jorge, J.M., Habr-Gama, A., and Wexner, S.D. Biofeedback therapy in the colon and rectal practice. *Appl Psychophysiol Biofeedback* 2003; 28(1):47–61.

61. Luca, A.D. Coupar, I.M. Insights into opioid action in the intestinal tract. *Pharmacol Ther* 1996;69:103–15.

62. Kromer, W. Endogenous opioids, the enteric nervous system and gut motility. *Dig Dis* 1990;8:361–73.

63. Fox-Threlkeld, J.E., Daniel, E.E., Christinck, F., Hruby, V.J., Cipris, S., and Woskowska, Z. Identification of mechanisms and sites of actions of mu and delta opioid receptor activation in the canine intestine. *J Pharmacol Exp Ther* 1994;268:689–700.

64. Maurer, A.H., Krevsky, B., Knight, L.C., and Brown, K. Opioid and opioid-like drug effects on whole-gut transit measured by scintigraphy. *J Nucl Med* 1996;37:818–22.

65. Thorpe, D.M. Management of opioid-induced constipation *Curr Pain Headache Rep* 2001;5(3):237–40.

66. Cherny, N., Ripamonti, C., Pereira, J., Davis, C., Fallon, M., McQuay, H., Mercadante, S., Pasternak, G., and Ventafridda, V. Expert Working Group of the European Association of Palliative Care Network. Strategies to manage the adverse effects of oral morphine: an evidence-based report. *J Clin Oncol* 2001;19(9):2542–54

67. Sykes N.P. The relationship between opioid use and laxative use in terminally ill cancer patients. *Palliat Med* 1998;12(5):375–82.

68. Radbruch, L., Sabatowski, R., Loick, G., Kulbe, C., Kasper, M., Grond, S., and Lehmann, K.A. Constipation and the use of laxatives: A comparison between transdermal fentanyl and oral morphine. *Palliat Med* 2000;14(2):111–9.

69. Fox-Threlkeld, J.E., Daniel, E.E., Christinck F., Hruby, V.J., Cipris, S., and Woskowska, Z. Identification of mechanisms and sites of actions of mu and delta opioid receptor activation in the canine intestine. *J Pharmacol Exp Ther* 1994;268:689–700.

70. Kurz, A. Sessler, D.I. Opioid-induced bowel dysfunction: Pathophysiology and potential new therapies. *Drugs* 2003;63(7): 649–71.

71. Choi, Y.S. and Billings, J.A. Opioid antagonists: A review of their role in palliative care, focusing on use in opioid-related constipation. *J Pain Symptom Manage* 2002;24(1):71–90.

72. Hawkes, N.D., Rhodes, J., Evans, B.K., Rhodes, P., Hawthorne, A.B., Thomas G.A. Naloxone treatment for irritable bowel syndrome — a randomised controlled trial with an oral formulation. *Aliment Pharmacol Ther* 2002;16(9):1649–54.

73. Liu, M. and Wittbrodt, E. Low-dose oral naloxone reverses opioid-induced constipation and analgesia. *J Pain Symptom Manage* 2002;23(1):48–53.

74. Stephenson, J. Methylnaltrexone reverses opioid-induced constipation. *Lancet Oncol* 2002;3(4):202.

75. Foss, J.F. A review of the potential role of methylnaltrexone in opioid bowel dysfunction. *Am J Surg* 2001;182(5A Suppl):19S–26S.

76. Yuan, C.S., Foss, J.F., O'Connor, M., Osinski, J., Karrison, T., Moss, J., and Roisen M.F. Methylnaltrexone for reversal of constipation due to chronic methadone use: a randomised controlled trial. *JAMA* 2000;283(3):367–72.

77. McNicol, E., Horowicz-Mehler N., Fisk R.A., Bennett, K., Gialeli-Goudas, M., Chew, PW., Lau, J., and Carr D American Pain Society. Management of opioid side effects in cancer-related and chronic noncancer pain: A systematic review. *J Pain* 2003;4(5):231–56.

78. Borowitz, S.M., Cox, D.J., Tam, A., Ritterband, L.M., Sutphen, J.L., and Penberthy, J.K. Precipitants of constipation during early childhood. *J Am Board Fam Pract* 2003;16(3):213–8.

79. Iacono, G., Cavataio, F., Montalto, G., Florena, A., Tumminello, M., Soresi, M., Notarbartolo, A., and Carroccio, A. Intolerance of cow's milk and chronic constipation in children. *N Engl J Med* 1998; 339(16):1100–4.

80. Roy, A. and Simon, G.B. Intestinal obstruction as a cause of death in the mentally handicapped. *J Ment Defic Res* 1987;31(Pt 2):193–7.

81. Betz, P., van Meyer, L., and Eisenmenger, W. Fatalities due to intestinal obstruction following the ingestion of foreign bodies. *Forensic Sci Int* 1994;69(2):105–10.

82. Jancar, J. and Speller, C.J. Fatal intestinal obstruction in the mentally handicapped. *J Intellect Disabil Res* 1994;38(Pt 4):413–22.

83. Dean A. The palliative effects of octreotide in cancer patients. *Chemotherapy* 2001;47 Suppl 2:54–61.

84. Mystakidou, K., Tsilika, E., Kalaidopoulou, O., Chondros, K., Georgaki, S., and Papadimitriou, L. Comparison of octreotide administration vs conservative treatment in the management of inoperable bowel obstruction in patients with far advanced cancer: a randomised, double- blind, controlled clinical trial. *Anticancer Res* 2002;22(2B):1187–92.

85. Di Lorenzo, C., Lucanto, C., Flores, A.F., Idries, S., and Hyman, P.E. Effect of octreotide on gastrointestinal motility in children with functional gastrointestinal symptoms. *J Pediatr Gastroenterol Nutr.* 1998;27(5):508–12.

86. Blasco, P.A. and Allaire, J.H. Sialorrhoea in the developmentally disabled: management practices and recommendations. Consortium on Sialorrhoea. *Dev Med Child Neurol* 1992;34(10):849–62.

87. Tahmassebi, J.F. and Curzon M.E. Prevalence of drooling in children with cerebral palsy attending special schools. *Dev Med Child Neurol* 2003;45(9):613–7.

88. Nunn, J.H. Drooling: Review of the literature and proposals for management. *J Oral Rehabil* 2000;27(9):735–43.

89. Tahmassebi, J.F. and Curzon, M.E. The cause of drooling in children with cerebral palsy—hypersalivation or swallowing defect? *Int J Paediatr Dent* 2003;13(2):106–11.

90. Tscheng, D.Z. Sialorrhea—therapeutic drug options. *Ann Pharmacother* 2002;36(11):1785–90.

91. Blasco, P.A. Management of sialorrhoea: 10 years after the Consortium on Sialorrhoea. *Dev Med Child Neurol* 2002;44: 778–81.

92. Lloyd Faulconbridge, R.V., Tranter, R.M., Moffat, V., and Green, E. Review of management of sialorrhoea problems in neurologically impaired children: A review of methods and results over 6 years at Chailey Heritage Clinical Services. *Clin Otolaryngol* 2001;26:76–81.

93. Mankarious, L.A., Bottrill, I.D., Huchzermeyer, P.M., and Bailey, C.M. Long-term follow-up of submandibular duct rerouting for the treatment of sialorrhea in the pediatric population. *Otolaryngol Head Neck Surg* 1999;120(3):303–7.

94. Duchateau, J., Heenen, M., and Sternon J. Les antihistaminiques H1.*Rev Med Brux* 2003;24(2):95–100.

95. Gwaltney, JM Jr, Winther B., Patrie, J.T., and Hendley, JO. Combined antiviral-antimediator treatment for the common cold. *J Infect Dis* 2002;186(2):147–54.

96. Zeppetella, G. Nebulised scopolamine in the management of oral dribbling: Three case reports. *J Pain Symptom Manage* 1999; 17(4):293–5.

97. Lewis, D.W., Fontana, C., Mehallick, L.K., and Everett, Y. Transdermal scopolamine for reduction of sialorrhoea in developmentally delayed children. *Dev Med Child Neurol* 1994;36(6):484–6.

98. Zeppetella, G. Nebulised scopolamine in the management of oral dribbling: three case reports. *J Pain Symptom Manage* 1999; 17(4):293–5.

99. Brei, T.J. Management of drooling. *Semin Pediatr Neurol* 2003; 10(4):265–70.

100. Strutt, R., Fardell, B., and Chye, R. Nebulised glycopyrrolate for drooling in a motor neuron patient. *J Pain Symptom Manage* 2002;23(1):2–3.

101. Mier, R.J., Bachrach, S.J., Lakin, R.C., Barker, T., Childs, J., and Moran, M. Treatment of sialorrhea with glycopyrrolate: A double-blind, dose-ranging study. *Arch Pediatr Adolesc Med* 2000;154(12): 121–48.

102. Bachrach, S.J., Walter R.S., and Trzcinski, K. Use of glycopyrrolate and other anticholinergic medications for sialorrhea in children with cerebral palsy. *Clin Pediatr (Phila)* 1998;37(8):485–90.

103. Ellies, M., Laskawi, R., Rohrbach-Volland, S., and Arglebe, C. Up-to-date report of botulinum toxin therapy in patients with sialorrhoea caused by different etiologies. *J Oral Maxillofac Surg* 2003; 61(4):454–7.

104. Ellies, M., Rohrbach-Volland, S., Arglebe, C., Wilken, B, Laskawi, R., and Hanefeld, F. Successful management of sialorrhoea with botulinum toxin A in neurologically disabled children. *Neuropediatrics* 2002;33(6):327–30.

105. Jongerius, P.H., Rotteveel, J.J., van den Hoogen, F., Joosten, F., van Hulst, K., and Gabreels, F.J. Botulinum toxin A: A new option for treatment of sialorrhoea in children with cerebral palsy. Presentation of a case series. *Eur J Pediatr* 2001;160(8):509–512.

106. Bothwell, J.E., Clarke, K., Dooley, J.M., Gordon, K.E., Anderson, R., Wood, E.P., Camfield, C.S., and Camfield P.R. Botulinum toxin A as a treatment for excessive sialorrhoea in children. *Pediatr Neurol* 2002;27(1):18–22.

107. Jongerius P.H., Joosten F., Hoogen F.J., Gabreels F.J., and Rotteveel J.J. The treatment of sialorrhoea by ultrasound-guided intraglandular injections of botulinum toxin type A into the salivary glands. *Laryngoscope* 2003;113(1):107–11.

108. Tan E.K., Lo Y.L., Seah A., and Auchus A.P. Recurrent jaw dislocation after botulinum toxin treatment for sialorrhoea in amyotrophic lateral sclerosis. *J Neurol Sci* 2001;190(1–2):95–7.

109. Hoon A.H. Jr., Freese PO., Reinhardt E.M., Wilson M.A., Lawrie WT Jr., Harryman S.E., Pidcock F.S., and Johnston M.V. Age-dependent effects of trihexyphenidyl in extrapyramidal cerebral palsy. *Pediatr Neurol* 2001;25(1):55–8.

110. Reddihough D., Johnson H., Staples M., Hudson I., and Exarchos H. Use of benzhexol hydrochloride to control sialorrhoea of children with cerebral palsy. *Dev Med Child Neurol* 1990;32(11):985–9.

111. Arglebe C., Eysholdt U., and Chilla R. Pharmacological inhibition of salivary glands: a possible therapy for sialosis and sialoadenitis. Effect of experimentally induced beta-receptor block on the rat parotid gland. *ORL J Otorhinolaryngol Relat Spec* 1976;38(4): 218–29.

112. Muether P.S. and Gwaltney J.M. Jr. Variant effect of first- and second-generation antihistamines as clues to their mechanism of action on the sneeze reflex in the common cold. *Clin Infect Dis* 2001;33(9):1483–8.

113. Peggs, J.F. and Shimp L.A. Opdycke R.A. Antihistamines: The old and the new. *Am Fam Physician* 1995;52:593–600.

114. Wilkie TF. The problem of sialorrhoea in cerebral palsy: A surgical approach. *Can J Surg* 1967;10(1):60–7.

115. Crysdale, W.S., Raveh E., McCann C., Roske L., and Kotler A. Management of sialorrhoea in individuals with neurodisability: a surgical experience. *Dev Med and Child Neurol*, 2001;43:379–83.

116. O'Dwyer, T.P. and Conlon B.J. The surgical management of sialorrhoea—a 15 year follow-up. *Clin Otolaryngol* 1997;22:284–87.

117. Shirley, W.P., Hill, J.S., Woolley, A.L., Wiatrak, B.J. Success and complications of four-duct ligation for sialorrhea. *Int J Pediatr Otorhinolaryngol* 2003;67(1):1–6.

118. Harriman, M., Morrison, M., Hay J., Revonta, M., Eisen, A., and Lentle B. Use of radiotherapy for control of sialorrhea in patients with amyotrophic lateral sclerosis. *J Otolaryngol* 2001;30:242–245.

119. Askenasy, J.J.M. About the mechanism of hiccup. *Eur Neurol* 1992;32:159–63.

120. Straus, C., Vasilakos, K., Wilson, R.J., Oshima, T., Zelter, M., Derenne, J.P., Similowski, T., and Whitelaw W.A. A phylogenetic hypothesis for the origin of hiccup. *Bioessays* 2003;25(2):182–8.

121. Federspil P.A., and Zenk J. Hiccup. *HNO* 1999;47(10):867–75.

122. Dickerman, R.D., Overby C., Eisenberg M. Hollis P., and Levine M. The steroid-responsive hiccup reflex arc: competitive binding to the corticosteroid-receptor? *Neuroendocrinol Lett* 2003;24(3–4):167–9.

123. Smith, H.S., Busracamwongs A. Management of hiccups in the palliative care population. *Am J Hosp Palliat Care* 2003;20(2):149–54.

124. Howard, R.S. and Charmers R.M. Causes and treatment of persistent hiccups. *Natl Med J India* 1996;9(3):104–6.

125. Friedman, N.L. Hiccups: A treatment review. *Pharmacotherapy* 1996;16(6):986–95.

126. Guelaud, C., Similowski T., Bisec J.L., Cabane J., Whitelaw W.A, and Derenne J.P. Baclofen therapy for chronic hiccup. *Eur Respir J* 1995;8(2):235–7.

127. Twycross, R. Baclofen for hiccups. *Am J Hosp Palliat Care* 2003;20(4):262.

128. Petroianu G., Hein G., Stegmeier-Petroianu A., Bergler W., and Rufer R. Gabapentin 'add-on therapy' for idiopathic chronic hiccup (ICH). *J Clin Gastroenterol* 2000;30(3):321–4.

129. Petroianu, G., Hein G., Petroianu A., Bergler W., and Rufer, R. Idiopathic chronic hiccup: Combination therapy with cisapride, omeprazole, and baclofen. *Clin Ther* 1997;19(5):1031–8.

130. Petroianu, G., Hein G., Petroianu A., Bergler W., and Rufer, R. ETICS-Studie: Empirische Therapie des idiopathischen chronischen Hiccup (ICS). [*ETICS Study: Empirical therapy of idiopathic chronic hiccup*] *Z Gastroenterol* 1998;36(7):559–66.

131. Cohen, S.P., and Lubin E., Stojanovic M. Intravenous lidocaine in the treatment of hiccup. *South Med J* 2001;94(11):1124–5.

132. Marhofer, P., Glaser C., Krenn C.G., Grabner C.M., and Semsroth M. Incidence and therapy of midazolam induced hiccups in paediatric anaesthesia. *Paediatr Anaesth* 1999;9(4):295–8.

133. Thompson, D.F., Landry J.P. Drug-induced hiccups. *Ann Pharmacother* 1997;31(3):367–9.

134. Calvo E., Fernandez-La Torre F, and Brugarolas A. Cervical phrenic nerve block for intractable hiccups in cancer patients. *J Natl Cancer Inst* 2002;94(15):1175–6.

135. Bruera, E. Anorexia, cachexia and nutrition. *Br Med J* 1997;315:1219–1222.

136. Plata-Salaman, C. R. Anorexia during acute and chronic disease. *Nutrition*, 1996;12: 67–78.

137. Schwartz, M.W. and Seeley R.J. Neuroendocrine responses to starvation and weight loss. *N Engl J Med* 1997;336:1802–1811.

138. Inui, A. Cancer anorexia-cachexia syndrome: Current issues in research and management. *CA Cancer J Clin* 2002;52(2):72–91.

139. Tisdale, M.J. Cancer anorexia and cachexia. *Nutrition* 2001;17:438–442.

140. Mitch, W.E., and Goldberg A.L. Mechanisms of muscle wasting. The role of the ubiquitin-proteasome pathway. *N Engl J Med* 1996;335:1897–905.

141. Fong, Y., Moldawer L.L., Marano M., Wei H., Barber A., Manogue K., Tracey K.J., Kuo G., Fischman D.A., Cerami A., *et al.* Cachectin/TNF or IL-1 alpha induces cachexia with redistribution of body proteins. *Am J Physiol* 1989;256(3 Pt 2):R659–65.

142. Kotler, D.P., Thea D.M., Heo M., Allison D.B., Engelson E.S., Wang J., *et al.* Relative influences of sex, race, environment, and HIV infection upon body composition in adults. *Am J Clin Nutr* 1999;69:432–9.

143. Inui, A. Cancer anorexia-cachexia syndrome: Are neuropeptides the key? *Cancer Res* 1999;59(18):4493–501.

144. Coats, A.J. Origin of symptoms in patients with cachexia with special reference to weakness and shortness of breath. *Int J Cardiol.* 2002;85(1):133–9.

145. Rosenbaum, K., Wang, J., Pierson, RN Jr, and Kotler, DP. Time-dependent variation in weight and body composition in healthy adults. *JPEN* 2000;24(2):52–5.

146. Dewys, W.D., Begg, C., Lavin, P.T., Band, P.R., Bennett, J.M., Bertino, J.R., Cohen, M.H., Douglass, HO Jr, Engstrom, P.F., Ezdinli, E.Z., Horton, J., Johnson, G.J., Moertel, C.G., Oken, M.M., Perlia, C., Rosenbaum, C., Silverstein, M.N., Skeel, R.T., and Sponzo, R.W., Tormey, D.C. Prognostic effect of weight loss prior to chemotherapy in cancer patients. Eastern Cooperative Oncology Group. *Am J Med* 1980;69(4): 491–7.

147. Azcona, C., Castro, L., Crespo, E., Jimenez, M., and Sierrasesumaga, L. Megestrol acetate therapy for anorexia and weight loss in children with malignant solid tumours. *Aliment Pharmacol Ther* 1996;10(4):577–86.

148. Eubanks, V., Koppersmith, N., Wooldridge, N., Clancy, J.P., Lyrene, R., Arani, R.B., Lee, J., Moldawer, L., Atchison, J., Sorscher, E.J., and Makris, CM. Effects of megestrol acetate on weight gain, body composition, and pulmonary function in patients with cystic fibrosis. *J Pediatr* 2002;140(4):439–44.

149. Miller, T.L. Nutritional aspects of HIV-infected children receiving highly active antiretroviral therapy. *AIDS* 2003;17 Suppl 1:S130–40.

150. Meacham, L.R., Mazewski C., and Krawiecki, N. Mechanism of transient adrenal insufficiency with megestrol acetate treatment of cachexia in children with cancer. *J Pediatr Hematol Oncol* 2003;25(5):414–7.

151. Orme, L.M., Bond, J.D., Humphrey, M.S., Zacharin, M.R., Downie, P.A., Jamsen, K.M., Mitchell, S.L., Robinson, J.M., Grapsas, N.A., and Ashley, D.M. Megestrol acetate in pediatric oncology patients may lead to severe, symptomatic adrenal suppression. *Cancer* 2003;98(2):397–405.

152. McKone, E.F., Tonelli, M.R., and Aitken, M.L. Adrenal insufficiency and testicular failure secondary to megestrol acetate therapy in a patient with cystic fibrosis. *Pediatr Pulmonol* 2002;34(5):381–3.

153. Stockheim, J.A., Daaboul J.J., Yogev R., Scully S.P., Binns H.J., and Chadwick E.G. Adrenal suppression in children with the human immunodeficiency virus treated with megestrol acetate. *J Pediatr* 1999; 134(3):368–70.

154. Di Marzo, V., Goparaju, S.K., Wang, L., Liu J., Batkai, S, Jarai, Z., Fezza, F., Miura, G.I., Palmiter, R.D., Sugiura, T., and Kunos, G. Leptin-regulated endocannabinoids are involved in maintaining food intake. *Nature* 2001;410(6830):822–5.

155. Meguid, M.M., Fetissov, S.O., Varma, M., Sato, T., Zhang, L., Laviano, A., and Rossi-Fanelli, F. Hypothalamic dopamine and serotonin in the regulation of food intake. *Nutrition* 2000;16(10):843–57.

156. Moertel, C.G., Kvols, L.K., and Rubin, J. A study of cyproheptadine in the treatment of metastatic carcinoid tumor and the malignant carcinoid syndrome. *Cancer* 1991;67:33–36.

157. Argiles, J.M., Meijsing, S.H., Pallares-Trujillo, J,, Guirao, X,, and Lopez-Soriano, F.J. Cancer cachexia: a therapeutic approach. *Med Res Rev* 2001;21(1):83–101.

158. Carroll, P.V. Treatment with growth hormone and insulin-like growth factor-I in critical illness. *Best Pract Res* Clin *Endocrinol Metab* 2001;15(4):435–51.

159. Ruokonen, E., and Takala, J. Dangers of growth hormone therapy in critically ill patients. *Curr Opin Clin Nutr Metab Care* 2002; 5(2):199–209.

160. Chlebowski, R.T., Herrold, J., Ali, I., Oktay, E., Chlebowski, J.S., Ponce, A.T., Heber D., and Block, J.B. Influence of nandrolone decanoate on weight loss in advanced non-small cell lung cancer. *Cancer* 1986;58(1):183–6.

161. Fanelli, M., Sarmiento, R., Gattuso, D., Carillio, G., Capaccetti, B., Vacca, A., Roccaro, A.M., Gasparini, G. Thalidomide: A new anti-cancer drug? *Expert Opin Investig Drugs* 2003;12(7):1211–25.

162. Okafor, M.C. Thalidomide for erythema nodosum leprosum and other applications. *Pharmacotherapy* 2003;23(4):481–93.

163. Marchand, V., Baker, S.S., Stark, T.J., and Baker, R.D. Randomised, double-blind, placebo-controlled pilot trial of megestrol acetate in malnourished children with cystic fibrosis. *J Pediatr Gastroenterol Nutr* 2000;31(3):264–9.

164. Meacham, L.R., Mazewski, C, and Krawiecki, N. Mechanism of transient adrenal insufficiency with megestrol acetate treatment of cachexia in children with cancer. *J Pediatr Hematol Oncol* 2003;25(5):414–7.

165. Hussey, H.J., Todorov, P.T., Field, W.N., Inagaki, N., Tanaka, Y., Ishitsuka, H., and Tisdale M.J. Effect of a fluorinated pyrimidine on cachexia and tumour growth in murine cachexia models: relationship with a proteolysis inducing factor. *Br J Cancer* 2000; 83(1):56–62.

166. Lissoni, P. Is there a role for melatonin in supportive care? *Support Care Cancer* 2002;10(2):110–6.

167. Lundholm, K., Gelin, J., Hyltander, A., Lonnroth, C., Sandstrom, R., Svaninger, G., *et al.* Anti-inflammatory treatment may prolong survival in undernourished patients with metastatic solid tumors. *Cancer Res* 1994;54:5602–6.

168. Umar, A., Viner, J.L., Anderson, W.F., and Hawk E.T. Development of COX Inhibitors in Cancer Prevention and Therapy. *Am J Clin Oncol* 2003;26(4):S48–57.

169. McMillan, D.C., O'Gorman P., Fearon K.C., and McArdle C.S. A pilot study of megestrol acetate and ibuprofen in the treatment of cachexia in gastrointestinal cancer patients. *Br J Cancer* 1997; 76:788–90.

170. Tayek, J.A., Bistrian, B.R., Hehir, D.J., Martin, R., Moldawer L.L., and Blackburn, G.L. Improved protein kinetics and albumin synthesis by branched chain amino acid-enriched total parenteral nutrition in cancer cachexia. A prospective randomised crossover trial. *Cancer* 1986;58(1):147–57.

171. Barber, M.D., Ross, J.A., Voss, A.C., Tisdale, M.J., and Fearon, K.C. The effect of an oral nutritional supplement enriched with fish oil on weight-loss in patients with pancreatic cancer. *Br J Cancer* 1999; 81(1):80–6.

172. Pereira, J., Bruera, E. Chronic nausea. In E. Bruera and I., Higginson eds. Cachexia-anorexia in cancer patients. Oxford: England: Oxford University Press;1996: pp.23–37.

173. Kawamura, I., Morishita, R., Tomita, N., Lacey, E., Aketa, M., Tsujimoto, S., Manda, T., Tomoi, M., Kida, I., Higaki, J., Kaneda, Y., and Shimomura, K., Ogihara, T. Intratumoral injection of oligonucleotides to the NF kappa B binding site inhibits cachexia in a mouse tumor model. *Gene Ther* 1999;6(1):91–7.

174. Fujita, J., Tsujinaka, T., Yano, M., Ebisui, C., Saito, H., Katsume, A., Akamatsu, K., Ohsugi, Y., Shiozaki, H., and Monden, M. Anti-interleukin-6 receptor antibody prevents muscle atrophy in colon-26 adenocarcinoma-bearing mice with modulation of lysosomal and ATP-ubiquitin-dependent proteolytic pathways. *Int J Cancer* 1996;68(5):637–43.

175. Llovera, M., Carbo, N., Garcia-Martinez, C., Costelli, P., Tessitore, L., Baccino, F.M., Agell, N., Bagby, G.J., Lopez-Soriano, F.J., and Argiles, J.M. Anti-TNF treatment reverts increased muscle ubiquitin gene expression in tumour-bearing rats. *Biochem Biophys Res Commun* 1996;221(3):653–5.

176. Eliaz, R., Wallach, D., and Kost, J. Long-term protection against the effects of tumour necrosis factor by controlled delivery of the soluble p55 TNF receptor. *Cytokine* 1996;8:482–7.

177. Szalkowski, D., White-Carrington, S., Berger, J., and Zhang, B. Antidiabetic thiazolidinediones block the inhibitory effect of tumor necrosis factor—on differentiation, insulin-stimulated glucose uptake, and gene expression in 3T3-L1 cells. *Endocrinology* 1995;136:1474–81.

178. Nomura, K., Noguchi, Y., and Matsumoto, A. Stimulation of decreased lipoprotein lipase activity in the tumor-bearing state by the antihyperlipidemic drug bezafibrate. *Surg Today* 1996; 26:89–94.

179. Ohara, M., Tsutsumi, K., and Ohsawa, N. Suppression of carcass weight loss in cachexia in rats bearing Leydig cell tumor by the novel compound NO-1886, a lipoprotein lipase activator. *Metabolism* 1998;47:101–5.

180. Jaskowiak, N.J., and Alexander, H.R. Jr. The pathophysiology of cancer cachexia. In: Doyle D., Hanks G.W.C., and MacDonald N ed., Oxford Textbook of Palliative Medicine, (2 edition), Oxford, New York., Tokio, Oxford University Press, 1998;534–47.

181. Hankard, R., Munck, A., and Navarro, J. Nutrition and growth in cystic fibrosis. *Horm Res* 2002;58 Suppl 1:16–20.

182. Dunphy, K., Finlay, I., Rathbone, G., Gilbert, J., and Hicks, F. Rehydration in palliative and terminal care: if not—why not? *Palliat Med* 1995; 9(3):221–8.

183. Ellershaw, J.E., Sutcliffe, J.M., and Saunders, C.M. Dehydration and the dying patient. *J Pain Symptom Manage* 1995;10(3):192–7.

184. Bernat, J.L. Ethical and legal issues in palliative care. *Neurol Clin* 2001;19(4):969–87.

185. Musgrave, D.R. Terminal dehydration: to give or not to give intravenous fluids? Cancer Nursing 1990;13:62–6.

186. Malone. N. Hydration in the terminally ill patient. *Nurs Stand* 1994;8(43):29–32.

187. Billings, J.A. Comfort measures for the terminally ill: Is dehydration painful? J Am Geriatr Soc 1985;33:808–10.

188. Bernat, J.L., Gert, B., and Mogielnicki, R.P. Patient refusal of hydration and nutrition: an alternative to physician-assisted suicide or voluntary active euthanasia. *Arch Intern Med* 1993;153: 2723–8.

189. Meisel, A. The legal consensus about foregoing life-sustaining treatment: its status and its prospects. *Kennedy Inst Ethics J* 1992;2:309–45.

190. Ferris, F.D., Von Gunten, C.F, and Emanuel, L.L.Ensuring competency In end-of-life care: Controlling symptoms. *BMC Palliat Care* 2002;1(1):5.

191. Wolfe, J., Grier, HE., Klar, N., Levin, S.B., Ellenbogen, J.M., Salem-Schatz, S., Emanuel, E.J., and Weeks, J.C. Symptoms and suffering at the end of life in children with cancer. *N Engl J Med* 2000;342 (5):326–33.

192. Angus, F. and Burakoff, R. The percutaneous endoscopic gastrostomy tube. Medical and ethical issues in placement. *Am J Gastroenterol* 2003;98(2):272–7.

193. Niv, Y. and Abuksis, G. Indications for percutaneous endoscopic gastrostomy insertion: ethical aspects. *Dig Dis* 2002;20(3–4):253–6.

194. Wollman B., D'Agostino, H.B., Walus-Wigle, J.R., Easter D.W., and Beale, A. Radiologic, endoscopic, and surgical gastrostomy: An institutional evaluation and meta-analysis of the literature. *Radiology* 1995;197(3):699–704.

195. Goretsky, M.F., Johnson, N., Farrell, M., and Ziegler, M.M. Alternative techniques of feeding gastrostomy in children: a critcal analysis. *J Am Coll Surg* 1996;182:233–40.

196. Mathus-Vliegen, E.M., Koning, H., Taminiau, J.A., and Moorman-Voestermans, C.G. Percutaneous endoscopic gastrostomy and gastrojejunostomy in psychomotor retarded subjects: a follow-up covering 106 patient years. *J Pediatr Gastroenterol Nutr* 2001;33(4):488–94.

197. Razeghi, S., L,ang T., and Behrens, R. Influence of percutaneous endoscopic gastrostomy on gastroesophageal reflux: a prospective study in 68 children. *J Pediatr Gastroenterol Nutr* 2002;35(1):22–4.

198. Samuel, M., and Holmes, K. Quantitative and qualitative analysis of gastroesophageal reflux after percutaneous endoscopic gastrostomy. *J Pediatr Surg* 2002;37(2):256–61.

199. Heine, R.G., Reddihough, D.S., Catto-Smith, A.G. Gastro-oesophageal reflux and feeding problems after gastrostomy in children with severe neurological impairment. *Dev Med Child Neurol* 1995; 37(4):320–9.

200. Cosentini, E.P., Sautner, T., Gnant, M., Winkelbauer, F., Teleky, B., and Jakesz, R. Outcomes of surgical, percutaneous endoscopic, and percutaneous radiologic gastrostomies. *Arch Surg* 1998; 133(10):1076–83.

201. Segal, D., Michaud, L., Guimber, D., Ganga-Zandzou, P.S., Turck, D., and Gottrand, F. Late-onset complications of percutaneous endoscopic gastrostomy in children. *J Pediatr Gastroenterol Nutr* 2001;33(4):495–500.

202. Kutiyanawala, M.A., Hussain, A., Johnstone, J.M., Everson, N.W., and Nour, S. Gastrostomy complications in infants and children. *Ann R Coll Surg Engl* 1998;80(4):240–3.

203. Gauderer, M.W. Percutaneous endoscopic gastrostomy and the evolution of contemporary long-term enteral access. *Clin Nutr* 2002;21(2):103–10.

204. Kimber, C.P., Khattak, I.U., Kiely, E.M., and Spitz, L. Peritonitis following percutaneous gastrostomy in children: management guidelines. *Aust N Z J Surg* 1998;68(4):268–70.

205. Rey, J.R., Axon, A., Budzynska, A., and Kruse, A., and Nowak, A. Guidelines of the European Society of Gastrointestinal Endoscopy (E.S.G.E.) antibiotic prophylaxis for gastrointestinal endoscopy. European Society of Gastrointestinal Endoscopy. *Endoscopy* 1998;30(3): 318–24.

206. Khattak, I.U., Kimber, C., Kiely, E.M., and Spitz, L. Percutaneous endoscopic gastrostomy in paediatric practice: complications and outcome. *J Pediatr Surg* 1998;33(1):67–72.

207. Fox, V.L., Abel, S.D., Malas, S., Duggan, C., and Leichtner, A.M. Complications following percutaneous endoscopic gastrostomy and subsequent catheter replacement in children and young adults. *Gastrointest Endosc* 1997;45(1):64–71.

208. Mercadante, S. Diarrhea in terminally ill patients: pathophysiology and treatment. *J Pain Symptom Manage* 1995;10(4):298–309.

209. Matheson, A.J. and Noble, S. Racecadotril. *Drugs* 2000;59(4): 829–35.

24 Feeding in palliative care

Angela Thompson, Anita MacDonald, and Chris Holden

Introduction

'Feeding in palliative care' brings to mind issues relating to artificial nutrition/hydration in the terminal stages, and the ethical dilemmas associated with these challenges. Artificial feeding refers specifically to interventions that bypass the swallowing process, such as nasogastric and gastrostomy tubes, in addition to parenteral forms of nutrition. Whilst these issues are real and relevant, they are *only one* aspect of the range of nutritional care considerations required for children with a life-limiting condition, whose palliative care needs may extend over months or years. Offering food to a child is one of the most basic of parental instincts. Artificial nutrition, on the other hand, may at times impose burdens on the child that outweigh the possible benefits. Attention to good nutritional care, offered either orally or artificially, has the potential to improve quality of life for both family and child, and should be a priority within their assessments, reviews, and care planning.

A review of ACT/RCPCH 1997 Guide [1] reveals the broad spectrum of conditions that may necessitate provision of palliative care to a child. These range from underlying cancer and irreversible organ failures, through neuromuscular disorders and metabolic disorders to severe multiple disabilities. Some have short and swift terminal-carestages, while others deteriorate steadily over time. Prognostic uncertainty exists in some cases with unpredictable time scales, compounding decision-making and bringing up ethical considerations. With such a range of diagnoses and time scales, what are the common principles that influence the approach to nutritional support? This chapter aims to support decision-making for individuals, based on the available relevant evidence relating to paediatric nutritional support, considered alongside specific palliative care issues, to inform and support sound nutritional care decision-making at the various stages of individual palliative care journeys. It does not ignore the place of 'common sense', non-technological approaches to improving children's nutritional intake, but seeks to add these to support planning, as the 'non-assisted' approaches become insufficient alone.

All children deserve that we acknowledge the relevance of attention to position [2] and seating, and provide them with encouragement, distraction, and extra snacks, as also with unhurried, small, frequent and colourful, temptingly presented and satisfying meals that are easy to swallow. Strongly aromatic foods should be avoided, especially when nausea and vomiting occur. Taste alteration associated, for example, with rapid cell turnover of the 10,000 taste discerning buds during chemotherapy, can be addressed by undertaking measures such as disguising metallic tastes with sharp or acidic flavours, like lemon juice, and salty tastes with sugar. When not contra-indicated, the use of calorie-dense additions to favourite meals by, for example, adding grated cheese to baked beans or mashed potato, lentils or cream to soups, and icecream to milk shakes provides family members with a way of feeling they are doing something positive to regain control of their child's care. It brings some normality to the child's situation, as does the use of carbohydrate-providing glucose polymers or nutritional supplements, and may do much to relieve tension, especially where artificial feeding brings more burdens than benefits.

Physical, psychological, and social influences upon feeding

Nutritional care decisions are affected not just by physical factors, but also by psycho-social influences. Societal attitudes to death have changed significantly, such that the death of a child is now often considered to be a medical failure within many societies [3]. Advances have increased the opportunity for technological support in nutritional care, compounding the dilemma at times when a means of nutritional intervention may appear to be available, but inappropriate. Consequently, decisions about whether interventions should be begun, and if so, for how long, and with what aims, as well as decisions about whether to withdraw, are required to be taken more frequently. This adds to the challenges of addressing changing nutritional requirements through the various stages of disease progression, for both families and staff.

Psychologically, strong forces influence attitudes towards nutritional care. A woman's maternal instinct is to nurture and feed her child, and this instinct is naturally strongest when the child is ill. This applies also to the mode of feeding; the desire to orally feed a child is a strongly emotive factor. This can influence both family and professionals to maintain attempts at oral feeding alone, beyond the stage when enteral feeding would have been of benefit to both child and exhausted family.

Whilst the evidence base supports artificial feeding, research suggests that the psychological factors affecting the decision to commence it may be 'replaced' by a different set of psycho-social issues after it commences. Not all families find the move to artificial feeding a positive one [4,5]. Complications in the procedure itself may occur, along with the possibility of rapid increase in weight gain, increase in the care burden on the family, and urgent needs for equipment provision and housing adaptations.

Poole [6] examined loss of weight and appetite as 'problems' experienced by patients with advanced cancer, and their carers. She suggested that anorexia may be more distressing for the carer than the patient. Holden [7] found that preparation and serving of food was an expression of love and caring, underpinned by the knowledge that 'intake is necessary for survival'. This perception will be recognised as familiar by those who work with families having children with palliative care needs. Holden noted that the consumption of food acted as a 'barometer' of a patient's condition, where a reduction of intake was equated with deterioration. Carers were frustrated that they could not influence the patient to eat, and saw it as a source of conflict. This is in contrast to the findings of Justice [8], who describes the 'natural' death, while not eating, as part of the Hindu culture in India. Here, acceptance that food intake will decline as death approaches reduces carer–patient conflict, as the patient prepares for a 'good', dignified death, with a reduced risk of incontinence. Hence, cultural and religious practices have an influence, and must be accommodated.

These attitudes will also influence decisions made for many children in the earlier stages of their palliative care needs, where prognosis may be months or years, or prognostic uncertainty may exist. The psychological factors influencing the carers' desire to 'build up' the child will be strengthened by the desire to avoid physical effects, witnessed or anticipated. Evidence relating to sub-optimal nutrition has been gathered in respect to children with neurological impairment. Sullivan [9] confirmed that feeding problems in this group were severe and common, citing prolonged feeding times. 38% of the members of this group were underweight, 56% choked on food, 22% experienced vomiting, 59% were constipated, and 31% had suffered at least one chest infection over the last 6 months, while 20% of the parents described feeding as unpleasant. Despite this, 64% of the patients had never had their feeding or nutrition formally assessed.

Sub-optimal nutrition has been shown to have many health consequences. Russell [10] showed a decrease in muscle strength, predisposing to ineffective cough reflex and aspiration pneumonia [11]. Poor circulation time results in limbs developing cold, mottled peripheries [12], and disturbances of the immune system, predisposing to infections, especially of the urinary and respiratory tract, along with reduced healing of pressure sores. Stallings [13] considered that poor nutrition may be associated with irritability, and decreased motivation and energy available for 'non-essential' activities such as play. Such effects are no longer considered inevitable and irremediable, but planned assessment is required to reduce their prevalence, and improve the quality of life of the child and family.

Case A 4-year-old-girl with a degenerative neurological condition was under regular multidisciplinary review. She developed a series of chest infections, during which she suffered associated weight loss and general deterioration. Her parents reported adequate nutritional intake. Referral was made for terminal-care support, but assessment revealed malnutrition, and a concern that malnutrition was the root cause of her rapid demise. Oral supplementation was replaced with nasogastric feeds, and she made an almost immediate and sustained improvement in energy levels, motivation, cognitive functioning, weight gain, skin condition, with reduction in severity and frequency of chest infections. She tolerated nasogastric (and subsequently, gastrostomy) feeds well, and the family's experiences with exhaustion over long pre-nasogastric feed periods ceased, reducing their stress and improving quality of life, replacing misery and distress with good-quality times in the later stages (years) of her disease progression.

When decisions have to be made

How can we best approach decision-making at different stages, from decisions to increase oral supplementation, through enteral/parenteral feeding, to issues of withholding or withdrawing artificial nutrition or hydration, for both families and professionals (see Chapter 4, Ethics, Larcher)?

No one professional group can support the nutritional care needs of a palliative care child. Support from a nutritional care team (including nutritionalists, nurses, paediatricians, dysphagia specialists, psychologists, etc), is essential [14], supplemented by access to information from those who know the child and family well. Many nutritional support teams are based in regional centres. As the number of children managed within the community with enteral/parenteral feeding is increasing rapidly, multidisciplinary forums are also developing within community settings, to support the delivery of care to children with life-limiting conditions. These work alongside the regional centre teams to ensure smoothly planned, timely transition of care between care settings, and to enable families' needs to be met locally. Since the number of professionals involved with any one family can be considerable, it is important that each has a key worker to coordinate and access care, and that the young people themselves are included in the decision-making, where appropriate.

Nutritional issues are rarely managed in isolation; their impact upon prognosis adds weight to the importance of including the young person in any decision-making.

Whilst decisions regarding nutritional intervention are required throughout the disease trajectory, decisions around the terminal phase involve challenging issues of artificial nutrition and hydration. A fierce debate has been held, primarily in the context of adult palliative care, on the subject of the need to withdraw or maintain hydration for comfort. Disadvantages of withdrawal may include thirst, dry mouth, nausea, postural hypotension, tachycardia, cognitive deficit, fever, constipation, and increased risk of tissue breakdown. However, symptomatic distress from oedema, respiratory secretions, urine output, etc, may occur when artificial hydration is continued in the terminal stage, as lower fluid volumes are required by terminal cancer patients than the average medical or surgical patient [15,16].

These decisions are no less taxing in paediatrics. Two guiding principles remain, however.

1. Assessment and consequent planning needs to be made for each child on an *individual basis.*

2. *No individual* should make such decisions alone.

Statements exist from national bodies and ethical committees, to steer and underpin these decisions.

The National Council for Hospice and Specialist Palliative Care Services [17], produced a statement concerning assisted artificial hydration. It emphasises that decisions of this nature should involve a multi-professional team and family, although the senior doctor has ultimate responsibility for the decision. It states that:

- A blanket policy regarding artificial hydration is ethically indefensible.

- When near death, a person's desire for food and drink diminishes. Artificial hydration in the imminently dying patient influences neither survival nor symptom control, and as such, may constitute an intrusion.

- Thirst or dry mouths may be caused by medication.

- Appropriate palliative care will consider using artificial hydration where dehydration results from potentially correctable causes, such as diuretics, sedation, vomiting, diarrhoea, and hypercalcaemia.

- The clinical team has responsibility for the decisions, which must be reviewed on a daily basis.

- Relatives often express concerns about lack of nutrition or hydration. Professionals should not be subordinate to relatives' anxieties, but should strive to address them.

The Royal College of Paediatrics and Child Health [18] drew up a framework for practice in withholding and withdrawing life-sustaining treatment. It states that 'the role of assisted feeding by nasogastric tube or gastrostomy should be considered very carefully and discussed fully with the family'. It suggests that whilst it may be appropriate in a child with a progressive neuro-degenerative-disease-related swallowing disorder, it would rarely be introduced in a child with a rapidly progressive, disseminated malignancy. It also places emphasis upon the inclusion of competent children in the decision-making process.

The United Kingdom's General Medical Council (GMC) produced good practice guidelines in 2002 [19]. Key points were:

- The benefits of artificial nutrition and hydration are different, and should be assessed separately.

- Agreed trial periods may be appropriate, where the balance of benefit/burden is unclear.

- Where death is imminent, it is not usually appropriate to start artificial nutrition or hydration, but artificial hydration by less invasive measures may provide symptom relief.

- Where death is imminent, and artificial hydration and/or nutrition are already in use, it may be appropriate to withdraw them if the burdens appear to outweigh the benefits.

- Where death is not imminent, it is usually appropriate to continue artificial nutrition and/or hydration. If the prognosis is poor, however, and it is felt that the artificial nutrition/hydration is causing suffering or an intolerable burden to the patient, it is best to seek independent consultation.
- Where significant conflicts/dissent arise, or may arise, legal advice should be sought as to whether the courts should be applied to for a ruling.

The British Medical Association (BMA) in 1999 [20] made some statements of clarity:

- Basic care should always be provided, including the offer of oral nutrition/hydration.
- Artificial nutrition/hydration refers specifically to techniques to bypass the pathology in the swallowing process—nasogastric tubes, gastrostomies, and total parenteral nutrition.
- Artificial nutrition/hydration is regarded as a medical treatment, and as such, may be withdrawn in some circumstances.
- Where nutrition and hydration are provided by ordinary means (cup, spoon or other method of delivering food or nutritional supplements into the patient's mouth)—or moistening of a patient's mouth for comfort—this forms part of basic care, and should not be withdrawn. It should be offered to, but not forced upon, the patient, so long as there are no significant risks of choking/aspiration of the food or fluid.

These points highlight the difficulties in paediatrics, where, for example, many of the children with neuro-degenerative disorders will already have artificial nutrition/hydration because of the high risk of aspiration, and withdrawal would not be followed by the option of oral nutrition/hydration. Hence, withdrawal may hold even greater significance and potentially ethical dilemmas than in adult oncology-based palliative care.

Managing the feeding of a child with palliative care needs

The management of a child with palliative care needs, therefore, begins at diagnosis, and includes input from a nutritional care team (where available), for assessment and nutritional planning according to anticipated energy and nutritional requirements. An approach of regular reassessment of nutritional intake according to need will enable an establishing of trust between the families and the professionals. This in turn paves the way for possible decision-making, including withholding/withdrawing artificial hydration/nutrition, as the family has witnessed

decisions being made in the child's best interest throughout the course of the disease progression.

The role of a nutritional care team can be illustrated by considering a child with a malignant disease. Malnutrition is not a significant finding in the majority of children with malignant diseases at presentation. The effects of cancer and its treatment can, however, result in malnutrition [21]. All three modalities of chemotherapy, surgery and radiotherapy are known to have significant negative effects on nutritional status. Careful attention to nutritional status has been shown to reduce complications of, and delays in, treatment. Chemotherapy, which may have taken its toll even before palliative stages are reached, or continue within them, can cause nausea, vomiting, anorexia, changes in taste, mucositis, diarrhoea, constipation, and liver damage, while steroids may cause muscle wasting and worsening of protein malnutrition. Disease-specific associations need careful consideration—children with brain tumours often have problems with swallowing when neurological deficits occur. The Cochrane review of post-BMT patients showed that reduced appetite, mucositis, and gastrointestinal failure often give rise to malnutrition, but that glutamine in association with parenteral nutrition may reduce the relative length of hospital stay and infection rates [22].

The nutritional assessment for an oncology patient contains the expected anthropometrics, biochemical indices, dietary intake details and clinical examination. Weight-for-height has been found to be one of the most useful parameters for assessment and monitoring of children with malignant diseases [21]. The history of weight change, treatment type, duration and intensity, and any infectious and surgical complications enables determination of the need for aggressive nutritional support. Careful nutritional assessment,using a battery of tests, thus has the aim of preventing the onset of malnutrition. Consequent potential benefits for families having children with palliative care needs are: the child's increased energy levels, decreased irritability, and greater motivation, and : a reduction in complications, resulting in an improved quality of life, within the knowledge that the child was supported in achieving his best nutritional status through active efforts to ensure access to appropriately intense, timely treatment.

Likewise, consideration of the underlying disease process will support nutrition management for children with non-malignant life-limiting illnesses. Those with neuro-muscular disorders may find small pieces of food moistened with sauces more manageable, and purees easier to swallow than liquids. Children with cardiac disease often develop hepatomegaly-related abdominal discomfort, nausea and vomiting, in relation to increased pressure on the stomach and compromised blood supply to the bowel. Frequent small-volume feeds may support, and a low-fat diet may ease stomach emptying and nausea. Those with renal disease may find that uraemic nausea is reduced by a high-carbohydrate diet [23]. A review of symptoms in the last month of life revealed substantial suffering, with poor nutritional status contributing to fatigue, the most commonly reported significant symptom [24]. Gastro-intestinal problem-related symptoms of poor appetite (80%), nausea and vomiting (57%), constipation (53%), and diarrhoea (45%), were all felt to warrant symptom control to improve well-being in the terminal month.

Whilst anorexia and dehydration are frequently reported in children nearing death, Goldman [23] reports that they naturally become less interested in food, and may survive many weeks with little nutrition, without discomfort. In such cases, it is important to ensure that there is no contributory nausea, vomiting, depression, constipation or sore mouth. Since steroids can produce significant mood swings in children, and rapid onset of Cushingoid appearance, they are not recommended as appetite stimulants in children. A sore mouth is the main symptom of dehydration observed in children, and may be managed with moistening and good attention to mouth care, with regular checking for candida, and treatment with nystatin. Chemotherapy-related mouth ulcers are common, and may significantly affect nutritional intake. Relief can be afforded by benzydamine hydrochloride spray. Management of other symptoms affecting nutritional intake are addressed elsewhere, but it should be remembered that nausea and vomiting in children with palliative needs is relatively common, and that anti-emetics according to presumed cause, for example, cyclizine in raised intracranial pressure, should be prescribed. Likewise, prophylactic regular laxatives should be used for opiate related constipation, and loperamide may be required to control diarrhoea in HIV/Aids.

Children with palliative care needs therefore require sound nutritional assessment, with application of good practice in nutritional care to their individual circumstances. This has to take account of treatment, disease, complications, and anticipated energy needs, placed within the psycho-social context of the family.

What then is evident as good practice in nutritional care in children with chronic and serious illnesses, which can be applied to children with palliative care needs? What is known about nutritional requirements, modes of delivery, care planning, training and support? These issues need application to the individual child's care, and will be addressed here.

Nutritional assessment

The three main functions of nutritional assessment are:

(1) to identify patients at risk of developing malnutrition;

(2) to quantify risk of developing malnutrition-related complications;

(3) to monitor adequacy of nutritional intervention.

There is no global 'gold standard' for determining nutritional status, because, (1) there is no universally accepted definition of malnutrition; (2) all current accepted parameters are affected by illness and injury; (3) it is difficult to isolate the effect of malnutrition from the disease on clinical outcome, and, (4) it is not clear which of the commonly used assessment techniques is the most reliable, because of the paucity of comparative data [25]. The clinical assessment of nutritional status should involve a focused history of physical examination, in conjunction with selected laboratory tests aimed at detecting specific nutrient deficiencies, and identifying patients who are at high risk of developing future nutrient abnormalities. The nutritional assessment should also include a psycho-social history, feeding history (Table 24.1), medication review for potential drug–nutrient interactions, and evaluation of ability to chew, swallow, digest and absorb adequate nutrients to meet nutrient requirements. Serial weight and height (length) are usually the main anthropometric measurements, but the adequacy with which these are carried out, documented, and interpreted is far from optimal [27].

Table 24.1 Important information from a feeding history (adapted from Coad [26])

- 3-day food record and food frequency questionnaire (including food preferences, food textures, typical food patterns, for example, number of meals, snacks, size or content);
- use of equipment for example, type of chair, utensils and cutlery;
- feeding skills, for example, finger foods, length of feeding;
- feeding behaviour, for example, length of mealtime, food refusal;
- any recent feed changes, such as reluctance with breast or bottle, regression of feeding patterns, or behaviour changes;
- dietary restrictions, or known allergies of the child or family;
- recent changes in body weight, such as weight loss or weight gain;
- parental/carer observations of feeding, including any concerns such as tiredness, breathlessness during feeding, or taking much longer time over feeding;
- awareness of any existing presence of an underlying condition, such as vomiting and diarrhoea;
- ability to self feed, chew or swallow food, and any oral or motor dysfunction;
- any additional dietary support, such as enteral feeding;
- cultural or religious food preferences;
- vitamin or mineral supplements or medications being taken, which may affect dietary intake, such as corticosteriods;
- reasons for changes in dietary and appetite patterns, including teething, dental or gum problems, and changes in taste, smell, or ability to chew or swallow food.

Nutritional requirements

In the United Kingdom, energy and nutrient requirements are detailed in the 1991 Department of Health document 'Dietary Reference Values for Food Energy and Nutrients for the United Kingdom' [28]. Dietary reference values (DRV's) are not just a single set of figures, but four sets of figures providing guidance on average needs, recommended intakes, minimum needs and safe levels of intake as appropriate for each nutrient. The reference nutrient intake (RNI) is the amount of a nutrient (EAR + 2 standard deviations), which is sufficient for almost all individuals (97.5%). By definition, it exceeds the requirement of most people, and habitual intakes above RNI are almost certainly adequate.

Requirements for energy and nutrients are thought to fulfill children's needs in proportion to the metabolically active tissue at various stages of development. The basal metabolic rate is the same for girls and boys until they enter puberty, when it increases more rapidly to meet the demands of their higher percentage of muscle mass. However, the RNIs do not cover additional needs, which arise from increased catabolism due to disease, malabsorption, or decreased utilisation from metabolic abnormalities, or the increased requirements necessary for catch-up growth to occur.

Energy requirements

To estimate an individual's true energy requirements, adjustments are necessary to account for special circumstances, such as activity levels, illnesses, and other factors. Individual requirements will vary widely, even for children of the same age and sex, who are afflicted with the same disease. For example, fever raises energy needs by 12% for each degree above 37°C. Illness, trauma, and recovery from malnutrition can almost double energy requirements. *However, decreased growth and activity during severe illness can decrease energy needs considerably. Children with disabilities are likely to have lower energy needs than healthy children.*

Therefore, individual energy requirements may only be determined on a trial and error basis, and regular monitoring of weight changes, growth and actual energy intake versus prescribed intake are important. Changes in clinical condition, such as increased seizure activity or infection, may affect requirements. Pragmatically, for infants and children who are underweight, it may be sensible to initially increase their usual energy intake by 20%, and evaluate the effect of this. For children with a low height or length-for-age, it may be better to calculate energy and nutrient intakes based on actual height-based age calculation, rather than chronological age. Children who have been chronically underweight may gain excessive weight when on tube feeds, sometimes to the point of obesity.

Protein requirements

This is a crucial determinant of linear growth, as it provides nitrogen and essential amino acid requirements for synthesis of body tissues. The protein-energy ratio is important, and normaly in infants, 7.5%–12% of the energy should be derived from protein, while at least 9% of energy for catch-up growth should be derived from protein.

Fluid requirements

In healthy children, fluid requirements vary from 150 ml/kg/day (0–3 month-old infants) to 50 ml/kg/day (teenagers). Water must be provided in sufficient quantities to replace fluid losses and allow for normal metabolism, although it is not known what the fluid requirements are in the terminal phase. Fluid requirements depend on many variables, including urine output, sweating, vomiting, fever, and stool output (constipation or diarrhoea). Constant drooling also contributes to fluid losses. *Many children appear to require much less than the usual amount of fluids at the end of life. At these times, it is important to maintain comfort by maintaining good mouth care and hygiene with local measures. Excess fluids can lead to increased secretions and respiratory distress, frequent urination, and at times, even heart failure.*

When to use tube feeding

Every effort should be made to optimise oral food intake before embarking on tube feeding. This may involve many measures, including change of posture, special seating, feeding equipment, oral desensitisation, food texture changes, thickening of liquids, increasing energy density of food, use of energy and nutritional supplements, and treatment of reflux or oesophagitis. However, tube feeding can play a role in both short-term rehabilitation and long-term nutritional management. The extent of its use ranges from supportive therapy, in which the enteral feed supplies a proportion of the needed nutrients, to primary therapy, in which the enteral feed delivers all of the necessary nutrients.

Some parents may find it difficult to consent to enteral feeding, and they need support and understanding. They may see artificial nutrition as a poor alternative to real food. It may arouse feelings of guilt, as the parents may feel that they have failed to provide nourishment to their child. However, most children receiving enteral feeds can continue to receive oral food and drink, and this should be actively encouraged so that they can enjoy the pleasurable and social aspects of eating.

Before initiation of enteral tube feeding, the child needs an assessment to: (1) ensure that there are no contra-indications for enteral feeding; (2) assess any possible gastro-intestinal problems (e.g gastro-oesophageal reflux, risk of aspiration); (3) determine the optimal delivery site for the feeding (i.e. stomach, duodenum, or jejunum), and (4), determine an appropriate oralmotor stimulation programme.

Tube feeding should be considered when one or more of the following factors are identified:

(1) unsafe swallowing and aspiration;

(2) inability to consume at least 60% of energy needs by mouth;

(3) total feeding time more than 4 hours per day;

(4) unpleasant feeding;

(5) weight loss or no weight gain for a period of 3 months (less for younger children and infants);

(6) weight-for-height (or length) less than 2nd percentile for age and sex.

Choice of tube feed

Choosing the best formula for paediatric patients depends on several factors, including:

- nutritional requirements
- gastro-intestinal function
- underlying disease
- nutrient restrictions
- age
- feed characteristics (nutritional composition, addition of novel components, viscosity, osmolality, availability and cost).

Standard, nutritionally complete polymeric formula can be divided into 3 groups, according to age or weight: (1) 0–1 year, (2) 1–6 years (8–20 kg), and, (3) 7–12 years (21–45 kg).

Children 0–1year. It has been traditional practice to tube feed term infants with normal gastro-intestinal function either breast milk or normal infant formula, during the first year of life. Energy supplements, in the form of glucose polymer and fat emulsion, were commonly added to increase energy density, but this has several disadvantages, including preparation errors, feed contamination, dilution of nutrient composition, and reduction of the protein: energy ratio. Another option is the use of high-energy, nutrient-dense infant formula, specially produced for infants who are failing to thrive. These provide approximately 1.0 kcal/ml, and are enriched with extra protein, vitamins and minerals. Initial evidence suggests that these formulas are well tolerated, and when compared with energy-supplemented normal infant formula, result in better growth in boys [30].

Children 1–6 years (8–20 kg). There is now a selection of standard, low-residue, nutritionally complete, ready-to use feeds, of 0.75, 1.0, and 1.5 kcal/ml, (with or without fibre, providing between 0.5–0.75 g fibre/100 kcal). They are all based on caseinates, maltodextrin, and vegetable oils, with or without added medium-chain triglyceride oil, and are clinically lactose-free, with a low osmolality. They are well tolerated and effective in improving nutritional status in this age group. Their long-term use also leads to a normal biochemical micronutrient profile[31]. Unfortunately, there is little data on fibre requirements in paediatrics, to help determine ideal feed composition. Initial data suggests that the high-fibre feeds are well tolerated, improve stool characteristics and reduce laxative usage. In a group of 20 developmentally disabled children, during a 2-month randomised crossover study, a high-fibre feed containing 10g/litre reduced use of laxatives, and had no abnormal effect on growth or biochemistry [32].

Children 6–12 years (21–45 kg). Standard nutritionally complete, 1.0 and 1.5 kcal polymeric feeds (with and without fibre) have recently been introduced for this age group. Their micronutrient composition is in between feeds designed for 1–6 years and adult feeds, but as yet, there is no published work demonstrating their efficacy and safety. However, feeds designed for younger ages or adult feeds are unsuitable. Feeds designed for 1–6 years are low in electrolytes, whereas adult formula contains excessive amounts of protein, electrolytes, vitamin, and trace minerals.

Energy density of whole protein feed

Whole protein tube-feeding formulae with varying energy densities are available. The choice of an appropriate energy density depends on energy requirements and tolerance. For children with cancer and cystic fibrosis, energy requirements may not be met by standard formula (1.0 kcal/ml), because of low infusion rates during initial days of feeding, feed interruptions due to medical procedures or illnesses, gastro-intestinal intolerance or sub-optimal prescribed volumes. In children with cancer, high-energy density formula (1.5 kcal/ml) has been shown to be more effective in improving nutritional status of children with cancer, during the intensive phase of treatment, than standard formula (1.0 kcal/ml)[33].

Route of feeding

The feeding tube is placed either nasally or surgically Table 24.2, and the choice of placement depends on many factors:

(1) preference of the caregiver(s);

(2) expected duration of the tube feeding;

(3) community support for enteral feeding;

(4) family's ability to learn the feeding technique;

(5) child's safety;

Table 24.2 Route of feeding

Indication	Problems/Complications	Contraindications
Nasogastric feeding		
Functioning GI tract, but is unable to meet total nutritional nutritional requirements orally	Misplacement (trachea/cranium/smallintestine) and aspiration pneumonia Accidental removal Occlusion Dysphagia/nausea/oral/nasal phobia Body image Trauma/ulceration/perforation	Persistent vomiting Severe delayed gastric emptying Complete intestinal obstruction Uncontrolled gastro-oesophageal reflux with a risk of pulmonary aspiration
Gastrostomy feeding As for nasogastric feeding, *plus*: • Congenital abnormalities such as oesophageal/choanal atresia or tracheo-oesophageal fistula • Requirement for long-term feeding • Oesophageal injury • Oesophageal dysmotility	Large bowel perforation/fistula Accidental displacement; can result in partial closure of the stoma Infection Over-granulation Occlusion Migration Body image	As for nasogastric feeding, *plus*: • Gross ascites/severe obesity • Clotting abnormalities

(6) development of 'normal' feeding behaviour;

(7) minimising trauma and discomfort.

Nasogastric feeding. The simplest and most obvious route for artificial enteral feeding. Selection of an appropriate size and type of nasogastric tube will depend on its material and the anticipated duration of feeding.

Types of tubes

For most children, the best method of enteral delivery is a fine bore nasogastric tube (FBT), generally made from soft *polyurethane* or *silicone elastomer*, with a diameter under 3mm. Polyurethane tubes are inserted using a guide wire, which is flexible enough to aid easy insertion and passage, avoids damage to the tube, and does not coil. This type of tube can be left in place for 4–6 weeks before needing to be changed.

A *polyvinyl chloride tube* may be considered if the child is likely to vomit frequently, as it is less likely to be vomited up. Unfortunately, this type of tube needs to be changed on a weekly basis, as it stiffens, over time, and is likely to cause more nasal irritation.

Techniques for insertion: Parents can be taught how to pass nasogastric tubes, but should not be pressurised into doing this. Information must be given by an experienced Nurse and Play Therapist, to decrease the anxiety of the parent and child and improve their ability to cope, by making the procedure understandable and less frightening.

Tips to maintaining integrity of tubes: Nasogastric tubes require flushing with 5 mls of cool, boiled or sterile water every 4h, to prevent occlusion of the tube and maintain the tube's integrity. A 50ml syringe must always be used (as per manufacturer's instruction) when flushing the tube, as smaller syringes create an increase in pressure, which can perforate the tube.

Gastrostomy feeding. Children who are likely to require feeding for more than 3 months should be considered for gastrostomy feeding. Percutaenous endoscopic gastrostomy (PEG), first reported by Gaurderer *et al.* [34] has become the preferred approach for children requiring prolonged tube-feeding support. Following the development of the gastrostomy button, skin-level gastrostomy devices are now frequently utilised when the PEG catheter is replaced. Although commonly used, it is not without mortality [35]. Complications include leakage at the site, tube displacement, stomal and gastro-intestinal infections and gastro-oesophageal reflux.

Children with poor gastric emptying and/or severe reflux or intractable vomiting are of particular concern. Such children have an increased risk of aspiration, and therefore, may be candidates for a simultaneous fundoplication.

Jejunostomy feeding. This can be achieved using naso-jejunal jejunostomy, or trans-pyloric jejunostomy, or trans-gastric jejunostomy placement. Jejunostomy feeding is rarely used in paediatrics, but may be indicated in children with persistent vomiting or severe delayed gastric emptying.

Feeding regimen

Feeds can be delivered by intermittent bolus feeds, continuous pump infusion, or a combination of the two (Table 24.3). Certain clinical situations dictate a specific regimen, but a

Table 24.3 Choosing a suitable feeding regimen (Adapted from Holden *et al.* [29])

Regimen	Example
Bolus top-up feeding	*Congenital heart disease*: Bottle feeds are not completed due to breathlessness and remaining feed is topped up via the nasogastric tube.
Exclusive bolus feeding	*Long-term feeding for children with a neurological handicap*: Daytime bolus feeding can allow flexibility and mobility, and provide a regimen that can fit in with the family mealtimes. *Post-fundoplication*: Bolus feeding is the method of choice for children following a surgical anti-reflux procedure (see text).
Combination of bolus and continuous feeding	*Chronic illness*: Children with anorexia associated with chronic illness may receive a large proportion of their nutrition via a nasogastric or gastrostomy tube. Daytime boluses allow for a normal meal pattern, and overnight feeding with a feeding pump reduces the time commitment at night for parents and ward staff.
Overnight feeding	*Supplementary nutrition*: Children who require enteral feeding to supplement their poor oral intake, or to meet their increased nutritional requirements, are usually fed overnight only. This allows the children to maintain a normal daytime eating pattern, whilst still providing the nutritional support they require.
Continuous feeding	*Primary disease management*: Gastro-oesophageal reflux. Malabsorption syndromes (e.g. short gut).

flexible approach to feeding should be taken wherever possible, and compromise is usually necessary. Priority should be given to the child's, parents' and siblings' quality of life, and the feeding regimen should be adapted to the family's routine and lifestyle as closely as possible. This enables the child to maintain his or her usual day-to-day activities. A regimen that keeps the parents up all night or demands that the parents spend all day feeding the child, is unlikely to be successful. In fact, in one small study (n = 10), all mothers described their prescribed feeding schedules as unrealistic and altered these to make them more compatible with their children's needs [37].

Bolus feeding. Bolus feedings are delivered three to eight times per day; each feeding lasting about 15–30 min. Bolus feeds do not interfere with the daily activity, are simple, and do not require a pump. They are more physiological than continuous feeds, and allow freedom of movement for the patient, so that the child is not 'tied' to a feeding bag. They are usually well tolerated when digestive function is normal. Their disadvantages include increased risk of aspiration, in some children, they may cause bloating, cramping, nausea, and diarrhoea. It may not be practical to bolus-feed a child when the volume of formula is large, and demands that the child needs to be fed around the clock.

Continuous feeding. Continuous drip feeding may be delivered without interruption for an unlimited period of time each day. However, it is best to limit feeding to 18 h or less. Feeding around the clock is not recommended as this limits a child's mobility, and may elevate insulin levels contributing to hypoglycemia. Commonly, it is used for 8–10 h during the night, and smaller bolus feedings or oral feeding may be used during the day, so that there is no interference with daytime activities.

Children who are sensitive to volume, at high risk of aspiration, or children who have gastro-oesophageal reflux, may tolerate continuous feeds better. Continuous feeds also increase energy efficiency, allowing more calories to be used for growth. This can be important for severely malnourished children. In addition, stool output is reduced: an important consideration for children with chronic diarrhoea. However, continuous feeding may interfere with serum concentration of some drugs, or the drugs may even reduce the even nutrient composition, for example, vitamin C concentration of the feeds [37].

Teaching home enteral feeding

Ideally, experienced professionals, who discuss both the social and mechanical aspects of feeding, should, administer training. Training programmes should be individually tailored, and parents should receive verbal and written information. Importantly, families should talk to other parents about their experiences of caring for a child on home enteral feeds, so that they can gain insight about the effects of tube feeding on daily social life.

Psychological preparation of a child pre- and post-feeding is essential, and experienced play therapists provide invaluable support to children. Imaginative and interactive training aids should be used. Videos and computer training, as well as written and pictorial guides for feeding, are helpful for families.

Teaching programmes should include technical aspects, and risks and complications and their prevention. Parents should also receive verbal and written information about the social and emotional impact feeding may have [38]. Fathers and other relatives should be encouraged to learn how to give enteral feeds, to lessen the burden on the maternal carer.

Any special needs of the child and family should be identified, and arrangements made to fulfil these needs, prior to hospital discharge. Ongoing 24-hour telephone support is essential for these families, particularly for children on overnight continuous feeds.

Holden [39,40] recommends that teaching sessions with the family or carer should be short, to minimise stress. Increasingly, pictorial teaching aids have been used to help non-English speaking parents and those unable to read and follow written guidelines [41,42].

Teaching programmes should include:

- reasons for home tube feeding;
- safety aspects of care;
- checking tube placement;
- hygiene principles;
- feed preparation;
- use of feeding equipment;
- psychosocial implications of feeding for the child and family;
- problem-solving advice, and what to do in an emergency;
- encouragement of oral stimulation during feeding;
- telephone contacts of hospital and community staff;
- how to obtain equipment, for example, via home delivery company, or from the community.

Home enteral feeding support and monitoring

Ongoing monitoring of children receiving home enteral feeding is essential, in order to assess the child's response to treatment, re-evaluate aims, ensure the feeding regimen and route are appropriate, and reduce the risk of complications which may lead to unnecessary hospital admissions. Regular monitoring of nutritional intake, growth, and biochemistry is essential. Enteral feeds are formulated to be nutritionally complete, but biochemical nutritional adequacy should be checked in children receiving long-term tube feeding. Annual or more frequent estimations of analysis of serum albumin, electrolytes, and haemoglobin are useful, as are as assessments of mineral and trace element status. These are particularly important in children with high requirements or malabsorption (e.g. children with cystic fibrosis).

Townsley and Robinson [43,44] have highlighted many weaknesses in home enteral nutritional support. Problems include lack of co-ordinated health care, with no single person carrying out a specific remit for home feeding, lack of enteral feeding knowledge and training amongst community staff,

funding confusion, inadequate family training, and families, unsure who to contact in the community, returning to specialist units for support. There may also be poor co-ordination, co-operation and communication between hospital and community settings, which can only disadvantage children and their families.

Problems and complications with home enteral nutrition

Holden [45] has identified that the practical, social, and emotional impact of tube feeding is often overlooked or grossly under-estimated by health and social care professionals. Families regularly experience sleep disturbance due to enuresis, diarrhoea, anxiety, and changes to overnight feeding equipment and other feed related problems. In the British Artificial Nutrition Survey [46], 25% of families said they received no practical help, in terms of domestic/laundry services. 25% said they received no help regarding respite facilities for their child. When a child was on a nasogastric feed, people stopped and stared when passing by, and so, parents were concerned about their child's physical appearance with a tube. Some avoided feeding outside in public places. They also commented that when their child eventually had a gastrostomy, they were happier due to the fact nobody needed to know. Many parents with children on long-term tube feeds may not seek professional health advice, preferring to devise their own strategies and solutions.

When families are asked about enteral feeding, their concerns include: finding a caretaker to tube feed their child; public ignorance about tube feeding; planning their social life around feeding schedules, and sadness over depriving a child of the pleasure of eating. Some parents find passing of a nasogastric tube distressing.

Common clinical complications associated with tube feeding include vomiting and aspiration; rapid feed delivery, gastro-oesophageal reflux, and tube displacement into the oesophagus are possible causes [47]. Diarrhoea, possibly due to high feed osmolarity or feed contamination, may cause dehydration, hypernatraemia, and hypoglycaemia.

Parenteral nutrition

Patients who are terminally ill with a severe immunodeficiency or malignancy may be considered for home parenteral nutrition. This is an invasive therapy with inherent risks, and is rarely required in palliative care. In 1998, of the 64 patients registered with the British Association for Enteral and Parenteral Nutrition (BAPEN), only one child was registered with a malignancy [48]. Ethical issues should be carefully thought through before embarking on treatment of such patients.

Parenteral nutrition needs careful supervision from a multi-disciplinary regional centre that has a member available 24 h a day, to give advice and support. Catheter related sepsis is one of the most common complications, and parents are taught about signs and symptoms, and closely monitor their child's temperature. Adjunctive nutritional support either enterally or parenterally, supports the patient during therapy with surgery, chemotherapy, or radiation. Many studies have now shown that a nutritionally replete patient tolerates therapy better, and in some paediatric malignancies, this may enhance survival.

Comfort eating

The social and psychological bonds maintained through mealtimes are very important to parents, and it is important that artificially fed children are still encouraged to enjoy the taste and feel of food, if this can be done safely [43,44]. Even if it is unsafe for a child to eat, it still should be possible to at least offer some form of oral stimulation, that is, by offering dummies to decrease hypersensitivity in the mouth. Advantages of oral stimulation include: bringing pleasure to the child through different tastes, fulfilling parental need to nurture, maintaining oral hygiene, preventing children from feeling excluded at mealtimes, promoting skill in managing secretions, and improving quality of life.

Conclusion

Children with palliative care needs present changing challenges in nutritional care as their disease progresses. Regular nutritional assessment, taking account of the psycho-social needs of the family, the child's underlying condition, the stage of progression, and treatment and associated complications as well as anticipated energy and nutritional requirements, should be undertaken. Where available, a nutritional care team, in conjunction with the child's specialist team, the family, the child (where appropriate), and the primary care and local palliative care teams, will be involved at various stages. The central aim is to support good quality life in the child's palliative care stages, and hence, the balance of benefit/ burden of any planned intervention should be carefully assessed for each child and family within their unique situation.

Addressing feeding issues in palliative care, therefore, begins at an early stage, from diagnosis, through progression,

to terminal care stages. It returns to families a means of some control within their child's devastating situation. The consequent building of trust that the child's nutritional needs are being managed appropriately, so affording the child with the best chance of a good quality life, can do much to improve the child's and family's ability to manage the trauma of the palliative care situation. It should be considered by staff as a high priority, at the heart of palliative care at all stages of care planning, to make practical solutions, determined by whether the goal is aggressive support or comfort and enjoyment of life, available to the family. It carries a tangible message to the child and family, which underpins the approach to their care, that their individual and unique life, and its quality, is valued and respected. It provides hope, and demonstrates that all those involved in their care are working together, despite many and changing challenges, to enable the child and family to live the best quality of life possible within their circumstances, acknowledging that the child is recognized and respected as 'having a lot of living to do'.

References

1. ACT/RCPCH. Guide to the Development of Palliative Care Services, Section 1.2, 1997.
2. Larnert, G. and Ekberg, O. Positioning improves the oral and pharyngeal swallowing function in children with cerebral palsy. *Acta Paediatr* 1995;84(6):689–92.
3. Evans, P.R. The management of fatal illness in childhood *Proceedings of the Royal Society of Medicine* 1969;62:549–50.
4. Darwish, H. Living with cerebral palsy and tube feeding: easier to feed but at what cost? *J Paediatr* 1999;135:272–3.
5. Day. A.S., Beasley. S.W., Meads. H., and Abbot. G. Morbidity associated with gastrostomy placement in children demands an ongoing integrated approach to care. *N Zea Med J* 2001;164–7.
6. Poole, K. and Froggat, K. Loss of weight and loss of appetite in advanced cancer: A problem for the patient, carer or health professional? *Palliat Med* 2002;16:499–506.
7. Holden, C.M. Anorexia in the terminally ill cancer patient: The emotional impact on the patient and the family. *Hosp J* 1991;7:73–84.
8. Justice, C. The natural death whilst not eating; a type of palliative care in Banares, India. *J Pall Care* 1995;11:38–42.
9. Sullivan, P.B., Lambert, B. Rose, M., Ford-Adams M., and Griffiths, P. Prevalence and severity of feeding and nutritional problems in children with neurological impairment: Oxford Feeding Study *Dev Med Child Neur* 2000;42:674–80.
10. Russell, D.M., Leiter, L.A., Whitwell, J. Marliss, E.B., and Jeejeebhoy K.N. Skeletal Muscle function during hypocaloric diets and fasting: A comparison with standard nutritional assessment parameters. *Am J Clin Nutrit* 1983;37:133–8.
11. Efthimiou, J., Fleming, J., and Spiro, S.G. The effect of supplementary oral nutrition in poorly nourished patients with chronic pulmonary disease. *Am Rev Resp Dis* 1998;137:1075–82.

12. Patrick, J., Boland, M., Stoski, D., and Murray, G.E. Rapid correction of wasting in children with cerebral palsy. *Dev Med Child Neurol* 1986:28;734–9.

13. Stallings, V.A., Charney, E.B., Davies J.C., and Cronk, C.E. Nutrition related growth failure in children with quadriplegic cerebral plasy. *Dev Med Child Neurol* 1993;35:126–38.

14. Puntis, J.W.L. Establishing a nutritional support team. In *Baillieres Clinical Paediatrics.* Bailliere Tindall,1997;5(2):177-187.

15. Steiner, N. and Bruera, E. Methods of hydration in palliative care patients. *J Pall Care* 1998; 14:2,6–13.

16. Fainsinger, R.L. and Bruera, E. When to treat dehydration in a terminally ill patient? *Support Cancer Care* 1997;5(3):205–11.

17. National Council for Hospice and Palliative Care Services/Ethics Committee of the Association for Palliative Medicine of Great Britain and Ireland. Joint Working Party. Ethics and Nutrition/Hydration, 2002.

18. Royal College of Paediatrics and Child Health. Withholding and withdrawing life sustaining treatment in children. A framework for practice, 1997.

19. General Medical Council. Withholding and Withdrawing Life-prolonging treatments: good practise in decision making. London, 2002.

20. British Medical Association. Withholding and withdrawing life-prolonging medical treatment. Guidance for decision making. *BMJ*, London, 1999.

21. Sheard, N. and Clarke, N. Nutritional management of paediatric oncology patients. In S.B. Baker, A.D. Baker, ed. *Paediatric Enteral Nutrition*, London: Hoddor Arnold, 1994; p. 387–97.

22. Murray, S.M. and Pindora, S. Nutrition support for bone marrow transplant patients. *Cochrane database Syst Rev.* 2002(2): CD002920.

23. Goldman, A. Life Threatening illnesses and symptom control in children. In D. Doyle, G. Hanks, N. Macdonald, ed. *Palliative Medicine, 2nd Edition*, 1998; p. 1033–43. Oxford: Oxford University Press.

24. Woolfe. J., Grier. H., Klar. N. *et al.* Symptoms and Suffering at the end of life in children. *N Eng J Med* 2000, 342 (5): 326–333.

25 Klein, S., Alpers, D.H., Grand, R.J., Levin, M.S., Lin, H.C., Mansbach, C.M., Burant, C., Reeds, P., and Rombeau, J.L. Advances in nutrition and gastroenterology: Summary of the 1997 A.S.P.E.N. Research Workshop. *JPEN J Parenter Enteral Nutr.* Jan-Feb 1998; 22(1):3–13.

26. Coad, J. and Moloney, B. Nutritional assessment of children's nutritional state during illness. In C. Holden and A. MacDonald *Nutrition and Child Health*. London: Baelliere Tindall, 2000, p. 251–264.

27. Bunting, J. and Weaver L.T. Anthropometry in a children's hospital: A study of staff knowledge, use and quality of equipment. *J Human Nutr Diet* 1997;10:17–23.

28. Department of Health. Dietary Reference Values for Food Energy and Nutrients for the United Kingdom. Report on Health and Social Subjects No 41, London: HMSO 1991.

29. Holden, C., Johnson, T., and Caney, D. Nutritional Support for children in the community. In C. Holden, A. MacDonald, eds. *Nutrition and Child Health*. London: Baelliere Tindall, p. 176–184.

30. Clark, S. MacDonald, A., and Booth, I.W. (1998) Abstract: Improved growth and nitrogen deficiency in infants receiving an energy-supplemented standard infant formula. Proceedings of the 2nd Annual Spring Meeting, Royal College of Paediatrics and Child Health 1998, p. 75.

31. Walsh, 1994.

32. Tolia, V., Ventimiglia, J., and Kuhns, L. Gastrointestinal intolerance of a pediatric fiber formula in developmentally disabled children. *J Am Coll Nutr* 1997;16:224–28.

33. den Broeder, E., Lippens, R.J., vant Hof, M.A., Tolboom, J.J., Sengers, R.C., van den Berg, A.M., van Houdt, N.B., Hofman, Z., and van Staveren, W.A. Nasogastric tube feeding in children with cancer: The effect of two different formulas on weight, body composition, and serum protein concentrations. *JPEN* 2000; 24:351–60.

34. Gauderer, M.W., Ponsky, J.L., and Izant, R.J. Jr. Gastrostomy without laparotomy: A percutaneous endoscopic technique. *J Pediatr Surg* 1980;15:72–5.

35. Kastner, T., Criscione T., and Walsh, K. The role of tube feeding in the mortality of profoundly disabled people with severe mental retardation. *Arch Pediatr Adolesc Med* 1994 May;148:537–8.

36. Spalding, K. and McKeever, P. Mothers' experiences caring for children with disabilities who require a gastrostomy tube. *J Pediatr Nurs* 1998;13:234–43.

37. Gorman, S.R., Armstrong G., Allen, K.R., Ellis, J., and Puntis J.W. Scarcity in the midst of plenty: Enteral tube feeding complicated by scurvy. *J Pediatr Gastroenterol Nutr* 2002;35:93–5.

38. Chaplen, C. Parents views of caring for children with gastrostomies. *British Journal of Nursing* 1997;6(1):34–8.

39. Holden, C.E. and Macdonald, A. Nutrition support at home: Emotional support and composition of feeds. *Current Paediatrics* 1997: 218–22.

40. Holden, C.E., Sexton, E., and Paul, L. Enteral nutrition for children. *Nurs Stand* 1997;11(32):49–56.

41. Shah, R. Practice with attitude: Questions in cultural awareness training. *Child Health* 1994;1:245–9.

42. Sexton, E., Paul, L., and Holden, C.E. A pictorial assisted teaching tool for families. *Paediatr Nurs* 1996;8:24–6.

43. Townsley, R. and Robinson, C. Comfort eating. *Nurs Times* 1997; 93:1997.

44. Townsley, R. and Robinson, C. Online support: Effective support services to disabled children who are tube fed. The Norah Fry Research Centre, Bristol, 1997b.

45. Holden, C. Implications for families: enteral and parenteral feeding. MSc University of Wolverhampton, 1994 (unpublished).

46. Bans, 2002.

47. Colomb, V. Home artificial nutritional support in gastrointestinal disease. *Curr Opin Clin Nutr Metab Care* 1998;1:395–9.

48. Elia, M., Russel, C., and Stratton, R. Trends in artificial nutrition support in the UK during 1996–2000. A report of the British Artificial Nutrition Survey (BANS), Maidenhead, Berks, 2001.

49. Cook, P. Family support in the community. Chapter 13; 177–187 in Supporting Sick Children and Their Families 1999. London: Baelliere Tindall.

50. Cronk, C., Crocker, A. C., Peusche, l. S. M. *et al.* Growth charts for children with Down's syndrome: 1 month to 18 years of age. *Paediatrics* 1998;81:102.

51. Hill S., and Long, S. Home enteral and parenteral nutrition for children. In J.Nigtingalr ed. Intestinal failure. Greenwich Medical Media: London, p. 438–446.

52. Johnson, T.E., Janes S.J., MacDonald, A., Elia M., and Booth, I.W. An observational study to evaluate micronutrient status during enteral feeding. *Arch Dis Child* 2002;86:411–5.

53. Kirk, J. Growth and nutritional assessment of children. In C. Holden, A. MacDonald eds. Nutrition and Child Health. Bailliere Tindall, London 2000; p. 161–176

54. Knowles, M.R. Diabetes and cystic fibrosis. New questions emerging from increased longevity. *Journal of Paediatr* 1988; 112:415–16.

55. Maynard, L., Barclay, S., Palmer, R., Todd, C., and Vickers, D. Families in need—the needs of families caring for children with life-threatening illnesses in Cambridge Health District. Cambridge Lifespan Healthcare NHS Trust, 1996.

56. Nardella, M. Early nutrition intervention with Williams syndrome and hypercalcaemia. *Nutrtio focus* 1996;11:1–8.

57. Wolley, H, Stein, A., Forest, G.C., and Baum, J. D. Imparting the diagnosis of life-threat illnesses in children. *BMJ* 1989;298:1623–26.

25 Depression, anxiety, anger and delirium

Renée McCulloch and Jim F. Hammel

Introduction

Despite numerous advances in paediatric palliative care over the past two decades, issues of a psychological, psycho-social, and psychiatric nature continue to experience a dearth of attention. Numerous reasons exist for the lack of evidence-based advances in the understanding and management of these areas. Firstly, clinicians in general might be hesitant to 'label' children—in any health context—with a socially stigmatising diagnosis, such as depression or anxiety. Froese [1] commented on this hesitancy in the arena of paediatric referrals to a general psychiatry service; in a study of 205 children seen by a psychiatric service, Froese noted that depression and adjustment reactions were less likely to be reported correctly in medical discharge diagnoses than psycho-physiological disorders and psychoses. Secondly, clinicians might shy away from viewing a child's psychological symptomatology as 'inappropriate' in the setting of the extraordinary life stresses inherent in life-limiting illness. Thirdly, the management of non-psychological symptoms may be the predominant concern of the clinician. Fourthly, although Paediatrics as a field is psychologically and holistically oriented, the specific issues in palliative care may be viewed as beyond the realm of expertise of the care-giver.

The timing as to when psychological symptoms may occur in the disease process is unclear, and subject to contradictory evidence in the literature. For example, a four-year prospective study of 39 children with cancer [2] found psychological problems most evident immediately after the diagnosis of cancer, only to have the symptoms gradually decline such that no difference existed between the study group and healthy controls at subsequent assessments. On the other hand, a study of 51 Swedish children with cancer showed the opposite pattern: 16 patients on treatment showed no difference in anxiety and depression compared with the healthy controls, while 35 off-treatment patients showed higher depression and anxiety than the control population [3]. With little firm data to establish the temporal pattern of psychological disturbance in paediatric palliative care, health care professionals must be aware that these symptoms may develop throughout the disease course.

Given these obstacles, it is perhaps not surprising that so little documented research exists on the subject of the identification, and particularly, the management of psychological symptoms in paediatric palliative care. Most of the studies that have been described have occurred in the paediatric oncology setting, with little work in other chronic, life-limiting, or terminal illnesses. Clearly, paediatric palliative care extends beyond the borders of oncology, yet, this is not reflected in the literature.

Extrapolating the available literature to include all paediatric palliative care patients is obviously unsound. Most oncology patients in these studies are receiving 'active' treatment in pursuit of cure and of course, living with a life threatening or life limiting illness (HIV, chronic disease) has different connotations to being in the palliative phase. However, tentative comparison might be drawn between these groups in that they share the 'burden' of undergoing intensive treatments and a significant number ultimately become palliative. Despite (indeed, because of) the notable absence of knowledge in this field, the clinician must be especially vigilant in identifying and treating these symptoms.

Depression

Features and diagnosis

Features and challenges

The clinical features of depression in the general paediatric population have been described as 'remarkably similar' to those of adult depression [4]; see also Kovacs [5]. Indeed, both populations depend upon essentially the same Diagnostic and Statistical Manual of mental disorder—version IV (DSM-IV) criteria for diagnostic purposes.

Despite obvious differences between healthy and ill paediatric patients, DSM-IV criteria frame the diagnosis of depression more than any other source. For diagnostic purposes, five or more of the following symptoms must have been present over a two-week period and represent a change from previous functioning (i.e. "cause clinically significant distress or impairment in functioning"), with at least one of the symptoms being either (1) depressed mood, or (2) loss of interest or pleasure:

- depressed mood;

- markedly diminished pleasure in all, or almost all, activities;

- significant weight loss when not dieting, or weight gain, or decrease or increase in appetite nearly every day;

- insomnia or hypersomnia nearly every day;

- psychomotor agitation or retardation nearly every day (observable by others, not merely subjective feelings of restlessness or being slowed-down);

- fatigue, or loss of energy, nearly every day;

- feelings of worthlessness, or excessive or inappropriate guilt (which may be delusional);

- diminished ability to think or concentrate, or indecisiveness (either by subjective account or as observed by others);

- current thoughts of death (not just fear of dying), recurrent suicidal ideation without specific plan, or a suicide attempt, or a specific plan for committing suicide (American Psychiatric Association [6]).

In the World Health Organization's ICD-10 classification (World Health Organization, The ICD-10 Classification of Mental and Behavioural Disorders: Diagnostic Criteria for Research, World Health Organization, Geneva, 1993), the criteria for 'depressive episode' are also defined as having a two-week duration, without any manic or hypomanic symptoms, and without a psychoactive substance or organic mental disorder etiology. The ICD-10 breaks-down depressive symptoms into two sets of 'criteria,' from which classification can be made for 'mild depressive episode' (at least two symptoms from Criterion B and one from Criterion C), 'moderate depressive episode' (at least two symptoms from Criterion B and four from Criterion C), or "severe depressive episode, with or without psychotic features" (all three symptoms from Criterion B and at least five symptoms from Criterion C.) Importantly, the ICD-10 criteria for 'severe depressive episode' note, 'If important symptoms, such as agitation or retardation, are marked, the patient may be unwilling or unable to describe many symptoms in detail. An overall grading of severe episode may still be justified in such a case.'

The DSM-IV and ICD-10 diagnostic criteria are compared in Table 25.1. Again, all of these depressive symptoms refer to adult patients, and are problematic, given the commonly encountered constellation of symptoms in the paediatric palliative care patient. One of the primary differences between the two systems is that mood disorders assessed as secondary to a general medical condition (e.g. hypothyroidism) are categorized under 'Organic mental disorders' in ICD-10, while in the DSM-IV they are listed as a sub-category of mood disorders. In neither case, though, are they considered in the specific context of either paediatric or palliative care patients.

While both DSM-IV and ICD-10 criteria have useful classification functions in the research setting, the clinician is best served by considering each paediatric palliative care patient on an individual basis, with the priority of evaluating the depressive severity and symptomatology within that patient's particular clinical milieu.

Attempts have been made to modify these criteria for children, so that they are more developmentally appropriate. For example, Luby et al. (2002)[7] have described modifications to the DSM-IV criteria specifically for the pre-school child, such as appending criteria 1 to include 'for a portion of the day for several days, as observed (or reported) in behaviour'. In a further study of 145 pre-schoolers, Luby et al. (2003)[8] have also shown that their modified depressive criteria identified a substantial proportion of children with clinically significant, but less severe, depressive symptoms 'missed' by the standard DSM-IV criteria; however, their modified criteria themselves failed to capture the most severely affected pre-schoolers.

In general, children often have difficulty recognizing, understanding, and then reporting depressive symptomatology. It is particularly challenging to accurately assess depression in the pre-school child, given the limitations in the child's understanding of affective state, time concepts, symptom course, and questions which require some form of judgment [4,9]. Birmaher et al. (1996)[10] found that depressed children and adolescents in the general paediatric population have fewer melancholic symptoms than adults, and children have more somatic complaints than adolescents. Furthermore, it was only with the use of developmentally adjusted DSM-IV criteria that the symptom of anhedonia was found to distinguish between depressed and non-depressed pre-school children [7].

The diagnosis of depression in children with life-limiting illness is especially challenging for several reasons. The DSM-IV does not contain criteria for depression (or anxiety) in children and adolescents with comorbid medical illnesses, life-limiting conditions, or palliative care needs. For many paediatric palliative care patients, the use of DSM-IV criteria is made particularly difficult, given the presence of disease symptoms that overlap with those of the depressive criteria. Specifically, neuro-vegetative symptoms (e.g., sleeplessness, anorexia, fatigue, and psychomotor slowing) may reflect

Table 25.1 Depressive symptoms criteria. Comparison of DSM-IV and ICD-10

DSM-IV Depressive symptoms[1]	ICD-10 Depressive symptoms[2]
• depressed mood • markedly diminished pleasure in all, or almost all, activities • significant weight loss when not dieting, or weight gain, or decrease or increase in appetite nearly every day • insomnia or hypersomnia nearly every day • psychomotor agitation or retardation nearly every day (observable by others, not merely subjective feelings of restlessness or being slowed-down • fatigue or loss of energy nearly every day • feelings of worthlessness, or excessive or inappropriate guilt (which may be delusional) • diminished ability to think or concentrate, or indecisiveness (either by subjective account, or as observed by others) • Current thoughts of death (not just fear of dying), recurrent suicidal ideation without specific plan, or a suicide attempt, or a specific plan for committing suicide	*Criterion B:* • depressed mood to a degree that is definitely abnormal for the individual, present for most of the day and almost every day, largely uninfluenced by circumstances, and sustained for at least two weeks • loss of interest or pleasure in the activities that are normally pleasurable • decreased energy or increased fatigability *Criterion C:* • loss of confidence or self-esteem • unreasonable feelings of self-reproach, or excessive and inappropriate guilt • recurrent thoughts of death or suicide, or any suicidal behaviour. • complaints or evidence of diminished ability to think or concentrate, such as indecisiveness or vacillation • change in psychomotor activity, with agitation or retardation (subjective or objective) • Sleep disturbance of any type • change in appetite (decrease or increase), with corresponding weight change

[1] American Psychiatric Association. Diagnostic and statistical manual of mental disorders Association © 2000. (Reprinted with permission from the Diapnosh. fourth edition. 1994, Washington, D.C.)
[2] World Health Organization. The ICD-10 Classification of Mental and Behavioural Disorders: Diagnostic Criteria for Research. 1993, Geneva.

disease or treatment effects, rather than depressive symptoms. This particular diagnostic challenge has been noted in the literature since 1955. In discussing 'the atmosphere of melancholia', often associated with the paediatric oncology patient, Richmond and Waisman commented:

Since the child's physical energy diminishes so significantly, it may be that most of the child's lack of emotional as well as physical response is due more to this factor, than to psychological awareness of the diagnosis[11].

Worchel *et al.* (1988)[12] have shown that somatic items are not good discriminators between depressed and non-depressed medically ill children; moreover, low self-concept (i.e. feeling that one is inferior to others, 'a bad person', feelings of self-blame) was present in paediatric oncology patients, regardless of their level of depression. In an attempt to address this issue, Phipps and Srivastava [13] recently devised an 'anhedonia scale' for use in children with cancer, but found no difference on this scale between children with cancer and healthy controls. In medically ill adults, Cavenaugh *et al.* [14] provided evidence that cognitive symptoms better discriminate

depression. Indeed, the DSM-IV criteria do caution 'Note: Do not include symptoms that are clearly due to a general medical condition …' They also provide the caveat that 'The symptoms are not better accounted for by bereavement, that is after the loss of a loved one.' Although written with the adult patient in mind, the issue of 'anticipatory grieving' also occurs in the paediatric palliative care population. Thus, for both of these reasons, the DSM-IV criteria might be especially inappropriate for evaluating the paediatric palliative care patient.

The appearance of depression in youth with chronic and life-limiting illness may, therefore, be less clear, due to the overlap of somatic and psychological symptoms, and may thus result in depression at the sub-clinical level. Of relevance to this point, Kovacs and colleagues [15,16] have shown that recurrent illness is seen in the majority of those with paediatric depression. In a meta-analysis of 60 studies on children and adolescents with chronic medical problems, Bennett [17] has concluded that while children with a chronic medical problem have a slightly greater risk of depressive symptoms, most are not clinically depressed.

Adjustment disorder

Many paediatric palliative care clinicians may consider whether their patients' symptoms most accurately reflect an 'adjustment disorder'. This diagnosis is considered when a patient develops 'emotional or behavioural symptoms' within 3 months of a significant life change, or as a result of a stressful life event, which can include the presence of serious physical illness. In the paediatric patient, adjustment disorder is often seen in the context of hospitalization. Children with adjustment disorder often display regressive symptoms, such as enuresis and thumb-sucking. Perhaps most importantly, the emotional or behavioural distress 'markedly exceeds what you would normally expect from such a stressor', and does not fulfil criteria for an Axis I disorder, or worsening of a pre-existing Axis I or II disorder. For DSM-IV coding purposes (which, again, are generally more applicable in the research, rather than the clinical, setting), adjustment disorders can be specified as 'with depressed mood' ('The patient is tearful, sad, hopeless'), 'with anxiety' ('the patient is nervous, fearful, worried'), or a combination of the two ('with mixed anxiety and depressed mood'). The distinction between adjustment disorder and depression can be also aided by the timing of the symptoms. As defined by both the DSM-IV and ICD-10, the symptoms of adjustment disorder occur within 3 months of a stressor, and do not last longer than six months after the end of the stressor, In the case of the paediatric palliative care patient, though, the life stressor does not 'end' as such. Moreover, the DSM-IV specifies that 'the symptoms are not caused by bereavement,' which can be problematic in the palliative care setting, given the prevalence of anticipatory grieving.

Risk factors

As with assessment of depression in the general paediatric population, it is important to identify factors that may place paediatric palliative care patients at risk of depression.

In paediatric palliative care, and especially in the case of the dying child, the potential for isolation and social neglect places the child at substantial risk of depression. Almost 25 years ago, Chapman and Goodall [18] commented on this, reporting, "We have heard this referred to as the dying child syndrome and such neglect is conducive to depression."

In considering depression in the paediatric palliative care patient, it is crucial to consider the possible role of co morbid pain. This relationship has been discussed in the chronic paediatric pain literature [19,20], where depression has been found to be strongly associated with chronic pain. The depression–pain linkage is particularly relevant in the paediatric palliative care setting. For example, a French study of 80 children with cancer, aged 2–6 years, found an association between disease-related pain and a depression-like reaction, which correlated with the pain's intensity. [21]. In a study of 43 in-patient paediatric oncology patients referred for psychiatric evaluation, Steif and Heiligenstein [22] found that 20% of the psychiatric consultations resulted in a primary recommendation for improved pain control. When assessing both depression and pain, it is imperative to bear in mind the symbiotic nature of these two common issues.

Depression is also more likely in the paediatric patient to whom diagnosis and health status are not disclosed. Last and van Veldhuizen [23] studied a sample of 56 children with cancer, aged 8–16 years, and showed significantly less depression if parents told them about their diagnosis and prognosis at the initial stage of the disease. In an Italian study of 30 leukaemic children in the first year of remission [23], children who received poor communication regarding their illness experienced more affective disturbances (including insecurity, irritability, poor self-perception, instability, and depression). A Finnish study of 53 patients who had electively discontinued treatment for leukaemia and lymphoma (mean age 12.8 at completion of study surveys) found that patients more

Table 25.2 Depressed mood compared with adjustment disorder

	Depressed mood	Adjustment disorder
Onset	Variable	Onset within 3 months of stressor
Duration	Generally at least 2 weeks	Does not last longer than 6 months after the end of the stressor or its consequences
Exclusionary criteria	Symptoms: (1) do not include manic or hypomanic symptoms; (2) are not attributable to psychoactive substance use, or to any organic mental disorder	Symptoms: (1) do not fulfil criteria for an Axis I disorder, and are not merely the worsening of a pre-existing Axis I or Axis II disorder; (2) are not caused by bereavement; (3) do not include separation anxiety disorder of chilhood

informed of their disease process were less depressed than poorly-informed children. [25].

Non-illness related psycho-social life events can also act as risk factors for depression. In a one-year longitudinal study of 38 children and adolescents with cancer, Kaplan et al. [26] found that depressive scores were highly related to psychosocial life events, but not related to the course of the oncologic illness (e.g. relapse or remission status, number of relapses, length of time since diagnosis, and number of weeks of treatment until remission).

The presence of maternal depression can also serve as a risk factor for depression in the child. Mulhern and colleagues [27] studied a sample of 99 children with cancer, and their mothers. They found that the severity of the mothers' self-reported depressive symptoms, assessed with the Beck Depression Inventory, was associated with higher levels of child depression by both child- and parent-reported measures. Similarly, maternal depression has been associated with poorer quality of life in children with cancer. In a study of 32 leukaemic children [28], children who self-reported poorer quality of life had mothers who were more depressed.

Diagnostic tools

All diagnostic tools for assessing paediatric depression have been developed for children and adolescents without the comorbidity of medical illness. Due to their low sensitivity, several screening tools (e.g. the Child Depression Inventory, the Pediatric Symptom Checklist, the Child Behaviour Checklist) may not be appropriate for use with chronically medically ill children and adolescents [29]. While highly specific (i.e. they may confirm the clinician's concerns), these tools are poorly sensitive (i.e. they may miss many disorders in chronically ill youth), and may thus undermine clinical judgment. The absence of assessment tools designed specifically for the paediatric palliative care patient further hampers the clinician's ease of diagnosis, as has already been noted in paediatric oncology [30].

One of the commonly cited deficiencies in screening tools for paediatric depression is the poor concordance on patient symptomatology. Many authors have reported low level, of agreement when comparing children's self-report scores and measures from parents [32–33], teachers, and peers. Andrews and colleagues [32] reported that a sample of general paediatric patients reported more depressive symptoms about themselves than their parents. Furthermore, Braaten et al. [31] have shown in a sample of 186 youth–mother pairs that youths reported a milder form of depression compared with that identified by parental reports.

In contrast to the general paediatric population, Challinor et al. [34] studied 43 paediatric oncology patients and found high positive correlations between scores from patients and their parents for depression, and high positive correlations between teachers and patients for depression; they also found that parents over-report depressive symptoms in their children. On the other hand, a study of 107 children with cancer and 442 healthy controls [13] found that both, a self-report depression inventory and a measure for anhedonia, were not significantly related to parental and physician ratings of depression. The contradictory findings between these studies are possibly due to the different measures used in each study, or to the health status of their respective patient samples. Thus, conclusions as to the concordance between parent–, child–, and teacher–symptom assessment are difficult to make.

The most commonly used diagnostic tool is the Children's Depression Inventory [CDI] [35]. This child self-report questionnaire utilises 27 items, each rated on a scale of 0–2, with more severe symptoms receiving higher ratings. In a direct comparison of the CDI and DSM-III in 231 child psychiatric patients [36], depressed and non-depressed children were shown to differ across all domains (including depressed-related symptoms, cognitive processes, and social activity). Nevertheless, many have questioned the validity of the CDI, given the poor correlations between CDI and non-self-report ratings from peers, parents, or teachers [37,38]. Kronenberg et al. [39] have found that non-interview techniques, such as the CDI and the Child Behaviour Check List, were less reliable in diagnosing affective disorders in general paediatrics, compared to a non-directive interview with psychological projective testing and a semi-structured psychiatric interview. The apparent superiority of diagnostic interviews over traditional survey evaluations has found additional support. In a study of 102 youth (ages 7–17), Carlson et al. [40] identified more children with sub-clinical and 'masked depression' using a systematic interview, than, with standard evaluative procedures. Similarly, comparison of the validity and reliability of the CDI and Depression Self-Rating Scale found both to have only moderate discrimination between depressed and non-depressed patients, with no significant relationship between teachers' assessments of classroom behaviour and the two scales; as an additional potential barrier to these tools, better agreement was seen in more verbally intelligent children, irrespective of age [41]. Finally, it must be emphasised that even if the CDI is used, a clinical or structured interview is necessary to determine diagnostic status [42].

As acknowledged previously, the presence of somatic items in paediatric depressive scales clouds the issue, and raises the question of whether it is truly depression, or rather, disease course being measured. Thus, the clinician may over-estimate the presence and severity of depression in using scales that incorporate somatic symptoms into the assessment. In a sample of 24 paediatric oncology patients referred for psychiatric assessment, Heiligenstein and Jacobsen [43] modified a common screening tool for depression (the Children's Depression Rating Scale—Revised or CDRS-R; [44] to eliminate items assessing somatic complaints. They found that this modified scale did not correlate with functional impairment, and also maintained the same level of diagnostic sensitivity in the clinicians' identification of depression severity.

Prevalence/Incidence

The prevalence and incidence of depression in the general paediatric population vary by age, assessment duration, and population. As thoroughly reviewed by Axelson and Birmaher [45], the prevalence of depression in children and adolescents from a 3-month assessment period is approximately 2.0%, while that from a 6–12 month period varied substantially between 1.6–18.0%. (Of note: all of these studies relied on DSM-III/III-R or IV criteria, included parent and/or child interviews, and had sample sizes between 222 and 3733). As reviewed by Son and Kirchner [46], depression affects 2% of pre-pubertal children, and 5–8% of adolescents in the general population.

Depression incidence has also been reported in children and adolescents with chronic illness. In a study of 44 epilepsy patients between the ages of 7–18 years, 26% exhibited significantly increased depression scores on the Child Depression Inventory [47]. The lifetime prevalence of depression in cystic fibrosis has been shown to be 11.5%, a marginally higher figure than that quoted previously in the general population; interestingly, though, the same study [48] also showed a significantly higher lifetime depression prevalence in Crohn's disease (29%) and ulcerative colitis (21). Thus, it appears that the prevalence of depression in youth with chronic illness is higher than in the general paediatric population, but cystic fibrosis—a chronic illnesses that is also life-limiting—does not appear to follow this pattern. Similarly, in a meta-analysis of 60 studies on paediatric chronic illness, Bennett [17] has reviewed the finding that depression is more likely in children with asthma and sickle cell anaemia than those with cystic fibrosis and cancer. In contrast, though, an Indian study [49] found depression (and anxiety) to be more common in 35 leukaemic children, compared with 35 children with chronic illness.

Other life-limiting illnesses that have a chronic deterioration in adolescence, such as Duchenne muscular dystrophy, may be unique in their manifestation of depression. These boys appear to develop depression over time. In a study of 23 Duchenne boys in Dublin, Fitzpatrick et al (1985)[50] found depression to be more common in

Duchenne patients than in matched healthy controls, and observed that this only occurred in boys older than nine years of age. This finding could be due to the previously discussed difficulty in diagnosing depression in younger children. It is also possible that depression in life-limiting illness may only become manifest as the illness progresses in severity, or as the child develops a greater understanding of the disease process and increasing limitations. Again, diagnosing depression in this particular group can be extremely challenging, due to the obvious overlap of symptoms that exist between depression and disease progression. Adolescents and young men with Duchenne muscular dystrophy frequently suffer from poor appetite, weight loss, weakness, headaches, and sleep disturbance, symptoms that occur within the spectrum of a depressive disorder. It is very likely that depression is under-diagnosed in this group. It should be considered and evaluated at appropriate intervals, in order to maximise well-being.

In children with cancer, the incidence of depression shows wide variability, with rates reported as high as 17% (using the DSM-III criteria; [51]) and as low as 7–8% [27]. Similarly, Dunitz et al. [52] studied depression prevalence in 34 children with newly-diagnosed paediatric oncology disease over a 14-month period, and found a 'clearcut depression' in six of the children. Although not specifically diagnosing depression, Collins et al. [30] found 36% of a sample of 159 children with cancer 'feeling sad,' (with 60% of those reporting the symptom severity between 'moderate' and 'very severe.') Worchel et al. (1992)[53] have discussed this wide variability in depression prevalence, and have shown that this might be explained by both the various measures used and patients' selective reporting of symptoms.

However, children with life-limiting illness and palliative care needs do not demonstrate depression as frequently as might be assumed. In a recent Taiwanese study, Chao and colleagues [54] found no difference on CDI scores between 24 paediatric cancer patients and a normative sample. Phipps and Srivastava [13] compared 107 children with cancer and 442 healthy controls, and found significantly fewer depressive symptoms in the children with cancer, and no difference between the two groups on the measure of anhedonia they designed. Bose et al. [55] found that children with HIV did not score as high on anxiety and depression scales when compared with the parental reports, and in fact, described low levels of depressive and anxious affect and generally positive self-regard. Worchel et al. [12] compared a paediatric sample of 72 oncology patients, 42 in-patient psychiatry patients, and 304 control schoolchildren. They found that the oncology group reported less depression than the psychiatric and control samples. Within the context of repressive adaptation (discussed further in this chapter), Canning et al. [56] also reported significantly lower levels of depression in 31 cancer patients, compared to 83 healthy controls. This contrary finding of 'lesser-than-expected' depression in paediatric oncology could be explained by the issue of repression.

The lower prevalence of depression might also simply be a reflection of the timing of depression assessment in the disease course. For example, in a study of 42 British adolescents with cancer compared with 174 healthy controls, Allen and colleagues [57] found that, contrary to the study's hypotheses, the adolescents with cancer were no more depressed than the controls, when assessed at the time of diagnosis.

Distinguishing from the normal range

As discussed, disease symptoms in the paediatric palliative care patient may result in a different clinical presentation from that seen in the general paediatric population. At the same time, though, the prevalence of depression may not necessarily be greater in palliative care than the norm. Indeed, few studies report greater depression in paediatric oncology than the healthy population (for an example, see [58]. Thus, studies showing greater depression in paediatric oncology patients, compared to the healthy paediatric population, are actually the exception rather than the rule.

In a study of 12 adolescents with end-stage renal failure, the incidence of depression, as well as anxiety and hostility, was described as no different from a healthy adolescent sample [59]. Noll and colleagues [60] compared 76 paediatric oncology patients with 76 case control classroom peers, and found no significant differences on measures of depression and loneliness. In a Brazilian study of 75 children (leukaemia = 21, blood dyscrasia = 21, controls = 33), no significant differences in depressive symptoms were found between the leukaemics and the two other groups of children[61].

Repression

Children with cancer and other life-limiting illnesses may report less depression than expected, due to the use of coping mechanism such as repression, denial, and defensiveness. As early as 1976, Kagan[62] described the use of denial as an appropriate coping mechanism in adolescents with bone cancer, resulting in a fluctuation between levels of denial and acceptance. Over the past decade, work has highlighted the attention being paid to repressive adaptation and defensiveness in children with cancer and other illnesses. Canning et al. [56] compared 31 adolescent cancer patients with 83 healthy high school students, and identified the feature of 'repressive adaptation' in those reporting low anxiety and high defensiveness; a significantly higher proportion of the cancer patients were identified as repressors, and, correspondingly, the cancer patients reported significantly less depression than the healthy

controls. Phipps and colleagues [63] conducted a study of 107 oncology patients aged 7–16 years, and compared measures of depressive symptoms, trait anxiety, defensiveness, and coping styles. They found a significant excess of children using a repressive coping style in the oncology group, and those who used this repressive coping style self-reported the lowest levels of depression. Moreover, repressive adaptation in the cancer patients was unrelated to duration of time since their diagnosis. In a subsequent study [64], a longitudinal assessment of children with cancer showed repressive adaptation to start at the time of diagnosis, and be maintained until 6-month and 1-year follow-ups post-diagnosis. Thus, repression seems to be a long-term phenomenon in children with cancer, and may explain why depressive symptoms may appear less commonly than expected [65]. Finally, Worchel et al. [12] have noted that the use of self-report measures is particularly problematic in paediatric oncology patients using denial or repressive adaptation as coping skills.

Non-pharmacological support

Open communication, informed choice on therapeutic options, and the provision of clear support to the patient and family are the non-pharmacological foundation to decreasing the presence of depression in paediatric palliative care patients. As early as 1980, Chapman and Goodall[18] emphasised the necessity of open communication with the child or adolescent as the initial management strategy in addressing depression in paediatric palliative care.

In the general child and adolescent population, depression has been treated non-pharmacologically, with diverse modalities. As reviewed by Findling et al. [66], these non-pharmacological approaches have even included light therapy and electro-convulsive therapy—modalities which would be of highly questionable use in the paediatric palliative care population. Of the psychotherapeutic approaches to depression in the general paediatric population, cognitive-behavioural therapy (CBT) has been shown to be the most useful. As might be expected, comorbidity with an anxiety disorder has been shown to be a predictor of poor response to CBT therapy for children with depression [67,68]

For children with chronic illness, some studies have hinted at the benefit of community-based support groups. Chernoff et al. [69] have described a randomised controlled trial of 136 children, aged seven to eleven years, with sickle cell anaemia, cystic fibrosis, diabetes mellitus, or moderate to severe asthma. After participation in a 15-month community support program, fewer children in the experimental group (19% at baseline, 10% post-intervention) scored in the "maladjustment range" (as measured by the Children's Depression Inventory, the Revised Children's Manifest Anxiety Scale, and the Self-Perception

Profile for Children); in the control population of children, there was an increase in these number, (15% vs. 21%).

Unfortunately, very few studies have examined the role of non-pharmacological support in the paediatric palliative care setting. In 1982, Nitschke and colleagues [70] described their unique hospital-based approach to decrease depression and psychological disorders in end-stage paediatric oncology patients. They organized a conference which emphasised 'patients' acknowledgement of the progression of the disease and the imminence of death' and patient-guided informed decision-making; subsequently, the majority of the 43 children who took part chose supportive care without chemotherapy, and 'severe depression and severe behavioural problems' were rarely seen to occur.

Pharmacological management

To date, there have been no reported studies on the specific use of any anti-depressants in paediatric patients with life-limiting illness or in the palliative care setting. Nevertheless, insight from adult palliative care practitioners is helpful in planning a therapeutic strategy in paediatric palliative care patients. For example, Block [71] has suggested that 'sometimes a short therapeutic trial can help clarify whether or not a patient suffers from depression.'

It is standard practice that prior to commencing several of these psychotropic medications (amitriptyline and some antipsychotics) an electrocardiogram (ECG) is performed. Despite the fact that these medications may be prescribed for palliative symptom control, it would be appropriate to exclude any underlying cardiac rhythm abnormality.

At present, the mainstay of treatment for paediatric depression involves the use of selective serotonin reuptake inhibitors (SSRI's). Many authors have studied the extensive prescribing of SSRI's for paediatric patients—even prior to any evidence-based research to support their use [72]. Rushton *et al.* [73,74] surveyed 453 general paediatricians and 306 family physicians, and found that 72% had prescribed an SSRI for a child or adolescent (with depression as the most common indication)—despite the lack of published randomised controlled trials on safety, efficacy, or guidelines in the paediatric population during the study period. As might be expected given the overlap with the adult population, more family physicians reported prescribing SSRIs for paediatric patients, compared to paediatricians (91% vs. 58%). In a finding related to the challenges inherent in the present discussion, more family physicians than paediatricians (22% vs. 11%) agreed that they were comfortable with the management of childhood depression.

Two large randomized controlled trials have now shown the efficacy of SSRI's—specifically, fluoxetine 20 mg daily and paroxetine 20–40 mg daily—as superior to placebo in the general paediatric population [75,76]. As of January 2003, the United States Food and Drug Administration approved the use of the fluoxetine for the treatment of obsessive-compulsive disorder and depression in paediatric patients of ages 7 to 17. While these results look promising, it should be added that at least a few clinicians have questioned the level of efficacy found.Improvement with SSRIs may take 4–6 weeks, and the dose should be maintained for at least 6 weeks, if the child shows a clinical response by 4 weeks [78]. 'As seen in adults', the adverse effects of SSRIs in "children and adolescents include nausea, tiredness", nervousness, dizziness, and difficulty concentrating [77,79]. All of these side effects are dose-dependent, and generally subside with time. After 19 weeks of treatment with fluoxetine in one clinical trial, children and adolescents weighed two pounds less, compared to those treated with a placebo[77]. Effects of fluoxetine on sleep parameters include disturbed subjective sleep, increased Stage 1 sleep, increased number of arousals, and increased rapid eye movement density [80].

Little research has been conducted on SSRI's in the management of dysthymic disorder, the second form of depression with which paediatric patients can be diagnosed. A small open trial of fluoxetine in 11 of 15 paediatric patients showed a reduction in symptoms, such that they no longer met criteria for dysthymic disorder or major depression [81]. Randomised controlled trials are clearly needed to further elucidate the efficacy of SSRIs in dysthymic children and adolescents.

SSRIs in children and adolescents: Emerging concerns and controversy

SSRIs have radically changed the treatment of depression and anxiety across the developmental spectrum. As early as 1991, however, concerns began to emerge regarding an association between SSRIs and self-harm [82]. In 2003, the Food and Drug Administration (FDA) in the United States received unpublished data from placebo-controlled trials which suggested that paroxetine, taken by paediatric patients with major depressive disorders, might be associated with a potentially elevated risk of 'suicide attempts' and 'possibly suicide-related' events. In the United Kingdom, the Medicines and Healthcare Products Regulatory Agency (MHRA) then issued a warning against prescribing paroxetine for depressed patients under 18 years of age. In December 2003, the MHRA in the United Kingdom issued similar contra-indications to the use of venlafaxine, sertraline, citalopram, and escitalopram, with the recommendation that fluoxetine was the only SSRI with a sufficiently favourable profile for use in the paediatric population [83].

In January 2004, the American College of Neuropsychopharmacology issued a report from its Task Force on SSRI's and Suicidal Behaviour in Youth. This task force studied the use of SSRIs (specifically, citalopram, fluoxetine, paroxetine, sertraline, and venlafaxine) in more than 2000 children and adolescents, and concluded, "After reviewing the evidence as a whole . . . taking SSRI's or other new generation antidepressant drugs do not increase the risk of suicidal thinking or suicide attempts and that the benefits of SSRIs for treatment of depression in youth outweigh the risks. There were no completed suicides in any of the trials." [84]. The task force also emphasized that "there were no completed suicides in any of the trials," and, using data from toxicology studies in autopsies, raised the suggestion that "suicide is more likely when depressed individuals do not take their medications, rather than when they take it."

On October 15, 2004, the United States FDA [85] Public Health Advisory issued a 'black box' warning in the United States for anti-depressants and youths:

Today the Food and Drug Administration (FDA) directed manufacturers of all anti-depressant drugs to revise the labeling for their products to include a boxed warning and expanded warning statements that alert health care providers to an increased risk of suicidality (suicidal thinking and behavior) in children and adolescents being treated with these agents, and to include additional information about the results of pediatric studies.

The risk of suicidality for these drugs was identified in a combined analysis of short-term (up to 4 months) placebo-controlled trials of nine anti-depressant drugs, including *inhibitor* SSRIs and others, in children and adolescents with major depressive disorder (MDD), obsessive compulsive disorder (OCD), or other psychiatric disorders. A total of 24 trials involving over 4400 patients, were included. The analysis showed a greater risk of suicidality during the first few months of treatment in those receiving anti-depressants. The average risk of such events on drug was 4%, twice the placebo risk of 2%. No suicides occurred in these trials. Based on this data, FDA has determined that the following points are appropriate for inclusion in the boxed warning:

- Antidepressants increase the risk of suicidal thinking and behaviour (suicidality) in children and adolescents with MDD and other psychiatric disorders.

- Anyone considering the use of an anti-depressant in a child or adolescent for any clinical use must balance the risk of increased suicidality with the clinical need.

- Patients who are started on therapy should be observed closely for clinical worsening, suicidality, or unusual changes in behaviour.

- Families and caregivers should be advised to closely observe the patient and to communicate with the prescriber.

- A statement on whether the particular drug is approved for any pediatric indication(s) and, if so, which one(s).

Among the antidepressants, only fluoxetine is approved for use in treating MDD in pediatric patients. Importantly, the following day the American Psychiatric Association (APA) released an "APA Statement on the FDA's Hearing on Antidepressant Use in Pediatric Patients." [86] The statement concludes: "It is key to note that the advisory committee's recommendation for 'black box' warnings was adopted by a split vote, with 15 committee members in favour, and eight opposed. The APA believes that several dissenters' concerns that such warnings, which limit access to care, are valid, and should be taken into account by the FDA as it proceeds . . . In addition, we will work with physicians—including pediatricians and general practitioners—to help them better understand their patients' needs, and properly monitor patients.'

In the past year, a multitude of studies have examined whether SSRIs are associated with an increased risk of suicidal behaviour in children and adolescents. Valuck *et al.* [87] studied more than 20,000 United States adolescents with major depressive disorder, and concluded, "anti-depressant medication use had no statistically significant effect on the likelihood of suicide attempt in a large cohort of adolescents across the US after propensity adjustment for treatment allocation and controlling for other factors." Jick *et al.* [88] studied 159,810 users of four antidepressant medications (fluoxetine, paroxetine, amitriptyline, and dothiepin (dosulepin), and concluded, "there were no significant associations between the use of a particular study anti-depressant and the risk of suicide." They also concluded, however, that "the risk of suicidal behaviour is increased in the first month after starting antidepressants, especially during the first 1 to 9 days." A recent study by Grunebaum *et al.* [89] found that the suicide rate among United States adults fell 13.5% from 1985–1999, with a four-fold anti-depressant prescription rate (mostly due to SSRI's) during the same period. A similar study by Olfson *et al.* [90] found an association between a 1% increase in use of anti-depressants by adolescents in the United States, and a decrease of 0.23 suicides per 100,000 adolescents per year. The authors found this inverse relationship particularly significant for male adolescents of age 15–19 years, and adolescents residing in lower socio-economic regions (all P<.001). In an August 2004 study from the *Journal of the American Medical Association*, March *et al.* [91] studied 439 depressed patients, between ages 12 and 17 years, and treated with fluoxetine alone, CBT, both fluoxetine and CBT, or placebo. They found that "clinically significant suicidal thinking, which was present in 29% of the sample at baseline, improved significantly in all four treatment groups," and that fluoxetine alone was superior to CBT alone in decreasing depressive scores; even further clinical efficacy was seen when fluoxetine was combined with CBT.

One of the primary difficulties inherent in this discussion comprises the distinctions between suicidal ideation, self-harm, attempted suicides, and completed suicides. Although such distinctions are beyond the scope of the present chapter, the reader should be aware that this is one of the most problematic methodological aspects of research in this area of risk assessment. As noted in the ACNP task force report, "Actual 'suicidal events' in the studies reviewed here are poorly defined. Attempts were defined by the treating clinician at the site, and therefore, varied not only across studies, but across sites within the study." Further confusing the picture, many of the studies evaluating the efficacy of SSRIs have not included unpublished data, or data from unpublished trials. For example, as reviewed by Whittington et al. [92], unpublished data on paroxetine and sertraline indicated that risks outweigh benefits in the use of these medications, while data from unpublished trials of citalopram and venlafaxine revealed unfavourable risk-benefit profiles. Thus, one of the primary means of clarifying the issue of SSRI safety is more widespread and translucent availability of data.

Further work is sorely needed on the use of antidepressants in the paediatric patient, and in the paediatric palliative care patient in particular. As in the field of general paediatrics, or child and adolescent psychiatry, the importance of close monitoring, frequent clinical contact, and multi-modal and multidisciplinary treatment cannot be emphasized enough. There is no doubting the understandable and inherent risk of depression, anxiety, and related psychiatric issues in paediatric palliative care; similarly, though, there is no excuse for not actively addressing, diagnosing, treating, and researching these same issues.

Tricyclic antidepressants and stimulant medication

Tricyclic antidepressants (TCAs) have been commonly used in adult palliative care (given their proven efficacy for treatment of both neuropathic pain and depression), but in the paediatric population this is not the case. TCAs have not been shown to be any more efficacious than placebo in the treatment of depression in children [76,93]. When used to treat paediatric neuropathic pain, the dose is far less than that prescribed for psychological disturbances. Moreover, the high side-effect profile of TCAs includes bothersome antimuscarinic effects, such as dry mouth, insomnia, night terrors, epigastric discomfort, constipation, tachycardia and

palpitations, blurred vision, and urinary retention. The most concerning side effects with TCAs of course, involve cardiac conduction disorders [76,94], with cardiovascular side effects manifesting as tachycardia, hypertension, and postural hypotension [95]. It is worth noting that cardiotoxic effects have occurred in depressed children receiving doses within the therapeutic range [96]. Thus, TCAs are not of proven therapeutic benefit for depression in the paediatric population [97,87]; given their side effect profile and need for close serum monitoring [99,100], they are especially inappropriate in treating depression in the paediatric palliative care patient.

The role of stimulants (e.g., dexamphetamine, methylphenidate) in the management of depressive symptoms in paediatric palliative care is unclear. This is despite their therapeutic history with attention deficit–hyperactivity disorder, and their use in adult palliative care, especially as an adjunctive treatment for depression and pain in cancer and HIV-positive patients [101,103]. As noted by House and Hughes (1996) [104], stimulants in these patients should not be first-line therapy, should be used in short courses, and only be prescribed after specialist psychiatric and medical assessment. Findling (1996) [105] has studied the co-administration of SSRIs and methylphenidate in 7 paediatric patients (ages 10–16) and 4 adults (ages 38–44) with comorbid depression and attention deficit-hyperactivity disorder. None of the patients developed suicidality, increased heart rate, increased aggressiveness, or mania, and only one patient developed a significant change in blood pressure (20 mm Hg increase in diastolic pressure). Findling reports that this combination therapy appeared efficacious in decreasing depressive symptoms. Further work is clearly needed on the use of SSRIs and psychostimulants in paediatric palliative care. Nevertheless, these studies illuminate a possible area of significant pharmacologic efficacy and benefit in depression management.

Anxiety

Features and diagnosis

Features and challenges

Anxiety in the paediatric palliative care patient usually takes the form of separation anxiety, loneliness, procedure-related anxiety, fear of abandonment and 'death anxiety.' It is important to recognise the difference between anxiety as a transitory 'state' dependent on the situation, and as a personality 'trait' less influenced by the situational milieu. For example, Kellerman et al. (1980)[106] noted that adolescents may understandably develop state anxiety related to painful procedures; nevertheless, their study of 168 adolescents with chronic medical illnesses (including cystic fibrosis, leukaemia, solid tumours, nephrotic syndrome, diabetes mellitus, systemic lupus, and congenital cardiac conditions) found no evidence of trait anxiety, compared with 349 healthy adolescent controls. Interestingly, prognosis did appear to influence the presence of trait anxiety, in the ill adolescents: those patients whose physicians rated their prognosis as 'improved,' 'uncertain,' or 'deteriorating' were all more likely to exhibit trait anxiety than those whose physicians rated their prognosis as 'stable.'

Using the Child Medical Fear Scale and the State-Trait Anxiety Inventory for Children (STAIC), Hart and Bossert (1994)[107] evaluated the fears of 82 hospitalised children (ages 8–11) from the general paediatric population. They found the fears with the highest mean scores to be: separation from the family, procedural-related anxieties ('having shots and finger sticks'), prolonged in-patient admission, and receiving bad news regarding their health.

The assessment of anxiety symptoms in the general paediatric population may be challenging, due to the lack of consensus regarding definitions, thresholds, and thus, what symptoms would qualify as 'disorders' [108]. In the paediatric palliative care setting, clinicians may be especially hesitant to label anxious symptoms as a 'disorder,' as they may appear entirely appropriate, given the stresses on the child.

Risk factors

As occurs in depression, anxiety has also been associated with paediatric chronic pain [20]. In a sample of 56 paediatric oncology patients, Last and van Veldhuizen (1996)[23] have shown that anxiety is reduced when parents provide their child with information regarding their diagnosis and prognosis. Frank et al. (1997)[109] reported on the psychosocial adjustment of 86 paediatric oncology patients, and found that children diagnosed at younger ages reported greater levels of anxiety. On the other hand, Grootenhuis and Last (2001)[65] found no association between anxiety and time since diagnosis, in a sample of 43 children with cancer in remission, and 41 children not in remission.

The ICU setting has been indicated as a risk factor for the development of anxiety and apprehension in the hospitalized paediatric patient. In a study of 43 hospitalized children (ages 6–17), Jones and colleagues (1992)[110] have concluded that anxiety and psychological trauma are more common in critically ill children in the intensive care unit, as well as in children with prolonged and repeated hospitalizations. These findings, of course, further support the traditional goals in paediatric palliative care of maximizing comfort and limiting traumatic experiences.

As in depression, the presence of maternal psychiatric disorder can serve as a risk factor for the same disorder in children. In a study of 61 leukaemic children and their mothers,

Brown et al. (1993)[111] have documented increased self-reporting of anxiety in the children of mothers meeting DSM-III-R criteria for any psychiatric disorder. Similarly, a study using the Children's State-Trait Anxiety Inventory and adult State-Trait Anxiety Inventory in 74 paediatric oncology patients (ages 9–18) found a positive association between the adjustment responses of children and those of their mothers [112].

This chapter has not addressed symptoms that may manifest themselves in siblings or even parents, although clearly, all family members have the potential to be vulnerable to the same symptoms presented here. Nevertheless, it is worth noting a specific population of family members who can, in a sense, come under the care of the clinician in the oncology setting: donor siblings. In a comparison of 23 donor- and 21 non-donor siblings (ages 6–18) of surviving paediatric bone marrow transplant patients, donors self-reported more anxiety than non-donors [114]. In addressing this unique population, programs have been described which provide support to donor siblings [114].

Diagnostic tools

Anxiety scales, while useful in providing an overall estimate of anxiety levels, are not sufficient to establish a concrete diagnosis of an anxiety disorder [108]. Greenhill et al. (1998)[115] have reviewed the many diagnostic tools and self-report instruments designed to identify anxiety symptoms and disorders in general paediatrics, and have discussed the problems of discriminant validity and reliability which they uncovered. Challinor et al. (1999)[34] studied 43 paediatric oncology patients, and found high positive correlations between scores from patients and their parents for anxiety, using the Behavioural Assessment System for Children. Ireland and Malgady (1999)[116] have created a unique scale, the Thematic Instrument for Measuring Death Anxiety in Children. They describe a culturally sensitive tool, specifically designed to assess death anxiety in children with AIDS. Recent work on the assessment of children's anxieties and fears has also included human figure drawings [117].

Prevalence/incidence

In the general paediatric population, anxiety disorders have a point prevalence estimated to range from 3–13% [118], making them the most common psychiatric disorders in children and adolescents [119].

In their study of 168 adolescents with chronic medical illnesses, Kellerman et al. (1980)[106] found no difference between the prevalence of anxiety in patients with cystic fibrosis, leukaemia, solid tumours, and congenital heart disease and those with diabetes mellitus, recurrent urinary tract infections, and rheumatic heart disease; moreover, these chronically ill adolescents, as a group, did not show higher anxiety than the 349 healthy controls. In 44 patients with epilepsy, 16% met the criteria for significant anxiety symptomatology, according to the Revised Child Manifest Anxiety Scale [47]. The prevalence of separation anxiety disorder in a sample of 26 dialysis-dependent children with end-stage renal failure has been reported as over 50% [120].

In a study of 35 children and adolescents with cancer, Kashani and Hakami (1982)[51] found separation anxiety in 12 (34%) of the children, while 13 children (37%) reported a related symptom of being frightened, scared, or fearful. Although not specifically diagnosing anxiety, Collins *et al.* (2000) [30] assessed symptoms in 159 children between the ages of 10–18 years. Thirty-six percent reported 'feeling nervous', and 35% reported 'worrying' (with 56% and 66%, respectively, rating the severity of the symptoms between 'moderate' and 'very severe').

Death anxiety

The presence of 'death anxiety' in children with palliative care needs is neither surprising nor new. Over three decades ago, Schowalter (1970)[122] observed that 'death anxiety' may be greatest at the age of 6–10 years, when the concept of terminal illness has first entered the child's awareness, but death is still poorly understood. Of importance, most studies concur that dying children over the age of 10 years have an awareness of their poor prognosis, whether or not this is disclosed to them [123]. 'Death anxiety' in the child younger than five years commonly manifests as separation anxiety, loneliness, and fear of abandonment. As early as 1955 [11], authors were discussing death anxiety and recognizing the role of repression:

Even among adolescents, who intellectually may know much about cancer, the question concerning diagnosis and the possibility of death usually was not raised, as it often is by the adult patient. Our suspicion is that this does not reflect an awareness, but rather represents an attempt at repression psychologically of the anxiety concerning death.

Regarding the 'efforts to keep the child with leukaemia from becoming aware of his prognosis,' Spinetta (1973)[123] concludes that the child 'somehow picks up a sense that his illness is very serious and very threatening. The fatally ill child is aware that his is no ordinary illness.' It is therefore not surprising that the paediatric palliative care patient may experience profound and appropriate anxiety—which may, ironically, be aggravated by the family's and caregiver's desire to 'protect' the child.

Non-pharmacological support

In the founding years of the field of paediatric palliative care, clinicians were already addressing the need for non-pharmacological support in decreasing anxiety symptoms. In their 1980 article, 'Symptom control in ill and dying children,' Chapman and Goodall[18] suggested that the first approach to treating anxiety centres on communication and allowing the paediatric palliative care patients to express their fears, anxieties, and concerns:

If personal discussion does not bring relief to the patient and family, anxiolytic drugs may be needed, but the second should not be prescribed without the first . . . We must provide opportunities for such anxieties to be spelled out if we are to hope to relieve them.

The importance of patient expression in reducing anxiety has continued in current non-pharmacological approaches to anxiolysis. Barrera *et al.* (2002)[124] have recently described the use of interactive music therapy as an efficacious means of reducing anxiety in 65 hospitalized children with cancer. Robb and Ebberts (2003)[125] have, similarly, shown anxiety reduction in a small study of bone marrow transplant patients, who participated in a song writing and digital video production intervention.

The non-pharmacological approach to anxiety disorders is largely dictated by whether the patient is experiencing separation anxiety, generalised anxiety, procedure-related anxiety, "death anxiety," or another form of the disorder.

In the case of separation anxiety, the initial approach should involve maximizing parent–child interaction. Such an approach is especially relevant in the pre-school population with life-limiting illness, where separation is a risk factor for the aetiology of both anxiety and depression (Hollenbeck *et al.*, 1980)[126].

Non-pharmacological support of the anxious toddler or pre-schooler in even the general paediatric setting can be especially challenging, and thus requires equally unique therapeutic approaches. For example, Olness and Gardner (1978)[127] posited that children are more receptive to using hypnosis than adults, since they engage in fantasy and imagination without the cognitive inhibitions of adults. Discussing the role of hypnotherapy, they note:

In addition to reduction of specific symptoms through hypnotherapy, children benefit by the sense of mastery which they acquire, a sense which is surely needed to overcome the feelings of hopelessness, loss of control, and depression induced by many diagnostic and therapeutic procedures in medicine.

Kohen *et al.* (1984)[128] subsequently described the use of 'relaxation mental imagery' ('self-hypnosis') in 505 children and adolescents—including children as young as three years old—with 51% reporting complete resolution of their presenting problems (including acute pain, chronic pain, and anxiety). Similarly, Ott (1996) [129] has described the use of guided imagery as an adjunct modality in the care of toddlers and pre-schoolers who are experiencing anxiety.

For the patient with procedure-related anxiety, amelioration of anxiety symptoms can occur through several means. An intervention that combined hypnosis with acupuncture in six weekly sessions has been shown to significantly decrease anticipatory anxiety in 33 chronic-pain youth (ages 6–18) [130].

As reviewed by Labellarte *et al.* (1999)[119] and Manassis (2000)[131], numerous controlled studies have shown CBT to be efficacious in treating anxiety disorders in the general paediatric population. In the specific area of procedure related anxiety, the efficacy of CBT has become increasingly evident. Cognitive-behavioural approaches have been used to decrease the anxiety associated with lumbar punctures and bone marrow aspirations [132]. In a study of 30 paediatric oncology patients (ages 5–15) undergoing bone marrow aspiration, Liossi and Hatira (1999)[133] have shown that CBT training and hypnosis result in decreased pain-related anxiety, when compared to both controls and the patients' own baselines. In a recent follow-up study [134], the authors have studied lumbar-puncture-associated anxiety in 80 paediatric oncology patients (ages 6–16 years), and found that patients in hypnosis intervention groups reported less anxiety and pain than controls. However, when patients where switched to self-hypnosis, the therapeutic benefit was observed to degrade. This finding thus suggests that the presence of the therapist trained in hypnosis may be necessary for the desired anxiolytic effect.

Pharmacological management

Despite being among the most common psychiatric disorders in children and adolescents, anxiety disorders have lacked substantial data on the efficacy of pharmacological options [135,72]. With the recent exception of SSRIs, the efficacy of anxiolytics has received only minimal support in the evidence-based literature. This dearth of research has been quickly changing in the past two years, though, with several well-designed studies in the general paediatric population [135].

Benzodiazapines are commonly used in the treatment of procedure-related anxiety, despite minimal research supporting their use as paediatric anxiolytics. The published studies of paediatric benzodiazepine use primarily address status epilepticus, rather than anxiety disorders. In critically ill infants and children, differences in plasma clearance and potential anxiolytic side effects must be taken into account. Finally, concern for both benzodiazepine dependence and withdrawal [136, 137] has reduced its use in clinical practice as a paediatric anxiolytic [131]. It is thus not surprising that benzodiazepine usage recommendations are limited to adjunctive medications in severe anxiety [138], short-term anxiolytics for specific anxiety-provoking situations, or as temporary anxiolytics when an SSRI has been started, but is not yet efficacious [131].

For procedure-related anxiety, Ljungman and colleagues (2000)[139] have studied the efficacy of intranasal midazolam in a randomised, double-blind, placebo-controlled trial of 43 children with cancer. Parents, nurses, and children reported significantly reduced anxiety and procedure problems, with no serious or unexpected side effects. The most common side effect was nasal discomfort, the primary reason for dropouts (8/43 patients), thus suggesting that its use may be limited without optional administration routes. Midazolam is now used buccally, and is available in some countries in a flavoured preparation. In order to elucidate potential hypersensitivity to midazolam, a small test dose (0.2 mg/kg) is recommended if the child is benzodiazepine naïve.

Intranasal, oral and buccal midazolam have also been used to decrease anxiety in dying children. Bentley and colleagues (2002)[140] have described the use of intranasal and oral midazolam in a sample of 4 dying patients of ages 8 months to 24 years. Symptoms treated were agitation, death anxiety, and 'extreme anxiety related to increasing pain.' In the dying child, the ease of administration and rapid onset of intranasal or buccal midazolam can greatly assist parents in the home setting.

Given the overlap between paediatric depression and anxiety, it should not be surprising that the pharmacological treatment of anxiety bears many similarities to that of depression. Nevertheless, as with depression, there have been no reported studies on anxiolytic pharmacotherapy in paediatric palliative care patients.

Following successful results from several open studies [141,142,143], SSRIs have recently been proven efficacious in two large randomised controlled trials of paediatric anxiety disorders. Walkup *et al.* (2001)[144] conducted a randomized controlled trial in 128 paediatric patients (ages 6–17), with diagnoses of social phobia, separation anxiety, or generalized anxiety disorder. After an eight-week course, the patients who received fluvoxamine were more likely to show a clinical response (as measured on the Pediatric Anxiety Rating Scale) than the placebo group (76% vs. 29%). Similarly, Birmaher *et al.* (2003)[145] recently reported on a randomized controlled trial on 74 anxious youth (ages 7–17), and found 'much' to 'very much' improvement in 61% of the fluoxetine group (vs. 35% in those taking placebo). The only side effects they reported were mild and transient headaches, and gastrointestinal disturbance. These trials are occurring in the general paediatric population, and not in the palliative care setting.

Depression–anxiety co-morbidity

Paediatric diagnosis and treatment of depression and anxiety are especially problematic, given the co-morbidity between the two conditions [146]. In an excellent review of the subject, Axelson and Birmaher (2001) [45] have noted that 10–15% of anxious youth have depression, and 25–50% of depressed youth also possess anxiety disorders. Furthermore, younger depressed children display higher rates of comorbid separation anxiety and phobias [147]. Moreover, Gurley *et al.* (1996)[138] showed that in children and adolescents with sub-clinical symptomatology, anxiety and depression were particularly difficult to identify as separate entities. Finally, it is important to note that a child experiencing a dysthymic disorder, rather than major depressive disorder, may display persistent irritability as the predominant mood, instead of depression. In order to meet the DSM-IV criteria for dysthymic disorder, this mood disturbance must last for one year (American Psychiatric Association, 1994)[6]. In a study of 159 children with cancer conducted by Collins and colleagues (2000)[30], 35% reported 'feeling irritable,' with 64% rating the symptom severity between 'moderate' and 'very severe.' Moreover, Hollenbeck *et al.* (1980)[126] have discussed a pattern of agitation preceding depression in pre-school children being treated for cancer.

Therapeutically, it is thus helpful that both sets of symptoms have been demonstrated as being responsive to SSRI's and CBT. In fact, randomised controlled trials of psycho-social therapies have only shown CBT to be efficacious in treating both paediatric depression [149–150] and anxiety [151–153]. In a review of depression in the general adolescent population, Parker and Roy (2001) [154] have observed that SSRI efficacy appears most clear in cases of 'anxious' or 'irritable' depression. This combination of depression, anxiety, fear, and even irritability is relevant to the paediatric palliative care patient, and would support the potential use of SSRIs in these patients.

Anger

The symptom of anger can be seen to accompany both depression and anxiety, and can be recognised as a manifestation of these disorders, or as a symptom in its own right. In the general paediatric population, Sherry and Jellinek [155] have described the manifestation of depression in preschoolers as aggressive or destructive behaviour. In chronic illness, patients may display a paradoxical pattern, with decreased expression of anger. For example, Meijer *et al.* (2000) [156] found that 107 chronically ill children were less likely to report aggressive behaviour than healthy children.

The appearance of anger as a psychological symptom has been examined in different paediatric oncology populations. Kashani and Hakami (1982)[51] noted that 17 of 35 of their patients demonstrated anger and irritability, based on self- and parental report. Kvist and colleagues (1991)[24] have described aggression as 'the dominant psychological response in children with malignant disease.' A study of 53 oncology patients who had electively discontinued treatment for leukaemia or lymphoma (mean age 12.8 years at completion of questionnaires) reported aggression in the form of irritation and anger, more common in girls than in boys. These dying patients also reported the co-morbidity of depression, hypersensitivity, phobic anxiety, death anxiety, and night terror. The child with cancer may not manifest aggression in all settings. Noll *et al.* (1999)[60] showed that peers and teachers reported less aggression in 76 children with cancer, compared with 76 classroom peers.

Agitation and delirium
Features and diagnosis

Agitation is a physical and psychological phenomenon that can exist in many forms. The causes of agitation are numerous, and in the paediatric population, are especially varied, and sometimes difficult to define. As referred to earlier in this chapter, agitation can be a feature of both depression and anxiety. It may also be a prominent characteristic of some neurodegenerative syndromes, such as Batten's and juvenile onset of Huntingdon's disease. In these conditions, changes in behaviour, movement patterns, or even sleep disturbance may be described as agitation. Occasionally, these changes can be more acute in nature, and agitation has been associated with the onset of visual and auditory hallucinations. Agitation manifests itself in many situations. In the young baby or toddler, it may purely be a reflection of a tired state of mind. When assessing agitation, the clinical context as a whole must be examined.

In more extreme forms, agitation may be associated with the dying process. Several terms have been used to describe this agitated state of mind at the end of life, including terminal agitation, terminal restlessness, or terminal delirium. Burke (1997) [157]defines 'terminal restlessness' as agitated delirium in a dying patient, frequently associated with impaired consciousness and multi-focal myoclonus. In contrast, the term 'terminal anguish' has been used to refer to the extreme emotional or spiritual turmoil that people may exhibit at the end of life [158]. The multiple synonyms used to describe this neuro-psychiatric state reflect the ubiquitous nature of the condition, rather than any diagnostic quandary.

In the adult literature, the term 'delirium' is frequently used to describe a form of agitation at the end of life, often in patients with advanced cancer. This neuro-psychiatric syndrome is described as 'a disturbance of consciousness, cognition and perception, with a course that may wax and wane over a period of hours' [6]. As an alteration in psychomotor activity, it has been specifically classified as hypermanic, hypomanic and mixed [159]. Classical features of delirium include an acute onset and fluctuating nature, and although it is described as being a transient and potentially reversible disorder, it frequently occurs as an irreversible event in the terminal phase of life [160]. Delirium causes extreme distress not only to the patient, but also to the family and carers. At a time when communication and clarity of thought are important, delirium hinders decision-making, and contributes added burden to suffering.

Causes of agitation and delirium

There has been much debate in the adult literature as to the possible causes of delirium in the terminally ill, and the potential for reversibility of these distressing symptoms. The causes of delirium are often multi-factorial [161,162], and include the presence of primary cerebral disease (cancer, cerebrovascular accidents) and other factors that may indirectly affect cerebral metabolism (sepsis, organ failure, electrolyte disturbance, psycho-active medication, nutritional deficiencies, drug withdrawal).

A leading study in 1992 by Bruera and colleagues [163] found a biological cause for cognitive failure in 44% of adult cancer patients at the end of life. Subsequent studies went on to identify opioid toxicity as a reversible cause of delirium, and recommended that opioid rotation could improve symptoms of delirium, whilst maintaining pain control [164,165]. Neuroexitatory features such as agitation, myoclonus, tactile hallucinations and hyperalgesia are symptoms suggestive of opioid toxicity. In some palliative care centers, opioid rotation and rehydration have become standard practice upon detection of cognitive failure; Bruera and colleagues have produced data to support this practice (1995)[166]. A small prospective study by Morita et al. (2002)[167] showed an increase in plasma morphine metabolites in eight patients, after the development of terminal delirium. Of note, all patients had clinical multi-organ failure.

Two recent well-designed prospective adult patient studies have identified precipitating factors of delirium, and the incidence of reversibility of symptoms in adult cancer patients receiving palliative care (Lawlor et al. 2000, Morita et al. 2001)[160, 168]. Lawlor found that 49% of delirium episodes in 71 patients were reversible, and that psycho-active medications (predominantly opioids) and dehydration were precipitating factors associated with reversibility. Lawlor specifies, however, that dehydration 'tends to act in association with other reversible factors such as opioid toxicity,' and in isolation, is not a primary cause of delirium. Hypoxic encephalopathy and metabolic factors were associated with non-reversibility.

Morita identified precipitating factors in 93% of the 153 cases of delirium studied, and specified the main pathologies as hepatic failure, medications, pre-renal azotaemia, hyperosmolality, hypoxia, disseminated intravascular coagulation (DIC), organic central nervous system damage, infection and hypercalcaemia. Interestingly, medication-induced delirium often showed a hyperactive clinical picture. Complete recovery of symptoms occurred in 20% of patients, and was most commonly achieved in cases with medication- and hypercalcaemia-induced delirium. In contrast, a low remission rate was achieved when hepatic failure, dehydration, hypoxia and DIC were present. The author states that the relatively low reversibility rate in this study might well be due to variability in patient selection, as most patients in this Japanese study were referred for terminal care, rather than symptom control.

Distinguishing delirium from other conditions

The diagnosis of delirium can be difficult. In adults, delirium is frequently misdiagnosed as depression or dementia. Several instruments are available to assess delirium and distinguish it from other psychiatric disorders, namely, the Confusion Assessment Method (CAM) [169], Delirium Rating Scale [170], and the Memorial Delirium Assessment Scale [171]. The CAM, devised by Inoue, has been validated as a diagnostic tool for the medically ill population, and is easy to use even for non-psychiatrists. The Memorial Delirium Assessment Scale, by Breitbart, is a ten-item scale specifically designed to measure the severity of delirium, and can, therefore, measure change, which the CAM does not. The Memorial Delirium Assessment Scale [171], the Communication Capacity Scale, and the Agitation Distress Scale [172] have been particularly validated to measure delirium in adult cancer patients. Unfortunately, there is no tool available to assess delirium in the paediatric population.

Prevalence/incidence

As with many symptoms in paediatric palliative care, the incidence of delirium (or terminal agitation) has not been evaluated. Anecdotally, it is not an uncommon feature of the dying process in children. Recent studies of adults dying, mostly of cancer, have revealed that 68–90% are delirious prior to death [160,163, 168,173,174].

Non-pharmacological support

Management of agitation, delirium and restlessness in patients at the end of life involves a thorough clinical assessment and an individual treatment plan. The goals of treatment should be discussed with the family, and should be appropriate to the situation. Any potentially reversible cause, of which there may be more than one, should be corrected, if possible. In clinical practice, however, priorities such as patient comfort, setting (home or hospice), and appropriateness of diagnostic procedures will limit the degree of investigation. The ability to rectify a problem with minimal burden to the patient and his or her family must also be considered. Relatively low-burden interventions, such as altering drug doses, discontinuing or changing psychoactive medication, and a trial of hypodermoclysis, might be considered.

All those nearing the end of life must be considered at risk of developing symptoms of agitation or delirium. Preventative measures, such as encouraging regular sleep through breathing and relaxation exercises, and quiet music or familiar stories to facilitate rest, may help the child feel calm. Treatment should be arranged to allow maximum periods of uninterrupted rest. Avoidance of sedative medications, such as antihistamines and choral hydrate, are advisable, as they do not relieve anxiety or fear, but paradoxically, may result in an agitated, confused and very tired child.

General environmental measures, aimed at reducing anxiety and disorientation, should be employed [175] at the first sign of symptoms. These include strategies such as familiarizing a room (i.e., using a child's own bedclothes and belongings), consistency in staff, reducing the level of noise stimulation, having adequate lighting with a clock visible, and, of course, the near presence of family members. It is extremely important to educate parents and family as to the nature of delirium and agitation, as the situation can be frightening and upsetting, and their reactions may exacerbate the patient's distress.

Pharmacological management

The pharmacological treatment of delirium and agitation should aim to alleviate symptoms, and bring the patient closer to his or her normal mental state. It is important to distinguish between medication that aims to 'clear the mind' and medication that aims to sedate the patient. Careful consideration as to the balance between sedation, suppression of symptoms, and the potential adverse side effects of medication must be made. For example, sedative medication may improve symptoms, but increase cognitive impairment, hindering communication and interaction.

Several agents are commonly used in the terminal phase in children, but as with most drugs in paediatric practice, they are off-licence, and little or no data exists to support their use. In adult palliative care, there is a similar lack of evidence-based protocols, however, the mainstay of treatment depends upon antipsychotic (neuroleptic) drugs, such as haloperidol and the benzodiazepines.

Haloperidol is a potent neuroleptic with antidopamine activity, but relatively few anti-cholinergic effects (potentially, it may cause extra-pyramidal side effects, but usually at higher doses). It improves cognition (onset of action is rapid; hours to days), and is sedative at high doses. Haloperidol can be administered through many routes (oral, subcutaneous, intravenous and intramuscular) [176]. It is the drug of choice in the treatment of delirium in adult patients [177], and is effective in relieving agitation, paranoia and fear.

Olanzapine and risperidone are new antipsychotic drugs that are less sedating than traditional neuroleptics, and are reported to have fewer extra-pyramidal side effects [178–183]. Of note: evaluation of the pharmacological treatment of delirium has been mostly in the elderly population, and these drugs are not currently available in the parental formulations for rapid onset. Olanzapine is available in a rapid orally disintegrating tablet, marketed in the USA as Zyprexa Zydis. Risperidone has recently been released as a two-week depot injection (marketed in the USA as Risperdal Consta). Nevertheless, neither of these formulations has been designed for, or tested in, the paediatric population.

Benzodiazepines are frequently used in paediatric practice for their anxiolytic effects, and ease of administration. Lorazepam, midazolam and clonazepam can all be administered via the sublingual or buccal routes, and are therefore valuable in the home setting. The therapeutic aim of benzodiazepine treatment must be explicit, as, in higher doses, sedative and hypnotic effects occur. Paradoxically, at higher doses, benzodiazepines can also cause agitation and delirium in some patients. However, many paediatric patients who have been taking regular benzodiazepines for the treatment of neurological disorders, such as seizures and spasm, can tolerate high doses of these agents, with perceived benefit, and little or no adverse effects. Lorazepam or midazolam are frequently used in combination with haloperidol for symptoms of agitated delirium. Benzodiazepines alone do not improve delirious symptoms, and actually worsen cognition, as shown by Breitbart in a double-blind randomized trail of haloperidol, chlorpromazine, and lorazepam in hospitalised AIDS patients [184]. As noted by Galloway and Yaster [185], some children remain agitated despite benzodiazepines and opioids, and it is preferable to switch to a different class of drugs, rather than continue with higher doses.

An alternative medication is the barbiturate phenobarbitone (Phenobarbital), used as a second line treatment in children and young people when symptoms remain uncontrolled, or drug side effects are intolerable. It has been shown to be a useful agent in controlling symptoms of agitation [186]. Phenobarbitone (Phenobarbital) is particularly beneficial when anti-convulsant action is also required. It should be considered in patients who are known to be suffering from CNS irritability, as it elevates seizure threshold [187], whereas phenothiazines lower seizure threshold. Phenobarbitone (Phenobarbital) should be administered by subcutaneous infusion (occasionally with an intramuscular or subcutaneous loading dose) as a single agent. It can cause skin irritation in some patients.

Induction of deeper levels of sedation is sometimes necessary in the management of agitated delirium or severe agitation. This may be a temporary treatment whilst a cause for the agitation is elicited, or may be on-going to control refractory symptoms, or where definite treatment is not possible [188]. When sedation is required, midazolam and levomepromazine are the agents most commonly used [189–194]. Levomepromazine (methotrimeprazine) is a phenothiazine with anti-dopaminergic properties that has been frequently used in children as an anti-emetic; at higher doses, it can be rapidly titrated to induce sedation. (See also Chapter 32, symptom control at the end of life.)

Conclusion

There is much we do not know about the assessment and management of psychological symptoms such as depression, anxiety, agitation, and delirium in paediatric palliative care, due to the lack of research into these issues. What we do know has been extrapolated from adult palliative care studies, as well as from the pediatric psychological and psychiatric literature. Symptoms of depression, anxiety, and anger are often present together in different degrees at different times in the course of illness of the child. The complexity of these difficult-to-quantify symptoms cannot be understated. At the same time, much can be done to help, if not eliminate, then at least reduce, the severity that these symptoms may have on the quality of life of

the child and family. First principles in the management of these symptoms are to get the best assessment possible by active listening and direct observation. In some cases the 'intervention' that is most needed and useful is the caring, active-listening professional. This approach, coupled with the judicious use of pharmacological and non-pharmacological management techniques, can serve to reduce the burden of suffering that these symptoms represent. The assessment and management of agitation and delirium has been well studied in adults at the end of life, and offers an initial approach that can be used in approaching these issues in children. By first reviewing possible iatrogenic causes (e.g., opioid toxicity), and investigating easy-to-treat and common physiological causes (e.g, hypercalcemia), the clinician may be able to alleviate symptoms with minimal interventions. Thus, although there is much that is still not known about the management of distressing psychological symptoms in palliative care for children, there is also much that is already known, that can effectively reduce the burden of suffering and improve quality of life. (See also Chapter 8, Psychological impact of life-limiting illness on the child.)

References

1. Froese, A.P. Pediatric referrals to psychiatry: III. Is the psychiatrist's opinion heard? *Int J Psychiatry Med* 1977;8(3):295–301.

2. Sawyer, M. *et al.* Childhood cancer: A 4-year prospective study of the psychological adjustment of children and parents. *J Pediatr Hematol Oncol* 2000;22(3):214–20.

3. von Essen, L. *et al.* Self-esteem, depression and anxiety among Swedish children and adolescents on and off cancer treatment. *Acta Paediatr* 2000;89(2):229–36.

4. Ryan, N.D. Diagnosing pediatric depression. *Biol Psychiatry* 2001; 49(12):1050–4.

5. Kovacs, M., Presentation and cause of major depressive disorder during childhood and later years of the lifespan. *J Am Acad Child Adolesc Psychiatr* 1996;35:705–715.

6. Association, A.P., *Diagnostic and Statistical Manual of Mental Disorders* (4th edition). Washington, D.C.: American Psychiatric Association 1994.

7. Luby, J.L. *et al.* Preschool major depressive disorder: Preliminary validation for developmentally modified DSM-IV criteria. *J Am Acad Child Adolesc Psychiatr* 2002;41(8):928–37.

8. Luby, J.L. *et al.* Modification of DSM-IV criteria for depressed preschool children. *Am J Psychiatr* 2003;160(6):1169–72.

9. Perez, R., Ascaso, L., Domenech Massons, J., and de la Osa Chaparro, N. Characteristics of the subjects and interview influencing the test-retest reliability of the Diagnostic Interview for Children and Adolescents-Revised. *J Child Psychol Psychiatry* 1998;39: 963–72.

10. Birmaher, B. *et al.* Childhood and adolescent depression: A review of the past 10 years. Part I. *J Am Acad Child Adolesc Psychiatr* 1996; 35(11):1427–39.

11. Richmond, J. and Waisman, H.A., Psychologic aspects of management of children with malignant diseases. A.M.A. *Am J Dis Child* 1955; 292: 42–47.

12. Worchel, F.F. *et al.* Assessment of depression in children with cancer. *J Pediatr Psychol* 1988;13(1):101–12.

13. Phipps, S. and Srivastava, D.K. Approaches to the measurement of depressive symptomatology in children with cancer: attempting to circumvent the effects of defensiveness. *J Dev Behav Pediatr* 1999; 20(3):150–6.

14. Cavanaugh, S., Clark, D., and Gibbons, R., Diagnosing depression in the hospitalized medically ill. *Psychosomatics* 1983;24:809–15.

15. Kovacs, M. *et al.* Depressive disorders in childhood. II. A longitudinal study of the risk for a subsequent major depression. *Arch Gen Psychiatr* 1984;41(7):643–9.

16. Kovacs, M. *et al.* Depressive disorders in childhood. I. A longitudinal prospective study of characteristics and recovery. *Arch Gen Psychiatry* 1984;41(3):229–37.

17. Bennett, D.S. Depression among children with chronic medical problems: a meta-analysis. *J Pediatr Psychol* 1994;19(2):149–69.

18. Chapman, J.A. and Goodall, J. Helping a child to live whilst dying. *Lancet* 1980;1(8171):753–6.

19. Kashikar-Zuck, S. *et al.* Depression and functional disability in chronic pediatric pain. *Clin J Pain* 2001;17(4):341–9.

20. Varni, J.W. *et al.* Chronic pain and emotional distress in children and adolescents. *J Dev Behav Pediatr* 1996;17(3):154–61.

21. Steif, B.L. and Heiligenstein, E.L. Psychiatric symptoms of pediatric cancer pain. *J Pain Symptom Manage* 1989;4(4):191–6.

22. Last, B.F. and van Veldhuizen, A.M. Information about diagnosis and prognosis related to anxiety and depression in children with cancer aged 8–16 years. *Eur J Cancer* 1996;32A(2):290–4.

23. Verri, A.P. *et al.* [The leukemic child after therapy. Psychological aspects]. *Pediatr Med Chir* 1985;7(4):545–8.

24. Kvist, S.B. *et al.* Aggression: The dominant psychological response in children with malignant disease. *Psychol Rep* 1991;68(3 Pt 2): 1139–50.

25. Kaplan, S.L. *et al.* Depressive symptoms in children and adolescents with cancer: A longitudinal study. *J Am Acad Child Adolesc Psychiatr* 1987;26(5):782–7.

26. Berard. Psychiatric symptomatology in adolescents with cancer. *Paediatr Heamatol and Oncol* 1998;15:211–21.

27. Mulhern, R.K. *et al.* Maternal depression, assessment methods, and physical symptoms affect estimates of depressive symptomatology among children with cancer. *J Pediatr Psychol* 1992;17(3):313–26.

28. Vance, Y.H. *et al.* Issues in measuring quality of life in childhood cancer: measures, proxies, and parental mental health. *J Child Psychol Psychiatry* 2001;42(5):661–7.

29. Canning, E.H. and Kelleher, K. Performance of screening tools for mental health problems in chronically ill children. *Arch Pediatr Adolesc Med* 1994;148(3):272–8.

30. Collins, J.J. *et al.* The measurement of symptoms in children with cancer. *J Pain Symptom Manage* 2000;19(5):363–77.

31. Andrews, V.C. *et al.* Mother-adolescent agreement on the symptoms and diagnoses of adolescent depression and conduct disorders. *J Am Acad Child Adolesc Psychiatr* 1993;32(4):731–8.

32. Angold, A. *et al.* Parent and child reports of depressive symptoms in children at low and high risk of depression. *J Child Psychol Psychiatr* 1987;28(6):901–15.

33. Braaten, E.B. *et al.* Methodological complexities in the diagnosis of major depression in youth: An analysis of mother and youth self-reports. *J Child Adolesc Psychopharmacol* 2001;11(4):395–407.

34. Challinor, J.M. *et al.* Somatization, anxiety and depression as measures of health-related quality of life of children/adolescents with cancer. *Int J Cancer Suppl* 1999;12:52–7.

35. Kovacs, M. Rating scales used to assess depression in school-aged children. *Acta Paedopsychiatrica* 1981;46:305–15.

36. Kazdin, A. Identifying depression in children: A comparison of alternative selection criteria. *J Abnorm Child Psychol* 1989;17(4): 437–54.

37. Asarnow, J.R. and Carlson, G.A. Depression Self-Rating Scale: Utility with child psychiatric inpatients. *J Consult Clin Psychol* 1985; 53(4):491–9.

38. Eason, L.J. *et al.* The assessment of depression and anxiety in hospitalized pediatric patients. *Child Psychiatry Hum Dev* 1985; 16(1): 57–64.

39. Kronenberg, Y., Blumensohn, R. and Apter, A. A comparison of different diagnostic tools for childhood depression. *Acta Psychiatr Scand* 1988;77(2):194–8.

40. Carlson, G.A. and Cantwell, D.P. Unmasking masked depression in children and adolescents. *Am J Psychiatry* 1980;137(4):445–9.

41. Fundudis, T. *et al.* Reliability and validity of two self-rating scales in the assessment of childhood depression. *Br J Psychiatr Suppl* 1991;11:36–40.

42. Fristad, M.A., Emery, B.L. and Beck. S.J. Use and abuse of the Children's Depression Inventory. *J Consult Clin Psychol* 1997;65(4): 699–702.

43. Heiligenstein, E. and Jacobsen, P.B. Differentiating depression in medically ill children and adolescents. *J Am Acad Child Adolesc Psychiatry* 1988;27(6):716–9.

44. Poznanski, E.O. *et al.* Preliminary studies of the reliability and validity of the children's depression rating scale. *J Am Acad Child Psychiatr* 1984;23(2):191–7.

45. Axelson, D.A. and Birmaher, B. Relation between anxiety and depressive disorders in childhood and adolescence. *Depress Anxiety* 2001;14(2):67–78.

46. Son, S.E. and Kirchner, J.T. Depression in children and adolescents. *Am Fam Physician* 2000;62(10):2297–308, 2311–2.

47. Ettinger, A.B. *et al.* Symptoms of depression and anxiety in pediatric epilepsy patients. *Epilepsia* 1998;39(6):595–9.

48. Burke, P. *et al.* Depression and anxiety in pediatric inflammatory bowel disease and cystic fibrosis. *J Am Acad Child Adolesc Psychiatry* 1989;28(6):948–51.

49. Rao, G.P., Malhotra, Malhotra, S., and Marwaha, R.K. Psychosocial study of leukemic children and their parents. *Indian Pediatr* 1992; 29(8):985–90.

50. Fitzpatrick, C., Barry, C., and Garvey, C. Psychiatric disorder among boys with Duchenne muscular dystrophy. *Dev Med Child Neurol* 1986;28(5):589–95.

51. Kashani, J. Hakami, N. Depression in children and adolescents with malignancy. *Can J Psychiatr* 1982;27(6):474–7.

52. Dunitz, M. *et al.* Depression in children with cancer. *Padiatr Padol* 1991;26(6):267–70.

53. Worchel, F.F. *et al.* Selective responsiveness of chronically ill children to assessments of depression. *J Pers Assess* 1992;59(3):605–15.

54. Chao C.C. *et al.*, Psychosocial adjustment among pediatric cancer patients and their parents. *Psychiatry Clin Neurosci* 2003;57(1): 75–81.

55. Bose, S. *et al.* Psychologic adjustment of human immunodeficiency virus-infected school-age children. *J Dev Behav Pediatr* 1994; 15(3):S26–33.

56. Canning, E.H., Canning, R.D., and Boyce, W.T. Depressive symptoms and adaptive style in children with cancer. *J Am Acad Child Adolesc Psychiatry* 1992;31(6):1120–4.

57. Allen, R., Newman, S.P., and Souhami, R.L. Anxiety and depression in adolescent cancer: Findings in patients and parents at the time of diagnosis. *Eur J Cancer* 1997;33(8):1250–5.

58. Cavusoglu, H. Depression in children with cancer. *J Pediatr Nurs* 2001;16(5):380–5.

59. Brem, A.S. *et al.* Psychosocial characteristics and coping skills in children maintained on chronic dialysis. *Pediatr Nephrol*, 1988; 2(4):460–5.

60. Noll, R.B. *et al.* Social, emotional, and behavioral functioning of children with cancer. *Pediatrics* 1999;103(1):71–8.

61. Michalowski, M. *et al.* Emotional and behavioral symptoms in children with acute leukemia. *Haematologica* 2001;86(8):821–6.

62. Kagan, L. Use of denial in adolescents with bone cancer. *Health Soc Work* 1976;1(4):71–86.

63. Phipps, S. and Srivastava, D.K. Repressive adaptation in children with cancer. *Health Psychol* 1997;16(6):521–8.

64. Phipps, S. *et al.* Repressive adaptation in children with cancer: a replication and extension. *Health Psychol* 2001;20(6):445–51.

65. Grootenhuis, M.A. and Last, B.F. Children with cancer with different survival perspectives: Defensiveness, control strategies, and psychological adjustment. *Psychooncology* 2001;10(4):305–14.

66. Findling, R.L. *et al.* Somatic treatment for depressive illnesses in children and adolescents. *Child Adolesc Psychiatr Clin N Am* 2002; 11(3):555–78, ix.

67. Brent, D.A. *et al.* Predictors of treatment efficacy in a clinical trial of three psychosocial treatments for adolescent depression. *J Am Acad Child Adolesc Psychiatry* 1998;37(9):906–14.

68. Clarke G., H.H., Lewinsohn P.M., and Andrews J. *et al.* Cognitive-behavioral group treatments of adolescent depression: prediction of outcome. *Behav Ther* 1992;23:341–354.

69. Chernoff, R.G., et al. A randomized, controlled trial of a community-based support program for families of children with chronic illness: pediatric outcomes. *Arch Pediatr Adolesc Med* 2002;156(6):533–9.

70. Nitschke, R., *et al.* Therapeutic choices made by patients with end-stage cancer. *J Pediatr* 1982;101(3):471–6.

71. Block, S.D. Assessing and managing depression in the terminally ill patient. ACP-ASIM End-of-Life Care Consensus Panel. American College of Physicians—American Society of Internal Medicine. *Ann Intern Med* 2000;132(3):209–18.

72. Kastelic, E.A., Labellarte, M.J., and Riddle, M.A. Selective serotonin reuptake inhibitors for children and adolescents. *Curr Psychiatry Rep* 2000;2(2):117–23.

73. Rushton, J.L., Clark, S.J., and Freed, G.L. Primary care role in the management of childhood depression: A comparison of pediatricians and family physicians. *Pediatrics* 2000;105(4 Pt 2):957–62.

74. Rushton, J.L., Clark, S.J., and Freed, G.L. Pediatrician and family physician prescription of selective serotonin reuptake inhibitors. *Pediatrics* 2000;105(6):E82.

75. Emslie, G.J. *et al.* Fluoxetine for acute treatment of depression in children and adolescents: A placebo-controlled, randomized clinical trial. *J Am Acad Child Adolesc Psychiatr* 2002;41(10): 1205–15.

76. Keller, M.B. *et al.* Efficacy of paroxetine in the treatment of adolescent major depression: A randomized, controlled trial. *J Am Acad Child Adolesc Psychiatry* 2001;40(7):762–72.

77. Prozac for pediatric use. FDA Consumer 2003;37(2):3.

78. Birmaher, B., Brent, D.A., and Benson, R.S. Summary of the practice parameters for the assessment and treatment of children and adolescents with depressive disorders. American Academy of Child and Adolescent Psychiatry. *J Am Acad Child Adolesc Psychiatr* 1998;37(11):1234–8.

79. Alderman, J. *et al.* Sertraline treatment of children and adolescents with obsessive-compulsive disorder or depression: pharmacokinetics, tolerability, and efficacy. *J Am Acad Child Adolesc Psychiatr* 1998;37(4):386–94.

80. Armitage, R., Emslie, G., and Rintelmann, J. The effect of fluoxetine on sleep EEG in childhood depression: A preliminary report. *Neuropsychopharmacology* 1997;17(4):241–5.

81. Waslick, B.D. *et al.* Open trial of fluoxetine in children and adolescents with dysthymic disorder or double depression. *J Affect Disord* 1999;56(2–3):227–36.

82. King, R.A. *et al.* Emergence of self-destructive phenomena in children and adolescents during fluoxetine treatment. *J Am Acad Child Adolesc Psychiatr*, 1991; 30(2): p. 179–86.

83. Sood, A., Weller, E., and Weller, R. SSRIs in children and adolescents: Where do we stand? *Current Psychiatry* 2004.3(3):83–89.

84. Neuropsychopharmacology, A.C.O., Preliminary Report of the Task Force on SSRIs and Suicidal Behavior in Youth, *Psychiatry* 2004; 31–4.

85. Advisory, F.P.H. Suicidality in Children and Adolescents Being Treated With Antidepressant Medications. United States Food and Drug Administration, 2004. http://www.fda.gov/cder/drug/antidepressants/SSRIPHA200410.htm.

86. Association, A.P. APA Statement on the FDA's Hearing on Antidepressant Use in Pediatric Patients. Arlington, Virginia. American Psychiatric Association: 2004.

87. Valuck, R.J. *et al.* Antidepressant treatment and risk of suicide attempt by adolescents with major depressive disorder: a propensity-adjusted retrospective cohort study. *CNS Drugs*, 2004;18(15): 1119–32.

88. Jick, H., Kaye, J.A., and Jick, S.S. Antidepressants and the risk of suicidal behaviors. *JAMA*, 2004;292(3):338–43.

89. Grunebaum, M.F. *et al.* Antidepressants and suicide risk in the United States, 1985–1999. *J Clin Psychiatry* 2004;65(11): 1456–62.

90. Olfson, M. *et al.* Relationship between antidepressant medication treatment and suicide in adolescents. *Arch Gen Psychiatry* 2003; 60(10):978–82.

91. March, J. *et al.* Fluoxetine, cognitive-behavioral therapy, and their combination for adolescents with depression: Treatment for Adolescents With Depression Study (TADS) randomized controlled trial. *JAMA* 2004;292(7):807–20.

92. Whittington, C.J. *et al.* Selective serotonin reuptake inhibitors in childhood depression: systematic review of published versus unpublished data. *Lancet* 2004; 363(9418):1341–5.

93. Kye, C.H. *et al.* A randomized, controlled trial of amitriptyline in the acute treatment of adolescent major depression. *J Am Acad Child Adolesc Psychiatry* 1996;35(9):1139–44.

94. Baldessarini, R. Drugs and the treatment of psychiatric disorders. In L.L. Hardman, J.G., Goodman, and Gilman, ed. *The Pharmacological Basis of Therapeutics.*, New York, McGraw-Hill, 1996, p. 431–59.

95. Wamboldt, M.Z., Yancey, A.G., Jr., and Roesler, T.A., Cardiovascular effects of tricyclic antidepressants in childhood asthma: A case series and review. *J Child Adolesc Psychopharmacol* 1997;7(1):45–64.

96. Popper C.W. E.G. Sudden death and tricyclic antidepressants: Clinical considerations for children. *J Child Adolesc Psychopharmacol* 1990;1:125–32.

97. Hazell, P. *et al.* Tricyclic drugs for depression in children and adolescents. *Cochrane Database Syst Rev* 2002;2:CD002317.

98. Kaplan, C.A. and Hussain, S. Use of drugs in child and adolescent psychiatry. *Br J Psychiatr* 1995;166(3):291–8.

99. Daly, J.M. and Wilens, T. The use of tricyclic antidepressants in children and adolescents. *Pediatr Clin North Am* 1998;45(5):1123–35.

100. Dugas, M, *et al.* Preliminary observations of the significance of monitoring tricyclic antidepressant plasma levels in the pediatric patient. *Ther Drug Monit* 1980;2(4):307–14.

101. Challman, T.D. and Lipsky, J.J. Methylphenidate: Its pharmacology and uses. *Mayo Clin Proc* 2000;75(7):711–21.

102. Fernandez, F. *et al.* Methylphenidate for depressive disorders in cancer patients. An alternative to standard antidepressants. *Psychosomatics* 1987;28(9):455–61.

103. Fernandez, F. *et al.* Effects of methylphenidate in HIV-related depression: A comparative trial with desipramine. *Int J Psychiatry Med* 1995;25(1):53–67.

104. House A., H.T. Depression in physical illness. *Prescribers' Journal* 1996;36(4):222–27.

105. Findling, R.L. Open-label treatment of comorbid depression and attentional disorders with co-administration of serotonin reuptake inhibitors and psychostimulants in children, adolescents, and adults: a case series. *J Child Adolesc Psychopharmacol*, 1996; 6(3):165–75.

106. Kellerman, J. *et al.* Psychological effects of illness in adolescence. I. Anxiety, self-esteem, and perception of control. *J Pediatr* 1980; 97(1):126–31.

107. Hart, D. and Bossert, E. Self-reported fears of hospitalized school-age children. *J Pediatr Nurs* 1994;9(2):83–90.

108. Klein, R., Pine, D.S. Anxiety Disorders. In M. Rutter, L. Hersov, and E. Taylor, ed. Child and Adolescent Psychiatry: Modern *Approaches* Oxford: Blackwell Scientific Publications. 2002;486–509.

109. Frank, N.C., Blount, R.L., and Brown, R.T. Attributions, coping, and adjustment in children with cancer. *J Pediatr Psychol* 1997; 22(4):563–76.

110. Jones, S.M., Fiser, D.H., and Livingston, R.L. Behavioral changes in pediatric intensive care units. *Am J Dis Child* 1992;146(3):375–9.

111. Brown, R.T. *et al.* Parental psychopathology and children's adjustment to leukemia. *J Am Acad Child Adolesc Psychiatr* 1993; 32(3):554–61.

112. Moore, J.B. and Mosher, R.B. Adjustment responses of children and their mothers to cancer: Self-care and anxiety. *Oncol Nurs Forum* 1997;24(3):519–25.

113. Packman, W.L. *et al.* Psychosocial consequences of bone marrow transplantation in donor and non-donor siblings. *J Dev Behav Pediatr* 1997;18(4):244–53.

114. Shama, W.I. The experience and preparation of pediatric sibling bone marrow donors. *Soc Work Health Care* 1998;27(1):89–99.

115. Greenhill, L.L. *et al.* Assessment issues in treatment research of pediatric anxiety disorders: What is working, what is not working, what is missing, and what needs improvement. *Psychopharmacol Bull* 1998;34(2):155–64.

116. Ireland, M. and Malgady, R.G. Thematic instrument for measuring death anxiety in children (TIMDAC). *J Pediatr Nurs* 1999; 14(1):28–37.

117. Carroll, M.K. and Ryan-Wenger, N.A. School-age children's fears, anxiety, and human figure drawings. *J Pediatr Health Care* 1999;13(1):24–31.

118. Costello, E., Angold, A. Epidemiology, in Anxiety Disorders in Children and Adolescents. *J. March. Editor* 1995, Guildford: New York. 109–24.

119. Labellarte, M.J. *et al.* The treatment of anxiety disorders in children and adolescents. *Biol Psychiatry* 1999;46(11):1567–78.

120. Fukunishi, I. and Kudo, H. Psychiatric problems of pediatric end-stage renal failure. *Gen Hosp Psychiatr* 1995;17(1):32–6.

121. Thompson, R.J., Jr., Hodges, K., and Hamlett, K.W. A matched comparison of adjustment in children with cystic fibrosis and psychiatrically referred and nonreferred children. *J Pediatr Psychol* 1990;15(6):745–59.

122. Schowalter, J. The child's reaction to his own terminal illness. In B. Schoenberger, A. Carr, and D. Peretz, ed. *Loss and Grief: Psychological management in medical practice.* New York: Columbia University Press, 1970.

123. Spinetta, J.J., Rigler, D., and Karon, M. Anxiety in the dying child, *Pediatrics* 1973;52(6):841–5.

124. Barrera, M.E., Rykov, M.H., and Doyle, S.L. The effects of interactive music therapy on hospitalized children with cancer: A pilot study. *Psychooncology* 2002;11(5):379–88.

125. Robb, S.L. and Ebberts, A.G. Songwriting and digital video production interventions for pediatric patients undergoing bone marrow transplantation, Part I: An analysis of depression and anxiety levels according to phase of treatment. *J Pediatr Oncol Nurs* 2003;20(1):2–15.

126. Hollenbeck, A.R. *et al.* Children with serious illness: Behavioral correlates of separation and isolation. *Child Psychiatry Hum Dev* 1980;11(1):3–11.

127. Olness, K. and Gardner, G.G. Some guidelines for uses of hypnotherapy in pediatrics. *Pediatrics* 1978;62(2):228–33.

128. Kohen, D.P. *et al.* The use of relaxation-mental imagery (self-hypnosis) in the management of 505 pediatric behavioral encounters. *J Dev Behav Pediatr* 1984;5(1):21–5.

129. Ott, M.J. Imagine the possibilities! Guided imagery with toddlers and pre-schoolers. *Pediatr Nurs* 1996;22(1):34–8.

130. Zeltzer, L.K. *et al.* A phase I study on the feasibility and acceptability of an acupuncture/hypnosis intervention for chronic pediatric pain. *J Pain Symptom Manage* 2002;24(4):437–46.

131. Manassis, K., Childhood anxiety disorders: Lessons from the literature. *Can J Psychiatr* 2000;45(8):724–30.

132. McCarthy, A.M. *et al.* Cognitive behavioral pain and anxiety interventions in pediatric oncology centers and bone marrow transplant units. *J Pediatr Oncol Nurs* 1996;13(1):3–12; discussion 13–4.

133. Liossi, C. and Hatira, P. Clinical hypnosis versus cognitive behavioral training for pain management with pediatric cancer patients undergoing bone marrow aspirations. *Int J Clin Exp Hypn* 1999;47(2):104–16.

134. Liossi, C. and Hatira, P. Clinical hypnosis in the alleviation of procedure-related pain in pediatric oncology patients. *Int J Clin Exp Hypn* 2003;51(1):4–28.

135. Kratochvil, C.J. *et al*. Pharmacotherapy of childhood anxiety disorders. *Curr Psychiatr Rep* 2002;4(4):264–9.

136. Yaster, M. *et al*. The management of opioid and benzodiazepine dependence in infants, children, and adolescents. *Pediatrics*, 1996; 98(1):135–40.

137. Hughes, J. *et al*. A prospective study of the adverse effects of midazolam on withdrawal in critically ill children *Acta Paediatr* 1994;83(11):1194–9.

138. Renaud, J. *et al*. Use of selective serotonin reuptake inhibitors for the treatment of childhood panic disorder: a pilot study. *J Child Adolesc Psychopharmacol* 1999;9(2):73–83.

139. Ljungman, G. *et al*. Midazolam nasal spray reduces procedural anxiety in children. *Pediatrics* 2000;105(1 Pt 1):73–8.

140. Bentley, R., Cope, J., Jenny, M., Hain, RDW. Use of intranasal/oral midazolam in paediatric palliative care. *Archives of Disease in Childhood* 2002;86:A76.

141. Birmaher, B. *et al*. Fluoxetine for childhood anxiety disorders. *J Am Acad Child Adolesc Psychiatr* 1994;33(7):993–9.

142. Dummit, E.S., III *et al*. Fluoxetine treatment of children with selective mutism: an open trial. *J Am Acad Child Adolesc Psychiatry* 1996;35(5):615–21.

143. Fairbanks, J.M. *et al*. Open fluoxetine treatment of mixed anxiety disorders in children and adolescents. *J Child Adolesc Psychopharmacol* 1997;7(1):17–29.

144. Walkup J.T., L.M., Riddle M.A., Pin D.P., Greenhill, L. Klein, R. Davies, M. Sweeney M., Abikoff H., Hack S., Klee B., McCracken J., Bergman L., Piacentini J., March J., Compton S., Robinson J., O'Hara T., Baker S., Vitiello B., Ritz L., Roper M., Fluvoxamine for the treatment of anxiety disorders in children and adolescents. *N Engl J Med* 2001;344(17):1279–1285.

145. Birmaher, B. *et al*. Fluoxetine for the treatment of childhood anxiety disorders. *J Am Acad Child Adolesc Psychiatry* 2003;42(4): 415–23.

146. Seligman, L.D. and Ollendick, T.H. Comorbidity of anxiety and depression in children and adolescents: An integrative review. *Clin Child Fam Psychol Rev* 1998;1(2):125–44.

147. Ryan, N.D. *et al*. The clinical picture of major depression in children and adolescents. *Arch Gen Psychiatry* 1987;44(10):854–61.

148. Gurley, D. C.P., Pine D.S., and Brook J. Discriminating depression and anxiety in youth: A role for diagnostic criteria. *J Affective Disorders* 1996;39:191–200.

149. Wood, A. R. Harrington, and Moore, A. Controlled trial of a brief cognitive-behavioural intervention in adolescent patients with depressive disorders. *J Child Psychol Psychiatry* 1996;37(6):737–46.

150. Brent, D.A. *et al*. A clinical psychotherapy trial for adolescent depression comparing cognitive, family, and supportive therapy. *Arch Gen Psychiatr* 1997;54(9):877–85.

151. Kendall, P.C. Treating anxiety disorders in children: results of a randomized clinical trial. *J Consult Clin Psychol* 1994;62(1): 100–10.

152. Kendall, P.C. *et al*. Therapy for youths with anxiety disorders: A second randomized clinical trial. *J Consult Clin Psychol* 1997; 65(3):366–80.

153. Barrett, P.M., Dadds, M.R., and Rapee, R.M. Family treatment of childhood anxiety: A controlled trial. *J Consult Clin Psychol* 1996; 64(2):333–42.

154. Parker, G. and Roy, K. Adolescent depression: a review. *Aust N Z J Psychiatr* 2001;35(5):572–80.

155. Sherry & Jellinece 1996.

156. Meijer *et al*. 2008

157. Burke, A.L. Palliative care: An update on "terminal restlessness". *Med J Aust* 1997;166(1):39–42.

158. Twycross, R. Symptom control: the problem areas. *Palliat Med* 1993;7(Suppl 1):1–8.

159. Liptzin B, L.S. An empirical study of delirium subtypes. *Br J Psychiatry* 1992;161:843–845.

160. Lawlor P.G., Mancini G.B. *et al* Occurrence, causes, and outcome of delirium in patients with advanced cancer: A prospective study. *Arch Intern Med* 2000;160(6):786–94.

161. Breitbart, W., Psychiatric aspects of palliative care. In H.G.D. Doyle, N. MacDonald ed. *Oxford Textbook of Palliative Medicine*, New York: Oxford University Press 1998;p. 933–956.

162. Breitbart, W, C.K., Delirium in the terminally ill. In B.W. Chochinov ed. *Handbook of psychiatry in palliative medicine*, New York: Oxford University Press 2000, p. 75–90.

163. Bruera, E. *et al*. Cognitive failure in patients with terminal cancer: A prospective study. *J Pain Symptom Manage* 1992;7(4):192–5.

164. Maddocks, I. *et al*. Attenuation of morphine-induced delirium in palliative care by substitution with infusion of oxycodone. *J Pain Symptom Manage* 1996;12(3):182–9.

165. de Stoutz, N.D., Bruera, E., and Suarez-Almazor, M. Opioid rotation for toxicity reduction in terminal cancer patients. *J Pain Symptom Manage* 1995;10(5):378–84.

166. Bruera, E. *et al*. Changing pattern of agitated impaired mental status in patients with advanced cancer: association with cognitive monitoring, hydration, and opioid rotation. *J Pain Symptom Manage* 1995;10(4):287–91.

167. Morita, T. *et al*. Increased plasma morphine metabolites in terminally ill cancer patients with delirium: an intra-individual comparison. *J Pain Symptom Manage* 2002;23(2):107–13.

168. Morita, T. *et al*. Underlying pathologies and their associations with clinical features in terminal delirium of cancer patients. *J Pain Symptom Manage* 2001;22(6):997–1006.

169. Inouye, S.K. *et al*. Clarifying confusion: The confusion assessment method. A new method for detection of delirium. *Ann Intern Med* 1990;113(12):941–8.

170. Trzepacz, P.B.R. and Greenhouse, J. A symptom rating scale for delirium. *Psychiatry Res* 1988;23:89–97.

171. Breitbart, W. *et al*. The Memorial Delirium Assessment Scale. *J Pain Symptom Manage* 1997;13(3):128–37.

172. Morita, T. *et al*. Communication Capacity Scale and Agitation Distress Scale to measure the severity of delirium in terminally ill cancer patients: A validation study. *Palliat Med* 2001;15(3): 197–206.

173. Minagawa, H. *et al*. Psychiatric morbidity in terminally ill cancer patients. A prospective study. *Cancer* 1996;78(5):1131–7.

174. Pereira, J., Hanson, J., and Bruera, E. The frequency and clinical course of cognitive impairment in patients with terminal cancer. *Cancer* 1997;79(4):835–42.

175. Meagher, D.J. *et al*. The use of environmental strategies and psychotropic medication in the management of delirium. *Br J Psychiatry* 1996;168(4):512–5.

176. Association, A.P. Practice guidelines for the treatment of patients with delirium. *Am J Psychiatry* 1999;156(suppl):1–20.

177. Adams, F., and Andersson, F.F., Emegency pharmacotherapy of delirium in the critically ill cancer patient. *Psychosomatics* 1986; 27:33–7.

178. Beuzen, J.N, Wesnes, T.N.K, and Wood A. A comparison of the effects of olanzapine, haloperidol and placebo on cognitive and psychomotor functions in healthy elderley volunteers. *J psychopharmacol* 1999; 13:152–9.

179. De Deyn, P.P. and Katz, I.R. Control of aggression and agitation in patients with dementia: Efficacy and safety of risperidone. *Int J Geriatr Psychiatry* 2000;15 Suppl 1:S14–22.

180. De Deyn, P.P. *et al*. A randomized trial of risperidone, placebo, and haloperidol for behavioral symptoms of dementia. *Neurology* 1999;53(5):946–55.

181. Sipahimalani, A.M.P. Olanzapine in the treatment of delerium. *Psychosomatics* 1998;39:422–30.

182. Sipahimalani A.S.R. and Masand P., Treatment of delirium with resperidone. *Int J Geriatr Psychopharmacol* 1997;1:24–6.

183. Conley, R.R. Risperidone side effects. *J Clin Psychiatry* 2000; 61 (Suppl) 8:20–3.

184. Breitbart, W. *et al*. A double-blind trial of haloperidol, chlorpromazine and lorazepam in the treatment of delirium in hospitalized AIDS patients. *Am J Psychiatry* 1996;153(2):231–237.

185. Galloway, K.S. and Yaster, M. Pain and symptom control in terminally ill children. *Pediatr Clin North Am* 2000;47(3):711–46.

186. Stirling, L.C., Kurowska, A., and Tookman, A. The use of phenobarbitone in the management of agitation and seizures at the end of life. *J Pain Symptom Manage* 1999;17(5):363–8.

187. Pritchard, J.W, R.B. Phenobarbital, mechanism of action. In M.R.a.M.B. Levy RH, ed. *Antiepileptic Drugs*, 1995, New York : Raven Press, p. 359–377.

188. Fainsinger, R., Treatment of delirium at the end of life: medical and ethical issues. In B.E. Portenoy R.K., ed. *Topics in Palliative care*, Oxford: Oxford University Press, 2000,pp.261–277.

189. Back, I. Terminal restlessness in patients with advanced malignant disease. *Palliat Med* 1992;6:293–298.

190. Bottomley, D.M. and Hanks, G.W. Subcutaneous midazolam infusion in palliative care. *J Pain Symptom Manage* 1990;5(4):259–61.

191. de Souza, E.J.B. Midazolam in terminal care. *Lancet* 1998; 1((letter)):67–68.

192. Oliver, D. The use of methotrimeprzine in terminal care. *Br J Clin Pract* 1985;39:339–340.

193. Power, D. and Kearney M. Management of the final 24 hours. *Ir Med J* 1992;85(3):93–5.

194. Stiefel, F., Fainsinger, R., and Bruera, E. Acute confusional states in patients with advanced cancer. *J Pain Symptom Manage* 1992; 7(2):94–8.

26 Neurological and neuromuscular symptoms

Kate W. Faulkner, Paul B. Thayer, and David L. Coulter

Introduction

Caring for children with life-threatening neurological or neuromuscular symptoms and conditions involves the art of palliative care much more than the science. For example, consider the challenge of pain assessment in non-verbal children whose development is regressing. Here, a working partnership with families is paramount, because often, it is the subtle deviation from children's baseline status that leads parents, and then practitioners, to the recognition of the presence of pain [1]. After a symptom is identified, the diagnostic art continues as caregivers attempt to identify the etiology, be it something physical (related or unrelated to the primary diagnosis), something in the environment, or even a side-effect of previous therapies. Again, since children with neurological impairments or symptoms often have a limited repertoire of responses, a symptom such as increased irritability could have a dizzying array of etiologies, each best approached in a different fashion.

Palliative care and hospice teams are unfortunately most often familiar with children in their last stages of life, when symptoms are rapidly progressive and usually require drug therapy to control. However, children may well live with prominent neurological and neuromuscular symptoms progressing slowly over a number of years. Though medication therapy might still be indicated, often there are other forms of treatment to consider, including surgery, physical and occupational therapy, integrative therapies, environmental interventions, and dietary manipulation. The palliative care team may help the family become aware of these options, serving an important educational and coordinating role. Even if drug therapy is indicated, the practitioner should be aware that few of the recommended drugs have been tested for safety or effectiveness in children. Again emanating from the art rather than the science of medicine, informal networking among physicians and pharmacists has led to a consensus about drugs, doses, effectiveness, and potential side-effects [2].

Chapter outline

This chapter addresses three aspects of palliative care for neurological and neuromuscular symptoms. The first section includes brief summaries of major life-limiting conditions, including synopses of their incidence, etiology if known, clinical presentation, prominent symptoms, general prognostic guidelines, current treatment options, and an indication of sources for more detailed information. This section should help the team provide a 'roadmap' of possible illness trajectories, future symptoms, and therapeutic options to affected children and their families.

The second section reviews the most common or problematic neurological and neuromuscular symptoms palliative care practitioners may encounter, along with a discussion of etiology (where known) and the range of therapeutic approaches to ameliorate the symptoms.

The third and final section highlights the global impact of these symptoms on children and their families. Several families have been willing to share their stories, so that the palliative care team might come to better appreciate the experience of living with these conditions and symptoms.

Neurological and neuromuscular conditions

Dramatic changes in the incidence and etiology of childhood death have occurred over the last century in developed countries, as better public health policies have led to improvement in infection prevention and control. After the first year of life, the current greatest threats to children's lives in these countries are unintentional and intentional injuries [3,4]. Yet, substantial numbers of children still die of complex chronic conditions or diseases, including malignancies.

More deaths occur in the first year of life than all other years of childhood combined, and two-thirds of these deaths occur in the first month of life [6]. The leading cause of infant mortality in the United States in 1999 was 'congenital anomalies', which include malformations, deformations, and chromosomal abnormalities. A review of two decades of mortality data in the United States showed that malignancies accounted for 2% of infant deaths, neuromuscular diseases for 15%, genetic conditions for 22%, and metabolic defects for 1% [5]. The overall steady decline in infant mortality in most developed countries has traditionally been linked to improved pre- and perinatal care [7]. However, increased use of prenatal testing, and diagnosis of lethal anomalies, leading to elective pregnancy termination prior to the birth of the affected infant, may also be contributing to the decreased number of deaths due to congenital anomalies [8].

During the middle years of childhood, a little over one-third as many deaths occur from life-limiting conditions, as occur in infancy. From one to nine years of age, malignancies account for 36% of deaths, neuromuscular for 21%, genetic for 5%, and metabolic for 3% of all life-threatening illnesses [5]. This proportion changes again in a modest way for 10- to 24-year-old adolescents and young adults. Cancer accounts for 48% of deaths from complex chronic conditions, neuromuscular for 17%, genetic for 13%, and metabolic for 1%. The total number of deaths in this age group work out to about 60% of the total number of deaths that occur in the first year of life.

These statistics are helpful in predicting where palliative care interventions are likely to be most needed and beneficial. Certainly, the team should have a large focus on infants who are newly diagnosed, very symptomatic, and having a prognosis of days to weeks. But at the other end of the spectrum, care is needed for children with neurological and neuromuscular symptoms, and disorders whose course may last for years. Some of these children may have a steady downward course, while others may have waxing and waning of their symptoms [9]. The challenges of supporting this diverse group of children require ongoing assessment and flexibility on the part of parents and professionals alike.

Synopses of major life-threatening conditions with prominent neurological or neuromuscular symptoms follow. Their representation in any given palliative care census may well depend more on the relationship of the team with different referrers, than on the absolute number of children afflicted.

Malformations of the central nervous system

Neural tube defects account for most congenital anomalies of the central nervous system, and result from the failure of the neural tube to close spontaneously between the third and fourth week of gestation [10]. Both genetic predisposition and environmental insults may be responsible for these conditions, including a variety of drugs, infections, maternal diabetes, folic acid deficiency, and irradiation [11]. The most devastating of these disorders is anencephaly. The incidence of this universally fatal condition varies in different populations, but occurs in approximately one in 1,000 live births [12]. In the United States, mandatory folic acid fortification of all enriched cereal grain products since 1996 has led to a 21% decline in the incidence of anencephaly [13]. Increased prenatal surveillance, with elective termination of pregnancy, has also led to a decreased incidence in developed countries [14].

A number of elements contribute to the lethality of the condition. Failure of the cephalic neural folds to fuse into a tube exposes brain cells to the degenerative effects of amniotic fluid. Additionally, mutual induction of the three primary germ layers of ectoderm, endoderm, and mesoderm fails, resulting in deformities of both nervous tissue and supporting axial bone. Clinically, therefore, the calvarium of the anancephalic infant fails to develop, forebrain germinal cells degenerate so no cortex exists, and descending spinal cord tracts as well as the pituitary and optic nerves are absent [11].

Anencephalic babies almost never survive infancy. During the days to weeks that they live, they exibit slow, stereotyped movements, and frequent decerebrate posturing. These movements can occur spontaneously, or in response to pain. Seizures sometimes occur. Brainstem reflexes, such as sucking and rooting, can be more prominent than in normal infants [11]. Palliative supportive care is generally indicated, though there may also be difficult ethical considerations of organ harvesting and extraordinary life support measures. Since anencephaly is difficult to diagnose histopathologically because of the presence of both primary and secondary destructive processes, it is hard to gauge the importance of the rare reports of survival for several years in a few cases of hydranencephaly [15].

Spina bifida in its many presentations is the second most prevalent neural tube defect. It represents a fusion failure of the posterior vertebral arches, sometimes with accompanying herniation of just the meninges (meningocele), or of the meninges and spinal cord parenchyma and nerve roots (myelomeningocele). In rachischisis, the most severe variant, an extensive defect of the cranio-vertebral bone exposes the brain, spinal cord and meninges. Although the etiology of the disorder is incompletely understood, it is influenced by socio-economic status, gender, ethnicity, prior offspring with neural tube defects, and maternal age and parity [16]. The overall incidence of all forms approaches one in 1000 births [12].

Historically, nearly half of the infants with meyelomeningoceles who were not treated surgically died within the first year of life, as a consequence of hydrocephalus or central nervous system (CNS) infections [17]. Medical and surgical advances have reduced the mortality rate to 10–15%, with most of these children dying before entering school, of urinary tract infection leading to sepsis and renal failure [12,18]. However, considerable morbidity exists in survivors that may be improved with palliative support. By adolescence, two-thirds will be wheelchair bound, incontinent of bowel and bladder, and have visual defects. Nearly half will have IQs below 80, and a quarter will have seizure disorders and develop precocious puberty. Nearly all will experience pressure sores and fractures [19].

The other major category of devastating CNS disorders likely to be encountered by the palliative care practitioner is defects of cell migration, including lissencephaly, schizencephaly, and porencephaly. Migratory disorders develop when neuroblasts of the germinal matrix, which forms the wall of the lateral ventricles, fail to reach their intended destination in the cerebral cortex [20]. This results in focal or generalized structural deformities of the cerebral hemispheres. Neuronal migration disorders are associated with a variety of other conditions, including metabolic diseases, chromosomal anomalies, neuromuscular conditions, and neurocutaneous syndromes. A variety of prenatal insults can lead to these disorders, only a few of which, including cytomegalovirus infection, fetal exposure to alcohol, carbon monoxide, radiation, mercury, and isoretinoic acid, have been identified [20].

The clinical presentation varies with the underlying abnormalities, but usually includes massive seizures, hypotonia, microcephaly, optic atrophy, a characteristic facies, spastic quadriparesis or hemiparesis, and profound developmental delay [21]. No treatment of the underlying brain development disorder is possible. This group of disorders is life-limiting, but prognostic variation is great, depending on the extent of the migratory defect and complications that arise.

Chromosomal anomalies

Human diploid cells contain 22 chromosome pairs called autosomes, and one pair of sex chromosomes. Genes, consisting of DNA coding sequences, are arranged in linear order on the chromosome, and contain most of the genetic information that is passed from one generation to the next. Maternal mitochondria also contribute DNA that transmits genetic information [22]. Constitutional chromosomal anomalies generally occur early in embryo-genesis, affecting all or most of children's cells. These mistakes occur more commonly with advancing maternal age [23].

Approximately one-third of recognized genetic disease shows phenotypic expression in the nervous system, reflecting the fact that more than 30,000 genes are expressed in children's brains [24, 25]. This section will consider conditions caused by duplication of an entire chromosome; the subsequent section on metabolic conditions reviews those caused by gene or mitochondrial DNA point mutations.

Studies have shown that major duplications or deficiencies in autosomes tend to be lethal, with death occurring either *in utero* or soon after birth [26]. Of the autosomal trisomies, only trisomy 21 (Down syndrome) is compatible with a survival of years. Even then, a review of spontaneous abortions reveals that less than a quarter of trisomy 21 cases are live born. No children with the most common trisomy, chromosome 16, are live born; only 2.8% of trisomy 13 cases, and 5.4% of trisomy 18 cases, are live born [27]. Overall, chromosomal anomalies occur in 0.4% of live births [23].

Trisomy 18 (Edwards syndrome) is the most common fatal anomaly, with an incidence of one out of 6,000 births [23]. Affected females are four times more common than males. The clinical presentation is that of a low-birth-weight infant, with a long, narrow skull and prominent occiput, low-set, malformed ears, closed fist with overlapping fingers, and rocker-bottom feet. Often, there are co-existing cardiac and renal defects. Neurological manifestations include a small brain and profound developmental delay [23,28]. Although the vast majority of children will die in the perinatal period, survival beyond the first year of life is possible. A recent mortality review, using United States death certificates from 1979 through 1997, noted that median survival time was 10 days, but 5.6% of children lived longer than one year. Median ages were higher among females and children of African-American origin. The age at death was unaffected by the presence of concurrent cardiac malformation [29].

Trisomy 13 (Patau syndrome) occurs in one out of 10,000 births [23]. Median facial anomalies are prominent in this condition, including cleft lip and palate, and micrognathia. Ears are low-set and malformed, with many infants being deaf. Polydactyly and flexion deformities of the fingers are common. Cardiac abnormalities are frequent, as are polycystic kidneys, omphaloceles, and neural tube defects. The majority of children have small brains, small eyes, and profound neuro-developmental delays. Their clinical course is characterized by feeding difficulties and apneic spells [28]. The median age at time of death is also 10 days; however, slightly over 5% of children survive longer than one year. Race, gender, and the presence of a cardiac defect do not affect survival [29].

Numerous other chromosomal trisomies and deletions have been described and clinically characterized, though not all of them are certain to cause death in childhood [30]. There have been recent, encouraging examples of involvement of the hospice team in the care of these infants and families [31].

Metabolic diseases of the nervous system

Inborn errors of metabolism may be static, chronic and non-progressive (such as many disorders of amino acid metabolism), or they may be progressive and degenerative (such as most lysosomal enzyme disorders). Progressive metabolic disorders generally arise from a mutation (or set of mutations) in a single gene coding for an enzymatic protein that is usually involved in a catabolic pathway. Over 500 of these disorders have been described, most with an autosomal recessive pattern of inheritance. The overall incidence is approximately one in 5,000 live births. The mechanism by which inborn errors of metabolism produce brain dysfunction remains incompletely understood; however, it may be that products 'upstream' of the enzymatic defect accumulate after birth in toxic amounts in brain tissue. Additionally, there may be a decrease in critical components 'downstream'

of the defect, so that appropriate neuro-development is not possible. The neuro-degenerative process can involve primarily the gray matter of the brain cortex itself, or the white matter of myelination [32].

Common neonatal symptoms of metabolic disorders include poor feeding, hypotonia, lethargy, respiratory difficulties, failure to thrive, psychomotor delay, seizures, and prominent vomiting. Rapid progression to death is the rule, unless prompt diagnosis and treatment are available [33]. Table 26.1 summarizes the symptoms for a select group of lethal point mutations. Diagnosis usually depends on specific enzyme assays, or on molecular genetic analysis [34]. Many nations have instituted newborn screening programs to detect more prevalent, treatable conditions. The recent introduction of tandem mass spectrometry has allowed rapid and inexpensive screening for a number of very rare disorders, but the yield and clinical utility of the procedure is still being defined [35].

In older infants and children, metabolic disorders present with chronic encephalopathy and the progressive loss of previously acquired abilities in mental and neurological function. Hallmarks include loss of developmental milestones, vomiting, irritability, seizures, myoclonus, tremors and either spasticity or hypotonia. Depending on the metabolic error, there may be changes in hair color and texture, skin dryness and texture, the development of coarse facial features, and a distinctive body odor. Again, without specific diagnosis and therapeutic intervention if available, many of these conditions will result in death in childhood. Besides assays, biopsies of liver or muscle may be helpful, as are neuro-imaging studies and genetic analysis [36].

Careful, specific diagnosis can lead to genetic counseling at a minimum, and treatment of the disorder, if treatment is available. Therapies are limited, and have as their goals correction of the metabolic abnormalities, removal of toxic metabolites, and treatment of other life-threatening conditions, such as cardiac arrythmias. For example, in the disorder phenylketouria (PKU), life-long dietary reduction of phenylalanine intake prevents neurological decline. A more definitive therapeutic approach to correcting genetic disease has been to transplant bone marrow or liver from a normal donor into affected children. Transplantation is effective only if the defective enzyme is normally expressed and active in the transplanted tissue, as stem cells are for several storage diseases [37]. Another possible therapy involves the periodic infusion of fully functional enzyme into children, if it can be identified, purified, and made affordable for a lifetime of therapy [38]. Finally, efforts to develop human protein drugs by cell culture or production in milk of transgenic animals are ongoing [39].

Table 26.1 Selected incurable point mutation disorders

Aminoacid disorders
NKH—nonketotic hyperglycinemia (Glycine encephalopathy)
  presents in the neonatal period;
  intractable seizures/profound hypotonia;
  frequent hiccups;
  progressive obtundation with coma;
  apnea/respiratory arrest in the neonatal period.

Ataxia disorders
Ataxia-telangiectasia
  presents in infancy/early childhood with ataxia;
  telangiectases bridge of nose/ears/neck/elbows/conjunctiva;
  choreoathetosis/eye apraxia/nystagmus;
  high incidence of leukemia/ lymphoma;
  diabetes in adolescence;
  death variable from bronchopulmonary infection/ cancer.

Carbohydrate disorders
Pompe's disease-infantile (Infantile acid maltase deficiency)
  presents in first weeks/months;
  diffuse hypotonia/weakness;
  macroglossia/increased muscle bulk;
  cardiomegaly/heart failure;
  respiratory insufficiency leading to death by age 1–2 years.

Degenerative disorders
Canavan's disease (Spongy degeneration of the cerebral white matter)
  presents at 2–4 months of age;
  developmental arrest/macrocephaly;
  optic atrophy/blindness/nystagmus;
  hypotonia/spasticity;
  irritability/sleep disturbance/seizures;
  intermittent fevers;
  gastroesophageal reflux/bulbar weakness;
  death often in first decade.

Genetic epilepsies
Batten's disease (Neuronal ceroid lipofuscinoses)
  presents at 9–19 months of age;
  developmental regression/microcephaly;
  generalized, persistent seizures;
  optic atrophy/blindness/brown macular pigmentation;
  death variable.

Lysosomal disorders
Hurler's syndrome (Mucopolysaccharidosis type I)
  normal at birth/coarse facial features develop after 6 months;
  chronic rhinorrhea/recurrent infections;
  organomegaly/hernias;
  bony changes (dystosis multiplex)/kyphosis;
  mental regression to vegetative state;
  death from airway obstruction/bronchopneumonia mid-childhood.
Sanfilippo's syndrome (Mucopolysacchaidosis type III)
  normal at birth/delayed development between 2–5 years of age;
  neurologic regression/ataxia/tremor/spasticity/bulbar palsy;

  coarse facial features/mild hepatosplenomegaly;
  loss of extension of the interphalangeal joints;
  hydrocephalus;
  death in adolescence.
Niemann-Pick disease type A (Sphingomyelin lipidosis)
  presents in first year of life;
  massive hepatosplenomegaly/diarrhea;
  persistent neonatal jaundice with brown/yellow skin;
  generalized lymphadenopathy/pulmonary infiltrates;
  macular degeneration with cherry-red spot;
  cognitive regression;
  death by 5 years of age.
Krabbe disease-infantile (Globoid cell leukodystrophy)
  presents at 4–6 months of age;
  restlessness/irritability/progressive stiffness;
  increased muscle tone/tonic spasms/seizures;
  fever without infection;
  mental/motor regression;
  death by 15 months with terminal flaccidity/bulbar signs.
Tay–Sachs disease (GM2 gangliosidosis)
  presents at 4–6 months of age;
  listlessness/irritability/hearing loss;
  developmental regression/lethargy/immobility;
  spasticity/myoclonus/generalized seizures/opisthotonus;
  progressive enlargement of the head;
  macular degeneration with cherry-red spot;
  death by 2–5 years of age.

Metal metabolism disorders
KHD—Kinky hair disease (Menkes disease)
  presents most often in neonatal period;
  hypothermia/hypoglycemia/poor feeding/poor weight gain;
  marked hypotonia/neurological deterioration/seizures;
  facies cherubic appearance/hair colorless and friable;
  radiographic abnormalities/hydronephrosis;
  enlargement intracranial vessels/subdural hematomas;
  course variable/death during childhood most often.

Mitochondrial disorders
Leigh syndrome (Subacute necrotizing encephalomyelitis)
  maternal transmission with presents in infancy/childhood;
  variable course/some survive to adulthood;
  psychomotor regression/somnolence;
  myopathy/hypotonia;
  optic atrophy with blindness/ophthalmoplegia;
  movement disorders/ataxia/peripheral neuropathies;
  disturbances of respiration.

Peroxisomal disorders
Zellweger syndrome (Peroxisomal assembly deficiency)
  intrauterine growth retardation/ typical high, flat facies;
  profound weakness/hypotonia;
  optic atrophy/cataracts/chorioretinities;
  hepatomelagy/cirrhosis/renal cysts;
  death by 1 year of age.

Source: Derived from Rosenberg, R.N., Prusiner, S.B., DiMauro, S., and Barchi, eds. *Clinical Companion to the Molecular and Genetic Basis of Neurological Disease (Second edition)*. Boston: Butterworth Heinemann, 1998 and Menkes, J.H., Sarnat, H.B., eds. *Child Neurology*. Philadelphia, PA: Lippincott Williams & Wilkins, 2000.

Neuromuscular disorders

Neuromuscular diseases affect the motor neuron unit in one of four places: the motor neuron, its axon, the neuromuscular junction, or the muscle fibers innervated by the neuron. These conditions have a limited clinical expression with considerable overlap of signs and symptoms, making definitive diagnosis challenging. Diagnostic tools include muscle enzyme assay, electromyography, nerve conduction studies, and muscle biopsy [40]. Since the identification of the specific gene responsible for Duchenne muscular dystrophy was made 15 years ago, research on the molecular pathogenesis has revealed a number of closely connected disorders, allowing for genetic counseling and the potential for replacement gene therapy [41].

The most common and clearly defined of the muscular dystrophies is Duchenne muscular dystrophy, an x-linked recessive disease with a prevalence of one in 25,000. The disease becomes apparent in early childhood, when affected boys exhibit pelvic muscle weakness, resulting in lordotic posture, and experience difficulty in climbing stairs or in getting up from the ground. Striking enlargement of the calf muscles occurs, as collagen and fat accumulate between muscle cells. Hamstring contractures are common. Confinement to a wheelchair generally occurs by the teenage years, accompanied by rapidly progressive scoliosis. Death tends to occur in young adulthood, either from respiratory failure or from cardiac myopathy. Supportive care from a physical medicine and rehabilitation team can prolong functional survival. Palliative therapies include orthotic bracing, physiotherapy, and surgery to release contracted tendons [42].

Non-invasive oral and nasal intermittent positive-pressure ventilation, in conjunction with mechanically assisted coughing, has led to a steady improvement in life expectancy in the muscular dystrophies [43]. Over half of those adolescents using nocturnal home external ventilation since the 1990's have achieved a mean age of over 25 years [44]. Although assisted ventilation can lead to better clinical status in terms of sleep improvement, energy levels, and headaches, some patients find it physically or psychologically objectionable. It does not prevent the development of fatal cardiomyopathy, so its use is truly palliative. Both patient and family will benefit from anticipatory information and support from the team, in making the decision on adopting non-invasive ventilation.

As in all diseases with a single gene defect, considerable effort is being devoted to develop gene therapies. Different researchers are attempting cell transfer therapy using viral vectors, drugs designed to 'up-regulate' compensatory muscle proteins, and strategies to repair the mutation *in vivo*. As yet, none of these approaches have entered the phase of human testing [45,46].

The second most common group of hereditary neuromuscular disorders is the spinal muscular atrophies (SMA's). These are transmitted by an autosomal recessive gene with an overall incidence of one in 10,000 to 25,000. The type 1 infantile form of SMA, commonly known as Werdnig-Hoffmann disease, generally presents before the age of 6 months with severe hypotonia, generalized weakness, muscle atrophy, absent tendon reflexes, and fasciculation of the tongue. Cardiac and smooth muscle remain unaffected, as does sphincter control. Children generally are unable to feed; over two-thirds die of respiratory involvement before two years of age [47].

Non-invasive nocturnal ventilation can confer numerous benefits, not only by prolonging life, but also by improving the quality. Symptoms related to hypoventilation, such as early morning drowsiness, headaches and feelings of 'heaviness' can all be relieved by non-invasive ventilation. However, for many families this represents a burden they are not prepared to consider. Patients may find the mask intolerable. Many families do not want hospital technology to invade their home. Palliative care paediatricians may find themselves paradoxically advocating against this palliative intervention, on behalf of the patient [48,49].

Lastly, it is important to remember that many patients who are offered interventions such as non-invasive ventilation, are old enough or mature enough to give or withhold consent for them. Boys with Duchenne muscular dystrophy, in particular, are often offered non-invasive nocturnal ventilation as they reach late teenage. It is important to consider the legalities of overriding the expressed wishes of these older children.

Cerebral palsy

Cerebral palsy (CP) is a neurological syndrome, rather than a specific disease entity. It is characterized by a group of motor syndromes resulting from disorders of early brain development. It is the most common form of chronic motor disability that begins in childhood. CP is often associated with epilepsy and abnormalities of speech, vision, and intellect [50]. Causes of CP include perinatal hypoxic-ischemic encephalopathy, intra- or periventricular hemorrhage, cerebral dysgenesis, and intracranial infection. The prevalence ranges from 1.5 to 2.5 per 1,000 live births, with the risk highest among very preterm and low-birth-weight babies [51]. The clinical feature common to all CP syndromes is the presence of pyramidal or extra-pyramidal signs. The syndromes may be classified by the predominant type of motor disturbance, for example, quadriplegia (four affected extremities), diplegia (legs more than arms), hemiplegia (one side), ataxic (incoordination of voluntary movement), or dyskinetic (involuntary movements).

The clinical presentation is one of a gradual change from generalized hypotonia of the newborn period to spasticity in childhood, along with an abnormal evolution of postural reflexes. Over time, the increased tone leads to contractures, with resultant limb deformities such as scissoring, and scoliosis [52]. In children with ataxic and dyskinetic forms of CP, however, the hypotonia of infancy persists. Once the diagnosis of CP is made on the basis of the clinical picture, a complete investigation of possible etiologies should be undertaken. Sometimes, underlying disorders have made children more susceptible to the effects of perinatal trauma and asphyxia. Many neurological, neuromuscular, and metabolic disorders cause increased vulnerability to the stresses of delivery and extra-uterine life [51].

Although CP has no cure, many palliative measures are available to aid children in becoming as highly functional as possible. Depending on the clinical presentation, these may include communication devices, physiotherapy, bracing, speech therapy, and involvement of other team members. The various treatments available for spasticity will be discussed in the next section.

Palliative care practitioners should be particularly familiar with spastic quadriplegia, the most severe form of CP. This syndrome, which accounts for about 20% of all CP cases, is characterized by marked motor impairment of all extremities and a high incidence of mental retardation and seizures. Swallowing difficulties are common, owing to supranuclear bulbar palsies, and often lead to aspiration pneumonia [50]. Nearly all deaths from CP during childhood will occur in this most severe group, with pneumonia frequently being the immediate cause of death [53,54].

Central nervous system cancer

After the first year of life, cancer is the leading cause of disease-related mortality in childhood [55]. Cancers of the brain and central nervous system are the most common type of solid tumor in childhood, and are second only to leukemia in overall incidence. They account for approximately 20% of all pediatric cancers [56]. Leukemia and CNS cancer are also the most frequent cause of cancer deaths in children and adolescents. Although overall survival rates for most childhood cancers have improved dramatically since 1975, as reflected in the 44% drop in age-adjusted mortality, the improvement in prognosis for brain tumor patients is less dramatic, at 24% [55].

The overall annual incidence of tumors of the central nervous system is approximately three cases per 100,000 children. The incidence peaks in the first decade of life, then declines steadily through adolescence. About 10% of children with a brain tumor have a syndrome that has placed them at increased risk, such as neurofibromatosis or tuberous sclerosis. Other known pre-disposing factors include radiation, immuno-suppressive disorders, rare familial clusters, and previous cancer [56].

Different types of tumors predominate at different ages. In the first two years of life, cerebral cancer occurs more commonly, including low-grade gliomas, primitive neuroectodermal tumors (PNET), and choroids-plexus tumors. In older children, posterior fossa lesions predominate, including diagnoses such as medulloblastoma, cerebellar and brainstem astrocytomas, ependymoma, and brainstem glioma [57]. It is this predominance of midline tumors of the posterior fossa that makes the clinical presentation of brain tumors in children so different from those in adults. In addition to focal neurological deficits, children often present with protean manifestations of increased intercranial pressure. Major clinical symptoms are presented in Table 26.2.

Treatment of pediatric brain tumors involves varying combinations of surgery, radiation, and chemotherapy, depending on the age of the child and the type of tumor [58]. The value of extensive tumor resection has been established in a number of childhood CNS tumors as a means of cytoreduction of the cancer, prior to other forms of therapy. Advances in microsurgical technique have made more extensive surgery possible, without increased morbidity. Several of the most common brain cancers respond well to radiotherapy, but radiation of the growing brain and spine carries more risk of negative side-effects, including decreased intelligence, short stature, and secondary bone cancers. For this reason, radiation is normally not administered to infants and very young children, except as a last resort. Pediatric brain tumors tend to be more responsive to chemotherapy than do adult tumors, with various regimens being studied in efforts to improve survival [56,58]. Considerable long-term sequelae of both cancer and cancer treatment are reported in survivors, including visual impairment, epilepsy, and cognitive and motor impairment [59].

In addition to primary brain cancer, neurological symptoms arise when other pediatric tumors metastasize to the brain or spinal fluid. Without specific chemotherapeutic or radiation therapy to prevent tumor spread, both leukemia and lymphoma have a high incidence of seeding the cerebral spinal fluid [60]. Neurological complications can occur in almost one-third of solid tumors as well, most often in association with neuroblastomas and sarcomas. Complications include brain space-occupying lesions, spinal cord compression, peripheral or cranial neuropathies, and seizures [61].

Table 26.2 Clinical manifestations of pediatric brain tumors

Signs and symptoms

Headache
  recurrent and progressive;
  in frontal or occipital areas;
  usually dull and throbbing;
  worse on arising, less during day;
  intensified by lowering head and straining, such as during bowel
    movement;
  coughing, sneezing.

Vomiting
  with or without nausea or feeding;
  progressively more projectile;
  more severe in morning;
  relieved by moving about and changing position.

Neuromuscular changes
  incoordination or clumsiness,
  loss of balance (use of wide-based stance, falling, tripping,
    banging into objects);
  poor fine motor control;
  weakness;
  hyporeflexia or hyperreflexia;
  positive Babinski sign;
  spasticity;
  paralysis;

Behavioral changes
  irritability;
  decreased appetite;
  failure to thrive;
  fatigue (frequent naps);
  lethargy;
  coma;
  bizarre behavior (staring, automatic movements).

Cranial nerve neuropathy varies by tumor location, but can
include
  head tilt;
  visual defects (nystagmus, diplopia, strabismus, episodic 'graying
  out' of vision visual field defects).

Vital sign disturbances
  decreased pulse and respiration;
  increased blood pressure;
  decreased pulse pressure;
  hypothermia or hyperthermia.

Other signs
  seizures;
  cranial enlargement (before sutures close);
  tense, bulging fontanel at rest (in infants);
  nuchal rigidity;
  papilledema.

(Adapted with permission from (2000) Wong D.L. and Hess C.S., eds.
Clinical manual of pediatric nursing, fifth edition, p. 498. Mosby, St. Louis).

Coma and the vegetative state

Unintentional injuries remain the leading cause of death in childhood after the first year of life [55]. Traumatic brain injury accounts for 70% to 80% of these deaths, with a particularly high incidence among adolescent males [62]. Many survivors have life-long disability. The most common cause of accidents in children is involvement in motor vehicle crashes. Other leading causes of traumatic brain injury include pedestrian accidents, bicycle accidents, and drowning [63].

While the most effective resuscitative techniques in the field and emergency room for a child with severe head trauma or anoxia have been debated for decades, attention has only recently turned to considering optimal palliative care for injured children and their families [64,65]. Teams can be effective in complementing the medical care by sensitive and effective communication with families, interpretation of diagnostic procedures, identification and coordination of the health care providers, and anticipatory guidance with families facing decisions about the course of further treatment.

Ongoing efforts to effectively prognosticate in children with severe traumatic brain injury involve refinement in clinical assessment and rating, with scales such as the Glasgow Coma Scale and Outcome Scale-Extended, and the use of tests such as the electroencephalogram (EEG) and somatosensory-evoked potentials (SEPs) [66,67]. Both medical and neurosurgical treatment advances have improved survival by careful attention to airway maintenance, circulation, fluid and electrolyte imbalances, increased intercranial pressure, coagulapothies, and seizures. Treatment often involves prolonged stays in pediatric intensive care units. In general, children with comparable injuries have better outcomes than do infants or adults [68].

Children who survive acute injuries sometimes lapse into what has been called a 'vegetative state,' as in the eighteenth century Oxford English dictionary definition, 'to live a merely physical life, devoid of intellectual activity or social intercourse [69].' The vegetative state is characterized by the combination of periods of wakeful eye opening, without any evidence of a working mind either receiving or projecting information, so there is a dissociation between arousal and awareness. After acute CNS insults, the eyes open spontaneously, after a period that varies according to the mechanism of the insult. In concussive head injury, it usually takes two to three weeks, and sometimes, as long as 12 weeks, before the eyes open and coma ends. The interval is much shorter in non-traumatic head injury. Some children can eventually regain a wide repertoire of reflex responsiveness without any evidence of awareness, while others regain some degree of recognizable consciousness. The term 'minimally responsive state' has been used to differentiate this condition [70].

The Multi-Society Task Force of adult and pediatric neurologists and neurosurgeons in the United States has summarized extensive outcome data on the vegetative state, and concluded that it could reasonably be declared permanent three months after non-traumatic injury, and 12 months after traumatic head injury in children. Out of children in a vegetative state one month after traumatic head injury, 9% were dead after one year, 27% were independent, with good recovery to moderate disability, and the rest were in a vegetative or minimally conscious state. For those with non-traumatic CNS injury, 22% had died after one year, and 6% were independent. The main causes of death were pulmonary or urinary tract infections, and "systemic failure" [71]. The type of palliative care that children receive, and the location of that care, also has some effect on survival [72].

There is no known cure for coma or the vegetative state, however, a wide range of palliative options, including feeding, physical therapy, environmental stimulation, and skin care are possible. Palliative care practitioners may become involved in the discussion of to what extent, and for how long, these supportive measures should be continued. Ongoing efforts to improve functional survival include the administration of bromocriptine, systematic neuropsychological testing, sensory stimulation, and comprehensive rehabilitation, with physical therapy, occupational therapy, and speech therapy [73].

Other life-threatening conditions with a neurological component

Neurological symptoms may complicate the process of other systemic life-threatening conditions. Although the brain and nervous system are not the initial targets, sometimes their involvement drives decisions to concentrate on comfort care, rather than further curative efforts. Several of these conditions are mentioned below.

Extreme prematurity

In the past decades, advances in the care of extremely premature infants (those born at 20–25 weeks of gestation, weighing 500–1000 g) have led to steady improvement in survival. However, neuro-developmental morbidity has been high, and includes impaired health, recurrent hospitalizations, educational problems, and adverse effects on the family [74]. Approximately 30% to 50% of surviving children who weigh less than 750 g at birth, or whose gestational age was less than 25 weeks, had moderate or severe disability, including blindness, deafness, and cerebral palsy [75,76].

No consensus exists at present in developed countries, as to which babies might be candidates for palliative care rather

than intensive care. Nor is there agreement on whether the final decision should come from the physician or the family. Physicians' attitudes tend to reflect those of the country and culture in which they live [77]. Parents tend to be more reluctant than physicians or nurses to withdraw life support from their extremely pre-term infants, even if the babies are likely to have moderate disabilities [74]. A palliative care consultation service in the neonatal intensive care setting can help facilitate the process of shared decision-making, and have a positive impact on the quality of ICU life for the infants who die [78].

Complex congenital heart disease

The interrelationship of neurological and cardiac disease occurs in at least two forms. The first is that some children are born with, or develop, both disorders as part of their disease process. In a recent review of cardiomyopathies, for instance, a number of co-existing conditions were identified, including inborn errors of metabolism, malformation syndromes and chromosomal defects, and neuro-muscular disorders [79]. Estimates are that about a third of the neurological complications associated with heart disease fall into this category. However, the other two-thirds occur following cardiovascular surgery. The majority of these were motor handicaps, that is, hemiplegia, tetraplegia, and paraplegia [80].

Even with improvements in surgical and medical care, children who have undergone repair or palliation of congenital heart defects have lower IQ scores and achievement tests, delays in reaching motor milestones, and higher frequencies of learning disabilities and use of special services, as well as speech, language, and behavioral abnormalities [81]. Helping families become aware of the prognosis and future course may assist them in making decisions about treatment [82].

Human immunodeficiency virus

The HIV virus is known to enter and replicate within the central nervous system shortly after initial systemic infection. Perinatally acquired HIV infection has a high association with neurological abnormalities, which seem to be associated with the release of various toxic factors by macrophages and microglia, or certain viral proteins, rather than through direct infection of neurons by HIV [83].

A wide range of CNS manifestations of HIV disease have been reported, including developmental decline in both fine and gross motor skills, cognitive delay or deterioration, language deficits, and delayed psychomotor speed [84]. The most severe and pervasive neurological problems occur in those children who have early serious HIV clinical disease [85]. Effective antiviral treatment shows promise in delaying and improving the neurological complications of HIV infection [83]. This should allow for better quality of life, as children can lead a more normal existence in school and with their peers.

Neurological and neuromuscular symptoms

Pediatric palliative care practitioners will encounter a wide variety of neurological and neuromuscular symptoms in their practice. The constellation of symptoms seen will depend on the underlying diagnoses of referred children, and their positions in the trajectory of their disease. This section of the chapter will explore the most common or urgent of these symptoms, examining possible etiologies, diagnostic approaches, and a range of therapeutic options.

Incidence of symptoms

The most important determinant of the prevalence and type of neurological symptoms is the underlying diagnosis. To illustrate this, it is useful to look at the epidemiology of neurological and neuromuscular symptoms in children with neuro-degenerative disorders, compared to that of children with cancer. The largest published series of the former is that of Helen House, an English pediatric hospice [86]. Over 40% of the children admitted in an 11-year period suffered from neuro-degenerative conditions, chiefly inherited metabolic diseases. Examining the clinical course of the 45 children admitted in the last study year, communication disorders and feeding problems were found in over 70% of the children. Respiratory infections and dyspnea were recorded in 38% of the children, exacerbated by limited mobility, swallowing difficulty, muscular weakness, and kyphoscoliosis. A third had problems swallowing their own secretions. Seizures occurred in 60% of the children. Constipation was an ongoing symptom in 44% of the children. A little over a third of the children were identified as experiencing pain, with the most common etiology being muscle spasm. Other causes included constipation, gastritis, and esophagitis from reflux. Only three children, out of those having pain, required an opioid for relief. Movement disorders, including ataxia, dystonic posturing, and jerky uncontrolled movements, were found in over a third of the children. About the same number of children, particularly those with mucopolysaccharidoses, experienced sleep disorders. Though the great majority of the children were immobile, requiring assistance to turn or get up, and were incontinent of bladder and bowel, none developed skin breakdown.

The most important group of children with cancer who experience neurological symptoms, is those with tumors of the central nervous system. Weakness, immobility, motor and sensory loss, pain and seizures are the commonest neurological symptoms.

Neurological symptoms are not, however, restricted to children with brain tumors [87]. On reviewing the consult histories of over 150 children, headache and seizures were found to be the most frequent symptoms prompting consultation. Structural lesions were found in over 84% of the children with headaches, and in 37% of the children with seizures. There was an approximately equal distribution between lesions attributable to the cancer, to the treatment for the cancer, or from an cause unidentified. Leukemias and lymphomas were represented most often, followed by neuroblastoma, Ewing's sarcoma, and rhabdomyosarcoma. In following a more recent group prospectively, headache was still seen to be the most common complaint, followed by altered mental status, and back pain [88,89].

Headache was more often reported by children with leukemia and lymphoma, and back pain by children with solid tumors. Iatrogenic complications, related to chemotherapy, accounted for over a quarter of the identifiable etiologies. Again, a high percentage of the neuroradiologic examinations were abnormal, and helped to identify the etiology of the symptom. A recent review limited to children with solid tumors showed that 31% presented with, or developed, neurological symptoms, including brain metastases, spinal cord compression, peripheral or cranial neuropathies, and seizures [61]. Children with neuroblastoma and sarcomas had the highest incidence of symptoms.

Neurological complications of chemotherapy have been examined in detail, and include acute alterations in consciousness, leukoencephalopathy, seizures, cerebral infarctions, paralysis, neuropathy, and ototoxicity [90]. Complications have been most often attributed to methotrexate, cyclosporin (ciclosporin), and platinum compounds. Radiation therapy on the central nervous system has also been associated with neurological toxicity, particularly in children less than three years of age, or in children receiving high dosages. Complications include an overall decrease in IQ, neuropsychological deficits, blindness or visual impairments, progressive necrotizing leukoencephalopathy, radionecrosis, intracerebral calcification, dilatation of the ventricular and subarachnoid spaces, and white-matter hypodensity [91].

A recent comprehensive review of symptoms experienced by all children dying in hospital during a nine-month period, identified six symptoms which occurred in over half of the children: lack of energy, drowsiness, skin changes, irritability, pain, and swelling of arms/legs [92]. The prevalence of neurological symptoms was less. Headaches occurred in slightly over a quarter of the children, insomnia in 20%, and numbness/tingling of the extremities in 10%.

Assessment tools

Though assessment is discussed in depth elsewhere in this book, palliative care practitioners should be cognizant of the different types of tools available to assess children with neurological and neuromuscular symptoms. One type of assessment focuses on physical symptoms, sometimes with a psycho-social component. Neurological symptoms were under-represented in two of the most recent studies using tools in this category. One retrospective survey of pediatric cancer deaths in the United States assessed fatigue, pain, dyspnea, poor appetite, constipation, nausea and vomiting, and diarrhea [93]. Validation of the Memorial Symptom Assessment Scale in children looked at lethargy, pain, insomnia, itch, lack of appetite, worry, nausea, and sadness [94]. Several other physical assessment tools have been developed to assess specific symptoms in children, including fatigue and delirium [95,96].

Another approach to assessment has been to look at the global functioning level of children studied. This has been attempted in children with cancer, via development of the play-performance scale [97]. A number of tools are available to assess the functional status of children with developmental disabilities, compared with normal controls. These adaptive–functional instruments include the Pediatric Evaluation of Disability Inventory, the Vineland Adaptive Behavior Scales, and the Battelle Developmental Inventory [98]. These assessment tools are maximum data sets, and involve detailed and extensive queries of self-care, mobility, communication, and social items. The Functional Independence Measure (WeeFIM) gives clinicians a shorter version of the same type of tool. Considerable validation has been done across cultural and geographic settings [99,100]. The US National Center for Medical Rehabilitation Research has developed a model of disablement assessing five dimensions of human functioning: patho-physiology, impairment, functional limitations, disability, and societal limitations, which can be used to describe the functional strengths and challenges in children with a variety of genetic and metabolic syndromes [101].

A comprehensive review of health-related quality of life assessment tools in pediatric palliative care supports the assumption that unrelieved disease-specific symptoms are predictive of generic Health Related Quality of Life (HRQ), and reinforces the necessity for practitioners to assess and address symptoms [102]. Functional limitations not only impact children's lives, but those of their family caregivers. It has been established that care needs of children with severe disabilities have significant time costs to the family, do not decrease as children grow, and may prevent the caregiver from working outside the home, thus reducing total family economic resources [103]. In addition, depression and anxiety in caregivers closely correlate with demands on care-time, particularly in the case of children who are disabled on the basis of a terminal neurodegenerative disease, as opposed to a static handicap [104]. This burden on the family will be discussed further in the next section, but it should give added impetus to the clinician to aggressively approach symptom management of neurological conditions.

Movement and paroxysmal disorders

A movement disorder typically is defined as 'dysfunction in the implementation of appropriate targeting and velocity of intended movements, dysfunction of posture, the presence of abnormal involuntary movements, or the performance of normal-appearing movements at inappropriate or unintended times. The movement abnormalities are not due to weakness or abnormal muscle tone, but may be accompanied by weakness or abnormal tone [105].' The first major category of movement disorders is the hyper-kinetic disorders, often referred to as dyskinesias. This category of abnormal, repetitive, involuntary movements encompasses tics, chorea, dystonia, myoclonus, stereotypies, and tremors. Hypokinetic movements constitute the second major category, sometimes referred to as akinetic, or rigid, disorders. The primary movement disorder in this category is Parkinsonism. This second category is much less common in children. Only a few of the movement disorders are seen with any frequency in palliative care.

Chorea

Chorea is characterized by frequent, brief, purposeless movements that tend to flow from body part to body part chaotically and unpredictably [105]. They last longer than myoclonic jerks, but not so long as the sustained contraction of dystonia. The movements can be sudden and abrupt, but are more often continuing and flowing. The term chorea-thetosis is used for the latter case. The disorder is commonly exacerbated by emotion and fatigue. Primary chorea is almost always attributable to acute rheumatic fever, and does not present in palliative care. However, secondary chorea is associated with a number of neuro-degenerative diseases, including ataxia telangiectiasia, Niemann-Pick, gangliosidoses, Lesch-Nyhan, perinatal asphyxia, and certain gene mutation syndromes. It can occur in hepatic and renal encephalopathy, hypo- and hypernatremia, and protein–calorie malnutrition. Numerous drugs, notably, haloperidol, isoniazid, reserpine, phenytoin, or phenothiazines, can also induce choreiform movements [105,106]. If the chorea is symptomatic and warrants treatment, bed rest in a darkened, quiet room can greatly help in the short term. A number of drugs are also available as treatment, including sodium valproate (15 to 25 mg/kg p.o. per day), which generally controls the movements in 5 to 10 days. The drug can gradually be withdrawn after two to six months, to see if it is still needed [106].

Dystonia

Dystonia is a syndrome of sustained muscle contractions, frequently causing twisting and repetitive movements, or abnormal postures [105]. In palliative care, secondary causes dominate. Heredo-degenerative disorders associated with dystonia include ataxia telangiectasia, gangliosidoses, glutaric aciduria, Lesch-Nyhan, metachromatic leukodystrophy, mitochondrial disorders, Neimann-Pick, and methylmalonic academia. Certain classes of drugs are commonly associated with acute dystonic reactions in children [107]. These include the older dopamine, antagonist anti-psychotics like haloperidol, and the anti-emetics, notably metoclopramide, and to a lesser degree, ondansetron and chlorpromazine. Other palliative care drugs that may cause acute dystonias include the tricyclic and SSRI antidepressants, and the anti-epileptics phenytoin, carbamazepine, and sodium valproate. Drug induced dystonias manifest with abnormal positioning of head and neck (torticollis), spasms of jaw muscles (trismus, grimacing), tongue dysfunction (dysarthria, protrusion), dysphagia, laryngo–pharyngeal spasm, dysphonia, and upward/ downward/sidewise deviation of eyes (oculogyric crisis), as well as abnormal positioning of limbs or trunk. These movements, also referred to as extrapyramidal reactions, are frequently accompanied by high levels of anxiety in the affected children. They respond quickly and completely to treatment with anticholinergic medications such as diphenhydramine (1 mg/kg per dose p.o. q.6 h.) and benztropine (benzatropine) (0.5–2 mg per day p.o. divided b.i.d.) [105,107]. These medications can be co-administered with the offending drug if it needs to be continued for symptom relief, but sedation can be expected. It may be necessary to continue the anticholinergic medication for a day or two after the offending drug is discontinued, in order to prevent the extrapyramidal reaction from reoccurring.

Akathisia

Acute akathisia is a form of motor restlessness, in which children feel compelled to pace up and down, or to change body position frequently [107]. It almost always occurs secondarily to a drug, with haloperidol and prochlorperazine carrying the highest risk. Concurrent administration of morphine or sodium valproate may add to the incidence of akathisia. It commonly develops within days of starting the drug, and may continue to Parkinsonism, if the offending drug is not recognized and discontinued. If drug therapy is needed to obtain relief, a lipophilic beta-adrenoceptor antagonist may be used with good effect, such as propranolol (0.5–4 mg/kg/day p.o. divided q. 6–8 h.) [107].

Myoclonus

Myoclonic movements are very brief, abrupt, involuntary, non-suppressible, and jerky contractions involving a single muscle or muscle group [105]. These shock-like movements can be focal, multi-focal, segmental, or generalized. They are present in normal situations (associated with sleep onset, exercise, and anxiety), and also occur in a variety of pathological situations. The most significant one in palliative care is the myoclonus associated with opioid therapy. It is usually seen in the setting of high-dose and long-term therapy, or spinal opioid, or in cases of rapid dose escalation [108]. If the myoclonus is frequent and distressing to the child, lessening the dose of opioid, or rotating to a different one, may be tried. If neither of these options appears optimal, the myoclonic jerks can be ameliorated by adding a benzodiazepine, such as clonazepam (0.01 mg/kg/dose p.o. q. 12 h.), lorazepam (0.02–0.05 mg/kg/dose p.o, s.l., pr., or i.v. q. 4–8 h.), or diazepam (0.5 mg/kg/dose p.o., p.r., or i.v. q. 4–8 h.) [108,109].

Seizures

Epilepsy may be defined as 'recurrent convulsive or non-convulsive seizures caused by partial or generalized epileptogenic discharges in the cerebrum [110].' Seizures are the principal neurological manifestations of many of the metabolic and neuro-degenerative conditions seen in palliative care. Generalized tonic-clonic seizures are the most common epileptic manifestation of childhood. They are sometimes preceded by non-specific premonitory feelings, such as a sensation of dizziness, or an unusual feeling of ascending abdominal discomfort. Specific neurological symptoms (such as focal somato-sensory feelings, olfactory sensations, focal motor activity, vertigo and odd psychic feelings) may reflect focal onset of seizure activity in one part of the brain, which then spreads to cause a secondarily generalized tonic-clonic seizure. The occurrence of these focal neurological symptoms should alert the clinician to the potential presence of a focal lesion in the brain. These feelings are typically followed by rolling up of the eyes and loss of consciousness. A generalized tonic contraction of the entire body musculature occurs, and children can utter piercing, peculiar cries, followed by apnea and cyanosis. With the onset of the clonic phases of the convulsion, the trunk and extremities undergo rhythmic contraction and relaxation. The end of the seizure is signaled by a decrease in the rate of clonic contraction. After they cease altogether, children remain semi-conscious and confused for several hours. They may vomit and complain of a severe headache, and appear uncoordinated and confused. Attacks can occur at any time, although their frequency is somewhat greater shortly before, or after, children fall asleep, or wake up [111].

In palliative care, seizures may occur in a variety of clinical settings. Seizures occur in over half of children with neuro-degenerative and metabolic disorders, as part of the terminal symptomatology [86]. They can be due to progression of the underlying condition, non-therapeutic levels of anticonvulsant medications, increased sensitivity due to systemic illness such as fever or electrolyte imbalance, or a medication side-effect [112]. In children with cancer, seizures occur most frequently in primary CNS tumors and leukemia, with toxic-metabolic disturbances being the most common identifiable etiology. In children with solid tumors, seizures are statistically most often caused by metastases. Children undergoing bone marrow transplant are particularly susceptible to seizures [113]. Slightly over a third of children with cerebral palsy may have epilepsy, with over 40% of children with quadriplegia being affected. It is often severe and difficult to control, especially in children with associated intellectual delay or cognitive impairment [114].

There is ongoing discussion of whether seizures, in and of themselves, can damage to children's brains. The emerging perspective is that seizure-induced damage does lead to neuronal loss, and thus, has adverse long-term behavioral and cognitive consequences [115]. In addition, seizures themselves can cause death in some children. Sudden and Unexplained Death in Epilepsy (SUDEP) may be a risk for as high as 10% of children with epilepsy [116]. The exact cause and mechanism of death in these cases remain undetermined, though there is clinical evidence showing that the death is a seizure-mediated event [117,118].

If children who are receiving palliative care have a generalized seizure, it may be appropriate to perform a diagnostic workup, to identify a specific etiology. The diagnostic approach will vary considerably, based on the underlying condition, but may include neuro-imaging studies, examination of cerebral spinal fluid, electroencephalography (EEG), blood chemistries (especially glucose and calcium), and metabolic and cytogenetic exams, if they have not previously been performed. If the underlying condition can be identified and treated, seizure control will be easier. If no etiology is found, or if the pathology cannot be corrected, most clinicians would institute anti-convulsant medication, particularly in children who have had more than one *grand mal* seizure in a year [119].

For many children, particularly those with known neurological abnormality, investigations will not be appropriate, and empirical treatment with an anticonvulsant should be considered.

Even if children have been diagnosed, and are on drugs, it helps if the palliative care practitioner understands the therapeutic principles of drug therapy [119–121]. These are summarized below:

- The selection of the preferred drug is based on the type of seizure, and on the potential toxicity of the drug, in other words, on the balance of likely benefit and possible cost to the patient.

- Treatment should begin with one drug, and the dosage should be increased until the seizures stop, or clinical toxicity ensues. If toxicity occurs before seizures are controlled, the first drug should be tapered, and a second single drug started.

- The selection of anticonvulsant drugs varies among practitioners; however, the most frequently used drugs for generalized tonic-clonic seizures are carbamazepine, phenytoin, and valproate. Although phenobarbital is highly effective and useful in the terminal phase, there is the risk of adverse effects on behavior and cognition of children who are likely to need it for some time.

- Adverse effects may reduce the benefits of anticonvulsants on quality of life, and it is helpful to be familiar with them. Diplopia is the most common side reaction to carbamazepine, followed by transient drowsiness, incoordination, and vertigo [122]. Toxicity with phenytoin may present as nystagmus, with lateral or upward gaze, lethargy, or aggravation of seizures. A syndrome of fever, rash, and lymphadenopathy may develop. Valproic acid causes gastrointestinal upset as the most frequent side effect. Increased appetite, with accompanying weight gain, is also seen. Thinning of hair is encountered less commonly.

- It is particularly important to recognize the possible neurological complications of anticonvulsant therapy, lest their onset be confused with disease progression in children receiving palliative care. These are summarized in Table 26.3.

- Alterations in dose should be made gradually, usually not more frequently than once every 5 to 7 days. If anticonvulsant medication is withdrawn, it should also be done gradually, as sudden discontinuation is one of the most common causes of status epilepticus [119].

- Drug blood levels are often unhelpful. A great deal of information can be learned by talking with the parents, and examining children on the drug. Monitoring of hematologic and hepatic status has been recommended for some

Table 26.3 Neurological complications of commonly used antiepileptic drugs

Drug	Most common neurological complications
Phenobarbital	Hyperkinetic behavior, drowsiness
Methylphenobarbital	Hyperkinetic behavior, drowsiness
Primidone	Drowsiness, ataxia, dizziness, dysarthria, diplopia, nystagmus, personality changes
Phenytoin	Nystagmus on vertical and horizontal gaze, truncal ataxia, intention tremor, dysarthria, aggravation of seizures, permanent cerebellar degeneration, personality disturbances
Ethosuximide	Headache, dizziness, hiccups, personality disturbances
Diazepam	Drowsiness, ataxia, hallucinations, blurred vision, diplopia, headaches, slurred speech, tremors, extra-pyramidal movements
Clonazepam	Ataxia, drowsiness, dysarthra, irritability, belligerence, other behavior disturbances
Carbamazepine	Diplopia, disturbed coordination, drowsiness, headaches, visual hallucinations, peripheral neuritis or paresthesias, extra-pyramidal movements
Valproic acid	Ataxia, tremor, asterixis, drowsiness, or stupor (when give with phenobarbital)
Vigabatrin	Dyskinesias, visual field defects
Topiramate	Dizziness, ataxia, somnolence, psychomotor slowing, impaired memory
Lamotrigine	Dizziness, ataxia, somnolence, diplopia, blurred vision
Gabapentin	Somnolence, diplopia, blurred vision
Felbamate	Insomnia, somnolence, mononeuritis, choreoathetosis

(Used with permission from Menkes J.H. and Sankar R. Paroxysmal disorders. In J.H. Menkes and H.B.Sarnat, eds. *Child Neurology, sixth edition* Lippincott Williams and Wilkins 2000, p.952.)

anticonvulsants, but this should be considered discriminatingly in the context of palliative care. Children often exhibit clinical symptoms at the same time they develop blood chemistry abnormalities.

• Renal and hepatic disease may affect blood levels of anti-epileptic drugs. Carbamazepine levels are altered in hepatic disease, but not in renal failure [123]. In cirrhosis and renal failure, the free fraction of valproic acid increases, but the drug's metabolism is reduced, so that the net effect is nearly normal clearance rates. The metabolism of the benzodiazepines, and newer anti-epileptic drugs such as gabapentin, topiramate and lamotrigine, is relatively unaffected by hepatic or renal failure.

Even after carefully following the approach outlines above, as many as 25% of children may continue to have seizures [119]. Addition of a second drug may improve seizure control. A newer anti-convulsant drug may also be considered. A number of new anti-convulsant drugs are available, including felbamate, gabapentin, tiagabine, lamotrigine, topiramate, oxcarbazepine, levetiracepam, and zonisaminde. Clobazam, nitrazepam, and vigabatrin are also available in many countries. Each of these drugs has specific patterns of efficacy and toxicity, so clinicians unfamiliar with them should consult with a neurologist, or an epilepsy specialist, before prescribing one of these drugs for children receiving palliative care [120,124].

The ketogenic diet is a dramatic, but sometimes effective, way to reduce seizures in some children refractory to traditional drug therapy, or in those with multiple allergies [120]. This diet, which attempts to reproduce the ketosis and acidosis of starvation by restricting protein and carbohydrate intake, and supplying 80% of caloric intake through fats, was introduced in 1921. Though the biochemical mechanism of effectiveness is unknown, 30–50% of children who successfully maintain a ketotic state will have improvement in their seizure control, though at the cost of significant increases in atherogenic lipoproteins [120,125,126].

Surgical management of intractable pediatric epilepsy continues to become more attractive, as microsurgical techniques lessen the morbidity of the procedures. In children with brain tumors, the surgical approach has been a mainstay of treatment for cancer and for associated seizures [127,128]. In children with other etiologies of their epilepsy, attempts are made to localize and remove the seizure focus, if possible. More non-specific surgery may also be successful, including corpus callosotomy, subpial transection, unilateral hemispheric removal, and temporal lobectomy [120,128,129].

Status epilepticus

Children are said to be in status epilepticus when 'seizures occur so frequently that over the course of thirty or more minutes, they have not recovered from the coma produced by one attack, before the next attack supervenes [130].' Unrelieved, continuous generalized tonic-clonic seizures lead to hypoxia, brain damage, and death. Management of children in status begins with maintenance of vital functions, chiefly, maintaining an airway, preventing aspiration, and protecting them from injury induced by violent movements.

Next, drug therapy is instituted to control the seizures. Although many drugs have been shown to be efficacious, the most commonly used class in palliative care medicine has been the benzodiazepines [131]. Lorazepam may be administered i.v., p.r., p.o., or s.l., in doses of 0.06–0.1 mg/kg/dose, and has been shown to be highly effective in relieving status [132,133]. If given i.v., infusion should be over several minutes, to lessen the risk of apnea. Doses may be repeated after 10 min if seizures persist. Diazepam may be administered i.v., p.o., or p.r., at 0.3–0.5 mg/kg/dose [109,130]. A rectal gel is available, or the i.v. solution may be used by attaching a tube to the syringe, so that the drug can be inserted 4 to 5 cm. beyond the anus [132,134]. Midazolam is being used with increasing frequency, administered most often as a continuous infusion [135]. An initial bolus of 0.15 mg/kg over a minute is given, followed by infusion of 1–7 µg/kg/min [136]. Midazolam may also be administered rectally, at a dose of 1 mg/kg (max. 20 mg), or p.o., via the buccal mucosa, at a dose of 0.5–0.7 mg/kg/dose [137]. A recent study examining treatment of prolonged seizures in a group comprised chiefly of adolescents, showed 10 mg (2 ml) of buccal midazolam to be equally effective as 10 mg rectal diazepam [138]. Both acted within 6–8 min, but the buccal route was preferred by patient and staff.

Respiratory depression is a rare, but feared, complication of benzodiazepine therapy. It can be reversed with flumazenil, administered initially at a dose of 0.1 mg/kg i.v. [139]. If no response occurs after a couple of minutes, may be repeated doses at one-minute intervals, upto a maximum dose of 1 mg.

If seizures are uncontrolled with benzodiazepine therapy, other anti-epileptic drugs may be used, such as fosphenytoin, i.v. phenobarbital, or intravenous anesthetic agents. However, close monitoring and aggressive maintenance of the airway and blood pressure usually necessitate transfer to an in-patient intensive care setting [140,141].

Terminal seizures

In a terminal phase, seizures may occur with increasing frequency, even when they do not merge into a continuous seizure. Underlying causes can include progression of the underlying condition, intercurrent illness, or children's inability to swallow or absorb their usual anti-epileptic medications. When this occurs, intervention and treatment should be consistent with the goals set by children and their families, to maximize their quality of life. Small, self-limiting seizures that do not distress the patient may not need treatment. If treatment is desired, the mainstays of seizure management in the terminal phase are phenobarbital (enterally or by subcutaneous infusion), and midazolam, by infusion. Phenobarbital, given at an initial dose of 10–20 mg/kg, followed by 3–5 mg/kg/day i.v. or p.o. in two divided doses, offers good seizure control, as well as anxiolysis [112]. In some children, it is quite sedating. While for many this is a desirable effect, for others it is not.

Phenobarbital cannot be combined with any other drug in a syringe driver. Midazolam is also anti-convulsant and anxiolytic. Although it too carries a risk of sedation, it is more easily titrated than phenobarbital, because of its very short half-life. Pentobarbitol, a shorter acting barbituate, has also been used, at a dose of 4 mg/kg/ p.r. q. 12 h, to control frequent or intractable seizures [142].

Like all symptoms in the terminal phase, it is important to have medication in the home, if terminal seizures are anticipated. They are particularly likely when children have a pre-existing seizure disorder, brain cancer, or are at high risk of cerebral hemorrhage.

Nerve pain and its treatment

Neuropathic pain arises from injury, disease, or altered excitability of portions of the peripheral, central, or autonomic nervous system. It is one of the few types of pain that is not protective, since the painful sensation persists independent of ongoing tissue injury or inflammation [143]. Common features of neuropathic pain conditions include sensory disturbances, such as allodynia, cold hypersensitivity, paresthesias and sensory deficits. Sometimes, there are motor findings, such as spasm, tremor, weakness and atrophy. Possible autonomic abnormalities include cyanosis, erythema, mottling, edema, and increased sweating. Neuropathic pain is frequently described by verbal children as having shock-like characteristics of burning, stabbing, and shooting [143,144].

Incidence and etiology

Current estimates suggest that 1–1.5% of the general adult population suffers from some sort of neuropathic pain, including the most common conditions of diabetic neuropathy, trigeminal neuralgia, post-herpetic neuralgia and spinal cord injury [144]. The incidence is unknown in the pediatric population, and the most common adult etiologies are rarely found in children. Practitioners can expect that children with neuropathic pain will be over-represented in the palliative care population. A review of the children seen at one large pediatric pain service showed that 40% of out-patient referrals included disorders with a neuropathic component [143]. The most common conditions in this group were post-traumatic and post-surgical peripheral pain, complex regional pain syndromes, and pain due to tumor involvement of peripheral or central nervous system. Metabolic and toxic neuropathies, neurodegenerative disorders, and pain after CNS injury were represented less frequently. Approximately 6% of children dying of cancer require extraordinary doses and means to control their pain, and in this group, most children had solid tumors metastatic to spine and major nerves [145]. In yet another review of terminal children with cancer, those with neuropathic pain in addition had higher baseline requirement of opioids and benzodiazepines, and also required rapid increases of both drugs in the last few days of life [146].

Assessment

Though pain assessment is considered in detail in other chapters of this book, it is worth noting that assessment of neuropathic pain is particularly challenging, because of the sophistication needed by children to recognize and characterize this type of pain. As a result, parents often feel as if their children have learned to live with significant levels of discomfort, without it being recognized by medical caregivers [147]. In non-communicative children, or in those with delayed development, the problem is exacerbated [1]. Development and standardization of assessment tools for children with cognitive impairments and the inability to verbally communicate has begun, and relies heavily on the parents' interpretation of children's perceptions [148,149]. The 'Paediatric Pain Profile', a behavior rating scale to assess pain in children with severe neurological disability, has been validated in children undergoing gastro-intestinal or orthopedic surgery [148]. Another tool, the 'Non-Communicating Children's Pain Checklist' has recently been used to help characterize subtle variations in patterns of self-injurious behavior of children, with and without chronic pain [150].

Treatment of neuropathic pain

An interdisciplinary approach works best with neuropathic pain, as it is rarely possible to achieve resolution of the pain with any one therapy [143]. Depending on the etiology of the pain, different types of approaches may be emphasized. Physical therapy and rehabilitation play a main role, and many children find cognitive-behavioral treatments helpful in decreasing pain, improving strength, and promoting functional improvement. Neurosurgical interventions or nerve blocks may be indicated for some problems. Acupuncture and hypnosis have been successfully used to treat chronic pediatric pain [143,151].

Several mechanisms exist to explain effective drug therapy of neuropathic pain. Some classes of drugs act as modulators of peripheral sensitization. These include a number of the anti-epileptic drugs that are sodium channel modulators (carbamazepine, oxcarbazepine, phenytoin, topiramate, and lamotrigine), as well as membrane stabilizing agents (lidocaine and mexiletine). Other classes of drugs act as modulators of the descending inhibitory pathways. These include the antidepressants (tricyclics, selective serotonin re-uptake inhibitors,

and serotonin and norepinephrine re-uptake inhibitors), and tramadol. The opioids also have this mechanism of action, though they exert their analgesic effect predominately as modulators of central sensitization, which is the third important mechanism. Some drugs inhibit central sensitization by blocking calcium channels (gabapentin, levetiracetam, oxcarbazepine, and lamotrigine), while others exert their effect via N-methyl-D-aspartate (NMDA) antagonism (ketamine, dextrometorphan, memantine, and methadone) [152]. Table 26.4 contains sample dose-titration schedules for therapy for pediatric neuropathic pain involving notriptyline and gabapentin, the non-opioids most often used in pediatrics.

Traditional teaching that neuropathic pain does not respond as well to opioid therapy as does nociceptive pain is controversial, because opioids are clearly effective in the treatment of some adults and children with neuropathic pain syndromes [153,154]. Prolonged, high-dose opioid therapy has been associated with the development of tolerance, hormonal effects, and immuno-suppression, but low-dose chronic therapy can relieve pain, and improve mood and functioning, without significant side-effects [155].

Increased intracranial pressure

While not normally considered a neuropathic pain syndrome, increased intracranial pressure (ICP) in palliative care often occurs because of the underlying involvement of brain or nerve tissue. Raised ICP is seen in several different scenarios. In infants, it can be a result of post-hemorrhagic hydrocephalus, asphyxia with subsequent brain swelling, cerebral edema from metabolic derangements, or hydrocephalus due to CNS malformations [156]. Treatment normally takes place in neonatal intensive care units, and includes careful attention to positioning, suppression of any neck, skull and abdominal compression, stimuli limitation, and fluid restriction. Babies may benefit from mechanical ventilation, hypothermia, surgical ventricular shunting, and enteral nutrition. A variety of drugs are used to decrease pressure, such as diuretics, sedatives and analgesics, barbiturates, anti-epileptic drugs, and steroids [156,157].

The same types of interventions and supports are used in older children, whose increased ICP most commonly is the result of trauma [158]. Though the treatment normally also takes place in the intensive care unit, the palliative care team may be involved because of the life-threatening nature of the condition. It is important to acknowledge that some of the treatments for raised ICP limit the contact between children and their families, and both will need support around this issue while therapies continue. It is also common for families to misinterpret news about success in controlling the ICP,

Table 26.4 Nortriptyline and gabapentin dose titration regimen for neuropathic pain

Nortriptyline dosage escalation schedule

A. For ambulatory patients

		<50 kg	>50 kg
	Day 1–4	0.2 mg/kg q.h.s.	10 mg q.h.s.
	Day 5–8	0.4 mg/kg q.h.s.	20 mg q.h.s.

Increase as tolerated every 4–6 days until:
1. good analgesia is achieved;
2. limiting side effects occur, or;
3. dosage reaches 1 mg/kg/day (<50 kg) or 50 mg (>50 kg).

B. For in-patients or others with severe and uncontrolled pain, begin with the above doses but titrate upwards every 1–2 days.

Gabapentin dosage escalation schedule

A. For ambulatory patients

		<50 kg	>50 kg
	Day 1	2 mg/kg q.h.s.	100 mg q.h.s.
	Day 2	2 mg/kg b.i.d.	100 mg b.i.d.
	Day 3	2 mg/kg t.i.d.	100 mg. t.i.d.
	Day 4	2 mg/kg a.m. and midday,	100 mg a.m. and midday,
		4 mg/kg q.h.s.	200 mg q.h.s.

Continue to increase by 2 mg/kg (<50 kg) or 100 mg (>50 kg) each day, alternating the timing of the increased dose, so that at least half the daily dose is at night-time. Dose escalation should continue until:
1. good analgesia is achieved;
2. side effects occur, or;
3. dosage reaches 60 mg/kg.

B. For in-patients or others with severe and uncontrolled pain, a similar scheme is used, but triple the dose given at each increment.

(Adapted with permission from Berde C.B., Lebel A.A., Olsson G. Neuropathic pain in children. In N.L. Schechter and C.B. Berde, eds. *Pain in Infants, Children, and Adolescents, second edition*, Philadelphia Lippincott Williams & Wilkins, 2003, p. 626.)

thinking that the underlying pathology is also being treated [158,159].

In children with primary or metastatic brain cancer, increased ICP may occur directly, from tumor infiltration, or compression of normal brain tissue, or indirectly, from obstruction of CSF pathways. Initial clues to increasing pressure are often subtle, with intermittent headaches, personality changes, and poor school performance. Over time, morning headaches, vomiting, and lethargy ensue [160]. There may come a point in palliative care of these children that surgical intervention, radiation therapy, and chemotherapeutic treatment of the underlying tumor will not be beneficial, or are no longer desired by children and their families. At this point, drug treatment with a corticosteroid is often offered, because of its effectiveness in relieving headache, pain, and other symptoms of the expanding lesion. A loading dose of 1–2 mg/kg of dexamethasone p.o. or i.v., followed by a maintenance dose of 0.1 mg/kg p.o., can often be dramatically effective [161]. However, the projected time course and expected dosage of continued therapy should be evaluated carefully, because of the many undesireable side-effects of prolonged, or

high dose, steroid therapy [162]. Personality changes can be prominent, and can include voracious appetite with associated weight gain, mood swings, aggressiveness, confusion and inability to concentrate, and interference with sleep. Besides weight gain, other significant physical complications may be edema, fat deposits on shoulder and hips, gastrointestinal ulceration, the development of diabetes, increased susceptibility to infection, hypertension, and muscle weakness. After prolonged usage, adrenal suppression occurs, requiring additional steroid support during times of physical stress, and a gradual tapering of the drug when discontinued. Older children, in particular, may choose to forego escalation of steroid therapy, because of the side effect profile [163].

Spinal cord compression

Acute compression of the spinal cord occurs in 3–5% of children with cancer [164]. Sarcomas, especially Ewing's sarcoma, account for most spinal metastases, followed by neuroblastoma, germ cell tumors, lymphoma, and metastases from primary CNS tumors. Clinical presentation depends on the location of disease, but often includes weakness/paralysis, sensory deficits, loss of bowel and bladder control, and central back pain. Therapeutic options include surgical decompression and tumor removal, radiation therapy, or drug treatment using chemotherapy or steroids. Dexamethasone is the corticosteroid used most often, at an initial dose of 1–2 mg/kg p.o or i.v. [161]. In some centers, palliative care practitioners have used maintenance doses of 6–10 mg three or four times a day, in older ambulatory patients [165]. Others limit doses of dexamethasone to 16 mg daily, because of the increased incidence of side-effects with very high-dose steroids [166]. Each treatment has its advantages and disadvantages, as discussed above, and each clinical situation will have to be evaluated with affected children and their families. Left untreated, compression leads to permanent neurological deficits [164].

Phantom limb pain

Phantom limb pain is the unpleasant sensation children feel after a body part is removed surgically or traumatically. The indication for amputation may be a congenital deformity, infection or trauma, or cancer. The sensation is as if the body part continues to be there; the pain may be described as stabbing, squeezing, tightness, burning, shooting, cramping, itching, or an unnatural position of the limb [167]. The incidence varies greatly from series to series, but occurs at least half the time. In all series, it tends to diminish over time [168,169]. A variety of treatments have been tried to impact this type of neuropathic pain, including afferent block of the nerves to be severed prior to amputation, and physical therapy with early and vigorous use of a prosthesis. Different classes of drug therapy have been employed, including NMDA antagonists, opioids, anti-depressants, and anti-epileptic drugs, particularly gabapentin [167,170].

Peripheral neuropathy

The two sub-types of extremity sensory neuropathy have different clinical presentations [171]. Involvement of small nerve fibers results in sharp pain, burning or shooting sensations, and aching in fingers and toes. It occurs most often in the elderly. When large nerve fibers are involved, pain is usually not a central feature. Instead, decreased proprioception, vibratory sensation, muscle-stretch reflexes and muscle strength are affected. Thus, although many chemotherapeutic agents cause peripheral neuropathy, it is uncommon for them to cause pain in the extremities [172,173]. Similarly, a review of children with human immunodeficiency virus infection indicates that approximately one-third have symptoms or signs of peripheral nerve involvement [174]. In general, however, the features

are less severe than the distal sensory polyneuropathy described in adults. When neuropathy does occur, the etiologies are diverse, and may include distal sensory or sensorimotor axonal neuropathy, median nerve compression at the carpal tunnel, demyelinating neuropathies, and occasionally, lumbosacral polyradiculopathy [175]. Less than one-fourth of the affected children have pain [174]. Although this type of pain responds variably to therapy, drug administration of an anti-depressant or anti-convulsant is warranted [171].

Peripheral neuropathies are also seen in the context of heredodegenerative diseases [176]. The most common of these are the different forms of Charcot-Marie-Tooth Disease, inherited generally in an autosomal dominant fashion. They are characterized pathologically by extensive segmental demyelination and remeylination of peripheral nerves, leading to muscle weakness and atrophy. The congenital neuropathies are generally not fatal in childhood.

Neuroirritability

The incidence of pain in children with metabolic diseases and other types of neuro-degenerative disorders remains unknown [177]. Clinicians recognize that many of these children may present with, or develop, a syndrome of long-standing severe irritability, or persistent crying and screaming [86,177]. These symptoms may be particularly prominent in children with leukodystrophies and mitochondrial disorders. Identifiable etiologies for the irritability include pain from muscle spasm, joint involvement, and spasticity. Sources of neuropathic pain in this population include visceral nerve involvement, with associated gastrointestinal dysmotility, and peripheral demyelination. However, often a treatable etiology remains unrecognized. A trial of anti-convulsant therapy is probably indicated in these situations, since there have been anecdotal reports of improvement [177,178]. Phenobarbital, with its combined anti-convulsant, sedative and anxiolytic effect, is a useful first line, but should not be continued indefinitely, due to the incidence of long-term side effects. An increase in understanding of the nerve damage in these disorders, coupled with a more complete understanding of the drug mechanism of action, may improve the possibilities for effective therapy [152].

Anesthetic and neurosurgical approaches to pain treatment

Regional anesthesia is most commonly used in pediatrics for pain relief during surgery and procedures. In palliative care, there is a limited role for epidural or subarachnoid (intrathecal) infusions in the treatment of severe neuropathic pain in those children whose pain cannot be relieved with oral or parenteral opioids plus adjuvants, or in those who suffer intolerable side-effects [177]. Most often these children have solid cancers, metastatic to the spine, or to nerve plexi. A large retrospective review of severe pain in childhood malignancy found that 4% of such children needed regional anesthesia to relieve their pain [145]. Effective long-term pain control can be achieved in these children by the infusion of either narcotics such as fentanyl and morphine, or local anesthetic agents such as bupivacaine, or α2 agonists such as clonidine [179]. In palliative care, these agents are typically administered via an implantable catheter, alleviating the necessity of repeated punctures. Intraspinal agents produce selective analgesia, without affecting non-nociceptive sensory modalities, and motor or autonomic reflexes [179].

Potential complications of regional anesthesia include dural puncture headache, mild respiratory depression, and infection [180]. These modalities can be safely used in the home setting, with proper training of staff, children, and their families. Both regional anesthesia and the neurosurgical treatments outlined below generally require evaluation and institution of care at a hospital or inpatient facility, which may limit their usefulness for some children.

Neurosurgical ablative procedures permanently interrupt the connection of afferent pain fibers with the spinal cord and brain. Different procedures have been developed to destroy principal pain pathways [181]. These include: neurectomy (division of a peripheral nerve), rhizotomy (division of a dorsal root), dorsal root entry zone (division at the point of entry into the substantia gelatinosa), myelotomy (midline interruption of crossing fibers in the anterior commissure), and cordotomy (ablation of the lateral spinothalamic tract). The major benefit of these procedures is permanent relief of pain, without further need of narcotics or adjuvant medication. However, sometimes it is difficult to cut all of the fibers communicating pain signals, and only those fibers. Therefore, pain relief is sometimes incomplete, or a new symptom, such as motor weakness, develops. Steady progress has been made in the 50 years that these procedures have been used, to maximize their effectiveness and minimize their unintended side-effects [181].

Other neurologically based symptoms

A number of other symptoms attributable to nerve or brain involvement may be problematic for children receiving palliative care. Some of these, such as swallowing disorders and bowel motility issues, are covered elsewhere in this book. Two other common concerns are discussed below.

Spasticity

Spasticity is characterized by an initial resistance to passive movement, followed by a sudden release call the 'clasp-knife' phenomenon [182]. Spasticity is most apparent in the upper extremity flexors and lower extremity extensor muscles. It is often associated with increased tone, spasms, increased deep tendon reflexes, and clonus. These signs are coupled with the negative signs of weakness and loss of dexterity. It can be a significant source of discomfort and pain for children [86,183]. If left untreated, spasticity not only interferes with motor function, but also contributes to the development of deformities (arched body with pointed toes). This adversely impacts care, positioning, and comfort [184]. This symptom may occur in any condition affecting the motoneuron, including brain hemorrhage, tumors, anoxia, and the vegetative state. Spasticity is the most important disorder of motor control in children with cerebral palsy [185].

The management of spasticity can be challenging, and is often best accomplished through an interdisciplinary team using a combination of medical and surgical approaches [184]. The goals of the affected children and their families must be considered. For non-ambulatory children, the principal challenges are improving comfort, reducing pain, easing the burden of caregivers, slowing the progression of deformities, and perhaps, improving function. For those children who can ambulate, the functional and performance goals tend to dominate.

Physiotherapy and bracing are the most traditional and principal non-surgical forms of treatment; however, despite early, appropriate and intensive intervention, approximately half of children with cerebral palsy will require surgery or other therapy [185]. Children with spastic quadriplegia, in particular, have a high incidence of spinal deformities, as well as progressive hip displacement or dislocation. Many of these children have traditionally required surgery between 4 and 8 years of age, to lengthen or release muscles and tendons [185].

Various neurosurgical techniques have been developed to reduce the excessive hypertonia, without suppressing the muscle tone and limb functions [186]. These include the neuroablative techniques of peripheral neurotomies, dorsal rhizotomies, and dorsal root entry zone-otomies (DREZotomy) [186,187]. In addition, implanted pumps may be used for the administration of intrathecal baclofen [188,189]. Spasticity in both upper and lower extremities decreases significantly with this therapy, which continues to be effective even when administered for years. Baclofen doses often have to be titrated upward initially, but after two years, a stable mean dose of 300 mg/day is usually achieved [189]. Complications are frequent initially. Adverse symptoms from the baclofen include lethargy and hypotonia; surgical complications include catheter-related problems, seromas, and cerebrospinal fluid leaks [189]. If the palliative care team is involved with these children and families during this time of intensive treatment, it can facilitate communication and pain management. It can also help with some of the technical issues that arise when children with terminal illnesses, and possibly do-not-resuscitate orders, come to the operating room for surgery or procedures [190].

A technique of reversible chemodenervation is the injection of botulinum A toxin into the spastic muscle, in order to neutralize neuro-muscular junction activity [191]. The toxin significantly reduces spasticity in about three-quarters of those treated. The effect lasts for months in almost all children, and in 1–2 years, is approximately halved [191,192]. Although the dose used varies considerably from center to center, nearly all children are able to receive treatment without general anesthesia [193].

Drug therapy for spasticity has been disappointing. Baclofen, diazepam, and tizanidine act principally on spinal and supraspinal sites within the central nervous system, while dantrolene and quinine act on muscle [194]. In children, the most frequently used drugs have been benzodiazepines, baclofen, dantrolene, α2-adrenergic agonists, and gabapentin [195]. Oral baclofen is often tried first, at a flat dose of 5 mg two to three times a day. It can be increased in 5 mg increments every 3 days until efficacy, or intolerable side-effects (sedation and hypotension are most common) occur. Effective doses for spasticity are generally in the range of 20 mg or less, three times a day (100 mg/day maximum dose). If no improvement occurs within 6 weeks with the maximally tolerated dose, the drug should be tapered slowly, since abrupt discontinuation may cause seizures [194].

Sleep disturbances

More than 20% of a general pediatric practice concerns issues relating to sleep, so it is no surprise that sleep disorders come up frequently in palliative care [196]. Sleep-related disorders have a profound impact on daily living, for both children and their families. Lack of restful sleep can lead to daytime drowsiness and inattention, headaches, depression, and school or work problems, for children and parents alike [197]. Since the underlying etiologies and associated therapies vary so greatly, it is important for the practitioner to obtain a clear and complete history, including a sleep diary, for complex cases.

An understanding of normal developmental changes in children's sleep patterns is helpful for practitioners and families. Newborns start out sleeping 16–20 h/day, with 1–2 h awake periods alternating with 1–4 h sleep periods around the clock. Between 6 weeks to 3 months, night differentiation develops, and by 9 months, about three-quarters of infants sleep through the night. Total sleep needs decline to 11–12 h/day by school entry, and most children give up naps by age five. Most children sleep about 10 h/day during the middle childhood years, and most adolescents should sleep 9 h/day [198]. Common sleep disturbances in well and sick children alike include: increased latency (the time it takes to fall asleep), parsomnias (sleepwalking, night terrors, nightmares, and rhythmic movement disorders), and night awakenings, in which children need parental intervention to re-establish sleep [199].

Anatomic pre-requisites exist for the development of a normal circadian cycle. States of wakefulness are thought to be regulated by diencephalic and brainstem nuclei, whereas the establishment of circadian rhythms require the development of the suprachiasmatic nucleus of the hypothalamus and its connections [196]. Therefore, children with midline brain maldevelopment are at high risk of sleep disorders. Some portions of the cerebral hemispheres also contribute to sleep-wake cycles, because children with hydranencephaly, lacking cerebral hemispheres, but having an intact brainstem and cerebellum, also have profound sleep disturbances.

Sleep-related breathing disorders may also be associated with anatomic abnormalities [200]. Cranio-facial deformities, common in children with trisomy defects and myelomeningocele, can lead to night-time obstructive apnea. The hypercapnic ventilatory and arousal response is also frequently blunted. Centrally mediated apnea may be identified with polysomnographic studies [197]. Central and obstructive apneas are also common complications for children with myopathies and neuro-muscular disease [197]. In addition, they face the real risk of ventilatory muscle fatigue, particularly in the latter hours of the night. This hypoventilation leads to arousal, daytime sleepiness, and headaches [200]. Yet another anatomical source of sleep disorders are seizures. Sleep-related epilepsy accounts for 30% of seizure disorders in children [197]. Frequent nocturnal seizures can fragment sleep, and negatively affect daytime performance.

Establishment of circadian rhythm also benefits from children's perceptions of environmental cues, known as "zeitgebers" [196]. Disturbed sleep can arise from blindness or poor vision, therefore, because of children's inability to distinguish light–darkness cycles. In general, children who are moderately or profoundly mentally challenged have difficulty in interpreting the social cues families use to promote healthy sleep cycles. Infants who are exposed to constant light, as in some neonatal intensive care units, can also suffer from lack of circadian rhythmicity [201].

A variety of other medical conditions frequently associated with neurological disorders may also hamper restful sleep. These include reflux, colic, hypoxia, and pulmonary edema associated with cardiac disease, pain, muscle spasm, headaches, and movement disorders [196,199]. In addition, many of the therapeutic drugs used in pediatric palliative care can disrupt normal sleep patterns. These include opioids, anti-epileptic drugs, stimulating agents, and anti-asthmatic medication [196]. Hospitalization and episodic illness can also interfere with consistent sleep, because of disruption of normal routines [196,199].

Psychologic stressors that hinder sleep onset are common in palliative care. Children may have worries about their situation, fears of the dark, compounded by fears of death, extreme separation anxiety, or a variety of other legitimate concerns that manifest by poor sleep patterns. They may also have negative associations with their bed, if it is linked with stressors, such as pain or procedures [197].

It should be clear that a complete history is always necessary, and a diagnostic workup sometimes necessary, to hope to successfully address sleep disorders in this group of children. The obstructive apnea of a child with trisomy may best be addressed via adenoidectomy; seizures, with anti-epileptic medication; headaches due to brain tumor growth, with steroids; muscle fatigue, with nighttime ventilatory assistance, and so forth. A number of studies have documented the effectiveness of melatonin in reducing sleep latency in many children with developmental disorders [202,203,204]. When melatonin is administered in doses ranging from 2 to 10 mg 2 h before bedtime, approximately three-quarters of children are able to fall asleep faster, and may stay asleep longer [202,203].

The use of hypnotics in children is less satisfactory [205]. Two benzodiazepines (flurazepam and delorazepam), one anti-histamine (niaprazine) and one phenothiazine (trimeprazine) (alimemazine), have been shown to be effective in the short-term treatment of insomnia in children, but none are officially approved. Tachyphylaxis precludes the long-term use of these medications [205]. If short-term therapy is indicated, hospices have tended to use drugs that might already be in the home for other reasons. Therefore, diphenhydramine, 1 mg/kg/dose p.o. at bedtime, with a repeat in an hour if necessary, or lorazepam, 0.05 mg/kg/dose p.o. q. 4–8 h, are commonly used, as is chloral hydrate 5–15 mg/kg/dose p.o. q. 6–8 h [206]. Several complementary and alternative treatments show promise for insomnia, including herbal therapy with valerian, and aromatherapy with bitter orange essential oil [207]. Anecdotal evidence from a palliative in-patient use promotes the use of lavender oils in a warm bath, and music therapy in selected cases [208].

The palliative care team would do well to teach and reinforce basic principles of sleep hygiene for children, since even ill children are likely to benefit [198]. These include keeping a child busy and active during the day, and limiting naps after mid-afternoon. Children sleep better after exercise, and after spending time outside each day. Even very sick children might benefit from having separate places in which to spend days and nights. Children hungry at bedtime are soothed more with a light snack, than with a full meal. A set bedtime should be established, along with a set bedtime routine. The hour before bedtime should be a quiet time for shared pleasures, with television, computer games, and other stimulating activities restricted. A cool, quiet, comfortable bedroom will promote sleep. Children are often comforted by a dim nightlight and a familiar transitional object, such as a stuffed animal. Finally, restful sleep is promoted by arising at about the same time each day, both on school days and weekends [198]. Simple measures such as these may go a long way in increasing restful sleep for the whole family, particularly if the palliative care team keeps nighttime medications and other interventions to a bare minimum.

Impact of neurological and neuromuscular conditions and symptoms on children and their families

A full consideration of the psychological consequences of life-threatening illness on children and their families may be found elsewhere in this book. No discussion of neurological and neuromuscular symptoms would be complete, however, without mentioning the particular stressors associated with these conditions. Parent voices heard by the authors over decades of care, as well as several studies, have helped identify these unique issues [209,210]. Several of these points have been highlighted by clinical vignettes to show the impact this group of disorders has on families.

- The diagnosis of neurological and neuromuscular diseases is often delayed, because of the vagueness and ubiquity of the symptoms, and the sophisticated, specialized laboratory testing necessary to confirm diagnoses. The diseases are often rare, and sometimes cannot be firmly established. Prognostic uncertainty often accompanies the scant diagnostic information, again because the condition is so rare, or expression of the defect is so variable from child to child.

- Families sometimes face the challenge of multiple children having the same fatal condition. Often the first child is not diagnosed (or even symptomatic) before other babies are born. Prenatal testing is available for some of the conditions, but even then, families have the burden of deciding whether they want to know, and how they will act on the knowledge.

- The guilt associated with having children die of inherited conditions cannot be underestimated. Mothers may feel guilty because of deferring childbirth until they were older, or having done something 'wrong' during pregnancy that caused the defect. The relationship between parents may be strained if one or the other carries the lethal gene.

- Having children with severe neurological or neuro-muscular symptoms often leads a family to social isolation. Children who are bedbound or require life-sustaining equipment may be difficult or impossible to transport out of the house. Others less severely affected may still look, smell, or act abnormal. Even a simple outing, such as going to a restaurant for dinner, can be difficult for children with poorly controlled seizures, unpredictable urinary or fecal incontinence, or extensive drooling.

- Families become extremely sensitized to medical jargon, and may find some expressions offensive. Terms commonly used to describe their children, such as 'neurodegenerative' or 'vegetative', may cause parental anger or suffering.

- For non-communicative children, the burden of "translation" may be heavy on parents and siblings. They often find themselves continually interpreting the needs of an affected child to professionals, and all too often, their experience is one of constantly struggling to be believed. Generally speaking, the people best qualified to understand the needs and problems of affected children are the family. When considering prescribing an analgesic, for example, the palliative care practitioner usually should not ask "do I believe the child is in pain?' but, 'why should I disbelieve it?"

- This can have the incidental effect of making the family carry the responsibility for medical decisions. It is important that reluctant doctors and nurses do not need to be persuaded to prescribe appropriate medications, but are proactive in offering them as the most appropriate medical intervention.

- Finally, there are special coordination and financial challenges in caring for children who may never be able to provide for themselves, or live independently. Parents sometimes spend the first couple of decades praying that their children will live, but then have to start worrying about who will continue the care when they themselves become frail, or die.

For all these reasons and more, easing the symptom burden of children with neurological or neuro-muscular disorders will make a difficult situation bearable. Identifying and anticipating symptoms, leading the family through a discussion of options, and listening to their goals and therapeutic decisions will help maximize children's potential. Hopefully, the palliative care team will employ both the art and the science of medicine, in mitigating neurological and neuromuscular symptoms.

Responding to family needs: Hope and reality

Our health coverage wouldn't pay for speech and occupational therapy services, because they were rehabilitative services. "Your daughter has a terminal illness, and is appropriate for palliative care only." Yes, we certainly wanted to keep her comfortable, but we also wanted to keep her in school as long as possible, and to be a part of our family as fully as possible.

Our nurse and physician became our advocates. They helped others understand the place of therapy services in her care. They helped the rehabilitation staff to incorporate anticipated declines into their goal setting. They helped us to explain these changes to her teachers, our relatives, and our other children. They helped us focus on obtainable goals, such as continuing school, and making a trip to see her grandparents.

Many people talked to us about hope vs. reality. Our team helped us understand that these do not need to compete with each other. We now understand our daughter's life as living out hope and reality.

Responding to family needs: Communication and language

The first physician we met with gave us the diagnosis. She explained how the brain worked, and what was wrong with our daughter's brain. I didn't understand half of what she said. She told us that our daughter had a 'neurologically degenerative disease.' All I heard was the word 'degenerative.' At the end, she asked us if we had considered an institution for her. We left the visit feeling hopeless and lost.

Next, we met with the developmental pediatrician. The first thing she asked us was, "What is your worst fear and how can I help you with it?" Rather than medical jargon, she addressed our fears that our daughter would never speak, be toilet-trained, or know us as her parents. She also helped us find the words to explain the illness to our other children. The visit didn't take any longer than with our first physician, but we left feeling listened to, and confident that we could care of her.

Many years later, we met with the same physician to talk about our daughter's progress in school. Now in the later stages of her disease, she was losing his ability to speak. I was going to school with her every day to help her write, using my hand over hers. The school staff began to question if the writing represented my thoughts, not hers. This wonderful physician responded," You are doing what parents always do when their child is not able to speak. You are her voice in the world."

Now that she has died, I find reassurance knowing that I gave voice to her life, that she made gains many thought were impossible, and that we found strength as a family that we never knew we had.

Responding to family needs: When there is no diagnosis

There were many parents in the Intensive Care Unit whose children had neurological conditions. Our son had some of the same symptoms, but no one could give us a diagnosis. Other parents talked about the wonderful support they found in the disease-specific support groups. We didn't have a support group where we fit in. We didn't know what to expect. We had no prognosis other than, "He probably won't live to adulthood." How were we supposed to prepare for the unknown?

The nurse carefully showed us how to care for his symptoms as they arose. She assured us that despite not yet understanding his underlying disease, we could keep him comfortable and happy.

The social worker connected us to two other families whose children also did not have definitive diagnoses. Even though their symptoms were different, we found comfort in having supportive relationships where we felt we belonged.

The physician ordered all available medical and genetic testing. Even though we never did receive a definitive answer, we did rule out many possibilities. We didn't need to carry around the weight of considering all the possibilities.

The chaplain talked to us about our child's life, his place in the world, and his value to us and others. He helped us see our son as more than a collection of symptoms.

The team understood our fear of not knowing what to expect because we didn't have a definitive diagnosis. One member of the team was assigned to call us weekly, to talk about our needs as they came up. By the time we were ready to go home, our planning was based not on the expected course of a known disease, but rather on a responsive team who understood our unique needs.

References

1. Hunt, A., Mastroyannopoulou, K., Goldman, A., and Seers, K. Not knowing—the problem of pain in children with severe neurological impairment. *Int J Nurs Stud* 2003; 40:171–83.

2. Roberts, R., Rodriguez, W., Murphy, D., and Crescenzi, T. Pediatric drug labeling. *JAMA* 2003; 290:905–11.

3. Committee on palliative and end-of-life care for children and their families. Patterns of childhood death in America. In M.J. Field and R.E. Behman, eds. *When Children Die: Improving Palliative and End-of-Life Care for Children and Their Families*. Washington, DC: The National Academies Press, 2003, p. 43.

4. Baum, D. Introduction: The magnitude of the problem. In A. Goldman, ed. *Care of the Dying Child*. Oxford: Oxford University Press, 1994, p. 43.

5. Feudtner, C., Hays, R.M., Haynes, G., Geyer, J.R., Neff, J.M., and Koepsell, T.D. Deaths attributed to pediatric complex chronic conditions: national trends and implications for supportive services. *Pediatrics* 2001;107:e99.

6. Committee on palliative and end-of-life care for children and their families. Patterns of childhood death in America. In M.J. Field, and R.E. Behman, eds. *When Children Die: Improving Palliative and end-of-life care for children and their families*. Washington, DC. The National Academies Press, 2003, p. 49.

7. Committee on palliative and end-of-life care for children and their families. Patterns of childhood death in America. In M.J. Field and R.E. Behman, eds. *When Children Die: Improving Palliative and End-of-Life Care for Children and Their Families*. Washington, DC: The National Academies Press, 2003, p. 42.

8. Liu, S.S., Joseph, K.S., Kramer M.S. *et al*. Relationship of prenatal diagnosis and pregnancy termination to overall infant mortality in Canada. *JAMA* 2002;287:1561–7.

9. Committee on palliative and end-of-life care for children and their families . Pathways to a child's death. In M.J. Field and R.E. Behman, eds. *When Children Die: Improving Palliative and End-of-Life Care for Children and Their Families*, Washington, DC: The National Academies Press, 2003, p. 72.

10. Johnston, M.V. and Kinsman, S. Congenital anomalies of the central nervous system. In R.E. Behrman, R.M. Kliegman, and H.B. Jenson, eds. *Nelson Textbook of Pediatrics*. Philadelphia, PA: Saunders, 2004, p. 1983

11. Menkes, J.H. and Sarnat, H.B. Malformations of the central nervous system. In J.H. Menkes and H.B. Sarnat, eds. *Child Neurology*. Lippincott Williams & Wilkins, Philadelphia, 2000, p. 307

12. Committee on palliative and end-of-life care for children and their families. Patterns of childhood death in America. In M.J. Field, and R.E. Behman, eds. *When Children Die: Improving Palliative and End-of-Life Care for Children and Their Families*. Washington, DC: The National Academies Press, 2003, p. 54.

13. Mathews, T.J., Honein, M.A., and Erickson, J.D. Spina bifida and anencephaly prevalence—United States, 1991–2001. *MMWR Recomm Rep* 2002;51:9–11.

14. Rankin, J., Glinianaia, S., Brown, R., and Renwick, M. The changing prevalence of neural tube defects: A population-based study in the north of England, 1984–96. *Paediatr Perinat Epidemiol* 2000;14: 104–10.

15. McAbee, G.N., Chan, A., and Erde, E.L. Prolonged survival with hydranencephaly: Report of two patients and literature review. *Pediatr Neurol* 2000;23:80–4.

16. Menkes, J.H. and Sarnat, H.B. Malformations of the central nervous system. In J.H. Menkes and H.B. Sarnat, eds. *Child Neurology*. Philadelphia, PA: Lippincott Williams & Wilkins, 2000, p. 311.

17. Menzies, R.G., Parkin, J.M., and Hey, E.N. Prognosis for babies with meningomyelocele and higher lumbar paraplegia at birth. *Lancet* 1985;2:993–7.

18. Menkes, J.H. and Sarnat, H.B. Malformations of the central nervous system. In J.H. Sarnat and H.B. Menkes, eds. *Child Neurology*. Philadelphia, PA: Lippincott Williams & Wilkins, 2000, p. 324.

19. Hunt, G.M. Spina bifida: Implications for 100 children at school. *Dev Med Child Neurol* 1981;23:160–72.

20. Menkes, J.H. and Sarnat, H.B. Malformations of the central nervous system. In J.H. Menkes and H.B. Sarnat, eds. *Child Neurology*. Philadelphia, PA: Lippincott Williams & Wilkins, 2000, p. 338.

21. Johnston, M.V. and Kinsman, S. Congenital anomalies of the central nervous system. In R.E. Behrman, R.M. Kliegman, and H.B. Jenson, eds. *Nelson Textbook of Pediatrics*. Philadelphia, PA: Saunders, 2004, p. 1987.

22. DiMauro, S. and Schon E.A. Mitochondrial respiratory-chain diseases. *N Engl J Med* 2003; 348:2656–68.

23. Hall, J. Chromosomal clinical abnormalities. In R.E. Behrman, R.M. Kliegman, and H.B. Jenson, eds. *Nelson Textbook of Pediatrics*. Philadelphia, PA: Saunders, 2004, p. 384.

24. Rosenberg, R.N. Molecular genetics and neurologic disease: An introduction. In R.N. Rosenberg, S.B. Prusiner, S. DiMauro, and R.L. Barchi, eds. *Clinical Companion to the Molecular and Genetic Basis of Neurological Disease (Second Edition)*. Boston, MA: Butterworth Heinemann, 1998, p. 1.

25. Menkes, J.H. and Falk, R. Chromosomal anomalies and contiguous gene syndromes. In J.H. Menkes and H.B. Sarnat, eds. *Child Neurology*. Philadelphia, PA: Lippincott Williams & Wilkins, 2000, p. 241.

26. Kuleshov, N.P. Chromosome anomalies of infants dying during the perinatal period and premature newborn. *Human Genet* 1976;31: 151–60.

27. Hook, E.B., Healy, N., and Willey, A. How much difference does chromosome banding make? *Ann Human Genet* 1989;54:237–42.

28. Menkes, J.H. and Falk, R. Chromosomal anomalies and contiguous gene syndromes. In J.H. Sarnat and H.B. Menkes eds. *Child Neurology*. Philadelphia, PA: Lippincott Williams & Wilkins, 2000, p. 250.

29. Rasmussen, S.A., Wong, L.C., Yang, Q., May, K.M., and Friedman, J.M. Population-based analyses of mortality in trisomy 13 and trisomy. *Pediatrics* 2003;111:777–84.

30. Menkes, J.H. and Falk, R. Chromosomal anomalies and contiguous gene syndromes. In J.H. Sarnat and H.B. Menkes, eds. *Child Neurology*. Philadelphia, PA: Lippincott Williams & Wilkins, 2000, p.252.

31. Tinkle, B.T., Walker, M.E., Blough-Pfau, R.I., Saal, H.M., and Hopkin, R.J. Unexpected survival in a case of prenatally diagnosed non-mosaic trisomy 22: Clinical report and review of the natural history. *Am J Med Genet* 2003;118A:90–5.

32. Rich, J. Degenerative central nervous system (CNS) disease. *Peds in Rev* 2001;22:175–6.

33. van den Hout, H., Hop, W., van Diggelens, O. *et al*. The natural course of infantile Pompe's disease: 20 original cases compared with 133 cases from the literature. *Pediatrics* 2003;112:332–40.

34. Sue, C.M., Hirano, M., DiMauro, S., and De Vivo, D.C. Neonatal presentations of mitochondrial metabolic disorders. *Semin Perinatol* 1999;23:113–24.

35. Wilcken, B., Wiley, V., Hammond, J., and Carpenter, K. Screening newborns for inborn errors of metabolism by tandem mass spectrometry. *N Engl J Med* 2003;348:2304–12.

36. Crumrine, P.K. Degenerative disorders of the central nervous system. *Peds in Rev* 2001;22:370–8.

37. Grewal, S.S., Shapiro, E.G., Krivit, W. *et al*. Effective treatment of α-mannosidosis by allogeneic hematopoietic stem cell transplantation. *Pediatr* 2004;144:569–73.

38. Charrow, J., Andersson, H.C., Kaplan, P. *et al*. Enzyme replacement therapy and monitoring for children with type 1 Gaucher disease, consensus recommendations. *J Pediatr* 2004;144:112–2.

39. Van den Hout, J.M.P., Kamphoven, J.H.J., Winkel, L.P.F. *et al*. Long-term intravenous treatment of Pompe disease with recombinant human α-glucosidase from milk. *Pediatrics* 2004;113: e448–57.

40. Menkes, J.H. and Sarnat, H.B. Diseases of the motor unit. In J.H. Menkes and H.B. Sarnat, eds. *Child neurology*, Philadelphia, PA: Lippincott Williams & Wilkins, 2000, p. 1027.

41. Tsao, C.Y. and Mendell, J.R. The childhood muscular dystrophies: Making order out of chaos. *Semin Neurol* 1999;1:9–23.

42. Sarnat, H.B. Muscular dystrophies. In R.E. Behrman, R.M. Kliegman, and H.B. Jenson, eds. *Nelson Textbook of Pediatrics*. Philadelphia, PA: Saunders, 2004, pp. 2060–4.

43. Gomez-Merino, E. and Bach, J.R. Duchenne muscular dystrophy: Prolongation of life by noninvasive ventilation and mechanically assisted coughing. *Am J Phys Med Rehabil* 2002;81:411–5.

44. Eagle, M., Baudouin, S.V., Chandler, C., Giddings, D.R., Bullock, R., and Bushby, K. Survival in Duchenne muscular dystrophy: Improvements in life expectancy since 1967 and the impact of home nocturnal ventilation. *Neuromuscul Disord* 2002;12: 926–9.

45. Rando, T.A. Artificial sweeteners–enhancing glycosylation to treat muscular dystrophies. *N Eng J Med* 2004;351:1254–6.

46. Escolar, D.M. and Scacheri, C.G. Pharmacologic and genetic therapy for childhood muscular dystrophies. *Curr Neurol Neurosci Rep* 2001;1:168–74.

47. Chung, B.H.Y., Wong, V.C.N., Ip, P. Spinal Muscular Atrophy: Survival pattern and functional status. *Pediatrics* 2004;114:e548–53.

48. Gilgoff, R.L. and Gilgoff, I.S. Long-term follow-up of home mechanical ventilation in young children with spinal cord injury and neuromuscular conditions. *J Pediatr* 2003;142:476–80.

49. Sritippayawan, S. Kun, S.S. Keens, T.G., and Davidson Ward, S.L. Initiation of home mechanical ventilation in children with neuromuscular diseases. *J Pediatr* 2003;142:481–5.

50. Johnston, M.V. Encephalopathies. In R.E. Behrman, R.M. Kliegman, and H.B. Jenson, eds. *Nelson Textbook of Pediatrics*. Philadelphia, PA: Saunders, 2004, pp. 2024.

51. Gupta, R. and Appleton, R.E. Cerebral palsy: Not always what it seems. *Arch Dis Child* 2001;85:356–60.

52. Menkes, J.H. and Sarnat, H.B. Perinatal asphyxia and trauma. In J.H. Menkes and H.B. Sarnat, eds. *Child Neurology*. Philadelphia, PA: Lippincott Williams & Wilkins, 2000, p. 425.

53. Reddihough, D.S., Baikie, G., and Walstab, J.E. Cerebral palsy in Victoria, Australia: Mortality and causes of death. *J Paediatr Child Health* 2001;37:183–6.

54. Williams, K. and Alberman, E. Survival in cerebral palsy: The role of severity and diagnostic labels. *Dev Med Child Neurol* 1998;40: 376–9.

55. Committee on palliative and end-of-life care for children and their families. Patterns of childhood death in America. In M.J. Field and R.E. Behman, eds. *When Children Die: Improving Palliative and*

End-of-Life Care for Children and Their Families. Washington, DC: The National Academies Press, 2003, p. 57.

56. Strother, D.R., Pollack, I.F., Fisher, P.G. *et al.* Tumors of the central nervous system. In P.A. Pizzo and D.G. Poplack, eds. *Principles and Practice of Pediatric Oncology* (4th edition). Philadelphia, PA: Lippincott Williams & Wilkins, 2002, p. 751.

57. Pollack, I.F. Brain tumors in children. *N Engl J Med* 1994; 331: 1500–7.

58. Pollack, I.F. Pediatric brain tumors. *Semin Surg Oncol* 1999; 16: 73–90.

59. Macedoni-Luksic, M., Jereb, B., and Todorovski, L. *Pediatr Hematol Oncol* 2003; 20: 89–101.

60. Margolin, J.F., Steuber, C.P., and Poplack, D.G. Acute lymphoblastic leukemia. In P.A. Pizzo and D.G. Poplack, eds. *Principles and Practice of Pediatric Oncology* (4th edition). Philadelphia, PA: Lippincott Williams & Wilkins, 2002, p. 510.

61. Weyl-Ben Arush, W., Stein, M., Perez-Nachum, M. *et al.* Neurolgic complications in pediatric solid tumors. *Oncology* 1995; 52: 89–2.

62. Johnston, B.D. and Rivara, F.P. Injury control: New challenges. *Ped in Rev* 2003; 24: 111–7.

63. Agran, P.F., Winn, D., Anderson, C., Trent. R., and Walton-Haynes, L. Rates of pediatric and adolescent injuries by year of age. *Pediatrics* 2001; 108: e45.

64. Greenberg, L.W., Ochsenschlager, D., O'Donnell, R., Mastruserio, J., and Cohen, G.J. Communicating bad news: A pediatric department's evaluation of a simulated intervention. *Pediatrics* 199; 103: 1210–7.

65. Wright, J.L., Johns, C.M.S., and Joseph, J.G. End-of-life care in emergency medical services for children. In M.J. Field and R.E. Behman, eds. *When Children Die: Improving Palliative and End-of-Life Care for Children and Their Families* 2004; Washington, DC: The National Academies Press, Appendix F, pp. 580–98.

66. Lew, H.L., Dikmen, S., Slimp, J., Temkin, N., Lee, E.H., Newell, D., and Robinson, L.R. Use of somatosensory-evoked potentials and cognitive event-related potentials in predicting outcomes of patients with severe traumatic brain injury. *Am J Phys Med Rehabil* 2003; 82: 53–61.

67. Mandel, R., Martinot, A., Delepoulle, F. *et al.* Prediction of outcome after hypoxic-ischemic encephalopathy: A prospective clinical and electrophysiologic study. *J Pediatr* 2002; 141: 45–50.

68. Levi, L. *et al.* Severe head injury in children—analyzing the better outcome over a decade and the role of major improvements in intensive care. *Child Nerv Syst* 1998; 14: 195–202.

69. Jennett, B. Features of the vegetative state. In B. Jennett, ed. *The Vegetative State.* Cambridge: Cambridge University Press, 2002, p. 4.

70. Jennett, B. A syndrome in search of a name. In B. Jennett, *The Vegetative State.* Cambridge: Cambridge University Press, 2002, p. 8.

71. The multi-society task force on PVS. Medical aspects of the persistent vegetative state (part 2). *N Engl J Med* 1994; 330: 1572–9.

72. Ashwal, S., Eyman, R.K., and Call, T.L. Life expectancy of children in a persistent vegetative state. *Pediatr Neurol* 1994; 10: 27–33.

73. Passier, M.A. and Biggs, R.V. Positive outcomes in traumatic brain injury—vegetative state: patients treated with bromocriptine. *Arch Phys Med Rehab* 2001; 82: 311–5.

74. Streiner, D.L., Saigal, S., Burrows, E., Stoskopf, B., and Rosenbaum, P. Attitudes of parents and health care professionals toward active treatment of extremely premature infants. *Pediatrics* 2001; 108: 152–7.

75. MacDonald, H. Perinatal care at the threshold of viability. *Pediatrics* 2002; 110: 1024–7.

76. Rijken, M., Stoelhorst, G., Martens, S. *et al.* Mortality and neurologic, mental, and psychomotor development at two years in infants born less than 27 weeks' gestation: The Leiden follow-up project on prematurity. *Pediatrics* 2003; 112: 351–8.

77. Rebagliato, M., Cuttini, M., Broggin, L. *et al.* Neonatal end-of-life decision making. *JAMA* 2000; 284: 2451–9.

78. Pierucci, R.L., Kirby, R.S., and Leuthner, S.R. End-of-life care for neonates and infants: the experience and effects of a palliative care consultation service. *Pediatrics* 2001; 108: 653–60.

79. Lipshultz, S.E., Sleeper, L.Y., Towbin, J.A. *et al.* The incidence of pediatric cardiomyopathy in two regions of the United States. *N Engl J Med* 2003; 348: 1647–55.

80. Puntis, J.W. and Green, S.H. Neurological complications of heart disease in childhood. *Br J Clin Pract* 1989; 43: 217–20.

81. Wernovsky, G. and Newburger, J. Neurologic and developmental morbidity in children with complex congenital heart disease. *J Pediatr* 2003; 142: 6–8.

82. Crawford, T.S., Olivero, W.C., and Hanigan, W.C. The prognosis of children with hydrocephalus and congenital heart disease. *Pediatr Neurosurg* 2000; 33: 12–5.

83. Raskino, C., Pearson, D.A., Baker, C.J. *et al.* Neurologic, neurocognitive, and brain growth outcomes in human immunodeficiency virus-infected children receiving different nucleoside antiretroviral regimens. *Pediatrics* 1999; 104: e32.

84. Pearson, D.A., *et al.* Predicting HIV disease progression in children using measures of neuropsychological and neurological functioning. *Pediatrics* 2000; 106: e76.

85. Belman, A.L., Muenz, L.R., Marcus, J.C. *et al.* Neurologic status of human immunodeficiency virus 1-infected infants and their controls: a prospective study from birth to two years. *Pediatrics* 1996; 98: 1109–18.

86. Hunt, A. and Burne, R. Medical and nursing problems of children with neurodegenerative disease. *Palliat Med* 1995; 9: 19–26.

87. Antunes, N.L. and De Angelis, L.M. Neurologic consultations in children with systemic cancer. *Pediatr Neurol* 1999; 20: 121–4.

88. Antunes, N.L. Acute neurologic complications in children with systemic cancer. *J Child Neurol* 2000; 15: 705–16.

89. Antunes, N.L. The spectrum of neurologic disease in children with systemic cancer. *Pediatr Neurol* 2001; 25: 227–35.

90. Reddy, A.T. and Witek, K. Neurologic complications of chemotherapy for children with cancer. *Curr Neurol Neurosci Rep* 2003; 3: 137–42.

91. Dreyer, Z.E., Blatt, J., and Bleyer, A. Late effects of childhood cancer and its treatment. In P.A. Pizzo and D.G. Poplack, eds. *Principles and Practice of Pediatric Oncology* (4th edition). Philadelphia, PA: Lippincott Williams & Wilkins, 2002, p. 1437.

92. Drake, R., Frost, J., and Collins, J.J. The symptoms of dying children. *J Pain Symptom Manage* 2003; 26: 594–603.

93. Wolfe, J., Grier, H.E., Klar, N. *et al.* Symptoms and suffering at the end of life in children with cancer. *N Engl J Med* 2000; 342: 326–33.

94. Collins, J.J., Devine, T.D., Dick, G.S. *et al.* The measurement of symptoms in young children with cancer: The validation of the Memorial symptom assessment scale in children aged 7–12. *J Pain Symptom Manage* 2002; 23: 10–6.

95. Hockenberry, M.J., Hinds, P.S., Barrera, P. et al. Three instruments to assess fatigue in children with cancer: The child, parent and staff perspectives. J Pain Symptom Manage 2003;25:319–28.

96. Turkel, S.B., Braslow, K., Tavere, C.J., and Trzepacz, P.T. The delirium rating scale in children and adolescents. Psychosomatics 2003;44:126–9.

97. Lansky, S.B., List, M.A., Lansky, L.L., Ritter-Sterr, C., and Miller, D.R. The measurement of performance in childhood cancer patients. Cancer 1987;60:1651–6.

98. Msall, M.E. Tools for measuring daily activities in children: promoting independence and developing a language for child disability. Pediatrics 2002;109:317–8.

99. Wong, V., Wong, S., Chan, K., and Wong, W. Functional independence measure (WeeFIM) for Chinese children: Hong Kong cohort. Pediatrics 2002;109:e36.

100. Custers, J.W., van der Net, J., Hoijtink, H., Wassengerg-Severijnen, J.E., Vermeer, A., and Helders, P.J. Discriminative validity of the Dutch pediatric evaluation of disability inventory. Arch Phys Med Rehab 2002;83:1437–41.

101. Msall, M.E. and Tremont, M.R. Measuring functional status in children with genetic impairments. Am J Med Genet 1999;89:62–74.

102. Bradlyn, A.S., Varni, J.W., and Hinds, P.S. Assessing health-related quality of life in end-of-life care for children and adolescents. In M.J. Field and R.E. Behman, eds. When Children Die: Improving Palliative and End-of-Life care for children and their families. Washington, DC: The National Academies Press, Appendix C, 2004, pp. 476–508.

103. Curran, A.L., Sharples, P.M., White, C., and Knapp, M. Time costs of caring for children with severe disabilities compared with caring for children without disabilities. Dev Med Chid Neurol 2001;43:529–33.

104. Labbe, E.E., Lopez, I., Murphy, L., and O'Brien, C. Optimism and psychosocial functioning in caring for children with Battens and other neurological diseases. Psychol Rep 2002;90:1129–35.

105. Schlaggar, B.L. and Mink, J.W. Movement disorders in children. Peds in Rev 2003;24:39–50.

106. Rust, R. and Menkes, J.H. Autoimmune and postinfectious diseases. In J.H. Menkes and H.B. Sarnat, eds. Child Neurology. Philadelphia, PA: Lippincott Williams & Wilkins, 2000, p. 656.

107. Twycross, R. Drug-induced movement disorders. In R. Twycross, A. Wilcock, S. Charlesworth, and A. Dickman, eds. Palliative Care formulary (2nd edition). Oxon: Radcliffe Medical Press, 2002, p. 339.

108. Berde, C.B. Billet, A.L., and Collins J.J. Symptom management in supportive care. In P.A. Pizzo and D.G. Poplack, eds. Principles and Practice of Pediatric Oncology (4th edition). Philadelphia, PA: Lippincott Williams & Wilkins, 2002, p. 1315.

109. Storey, P., Knight, C.F., and Schonwetter, R.S. The hospice/palliative medicine approach to caring for pediatric patients. In Pocket guide to Hospice/Palliative Medicine. Glenview: American Academy of Hospice and Palliative Medicine, 2003, p. 168.

110. Menkes, J.H. and Sankar, R. Paroxysmal disorders. In J.H. Menkes, and H.B. Sarnat, eds. Child Neurology. Philadelphia, PA: Lippincott Williams & Wilkins, 2000, p. 919.

111. Menkes, J.H. and Sankar, R. Paroxysmal disorders. In J.H. Menkes, and Sarnat H.B., eds. Child Neurology. Philadelphia, PA: Kippincott William & Wilkins, 2000, p. 932.

112. Hellsten, M.B., Hockenberry-Eaton, M., Lamb, D., Chordas, C., Kline, N., Bottomley, S. Central nervous system symptoms. In Texas Children's Cancer Center. End-of-Life Care for Children. Austin: Texas Cancer Council, 2000, pp. 47–53.

113. Antunes, N.L. Seizures in children with systemic cancer. Pediatr Neurol 2003;28:190–3.

114. Singhi, P., Jagirdar, S., Khandelwal, N., and Halhi, P. Epilepsy in children with cerebral palsy. J Child Neurol, 2003;18:174–9.

115. Sutula, T.P., Hagen, J., and Pitkanen, A. Do epileptic seizures damage the brain? Curr Opin Neurol 2003;16:189–95.

116. Harvey, A.S., Nolan, T., and Carlin, J.B. Community-based study of mortality in children with epilepsy. Epilepsia 1993;34:597–603.

117. Thom, M., Seetah, S., Sisodiya, S., Koepp, M., and Scaravilli, F. Sudden and unexpected death in epilepsy (SUDEP): Evidence of acute neuronal injury using HSP-70 and c-Jun imunohistochemistry. Neuropathol Appl Neurobiol 2003;29:132–43.

118. Donner, E.J., Smith, C.R., and Snead O.C. Sudden unexplained death in children with epilepsy. Neurology 2001;14:430–4.

119. Menkes, J.H. and Sankar, R. Paroxysmal disorders. In J.H. Menkes and H.B. Sarnat eds. Child Neurology. Philadelphia, PA: Lippincott Williams & Wilkins, 2000, p. 959–61.

120. Holmes, G.L. When the first drug does not work: Treatment options. J Pediatr 1997;131:794–6.

121. Pellock, J.M. Treatment considerations: traditional antiepileptic drugs. Epilepsy Behav 2002;3:18–23.

122. Menkes, J.H. and Sankar, R. Paroxysmal disorders. In J.H. Menkes and H.B. Sarnat eds. Child Neurology. Philadelphia, PA: Lippincott Williams & Wilkins, 2000, p.967–9.

123. Menkes, J.H. and Sankar, R. Paroxysmal disorders. In J.H. Menkes and H.B. Sarnat, eds. Child Neurology. Philadelphia: Lippincott Williams & Wilkins, 2000, pp. 975-6.

124. La Roche, S.M., Helmers, S.L. The new antiepilettic drugs. JAMA 2004;291:605–14.

125. Gilbert, D.L., Pyzik, P.L., Vining, E.P., and Freeman, J.M. Medication cost reduction in children on the ketogenic diet: data from a prospective study. J Child Neurol 1999;14:469–71.

126. Switerovich, P., Vining, E., Pyzik, P., Skolasky, R., and Freeman, J. Effect of a high-fat ketogenic diet on plasma levels of lipids, lipoproteins, and apolipoproteins in children. JAMA 2003;290:912–20.

127. Khajavi, K., Comair, Y.G., Wyllie, E., Palmer, J., Morris, H.H., and Hahn, J.F. Surgical management of pediatric tumor-associated epilepsy. J Child Neurol 1999;14:15–25.

128. Strother, D.R., Pollack, I.F., and Fisher, P.G., et al. Tumors of the central nervous system. In P.A. Pizzo, and D.G. Poplack, eds. Principles and Practice of Pediatric Oncology, fourth edition. Philadelphia, PA: Lippincott Williams & Wilkins, 2002, p. 766.

129. Sinclair, D.B. et al. Pediatric temporal lobectomy for epilepsy. Pediatr Neurosurg 2003;38:195–205.

130. Menkes, J.H. and Sankar, R. Paroxysmal disorders. In J.H. Menkes and H.B. Sarnat, eds. Child Neurology. Philadelphia, PA: Lippincott Williams & Wilkins, 2000, pp. 981–4.

131. Twycross, R. Benzodiazepines in palliative care. In R. Twycross, A. Wilcock, S. Charlesworth, and A. Dickman, eds. Palliative Care Formulary, second edition. Oxon: Radcliffe Medical Press, 2002, p. 66.

132. Crawford, T.O., Mitchell, W.G., and Snodgrass, S.R. Lorazepam in childhood status epilepticus and serial seizures: Effectiveness and tachyphylaxis. *Neurology* 1987;37:190–5.

133. Alldredge, B.K., Gelb, A.M., Isaacs, S.M. *et al*. A comparison of lorazeppam, diazepam, and placebo for the treatment of out-of-hospital status epilepticus. *N Engl J Med* 2001;345: 631–7.

134. Dreifuss, F.E., Rosman, N.P., Cloyd, J.C. *et al*. A comparison of rectal diazepam gel and placebo for acute repetitive seizures. *N Engl J Med* 1998;338:1869–75.

135. Holmes, G.L. and Riviello, J.J. Midazolam and pentobarbital for refractory status epilepticus. *Pediatr Neurol* 1999;20:259–64.

136. Koul, R., Chacko, A., Javed, H., and Al Riyami, K. Eight-year study of childhood status epilepticus: Midazolam infusion in management and outcome. *J Child Neurol* 2002;17:908–10.

137. Tobias J.D. Pain management for the critically ill child in the pediatric intensive care unit. In N.L. Schecter, C.B. Berde, and M. Yaster, eds. *Pain in Infants, Children, and Adolescents*. Philadelphia, PA: Lippincott Williams & Wilkins, 2003, p. 809.

138. Scott, R.C., Besag, F.M., and Neville, B.G. Buccal midazolam and rectal diazepam for treatment of prolonged seizures in childhood and adolescence: a randomized trial. *Lancet* 1999;353:623–6.

139. Wong, D.L. Management of opioid-induced respiratory depression. In: *Pediatric quick reference* (3rd edition). Mosby, St. Louis, 2000, p. 46.

140. Pellock, J.M. Use of midazolam for refractory status epilepticus in pediatric patients. *J Child Neurol* 1998;13:581–7.

141. Hanahn, U.A., Fiallos, M.R., and Orlowski, J.P. Status epilepticus. *Pediatr Clin North Amer* 2001;48:683–94.

142. Kenny, N.P. and Frager, G. Refractory symptoms and terminal sedation of children: ethical issues and practical management. *J Palliat Care* 1996;12:40–5.

143. Berde, C.B., Lebel, A.A., and Olsson, G. Neuropathic pain in children. In N.L. Schecter, C.B. Berde, and M. Yaster, eds. *Pain in Infants, Children, and Adolescents*. Philadelphia, PA: Lippincott Williams & Wilkins, 2003, pp. 620–4.

144. Chong, M.S. and Bajwa Z.H. Diagnosis and treatment of neuropathic pain. *J Pain Symptom Manage* 2003;25:S4–11.

145. Collins, J.J., Grier, H.E., Kinney, H.C., and Berde, C.B. Control of severe pain in children with terminal malignancy. *J Pediatr* 1995; 126:653–7.

146. Dougherty, M. and DeBaun, M.R. Rapid increase of morphine and benzodiazepine usage in the last three days of life in children with cancer is related to neuropathic pain. *J Pediatr* 2003;142: 373–6.

147. Carter, B., McArthur, E., and Cunliffe, M. Dealing with uncertainty: Parental assessment of pain in their children with profound special needs. *J Adv Nurs* 2002;38:449–57.

148. Hunt, A., Goldman, A., and Seers, K. *et al*. Clinical validation of the Paediatric Pain Profile, a behaviour rating scale to assess pain in children with severe neutological disability. *Dev Med Child Neurol* 2004;46:9–18.

149. Breau, L.M., McGrath, P.J., Camfield, C., Rosmus, C., and Finley, G.A. Preliminary validation of an observational pain checklist for persons with cognitive impairments and inability to communicate verbally. *Dev Med Child Neurol* 2000;42: 609–16.

150. Breau, L.M., Camfield, C.S., Symons, F.J. *et al*. Relation between pain and self-injurious behavior in nonverbal children with severe cognitive impairments. *J Pediatr* 2003;142:498–503.

151. Zeltzer, L.K., Tsao, J.C., Stelling, C., Powers, M., Levy, S., and Waterhouse, M. A phase I study on the feasibility and acceptability of an acupuncture/hypnosis intervention for chronic pediatric pain. *J Pain Symptom Manage* 2002;24:437–46.

152. Beydoun, A. and Backonja, M.M. Mechanistic stratification of antineuralgic agents. *J Pain Symptom Manage* 2003; 25: S18–30.

153. Rowbotham, M.C., Twilling, L., Davies, P.S., Reisner, L., Taylor, K., and Mohr, D. Oral opioid therapy for chronic peripheral and central neuropathic pain. *N Engl J Med* 2003;348:1223–32.

154. Klepstad, P., Borchgrevink, P., Hval, B., Flaat, S., and Kaasa, S. Long-term treatment with ketamine in a 12-year-old girl with severe neutopathic pain caused by a cervical spine tumor. *J Pediatr Hematol Oncol* 2001;23:616–9.

155. Ballantyne, J.C. and Mao, J. Opioid therapy for chronic pain. *N Engl J Med* 2003;349:1943–53.

156. Oriot, D. and Nassimi, A. Intracranial hypertension in the infant: from its physiopathology to its therapeutic management. *Arch Pediatr* 1998;5:773–82.

157. Libenson, M.H., Kaye, E.M., Rosman, N.P., and Gilmore, H. E. Acetazolamide and furosemide for posthemorrhagic hydrocephalus of the newborn. *Pediatr Neurol* 1999;20:185–91.

158. Palmer, J. Management of raised intracranial pressure in children. *Intensive Crit Care Nurs* 2000;16:319–27.

159. Committee on palliative and end-of-life care for children and their families. Pathways to a child's death. In M.J. Field and R.E. Behman, eds. *When Children Die: Improving Palliative and End-of-Life Care for Children and Their Families*. Washington, DC: The National Academies Press, 2003, p. 78.

160. Strother, D.R., Pollack, I.F., Fisher, P.G., *et al*. Tumors of the central nervous system. In P.A. Pizzo and D.G. Poplack, eds. *Principles and Practice of Pediatric Oncology* (4th edition). Philadelphia: Lippincott Williams & Wilkins, 2002, p. 758.

161. Rheingold, S.R. and Lange B.J. Oncologic emergencies. In P.A. Pizzo, D.G. Poplack, eds. *Principles and Practice of Pediatric oncology* (4th edition). Philadelphia, PA: Lippincott Williams & Wilkins, 2002, p. 1190.

162. World Health Organization. Adjuvant Therapy. In *Cancer Pain Relief and Palliative Care in Children*. Geneva: World Health Organization, 1998, p. 50.

163. McGrath, P. and Pitcher, L. 'Enough is enough': Qualitative findings on the impact of dexamethasone during reinduction/ consolidation for paediatric acute lymphoblastic leukaemia. *Support Care Cancer* 2002;10:146–55.

164. Rheingold, S.R. and Lange, B.J. Oncologic emergencies. In P.A. Pizzo and D.G. Poplack, eds. *Principles and Practice of Pediatric Oncology* (4th edition). Philadelphia, PA: Lippincott Williams & Wilkins, 2002, pp. 1193–4.

165. Storey, P., Knight, C.F., and Schonwetter, R.S. The hospice/ palliative medicine approach to caring for pediatric patients. In *Pocket Guide to Hospice/Palliative Medicine*. Glenview: American Academy of Hospice and Palliative Medicine, 2003, p. 101.

166. Hillier, R. and Wee, B. Palliative management of spinal cord compression. *Eur J Palliat Care* 1997;4:77–80.

167. Berde, C.B., Lebel, A.A., and Olsson, G. Neuropathic pain in children. In Schecter, N.L., Berde, C.B., Yaster, M., eds. *Pain In infants, Children, and Adolescents*. Philadelphia, PA: Lippincott Williams & Wilkins, 2003, pp. 628–30.

168. Krane, E.J. and Heller, L.B. The prevalence of phantom sensation and pain in pediatric amputees. *J Pain Symptom Manage* 1995;10: 21–9.

169. Wilkins, K.L., McGrath, P.J., Finley, G.A., and Katz, J. Phantom limb sensations and phantom limb pain in child. *Pain* 1998;78: 7–12.

170. Rusy, L.M., Troshynski, T.J., and Weisman, S.J. Gabapentin in phantom limb pain management in children and young adults: report of seven cases. *J Pain Symptom Manage* 2001;21:78–82.

171. Mendell, J.R. and Sahenk, Z. Painful sensory neuropathy. *N Engl J Med* 2003;348:1243–55.

172. Frisk, P., Stalberg, E., Stromberg, B., and Jakobson, A. Painful peripheral neuropathy after treatment with high-dose ifosfamide. *Med Pediatr Oncol* 2001;37:329–82.

173. Reddy, A.T. and Witek, K. Neurologic complications of chemotherapy for children with cancer. *Curr Neurol Neurosci Rep* 2003;3:137–42.

174. Prufer de QC Araujo, A., Nascimento, O.J.M., and Garcia, O.S. Distal sensory polyneuropathy in a cohort of HIV-infected children over five years of age. *Pediatrics* 2000;106:e35.

175. Floeter, M.K., Divitello, L.A., Everett, C.R., Dambrosia, J. and Luciano, C.A. Peripheral neuropathy in children with HIV infection. *Neurology* 1997;49:207–12.

176. Menkes, J.H. Heredodegenerative diseases. In J.H. Menkes, H.B. Sarnat, eds. *Child Neurology*. Philadelphia, PA: Lippincott Williams & Wilkins, 2000, pp. 198–209.

177. Berde, C.B., Lebel, A.A., and Olsson, G. Neuropathic pain in children. In N.L. Schecter, C.B. Berde, and M. Yaster, eds. *Pain in Infants, Children, and Adolescents*. Philadelphia, PA: Lippincott Williams & Wilkins, 2003, p. 635.

178. World Health Organization. Adjuvant Therapy. In *Cancer Pain Relief and Palliative Care in Children*. Geneva: World Health Organization, 1998, p. 51.

179. Smith, J.L. and Madsen, J.R. Neurosurgical procedures for the treatment of pediatric pain. In N.L. Schecter, C.B. Berde, and M. Yaster, eds. *Pain in Infants, Children, and Adolescents*. Philadelphia, PA: Lippincott Williams & Wilkins, 2003, p. 337.

180. Collins, J.J., Grier, H.E., Sthna, N.F., Wilder, R.T., and Berde, C.B. Regional anesthesia for pain associated with terminal pediatric malignancy. *Pain* 1996;65:63–9.

181. Smith, J.L. and Madsen, J.R. Neurosurgical procedures for the treatment of pediatric pain. In N.L. Schecter, C.B. Berde, and M. Yaster, eds. *Pain in Infants, Children, and Adolescents*. Philadelphia, PA: Lippincott Williams & Wilkins, 2003, pp. 330–7.

182. Haslam, R.H.A. Neurologic evaluation. In R.E. Behrman, R.M. Kliegman, and H.B. Jenson, eds. *Nelson Textbook of Pediatrics*. Philadelphia, PA: Saunders, 2004, p. 1978.

183. Oberlander, T.F. and Craig, K.D. Pain and children with developmental disabilities. In N.L. Schecter, C.B. Berde, and M. Yaster, eds. *Pain in Infants, Children, and Adolescents*. Philadelphia, PA: Lippincott Williams & Wilkins, 2003, p. 609.

184. Gormley, M.E., Krach, L.E., and Piccini, L. Spasticity management in the child with spastic quadriplegia. *Eur J Neurol* 2001; 8 suppl 5:127–35.

185. Menkes, J.H. and Sarnat, H.B. Perinatal asphyxia and trauma. In J.H. Menkes and H.B. Sarnat, eds. *Child Neurology*. Philadelphia, PA: Lippincott Williams & Wilkins, 2000, pp. 442–5.

186. Lazorthes, Y., Sol, J.C., Sallerin, B., and Verdie, J.C. The surgical management of spasticity. *Eur J Neurol* 2002;9(suppl 1):35–41.

187. Kim, D.S., Choi, J.U., Yang, K.H., and Park, C.I. Selective posterior rhizotomy in children with cerebral palsy: A ten-year experience. *Childs Nerv Syst* 2001;17:556–62.

188. Sgouros, S. and Seri S. The effect of intrathecal baclofen on muscle co-contraction in children with spasticity of cerebral origin. *Pediatr Neurosurg* 2002;37:225–30.

189. Albright, A.L., Gilmartin, R., Swift, D., Krach, L.E., Ivanhoe, C.B., and McLaughline, J.F. Long-term intrathecal baclofen therapy for severe spasticity of cerbral origin. *J Neurosurg* 2003;98:291–5.

190. Santos, K.G. and Fallat, M.E. Surgical and anesthetic decisions for children with terminal illness. *Semin Pediatr Surg* 2001;10:237–42.

191. Koman, L.A., Smith, B.P., and Balkrishnan, R. Spasticity associated with cerebral palsy in children: guidelines for the use of botulinum A toxin. *Paediatr Drugs* 2003;5:11–23.

192. Wong, V., Ng, A., and Sit, P. Open-label study of botulinum toxin for upper limb spasticity in cerebral palsy. *J Child Neurol* 2002;17: 138–42.

193. Bakheit, A.M. Botulinum toxin in the management of childhood muscle spasticity: comparison of clinical practice of 17 treatment centers. *Eur J Neurol* 2003;10:415–9.

194. Twycross, R. Skeletal muscle relaxants. In R. Twycross, A. Wilcock, S. Charlesworth, and A. Dickman, eds. *Palliative Care Formulary* (2nd edition). Oxon: Radcliffe Medical Press, 2002, p. 264–7.

195. Krach, L.E. Pharmacotherapy of spasticity: oral medications and intrathecal baclofen. *J Child Neurol* 2001;16:31–6.

196. Scher, M.S. Applying classification of sleep disorders to children with neurologic conditions. *J Child Neurol* 1998;13:525–36.

197. Kohrman, M.H. and Carney, P.R. Sleep-related disorders in neurologic disease during childhood. *Pediatr Neurol* 2000;23:107–13.

198. Owens, J.A. Sleep disorders. In R.E. Behrman, R.M. Kliegman, H.B. Jenson, eds. *Nelson Textbook of Pediatrics*. Philadelphia, PA: Saunders, 2004, pp. 75–80.

199. Ward, T. and Mason, T.B. Sleep disorders in children. *Nurs Clin North Am* 2002;37:693–706.

200. Zucconi, M. and Bruni, O. Sleep disorders in children with neurologic disease. *Semin Pediatr Neurol* 2001;8:258–75.

201. Rivkees, S. Developing circadian rhythmicity in infants. *Pediatrics* 2003;112:373–81.

202. Dodge, N.N. and Wilson, G.A. Melatonin for treatment of sleep disorders in children with developmental disabilities. *J Child Neurol* 2001;16:581–4.

203. Jan, J.E. and O'Donnell, M.E. Use of melatonin in the treatment of paediatric sleep disorders. *J Pineal Res* 1996;4:103–9.

204. Ross, C., Davies, P., and Whitehouse, W. Melatonin treatment for sleep disorders in children with neurodevelopmental disorders: an observational study. *Dev Med Child Neurol* 2002;44:339–44.

205. Younus, M. and Labellarte, M.J. Insomnia in children: when are hypnotics indicated? *Paediatr Drugs* 2002;4:391–403.

206. Levetown, M. Treatment of symptoms other than pain in pediatric palliative care. In R.K. Portenoy and E. Bruera, eds. *Topics in Palliative Care.* New York: Oxford University Press, 1998, pp. 60–1.

207. Ernst, E. Insomnia. In E. Ernst, ed. *The Desktop Guide to Complementary and Alternative Medicine.* Edinburgh: Mosby, 2001, pp. 290–5.

208. Lewis, C.R., de Vedia, A., Reuer, B., Schwan, R., and Tourin C. Integrating complementary and alternative medicine (CAM) into standard hospice and palliative care. *Am J Hosp Palliat Care* 2003;20:221–8.

209. Davies, H. Living with dying: families coping with a child who has a neurodegenerative genetic disorder. *Axone* 1996;18:38–44.

210. Steele, R.G. Experiences of families in which a child has a prolonged terminal illness: modifying factors. *Int J Paliat Nurs* 2002;8;418–34.

27 Respiratory symptoms

Stephen Liben, Richard Hain, and Ann Goldman

Introduction

A major goal of palliative care is to alleviate symptoms that cause suffering. Suffering may stem from conditions or events that threaten the integrity of a person as a complex psychological and social entity [1]. However, suffering is not simply related to the severity of unrelieved physical symptoms. It is also experienced by whole persons and can occur in relation to any aspect of their physical, psychological, social, or spiritual personhood. A sense of loss of meaning and purpose, helplessness, hopelessness, endlessness, and lack of control are major causes of suffering [2].

Respiratory symptoms require management when they are the cause of distress or discomfort to the child. At the same time there are therapeutic interventions that may serve to both alleviate one kind of suffering while imposing another, for example mechanical ventilation may alleviate some aspects of breathlessness but also result in the need for suctioning, frequent infections, and potentially life-threatening complications. As with all therapies the ultimate decision as to whether an intervention is indicated will be mandated by the balance between benefit versus burden of the treatment, taken together with the unique needs of the particular child.

Respiratory symptoms in children with life-limiting conditions are often life-threatening. Their management must be appropriate to the stage of the disease. Postponing death is not appropriate if prolonging life is counter to the child's best interests.

Healthcare professionals are generally well-trained in the management of acute cardio-respiratory failure. This expertise may be counterproductive in end of life care and when misapplied may compromise dignity and increase suffering of the dying child.

Dyspnoea

Breathlessness (dyspnoea) is described as a subjective, uncomfortable awareness of difficulty in breathing or of the need to breathe. Breathlessness can be one of the most frightening and distressing symptoms. It is often accompanied by considerable anxiety in both the child and the family. The vicious cycle in which anxiety aggravates breathlessness and breathlessness in turn creates further anxiety is experienced to some degree by most breathless patients. Some patients may experience a severe panic attack and become convinced that they are about to die. Such attacks may be more common than is acknowledged. Dyspnoea occurs in 40–65% of children with malignant conditions and there is evidence that the control of dyspnea may be less effective than that of pain in palliative care [3–5].

The precise origin of the sensation of breathlessness remains unknown. From a pathophysiologic point of view, dyspnoea is associated with three main abnormalities: (1) an increase in respiratory effort to overcome a certain load (e.g., obstructive or restrictive lung disease, pleural effusion), (2) an increase in the proportion of respiratory muscle required to maintain a normal workload, and (3) an increase in ventilatory requirements (hypoxemia, hypercapnia, metabolic acidosis, anaemia, and so forth). In many cancer patients, different proportions of the three abnormalities may coexist making the pathophysiologic interpretation of the intensity of dyspnoea complex. Although it is well recognised that both hypoxia and hypercapnia may cause severe dyspnoea, it is not clear if this occurs as a direct perception of altered chemoreceptor stimulation or if the distress is due to the combination of this stimulation and a significant effect of efferent muscle stimulation which results in an increase in ventilation [6].

Dyspnoea has been described as a 'synthetic sensation, like that of thirst or hunger' [7], that is the result of a complex interaction of signals arising from within the central nervous system, both from the automatic centres in the brain stem and from the motor cortex, and from a variety of receptors in the upper airway, lungs, and chest wall. Most conditions that cause breathlessness likely do so by more than one mechanism, and different conditions share common mechanisms. However, each condition probably has a unique combination of physiologic factors that determines the quality and intensity of dyspnoea in a particular patient at a given time.

Current hypotheses on the origin of dyspnoea emphasise the importance of respiratory muscle effort that reflects central motor command [8]. However, the role of the central mismatch between respiratory muscle effort and instantaneous feedback from sensory receptors throughout the respiratory system in the perception of dyspnoea has also been emphasised. This theory has its basis in the disparity between the respiratory motor output and the mechanical response of the system [9–11].

Both studies and clinical observations suggest that under a given set of conditions, the brain 'expects' a certain pattern of ventilation and associated afferent feedback and that deviations from this pattern cause or intensify the sensation of dyspnoea. Even patients receiving mechanical ventilation are often breathless, despite a reduction in the work performed by the respiratory muscles. The process that necessitated mechanical ventilation in the first place is often responsible for the symptoms, but additional factors may play a part. For example, unless the output of the ventilator is matched to the patient's requirements for flow and tidal volume they may not match those desired by a patient with heightened respiratory drive, in which case the afferent mismatch may intensify dyspnoea [12].

Causes and assessment of dyspnoea

Causes of breathlessness are diverse and include anxiety, airway obstruction, anaemia, bronchospasm, chest pain (musculoskeletal, pleuritic, post-thoracotomy or rib fracture), elevated diaphragm (secondary to ascites, hepatomegaly or phrenic nerve lesion), hypercapnia, hypoxemia, metabolic disorders, pleural effusion, pneumonia, pulmonary oedema, pulmonary embolism, respiratory muscle weakness, and thick secretions. The sudden development of dyspnoea, headache, swelling and distension of the veins of the face, chest and upper limbs suggests the development of superior vena caval obstruction in cancer patients.

Breathlessness, like pain, is a symptom not a sign. Measures of respiratory rate, oxygen saturation, blood gas levels, and professional and family members' perceptions do not necessarily correlate with the patient's perception of breathlessness. The only reliable measure of dyspnea is patient self-report which may be difficult or impossible to obtain from pre- and non-verbal children.

Dyspnoea is a difficult symptom to measure due to both its subjective and multidimensional nature. Because neither the initiation nor the perception of dyspnoea can be measured, assessment is based on the patient's self-report. The expression of the intensity of dyspnoea can be influenced by a number of factors such as cultural background, environment, life experiences, and psychological state [13,14]. Additionally, the assessment of dyspnoea is not always expressed directly by the patient but rather by the proxy caregiver or professional staff introducing a potential bias. Moreover, there is always the possibility of mistaking tachypnoea for dyspnoea. Tachypnoea simply refers to an increased rate of breathing and says nothing about subjective unpleasantness.

The visual analogue scale (VAS) was introduced by Aitken in 1969 for the assessment of the intensity of dyspnoea [15]. VAS is a horizontal or vertical line anchored with terms that characterise two extremes of a possible subjective status from 'no breathlessness' to 'worst possible breathlessness'. Individuals are asked to mark the portion of line (creating an interval scale) that best reflects the intensity of dyspnoea at a given time. The use of the VAS for the comparison of different populations is of limited value, rather it is best to use the VAS for repeated measurements with the same patient in order to quantify disease severity and the effects of therapeutic interventions.

For inter-individual comparisons the Borg Category Scale is more convenient than the VAS. The Borg modified scale consists of a vertical scale labelled 0–10, with corresponding verbal expressions of progressively increasing sensation intensity from 'nothing at all' to 'maximal' [16]. Other methods of dyspnoea assessment include both a Lickert-type scale and a verbal rating scale.

Pulmonary function tests can be particularly useful in the assessment of obstructive and restrictive pulmonary disorders, as well as neuromuscular weakness. The following tests are available: forced vital capacity (FVC), expiratory and inspiratory slow vital capacity (VC/IVC), and maximum voluntary ventilation (MVV). These tests are useful to select patients both for palliative care or ventilatory support programmes (depending on the patient's choice), and also for the assessment of the response to different therapies. However, they remain inadequate to assess the intensity of dyspnoea. In one study the age of patients with Duchenne muscular dystrophy (DMD) when vital capacity fell below 1 l was a strong marker of subsequent mortality (5-year survival 8%) [17].

Management of dyspnoea

The first principle of management is to identify and treat the underlying cause of dyspnoea. This may not always be possible or appropriate in the setting of palliative care and needs to be considered on an individual basis. In patients with advanced disease, the burden of investigations and disease-modifying interventions may outweigh any potential benefit. There are three widely used medical approaches for the symptomatic relief of breathlessness: oxygen, opioids, and anxiolytics.

Oxygen is prescribed for breathless patients because some respond with a decreased sense of breathlessness while others have no change in their level of comfort. Some dyspnoeic patients may benefit from compressed air delivered by nasal prongs or from a fan. This is likely due to physiologic effect of stimulating the V2 branch of the fifth cranial nerve that has a central inhibitory effect on the sensation of breathlessness [18–20]. One practical approach to determining the potential benefit of inhaled oxygen is a trial with direct observation and self-report to best assess if oxygen achieves the primary goal of making patients more comfortable, regardless of whether or not their measured oxygen saturation is affected.

Nocturnal hypoventilation in children with neuro-degenerative diseases and muscle dysfunction can lead to poor sleep, tiredness, lethargy, headache and reduced appetite. Nocturnal hypoxia is assumed to be one of the most important causative factors of morning headaches. In the intermediate phase of neuromuscular disease hypoxia is difficult to diagnose and requires empirical treatment. Morning headaches may be improved by oxygen therapy.

Case A 16-year-old girl diagnosed with juvenile amyotrophic sclerosis was admitted to a hospice for children. Slowly, progressive muscle weakness was observed from her 8th year of life until eventually she was incapable of moving by herself. On admission she had significant bulbar dysfunction with slurred speech, snoring and dysphagia requiring a gastrostomy.

She had symptoms of nighttime hypoventilation including nightmares, disturbed sleep, tiredness and daytime fatigue. Severe headaches appeared suddenly after awakening and receded partially in the afternoon/evening. Oxygen provided during the night that was discontinued in the morning did not provide relief. A trial of opioids was similarly unsuccessful. It was only after oxygen therapy was continued until midday that a dramatic improvement in her headache pain was obtained [21].

Opioids may relieve the distress of breathlessness in many patients without a measurable effect on their respiratory rate or blood gas. In a placebo-controlled crossover study of 10 dyspnoeic adult cancer patients on regular morphine the intensity of dyspnoea was significantly improved after a test dose of morphine, which was 50% of the regular dose [22]. In a randomized continuous sequential controlled trial to compare the efficacy of two supplementary dosing regimens of opioids (25% vs. 50% of 4-hourly analgesic dose) on dyspnoea in terminally ill adult cancer patients, 25% of the equivalent of the 4-hourly dose of opioid was sufficient to reduce both dyspnoea intensity and tachpnea for 4 h; there was no obvious advantage of using more than one quarter of the regular dose [23].

Opioids can be commenced at a low dose (half of the usual starting dose) and increased as required to reduce symptoms (e.g. for a child aged over 6 months, start with oral morphine 0.1–0.25 mg/kg/dose q 4 h orally). Nebulized morphine may be effective in some patients with dyspnoea and has the potential advantage of being rapidly effective while producing fewer systemic side-effects. The starting dose is 2.5–5 mg morphine (injectable solution) via nebulizer. Caution is needed in using nebulised morphine both because of limited experience in its use and potential for causing bronchospasm in some children.

Benzodiazepines are often used in combination with opioids for their sedative and anxiolytic effects. Benzodiazepines are a group of drugs that reduce anxiety and aggression, sedate and improve sleep, suppress seizures, and relax muscles.

Radiotherapy may have a valuable palliative role in dyspnoea due to malignant chest disease. Radiotherapy is likely to provide benefit only where symptoms are caused by tumour that is close to one of the bronchi or other major airways. Tumours that are elsewhere in the lung parenchyma are usually asymptomatic and radiotherapy is often unnecessary. Tumours near a bronchus can also cause haemoptysis. Major haemorrhage is unlikely but even small amounts of haemoptysis can be very distressing for patients. Radiotherapy may also have an important role in superior vena caval obstruction. The potential benefits of radiotherapy need to be weighed carefully against the fact that the child may need to come to the hospital repeatedly or even be admitted for such treatments. Finally, some children will already have received maximum doses of radiotherapy to the chest during previous attempts to cure their disease.

Bronchospasm may contribute to dyspnea and respiratory distress and is often responsive to bronchodilators. Steroids can also be useful in alleviating bronchospasm and may reduce inflammation around pulmonary metastases. The prolonged use of steroids over months requires a balancing of their benefits versus their long-term side-effects that include weight gain and behavioural changes.

Additional measures to help relieve dyspnea include attending to the psychological impact of breathlessness. Anxious children benefit from the presence of confident and reassuring family members and staff. Breathing exercises (e.g. long, slow breaths), appropriate positioning (i.e. upright) and relaxation training may also be helpful.

Neuromuscular diseases

Neuromuscular diseases (NMD) like Duchenne muscular dystrophy (DMD) and spinal muscular atrophy (SMA) are often associated with abnormalities of ventilatory control with associated hypoventilation, particularly during sleep, and a reduced ventilatory response to CO_2 and oxygen [24].

Patients with NMD exhibit a heightened neuromotor output [25,26]. The latter is sensed as an increased respiratory muscle effort and as such is likely to be the principal mechanism of dyspnoea in patients with uncomplicated NMD [27]. Alternatively, the association of an increased respiratory system impedance with respiratory muscle weakness increases the respiratory muscle load and may affect the coupling between respiratory effort and volume; therefore, a greater-than-normal dyspnoea sensation might be expected.

DMD is an X-linked condition that affects approximately one in 3300 live male births and is caused by the absence or disruption of the protein dystrophin. The majority of affected boys die from respiratory failure but the time to death is variable. DMD is the most common and most severe form of childhood muscular dystrophies, resulting in early loss of ambulation between the ages of 7 and 13 years and death in the teens and twenties. Despite advances made in the understanding of the molecular genetics of the disease, no definitive cure has been found.

SMA is a severe disease of childhood characterised by degeneration of lower motor neurons associated with muscle paralysis and atrophy that eventually leads to pulmonary complications and early death in those most severely affected [28,29]. Mutations of the SMN1 gene are responsible for SMA. On a clinical basis the subgrouping of three stages is now widely accepted [30]. Type I (Werdnig Hoffman) patients are the most severely affected, with symptoms presenting from birth to 6 months; they are never able to sit or stand. Children with the intermediate form, type II (Dubowitz), develop symptoms during the first 6–18 months. They are able to sit without support, but cannot walk. Type III (Kugelberg Welander) patients are able to stand and walk and the onset of symptoms before the age of 18 months are unusual. SMA type I is associated with impairment of respiratory function, which is probably caused by involvement of the intercostal muscles as well as the diaphragm [31]. Death as a result of respiratory insufficiency within the first 18 months of life is common. However, in one study 36 out of 349 SMA type I patients (10%) survived at least beyond their fifth birthday, in spite of total immobility and frequent respiratory infections [32]. Type II SMA is more heterogeneous than type 1, but respiratory function is the most important factor in determining prognosis. Type III affected children have no respiratory

problems. Both type I and type II patients tend to develop scoliosis and other vertebral deformities. Scoliosis contributes to the impaired lung function by physically impeding respiratory movement and thereby reducing vital capacity, as well as increasing ventilation/perfusion mismatch [33]. Spinal bracing (wearing a rigid jacket) delays the progression of the spinal deformity [34,35], however, bracing may also cause respiratory impairment.

Of important clinical significance is the fact that patients with certain NMD's may have significant changes in arterial blood gases without impressive symptoms. These patients increase their respiratory rate rather than tidal volume (TV) in response to hypercapnia and hypoxemia [36]. This rapid and shallow breathing response is thought to be an attempted compensation aimed at increasing ventilation with minimal increase in work of breathing. This is a particularly important feature of patients with chest wall deformities (kyphoscoliosis) in whom thoracic compliance is low. Accordingly, there is a less impressive increase in total alveolar ventilation due to increased dead space ventilation. This is in comparison with the normal response of increased TV in response to hypercapnia or hypoxemia. The tachypnoea may then cause worsening respiratory muscle fatigue leading to a further reduction in TV. Respiratory failure typically complicates advanced NMD by compromising effective respiratory muscle function. It is now known that nocturnal hypoventilation precedes resting daytime gas exchange abnormalities, probably accounting for the commonly presenting symptoms of disturbed sleep, increasing daytime hyper-somnolence, morning headaches, and features of cor-pulmonale, despite reasonably normal daytime gas exchange [37]. Regardless of the status of the associated muscle weakness, respiratory failure can be anticipated when the VC falls to <55% of predicted, and the maximum inspiratory force falls to <30% of predicted [38]. Death in these patients is usually caused by progressive respiratory failure and superimposed infections secondary to aspiration as a result of pharyngeal dysfunction [39].

Cystic fibrosis

Cystic fibrosis (CF) is a multi-system disorder affecting the respiratory, alimentary, hepatobiliary, and reproductive systems associated with a variety of endocrine and metabolic complications including diabetes and osteoporosis. With many therapeutic advances in the treatment of CF, the median survival in developed countries is now around 30 years [40]. Over 90% of deaths are from respiratory disease caused by a vicious cycle of infection, inflammation and progressive lung destruction leading to respiratory failure [41]. The terminal phase is usually heralded by increased frequency and severity of respiratory exacerbations, oxygen dependence and declining lung function. Patients who have already progressed to severe airflow obstruction with a forced expiratory volume in one second (FEV1) of less than 30% of the predicted value are much more likely to die, with an estimated 2-year mortality rate of approximately 50% [42,43]. The initiation of discussions regarding end-of-life care should be considered in all patients with CF, in particular in those with an FEV1 < 30% or a rapid decline in functional status. These criteria are similar to those for referral for consideration of lung transplantation, and clearly the issues of transplantation and end-of-life care are intertwined [44].

In a retrospective study of 44 patients who died of CF-related respiratory failure the mean FEV1 was 23% of predicted. All patients had been designated as do-not-resuscitate (DNR) for at least 24 h before death. The mean duration of DNR status was 25 days. Forty-three patients died in the hospital; five died in ICU, four of which had been listed for lung transplantation, received assisted ventilation by means of biphasic positive airway pressure (BiPAP). Only one patient died at home under hospice care. Length of stay in the hospital before death varied from 24 h to several months; the typical length of stay was 2–3 weeks. Thirty-eight patients (86%) received opioids at the time of death. Thirty-three patients (75%) received intravenous antibiotics 12 h before death [45]. In contrast to this U.S. study, data from South Africa reported that 56% of their CF patients died at home [46]. These cross-country disparities of place and mode of death remain to be fully explained as to what is best for an individual child and family.

Suggested treatments of dyspnoea in patients with CF include [47]:

- Physiotherapy to clear excessive secretions (fatigue and hypoxia may limit its use).
- Nebulised saline or bronchodilators to assist with expectoration.
- Nebulised amiloride and DNase as mucolytics.
- Oxygen if comfort improves with its administration
- Opioids for relief of dyspnoea.
- Relaxation techniques and small doses of anxiolytics such as benzodiazepines.

Home palliative care may be considered when bacterial pneumonia's become resistant to available antibiotics. Pseudomonas aeruginosa respiratory infection was found to be a major predictor of morbidity and mortality in children with CF [48]. In the terminal stage antibiotics, physiotherapy and mucolytics could be withdrawn, though for many children oxygen, nebulised morphine [49], and sedation if required should be considered.

Life-prolonging medical treatments in CF include medication and artificially or technologically supplied respiration, nutrition, and hydration [50]. The development of lung transplantation in the 1980s offers a therapeutic opportunity for some patients with CF. However, palliative care is often needed for patients on a transplant list as in developed countries up to 40% of accepted patients will die awaiting a lung transplant. In one study the survival in a group of 190 children who underwent isolated lung transplant was 77% at 1 year, 62% at 3 years, and 55% at 5 years. There were 25 early (< 60 days) and 61 late deaths. The most common cause of early death was graft failure (52%), while the most common causes of late death were bronchiolitis obliterans (57%), infection (21%), and post-transplant malignancies (18%)[51]. Clearly, palliative care issues remain relevant both pre- and post-transplant for the majority of patients with CF who are transplant candidates.

Invasive mechanical ventilation (via a tracheostomy or endotracheal tube) for respiratory failure in CF is generally considered ineffective and is not usually recommended unless a clearly reversible component to the respiratory compromise exists. Non-invasive ventilation refers to the delivery of mechanical ventilation to the lungs using techniques that do not require an endotracheal airway (e.g. via a tight-fitting mask on the face). Non-invasive positive pressure ventilation has been used in patients with end-stage CF, often as a bridge to lung transplantation [52]. The use of mechanical ventilation in children with NMD is complex and requires a careful balance between potential benefits versus the burden of suffering for each individual patient.

Cough

Cough is a physiological reflex designed to expel particles and excess mucus from the airways. An effective cough depends on the ability to generate an adequate expiratory airflow, estimated at >160 L/min [53]. Expiratory airflow is determined by lung and chest wall elasticity, airway conductance, and, at least at higher lung volumes, expiratory muscle force. By generating an adequate vital capacity (in adults >2.5 L) to take advantage of respiratory system elasticity, inspiratory muscle function also contributes to cough adequacy. In addition, an effective cough requires intact glottis function, so that explosive release of intrathoracic pressure can generate high peak expiratory cough flows [54].

Cough can result from irritation to the upper or lower airway, pleura, pericardium or diaphragm. It may be caused by respiratory infection, airways disease, malignant obstruction, oesophageal reflux, aspiration of saliva, or induced by drugs.

Cough is pathological when it is ineffective and when it adversely affects sleep, rest, eating, or social activity. Persistent cough can also precipitate vomiting, exhaustion, chest or abdominal pain, rib fracture, and syncope. The primary aim is to identify and treat the cause of the distressing cough but when this is not possible or is inappropriate a cough suppressant may be used. An example is a dry cough that is distressing to the patient, or a nocturnal wet cough that is disturbing sleep.

Tenacious or thick secretions can be loosened with nebulised saline allowing the child to then remove them by coughing. Use of nebulised saline, as well as other mucolytics can result in the production of copious liquid sputum, and this makes it unsuitable for those who are unable to expectorate. Physiotherapy can also be helpful. For upper airway irritation, it is worth seeing whether cough lozenges or a simple cough linctus can soothe the throat and alleviate a dry, irritating cough. Bronchospasm may also contribute to cough and treatment with salbutamol may be helpful.

Children with a persistent dry cough may benefit from opioids that are generally effective at reducing coughing and the distress associated with coughing. Children already receiving opioids for analgesia may need the dose increased.

In patients with neuromuscular disorders the diaphragm and intercostal muscles are often affected, causing hypoventilation and weak cough. Difficulty in clearing secretions, combined with aspiration due to problems in swallowing also predisposes these patients to chest infections. When weak expiratory muscles are combined with a markedly reduced vital capacity, as occurs in end-stage neuromuscular diseases, the cough mechanism is severely impaired. The inability to cough effectively is tolerable for patients who have minimal airway secretions and an intact swallowing mechanism, but an episode of acute bronchitis or aspiration of oral secretions can precipitate a life-threatening crisis. The simplest manoeuvre to augment cough flow is manually assisted or 'quad' coughing. This consists of firm, quick thrusts applied to the abdomen using the palms of the hands, timed to coincide with the patient's cough effort. The technique should be taught to caregivers of patients with severe respiratory muscle weakness with instructions to use it whenever the patient encounters difficulty expectorating secretions. With practice, the technique can be applied effectively and frequently, with minimal discomfort to the patient. Peak expiratory flows can be increased several-fold when manually assisted coughing is applied successfully [55]. To minimise the risk of regurgitation and aspiration of gastric contents, the patient should be placed semi-upright when manually assisted coughing is applied, and the technique should be used cautiously after meals.

Although manually assisted coughing may enhance expiratory force, it does not augment inspired volume. Patients with severely restricted volumes, therefore, may still achieve insufficient cough flows, even when assisted by skilled caregivers. To overcome this problem, the inhaled volume should be augmented [56]. One approach is to 'stack' breaths using glosso-pharyngeal breathing or volume-limited ventilation and then to cough using manual assistance. Another is to use a mechanical insufflator-exsufflator, a device that was developed during the polio epidemics to aid in airway secretion removal. This device delivers a positive inspiratory pressure of 30–40 cm H_2O via a facemask and then rapidly switches to an equal negative pressure. The positive pressure assures the delivery of an adequate tidal volume, and the negative pressure has the effect of simulating the rapid expiratory flows generated by a cough.

Excessive secretions/noisy breathing

Excessive secretions or difficulty clearing pharyngeal secretions may lead to noisy or 'rattly' breathing that commonly occurs during the terminal phase of the child's illness and is often associated with diminished consciousness. Positioning on the side or slightly head down will allow some postural drainage and this may be all that is required. Reassurance and explanation to the family is essential as the noise of the gurgling can be very distressing to the family, while the child is usually unaware and untroubled by the noise and sensation.

Anticholinergic drugs can be used to reduce the production of secretions and a portable suction machine at home may be of benefit for children with chronic conditions or for those who are unconscious. Hyoscine hydrobromide can be administered either subcutaneously as a bolus, via a continuous infusion, or via a transdermal patch. Glycopyrrolate (4–10 micrograms/kg q. 6 h; max 0.2 mg) also has anticholinergic properties and a selective and prolonged effect on salivary and sweat gland secretions. Consideration of the use of glycopyrrolate should be given if there is an inadequate response from hyoscine. Atropine can also be used but may lead to bradycardia with repeated dosing.

Haemoptysis

In studies of patients with haemoptysis a definite cause is established only half of the time. Even in patients with a proven malignancy, haemoptysis can be due to other causes. While lung cancer is the commonest cause of massive haemoptysis (>200 ml/24 h), non-malignant disorders such as acute bronchitis, bronchiectasis, aspergellosis, and pulmonary embolism can cause mild to moderate haemoptysis. It is important to establish that the blood or blood stained material has come from the chest and not the nose, upper respiratory tract, or gastrointestinal tract. Management depends on the cause and prognosis. Radiotherapy (endobronchial or external beam) and laser therapy are particularly effective in controlling bleeding from endobronchial tumours. Rapid sedation may be required for massive hemoptysis using a combination of a parenterally administered strong opioid and a benzodiazepine [57]. As with the possibility of any acutely potentially traumatic event, the management of acute hemoptysis should begin with a plan and anticipatory guidance before the event occurs.

In CF patients' recurrent haemoptysis has been managed with bronchial artery embolization (BAE). In one study the immediate success rate after embolization (i.e. no recurrent bleeding within 24 h) was 95% (36 of 38 BAEs). Eleven (55%) patients required more than one procedure, and the median time between first and second embolization was 4 months (range, 5 days to 61 months). Three patients died as a consequence of severe haemoptysis during induction of anaesthesia with intermittent positive pressure ventilation in preparation for the procedure. The median survival duration after the first embolization was 84 months [58].

Pleural effusion

A pleural effusion is an abnormal volume of fluid that has collected between the visceral and parietal pleura. Normally there is 10–20 ml of pleural fluid between these two layers of pleura. This is part of dynamic system that turns over 100–200 ml of pleural fluid a day. Fluid accumulation occurs when there is imbalance between fluid formation and resorption mainly due to a dysfunction of lymphatic drainage [59].

Mechanisms of malignant pleural effusion formation include:

- Tumour involving the pleura increases capillary permeability, which produces an excess of fluid, and decreases pleural resorption area.
- Low serum albumin decreases oncotic pressure.
- Lymphadenopathy leading to thoracic duct obstruction.
- Lymphangitic carcinomatosis leading to lymphatic system obstruction.

Non-malignant pleural effusions may be caused by heart failure, renal failure, pulmonary infection, and pulmonary infarction.

Thoracocentesis (insertion of a temporary or permanent chest drain to remove pleural fluid) is often of only marginal benefit. Although thoracentesis can relieve the symptoms of dyspnoea caused by pleural fluid, the procedure is uncomfortable and poorly tolerated by most children, especially if general anaesthetic is not available or appropriate. Furthermore, the benefit is typically limited to hours or days before the procedure needs to be repeated. It is possible to reduce the risk of this by pleurodesis in which the pleural membranes are made to adhere to one another by inducing inflammation. This is usually achieved by instilling an irritant such as tetracycline or talc. In general thoracocentesis should be reserved for those relatively few patients in whom the potential benefit is likely to outweigh the considerable discomfort of the intervention.

The management of distressing respiratory symptoms is a mainstay in palliative care for children. Assessment of respiratory symptoms begins by understanding and clarifying the difference between a comfortable child who with an increased respiratory rate (tachypnoea) versus the distressed or uncomfortable child with breathlessness (dyspnoea). Management strategies to help alleviate distressing respiratory symptoms are then evaluated in terms of what is best for the particular child and their family whilst balancing the benefits of an intervention with its possible burdens. As with the management of other symptoms, much can be gained by open discussion with the child and family about likely outcomes and risks and benefits of different therapies. Sensitive discussions with the child and family around advance care planning (e.g. 'these are some of the things we can do to make you comfortable if your breathing becomes difficult') may provide comfort and security both for the child/family as well as for involved professional and non-professional caregivers.

Current ethical controversies in the withdrawal or withholding of mechanical ventilation

In all cultures, paediatric palliative care must advocate for children. It is often difficult for medical teams to recognise the need to withhold or even to withdraw interventions that may prolong life. In some societies, this may be due to reluctance to give autonomy to patients and families, or to allow them to participate in treatment decisions. It is expected that the family will do only what they are 'permitted' to do by doctors. In other cultures, often where autonomy is given high priority, the same reluctance may be due to concerns about litigation that may follow if life is perceived to have been shortened deliberately. It can be a struggle even to persuade paediatric teams to allow a child to return home to die, or for paediatric oncology teams to discontinue chemotherapy even where it is recognised that cure is impossible.

In any society, therefore, paediatric palliative care may find itself having to take on a role of advocate, allowing the voices of child and family to be heard in pleading for invasive and futile interventions to be withheld or even withdrawn. Where necessary this may mean representing their needs to professional colleagues in ways that will not always be popular, and may even be seen by some as ethically questionable.

Use of mechanical respirators is one of these issues. There are many countries in which patients have as yet no legal right to be disconnected from a respirator, nor physicians any legal right to extubate. Freedom, dignity and autonomy of the patient, and the medical principle *primum non nocere* ('First, do no harm') are the most important ethical imperatives, rather than simply prolonging life. For patients in whom mechanical ventilation is not life-saving (such as those with DMD or SMA), there should be a free choice to withhold or even to withdraw this kind of treatment. Paediatric palliative care provides an active alternative that improves symptoms and quality of life for those patients who choose to reject mechanical ventilation. It is also important to remember that many boys in the terminal stages of DMD are adults in their own right, and do not need their parents' permission to make such a choice.

Where possible, futile or unwelcome ventilation should be avoided. This can best be done through repeated discussions and exploration of the issue with family and (where appropriate) the child. This can be a valuable role for those working in children's palliative care. The outcome of such discussions should always be clearly recorded and the record made accessible. This may mean allowing the family themselves to have a copy for presentation to ambulance drivers or emergency staff.

Despite such an approach, some children who are unlikely to benefit will find themselves undergoing mechanical ventilation. It can be difficult for staff to accept withholding ventilation as an option, even if it is clearly the family's wish, and at the moment a decision needs to be made, the child or family themselves may change their minds.

Actively withdrawing invasive mechanical ventilation needs to be done sensitively in an unhurried and considered manner. There are many protocols for approaching this which provide a practical and compassionate approach to relieving any symptoms associated with extubation. The tube may be withdrawn suddenly or gradually ('terminal weaning'), depending in part on the preferences of the patient, if known, as well as the family and staff. Terminal weaning, as the name suggests, involves a gradual reduction in ventilation parameters rate, inspiratory and expiratory pressures and inspired oxygen. Terminal weaning may be over as little as 30–60 min but can be much longer, and some patients may breathe spontaneously.

It is important that the needs of the family be considered during withdrawal. This may include playing music, the presence of a favourite toy, or simply enough physical space for family members to be present at the bedside. The paraphernalia of high-technology medicine, especially noisy and intrusive alarms, should be removed.

The two most common and feared physical symptoms associated with withdrawal of ventilation are breathlessness and anxiety. Both are readily managed with opioids and benzodiazepines. Prescription of medications at the time of extubation may cause concern among medical and nursing staff, who worry that they may cause respiratory depression and hasten death. The risks of respiratory depression are, in reality, small—properly titrated, it is usually possible to find a dose for most patients that eases anxiety and dyspnoea without significantly impairing respiration.

In the past, invasive ventilation using an endotracheal tube was the only option available to families of children with life-limiting respiratory illnesses such as DMD. Increasingly, however, families are being offered the alternative of non-invasive positive pressure ventilation (NIPPV) in the United Kingdom (BiPAP in the United States) using a face-mask, usually at night. For many, this provides a 'third way'; there is growing evidence that it can relieve symptoms and improve both quality and even duration of life, sometimes by several years.

Despite the fact that NIPPV is less invasive than traditional mechanical ventilation, the same ethical issues apply and patients who fully understand the issues need to be allowed the chance to decline. For some patients it is too invasive or intrusive, sometimes for physical reasons and sometimes for less obvious ones. The mask can be very uncomfortable, causing pain or feelings of claustrophobia, and some patients simply find the presence of a ventilator in the home intolerable.

In summary, for children with life-limiting respiratory conditions, the benefits of mechanical ventilation in terms of prolonged life need to be carefully weighed against the impact on its quality. Where families, or even patients themselves, understand these issues and request that ventilation be withheld or withdrawn, their voice should be heard and their view respected. Advocating for such families is an important role for paediatric palliative care.

References

1. Cassel, E. *The Nature of Suffering and the Goals of Medicine*. Oxford: Oxford University Press, 1991, p. 979.
2. Twycross, R. and Lichter, I. The terminal phase. In D. Doyle, G. Hanks , and N. MacDonald, eds. *Oxford Textbook of Palliative Medicine*. Oxford: Oxford University Press, 1998, pp. 977–92.

3. Hain, R.D.W., Patel, N., Crabtree, S., and Pinkerton, R. Respiratory symptoms in children dying from malignant disease. *Palliat Med* 1995; 9: 201–6.

4. McQillan, R. and Finlay, I. Facilitating the care of terminally ill children. *J Pain Sympt Manage* 1996;12:320–4.

5. Wolfe, J., Grier, H.E., Klar, N. *et al.* Symptoms and suffering at the end of life in children with cancer. *N Engl J Med* 2000;342: 326–33.

6. Ripamonti, C. and Bruera, E. Dyspnea: Patophysiology and assessment. *J Pain Symptom Manage* 1997;13:220–32.

7. Harver, A. and Mahler, D.A. The symptom of dyspnea. In D.A. Mahler, (ed.) *Dyspnea*. Futura, Mount Kisco, N.Y, 1990; pp. 1–53.

8. Killian, K.J. and Jones, N.L. Respiratory muscle and dyspnea. *Clin Chest Med* 1988;9:237–48.

9. Chonan, T., Mulholland, M.B., Leitner, J., *et al.* Sensation of dyspnea during hypercapnia, exercise and voluntary hyperventilation. *J Appl Physiol* 1990;68:2100–06.

10. Demediuk, B.H., Manning, H., Lilly, J., *et al.* Dissociation between dyspnea and respiratory effort. *Am Rev Respir Dis* 1992;146: 1222–5.

11. O'Donnel, D.E. Breathlessness in patients with chronic airflow limitation: Mechanisms and management. *Chest* 1994;106: 904–12.

12. Manning, H.L. and Schwartzstein, R.M. Mechanisms of Disease: Pathophysiology of Dyspnea. *N Engl J Med* 1995;333:1547–53.

13. McCord, M. and Cronin-Stubbs, D. Operationalizing dyspnea: Focus on measurement. *Heart Lung* 1992;21:167–79.

14. Gift, A. and Cahill, C. Psychophysiologic aspects of dyspnea in chronic obstructive pulmonary disease: A pilot study. *Heart Lung* 1990;19:252–9.

15. Aitken, R.C.B. Measurement of feelings using visual analogue scales. *Proc R Soc Med* 1969;62:989–93.

16. Borg, G.A.V. Psychophysical bases of perceived exertion. *Med Sci Sport Exerc* 1982;14:377–81.

17. Phillips, M.F., Quinlivan, R.C., Edwards, R.H., and Calverley, P.M. Changes in spirometry over time as a prognostic marker in patients with Duchenne muscular dystrophy. *Am J Respir Crit Care Med* 2001;164:2191–4.

18. Schwartzstein, R.M., Lahive, K., Pope, A., Weinberger, S.E., and Weiss, J.W. Cold facial stimulation reduces breathlessness induced in normal subjects. *Am Rev Respir Dis* 1987;136:58–61.

19. Simon, P.M., Basner, R.C., Weinberger, S.E., Fencl, V., Weiss, J.W., and Schwartzstein, R.M. Oral mucosal stimulation modulates intensity of breathlessness induced in normal subjects. *Am Rev Respir Dis* 1991;144:419–22.

20. Spence, D.P.S., Graham, D.R., Ahmed, J., Rees, K., Pearson, M.G., and Calverley, P.M.A. Does cold air affect exercise capacity and dyspnea in stable chronic obstructive pulmonary disease? *Chest* 1993;103:693–6.

21. Karwacki, M.K. and Dangel, T. Prolonged daily oxygenation alleviates severe morning headache in an adolescent with sporadic juvenal amyotrophic lateral sclerosis with dementia. *The Suffering Child* 2003; 4: http://www.thesufferingchild.net/issues/issue04/03/index.htm

22. Bruera, E., MacEachern, T., Ripamonti, C., and Hanson, J. Subcutaneous morphine for dyspnea in cancer patients. *Ann Intern Med* 1993;119:906–7.

23. Allard, P., Lamontagne, C., Bernard, P., and Tremblay, C. How effective are supplementary doses of opioids for dyspnea in terminally ill cancer patients? A randomized continuous sequential clinical trial. *J Pain Symptom Manage* 1999;17:256–65.

24. Johnson, D.C. and Homeyoun, K. Central control of ventilation in neuromuscular disease. *Clin Chest Med* 1994;15:607–15.

25. Begin, R., Bureau, M.A., and Lupien, L., *et al.* Pathogenesis of respiratory insufficiency in myotonic dystrophy. *Am Rev Respir Dis* 1982;125:312–18.

26. Spinelli, A., Marconi, G., and Gorini, M. *et al.* Control of breathing in patients with myasthenia gravis (MG). *Am Rev Respir Dis* 1992; 145:1359–66.

27. Manning, H.L. and Schwartzstein, R.M. Mechanisms of dyspnea. In Mahler, D.A. ed. *Dyspnea: Lung biology in health and disease series*. New York: Marcel Dekker, 1998, Vol 3: pp. 63–90.

28. Merlini, L., Granata, C., Bonfiglioli, S. *et al.* Scoliosis in spinal muscular atrophy: Natural history and management. *Dev Med Child Neurol* 1989;31:501–8.

29. Tangsrud, S. and Halvorsen, S. Child neuromuscular disease in Southern Norway. *Clin Genet* 1988;34:145–52.

30. Dubowitz, V. *Muscle disease in childhood*. Philadelphia., PA: Saunders, 1978, p. 253

31. Noble-Jamieson, C.M., Heckmatt, J., Dubowitz, V., and Silverman, M. Effects of posture and spinal bracing on respiratory function in neuromuscular disease. *Arch Dis Child* 1986;61:178–81.

32. Borkowska, J., Rudnik-Schoneborn, S., Hausmanowa-Petrusewicz, I., and Zerres, K. Early infantile form of spinal muscular atrophy (Werdnig-Hoffmann disease) with prolonged survival. *Folia Neuropathol* 2002;40:19–26.

33. Dollery, C.T., Gillam, P.M.S., Hugh-Jones, P. *et al.* Regional lung function in kyphoscoliosis. *Thorax* 1965;20:181A.

34. Schwentker, E.P. and Gibson, D.A. The orthopaedic aspects of spinal muscular atrophy *J Bone Joint Surg* 1976;58A:32–8.

35. Rodillo, E., Marini, M., Heckmatt, J., and Dubowitz, V. Scoliosis in spinal muscular atrophy: Review of 63 cases. *J Child Neurol* 1989;4: 118–23.

36. Baydur, A. Respiratory muscle strength and control of ventilation in patients with neuromuscular diseases. *Chest* 1991;99:330–8.

37. Guilleminault, C., Stoohs, R., and Quera, S.M.A. Sleep-related obstructive and non-obstructive apneas and neurological disease. *Neurology* 1992;42:53–60.

38. Braun, N.M.T., Arora, N.S., and Rochester, D.F. Respiratory muscle and pulmonary function in polymyositis and other proximal myopathies. *Thorax* 1983;38:616–23.

39. Caruana-Montaldo, B., Gleeson, K., and Zwillich, C.W. The control of breathing in clinical practice. *Chest* 2000;117:205–25.

40. FitzSimmons, S. Cystic Fibrosis Foundation Patient Registry Annual Data Report. Bethesda: Cystic Fibrosis Foundation, 1995.

41. Ramsey, B. Management of pulmonary disease in patients with cystic fibrosis. *N Engl J Med* 1996;335:179–88.

42. Kerem, E., Reisman, J., Corey, M., Canny, G., and Levison, H. Prediction of mortality in patients with cystic fibrosis. *N Engl J Med* 1992;326:1187–91.

43. Schluchter, M.D., Konstan, M.W., and Davis, P.B. Jointly modelling the relationship between survival and pulmonary function in cystic fibrosis patients. *Stat Med* 2002;21:1271–87.

44. Tonelli, M.R. End-of-life care in cystic fibrosis. *Curr Opini Pulmonary Med* 1998;4:332–36.

45. Robinson, W.M., Ravilly, S., Berde, C., and Wohl, M.E. End-of-life care in cystic fibrosis. *Pediatrics* 1997;100:205–9.

46. Westwood, A.T.R. Terminal care in cystic fibrosis: Hospital versus home? *Pediatrics* 1997;100:436–7.

47. Jefferson, M. and Davies, C. Adults with cystic fibrosis. *Eur J Palliat Care* 1998;5:107–11.

48. Emerson, J., Rosenfeld, M., McNamara, S., Ramsey, B., and Gibson, R.L. Pseudomonas aeruginosa and other predictors of mortality and morbidity in young children with cystic fibrosis. *Pediatr Pulmonol* 2002;34:91–100.

49. Cohen, S.P. and Dawson, T.C. Nebulized morphine as a treatment for dyspnea in a child with cystic fibrosis. *Pediatrics* 2002;110:38.

50. Dickey, N.W. Withholding or withdrawing life-prolonging medical treatment. *J Am Med Ass* 1986;256:471.

51. Huddleston, C.B., Bloch, J.B., Sweet, S.C., de la Morena, M., Patterson, G.A., and Mendeloff, E.N. Lung transplantation in children. *Ann Surg* 2002;236:270–6.

52. Hodson, M.E., Madden, B.P., Steven, M.H., Tsang, V.T., and Yacoub, M.H. Non-invasive mechanical ventilation for cystic fibrosis patients: A potential bridge to transplantation. *Eur Respir J* 1991;4:524–27.

53. Bach, J.R. and Saporito, L.R. Criteria for extubation and tracheostomy tube removal for patients with ventilatory failure: A different approach to weaning. *Chest* 1996;110:1566–71.

54. Leith, D.E. Cough. In J.D. Brain, D. Proctor, and L. Reid, (eds.) *Lung Biology in Health and Disease: Respiratory Defense Mechanisms.* New York: Marcel Dekker, 1977, Vol. 2, pp. 545–92.

55. Bach, J.R. Mechanical insufflation-exsufflation: comparison of peak expiratory flows and manually assisted and unassisted coughing techniques. *Chest* 1993;104:1553–62.

56. Bach, J.R. Update and perspective on noninvasive respiratory muscle aids. Part 2: The expiratory aids. *Chest* 1994;105:1538–44.

57. Davis, C.L. ABC of palliative care: Breathlessness, cough, and other respiratory problems. *BMJ* 1997;315:931–4.

58. Barben, J., Robertson, D., Olinsky, A., and Ditchfield, M. Bronchial artery embolization for hemoptysis in young patients with cystic fibrosis. *Radiology* 2002;224:124–30.

59. Stretton, F., Edmonds, P., and Marrinan, M. Malignant pleural effusions. *Eur J Palliat Care* 1999;6:5–9.

28 Skin symptoms

Gillian Watterson, Jacqueline Denyer, and Richard Hain

Introduction

The skin can in some ways be considered one of the largest organs of the body, and it can be involved in a wide range of conditions that limit life in childhood. Some are primary dermatological diseases that are ultimately fatal because of their effect on the skin itself. Among these, perhaps the most important is epidermolysis bullosa (EB), a painful, debilitating and disfiguring inherited condition of fragile skin. The range of symptoms experienced by children with EB is wide, reflecting both the diverse anatomical locations in which skin is found and the broader psychological and emotional impact of altered self-image.

Because skin is so widely distributed, it is not surprising that it is also involved as an incidental problem in many other, non-dermatological life-limiting conditions. A range of non-malignant and sometimes malignant LLC may be complicated by symptoms attributable to damage to or dysfunction of the skin. These include, for example pruritus associated with cholestasis, dry skin associated with mucopolysaccharidosis and pain or odour associated with pressure sores.

This chapter will consider both the symptoms associated with life-limiting dermatological disease, particularly EB, and those associated with other LLC that manifest in the skin.

Dermatological symptoms in children with life-limiting disorders

Fungating malignant tumours

Aetiology

Fungating tumours are rare in children but when they occur can be an extremely distressing, causing not only pain but emotional and psychological anguish as a result of disfigurement, bleeding and odour. They may occasionally arise from rhabdomyosarcomas, squamous cell carcinomas and lymphomas.

Pathology

Fungating malignant wounds result from infiltration of a tumour into the skin and it blood and lymphatic vessels. Extensive damage to the skin, progressing to necrosis can result, due to the loss of vascularity.

These wounds may produce copious exudate, permitting the invasion of the tissue by both aerobic and anaerobic organisms which can produce an offensive smell.

Thus the emergence of a fungating tumour can be a source of enormous distress producing both physical discomfort as a result of pressure symptoms and devastating psychological problems because of loss of altered body image and loss of dignity.

Management

Management of fungating tumours relies on an interdisciplinary approach for optimum symptom control of pain, irritation, infection and malodour and haemorrhage.

1. Pain: A combination of non-pharmacological approaches (such as guided imagery) and pharmacological methods such as those medications acting to reduce neuropathic pain and nociceptive pain should be considered. Case reports in adult patients describing topical diamorphine applied directly to the wound, suggest it can provide analgesia without systemic opioid adverse effects [1,2]. This form of topical analgesia would be ideal for the pediatric population and further controlled studies are awaited.

2. Irritation: Continual leakage of exudates is a cause for cutaneous excoriation in fungating tumours. Methods of prevention have included topical anaesthetic agents which had limitations. They did not provide an adequate barrier from the exudate and they contained alcohol which caused stinging. Two products are currently being trialled in adults: Lutrol which is a local anaesthetic gel with lignocaine (lidocaine) and Cavilon, an alcohol free agent [3].

3. Odour: Systemic antibiotics to treat the usual skin pathogens may be required, as well as metronidazole for anaerobic organisms. Topical metronidazole gel [4–6] may reduce the need for the systemic route, but it is not useful in larger tumours, due to inability to penetrate to the offending bacteria. Debridement of the necrotic tissue would be useful in reduction of malodour but this is a potential cause of spontaneous bleeding and this risk need to be assessed.

4. Haemorrhage: Practical methods of preventing bleeding include, appropriate cleaning techniques, use of non-fibrous materials, good dressing application/removal techniques and maintainance of humidity at the wound/dressing interface. Pharmacological agents used to control bleeding include oral fibrinolytics (such as tranexamic acid), radiotherapy and embolization. Topical adrenaline 1 : 1000 may be applied as an emergency measure.

5. Local wound management: This should be occlusive or semi-occlusive and permeable or semi-permeable. The function of the dressing is to act as a reservoir for the excess exudates and conserve the surface humidity and moisture in order to prevent adherence [1].

Pruritus

Itching (pruritus) is reported relatively uncommonly in children with life-limiting conditions. When it does occur it can be one of the most uncomfortable symptoms to experience and one of the most challenging to manage. This is partly because, until recently, relatively little was known about the pathophysiology, and therefore the most appropriate therapeutic approaches.

Pruritus has been defined as 'an unpleasant cutaneous sensation which provokes the desire to scratch' [7]. Identifiable causes can include, for example, renal failure, cholestatic jaundice or medications such as morphine itself. In children with life-limiting conditions, there may be no obvious cause. Like pain, it is an illustration of the need for a systematic and rational approach to diagnosis and management of symptoms. Such an approach may fail; pruritus is a difficult symptom to manage.

Mechanisms

The origins of pruritus have been classified as cutaneous, i.e. arising from the skin itself, neuropathic, i.e. caused by damage to the nerves, or neurogenic, i.e. caused by nerves that function well but are acted on by pruritogenic stimuli such as cholestasis. To that could be added pruritus which is of mixed origin, and that which has a largely psychogenic origin [8].

The itch of cutaneous origin shares much of its neural pathway with the sensation of pain. Like pain, pruritus of neurogenic origin is transmitted through C fibres. It is now clear that these are specifically evolved for the transmission of

itch. They do not respond, as pain fibres do, to mechanical stimuli but to a number of 'pruritogens' including histamine and acetylcholine. Itch can therefore be seen, not as a low level experience of pain, but a specific modification of it. Its evolutionary significance is not clear.

Another way to categorise types of pruritus is to distinguish between those that result from direct stimulation of these itch specific C fibres (by histamine itself or a small number of other transmitters [8] and causes that are indirect by causing histamine release. It is important to note that while histamine is an important direct stimulator of C fibres it is not the only one. Others include papain, kallikrein and interleukin-2. Even acetylcholine can cause itch through directly stimulating C fibres, though interestingly only in atopic individuals [9].

The observation that specific 5HT3 receptor antagonists such as ondansetron can relieve itch [10,11] revealed that serotonin can cause pruritus associated with opioid therapy. Peripherally, serotonin is known to act indirectly through the release of histamine in skin mast cells [12,13]. The extent to which histamine is involved in pruritus associated with opioids, if indeed it is involved at all, is far from clear [8,14].

Management

As with all symptoms, a rational approach to the management of pruritus requires a structured assessment based on history, examination and laboratory findings. Given their similar pathophysiology, it is perhaps not surprising that an assessment of pruritus should be along the same lines as that of pain. This should start with noting precipitating or relieving factors. The quality of the subjective experience can sometimes include, for example, a burning sensation or that of ants crawling over the affected area (formication). The location and any radiation of the sensation should be noted, and perhaps some measure of its severity. The timing of the symptom can be helpful, whether it is worse during the day or during the night, or whether intermittent or continuous. More specific causes may be identified by taking a thorough drug and travel history.

Examination findings that may point to a cause would include findings of eczema, scabies or jaundice. Psychogenic pruritus should also be considered.

Invasive laboratory investigations are often unnecessary or inappropriate in the palliative phase, but can for example confirm a presumptive diagnosis of pruritus due to cholestatic jaundice. Pruritus can be an early presenting sign of relapse in some lymphomas.

If there is an obvious cause, such as dry skin, this should be managed appropriately. Management can be considered under non-specific and specific approaches.

Specific measures

Opioid induced

Opioids can induce itch by at least two, apparently unrelated, mechanisms. Intradermal injection of some opioids, including morphine, will cause a typical histamine-like response that is not observed in opioids of a different class such as fentanyl [15]. This localized itch and response is suppressed by H1 antihistamines [16].

More generalized itch is a complication that occurs in some children receiving opioids systemically. In adults, the proportion has been put at 1% [17] but anecdotally it is more frequent in children. It is often manifest by the child repeatedly rubbing the tip of his or her nose. It is not clear why this should be the apparent location of opioid induced itching, nor why it should be commoner in children, but the phenomenon has also been observed in adults [18]. Pruritus is more likely in association with opioids given by the spinal route [17]. This is a relatively uncommon route in paediatric palliative medicine and there are no data yet to compare with other routes.

It is currently felt that pruritus associated with systemic opioids is not caused by histamine [8]. It may be that morphine can stimulate itch through mu receptors while at the same time suppressing it through kappa receptors [19]. Good evidence for the role of opioid receptors is the observation that naloxone will relieve the itch [20] but H1 antihistamines will not. Serotonin clearly plays a part, since serotonin antagonist ondansetron can prevent as well as relieve some opioid induced pruritus [10,21]. Given their familiarity to paediatricians, and their benign side-effect profile, it seems appropriate to consider serotonin antagonists early to treat the problem in children. Opioid antagonists will also improve pruritus [22] but most also reverse analgesia. Nalbuphine appears to be the exception [23].

The mechanism of pruritus associated with opioid therapy is therefore complex. The observation, however, is that ondansetron and opioid antagonists such as naloxone are more likely to be effective than our traditional approach using H1 antihistamines.

Hodgkin's lymphoma

Pruritus is relatively common in terminal Hodgkin's disease. Steroids and vinblastine or other relatively non-toxic chemotherapy have been reported to be effective [8].

Uraemia

Pruritus associated with uraemia is multi-factorial in nature, including the effect of dry skin, cytokines and immunological mechanisms [8]. Uraemic patients with pruritus demonstrate raised numbers of mast cells [24–26] and electrolyte imbalances [27]. 'Imbalances' in opioid receptor subtype expression have been postulated [19].

None of these explanations is entirely satisfactory on its own, and there is an apparent contradiction in the consistent observation that histamine levels and numbers of mast cells are high, while H1 antihistamines are ineffective unless they sedate.

The opioid antagonist naltrexone has been studied [28,29] with inconsistent results. It has been suggested [8,28,29] that it may have a place in severe itch associated with uraemia.

Cholestasis

Severe cholestasis as a cause of itch is rather rare in children. In adults, cholestatic pruritus is described as typically commencing on the soles of the feet and the palms of the hands. The mechanism is not clear but is believed to be central [14,30].

In adults, there has been considerable research which suggests that opioid antagonists may have a useful role [31–34]. As always, if given to patients who are also receiving opioids, there is a risk that control of pain can be lost. There is some evidence of a paradoxical response of itch to opioids [35,36]. Drugs that induce hepatic enzymes such as rifampicin [37] and phenobarbital [38] can be effective although both can interfere with hepatic metabolism of other drugs. Phenobarbitone (phenobarbital) is quite widely used in paediatric palliative care for seizures and sedation. Cholestyramine (Colestyramine) has been used in primary biliary cirrhosis [39] on slender evidence [8,40]. It's effect depends on an intact enteropathic circulation of bile acids and therefore it is ineffective if the bile duct is completely obstructed.

Non-specific measures

Many children with life-limiting conditions have dry skin, related partly to their hydration status and partly to the nature of the underlying condition. This can often be helped using simple topical moisturising creams. There is further benefit to be gained through engaging the family and from the counter irritation of rubbing the cream into the skin.

Damage to the skin due to scratching itch is common, particularly among children with neurodegenerative conditions. The child's nails should be kept short, or if necessary in mittens, to reduce the likelihood of skin damage. Itch can be made worse by an environment that is too warm and carers for children with life-limiting conditions should ensure they are not overdressed and that the room temperature is kept reasonably cool. Treatment with ultraviolet B has many different actions [8] and should be considered in children with HIV AIDS or uraemia [41–43].

The pendulum has somewhat swung away from the traditional approach of prescribing an H1 antihistamine, irrespective of the cause of itch. It has been suggested that H1 antihistamines are effective only if they are also significantly sedating, or if the itch is specifically histamine mediated. However, as always in paediatric palliative care, it is important to have an empiric approach to fall back on if more evidence-based approaches such as those outlined earlier in this section have failed.

Although calamine lotion (another paediatric favourite) is more reliably effective due to its phenol content, as it evaporates it can dry the skin which can make pruritus worse. Capsaicin cream is rarely used in children partly because of the mild burning sensation it causes when first used, but can be effective in some sorts of itch [44]. There are also a number of topical H1 antihistamines such as diphenhydramine.

Summary

An approach to pruritus is similar to many of the other symptoms considered in this book that complicate the palliative phase of children with life-limiting conditions. It is often possible to develop a rational and evidence based initial approach, taking into account the probable cause for itch and its pathophysiology. If this first line therapy fails, however, it is important to consider less specific and more empiric approaches such as topical drugs and H1 antihistamines, bearing in mind that these may carry only a small chance of success and bring with them inevitable side-effects.

Pressure sores

The skin is richly innervated, and when it becomes damaged is a powerful source of pain. Furthermore, the impact of skin breakdown on body image can have profound emotional and psychological impact [45]. Managing pressure sores is therefore of critical importance in maintaining good symptom control and quality of life in general in palliative care.

Evaluation of risk

Children with life-limiting conditions are particularly susceptible to skin breakdown. Six groups of factors that can influence the likelihood of a pressure sore have been identified in adults [46,47]. They include sensory perception, skin moisture, activity, mobility, risk of friction and shear, and finally nutritional status. The nature of life-limiting conditions in childhood means that children needing palliative care will be at risk simultaneously of many of these. Those with non-malignant diseases are typically relatively immobile, needing frequent changes of position by carers, each of which risks friction or shear damage to the skin (shear damage occurs

when the skin adheres to an external surface such as bedding while underlying tissue moves [46]. Prolonged moistness is also common: there may be contact with urine soaked nappies or bedding, and hyperhidrosis is a feature of many metabolic conditions in childhood. Furthermore, many children with life-limiting conditions suffer from mild nutritional deficiencies due to practical difficulties with oral or gastrostomy feeding.

Assessment of risk factors for pressure sores is an important step in reducing the likelihood that they will occur. Such an assessment has been formalized in a number of instruments, of which the Braden Scale is probably the best validated [46,48–50]. All these studies were carried out in an adult population, but the Braden Scale has been modified for use with children [51]. It has been observed [52] that this paediatric 'Braden Q Scale' does not always accurately identify those at risk in acute hospital paediatric settings.

Assessment of severity

The single term 'pressure sore' or 'pressure ulcer' is used to cover a wide range of damage, varying from the trivial to the life-threatening. The term is therefore of little practical help without further elaboration. A staging system has been devised [53]. Stage 1 simply describes intact skin which has become reddened and is distinguished from a normal response to pressure only in that the erythema is not blanchable.

At stage 2, there is partial thickness skin loss which involves the epidermis and dermis itself. The sore is very superficial, however, and may appear as a blister or shallow ulcer.

Stage 3 pressure sores have loss of the full thickness of skin and some damage or even necrosis to subcutaneous tissues. It looks like a deep crater but does not penetrate underlying fascia.

By the time stage 4 is reached, the most severe form of pressure sore, there is extensive destruction including tissue necrosis and damage to underlying tissues such as muscle, bone, tendons or joint capsules [2].

Clinical management

Where possible, it is clearly desirable to avoid pressure sores developing in the first place. Good nursing care, and in particular regular inspection of the skin over bony prominences and other pressure points, is essential. Prompt intervention to avoid prolonged moistness, infection or immobility can reduce the risk. Simple measures such as regular turning (as appropriate) of the patient and use of pressure relieving mattresses such as Spenco and sheepskin bedding should be considered as an essential part of the care programme. Where moistness of the skin is inevitable, barrier creams or ointments can be helpful to maintain an environment in which the skin can heal. Careful attention to the child's nutritional status in consultation with dieticians can be important.

During a prolonged palliative phase, a child will usually be at home for most of the time, and the main carers will be the rest of the family, particularly parents, rather than nursing staff. The family may need education in avoiding risk factors and prompt recognition of early skin problems.

The likelihood that a pressure sore will heal is related to the stage. Many stage 1 pressure sores will return to normal skin if carefully managed. This is less likely if the pressure sore has reached stage 4 [54]. Stage is probably less clearly related to the risk of severe symptoms: even superficial sores can be extremely painful.

Pressure sores may give rise to physical symptoms in two main ways:

i Pain: Even a superficial pressure sore can be extremely painful, to an extent that is often disproportionate to its size. In children who appear to be pain but are not able to express an exact location, such as those with impaired cognitive function, it is always important to consider an early pressure sore as the cause. The management of pain has been considered in detail in a separate chapter (cross ref Chapter 21, Pain). The pain of pressure sores is sharp, intense and well localised but there is often an area of hyperalgesia extending well beyond any obvious skin damage. The pain is usually responsive to simple analgesia and opioids, but these should always be offered alongside measures designed to promote skin healing.

There has been increasing interest over recent years in the use of topical analgesics, particularly major opioids, for managing the pain of more serious ulcers [1,2]. Typically, 2.5 mg–5 mg of diamorphine are mixed with the preferred topical base.

ii Odour: Superinfection of any skin lesion can cause odour. This can be extremely distressing for patient and family alike and should be rigorously treated if possible. Odour is often caused by anaerobic organisms and systemic metronidazole can be very effective. Metronidazole too has been used topically [4–6] with good effect and less risk of systemic toxicity such as nausea and vomiting.

Ordinary measures such as maintaining cleanliness, always avoiding extreme abrasion and soaps that are strongly alkaline, are also important in reducing the risk of skin damage and infection.

Epidermolysis bullosa and other life-limiting conditions of the skin

Life-limiting skin disorders include:

Restrictive dermopathy, which is a very rare, fatal autosomal recessive genodermatosis, in which tautness of a translucent thin skin is the major clinical sign. The skin is highly vulnerable to tears and all reported cases have been born prematurely. The appearance of skin at birth is thin and shiny and it restricts limb movements and respiratory effort. Early neonatal death results from respiratory insufficiency, as the chest is unable to expand due to constriction from the skin [55].

The ichthyoses are a group of diseases characterised by disorders of cornification. The most severe forms cause a restrictive encasement of skin and affected infants are referred to as 'collodion babies'. A severe form is the harlequin baby, which used to be incompatible with life due to restriction of respiratory effort by the skin. However it has been found to respond to treatment with oral acitrecin and indeed early management could prevent life-threatening events such as temperature dysregulation, disturbance in electrolytes and serious infections [56].

Neu-laxova syndrome is a rare disorder characterised by microcephaly, limb contractures and ichthyosis. Other frequently found features include pulmonary, renal and cardiac abnormalities. Neu-Laxova is a lethal condition; most of the infants have been stillborn or died within the first few days. Those surviving the neonatal period have not lived more than four months with death resulting from pneumonia or respiratory failure [57].

The main focus of this section will be to discuss the largest of this group, EB, but many of the principles can be applied to the care of other serious skin conditions.

EB sub-types and their prognosis

Epidermolysis bullosa is characterized by extreme fragility of the skin and mucosa and its susceptibility to blister and separate from the underlying tissue in response to minimal every day friction and trauma (Figure 28.1).

There are three main categories within the group: simplex, junctional and dystrophic, each varying in severity.

The recessively inherited types of EB, include junctional EB and recessive dystrophic EB and are the most severe. Although there is a wide spectrum of severity within this group many children are severely affected leading to serious morbidity and mortality. The incidence of recessively inherited EB is 1 : 175000 [58].

The most serious type of junctional EB is the Herlitz form. Blistering is generally present at birth or develops within the first few days of life and initially this often presents as a mild form of EB but disease progression can be rapid. It is important that, before the parents are informed, diagnosis is confirmed by analysis of a skin biopsy at a centre experienced in this investigation. Death usually occurs within the first few years of life, with many not surviving beyond the first few months. In this group of children, a support network should

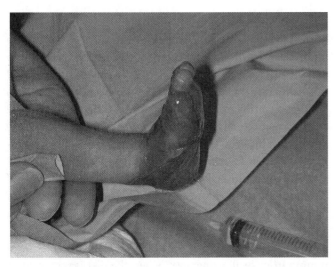

Fig. 28.1 Intrauterine damage in a neonate with a severe bullous skin disorder.

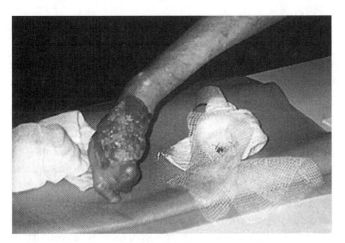

Fig. 28.2 Advanced squamous cell carcinoma in an adolescent.

be formed with the community team, in order to initiate palliative care at the onset of diagnosis.

Recessive dystrophic EB in its severe form, Hallopeau-Siemens results in multiple complications. There is a tendency for blistered areas and wounds to heal with scarring leading to the development of contractures.

Although it is unusual for those affected to die in infancy, the contractures lead to progressive and permanent disability. The survivors of childhood are also at risk of an aggressive form of squamous cell carcinoma as young adults and indeed it has been reported in a child of 13 years [59] (Figure 28.2). There are often multiple primary tumours and the average life expectancy after the tumour diagnosis is 5 years. In this subtype, our approach in the United Kingdom is to establish links with the community multi disciplinary team from diagnosis, including respite provision at a children's hospice.

When required, palliative care can be offered from those who know the child and their family. It is extremely beneficial, if a videotape of the dressing techniques specific for each individual child is supplied as part of their care plan, when admitted for hospice care. It is important that genetic counselling is offered to families following diagnosis, in order that they are aware of prenatal diagnosis for future pregnancies.

Symptoms and their management in EB

Children with life-limiting skin disorders such as EB experience a variety of symptoms which present in a multi-system manner.

Pain

From animal studies of EB, it appears that even in the fetal period, repeated disruption to the skin from minimal trauma within the uterus, leads to skin nerve damage and increased production of nerve growth factor (NGF). This subsequently produces hyperinnervation of the peripheral sensory nerves and hyperalgesia ensues (an exaggerated response to a normal noxious stimulus [60]). Hyperalgesia means that minimal trauma and normal tactile actions, such as hugging, can lead to both acute and chronic inflammatory pain in children with skin disorders.

Pain (see also Chapter 21, Pain management) is individual and encompasses not only the physical sensation but also cultural, social, emotional aspects [61]. This needs to be considered when assessing a baseline pain score of any child who has a chronic illness.

Procedural pain in patients with EB is a major source for pain. In addition, for procedures such as the dressing change or baths, which may occur on a daily basis, the patient appears to have enormous anticipatory fear, which needs to be considered in addition to the actual pain experienced. In fact in some children, bathing is impossible even with adequate analgesia because the exposure of all the wounds simultaneously and pain from being lifted in and out of the bath is unbearable.

Table 28.1 Sources of pain in EB

Acute	Chronic
Bullae/Wounds	Inflammatory pain
Reflux	Neuropathic pain
Dental	Osteoporosis
Corneal ulcers	Constipation
Anal fissures	Contractures
Procedural	

The first steps of managing pain, is to assess and formulate a baseline pain score. Prevention of the symptoms such as constipation, osteoporosis and gastroesophageal reflux may be possible with appropriate medication as discussed under the symptoms. Treating superficial skin infections, which seem to exacerbate acute pain, with topical or oral antibiotics is important. Good dressing techniques and regular dressing changes are necessary.

When analgesia is required for mild pain, for example, small blisters requiring a quick dressing change, combining simple analgesia such as paracetamol with a non-steroidal, for example, ibuprofen or piroxicam melt (which just requires once daily administration: 20 mg/melt), is usually sufficient. However with more severe pain associated with dressing changes or baths, opioid analgesia and anxiolytic sedation such as midazolam is usually necessary. In this case, doses of oral morphine should be in the range of 0.3–0.6 mg/kg and midazolam, 0.5 mg/kg given around 30–45 min prior to the procedure [62]. Procedural pain has also been managed by novel methods of analgesia such as Entonox [63] and fentanyl lozenges [64]. Both approaches have the advantage that the child should be able to administer the analgesia to him or herself.

However with Entonox, (nitrous oxide) there have concerns regarding potential for abuse because it is known to be a habit forming drug [65]. It is also known to inactivate vitamin B12 and repeated use affects folate metabolism, impairing DNA synthesis and causing megaloblastic changes in the bone marrow [66].

For the chronic background pain administration of long acting morphine (MST or) on a daily basis may be required . Pain in EB is partly neuropathic in origin and may be relatively opioid-resistant. It may respond to a low dose of amitriptyline, nocte (0.5 mg /kg) [67]. It may take up to two weeks to be effective, it is anticholingergic and there have been reports of blurred visions as an adverse effect. Gabapentin [68], an anticonvulsant drug used in epilepsy, has also been used to manage the neuropathic pain in children. This has an advantage over amitriptyline as it has no interaction with any other medication and it has virtually no reported adverse effects. Well controlled randomised studies are necessary to investigate the efficacy and safety of these agents against pediatric neuropathic pain. Children with lethal skin conditions may also require opioid analgesics, anxiolytic and sedative drugs, often via a syringe driver, when they reach the terminal phase of their illness.

It is essential that as well as the above pharmacological therapies physical treatments such as physiotherapy and hydrotherapy, visualisation and guided imagery should be offered in combination to manage a child's acute and chronic pain.

Gastrointestinal

Blistering may form internally throughout the entire gastrointestinal tract, extending from the oropharyngeal region making eating an unpleasant and painful experience. The oral mucosa is very fragile and blisters readily occur in response to sucking or eating even soft foods. Breast—feeding is possible and causes minimal trauma to the mucosa, but friction of the face against the breast can result in blistering. Feeding is therefore a major problem from a very young age.

In dystrophic EB, the tongue becomes fused to the base of the mouth making mastication and removal of debris from the teeth difficult. In time, the repeated blistering and scarring lead to loss of the labial sulcus and microstomia.

Blistering in the lining of the oesophagus, results from trauma from swallowing, even when the diet is restricted to soft foods. This is acutely distressing for the child and gastro-oesophageal reflux as well as the formation of webs and strictures ensues.

In the Herlitz subtype, in addition to the problem with feeding, affected infants suffer malabsorption leading to profound failure to thrive even when intake is optimal. This is one of the most distressing components of the disease, as parents watch their child starve. It is not unusual for infants of several months old to die weighing less than their birth-weight.

Measures to improve eating and nutrition include use of specialised teats such as those recommended for infants with cleft lip and palate reduce the need for vigorous sucking and limit trauma to the oral mucosa.

Despite such measures infants often remain reluctant to feed due to pain from intra oral blisters and require analgesia prior to feeding. Use of teething gels can improve comfort. In order to provide adequate nutritional support needed because of the increased requirements and competition for nutrients between wound healing and growth, the insertion of gastrostomy tubes may be necessary in those with severe dystrophic EB [69]. In the longer-term survivors of junctional EB, feeding via a gastrostomy has led to breakdown of the skin on the abdomen with exacerbation from leakage of acid gastrointestinal contents around the device.

Gastroesophageal reflux occurs in severe EB and is usually managed by a combination of medication including, gaviscon, ranitidine or omeprazole and domperidone. Oesophageal strictures are also a feature of dystrophic EB and these can be exacerbated by reflux. Strictures may be successfully relieved using balloon dilatation under expert radiological guidance [70].

At the lower end of the gastrointestinal tract, pain from perianal blistering leads to withholding of stool and faecal retention. This is a common feature in all types of EB. Management is by use of stool softeners and laxatives and adding soluble fibre to supplementary feeds (Figure 28.3).

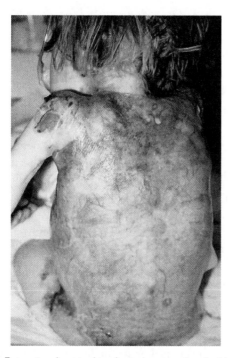

Fig. 28.3 Extensive chronic skin ulceration associated with cachexia.

Respiratory

Herlitz junctional EB may also affect the larynx with bullae formation [71]. This is characterised by a hoarse cry in the first few days or weeks of life and subsequently recurrent attacks of stridor occur, each episode carrying a great risk of asphyxiation. Acute stridor responds to nebulised budesenide and oral dexamethasone. However, this is a palliative measure to reduce respiratory distress and has no effect on survival.

Tracheostomy has successfully been carried out in severely affected infants, and may be considered a palliative measure to provide comfort. In the presence of failure to thrive, it is unlikely to alter outcome. Ulceration commonly occurs around the tube and beneath the securing ties. Respiratory tract infections are common in this group of children and may lead to death from pneumonia. Short courses of oral antibiotics may provide short-term resolution of symptoms.

Cardiac

A small number of children with severe EB develop a fatal dilated cardio myopathy [72]. The cause for this is unclear and routine echocardiograms are carried out at regular intervals to monitor the progress.

The child may become tired and tachypnoeic due to a decrease in flow of oxygenated blood from the heart, associated with peripheral oedema. This is exacerbated by fragility of the skin, leading to a progression in the number of open wounds, providing much distress for the child and family.

Occasionally acute chest pain secondary to ischemia may ensue.

This can be managed with conventional diuretics, low flow oxygen therapy and often may require the use of strong analgesia such as morphine. It is often important to reduce anxiety in the patients by providing adequate sedation or an anxiolytic such as diazepam.

Anaemia

This is a common and troublesome symptom in children with a skin disorder, in which there is inadequate nutritional intake, but also as a result of chronic blood loss from skin and mucosa. It is most commonly iron deficiency anaemia but normocytic normochromic anaemia may also exist. Symptoms include fatigue, pallor and if it is acutely severe, the child may have signs to suggest a hyperdynamic circulation such as tachycardia and a systolic cardiac murmur. Treatment can include dietary advice, oral iron supplements, intravenous iron and blood transfusions. It is important to judge the management of each patient individually in conjunction with the family; the use of repeated transfusions of blood and iron may not be appropriate.

Renal

Renal complications, although rare, have been described in dystrophic and junctional EB.

Chronic post—infectious glomerulonephritis most probably secondary to streptococcal skin infection has been described in dystrophic EB. Nephropathy is a recognised complication of recessive dystrophic EB and this may be secondary to renal amyloidosis and can be fatal [73].

End-stage renal failure is when the glomerular filtration rate is < 10 ml /min/1.73 m^2. Clinically, the main features are growth failure, anaemia, osteodystrophy leading to severe bone pain and hypertension.

Management of these symptoms include expert nutritional advice, which is mainly protein restriction; 1-alpha—hydroxycholcalciferol (hydroxycholecalciferol) supplement for the renal osteodystrophy and sodium bicarbonate if metabolic acidosis persists. Eyrthropoietin and growth hormone injections can also be considered to manage the anaemia and growth failure.

Peritoneal dialysis and haemodialysis is used to achieve control of biochemical abnormalities but the ultimate control of renal failure is transplantation. Children who receive live donor transplants usually have 90% 1-year-graft survival.

Following transplant, growth is improved and indeed the overall quality of life. However a renal transplant is not a cure and in children who have already a life limiting skin disorder, it is vital to give an alternative active choice of symptom control.

Psychological distress

The birth of a child with severe skin disease can be a distressing perinatal experience. For the family to survive emotionally the initial shock of seeing their baby with open wounds, and the guilt of passing on a previously unknown disease requires support and understanding from all those in contact with them. In view of this, parents of children with rare conditions such as EB should attend a designated centre where questions can be answered and staff has knowledge of the condition, its complications and recommended treatments.

Paediatric community nurses can offer support with dressing changes, but the child often prefers family help to professional help. Large quantities of expensive dressing and enteral feeding materials need to be stored in the family home. Parents are typically in a state of constant anxiety, both about the cost and that there will be disruption in their supply of dressings, with disastrous consequences.

Even from an early age, children with any dermatological disorder are conscious that they are different from their peers because of their physical appearance. In those with dystrophic EB the knowledge that their condition is progressively disabling can lead to depression as they realise loss of previously mastered skills and developmental milestones. They become anxious about school and socialising and it may even cause depression, to such an extent that compliance, especially during the adolescent period, can be a huge problem. In this group of patients, screening for squamous cell carcinoma may not be permitted in a hospital setting and home visiting, in order to allow dressings to take place in familiar surroundings, with respect for privacy is often necessary.

Education

Prior to entry of a child with fragile skin into playgroup or school, everyone who will be in contact with the child should receive advice regarding handling. This must include those involved in transporting the child to and from school.

Children with severe skin disease generally attend mainstream schools, but require input from a non-teaching assistant in order to achieve their full potential and to avoid any unnecessary trauma.

Simple measures such as leaving the classroom immediately before or after the end of the lesson reduce the risk of knocks or shearing forces in crowded corridors. Care-assistants can carry heavy books for the mobile child or are required to push wheel-chairs for more severely affected children.

Provision of a lap top computer or a scribe ensure work is recorded even when the child's hand function may be impaired.

Carers should be trained to apply dressings if the child has an accident during school hours and this releases the burden on parents who may otherwise be called to the school.

Prior to school entry, teaching and non-teaching staff should be offered training by a specialised nurse and written guidelines given.

Mobility

Severe hand deformity in recessive dystrophic EB results from repetitive trauma leading to scarring, contractures and pseudo-syndactyly [74]. Functional improvement of the hand can be achieved by surgical release and application of skin grafts. Following surgery light-weight splints are given to try to maintain function. Unfortunately the effects of surgery are often short-lived before the hand contracts again. Children often become disenchanted with surgery and refuse further intervention.

Progressive scarring in those with dystrophic EB gradually reduces mobility and in combination with a reluctance to move and weight-bear due to pain, children may suffer with osteoporosis [75]. Severe bony pain has been treated with intravenous pamidronate along with calcium supplementation but the efficacy of bisphosphonates in this context has not yet been definitively shown. Children may become dependent on a wheel-chair and it is important that the child is encouraged to retain some mobility, for example being able to transfer in order to avoid excessive lifting at a risk of further skin damage (Figure 28.4).

General principles of skin care in EB

Dressings

Children with severe skin disorders form develop large areas of chronic ulceration, which are often difficult to heal. Whilst wound management is always with the intention of healing, in reality this is often not achievable. In reality dressings should be chosen which would not lead to further ulceration and cause no harm to the surrounding skin.

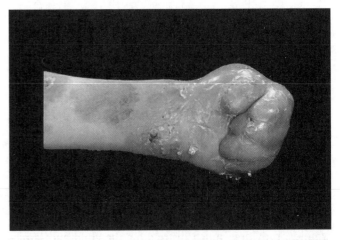

Fig. 28.4 Typical distal skin limb deformity in a child with dystrophic EB.

The correct dressing should cause minimal pain on removal. Whilst many dressings are advertised as non-adherent there are only a small number, which are truly atraumatic when used on children with fragile skin.

Dressing changes can take several hours and should be kept to a minimum in order to limit pain and distress. If there is copious exudate, this can be managed by leaving a primary dressing in place and changing the secondary dressing more frequently.

Some children or their carers prefer to use Vaseline gauze or tulle dressings, but these require changing daily as this carries the risk of removal of new epithelium if there has been any adherence and additional distress due to frequent changes of dressing.

Even if removal of dressing is pain free, exposure of the wound is painful and changes of dressings should be done as quickly as possible. When the pattern of the wounds is known, dressings can be pre-cut to speed the procedure.

Dressing changes are considered to be a 'clean' rather than 'sterile procedure'. Wearing gloves can drag on the skin and cause unnecessary trauma, as well as carrying the risk of distressing the child and making them feel dirty and unattractive.

Infection is a common problem with resistant infections being increasingly seen. Surprisingly septicaemia is rarely described in this group of children unless this is secondary to infection from an indwelling central line.

Handling the child with severe skin disease

Handling should be kept to a minimum whilst enabling contact with the infant or child. Parents and other carers should be taught how to lift the children without causing skin damage from friction or shearing forces. Small infants should be lifted using a 'roll and lift technique'. The infant is rolled onto his side, one hand placed on the buttocks, and the other behind the head, or neck if scalp lesions are present; the infant is then rolled back onto the carer's hands and lifted in one movement.

Older children can be lifted with one hand under their bottom and the other behind the head or neck. The children prefer to move themselves and this should be encouraged when ever possible to avoid skin damage.

No child with fragile skin should ever be lifted under the arms, as this leads to skin loss in an area, which is difficult to dress and has a tendency to heal with stricture formation in those with dystrophic EB.

Name bands cannot be worn as these cause friction and denudes the skin over the ankle or wrist; however labels can be applied over clothing or on the cot or bed.

Despite their skin fragility, children should be able to enjoy gentle cuddles, and kisses will do no harm (Figure 28.5).

Conclusion

Caring for children with life-limiting skin disorders poses a challenge for all involved in their management. It is essential that all professionals involved are familiar with the disease process and the particular symptoms which may arise, in order to provide multidimensional care in accordance with the child and family's request.

Most professionals working in paediatric palliative care will encounter such primary skin diseases only relatively infrequently. Much more often, they will be faced with the need to manage symptoms in the skin that arise from other, more general systemic LLC. The range of these is very wide: this chapter has provided an overview of the pathophysiology and management of some of the commoner symptoms that may manifest in the skin.

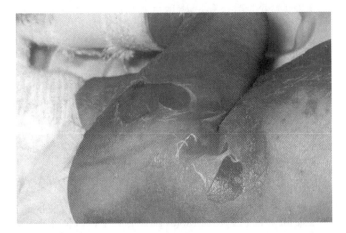

Fig. 28.5 Trauma secondary to minimal handling in an infant with fragile skin.

References

1. Grocott P. Palliative management of fungating malignant wounds. *J Commun Nurs* 2000;14(3):31–40.

2. Flock P. Pilot study to determine the effectiveness of diamorphine gel to control pressure ulcer pain. *J Pain Symptom Manage* 2003; 25(6):547–54.

3. Beynon T., Laverty, D., Baxter, A., *et al*. Lutro gel: A potential role in wounds? *J Pain Symptom Manage* 2003;26(2):776–80.

4. Poteete, V. Case study: Eliminating odors from wounds. *Decubitus* 1993;6(4):43–6.

5. Gomolin, I.H. and Brandt, J.L. Topical metronidazole therapy for pressure sores of geriatric patients. *J Am Geriatr Soc* 1983; 31(11):710–2.

6. Haisfield-Wolfe, M.E. and Rund, C. Malignant cutaneous wounds: A management protocol. *Ostomy Wound Manage* 1997;43(1): 56–60, 62, 64–6.

7. Haffenreffer, S., and Rothman, S.F. Physiology of itching. *Physiological Reviews* 1941;21:357–81.

8. Twycross, R., Greaves, M.W., Handwerker, H., Jones, E.A., Libretto, S.E., Szepietowski, J.C., et al. Itch: Scratching more than the surface. Q J Med 2003;96:7–26.

9. Heyer, G.R. and Hornstein, O.P. Recent studies of cutaneous nociception in atopic and non-atopic subjects. J Dermatol 1999;26:77–86.

10. Borgeat, A. and Stimemann, H.-R. Ondansetron is effective to treat spinal or epidural morphine-induced pruritus. Anesthesiology 1999;90:432–6.

11. Kyriakides, K., Hussain, S.K., and Hobbs, G.J. Management of opioid-induced pruritus: a role for 5Ht antagonists? Br J Anaesthesia 1999;82:439–41.

12. Hagermark, O. Peripheral and central mediators of itch. Skin Pharmacol 1992;5:1–8.

13. Weisshaar, E., Ziethen, B., Rohl, F.W., and Gollnick H. The anti-pruritic effect of a 5HT3 receptor antagonist (tropisetron) is dependent on mast cell depletion: An experimental study. Exp Dermatol 1999;8(254–60).

14. Jones, E.A. and Bergasa, N.V. The pruritus of cholestasis. Hepatology 1999;29:1003–6.

15. Hermens, J.M., Ebertz, J.M., Hanifin, J.M., and Hirshman C.A. Comparison of histamine release in human skin mast cells induced by morphine, fentanyl, and oxymorphone. Anesthesiology 1985; 62:124–9.

16. Saucedo, R. and Erill, S. Morphine-induced skin wheals: A possible model for the study of histamine release. Clin Pharmacol Therapeut 1985;38:365–70.

17. Ballantyne, J.C., Loach, A.B., and Carr, D.B. The incidence of pruritus after epidural morphine. Anaesthesia 1989;44:863.

18. Ballantyne, JC, Loach, A.B., and Carr, D.B. Itching after epidural and spinal opiates. Pain 1988;33:149–60.

19. Kumagai, H., Utsumi, J., and Suzuki, T. Endogenous opioid system in uraemic patients. Br J Clinical Pharmacology; abstracts of the joint meeting of VII World Confe Clin Pharmacol Therapeut IUPHAR 2000;282.

20. Kuraishi, Y., Yamaguchi, T., and Miyamoto, T. Itch-scratch responses induced by opioids through central mu opioid receptors in mice. J Biomed Sci 2000;7:248–52.

21. Yeh, H.M., Chen, L.K., Lin, C.J., Chan, W.H., Chen, Y.P., Lin, C.S., et al. Prophylactic intravenous ondansetron reduces the incidence of intrathecal morphine-induced pruritus in patients undergoing cesarean delivery. Anesth Analg 2000;91:172–5.

22. Kjellberg, F. and Tramer, M. Pharmacological control of opioid-induced pruritus: A quantitative systematic review of randomized trials. Eur Anaesthe 2001;18:346–57.

23. Cohen, S., Ratner, E., Kreitzman, T., Archer, J., and Mignano, L. Nalbuphine is better than naloxone for treatment of side effects after epidural morphine. Anesthes analg 1992;75:747–52.

24. Matsumoto, M., Ichimam, K., and Horie, A. Pruritus and mast cell proliferation of the skin in end stage renal failure. Clin Nephrol 1985;23:285–8.

25. Leong, S.O., Tann, C.C., Lye, W.C., Lee, E.J., and Chan, H.L. Dermal mast cell density and pruritus in end-stage renal failure. Ann Acad Med Singapore 1994;23(327–9).

26. Szepietowski, J.C., Thepen, T., vanVloten, W.A., Szepietowski, T., and Bihari, I.C. Pruritus and mast cell proliferation in the skin of haemodialysis patients. Inflam Res 1995;44(Suppl.1):S84–5.

27. Blachley, J.D., Blankenship, D.M., Menter, A., Parker, T.F., and Knochel, J.P. Uremic pruritus: Skin divalent ion content and response to ultraviolet phototherapy. Am J Kidney Dis 1985; 5:236–41.

28. Pauli-Magnus, C., Mikus, G., Alscher, D., Kirschner, T., Nagel, W., Gugeler N., et al. Naltrexone does not relieve uremic pruritus. J Am Soc Nephrol 2000;11:514–9.

29. Peer, G., Kivity, S., Agami, O., Fireman, E., Silverberg, D., Blum M., et al. Randomised crossover trial of naltrexone in uraemic pruritus. Lancet 1996;348:1552–4.

30. Bergasa, N.V. and Jones, E.A. The pruritus of cholestasis: Potential pathogenic and therapeutic implications of opioids. Gastroenterology 1995;108:1582–8.

31. Bergasa, N.V., Alling, D.W., Talbot, T.L., Swain, M.G., Yurdaydin, C., Turner M.L., et al. Effects of naloxone infusions in patients with the pruritus of cholestasis. Ann Intern Med 1995;123:161–7.

32. Bergasa, N.V., Talbot, T.L., Alling, D.W., Schmitt, J.M., Walker, E.F., Baker, B.L., et al. A controlled trial of naloxone infusions for the pruritus of chronic cholestasis. Gastroenterology 1992;102:544–9.

33. Bergasa, N.V., Schmitt, J.M., Talbot, T.L., Alling, D.W., Swain, M.G., Turner, M.L., et al. Open-label trial of oral nalmefene therapy for the pruritus of cholestasis. Hepatology 1998;27:679–84.

34. Bergasa, N.V., Alling, D.W., Talbot, T.L., Wells, M.C., and Jones, E.A. Oral nalmefene therapy reduces scratching activity due to the pruritus of cholestasis: A controlled study. J Am Acad Dermatol 1999;41:431–4.

35. Zylicz, Z. and Krajnik, M. Codeine for pruritus in primary biliary cirrhosis. Lancet 1999;353:813.

36. Juby, L., Wong, V., and Losowsky, M. Buprenorphine and hepatic pruritus. Br J Clin Pract 1994;48:331.

37. Ghent, C. and Carruthers, S. Treatment of pruritus in primary biliary cirrhosis with rifampin: Results of a double-blind crossover randomized trial. Gastroenterology 1988;94:488–93.

38. Bloomer, J. and Boyer, J. Phenobarbital effects in cholestatic liver disease. Ann Intern Med 1975;82:310–17.

39. Carey, J. Lowering of serum bile acid concentrations and relief of pruritus in jaundiced patients fed a bile acid sequestering resin. J Lab Clin Med 1960;56:797–8.

40. Datta, D. and Sherlock, S. Cholestyramine for long term relief of the pruritus complicating intrahepatic cholestasis. Gastroenterology 1966;50:323–32.

41. Saltzer, E. and Grove, G. Relief from uremic patients: A therapeutic approach: Cutis 1975;16:298–9.

42. Gilchrest, B., Rowe, J., Brown R., Steinman, T., and Arndt, K. Relief of uremic pruritus with ultraviolet phototherapy. N Engl J Med 1997;297:136–8.

43. Lim, H., Vallurupalli, S., Meola, T., and Soter, N. UVB photo-therapy is an effective treatment for pruritus in patients infected with HIV. J Am Acad Dermatol 1997;37:414–17.

44. Breneman, D., Cardone, J., Blumsack, R., Lather, R., Searle, E., and Pollack, V. Topical capsaicin for treatment of hemodialysis-related pruritus 1992.

45. Magnan M.A. Psychological considerations for patients with acute wounds. Crit Care Nurs Clin No Am 1996;8(2):183–193.

46. Bergstrom, N., Braden, B., Laguzza, A., and Holman V. The Braden scale for predicting pressure sore risk. Nurs Res 1987;36(4):205–209.

47. Horn, S.D., Bender, S.A., Ferguson, M.L., Smout, R.J., Bergstrom, N., Taler, G., et al. The National Pressure Ulcer Long-Term Care

Study: Pressure ulcer development in long-term care residents. *J Am Geriatr Soc* 2004;52(3):359–67.

48. Bergstrom, N., Braden, B. Kemp, M. Champagne M. and Ruby E. Multi-site study of incidence of pressure ulcers and the relationship between risk level, demographic characteristics, diagnoses, and prescription of preventive interventions. *J Am Geriat Soc* 1996;44:22–30.

49. VandenBosch, T., Montoye, C., Satwicz, M., Durkee-Leonard, K., and Boylan-Lewis, B. Predictive validity of the Braden scale and nurse perception in identifying pressure ulcer risk. *Appl Nurs Res* 1996;9(2):80–6.

50. Lyder, C.H., Yu, C., Emerling, J., Mangat, R., Stevenson D., Empleo-Frazier O, *et al.* The Braden Scale for pressure ulcer risk: Evaluating the predictive validity in Black and Latino/Hispanic elders. *Appl Nurs Res* 1999;12(2):60–8.

51. Quigley, S.M. and Curley, M.A. Skin integrity in the pediatric population: Preventing and managing pressure ulcers. *J Soc Pediatr Nurs* 1996;1(1):7–18.

52. Pallija, G., Mondozzi, M., and Webb A.A. Skin care of the pediatric patient. *J Pediatr Nurs* 1999;14(2):80–87.

53. Panel NPUA. Statement on pressure ulcer prevention. Silver Spring, MD: Agency for Health Care Policy and Research, 1992.

54. Cole L. and Nesbitt C. A three year multiphase pressure ulcer prevalence/incidence study in a regional referral hospital. *Ostomy Wound Manage* 2004;50(11):32–40.

55. Nijsten, T., De Moor, A., Colpaert, C., *et al.* Restrictive dermopathy: A case report and a critical review of hypotheses of its origin. *Pediatr Dermatol* 2002;19(1):67–72.

56. Saracoglu, Z., Tekin, N., Urer, S., *et al.* Oral acitretin treatment in severe congenital ichthyosis of the neonate. *Turk J Pediatr* 2002; 44(1):61–4.

57. Hickey, P., Piantanida, E., Lentz-Kapua, S., *et al.* Neu-laxova syndrome: A case report. *Pediat Dermatol* 2003;20(1):25–7.

58. Fine, J., Eady, R., Bauer E., *et al.* Revised classification system for inherited epidermolysis bullosa; report of the Second International Consensus Meeting on diagnosis and classification of epidermolysis bullosa. *J Am Acad Dermatol* 2000;42:1051–66.

59. Ayman, T., Yerebakan, O., Ciftcioglu, M., *et al.* A thirteen year old girl with recessive dystrophic epidermolysis bullosa presenting with squamous cell carcinoma. *Pediatr Dermatol* 2002;19: 436–8.

60. Constantinou, J., Reynolds, M., and Woolf C. Nerve growth factor levels in developing rat skin: up-regulation following skin wounding. *Neuroreport* 1994; 5: 2281–4.

61. IASP. Pain Terms: A list of definitions and notes on usage. *Pain* 1979;6(249–252).

62. Herod, J., Denyer, J., Goldman, A., *et al.* Epidermolysis bullosa in children: Pathophysiol, anaesthesia and pain management. *Paed Anaesthesia* 2002;12:388–97.

63. Kalach, N., Barbier, C., and Kohen, R., *et al.* Tolerance of nitrous oxide—oxygen sedation for painful procedures in emergency pediatrics. *Arch Pediatr* 2002;9(11):1213–5.

64. Prosser D., Allman M., and Grassby P. Oral transmucosal fentanyl. *Anaesthesia* 1998;53:1030.

65. Bruce, E. and Franck, L. Self-administered nitrous oxide for the management of procedural pain. *Paed nursing* 2000;12:15–19.

66. Nunn J. Clinical aspects of the interaction between nitrous oxide and vitamin B12. *Brit J of Anaesthesia* 1987;59:3–13.

67. Collins, J., Kerner, J., Sentivany, S., *et al.* Intravenous amitriptyline in pediatrics. *J Pain Sympt M* 1995;10:471–5.

68. Wheeler, D., Vaux, K., and Tam, D. Use of gabapentin in the treatment of childhood reflex sympathetic dustrophy. *Paed neurol* 2000;220–221.

69. Haynes, L., Atherton, D., Ade-Ajayi, N., *et al.* Gastrostomy and growth in dystrophic epidermolysis bullosa. *Br J Dermatol* 1996; 134(5):872–9.

70. Naehrlich L., Lang T., Schamberger U., *et al.* Balloon dilatation of an esophageal stenosis in a patient with recessive dystrophic epidermolysis bullosa. *Pediatr Dermatol* 2000;17(6):477–9.

71. Kenna M., Stool S., and Mallory S. Junctional epidermolysis bullosa of the larynx. *Pediatrics* 1986;78:172–4.

72. Sidwell R., Yates R., and Atherton D. Dilated cardiomyopathy in dystrophic epidermolysis bullosa. *Arch Dis Child* 2000;83(1):59–63.

73. Mann J., Zeier M., Zilow E., *et al.* The spectrum of renal involvement in epidermolysis bullosa dystrophica hereditaria: A report of two cases. *Am J Kidney Dis* 1988;11(5):437–41.

74. Fine, J.D., Johnson, L.B., Weiner, M., *et al.* Pseudosyndactyly and musculoskeletal contractures in inherited epidermolysis bullosa: experience of the National Epidermolysis Bullosa Registry 1986–2002. *Journal of Hand Surgery* 2005;30:14–22.

75. Kawaguchi M., Mitsuhasi Y., and Kondo S. Osteoporosis in a patient with recessive dystrophic epidermolys bullosa. *Br J Dermatol* 1999; 141(5):934–5.

29 Haematological symptoms

Erica Mackie and Marie-Louise Millard

Introduction

One of the principles that should underpin good palliative medicine in children, is that investigations and treatment should be used discriminatingly. In deciding what medications to prescribe, or investigations to order, we need to consider whether the net effect will be to the child's benefit.

The decision is often clear-cut. In prescribing morphine, the burden to most patients is small and the potential benefit, very significant. In managing haematological symptoms, however, things are not always as straightforward. For example, anaemia can have a profound impact on the quality of some children's lives, preventing them from socialising through its effect on fatigue, and even contributing to other symptoms such as shortness of breath. On the other hand, embarking on blood transfusion will often mean additional trips to the hospital, and blood tests that would, otherwise, be unnecessary.

The cellular components of blood are synthesized in the bone marrow. Bone marrow failure is a common, late complication of many life-limiting conditions, particularly malignancies. This chapter considers how the symptoms caused by bone marrow failure can be identified, investigated, and treated. The chapter also considers the balance of burden and benefit to patients and how this should influence our approach to such symptoms.

Anaemia

Anaemia is a challenging and not infrequent problem in children with life-limiting conditions and is the most common haematological abnormality identified in those with a malignant disorder. However, the underlying mechanism in the terminal period is usually multifactorial for each child [1]. Equally, with the wide-ranging disorders that are managed in the palliative setting, from a child with a neuro-degenerative disease to one with underlying bone marrow dysfunction, decisions about how to manage anaemia become particularly complex.

Many children who are life-limited, have potentially long periods of good quality living and this may affect decision making for this group, compared to children who are reaching the end-stages of their lives. Indeed, there is a significant number of studies that demonstrate lower survival, and poorer growth and development in children with iron deficiency anaemia, sickle cell disease, and thalassaemia [2–5]. Relating the contribution of the underlying disease process from the anaemia to poor outcome, however, is not always possible.

Definition

It is generally agreed that in the palliative setting, the absolute haemoglobin concentration is less critical than the symptoms that are experienced by the child or the young person [6,7]. Normal ranges for haemoglobin levels are documented for reference, however, in Table 29.1.

Symptoms of anaemia

Clearly, many of the symptoms secondary to anaemia are non-specific and often impossible to separate from other difficulties experienced by the terminally ill young person. Fatigue and dyspnoea, classically associated with anaemia, have rarely been studied in relation to the anaemia of the terminally ill, with little evidence-based guidelines in the literature, to inform management [8]. Many children with long standing

Table 29.1 Normal haematological values

Age	Haemoglobin (gms/dl) Mean(Range)	Hematocrit %(Range)	MCV (fl) Range
Birth	17 (14–20)	55 (45–56)	94–118
2 weeks	16.5 (13–20)	50 (42–66)	86–106
6 months-6 years	12 (10.5–14)	38 (33–42)	76–88
Adult female	14 (12–16)	42 (37–47)	76–98
Adult male	16 (14–18)	46 (42–52)	76–96

Source: Reprinted *from Textbook of Pediatrics,* © 1998 Elsevier Inc, with permission from Elsevier [36]. *Forfar and Arneil 5th Edition* [24].

anaemia adapt physiologically to low haemoglobin levels, experiencing few symptoms. Equally, as the child becomes more unwell, adjustment is made to daily activities and consequently, the child may not necessarily complain of new problems. Symptoms that are commonly identified in a child with anaemia include weakness, dyspnoea, and dizziness [6,9] (Box 29.1).

Causes of anaemia in paediatric palliative care

The underlying mechanisms resulting in anaemia in a life-limited child or young person, depend on the underlying disease process. The common causes during the palliative period are given below (Box 29.2).

Anaemia of chronic disorder

Characteristic features are a relatively mild, and non-progressive anaemia, which is unresponsive to iron therapy. Morphologically, there is a normochromic, normocytic picture or a mild hypochromia. This anaemia presents in response to an underlying chronic inflammatory or malignant process. Typically, a low haemoglobin count will be identified alongside a low reticulocyte count and low circulating levels of iron. Conversely, however, tissue-storage forms of iron, such

as ferritin, are high [10]. The pathophysiology of anaemia of chronic disorder can be explained by the inability of the bone marrow to respond adequately to a relative decrease in red cell survival. This occurs because of both impaired iron utilisation, resulting in diminished red cell production, and also a blunted erythropoietin (EPO) response to the developing anaemia. Inadequate response of EPO has been identified in cohorts of adults with anaemia, secondary to both malignancy [11] and acquired immunodeficiency syndrome [12].

Inadequate nutrition

Maintaining appropriate nutrition in children with a life-limiting condition, can pose an enormous challenge for both the parents and health professionals. The contributors to malnutrition are many and include poor food intake as well as cancer-cachexia syndrome (Chapter 23, Gastrointestinal symptoms). Normal red cell production can be impaired as a consequence of the deficiencies secondary to malnutrition (Box 29.3).

Bone marrow dysfunction

Bone marrow failure, resulting in pancytopenia, is a common end-stage of both haematological malignancy and solid tumours such as neuroblastoma and rhabdomyosarcoma. Most commonly, this is secondary to marrow infiltration with malignant cells, although bone marrow suppression following palliative chemotherapy must also be considered. A primary bone-marrow disorder, such as aplastic anaemia, can also

Box 29.1 Common symptoms of anaemia in palliative care

- Weakness
- Fatigue
- Dizziness secondary to postural hypotension
- Dyspnoea
- Anorexia
- Tachycardia
- Headache

Box 29.2 Common causes of anaemia in palliative care

- Anaemia of chronic disease
- Inadequate nutrition
- Haemorrhage
- Bone marrow dysfunction
- Chronic renal failure

Box 29.3 Required for red cell production

- Metals
  - Iron
  - Manganese
  - Cobalt
- Vitamins
  - Vitamin B_{12}
  - Folate
  - Vitamin C
  - Vitamin E
  - Pyridoxine
  - Thiamine
  - Riboflavin
- Aminoacids
- Hormones
  - Erythropoietin
  - Androgens
  - Thyroxine

cause a pancytopenia. The use of blood products for these children is controversial and is discussed later.

Haemorrhage

Chronic haemorrhage can occur due to bleeding, often occult, from a neoplastic lesion. This is usually characterized by a microcytic, hypochromic blood picture, and associated iron deficiency. It is essential to identify the underlying source, which can include lesions in the gastrointestinal tract, liver, brain, and pathological fractures. Surgery, radiotherapy, or topical adrenaline may be required to achieve local control. Blood loss secondary to gastric irritation or peptic ulceration can be managed with an H2 antagonist, such as ranitidine or other alternatives, including sucralfate, and omeprazole.

Chronic renal failure

There is evidence that correction of anaemia in chronic renal failure enhances both quality of life and functional status [2,13]. Improved school attendance, physical wellbeing and growth have been reported in children with partially treated anaemia [4,5]. Improved cardiovascular status has also been documented in children with end-stage renal failure, who have been treated successfully with recombinant human erythropoietin (rHuEPO) [14]. Unfortunately, a prospective, multi-centre, crossover trial comparing outcome data, such as exercise capacity, and cognitive function with partial haematocrit correction is still necessary [2]. However, rHuEPO has been shown to be effective in children with chronic renal failure and dialysis and also in those with failing transplants [5]. Dosage of rHuEPO is comparable to adult requirements [15], with optimal bio-vailability via the subcutaneous route. The Renal Association and the Royal College of Physicians of London published a standards and audit document in August 2002, part of which outlines the standards and recommendations for anaemia in children with chronic renal failure [16] (Box 29.4).

When a child ceases active therapy for end-stage renal failure, the approach towards the management of anaemia also becomes less aggressive. However, it is generally thought that rHuEPO still has a role to play in improving the quality of life for some children during this period.

Management of anaemia in palliative care

In considering the management of any child in the palliative phase, it is essential to consider the overall objectives of interventional therapy. The physical wellbeing of the child must be reviewed alongside the emotional and social needs at any individual point in time. The role of different factors in decision making will vary from one family to another and may include the stage of the child's illness, whereby active interventions

Box 29.4 Anaemia in Children with Chronic Renal Failure (The Renal Association)

Standards

Target haemoglobin is age-specific:
- Children under 6 months > or = to 9.5 gms/l
- Children aged 6 months to 2 years > or = to 10.0 gms/l
- Children over 2 years > or = to 10.5 gms/l

Children should achieve a serum ferritin between 100–800 µg/l

Recommendations

Evaluate of anaemia when the haemoglobin falls:
- Children under 6 months < 10.0 gms/l
- Children aged 6 months to 2 years < 11.0 gms/l
- Children over 2 years < 12.0 gms/l

Low ferritin, despite oral supplements, is an indication for intravenous iron therapy. Haemoglobin concentration should be monitored every 1–2 months. Iron status should be monitored every 3 months.

become less appropriate as the child reaches the terminal phase. Equally, the proximity to a healthcare facility, such as the hospital or a local hospice, and the skill mix of the community team can potentially influence decisions regarding the type of treatment offered. The family and the child may have lifestyle or cultural commitments that effect the management options. For instance, a Jehovah's Witness would not consider the administration of blood products for religious reasons, or a family may simply live at a distance too great to consider travelling for interventional or time consuming therapy, as their child reaches the end stages of life.

To treat or not to treat?

Whatever the factors involved, it is clear that in the terminal phase of a child's illness, active treatment of anaemia should only be considered if the child is symptomatic or if it is felt that the quality of the child's life will be enhanced. Equally, if therapy is to be considered, an understanding of the underlying cause is essential and clearly, it is inappropriate to initiate investigations, without intent to treat. A child with a life-limiting condition, but who has not yet reached the terminal phase, may for instance, require careful nutritional evaluation, with appropriate dietary supplementation recommended. With chronic blood loss, on the other hand, control of the haemorrhage remains the most important aspect of management, with the possibility of blood transfusions reserved for those cases where local therapy has failed.

To transfuse or not to transfuse?

As a child makes the transition from active to palliative management, the role of supportive therapy also shifts. Red cell transfusions during treatment for children receiving chemotherapy, are routinely based on a full blood count result and indeed, even parents will become experts at monitoring the haemoglobin indices, with a corresponding expectation for transfusions at a certain level. The change in emphasis during the palliative phase can, not surprisingly, be a significant challenge for families. The regular blood counts, on which so much previously depended, become a much lower priority in the child's management. Together with the often-controversial debate about the role of the blood transfusion in this new phase, families can feel vulnerable and uncertain about what is now best for their child.

So, what is the evidence that red cell transfusions benefit patients in the palliative phase? The adult literature suggests that blood transfusions can improve quality of life in certain situations [7,17]. The UK South West Thames Palliative Medicine Collaborative Audit Group assessed 97 patients with malignant disease, over one year, in whom transfusion was felt appropriate. In the three parameters of weakness, dyspnoea and overall well being, a significant proportion demonstrated an improvement following transfusion. This was particularly documented in those presenting with weakness as a symptom [18]. However, a National Hospice Study from North America, examining the use of transfusion in terminal care patients, identified that those in conventional care settings were ten times more likely to be transfused than patients in home-care hospices. As the outcome, in terms of comfort and satisfaction, was similar for both groups, the authors suggested that red cell transfusions tend to be over-prescribed in the terminal phase [19]. Transfusions administered during the last four weeks of life are unlikely to influence the quality of life [8], but when it is felt clinically appropriate, both blood and platelet transfusions can be successfully administered in the home with no complications [20].

Is it ethical to transfuse in the terminal phase?

As with all symptom control in palliative care, an assessment of the risks, burdens and benefits should be made for each intervention. Treatment should only be offered which contributes to the child's overall good and where the clinician feels that it will be physiologically effective. Potential burdens must be identified and discussed with the child and the family and it is the professional's duty to explain the situation, where the burdens and the risks may outweigh the benefit [21].

In the case of a blood transfusion, it may be that life is temporarily prolonged, but at the expense of different and more challenging symptoms emerging. As always, a balance needs to be found where the benefits/risks calculus is in favour of enhancing the child's life. At the beginning of the terminal phase, a blood transfusion may improve symptoms of anaemia, allowing a child to participate in a special trip, or family event (Case Study 1). However, as time progresses, the symptomatic benefit from a transfusion may diminish, with an increasing risk of symptoms developing secondary to progressive disease.

Transfusing red blood cells

When a decision has been made to prescribe a blood transfusion, it is essential that all necessary precautions be taken to maximise the safety of the child. It is not acceptable to consider the transfusion of un-cross matched blood in the palliative setting. A blood sample must be taken from the patient to test red cell compatibility. It is essential that the blood sample is accurately labelled; at least 5% of samples arriving at the laboratory bear a labelling error, leading to delays, and potentially serious complications [22].

Red cell compatibility

The ABO type must be determined and compatibility tested as illustrated in Table 29.2. Ensuring Rhesus compatibility is not mandatory in palliative care, although the child's serum should be tested by the local transfusion department against the red cells to be transfused.

If red cells with the incorrect group are transfused, the child's antibodies will bind to these cells, leading to complement activation and consequent damage to the red cells. Released haemoglobin may lead directly to acute renal failure, whilst cell membrane fragments may activate the coagulation pathway, causing disseminated intra-vascular coagulation. An error such as this, could be disastrous and is clearly avoidable.

Table 29.2 To demonstrate the ABO blood groups and compatible donor blood groups

Patients blood groups	Antibody present	Donor blood groups
Group A	Anti B antibody	Groups A and O
Group B	Anti A antibody	Groups B and O
Group O	Anti A and Anti B antibody	Group O
Group AB	Neither Anti A or Anti B	Groups AB, A, B and O

Box 29.5 Signs and symptoms of an acute haemolytic transfusion reaction

- Feeling 'uncomfortable' or 'agitated'
- Flushed
- Pain in abdomen, flank, chest or infusion site
- Fever
- Hypotension
- Generalized oozing from wounds

[23] If incorrect red cells are administered by mistake, there is an approximately 1 in 3 chance of ABO incompatibility. The reaction is most severe if Group A cells are received by a Group O child [22].

Management of transfusion reactions

Prevention, with close attention to all safety measures must be the most important aspect in the management of any potential transfusion reaction. The child should, if possible in the palliative setting, be observed for at least the first fifteen minutes of a blood transfusion. Both allergic and acute haemolytic reactions can occur within minutes of initiating the transfusion. Whereas an allergic reaction is usually characterised by pruritis and urticaria, the symptoms of an acute haemolytic reaction are more diverse (Box 29.5). If the latter is suspected, the blood transfusion must be stopped immediately, the blood returned to the blood bank, along with appropriate blood samples from the child. If this diagnosis or possible bacterial contamination is confirmed, treatment must be considered that is relevant and ethical for the child's situation.

In the case of an allergic reaction, it is usually sufficient to slow the transfusion and administer an antihistamine. When a child has previously experienced an allergic reaction, an antihistamine such as oral chlorpheniramine (chlorphenamine) should be given thirty minutes prior to the transfusion (Box 29.6).

Anaphylaxis is extraordinarily rare, but should be managed in the usual way with fluid boluses, oxygen, and appropriate medication, dependant on where the transfusion is being delivered. Adrenaline, hydrocortisone, and chlorpheniramine (chlorphenamine) should however, be available even in the home or hospice setting (Box 29.7).

Safety measures

Labelling

Along with the accurate labelling of the initial blood sample, the UK Blood Transfusion and Tissue Transplantation

Box 29.6 Dosage of drugs commonly used in the management of transfusion reactions

Chlorpheniramine

Oral

Age	Dose
1 month – 2 years	1 mg
2–5 years	1–2 mg
6–12 years	2–4 mg
Over 12 years	4 mg

Given 30 min prior to transfusion

Intravenous

Age	Dose
1 month – 1 year	250 µg/kg
1–5 years	2.5–5 mg
6–12 years	5–10 mg
Over 12 years	10 mg

Must be given slowly over at least 1 min

Hydrocortisone

4 mg/kg intravenously

Adrenaline

0.1 ml/kg	1:10,000	intramuscular
0.01 ml/kg	1:1000	intramuscular

Source: Transfusion Guidelines for Neonates and Older Children (www.bbts.org.uk)
Medicines for Children 2003 Royal College of Paediatrics and Child Health

Box 29.7 Doses of tranexamic acid [35]

Oral

1–12 years	25 mg/kg/dose tds
>12 years	1–1.5 g tds-qds

Intra-venous

All ages	15 mg/kg/tds
All ages	Continuous infusion 45 mg/kg over 24 h

Guidelines outline the labelling required for each unit of red blood cells. This includes the ABO group, the date of collection and expiry date, the unique donation number, and the details of the type of blood product. In addition to the careful scrutiny of this documentation, the compatibility label must be checked, together with a general inspection of the blood pack for signs of any damage [23].

Infusion procedure

Due to the risk of bacterial proliferation, the red cells should only be removed from the refrigerator when the unit is ready to be checked and transfused. The whole procedure, from start to completion of the transfusion, should take no longer than four hours. If for some reason the transfusion is delayed by more than 30 min, the unit of blood must be returned to the blood bank, and labelled with this detail.

Case Dan was a 6-year old boy who relapsed 16 months after completing treatment for a Stage IV neuroblastoma. Apart from a short history of leg pain and a recent nosebleed, he had been exceptionally well and leading a normal life. Investigation revealed distant relapse, with widespread bone metastases and neuroblastoma infiltration of the bone marrow. A full blood count confirmed bone marrow involvement, with a Hb of 8.1 gm/dl, WCC of $3.2 \times 109/l$, with neutrophils of $1.1 \times 109/l$, and a platelet count of $45 \times 109/l$. After discussions with Dan and his parents, it was accepted that no further curative therapy was available. A decision was, therefore, made to proceed to symptom control alone, enabling Dan to return to school and enjoy some time at home.

Over the following month, Dan became increasingly tired and the family were concerned that he would not manage the long awaited trip to see his favourite football team at their home ground. A haemoglobin count at this time was 5.8 gm/dl, and after careful discussion with the family, a single blood transfusion was arranged at Dan's local hospital.

Dan achieved a good qualitative response and the family had a memorable weekend away together. Subsequently, Dan deteriorated quickly, requiring increasing analgesia for bone pain. It was felt at this stage, that a further blood transfusion would not be helpful, as new symptoms were emerging, the procedure would be interventional and take Dan away from his home. Dan died peacefully amidst his family several weeks later.

Thrombocytopenia

For a small number of children, in particular those with malignant disease, symptoms, secondary to a low platelet count, may warrant intervention.

Thrombocytopenia is defined as a platelet count $<150 \times 10^9/l$ [24]. Symptoms are unlikely to occur until the count is $<50 \times 10^9/l$ and the risk of bruising and spontaneous bleeding increases significantly only with platelets $<20 \times 10^9/l$. Children, most likely to develop low platelets, are those with marrow infiltration (i.e. malignancy or storage diseases). Less commonly, platelet consumption secondary to hypersplenism or disseminated intra-vascular coagulation (DIC) may occur.

Symptoms and signs of thrombocytopenia include petechiae, bruising and bleeding, principally from mucosal surfaces.

Management

In the palliative phase, thrombocytopenia requires no treatment unless symptomatic. In the event of significant bruising or bleeding, intervention may be considered, that is: platelet transfusion or medication. The threshold for intervention will vary between patients, but episodes of bleeding such as haemoptysis or epistaxis, usually warrant treatment.

If platelet transfusion is considered, the risks associated with transfusion and the need for the patient, in some cases, to attend hospital must be weighed up against the possible benefits [20]. The decision to transfuse will also depend upon the child's overall condition and degree of activity. In the event of platelets being given, standard transfusion guidelines still apply (see above). The lifespan of transfused platelets is only a few days and a commitment to maintaining platelets can mean frequent transfusions.

Oozing and minor haemorrhage

Oozing and bleeding may also occur in the presence of normal platelet numbers, as a result of dysfunctional platelets or the influence of some medications such as aspirin.

Visible bleeding can be very distressing for the patient and the family and should be vigorously treated, if possible.

Unfortunately, there are few therapeutic options available for the management of acute bleeding in a palliative care context. Essentially, there are, generally, three means by which bleeding can be controlled: by impeding vascular flow to the area, by increasing the effectiveness of platelets, or by increasing the effectiveness of the coagulation cascade. If the bleeding point is easily accessible, as in epistaxis, local vasospasm may be induced using cautery, if the patient is stable enough for an otorhinolaryngology opinion. Packing the nose with an alginate dressing such as Sorbisan, or with gauze soaked in adrenaline may achieve the same object.

Platelet function may be compromised by metabolic disturbances such as uraemia. Bleeding is particularly likely if it was a significant feature at diagnosis, for example often in M3 promyelocytic leukaemia. It is not known whether a megakaryocyte stem-cell defect may arise in children who have been heavily treated for other forms of relapsed leukaemia, either as a result of the disease or the effect of myelotoxic drugs. Certainly, distressing bleeding during the terminal phase appears to be more common in this group of patients. Functional platelets may be transfused. In the presence of normal numbers of platelets, platelet function may, in principle be improved by the use of etamsylate. In practice, however, it seems not to help [25,26].

Tranexamic acid (TA) is an antifibrinolytic agent, which helps to stabilize clots. It can be used to stop bleeding from mucosal surfaces or ulcerated, oozing lesions [24,27,28]. TA comes in oral and i.v. forms and can also be administered topically, as a solution of the i.v. preparation. Treatment should start with the onset of bleeding and be continued for a few days after bleeding has stopped. Evidence to support its use prophylactically is lacking.

More occult haemorrhage, such as intracranial bleeding, should usually be managed symptomatically. Seizures (see also Chapter 26, Neurological and neuromuscular symptoms) and pain (see also Chapter 21, Pain) are the most common symptoms.

Management of terminal haemorrhage

Catastrophic haemorrhage can be a terrifying event for the child, the family and the health professionals. Uncontrollable bleeding, usually, occurs from the site of a malignancy and commonly presents as a haematemesis, haemoptysis, or erosion of the tumour into a major artery, such as the carotid. In the terminal phase, it is essential to maintain a calm and reassuring environment for the child. Death can occur within minutes and it is more important to remain with the child, than leave the patient in search of medication, or the telephone. Anticipating the possibility of a terminal bleed can enable helpful preparation. Dark sheets and towels will mask the colour and quantity of blood and should be readily accessible. Symptom management must focus on controlling the fear experienced by the child. As time is usually limited and the situation potentially dramatic, it is essential to ensure that the necessary medication, syringes and clearly written prescriptions are readily available in the home. For some families, it can be appropriate to draw up a syringe with the correct drug dosage in advance. Distress in these situations is most effectively managed with either an analgesic or sedative drug, such as diamorphine, or midazolam [24,29,30,31] (Box 29.8).

Thrombosis

Deep vein thrombosis is uncommon in the paediatric palliative setting. However, it is most likely to occur secondary to tumour mass effects, particularly in the pelvis, as a paraneoplastic phenomenon, or following prolonged immobilization or inactivity.

The symptoms associated with thrombosis can make a significant adverse impact on the quality of a child's life. Deep vein thrombosis of the calf can cause severe pain and immobility and, of course, carries the risk of pulmonary embolism. This, in turn, can cause pain, shortness of breath, and frightening haemoptysis. Heparin not only reduces the risk of pulmonary embolism, but also is, probably, analgesic because of its effect

Box 29.8 Management of terminal bleeding

- Maintain a calm and reassuring environment
- Use dark sheets and towels
- Prescribe the following medication in advance, to be given subcutaneously (or, if appropriate, buccally):

Midazolam

Age	Dose
1–12 years	0.05–0.1 mg/kg as a single dose
>12 years	2 mgs as a single dose

Diamorphine

Age	Dose
1–3 months	20 μg/kg
3–6 months	25–50 μg/kg
6–12 months	75 μg/kg
>12 months	75–100 μg/kg
12–18 years	2.5–5 mg

on the surface of the clot and its contact with the sensitive vascular endothelium. There is, therefore, a good case for treating thrombosis, should it occur.

On the other hand, traditional approaches to the management of thrombosis have required numerous blood tests, which should, if possible, be avoided in the palliative phase. Although full anticoagulation with intravenous heparin and warfarin remains an option, it is likely to be undesirable in this patient group. However, the advent of low molecular weight heparin (LMWH) has removed the need for repeated monitoring of drug levels and so presents a real alternative in the management of clot related symptoms such as swelling and pain [32–34]. (Case below).

LMWH is administered subcutaneously, once a day and in older children and young adults, no drug level monitoring is required [35]. In younger, non-palliative children, some monitoring is currently undertaken.

Case A 15-year-old boy known to have an extensive pelvic tumour, presented with swelling, tenderness and bluish discolouration of the thigh of the right leg. Imaging revealed the presence of a deep vein thrombosis. In combination with appropriate levels of analgesia, subcutaneous low-molecular weight heparin was commenced. Within 3 days, there was significant reduction in swelling and tenderness, so allowing improved mobility during the last 2 weeks of this young man's life.

Summary

The management of symptomatic anaemia, thrombocytopenia, haemorrhage, and thrombosis in the palliative phase, illustrate very well, the challenging decisions that face professionals working with dying children. On the one hand, modern medical interventions have the capacity to relieve some of the symptoms haematological abnormalities can cause. On the other, the interventions themselves carry morbidity and can cause not only symptoms related to physical reactions, but also often emotional and psychological ones related to otherwise avoidable hospital attendance.

The best clinical decision can only be made by considering the needs of the individual child and the family, giving appropriate weight to the risks of giving, and those of withholding an intervention, both physical and otherwise. In this respect, management of haematological symptoms is typical of thoughtful and skilled childhood palliative care in general.

References

1. Doll, D.C. and Weiss, R.B. Neoplasia and the Erythron. *J Clin Oncol* 1985;3(3):429–46.

2. Yorgin, P.D., Belson, A., Al-Uzri, A.Y., and Alexander, S.R. The Clinical Efficacy of Higher Hematocrit Levels in Children with Chronic Renal Insufficiency and Those Undergoing Dialysis. *Sem Nephrology* 2001;21(5):451–62.

3. Singhal, A., Morris, J., Thomas, P. *et al*. Factors affecting prepubertal growth in homozygous sickle cell disease. *Arch Dis Child* 1996; 74:502–6.

4. Morris, K.P., Sharp, J., Watson, S., and Coulthard, M.G. Non-cardiac benefits of human recombinant erythropoietin in end stage renal failure and anaemia. *Arch Dis Child* 1993;69:580–6.

5. Jabs, K. The effects of recombinant human erythropoietin on growth and nutritional status. *Pediatr Nephrol* 1996;10:324–7.

6. Salt, S. Anaemia and blood transfusions in palliative care. *Eur J Palliat Care* 2003;10(2):49—53.

7. Beardsmore, S. and Fitzmaurice, N. Palliative care in paediatric oncology. *E J Cancer* 2002;38:1900–07.

8. Monti, M., Castellani, L., Berlusconi, A., and Cunietti, E. *et al*. Transfusions in terminally ill patients admitted to a palliative care unit. *J Pain Symp Manag* 1996;12(1):18–22.

9. Wolfe, J., Friebert, S., and Hilden, J. Caring for children with advanced cancer; Integrating palliative care. *Pediatr Clin N Am* 2002;49:1043–62.

10 Henry, D.H. Changing patterns of care in the management of Anaemia. *Sem Oncol* 1992;19(3)(Suppl 8):3–7.

11. Miller, C.B., Jones, R.J., Piantadosi, S., Abeloff, M.D., and Spivak, J.L. Decrease erythropoietin response in patients with the anaemia of cancer. *N Engl J Med* 1990;322:1689–92.

12. Fischl, M., Galpin, J.E., Levine, J.D. *et al*. Recombinant human erythropoietin for patients with AIDS treated with zidovudine. *N Engl J Med* 1990;322:1689–92.

13. Moreno, F., Sanz-Guajardo, D., Lopez-Gomez, J.M. *et al*. Increasing the hematocrit has a beneficial effect on quality of life and is safe in selected hemodialysis patients. Spanish Co-operative Renal Patients Quality of Life Study Group of the Spanish Society of Nephrology. *J Am Soc Nephrol* 2002;11:335–42.

14. Martin, G.R., Ongkingo, J.R., Turner, M.E. *et al*. Recombinant erythropoietin (Epogen) improves cardiac exercise performance in children with end-stage renal disease. *Pediatr Nephrol* 1993; 7:276–80.

15. Brandt, J.R. Safety and efficacy of erythropoietin in children with chronic renal Failure. *Pediatr Nephrol* 1999;13:143–7.

16. Treatment of adults and children with renal failure: Standards and audit measures. Royal College of Physicians of London and the Renal Association. 2002;105(7).

17. Himelstein, B.P. Commentary. *Eur J Cancer* 2002; 38: 1908–10.

18. Gleeson, C. and Spencer, D. Blood transfusion and its benefits in palliative care. *Palliat Med* 1995;9:307–13.

19. Wachtel, T.J. and Mor, V. The use of transfusion in terminal cancer patients: Hospice versus conventional care setting. *Transfusion* 1985;25:278–9.

20. Stockelberg, D., Lehtola, P., and Noren, I. Palliative treatment at home for patients with haematological disorders. *Supp Care Can* 1997;5:506–8.

21. Randall, F. and Downie, R.S. Process of clinical decision making. In F. Randall and R.S. Downie, *Palliative Care Ethics: A Good Companion*. eds. Oxford: Oxford University Press,1996, pp. 109–37.

22. McClennand, B. Handbook of Transfusion Medicine (3rd edition). London: HMSO, 2001.

23. www. transfusionguidelines.org.uk

24. Goldman, A. and Burne, R. Symptom Management. In Goldman, A. ed. *Care of the Dying Child*. Oxford: Oxford University Press, 1998, pp. 71–2.

24. Tranexamic acid. In Martindale, ed. *The Extra Pharmacopoeia* (31st edition) 1996; 771–2.

25 Ritter, L., Schlosser, H., Boos, J., and Heyen, P. Effect of Ethamsylate on haemorrhagic diathesis of children with oncologic diseases. *Klin Paediat* 1991;203(4):296–301.

26. Bonnar, J. and Sheppard, B.L. Treatment of menorrhagia during menstruation: Randomised controlled trial of ethamsylate, mefenamic acid and tranexamic acid. *BMJ* 1996;313:579–82.

27. Seto, A. and Dunlap, D. Tranexamic acid in oncology. *Anna Pharma* 1996;30:868–70.

28. Dean, A. and Tuffin, P. Fibrinolytic Inhibitors for Cancer-Associated Bleeding Problems. *J Pain Symptom Manage* 1997;13:20–4.

29. Goldman, A. Life threatening illnesses and symptom control in children. In *Oxford Textbook of Palliative Medicine* D. Doyle, G.W.C. Hanks, and N. MacDonald, eds. Oxford: Oxford University Press, 1998, pp. 1038–39.

30. Smith, A.M. Emergencies in Palliative Care. *Ann Acad Med Singapore* 1994;23(2):186–90.

31. Provan, D., Chisholm, M., Duncombe, A., Singer, C., and Smith, A. Reduced platelet count. In *Oxford Handbook of Clinical Haematology*. Oxford: Oxford University Press, 2003, p. 20.

32. Hirsh, J., Siragusa, S., Cosmi, B., and Ginsberg, J.S. Low molecular Weight Heparins in the treatment of patients with acute thromboembolism. *Thromb Haemost* 1995;74(1):360–3.

33. Hirsh, J. and Crowther, M. Low molecular weight heparin for the out-of—hospital Treatment of venous thrombosis: Rationale and clinical results. *Thromb. Haemost* 1997;76(1):689–92.

34. Garon, J.E. Monitoring low molecular weight heparins. *Clin Leadersh Manag Rev* 2003;17(1):47–50.

35. British National Formulary. British Medical Association & Royal Pharmaceutical Society of Great Britain, *March* 2003.

36. Adam, J. The last 48 hours. In M. Fallon and B. O'Neill, eds. In *ABC of Palliative Care*. London: BMJ books, 2001, pp. 39–42.

30 HIV/AIDS

Debbie Norval, Bernadette O'Hare, and Rodica Matusa

Introduction

The management of children with human immunodeficiency virus (HIV) or AIDS (acquired immunodeficiency syndrome) presents problems that are, in many ways, rather different from other life-limiting conditions. Even in adult palliative medicine, it has long been recognized that the needs of patients with HIV/AIDS present particular challenges that are quite distinct from the needs of patients with cancer. One author [1] observed that, in the United Kingdom, adult palliative care in HIV/AIDS differs from 'mainstream' adult palliative medicine in four major ways:

- It is a disease of the young rather than the elderly.
- There may be multiple pathologies, so that cure and palliation may become indistinguishable earlier than in cancer.
- Within a progressive and ultimately fatal syndrome, there may be curable components.
- The patient is characteristically informed, vocal, and assertive.

It seems from this that palliative medicine in HIV/AIDS may have more in common with the speciality in children. Much of what is described here, could equally be said of many conditions that limit life in childhood. One principle in particular, seems common to HIV/AIDS and paediatric palliative medicine; the co-existence of conditions (such as chest infection) that impose a heavy symptom load, and which are themselves potentially curable, but occur within a relentlessly progressive condition. Treating these can contribute significantly, to good symptom management, so that within palliative care there are elements of a curative approach.

The clinical course of HIV/AIDS in children has been dramatically changed by the introduction of antiretroviral agents, where they are available. It has become for many, a chronic illness in which many acute 'curable components' may occur. These include infections and, less commonly, malignancy.

This chapter will be in two sections. One, based largely on clinical experience from Africa, will consider the active management of HIV/AIDS itself and some of the curable components within it. The second, based on clinical experience from Romania, will consider common symptoms among children with HIV/AIDS and how they can be approached.

Management of HIV/AIDS: The African experience

Ninety-five per cent of children infected with human immunodeficiency virus (HIV) in Africa, will have acquired their infection by vertical transmission from mother to child (MTCT). Sexual abuse, transfusion of blood and related products, and other forms of horizontal transmission (expressed breast milk, rare nosocomial spread in nurseries) account for the remainder.

Perinatal HIV transmission in this population [2] can be reduced to 12%, but the infrastructure to make these interventions available to all does not exist. Nevirapine and HIV rapid testing has been made free to eligible countries as of 2000 and 2002 [3] and hopefully interventions will become more widely available.

There are 2.5 million children aged <15 years living with HIV/AIDS in sub-Saharan Africa. During 2003, there were 700,000 newly infected children and up to 540,000 died. One thousand five hundred children died each day as opposed to fewer than 100 per year in either USA or Europe [4]. In the absence of antiretroviral intervention or caesarian section, between 25–39% of infected African women transmit HIV to their offspring [5] but the number of children living with

HIV/AIDS is lower than one would expect due their high mortality in early infancy.

In regions of high HIV prevalence, up to 50% of all admissions to regional and specialist paediatric hospitals are HIV-related. These children have a mortality rate at least three times, as high as, that of HIV-negative children.

The natural history of HIV-related disease in children with perinatal infection.

In the absence of anti-retroviral therapy (ART), survival of HIV-infected children is dependent on access to programmes providing comprehensive and intensive health care.

Prior to access to ART, fewer than 10% of vertically infected children in developed countries were likely to die before they were a year old, and median survival from the time of diagnosis was 38 months. Experience regarding the natural history of HIV/AIDS in developing countries, shows that 25% of children die before they are a year old [6] and 90%, by the time they are three years old [7]. This difference in mortality points to disparities in resources and access to care.

Early death is due to the common causes of morbidity and mortality among all children in developing countries. In children first diagnosed as HIV-positive under 6 months of age, a combination of diarrhoea, pneumonia, failure to thrive, and neurological abnormalities should alert one to the possibility of rapidly progressive disease and death. Yet, as is suggested by the far lower annual death rates observed in developed countries, many early deaths are preventable. In both resource-rich and resource-poor scenarios, children may remain asymptomatic and without significant symptoms or signs for many years.

Features of HIV/AIDS

Table 30.1 describes signs, symptoms and investigations that are suggestive or diagnostic of HIV/AIDS in childhood.

Particular clinical issues include attention to nutrition and growth, prescription of anti-retroviral therapy where its is available, and management of diarrhoea, respiratory conditions, skin conditions, and fever that can all complicate HIV/AIDS itself. Prompt recognition and intervention of these intercurrent problems can make a significant impact on the symptoms experienced by the child.

Growth

The majority of children who are diagnosed with HIV-1 infection in the first few years of life, grow poorly and may present with or continue to suffer from, varying degrees of failure to thrive. The mean birth weight and length of HIV-positive infants is less than that of HIV-negative infants [8]. The body

Table 30.1 Signs, symptoms, and investigations in the diagnosis of HIV/AIDs in children

'Classical' disease complex suggesting HIV infection:
    Failure to thrive
    Recurrent or chronic diarrhoea
    Pneumonitis in the first year of life
    Oral candidiasis
    Recurrent upper respiratory infections
    Recurrent invasive infections (meningitis, septicaemia, osteitis, mastoiditis)
    Unexplained anaemia or thrombocytopaenia
    Tuberculosis
    Severe herpes simplex stomatitis, herpes zoster or chicken pox

Physical signs commonly seen and suggestive of HIV infection. These clinical features are not specific, either in respect of making the diagnosis of HIV infection or in determining prognosis:
    Malnutrition
    Generalized lymphadenopathy
    Hepatomegaly with or without splenomegaly
    Severe papular acrodermatitis or papular urticaria
    Unexplained encephalopathy
    Chronic otorrhoea
    Parotid gland enlargement
    Digital clubbing
    Rectovaginal or rectovesical fistula (an uncommon sign)

Diagnosis in a child suspected of having HIV/AIDS:
    If the child is >18 months ELISA confirmed with Western Blot
    If the child is <18 months HIV PCR is required as the antibodies may reflect his mother's status and not his own

mass index of HIV-infected infants is lower than that of uninfected children in the first 6 months of life, perhaps because their energy and nutrient requirements are higher than those of uninfected children [9]. HIV-infected infants continue to grow poorly, as reflected by a significant deficit in weight, length, and head circumference for age at 24 months of age [10].

While weight and length/height for age continue to fall below the normal growth percentiles, weight for length does not, and children may not appear wasted. The reason for the disproportionate short stature amongst HIV-positive children has yet to be established; indeed, the pathogenesis of poor growth in HIV/AIDS in general is poorly understood.

Failure to thrive in HIV-infected children is generally multifactorial. Poor growth may be the consequence of one or more of the following:

- poverty-related malnutrition

- malabsorbtion

- recurrent or chronic diarrhoea

- the consequences of concurrent chronic infections
- increased energy expenditure
- the effects of HIV infection itself (6)—HIV wasting syndrome
- poor feeding related to recurrent and severe oral thrush, oesophagitis, encephalopathy, etc.

In a Rwandan prospective cohort study of infants born to HIV-positive mothers, mean weight, height and head circumference for age, were lower among HIV-1 infected infants than among HIV-negative infants [11].

Weight velocity is of prognostic utility in HIV-positive children. Those with significant deficits in weight velocity have a poorer prognosis, correlating with more rapid falls in CD4+ counts and higher viral loads [12]. Significantly, low weight for age prior to the onset of monotherapy with Zidovudine, or a failure to gain weight to the 25th percentile *prior* during the first 6 months of therapy, are significant predictors of early death [13].

Highly active anti-retroviral therapy (HAART) has a positive effect on the growth of HIV-infected children. Height and weight are favourably influenced in children in whom HAART reduces viral load by at least 1.5 log or to less than 500 copies per ml and increases the CD4+ count [14]. The palliative effect of HAART for children, therefore, extends beyond an improvement in immune status and fewer intercurrent infections to better growth in respect of both height and stature.

Antiretroviral treatment

Goals of antiretroviral therapy

The goal of antiretroviral therapy for children is to decrease HIV-related morbidity and mortality.

- The child's CD4 count should rise to near normal values for age and remain above the baseline count.
- The child's viral load should become undetectable (<400 copies/ml) and remain undetectable on ARV therapy.
- In some children, a suppressed though detectable viral load, with sustained elevation in CD4 count and absence of intercurrent and/or opportunistic infection, may be the best achievable goal.

Who should receive therapy?

In addition to medical criteria based on number of admissions and stage of disease, patients need to fulfil certain social criteria including:

- an identifiable adult who is able to administer medication;
- demonstrated reliability in adult caregiver that is, the adult has attended three or more scheduled visits to an HIV clinic. Immunization record up to date;

- previous record of adherence to nutritional supplements/other chronic care regimens such as TB drugs;
- able to attend the antiretroviral centre on a regular basis (transport may need to be arranged for patients in rural areas or for those remote from the treatment site).

The decision to start antiretroviral therapy should be made on the basis of a multi disciplinary group that includes medical, nursing and counselling staff, as well as, the child's mother, and other main care giver.

Prophylaxis in HIV/AIDS

Pneumocystis carinii pneumonia prophylaxis

Cotrimazole is a potent preventer of PCP in children with HIV/AIDS. The dose of cotrimoxazole depends on the size of the child. Children less than 5 kg should receive a dose of 20/100 (trimethoprim/sulphamethoxazole (sulfa methoxazole) dose in mg) twice daily, those between 5 and 10 kg 40/200, and those over 10 kg 80/400.

An alternative, for those who are allergic to or cannot tolerate cotrimoxazole, is Dapsone 1 mg/kg/day.

Vitamins

Multivitamin supplements can reduce symptoms among poorly nourished children. If there is any evidence of poor nutrition, administer one tablet or 5 ml suspension of multivitamin preparation daily.

Vitamin A deficiency imposes a particular risk of corneal damage, including ulceration, so should be treated prophylactically. Administer 6 monthly (age 6–12 months: 100,000 IU, age 1–6 years: 200 000 IU). In symptomatic children, or those with corneal ulceration on staining, give 10 000 IU/kg for 3 days.

Vitamin A supplementation is also reported to be of benefit in preventing or reducing the severity of diarrhoea in vitamin deficient populations. There is no evidence that this intervention is of benefit in Vitamin A-replete populations [15], but it would seem to reduce the diarrhoea-related morbidity in malnourished children, with or without HIV/AIDS [16,17]. Zinc supplementation (1 mg/kg/day elemental zinc) reduces the duration of acute and chronic diarrhoea [18].

Tuberculosis prophylaxis

Infants and children of mothers who have tuberculosis are at high risk of infection and disease. They should receive Isoniazid (INH) + Pyrazinamide (PZA) and Rifampicin (Rif) as prophylaxis for a minimum of three months. Children under the age of five years with known exposure to tuberculosis, should receive INH + PZA + Rif for three months. It is recommended that all HIV-positive children living in areas where pulmonary tuberculosis is highly prevalent, should receive INH prophylaxis at a dose of 5 mg/kg/day, once daily. However, there is currently a high level of resistance to INH and it may be necessary to consider prophylaxis with INH and Rifampicin together.

Ascaricides, (mebendazole)

Prophylactically, administer 3 monthly (age < 5 years: 2 tablets (200 mg), age > 5 years: 5 tablets (500 mg). Alternatively, use Albendazole suspension : > 2 years : 400 mg (20 ml), <2 years or <10 kg : 200 mg (10 ml)

Diarrhoea

Diarrhoea and wasting are common features of HIV/AIDS in Africa [19]. It is associated with the common bacterial pathogens [46] encountered in HIV-negative children [20], but HIV infected children are more likely to be malnourished, to have prolonged diarrhoea, and to have co-morbid pneumonia than HIV-negative children.

Aetiology

Water-borne infection is a common source of enteric infection in developing countries, but there is no published account of benefit derived from interventions designed to improve water-related hygiene. Families that do not have tap water in their homes, tend to store water in buckets. Water is then dispensed from the reservoir bucket by dipping into it with a pitcher or a cup. Each dipping event is likely to contaminate the water in the bucket with whatever organisms the person is carrying on his/her hand at the time. In summer, it is likely that enteropathic organisms will flourish under these circumstances and that this form of water storage is a cause of bacterial diarrhoea. One prophylactic intervention would be to provide families with a 25 l, polyethylene water container with a spigot, so as to rule out contamination of water as described above. While this is intuitively an appropriate intervention, there is no trial-based evidence that it has positive effects.

Investigation

The nature of palliative care in children with HIV/AIDS means that, even aggressive investigation and management may be justified. For example, the acid-base state should be established in tachypnoeic children with acidotic breathing, and those with features suggesting shock. Serum electrolytes, including serum calcium should be measured, since malnourished children are frequently hypokalaemic, and

because hypocalcaemia is relatively common in HIV-positive patients [21]. A full blood count should be performed, because anaemia and thrombocytopenia are relatively frequent complicating factors and should be taken into account in the management plan.

Stool specimens must be collected and delivered to the laboratory promptly and repeatedly if they remain negative in persistent diarrhoea. Antimicrobial therapy should be directed by the results of stool microscopy and culture.

Invasive investigation by sigmoidoscopy may be of value where a cause for colitis cannot be determined and in children with rectal fistulae [22] although, in the developing world, this is not usually provided. Bacterial overgrowth of the upper small bowel may be confirmed by aspiration of duodenal fluid by upper gastro-intestinal endoscopy.

Treatment

Patients presenting with diarrhoea may initially be managed as ambulatory patients provided they are not shocked (showing signs of intra-vascular dehydration) and do not have intractable vomiting. Either of these complications is an indication for admission and intravenous rehydration. Ambulatory care of diarrhoea in HIV-infected children includes a course of Metronidazole as treatment for presumed Giardia lamblia infestation, Albendazole for intestinal worms and microsporidium, and a supply of a packaged salt and electrolyte mixture for suspension in water. Mothers should be advised to return to the clinic if the child becomes drowsy or if vomiting prevents fluid retention. Be aware of treating for intestinal worms in a patient with acute diarrhoea as a worm bolus can result in an acute intestinal obstruction.

In children who are not shocked, but in whom hydration is felt to be necessary, oral rehydration is safe and efficient. Feeds should be introduced as soon as shock has resolved. In malnourished children with chronic diarrhoea, lactose intolerance is likely and the benefit of lactose-free milk should be assessed in management. Intravascular resuscitation may be indicated in children with shock.

Specific issues influencing management in African children

- Clean water supplies may not be easily accessible. Families should be advised to drink more fluids than usual from the onset of diarrhoea

- Oral rehydration solution:
  — 8 tsp sugar
  — 1 level tsp salt r
  — 1 litre boiled water

— Mix well and store covered in a cool place. Make a fresh solution every day
— Water, unsweetened juice, weak tea, can be used as maintenance, but should not be used for rehydration
— Rice water (see below)
— Dilute maize/millet/sorghum pap
— Maize-based ORS (see below)

• Children should be encouraged to drink as much as possible. Often, they will not feel thirsty, so encourage them to keep a glass nearby and take small sips every five minutes. If the child is breast-feeding, this should continue, but more frequently than before (at least every 3 h).

• Continue to eat. If children stop eating when they have diarrhoea, this can cause malnutrition, or make existing malnutrition, worse. Stopping oral feeds is unnecessary except in severe dehydration when it may be necessary for the carer to concentrate on rehydration for four to six hours (50–100 ml/kg).

• Prepare food, for example, porridge more watery than usual, so the child gets both nutrition and fluids.

• Eat small amounts of nutritious and easily digestible food frequently.

• After the diarrhoea has stopped, an extra meal each day for two weeks will help regain any weight lost during the illness.

• Preparation of Rice-based Oral Rehydration Solution
— Fistful of dry rice grain (25 g)
— Wash and soak until soft
— Grind to paste
— Put 2 cups of water in pan and mix with paste
— Heat and stir until bubbling
— Use within 6–8 hrs

• Preparation of Maize-based Oral Rehydration Solution
• Add 50 g maize to l water
• Cook for 5–8 min
• Add 1 tsp salt once cooled

In addition to specific antimicrobial and antiviral therapy as indicated by stool culture, 'Bowies regimen' may be tried although there is inadequate evidence that it is effective: Cholestyramine (colestyramine) 1 g 6 hourly × 5 days and Gentamicin 50 mg/kg/day 4 hourly for 3 days given orally. Lactose-free milk. Small doses of oral morphine solution may be useful for intractable diarrhoea.

Management of skin conditions

Skin lesions (Table 30.2) are common in children with HIV/AIDS and may cause them great discomfort. When correctly diagnosed, they are often easily treated.

Table 30.2 Skin infections in HIV/AIDS

Common skin conditions in HIV-infected children
Herpes simplex
Seborrhoeic eczema
Tinea of the head and body
Fungal nail infections
Dry skin
Scabies
Drug hypersensitivity
Molluscum contageosum
Warts
Pruritic papular eruption of HIV
Varicella Zoster
Varicella (chicken pox)
Bacterial skin infections

Herpes simplex

Vesicles and erosions around the mouth and other mucocutaneous surfaces such as penis and vagina. Treat with Acyclovir 10 mg/kg/dose 5 times a day for 7 days. Topical and oral analgesia.

Seborrhoeic eczema

Seborrhoeic eczema occurs in the axillae, neck, groin and scalp. It may complicate fungal napkin dermatitis. A potent topical steroid (betamethasone valerate 0.1%) should be used as lotion in the hair and body folds. On the face, 1% hydrocortisone lotion is appropriate. Secondary infection should be treated with flucloxacillin. Topical therapy should be followed-up with an anti-dandruff shampoo. Should the condition persist, an azole anti-fungal agent may be of benefit.

Tinea capitis

This may present as grey balding patches, as alopecia areata, as seborrhoeic dermatitis or as patches of hair loss with crusting and pustulation.

Clotrimazole cream should be used for localised infection and griseofulvin for extensive disease and involvement of the nails.

Fungal nail infections

Griseofulvin 10 mg/kg/day once each day with fat containing meal. Treat for 4–6 weeks.

Dry skin

Dry skin is a common complaint. Mothers should be encouraged to bathe children by first applying aqueous cream (UEA) and then rinsing this off in the bath, rather than to use soap. Petroleum Jelly should be avoided.

Scabies

This may be confused with papular urticaria and the pruritic papular eruption of HIV. Finding a typical burrow will avoid confusion and the diagnosis may be confirmed by identifying mites in skin scrapings. Children who have raw lesions and those under 6 months of age, should be treated with 2% sulphur ointment, three times daily, for three days. Benzyl benzoate lotion stings on open lesions. However, Benzyl Benzoate can be used on infants if diluted and it is more effective than sulphur. All members of the household other than specified above, should be treated by the application of lotion to the whole body overnight and a repeat application after 72 h.

Prevention of scabies is also important and includes the use of heat in the form of the hot sun or ironing of linen and Tetmosol (Monosulfiram) soap for all family members.

Bacterial skin infections

Impetigo, folliculitis, furunculosis and abcesses are caused by Staphylococci and streptococci. Treat with Cloxacillin 25 mg/kg/dose, four times, each day (on an empty stomach) for 7 days or until healed. If severe, treat for two weeks initially. For recurrent problems, topical application of mupirocin 2% may be effective. Nasal irradiation of bacteria using Mupirocin is also important.

Drug reactions

The number of medications they can be taking means that drug reactions are common in children with HIV/AIDS. Patients present with a generalised erythema and systemic signs within two to four weeks after starting a drug. Co-trimoxazole, phenytoin, carbamazepine, anti-tuberculous drugs, and importantly, non-nucleoside reverse transcriptase inhibitors are the most frequent causes. Stop therapy with the suspected drug. Use topical steroid ointment in the absence of secondary skin infection.

Molluscum contagiosum

Though often considered a trivial infection, molluscum causes significant morbidity through disfigurement (Figure 30.2) when lesions are extensive. Repeated application of liquid nitrogen or silver nitrate may be required, but this may not be effective and can result in spread. Lesions regress on anti-retroviral therapy. Molluscum contagiosum is often best left alone.

Warts

Warts may be large and extensive in the ano-genital region, particularly in babies and young children. Treatment is with podophyllin 25% applied weekly and washed off, after 4 h to prevent irritation. Lesions frequently recur, even after cautery or the application of liquid nitrogen. Other treatments include radiotherapy and, of course, antiretroviral therapy.

The pruritic papular eruption of HIV

This presents on the limbs and the trunk and may be the manifestation of several disorders. Papular urticaria in response to insect bite, folliculitis and a form of the Gianotti–Crosti syndrome [23], may contribute to the underlying pathology. Children suffer severe discomfort because of itching. Scratching leads to secondary impetigo. Symptoms are relieved by application of a potent topical steroid, treatment of secondary bacterial infection and a sedative anti-histamine, such as promethazine 25 mg at night.

Varicella (chicken pox)

In the child with HIV/AIDs, systematic varicella may be fatal. Symptomatic treatment with topical calamine lotion. IV Acyclovir 20 mg/kg/dose, five times, daily for seven days. If IV therapy is not available, use oral formulation.

Varicella zoster

Zoster eruptions are a cause of severe pain and carry a high mortality rate in severely immuno-compromised patients. Children with low CD4+ counts may have extensive mucocutaneous disease with persistent vesicle formation [24]. Treatment is according to the WHO approach [25], with analgesia 'by-the-ladder' and 'by-the-clock' (i.e. regularly around the clock to prevent recurrence of pain). The first step is often a paracetamol and codeine combination 6 hourly, a soothing topical anti-bacterial cream or calamine lotion and Aciclovir 20 mg/kg/dose 800 mg 5-hourly, for 7 days. The best response is obtained by starting Aciclovir within 72 h of the onset of symptoms. An evening dose of amitriptyline is recommended for post-herpetic neuralgia in Herpes Zoster.

Candidiasis

Cutaneous candidiasis is typically found in the nappy area, armpits or neck folds. Topical gentian violet 1% aqueous solution twice daily for 7 days or topical clotrimazole twice daily for 7 days.

Measles

Treat symptomatically. Ensure vitamin A has been administered within the last 3 months, if not, administer. If any signs of pneumonia, treat.

Respiratory complications (see also

Chapter 27, Respiratory symptoms)

Lower respiratory tract infections

A number of acute and chronic disease processes give rise to lower respiratory symptoms in children with HIV/AIDS. Chief amongst these symptoms are shortness of breath, cough and effort intolerance. The management of these symptoms depends on the underlying cause.

Pneumocystis carinii pneumonia (PCP) is common amongst HIV-infected children, not on chemoprophylaxis children, and may be the presenting illness in infants [26]. PCP presents in a non-specific fashion, with tachypnoea, fever, cough, and dyspnoea. The cough is non-productive and the chest may be clear to auscultation, except for scattered crepitations and rhonchi. Arterial oxygen saturation is low, measured by pulse oxymetry, or by blood gas analysis. The serum lactate dehydrogenase (LDH) concentration may be markedly elevated, although this is non-specific. The chest radiograph may show a diffuse interstitial infiltrate with 'bat wing' appearance, may be normal, or show features of concomitant chronic lung disease.

The organism is rarely isolated from children. Adequate sputum samples require broncho-alveolar lavage or sputum induction. Giemsa, modified silver methenamine, or toluidine blue staining of sputum or lung tissue will confirm the diagnosis.

A presumptive diagnosis based on symptoms, signs, hypoxaemia, a chest-suggestive radiograph and an elevated serum LDH, indicates a need for treatment. Intravenous co-tromoxazole at 10 mg/kg of the trimethoprim base as a loading dose, followed by 20 mg/kg in four divided doses for three weeks, is the treatment of choice. Co-administration of prednisone 2 mg/kg for seven days followed by a 14 day tapering-dose-reduction over 14 days, is reported to improve survival [27].

Prophylaxis against PCP is indicated in infants from six weeks until one year of age. Children over the age of one year, should receive prophylaxis if their CD4+ counts fall below an absolute count of 500 per micro-litre or if the CD4+ cells count is less than 15 per cent of the total lymphocyte count. All children with prior PCP should receive life-long chemoprophylaxis. Cotrimoxazole is the chemo-prophylactic agent of choice and should be given at a dose of 5 mg/kg of the trimethoprim component. Guidelines for dosing vary between a single dose daily and a twice-daily dose on three days of the week. PCP prophylaxis may be discontinued in children over the age of one year with CD4+ counts over 15 per cent. Because co-trimoxazole is useful in preventing recurrent bacterial infections, it may be advisable to continue, regardless of CD4+ count, even in children with good immunological recovery on HAART. In the absence of CD4 monitoring, consider life-long prophylaxis.

HIV-positive children are at risk of recurrent severe bacterial pneumonia, presenting with fever, cough, intercostal recession and hypoxia that is mild—relative to that associated with PCP. Streptococcus pneumoniae and Haemophilus influenzae are most frequently the causative agents. Blood culture is positive in 15–20 per cent of cases. Sputum microscopy will provide evidence of a preponderant organism and is more useful than culture, which will not distinguish between pathogenic and commensal organisms. A blood count is useful to determine oxygen carrying capacity in hypoxic patients, but the differential count is not sufficiently sensitive to distinguish between bacterial, viral, or mixed infections. The chest radiograph may show lobar, segmental, or broncho-pneumonic consolidation and is more useful in detecting complications of infection than in altering management.

Treatment of acute lower respiratory infection is in accordance with guidelines from Integrated Management of Childhood Illness [28]. Immunofluorescent staining of sputum or nasopharyngeal aspirate may identify viral agents of lower respiratory infection. The burden of disease due to respiratory syncytial virus (RSV), adenovirus influenza, and Para influenza viruses is increased in HIV-positive children. RSV infection in HIV-positive children is associated with increased morbidity and mortality [29].

Lymphoid interstitial pneumonitis

Between 16% and 50% of HIV-1 infected children, acquire lymphoid interstitial pneumonitis (LIP), most often in the second or third year of life [30]. In this age group, LIP is strongly associated with progression to AIDS and is listed in clinical category B in the clinical classification of HIV/AIDS in children under 13 years of age [31]. Although a lung biopsy is generally thought necessary to differentiate between LIP and infectious aetiologies [32], this procedure is rarely performed in children, and the diagnosis is generally made on clinical and radiological findings.

Children with LIP present, in their second and third years, with respiratory distress, radiological lung infiltrates and failure to thrive. Symptoms suggestive of small airways disease (air trapping, with or without reversible airways obstruction) and cough, may present long before any radiological abnormality [32]. Acute lower respiratory tract infections occur more frequently in LIP [30], a finding that confounds the analysis of symptoms associated with LIP and contributes to an understanding of the aetiology of both bronchiectasis and cor-pulmonale associated with LIP. Finger clubbing, parotid gland enlargement, and prominent generalised lymphadenopathy are commonly associated with LIP.

The classical chest radiograph in LIP has bilateral, predominantly lower zone reticular or reticulo-nodular opacities. While this pattern is also seen in miliary tuberculosis and Cytomegalovirus pneumonia, in LIP, it is indolent and does not respond to standard therapy for these conditions. In children, a resolution of this infiltrate has been correlated with a declining CD4+ count and advancing immunosuppression [33], although the association is not absolute. Resolution of the pulmonary infiltrate has also been observed in response to anti-retroviral therapy and to glucocorticoids.

There are no randomized, controlled clinical trials of glucocorticoids therapy in LIP, but case reports support this treatment, and also indicate a favourable response to single and multiple anti-retroviral drug regimens [34]. Indications for steroids in LIP include hypoxia and cor-pulmonale. Most patients with LIP and no access to anti-retroviral agents, die from infections related to immunosuppression and progressive pulmonary fibrosis. Cor-pulmonale and cardiac failure are frequently observed complications. While some studies have reported a shorter survival for children with LIP, other reports indicate a substantially better prognosis for these children compared with those who have other AIDS-defining conditions [35].

If a child does not have access to HAART, then pulsed steroid (2 mg/kg for 7 days, tailed to 5 mg daily over a month) offers appropriate palliative therapy for symptomatic LIP. If HAART is accessible, then triple therapy is the most appropriate and effective treatment.

Bronchiectasis

Children with AIDS and pulmonary disease, frequently, also have bronchiectasis; those who have LIP, also have recurrent or unresolved pneumonia and CD4+ counts below 100 per cubic millimetre [36]. This problem emerges particularly in children who, because of intensive and comprehensive management, survive for longer periods of time, and may occur in up to 15% of children with HIV and chronic chest illness [37].

The diagnosis of bronchiectasis in children is suggested by a history of recurrent, febrile, productive lower respiratory tract infections, recurrent signs of lower respiratory tract consolidation, and finger clubbing. Recurrent infections and increased work of breathing, contribute to failure to thrive. Plain chest radiography is not the gold standard for bronchiectasis, but recurrent consolidation in the same anatomical distribution, sometimes associated with lobar or segmental collapse is suggestive, in the presence of the other features mentioned above. In the absence of bronchography (where late films indicate poor clearance of radio-opaque dye), high-resolution computerised tomography is a convenient diagnostic aid [38]. Radioisotope ventilation perfusion scan is also useful in the diagnosis of bronchiectasis.

In some children, radiographic features of LIP coexist with persistent consolidation, and features suggestive of bronchiectasis. Since both these conditions may present with similar clinical histories, with recurrent infections and clinical findings such as finger clubbing, it is difficult to tease out features of individual pulmonary disease processes. Consequently, a substantial number of children are thought to have both these conditions concurrently.

In the absence of access to HAART, the palliative care of bronchiectasis in children with HIV/AIDS includes the use of antibiotics to treat acute bacterial super-infection of lower respiratory tract disease and a rotating antibiotic regimen as prophylaxis against progression of bronchietasis-related lung damage. Children also benefit from vigorous physiotherapy with dependent drainage, should damage be focused, in a particular and anatomical area. Bronchiectatic change in HIV/AIDS is generally diffuse and not amenable to surgery. Where it is localised, and if thoracic surgeons are amenable to operate on HIV positive children without access to HAART, surgery would be an appropriate element of the palliative management of bronchiectasis in such children. HAART does not reverse established bronchiectasis.

Cor-pulmonale

Cor-pulmonale is defined as hypertrophy of the right ventricle resulting from disease affecting the function and /or structure of the lung—excepting causes related to primary left ventricular or congenital heart disease.

In children with HIV/AIDS, right ventricular hypertrophy is associated with recurrent pulmonary infections [37], and is observed in children with bronchiectasis and/or LIP. Chronic hypoxia, caused by interstitial pneumonitis or parenchymal lung disease, is likely to play a part in the pathogenesis of cor-pulmonale. A large proportion of children with a chronic cough and a persistent pulmonary infiltrates, have right ventricular hypertrophy and dilatation on echocardiography.

Cor-pulmonale responds to anti-failure therapy with diuretics and digoxin and these are appropriate in the palliative care of affected children who do not have access to HAART. Patients with chronic lung disease who are oxygen dependent, often spend protracted periods as in-patients. Home-oxygen can be arranged for children living in houses with electricity by means of an oxygen concentrator; or a supply of oxygen cylinders where there is no access to electricity.

Experience in the effects of anti-retrovirals on children with cor-pulmonale, has revealed unexpected and gratifying benefits in cardiac function. Children who have been oxygen dependent and on treatment with digoxin, diuretics, and alpha blockers have first been weaned off home-oxygen and subsequently off treatment of cardiac failure. The basis of therapeutic response is uncertain, but is likely to be the effect of anti-retrovirals at several sites: On retroviral myocarditis, on lymphoid interstitial pneumonitis, and possibly because with an improvement in immune function. On HAART, these children have fewer episodes of intercurrent lower respiratory tract infections, and fewer episodes of infection with associated increase in metabolic rate.

Tuberculosis in children with HIV/AIDS

Tuberculosis is a common opportunistic infection amongst children with HIV/AIDS. The risk of tuberculosis in HIV-infected individuals who have been exposed to tuberculosis, is approximately 10% per annum [39] and tuberculosis occurs with increasing frequency as patients become more immuno-suppressed [40]. Most frequently, the child acquires M tuberculosis infection from an adult. In the case of an HIV-positive child, this is usually, from an adult living in his home with HIV/AIDS and reactivation of tuberculosis. HIV-positive children in contact with tuberculosis should receive preventive therapy, regardless of whether the sputum smear is negative or positive in the index case.

Tuberculosis in an HIV-infected child, usually presents with prolonged fever, chronic cough, and a history of contact with an active case and weight loss. Some children present with less specific symptoms and an abnormal chest radiograph, that does not respond to antibiotics. Unusual presentations include extra-pulmonary disease with hepato-splenomegaly, lymphadenopathy, anaemia, and weight loss in children with more advanced immuno-suppression. It is difficult to distinguish this presentation from that of advanced HIV/AIDS itself [41], lymphoma, deep mycosis, or infection by atypical mycobacteria.

Children with HIV and M tuberculosis co-infection have a shorter life expectancy than children with HIV alone [42,43], but respond to conventional anti-tuberculosis therapy both in the acute and the maintenance phase of the treatment.

Anti-retroviral, anti-fungal and anti-tuberculosis drugs interact with one another. 39 Ketoconazole and fluconazole inhibit the absorption of Rifampicin, which is a regular first-line agent in the treatment of tuberculosis. Rifampicin in turn reduces the serum concentration of these anti-fungal agents and accelerates the metabolism of some Protease Inhibitors (PIs) and the non-nucleoside reverse transcriptase inhibitor (NNRTI) Nevirapine. When a Rifampicin-containing regimen for tuberculosis and HAART are indicated simultaneously, the non-nucleoside reverse transcriptase inhibitor NNRTI Efavirenz or the PI Ritonavir may satisfactorily be combined with two nucleotide reverse transcriptase inhibitors.

Paradoxical reactions to HAART are defined as transient worsening of signs, and symptoms or the appearance of new signs, symptoms or radiographic features of tuberculosis that occur after the initiation of treatment. They are not a sign of treatment failure, but are thought to be a manifestation of an immune reaction to tubercle bacilli, previously inert because of immune suppression. Such paradoxical reactions are reported in up to 36% of patients starting treatment [44].

Immune reconstitution symptoms occur within days to weeks, after starting HAART [44]. Initiation of HAART within the first 2 months of starting anti-tuberculosis therapy is associated with an increased risk of a paradoxical reaction.

Common presenting signs include fever, enhanced adenopathy, serositis, cutaneous lesions, and new or expanding central nervous system lesions. Most patients who present paradoxical reactions have advanced HIV infection with CD4+ counts below 50 cells and very high viral loads [45]. Treatment includes non-steroidal anti-inflammatory agents and reassurance. High dose corticosteroids (prednisone 2 mg/kg for 7–10 days) are indicated in the case of lymphadenopathy with life-threatening airway compression.

Symptomatic pyrexia

Causes for fever in children with HIV/AIDs are many and varied. Management (Figure 30.1) will often require anti-infective treatment, which may need to be empirical if no specific cause can be found. HIV itself can be a cause of fever.

Symptoms in HIV/AIDS: The Romanian experience

Between 1989 and 2004, there were 1800 children under the paediatric HIV/AIDS service based in Constanza, Romania. This cohort of children, unique in Europe, were infected as a result of blood transfusion or dirty needles, at a time when blood transfusion was often seen as a 'tonic' to help children who were lethargic or failing to thrive. The stigma of the diagnosis was intolerable for some families, and many children continue to live in communal residential-respite facilities. While these are valuable providers of social and psychological support, living in close proximity can also encourage transmission of

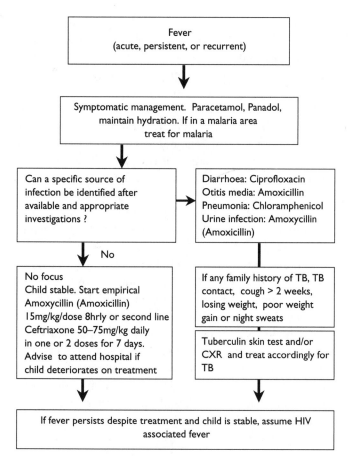

Fig. 30.1 Management of symptomatic pyrexia in children with HIV/AIDS.

contagious diseases; and tuberculosis in particular is a common problem.

In adults, the two main causes of symptom complications in HIV/AIDS are, malignancy and infection [46]. Our experience suggests that malignancy is much less often a problem in children. Of 1800 cases, only 20 have suffered from a malignancy (14 Kaposi's sarcoma, 4 NHL and 2 Burkitt's lymphoma). Infective problems (including tuberculosis, toxoplasmosis, CMV and zoster) seem to be equally common in children. Even here, there are differences in incidence; for example, pneumocystis carinii pneumonia is rather rare among our patients.

Antiretroviral agents were introduced in Romania in 1996. They have resulted in a dramatic change in the problems presented by children with HIV/AIDS. Many can live normal or near normal lives, but for others, the drugs themselves may have an impact. The occurrence of symptomatic infections remains relatively common and correlates closely with falls in CD4 count or rises in viral load.

This section will consider 'clusters' of symptoms that can occur.

Consequences of poor nutrition

Even before the arrival of antiretroviral drugs, it was possible to observe a dramatic improvement in a child's general condition, simply by attention to good nutrition. Muscle wasting and weakness can lead to pain directly [1] or by causing osteoporosis. Poor skin quality and ulceration of skin or mouth can be sources of severe pain.

As children are surviving into teenage, poor nutritional status increasingly carries with it, the problems of self-image. Normal pubertal development can be delayed by poor nutrition and final adult height may be significantly reduced. Many children with HIV/AIDS in Romania attend normal schools and their classmates may be unaware of the diagnosis. Changes in appearance that mark them out as different, can carry great stigma.

The pain of muscle wasting is musculoskeletal in nature and may well respond to a non-steroidal anti-inflammatory drug. Currently, major opioids are not yet available for prescription to children in Romania, but where they are available they too, can be effective in managing pain.

Gastrointestinal symptoms

Appetite is often affected. Although many children lose their appetite, it is less well recognized, that others can develop a form of hyperphagia. Diarrhoea is also common, often with an infective aetiology (see above).

There are a number of potential gastrointestinal sources for pain. Candidiasis of the mouth and oesophagus, or colonising the entire bowel from mouth to anus, can cause considerable discomfort.

Painful stomatitis or frank mouth ulcers can occur, due often to CMV or anaerobic infections. Multiple infections are common.

Less commonly, abdominal pain can be caused by atypical infections such as mycobacterium avium intracellulare (MAI). The lymphadenopathy of MAI is particularly uncomfortable but will often respond well to straightforward measures such as simple analgesics or opioids. Where intestinal spasm is a cause for pain, adjuvants such as buscopan should be considered (see also Chapter 23, Gastrointestinal symptoms).

Otherwise, treatment is often that of the underlying condition. Specific approaches (see above) include antibiotics, antivirals and antifungals. Malignant conditions can and should be treated, where it is likely that the benefit of doing so will outweigh the burden. Lymphoma in childhood, even in HIV/AIDS, is often curable and the treatment can be well tolerated.

Respiratory symptoms

Pneumocystis carinii pneumonia is relatively rare in children. Tuberculosis, on the other hand, is commonly seen. It is usually treatable but can spread to involve meninges, pericardium, liver, spleen, or to form cold abscesses.

TB meningitis, which is very difficult to treat, can also cause nausea and vomiting. Again, symptomatic treatment using appropriate antiemetics for centrally mediated emesis (see also Chapter 23, Gastrointestinal symptoms) should be accompanied by attempts to treat the underlying condition.

The dyspnoea associated with TB in children with HIV/AIDS does not tend to be painful. Rather, the child will become agitated and struggle for breath. There is an objective rise in respiratory rate. In our experience, excessive secretions are a relatively uncommon problem. Oxygen is rarely helpful, suggesting that most children are not hypoxaemic. The usual measures to relieve dyspnoea, may be of value. In addition, we have found good effect from short courses of steroids. This can be effective not only in TB, but in the dyspnoea associated with LIP (lymphocytic interstitial pneumonia), and pneumocystis pneumonia. The mechanism is presumably, reduction of interstitial oedema.

We have also used bronchodilators with some effect. Even in patients who are not asthmatic, there may be a reversible element to bronchospasm associated with pulmonary pathology.

Skin problems

Most problems with the skin are associated with infections and, again, symptomatic treatment should be combined with treatment of the underlying cause where this is possible.

Herpes, simplex and zoster are common and can cause considerable pain, pruritus or both. Approaches to pruritus are considered elsewhere in this book (see also Chapter 28, skin sypmtoms). The conditions can be recurrent over many years or even decades, and treatment with acyclovir seems to be progressively less effective over time.

Atypical tuberculosis, or other infections with anaerobes or staphyloccus aureus can cause cutaneous or subcutaneous infection. Cellulitis can be extremely painful, not only in the infected area but elsewhere in skin and joints. Staphylococcal infection in particular can cause a syndrome of severe myalgia.

Scabies is common among our children, due to a combination of close living contact and poor skin condition. Before the introduction of antiretrovirals, this was a particularly uncomfortable condition that could be very difficult to treat. Norwegian scabies (sc. norvegium) resulted in hyperkeratotic clusters that could be intensely pruritic and painful. Again, symptomatic treatment should be accompanied by management of the underlying condition.

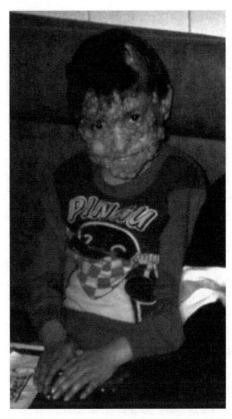

Fig. 30.2 Facial molluscum contagiosum in an 8-year old girl with HIV/AIDS (reproduced by kind permission of Children in Distress).

Molluscum contagiosum can present in children with HIV/AIDS as a widespread and disfiguring disease (Figure 30.2). Management is complicated by issues of self-image, and by problems associated with odour, as infections develop between the lesions. Management of odour, which is often caused by anaerobes, can include topical or systemic metronidazole.

Neuropsychiatric problems

At presentation, children with HIV/AIDS tend to be mildly developmentally delayed and to be mentally slower than their peers. The cause for this is unclear, and may not be related directly to infection with HIV/AIDS itself but to the poor social and family circumstances of the child at the time. Once children are well cared for, and their nutritional and emotional needs are met, there is often a rapid recovery. Some will go on to function normally. It appears therefore, that this syndrome of mild delay may be related more to circumstances, than to HIV/AIDS itself.

In our experience, 4–5% of children with HIV/AIDS will develop a syndrome analogous to the AIDS/dementia complex seen in adults. This may be characterized by lethargy, absent-mindedness or psychoretardation, or by seizures or pseudoseizures comprising repetitive movements and absences. It may be accompanied by dramatic loss of some skills including facial expression, speech, and recognition of family members.

Other than maintaining a safe and caring environment, there is little treatment available for this syndrome. Management of seizures is often difficult but is important for child and family.

Kaposi's sarcoma

Malignancies are less common in children with HIV/AIDS than in adults. Nevertheless, when they occur they can impose a heavy symptom load. Among our children, Kaposi's sarcoma was most common in the skin of the face, usually the nose or the ear, and then on the abdomen. The lesions themselves are tender, particularly the less superficial ones, but only mildly so.

Kaposi's sarcoma can develop or metastasise to meninges or lung. Pulmonary Kaposi's sarcoma is another cause for dyspnoea, and can cause significant haemoptysis.

Toxoplasmosis

Toxoplasmosis can occur at many sites, including intracerebral, ocular and pulmonary. Intracerebral and ocular toxoplasmosis can be very painful. Indeed, toxoplasmosis is the only condition other than cancer, for which major opioids can be prescribed in Romania. In our experience, pain is pulsatile and characterised by a relatively short response to morphine. The pain appears to be related to raised intracranial pressure and is particularly severe when the patient presents with visual disturbance.

Intracerebral toxoplasmosis can also cause nausea and vomiting, though this seems to be less of a problem than with TB or cryptococcal meningitis.

Our experience suggests that in contrast to tuberculosis and cryptococcosis which can be treated successfully even after recurring many times, toxoplasmosis becomes increasingly difficult to treat. This is particularly true of intracranial toxoplasmosis.

Cryptococcosis

Since the advent of antiretroviral drugs, generalized cryptococcosis or cryptococcal meningitis has become much rarer. Cryptococcosis is associated with severe headaches which seem to be made worse on movement, but can otherwise be of any type. Nausea and vomiting can be a major problem, leading to significant loss of weight. Torpor is another common symptom.

Management is, where possible, that of the underlying condition. This should be accompanied by careful attention to symptom management with appropriate analgesics and antiemetics.

Summary

In contrast with many other life-limiting conditions in childhood, in HIV/AIDS, the causes of pain and other symptoms themselves, are often a result of potentially curable conditions rather than directly to HIV/AIDS itself. In children, malignancy is relatively rare but infections are common. When it occurs, malignancy can cause significant symptoms. The main causes of pain in our experience, have been cerebral toxoplasmosis, cerebral lymphoma, cellulitis, visceral Kaposi's sarcoma and herpes zoster infection.

In parallel to curative approaches, the principles of good palliative care remain applicable to children with HIV/AIDS. Simple analgesia, opioids and appropriate adjuvants should be considered in the management of pain. Pain from zoster, for example, will often have a neuropathic component. Headache associated with lymphoma or toxoplasmosis may have an element of oedema, which can respond to short courses of sterioids or non-steroidal anti-inflammatory drugs, as well as, more usual measures. Other symptoms, such as nausea and vomiting, should be approached in the usual rational way, by considering the likely mechanism for the symptom.

It seems likely that children who have access to antiretroviral drugs will often survive into adulthood. The role of those working in paediatric palliative care, therefore, may be to ensure that a curative approach to intercurrent illness is always accompanied by a systematic approach to good symptom management.

References

1. Jennings, A. and George, R. HIV/AIDS, palliative care of HIV disease and AIDS. Themed Review Series. *Progr Palliat Care* 1996; 4:44–7.

2. Guay, L. *et al.* Intrapartum and neonatal single-dose nevirapine compared with zidovudine for prevention of mother-to-child transmission of HIV-1 in Kampala, Uganda: HIVNET 012 randomised trial. *Lancet* 1999;354(9181):795–802.

3. www.pmtctdonations.org/en/welcome.

4. UNAIDS, AIDS epidemic update: December 2003. www.unaids.org/en/resources/epidemiology/epidemicupdateslides.asp, 2003.

5. Dabis, F. *et al.* Estimating the rate of mother-to-child transmission of HIV. Report of a workshop on methodological issues Ghent (*Belgium*), 17–20 February 1992. The Working Group on Mother-to-Child Transmission of HIV. *AIDS* 1993;7(8):1139–48.

6. Bobat, R. *et al.* Mortality in a cohort of children born to HIV-1 infected women from Durban, South Africa. *S Afr Med J* 1999;89: 646–8.

7. Taha, T. *et al.* Morbidity among human immunodeficiency virus-1-infected and -uninfected African children. *Pediatrics* 2000; 106(6):E77.

8. Bulterys, M. *et al*. Maternal human immunodeficiency virus 1 infection and intrauterine growth: A prospective cohort study in Butare, Rwanda. *Pediatr Inf Dis J* 1994;13:94–100.

9. Agostoni, C. *et al*. Body mass index development during the first six months of life in infants born to human immunodeficiency virus-seropositive mothers. *Acta Pediatr* 1998;87:378–80.

10. McKinney, R., Robertson, W., *et al*. Effect of human immunodeficieny virus infection on the growth of young children. *J Pediatr* 1993;123:579–82.

11. Lepage, P. *et al*. Growth of human immunodeficiency type 1 infected and uninfected children: A prospective cohort study in Kigali, Rwanda, 1988 to 1993. *Pediatr Infect Dis J* 1996;15:479–85.

12. Carey, V., Yong, F.H., Frenkel, L.M., and McKinney, R.E. Pediatric AIDS prognosis using somatic growth velocity. *AIDS* 1998;12: 1361–9.

13. McKinney, R., Wilfert, C., *et al*. Growth as a prognostic indicator in children with human immunodeficiency virus infection treated with Zidovudine. *J Pediatr* 1994;125:728–33.

14. Verweel, G. *et al*. Treatment with highly active antiretroviral therapy in human immunodeficiency virus type-1-infected children is associated with a sustained effect on growth. *Pediatrics* 2002; 109(2):25.

15. Grotto, I. *et al*. Vitamin A supplementation and childhood morbidity from diarrhoea and respiratory infections: A meta-analysis. *J Pediatr* 2003;142:297–304.

16. Fawzi, W. *et al*. Vitamin A supplements and diarrhoeal and respiratory tract infections among children in Dar es Salaam, Tanzania. *J Pediatr* 2000;2003;137:142:660–7;297–304.

17. Barreto, M. *et al*. Effect of vitamin A supplementation on diarrhoea and acute lower respiratory tract infections in younger children in Brazil. *Lancet* 1994;344:228–31.

18. Baqui, A., Black, R., and Afeen, E. Effect of zinc supplementation started during diarrhoea on morbidity and motality in Bangladeshi children: Community randomised trial. *BMJ* 2002;325:1095.

19. *Quinn*, T. *et al*. AIDS in Africa: An epidemiological paradigm. *Science* 1986;234:955–63.

20. Johnson, S. *et al*. Effect of human immunodeficiency virus infection on episodes of diarrhoea among children in South Africa. *Pediatr Inf Dis J* 2000;19:972–9.

21. Kuehn, E. *et al*. Hypocalcaemia in HIV infection and AIDS. *J Intern Med* 1999;245:69–73.

22. Wiersma, R. HIV-positive African children with rectal fistulae. *J Pediatr Surg* 2003;38:62–4.

23. Blauvelt, A. and Turner, M. Gianotti–Crosti syndrome and human immunodeficiency virus infection. *Arch Dermatol* 1994;130:481–3.

24. Pediatrics, A.A.O. Varicella-zoster infections. In (25th edition) L. *Pickering* Red Book Elk Grove Village, IL: American Academy of Pediatrics;2000, p. 636.

25. World Health Organization, Guidelines for analgesic drug therapy. In Cancer Pain Relief and Palliative Care in Children. Geneva: WHO/IASP, 1998, pp. 24–8.

26. Pediatrics, A.A.O., Pneumocystis carinii infections. In L. Pickering, Red Book 25th edition, Elk Grove Village, IL: American Academy of Pediatrics 2000, pp. 460–5.

27. McLaughlin, G. *et al*. Effect of corticosteroid on survival of children with acquired immunodeficiency syndrome and Pneumocystis carinii-related respiratory failure. *J Pediatr* 1995;127:1007–8.

28. World Health Organisation. Cough or Difficult Breathing, in Management of the Child with a Serious Infection or Severe Malnutrition: Guidelines for Care at the First-Referral Level in Developing Countries. Geneva: WHO, 2000.

29. Mahdi, S. *et al*. Increased burden of respiratory viral associated severe lower respiratory tract infections in children with human immunodeficiency virus type-1. *J Pediatr* 2000;137:78–84.

30. Sharland, M., Gibb, D., and Holland, F. Respiratory morbidity from lymphocytic interstitial pneumonitis (LIP) in vertically acquired HIV infection. *Arch Dis Child* 1997;76:334–6.

31. Control, C.f.D. 1994 revised classification for immunodeficiency virus infection in children less than 13 years of age. *Morb Mort Wkly Rep* 1994;43:1–10.

32. Swigris, J. *et al*. Lymphoid interstitial pneumonia. *Chest* 2002;122: 2150–64.

33. Prosper, M. *et al*. Clinical significance of resolution of chest X-ray findings in HIV-infected children with lymphocytic interstitial pneumonitis (LIP). *Pediatr Radiol* 1995;25 (Suppl. 1):S243–6.

34. Bach, M. Zidovudine for lymphocytic interstitial pneumonia associated with AIDS (letter). *Lancet* 1987;2:796.

35. Tovo, P. *et al*. Prognostic significance of immunologic changes in 675 infants perinatally exposed to HIV infected individuals. *Lancet* 1992;339:702–9.

36. Sheikh, S. *et al*. Bronchiectasis in pediatric AIDS. *Chest* 1997;112: 1202–7.

37. Bannerman, C. and Chitsike, I. Cor pulmonale *in* children with human immunodeficiency virus infection. *Ann Trop Paediatri* 1995; 15:129–34.

38. Chang, A. *et al*. Non-CF bronchiectasis: Clinical and HRCT evaluation. *Paed Pulmon* 2003;35:477–83.

39. Africa, H.C.S.O.S. Guidelines for tuberculosis preventative therapy in HIV infection. *South Afr Med J* 2000;90:592–4.

40. Wood, R., Maartens, G., and Lombard, C. Risk factors for developing tuberculosis in HIV-1 infected adults from communities with a low or very high incidence of tuberculosis. *J Acquir Immune Def Syndr Hum Retrovirol* 2000;23:75–80.

41. Jeena, P. *et al*. Impact of HIV-1 co-infection on presentation and hospital-related mortality in children with culture proven pulmonary tuberculosis in Durban, South Africa. *Int J Tuberc Lung Dis* 2002;6:672–8.

42. Palme, I. *et al*. Impact of human immunodeficiency virus 1 infection on clinical presentation, treatment outcome and survival in a cohort of Ethiopian children with tuberculosis. *Pediatr Infect Dis J* 2002;21:1053–61.

43. Blusse van Oud-Alblas, H., van Vliet, M., and Kimpen, J. Immunodeficiency virus infection in children hospitalised with tuberculosis. *Ann Trop Paediatr* 2002;22:115–23.

44. Furrer, H. and Malinverni, R. Systemic inflammatory reaction after starting highly active antiretroviral therapy in AIDS patients treated for extrapulmonary tuberculosis. *Am J Med* 1999;106:371–2.

45. Narita, M. *et al*. Paradoxical worsening of tuberculosis following antiretroviral therapy in patients with AIDS. *Am J Resp Crit Care Med* 1998;158:157–61.

46. Winter, H. Gastrointestinal and nutritional problems in children with immunodeficiency and AIDS. In T. Chang, ed. *Pediatr Clini N Am*. 1996;43:573–90.

31 Complementary and alternative medicine

David M. Steinhorn and Michelle Rogers

Introduction to complementary therapies

The purpose of this chapter is to familiarize the reader with the wide range of modalities contained under the rubric of Complementary and Alternative Medicine (CAM). Given the diverse nature and history of the field, it is impossible to mention all known disciplines, but an effort has been made to address those most commonly encountered in practice by western medical physicians and nurses.

In the past, there have often been misunderstandings, and pre-conceived biases associated with other terminology, and the term, 'complementary therapies', or CAM, will be used throughout this chapter, to refer to a wide range of therapeutic and treatment modalities that are not widely taught in medical schools. The term has been chosen for its neutral meaning. By contrast, therapeutic approaches practiced by most western physicians will be referred to as 'Western' or 'allopathic', a term commonly used in North America. The derivation of these terms will be considered later in the chapter. It should be recognized that each school or philosophy of healers tends to view its own approach to healing as the more traditional one.

Background

From time immemorial, societies and cultures have found ways to care for injured and ill individuals. Such efforts stem from a universal desire to extend both the quantity and quality of life, to protect individuals from harm, and to relieve suffering. The concept of, and approach to, illness and its treatment have changed dramatically. The earliest civilizations must have viewed the body as a mysterious, unfathomable entity, and disease as an inexplicable process, mediated by invisible forces or spirits. Healing was equally mysterious, with prayer, dancing, chanting, and herbal remedies the primary tools of early healers. Out of this early existential view of health, disease, and healing, a mechanistic model of disease began to evolve. Patterns of disease were gradually identified, and healers found more reliable herbal or chemical remedies for various symptoms and ailments. These developments laid the foundation for understanding disease as a disruption in natural processes, which could be rectified through appropriate intervention. However, throughout history, prayer, sacrifice, and supplication of higher powers continued to be important routes to healing, in an attempt to placate the invisible world thought to be responsible for ill health. Little attempt was made to distinguish the individual from his or her physical ailments. With the renaissance and age of enlightenment in the West, western physicians began to separate the physical from the psychic components of the individual. The development of science, and the elevation of reason over emotion in the West over the last few centuries, have led to a still greater separation between physical disease and the inner, psychological, or spiritual condition of the individual. Contemporary medical science has only recently begun to recapture the earlier vision of wholeness, and to appreciate again the inextricable connection between one's inner state and somatic disease [1–6].

Thus, the movement in western societies towards a more integrated view of a patient's state of health, espoused by palliative medicine, in many ways represents a rebirth, and a renewed exploration of approaches that often have their roots in ancient systems of medicine. A common theme is the identification of disease with a disruption in some form of natural 'balance' that occurs in health. This is a principle that has echoes of modern understanding about the importance of a normal internal milieu maintained through homoeostasis, but often extends it well beyond the merely physical.

Herbal medicine has always been an important part of healing for African, South American, and Native American shamans, and healers from the Far East to Europe. In Europe, homeopathy was developed in the eighteenth century by the German physician Samuel Hahnemann, who formulated a set of laws and principles governing health and disease. Homeopathy is still widely used in Germany, India (in conjunction with Ayurvedic medicine), and elsewhere in western Europe and North America. There is a national Homoeopathic Hospital in London.

Acupuncture has a 3500 year history, with its inception in China. The Huang Di Nei Jing, a collection of writings that serves as the primary foundation for Traditional Chinese Medicine theories, is over 2000 years old. It was the first book to discuss anatomy, physiology, pathology, diagnosis, treatment, and prevention of diseases. The concept of Yin and Yang developed during the Yin (1600–1046 BC) and Zhou (1046–221 BC) Dynasties. This concept sees two opposite, but complementary, principles in all phenomena of the natural world. Yin and yang provide the conceptual foundation and framework for present Traditional Chinese Medicine, which is still widely used in China. Many medical schools there teach this traditional medicine, alongside modern pharmacological and technological based medicine.

Commonly used herbal and naturopathic medicine have rich traditions in western Europe. Modalities used included herbal and homeopathic medicines, hydrotherapy, diet and nutrition recommendations, massage, and energy work, in programs designed for the needs of the individual patient.

While health care traditions in some places have continued largely unchanged over many generations, western medicine has made significant technological strides over the past 150 years. The last half of the twentieth century witnessed improved survival rates, and reductions in morbidity for many congenital and acquired diseases of childhood. At the same time, this period brought a growing awareness that science alone may not be able to provide all the answers to alleviate suffering, for humankind as a whole, or for individuals. Patients hospitalized in western medical institutions who receive state-of-the-art medical care, may nevertheless, feel that many of their wider needs go unmet [6,7]. One expression of this is that parents are requesting the incorporation of complementary therapies into their child's care, in the hope that they will more fully address spiritual, emotional, and other needs. Such requests seem to be most common for children suffering from conditions which western medicine continues to be unable to cure, or to treat adequately [8]. These are the same outcome priorities, and the same patient group addressed by palliative care services in children; it is not surprising that most professionals working with dying children will encounter families who would like to access CAM.

As in most fields of research, the use of complementary medicine has been more thoroughly studied in adults, both as in-patients and out-patients, than in children. An important report of CAM use by 2055 adults in the United States found that that the use of some kind of alternative therapy had risen, from 34% in 1990 to 41% in 1997 [9,10]. More than US$21 billion was paid for alternative medicine services during 1997, with more than half of this coming from patients themselves. Third-party payers provided reimbursement for a large number of therapies, but the willingness of private individuals to pay directly for non-reimbursed CAM services was an eye-opening, unexpected finding. 96% of the survey respondents, who consulted an alternative practitioner for a primary complaint, had also seen a conventional physician in the preceding 12 months. Only 38.5% acknowledged discussing these therapies with their physicians, the others indicated either embarrassment, or fear of offending their physician, as the reason for not informing them [11]. This study suggests that many patients will access CAM's, whether their physicians, want them to or not, and that unless encouraged to discuss it, they will often keep such contact secret.

CAM Therapies as adjuncts in palliative care

One of the underlying principles of palliative care is that of 'holism'—the recognition that all human experience takes place not only in a physical dimension, but also in the emotional, social and spiritual ones. Conventional western medical approaches may not be enough to alleviate the wider suffering of approaching death, and for many, the use of CAM therapies to augment conventional care is very attractive [12,13]. A recent report on the prevalence of inadequately relieved end-of-life symptoms in children reinforces the importance of this issue for the paediatric palliative care team[14]. As in other situations, problems which they feel are inadequately relieved by conventional approaches, are the ones for which families frequently seek out CAM interventions. These symptoms fall into two groups: physical symptoms, such as nausea and pain, that have not been adequately controlled, and emotional-spiritual symptoms of depression, fear, and existential dilemmas that have not been adequately explored, and remain unresolved. Ironically, some of these symptoms go unrelieved, not because of a failure of conventional medicine *per se*, but because of a lack of expertise available to the child or family in practice.

CAM Worldwide

In 2001, the World Health Organization (WHO) published a report assessing the current use of CAM therapies, the state of legislation and regulation, education/training of CAM practitioners, and the state of health insurance coverage for 123 of its 191 member states [15]. Although it remained incomplete, due to repeated legislative and educational policy changes, the report provides an excellent summary of CAM worldwide in 2000. A second document entitled, *World Health Organization Traditional Health Strategy 2002–2005* sets out strategies for the worldwide development of CAM therapies [16]. By providing these guidelines, the WHO has begun to set international standards for training and licensing of providers (Table 31.1).

Table 31.1 Resources for CAM therapies

Acupuncture- website (http://wfas.acutimes.com/index.htm) Established in 1987, the World Federation of Acupuncture-Moxibustion Societies (WFAS) has nearly 60,000 members from 73 acupuncture organizations from 40 countries in several regions.

Homeopathy- website (www.lmhi.net) The Liga Medicorum Homeopathica Internationalis (International Homeopathic Medical League) (LMHI) was established in 1925, and represents about 8000 homeopathic practitioners in 50 countries.

Chiropractic Medicine- website (www.wfc.org/) The World Federation of Chiropractic (WFC) works with national and international organizations to provide information and other assistance in the fields of chiropractic and world health; promotes uniform high standards of chiropractic education, research and practice; works to develop an informed public opinion among all peoples with respect to chiropractic; and upon request, provides advice on appropriate legislation for chiropractic in member countries.

Islamic Medicine- website (www.islamset.com/) The Islamic Organization for Medical Sciences (IOMS) works with WHO on preparation of a manual on the use of medicinal plants. Islamic medicine, incorporates modern Western medicine, but its fifth criterion of 'utilizing all useful resources' means that it is also willing to consider any potentially useful treatment.

UK Research Council on CAM- website (www.rccm.org.uk) An excellent resource, especially for the United Kingdom, with information on CAM topics, and links to large CAM databases, search engines, etc.

Association of Bodywork and Massage Professionals- Their website (www.abmp.com/) provides useful information and links to state licensing agencies, schools, etc., in North America, which deal with many commonly used body therapies, e.g., Rei Ki, Feldenkrais, cranio-sacral manipulation, massage, etc.

National Health Information Center- Website (www.health.gov/NHIC/) provides extensive background information on numerous topics related to CAM and other medical issues. Links to professional organizations.

NIH—National Center for Complementary and Alternative Medicine (NCCAM)- (www.nccam.nih.gov/) Provides excellent background information, evidence based results, links to other information.

Integrative Therapies Program for Children with Cancer (www.integrativetherapiesprogram.org). A well-maintained academic website dedicated to CAM therapies often requested for children with cancer, including herbal remedies, drug-herb interactions, accupuncture, massage, etc.

The recent attention on CAM therapies has served to highlight the differences that exist in health care delivery in various regions of the world. Systems for the delivery of medical care range from the shamans of various indigenous tribes worldwide, to the most technologically complex systems of the industrialized countries. Within this broad spectrum, one finds a large variety of health care providers, including the many CAM providers, practicing in all areas of high population density. The philosophical roots of conventional western medicine grew out of a rationalist approach, which explained disease by identifying a problem, studying it, and accumulating a body of knowledge and understanding, from which specific treatments could be developed. According to this model, medicine is seen as the source of healing for a body and nature which have 'gone wrong'. Because treatment is applied from outside, this approach is sometimes referred to as *allopathic*.

By contrast, the *vitalist* or *empiric* approach is that exemplified by some CAM practitioners. Vitalists see the entire individual as an integrated entity that interacts with its environment, whereas western medicine has a recent history of seeing the patient's physical illness separate from the many other human dimensions. Of great importance in the vitalist view is the capacity of the body to heal itself. This view of disease and healing, which is the basis of *homeopathy*, naturopathy, and some schools of chiropractic medicine, sees the physician as an adjunct or facilitator of the body's ability to heal, rather than as the primary agent of healing.

In the European Union, North America, and other regions, two principal problems face CAM therapies, pertaining to the licensing to practise complementary medicine, and the reimbursement of treatment by both social health insurance systems and private insurance. In all countries of the EU, access to medical practice is regulated by specific laws; however, legislation appears to vary widely between the EU countries. Similarly, reimbursement is different between countries, with many providing insurance coverage only when CAM therapies are provided under the supervision of a physician. In many countries, CAM practitioners are viewed as allied health care providers, and frequently work under the direction of a licensed physician, rather than having independent practices, as occurs often in the United States.

In the United Kingdom, a government committee was charged with evaluating the state of CAM therapies, and found that a lack of regulation of CAM might put the public at risk of poor, or possibly harmful, treatment by unqualified practitioners [17]. The Committee concluded that acupuncture, herbal medicine, and possibly, non-medical homeopathy, should be subject to statutory regulation. They recommended regulation of herbal medicines. A recommendation was made for standardized training of CAM practitioners with independent accreditation. Registered conventional health professionals are encouraged to become more familiar with CAM, and those working in the best regulated CAM professions should strive for closer integration with conventional medicine. The dissemination of information to the public and health professionals was found to be inadequate, and recommendations have been made for improving this situation. Information is available from the Research Council on Complementary Medicine (Table 31.1)

In North America, there are also regional differences for CAM practitioners. Even within the United States, individual states differ widely in their approach to licensure of specific CAM therapists. There are, of course, well-established licensing mechanisms in all states for the major medical providers, which in the United States include chiropractors and osteopaths, as well as allopathic physicians. Licensing arrangements for other practitioners are much less consistent. Patients and referring physicians must contact their local professional boards, or licensing agencies, to find practitioners who have achieved basic standards of training and credentialing recognized by their respective professional boards.

In the United States, medical curricula for osteopaths are similar to those of allopathic physicians. Osteopaths are licensed to prescribe medications, and many complete additional training in traditional allopathic residencies and fellowships. Other health care providers function as allied health care workers, rather than as physicians. There are training and licensing standards in many states for many CAM practitioners. Worldwide, professional certifying boards with training programs for many CAM therapies are available. Many of these programs fall under the banner of Traditional Chinese Medicine (TCM) which includes a wide range of modalities, such as acupuncture, life-style changes, herbal and dietary manipulations, and massage. Schools of TCM can be found in most industrialized countries, and can be helpful in providing information to physicians.

General paediatric use of complementary therapies

Comprehensive clinical studies regarding the use and effectiveness of CAM in children are lacking. However, approximately 20% to 30% of paediatric patients have received one or more CAM therapies, and in teenagers, the proportion reaches 50 to 75% [18–22]. In children, these interventions have been used for acute and chronic conditions alike. The most common pediatric conditions for which complementary therapies were used include symptoms of common colds and influenza, irritable bowel disease, asthma, juvenile rheumatoid arthritis, and cystic fibrosis. Symptom relief during oncology treatment [19,23] [24] was another common cause. Use of complementary therapies among pediatric patients, including infants with chronic, recurrent, or incurable conditions such as cancer,

asthma, rheumatoid arthritis, and cystic fibrosis, range from 30 to 70% [8]. Complementary therapies have been used with varying levels of validation, for a wide variety of common pediatric conditions, including disordered sleep, perioperative nausea, allergies, attention deficit hyperactivity disorder, depression, and similar chronic distressing symptoms. A number of reports indicate potential benefits from the use of complementary modalities in the newborn period, including sick premature infants receiving intensive care therapies [25,26]. A recent survey of the use of CAM by children with cancer demonstrates that 75% use at least one modality [27]. Traditional folk remedies also continue to be important in many ethnic and cultural groups [28–31].

Use of CAM is, therefore, widespread among families of children with life-limiting conditions. It is clearly important for health care workers to inquire sensitively into the use of such therapies, and the belief-systems that may underlie them [32].

Definition of terms

Integrative medicine

When complementary therapies are included in an intentional blend of western and non-western methods, the approach is sometimes referred to as *integrative*. Integrative medicine describes an approach that considers a broad range of therapies, therapeutic modalities, and approaches selecting those that have the best evidence of *safety* and *efficacy* within the context of holistic care [33]. The term, therefore, describes good palliative care in children.

Alternative vs. complementary therapies

It is worthwhile, at this juncture, to discuss the distinction which has been made between alternative and complementary therapies. It could be argued that, much as the adult hospice movement began as a counter-cultural response to perceived inadequacies in caring for dying adults, the field of alternative medicine grew out of the dissatisfaction patients experienced with conventional medical care for acute illnesses. Alternative approaches were seen as equivalent substitutes for conventional therapies, in spite of the frequent absence of convincing data to support the efficacy of the therapy. While western medicine increasingly demands reproducible, objective outcomes, alternative therapies are often based upon historical traditions or anecdote, lacking rigorous validation.

Despite medical progress, there remain many conditions for which standard 'curative' approaches are unlikely to be effective in substantially increasing the quality or duration of a child's life. These include, for example, some conventional treatments for progressive brainstem glioma, leukaemia that recurs after successful bone marrow transplant, and many of the inherited neuro-degenerative disorders, such as Tay-Sachs disease. It can be argued that for patients with these conditions, it is acceptable to try an alternative, providing this does not itself cause suffering (see case study of DM below), and can offer results as good as or better than those obtained through the conventional recommendation.

Where conventional therapy offers demonstrable benefit to patients, e.g. insulin for Type-I diabetes, or treatment of most forms of childhood cancer, health care providers have a legal, as well as a moral, responsibility to act in the best interests of the child. Indeed, in most countries, to withhold such treatments would constitute a breach of parents' legal responsibilities to their child. At the same time, it is usually important to support a family's desire to explore additional options, if they so choose. The term *complementary* has come into more common usage, to indicate therapies which are used as potential adjuncts to conventional therapy.

Case *Supporting the family.* DM was a 8-year-old male of eastern European descent, admitted for loss of developmental milestones and seizure activity. An idiopathic degenerative CNS process was diagnosed, after many weeks of evaluation for known metabolic and infectious aetiologies. The seizures became progressive and intractable, in spite of attempts at control with drug induced coma, and supplementation with coenzyme Q10 and pyridoxine, in addition to conventional anticonvulsants. The family sought additional help, and requested massage therapy sessions, acupuncture, energy healing sessions, magnet therapy, and bee venom injections, as well as other folk remedies. The medical team made decisions regarding the potential risk of each requested complementary intervention, and permitted the family's chosen therapist to provide those interventions with courtesy privileges, in the presence of the hospital nurse and, often, the physician. The physicians refused to permit the administration of bee venom, due to the known potential risk and the profound degree of cerebral atrophy apparent on MRI studies, suggesting irreversible loss of brain tissue and metabolic activity. The hospital team felt that permitting the therapies provided an indication of good-faith, in leaving no stone unturned in attempting to improve DM's condition. Rather than refuse the family's requests, which would likely have driven them to seek out other medical care, an effort was made to work with them. The family often became demanding and, many felt, unreasonable, in the requests for the administration of supplements brought in from the outside. In spite of the frequent conflicts between the health care team and the family's unusual requests, the family continues to see our institution as the one to turn to when help is needed, suggesting ongoing trust. The child remains in a vegetative state, on a respirator, after four years. It is of interest to note that the magnet therapist brought in by the family refused to treat the patient, due to the presence of advanced cerebral atrophy, which she felt would not respond to her interventions (*note*- her practice of magnet therapy was primarily used in adults, following hemorrhagic stroke, which she believed could respond well to her interventions).

Goals of therapy

When considering all therapeutic and palliative interventions, whether for acute illness or the relief of distressing symptoms in life-limited patients, it is important to recognize that multiple goals may co-exist. Although medicine continues to see curing disease as a primary mandate, and it is often the one for which patients seek attention, there remains a range of valid options, even when a cure is not possible. It is just these additional options which are most relevant to patients at the end of life, and are often well established in palliative care practice. Practitioners of complementary therapies share similar goals in planning healing interventions. Many non-western traditions, which place great importance on the effect of the inner psychic, or spiritual, state on somatic disease, will focus more heavily on treatment options which aim to create a deeper sense of inner peace, tranquillity, and harmony with life. Improving the sense of inner tranquillity is an important goal for contemporary palliative care for children. Thus, complementary approaches may be beneficial adjuncts in the care of dying patients.

Suffering in children

There is little authoritative literature regarding the nature of suffering in children. A major component of suffering experienced by dying children comes from distressing physical symptoms [14], but it is an axiom of good palliative care that the physical dimension is only one aspect of suffering. While there are differences in the logistics of palliative care delivery across different cultures, the wider issues that can hinder personal happiness and individual fulfilment are similar worldwide [34]. Contemporary palliative care recognizes that lingering existential uncertainties, for example, may contribute to overall suffering, as death approaches. Resolving relationships, dealing with feelings of guilt or loss, a sense of unfulfilled desires, reconciling spiritual conflicts and achieving a sense of 'having put one's affairs in order', are common challenges for patient, family and palliative care team [32].

Such issues obviously depend upon the developmental stage of the child [35]. Very young children depend upon the comforting touch of familiar individuals, to feel safe and peaceful, with the same holding true for many older patients as well. In younger children, pre-verbal children and patients with encephalopathy due to medications or advanced disease, it is much more difficult to determine the existential needs. Yet, if we accept that conscious individuals suffer from 'unfinished business' at the end of life, we must consider that patients with altered consciousness may also have unfinished life tasks, even if they cannot manifest the suffering, or do not seem aware of it. It is in addressing the difficult-to-determine inner needs of such patients that complementary techniques may provide significant comfort.

Case *Relief of general suffering.* SA, a 10-year-old girl with meningomyelocele, ventriculoperitoneal shunt, and paraplegia, developed Acute Respiratory Distress Syndrome, due to RSV pneumonitis. Her recovery was prolonged, and she required tracheostomy and chronic ventilation for respiratory support. This alert, bright child had numerous re-admissions to the paediatric ICU for various medical conditions. As part of her care, a hospital chaplain, who practised Reiki and aromatherapy, visited her and provided these therapies. SA indicated that the treatments made her feel 'warm' and comfortable. Aromatherapy too produced a sensation of warmth through her body, in spite of the fact that she was ventilated via tracheostomy, and had no nasal air flow. She requested visits from the chaplain whenever she was in hospital, and saw her support as an integral part of her experience in the ICU.

Commonly utilized complementary therapies

The US National Institute for Health established the National Center for Complementary and Alternative Medicine (NCCAM), in 1992, to deal with the increasing utilization of complementary therapies in the United States, and to oversee the allocation of national funding resources for high quality research. In an attempt to reduce confusion, and to understand the potential place of various complementary therapies, expert panels established by NCCAM have defined several major categories of complementary therapy (Table 31.2). Given the thousands of non-allopathic healing traditions and techniques that are used throughout the world, it is important, but difficult, to identify unifying principles. For example, conventional surgery, massage therapy and Rolfing have in common a focus on physical manipulation of tissue, while some acupuncture and energy healing techniques strive to re-balance and enhance putative subtle energy derangements, which can lead to psychic or somatic disease.

Further confusion arises in trying to interpret the several mechanisms by which individual complementary techniques may affect patients. For example, aromatherapy may be considered to be a biophysical intervention in the case of pure aromas that work through pure olfactory effects, but as an energy healing modality when flower essences are utilized. In order to perform meaningful research, and to compare the effects of various techniques, it is critical to have a standardized

Table 31.2 Major branches of complementary therapies—NCCAM

Energy therapies
    Acupuncture
    Biofield therapies: Reiki, Qi Gong, Therapeutic Touch
    Bioelectromagnetic-based therapies

Mind–body interventions
    Meditation, prayer, music

Biologically based therapies
    Herbs, foods, vitamins, supplements

Manipulative and body-based methods
    Massage, Physical Manipulation, e.g. chiropractic, surgery

Alternative medical systems
    Homeopathy, naturopathy, Chinese medicine, Ayurveda

vocabulary and concept of how each technique might facilitate healing. It should be further recognized that general life-style issues, such as diet, exercise, weight management, and time to relax, play a role, not only for patients, but for health care workers themselves—'Health care system, heal thyself! [23].'

Research into the application of complementary approaches for children continues to lag behind that for adults. There are many unmet needs and unanswered questions [36]. The literature on the use of complementary therapies in children with life-limiting conditions is even more limited [37–39]. The following brief overview will focus on the major modalities utilized with children. It is not meant to be exhaustive, but emphasizes those techniques with demonstrated efficacy, or those in most common use.

Energy based therapies

Acupuncture

Acupuncture is probably the one energy-based therapy that is most widely recognized by most western health care providers. It is a complementary therapy, which has experienced remarkable attention in western medicine over the last several decades, after a history spanning several millennia in the Far East [40–42]. The term acupuncture represents a family of different approaches, which stimulate specific areas of the skin, either through piercing with needles, or by applying pressure, heat, etc. Traditional explanations for its efficacy refer to the balancing of subtle energy (*Qi* or *Chi*) in the body, which is not easily measurable by western techniques. Scientific investigations suggest that the acupuncture points correspond to areas of the skin with low electrical resistance, and proximity to nerve endings. It is speculated that the release of various neurotransmitters may produce the beneficial effects reported. Recent basic research has demonstrated an increase in nitric oxide generation in areas of the skin over the acupuncture meridians [43].

A growing number of acupuncture practitioners are specifically trained to treat children [44]. It is now provided as a treatment option in approximately one-third of paediatric pain treatment programs at academic medical centres in North America. Parents and children tend to find the procedure acceptable, and not overly threatening [45]. In a retrospective analysis of 50 eligible patients treated with acupuncture for chronic pain, acupuncture therapies included needle insertion (98%), heat or moxabustion (85%), magnets (26%), and cupping (26%). Most patients and parents rated the therapy as pleasant (67% children/60% parents), and most (70% children/59% parents) reported improvement in pain, with few adverse outcomes. Some children with chronic, severe pain found acupuncture treatment to be pleasant and helpful. Additional, prospective studies with appropriate controls are needed, to quantify the costs and effectiveness of acupuncture treatment for paediatric pain. To this end, criteria have been established to evaluate the outcomes of acupuncture trials, and to increase the scientific validity of future studies [46]. In addition to an attempt to increase the rigor of clinical trials, basic research has begun to demonstrate a cellular basis to the effects of acupuncture mediated through postulated mechanisms, e.g. nitric oxide, which are receiving much attention in other clinical settings [43].

Perhaps the best documented evidence for acupuncture has been shown for the treatment of chronic pain and nausea [45, 47–49]. Considerable discussion continues to be held, on whether predetermined regimens of needle placement are as effective as the more traditional eastern approach of selecting points based upon the unique needs and nature of the individual patient. Because the field known as 'Traditional Chinese Medicine' is both complex, and utilizes different criteria for physical examination and diagnosis than western medicine, it is difficult for western trained practitioners to fully understand and embrace those concepts, without significant additional education and experience [50]. In many industrialized countries, there are schools of Traditional Chinese Medicine and acupuncture, that can serve as resources for physicians. The certification of competency for acupuncturists is generally based upon successful completion of a standardized curriculum, completion of numerous hours of supervised treatment and, where available, licensing by local professional boards.

The use of acupuncture [27]as an adjunct in pain control [51] [45, 47] and nausea and vomiting [49,52] demonstrates benefits in children. When successful as an adjunct, acupuncture has permitted the use of lower doses of sedating analgesic agents, thus permitting greater alertness in patients. Additional uses have been directed at emotional and spiritual interventions in adults [53], however, reliable evidence in children is lacking at present.

Energy via touch

Further modalities which rely upon manipulation of a putative subtle energy, *Qi*, in the body, include the western technique of Therapeutic Touch, introduced several decades ago into the nursing curriculum, as well as a wide range of other techniques which aim to balance the *Qi*. While Therapeutic Touch has been widely accepted in traditional, institution-based western medicine, the other techniques have found more acceptance in the outpatient setting. In contrast to acupuncture, for which licensing standards exist in many regions, the other forms of energy techniques are much less standardized, in terms of training without a formal credentialing process. A number of reputable schools exist in every community which teach such techniques. Rigorous controlled studies of energy healing techniques are limited, however, it is clear that many patients derive a general, often profound, sense of well-being from such treatments. A typical session may last for 30–60 min, during which the practitioner will move his or her hands in a gentle motion around the body. Light touch may also be used. Many practitioners focus on the intention for the energy to be used for the highest good of the patient. The highest good of the patient may include both spiritual enlightenment, as well as healing of somatic or psychological disease. Healing touch is believed to work with the energy of the body, to induce deep relaxation and promote self-healing. Patients report that it can help in reducing pain, promoting relaxation, managing stress, acceleration of tissue and bone healing, and strengthening of the immune system; however, conclusive evidence for its efficacy in paediatric conditions is presently anecdotal. By inducing a state of deep relaxation, one might anticipate that so-called 'relaxation response' may be elicited in the patient, even when the patient lacks the ability to participate in creating the state of relaxation [54, 55].

For many practitioners of energy healing techniques, qualifications are less well defined than for acupuncturists. Many have no formal training, having come by their skill through serendipity or personal study. Beyond attendance in a school or training workshops anyone may claim to be so skilled; little proof is required to open a practice. Professional licensing boards do not generally offer credentials; most do not acknowledge this branch of healing. Each physician considering referring patients to such healers must, therefore, develop a network of collaborators.

It is not clear whether skills in energy healing that are utilized for adults and teenagers can be applied to younger children. There has been a dearth of controlled, scientific investigation, a lack of standardization of training, and a paucity of information on applicability to children. Nonetheless, many patients and families report dramatic improvement in their sense of wellbeing and inner peace, and a reduction in adverse symptoms, following skilled treatment by adjunctive healers utilizing energy techniques. While it is generally true that those techniques which are minimally invasive tend to have few adverse effects, lack of risk alone should not be taken as an indication for their use. Good care of a child must always be based upon the best possible evidence for benefit, rather than an absence of harm.

Many energy healing techniques include aspects of 'prayer', a laying on of hands, specific regimented exercises and homeopathy. Some (e.g., Reiki Qi Gong, or homeopathy) can be performed on behalf of a sick child, while others (e.g., Tai Chi) require greater understanding, training, and maturity to be effective. As with allopathic interventions, there is an ethical issue to be considered in the child whose parents request a technique to which the child does not, or cannot, consent. Much of the consideration for which modality to choose depends upon the availability, skill and willingness of local complementary healers to work with the existing health care team.

Case *Energy healing.* MS was 17 years old, with neuroblastoma and tumour recurrence following stem cell transplant. He was referred to the Integrative Medicine team for help managing headache, nausea, chronic fatigue, and pain at the site of primary tumor and the radiation site. He received several treatments initially, and reported feeling a tingling sensation in his leg, with a significant reduction in pain and nausea. He requested treatments whenever he was in the hospital, receiving a total of eight treatments over several months. On one occasion, he was having nausea, pain and fever, and the energy healer was asked to visit him. Following the treatment, his headache was gone, his nausea had reduced and the fever had abated, eliminating the need for further pharmacologic intervention. MS attributed this response to the energy healing session.

Energy healing in palliative care

Touch should be encouraged as part of palliative care where it is culturally acceptable,. Energy healing techniques can provide comfort through the presence of another human being, and the communication of that person's good will and caring through touch. The other value of touch derives from the subtle energy which, according to its practitioners, can flow at a level far deeper than that of a patient's normal consciousness. The healer's intention for a peaceful death, and his or her willingness to be present for the patient through that journey can, it is believed, be transmitted without words, through touch. Given the wide acceptance of touch in adult palliative care

[50,56], and the comfort provided to children by parental and adult touch, all care of children with life-limiting conditions should include human contact and touch as central components. In this context, touch may be through traditional massage, therapeutic touch or energy healing techniques [25,57,58].

Biologically based therapies

Herbal remedies/dietary supplements

Few well-performed studies, with appropriate controls and blinding, have examined the use of dietary or herbal supplements for the treatment of childhood conditions. In the United States, herbal preparations and most supplements are not subjected to the rigorous process of approval demanded by the Food and Drug Administration. They enter the marketplace without the same quality assurances to which conventional medicines are subjected. Documentation of efficacy, analysis of how much active substance is contained in the preparation, and proof of purity, are commonly absent from such preparations.

Herbal remedies include a staggering range of materials, ranging from simple teas to exotic plant and animal extracts indigenous to isolated areas of the world, which patients find in ethnic health care stores or apothecaries. Perhaps the best documented beneficial effects are seen with the use of probiotics, such as yogurt and *lactobacillus*, for diarrheal conditions [59–61]. They may also have utility in children with antibiotic associated diarrheal states, as is frequently experienced by patients with immuno-suppression. For other common therapies, such as *Echinacea* and *St John's wort* [62,63], reliable studies are lacking. Adverse interactions with a wide range of medications have been reported, from immune suppressants prescribed following organ transplantation [64], to antiviral therapies and digoxin. These reports raise serious concerns about uncontrolled use of herbal preparations, without knowledge of possible drug–herb interactions [64–66]. Symptomatic management in children with terminal illnesses also is lacking in rigorous clinical investigation. Milk thistle (*Silybum marianum*) has been studied in adults, for the indications of cirrhosis and prostatic cancer. Its use in adults was recently reviewed, but indications in children remain anecdotal at present [67]. Similarly, there is little evidence for many other supplements, such as coenzyme Q10 and pyridoxine, which are often used for degenerative CNS disease, intractable seizures, cardiomyopathy, and other conditions that often respond only poorly to conventional allopathic treatment.

While many such compounds available through community outlets have relatively low toxicity, numerous case reports document the presence of contaminating substances, ranging from lead to cyanide [68]. Recent reviews of the subject recommend that parents inform clinicians of the use of herbal supplements, and that they be used with circumspection, given the many unknowns that exist [69,70]. As with many other popular remedies, the apparent absence of harm alone does not warrant their use. Clinicians should seek out competent local practitioners to serve as resources on such topics. Diplomates of schools of Traditional Chinese Medicine or graduates of recognized programs in Naturopathic Medicine tend to be well-versed in herbal remedies and supplements. Additionally, many good sites exist on the Internet, which provide information on this changing subject for both consumer and health care professionals [71].

Vitamin therapy

Beyond the established, known deficiency states or conditions known to affect vitamin absorption (e.g., short bowel syndrome leading to potential B_{12} deficiency, and fat malabsorption syndromes), there is little reliable information to support the use of either herbal or nutritional supplementation in chronic and potentially life-threatening conditions of children. Conventional supplements of individual vitamins may be of value in conditions of impaired dietary intake, such as, for example, cancer-induced anorexia, or states of altered taste. The wide availability and relative safety of vitamin supplements has led to an enormous industry, supplying products of uncertain purity and little demonstrated value to often desperate, suffering patients of all ages. Numerous cases of hypervitaminoses have been reported, following the unsupervised use of vitamin preparations, raising concern amongst health care providers in regards to potential harm for users.

Aromatherapy

Aromatherapy can be defined as the utilization of naturally extracted aromatic essences from plants, that seeks to achieve physiologic effects that can calm, balance, and promote the health of body, mind and spirit. It appears to have few potential adverse effects on patients, with the exception of rare cases of mild allergic reactions to some of the components. Proposals for the use of aromatherapy, often as part of therapeutic massage, exist for a wide range of indications; however well designed studies do not exist, with little evidence for determining its efficacy [57,72–74]. As with other therapies, there are reports of initially encouraging results, with subsequent failure to sustain a response [75]. Anecdotal reports indicate the use of various aromas by pediatric facilities to assist in the treatment of anxiety, depression, grief, panic attacks, and multiple other psychological diagnoses. The effectiveness of aromatherapy appears to depend partly upon primitive aspects of the limbic system, which respond to conditioning very early in life. A study of pre-term infants' responses to phlebotomy in the presence of a familiar odor indicates that even pre-term infants may achieve comfort through the use of suitable aromas [76]. Practitioners of flower essence therapy also believe that these remedies exert their effect through alterations in subtle energy, as discussed above.

Aromatherapy has aided patients with disordered sleep [77], and has alleviated anxiety, when compared with control measures [27,50,57,58,73]. Reliable studies of aromatherapy in children with life-limiting conditions are not available, but it is worth considering the use of aromatherapy as an adjunctive measure for both calming, and improving sleep in, children in palliative care programs. The selection of aromas is best made in conjunction with a reliable local practitioner, who can also direct families to a reliable source for the herbal materials.

Aromatherapy represents one of the complementary therapies which have such a low risk of toxicity for most patients (except for some patients with pre-existing hypersensitivity to various components of the aromatic mixtures) that it can be legitimately supported by clinicians, when families request it. Support for the family's pursuit of complements to conventional therapy reinforces trust and bond between the health care team and the family, which is essential in facilitating communications as disease progresses.

Homeopathy

Homeopathy, a centuries-old school of diagnostic and therapeutic approach, is in many ways the antithesis of allopathic medicine, in that its basic premise is that healing comes from within the body, rather than from outside it. It holds that people have a vital force which, if disrupted, leads to health problems. Homeopathy aims to stimulate the body's own healing process by the administration of extremely small doses of substances (called 'remedies'), which produce characteristic symptoms of illness when given in larger doses. Treatments must be tailored to the unique circumstances of each patient, based on symptoms, personality, life-style and other factors. Research findings on the benefits of homeopathy have been contradictory [78,79]. Where a response has been shown, it is not easily explained by conventional allopathic understanding of disease pathogenesis. It is important for both homeopathic and allopathic physicians to be aware of the various treatments being used by patients, when different approaches are used simultaneously.

Mechanical/manipulative interventions

Conventional surgery

Contemporary practitioners of integrative medicine view surgery as one of several tools available to treat disease.

For example, complementary techniques may hasten callus formation in bone fractures in some individuals, but the application of contemporary orthopaedic technique may provide additional improvement to functional recovery. Various congenital malformations mandate surgery as a life-saving measure. In patients with cancer, for example, surgery or radiation may provide symptomatic improvement, and should be considered as part of the overall care to improve the quality of life. Complementary means may serve as adjuncts to traditional surgery, by reducing distressing symptoms, or as one way of improving the overall sense of well being.

Osteopathic medicine

Osteopathy in the United States developed in the early nineteenth century, at a time when western medicines were often crude extracts, anaesthesia had not been developed, and surgery was limited in scope. While the origins grew out of primary attention to the musculo-skeletal system, modern osteopathy incorporates many diagnostic and therapeutic tools used by allopathic medicine.

Massage therapy

Massage has been studied in pediatric populations for indications such as low birth weight, pain, asthma, attention deficit hyperactivity disorder, and depression [25,80,81]. Massage therapists traditionally undergo established curricula of education, training, and supervised practice. There are licensing boards in many localities, for assuring the successful completion of standard training. Additional training is available for infant massage, and massage in medically fragile children. Massage benefits patients through several different mechanisms, which have been only superficially characterized in the medical literature. The act of physically manipulating tissue may influence circulation and lymphatic flow, and also alter connective and supportive structures. In addition, the human touch, and the proximity of another individual focused directly on the patient, usually confer additional comfort and benefit. Massage has found a place in adult and pediatric palliative care practice [57,58,75].

Chiropractic medicine

In the United States, chiropractic medicine is one of the more popular forms of CAM. There are few rigorous studies available to support its routine use in children with life-limiting conditions. Chiropractic medicine represents a different philosophical approach to disease, based on the relationship of the nerve roots emerging from the spinal cord. It may have a greater role in chronic, out-patient care, than in a more acute in-patient setting. One advantage in the United States is that it is one of the CAM's that is usually reimbursed under the health care system [82].

Many allopathic physicians remain wary of chiropractors, but again, many families of children with life-limiting conditions will choose to consult them anyway. As with other forms of manipulation, the chiropractic approach offers an intimate, individual relationship with a caring practitioner, that many patients find comforting. Acknowledging this, and where appropriate, facilitating it can benefit the relationship of allopathic professional with the family.

Mind-body techniques

This category of therapies involves a wide range of activities, which include well known techniques such as relaxation imagery and hypnosis, to music therapy and meditation [55, 83–85]. The responses they elicit may be equivalent to the state of calm and inner peace popularized in recent times by Benson and others [54,55,86]. As one may see with all palliative care techniques, treatment goals depend upon the timing of their introduction in the course of the disease. For example, at some stages, they may provide opportunities for developing insight, becoming aware of deep seated feelings, and becoming more active in the approach to their lives (a difficult task for some patients and families, who can feel 'victimized' by their disease). When applied later in the disease, the intended effect may be comfort and palliation of symptoms.

Mind-body techniques require varying degrees of cognitive capacity, maturity, and understanding in the patient, as well as expertise on the part of the therapist, teacher or guide to be effective. *Meditation* and relaxation imagery, in particular, require the active engagement of the patient, and an ability to focus the attention—a task which may be difficult for children in significant discomfort, or impossible for children with encephalopathy and delirium. Meditation in adults is reported to be effective in inducing a greater sense of calm [87]. This state can be produced by a wide range of techniques, such as traditional eastern forms of meditation, states of deep prayer, breath awareness, and the recently popularized 'relaxation response' of Benson and others [54,86]. Young children can often be guided directly to awareness of bodily sensations, or of breathing ('following it in and out through the nose', for example), which can help them to relax or fall asleep. For young children, guided imagery, or developmentally appropriate hypnosis techniques, are usually more suitable than traditional meditation. The active imagination of young children makes them ideal candidates for guided imagery. Success depends largely upon the skill of the therapist.

These approaches to self-calming can often be effectively taught to older children and their parents, and provide additional tools for management of some symptoms, for example, acute dysnpnea, when medical attention is not immediately available. For many patients, such techniques provide a reduction in pain perception and anxiety in many distressing conditions, including invasive medical procedures, during the perioperative period, as well as during moments of fear and anxiety [83]. Although recorded tapes for both meditation and guided imagery can be of benefit, a human therapist is preferable. Hypnosis has also been proposed for adults as a method for working through 'developmental tasks' at the end of life [88]. Its primary use in children has been as an adjunct in symptom control [89,90].

Music therapy

Music therapy is a time-honoured approach, with a history reaching back to ancient eras. Music is used both as a technique for esoteric teaching, and for its profound effect on the inner state, and is almost universally recognized as a method for affecting a person in a non-verbal fashion, on an emotional and/or spiritual level.

The application of music in the medical setting has received increasing attention over the last several decades, with formal training programs established in many universities, often under the aegis of departments of social service or counselling. Its use as an adjunctive therapy for patients with life-limiting conditions is well established in adult palliative care to improve quality of life [91], it has also been reviewed in paediatrics [92]. An intriguing recent report regarding the potential power of music, indicates earlier time to engraftment of bone marrow transplantation in patients receiving music therapy [93]. Early in the course of the disease, the music therapist can become an ally to the patient and family, a friendly face in what can seem to families to be the foreign environment of a medical institution. Support, encouragement, and validation of self may be achieved through the patient's choice of music, and the composing of lyrics to existing melodies. During times of acute distress, music can provide solace, and allow a patient to move inwardly to a place of greater peace and familiarity, without significant volitional involvement. In more terminal phases, music may touch the patient's inner psyche, allowing some contact even with non- or pre-verbal children, and can provide support to parents and siblings, as well as patients themselves. The use of chanting, rhythm and prayer, in conjunction with melody, is essential in many cultures for the orderly departure of the soul from the body.

Play therapy

Play is a child's natural method of learning, developing, and expressing feelings. Play therapy is based on the premise that children lack the cognitive maturity to process their problems in the same manner adults do. It has a long history in child

psychiatry and psycho-analysis. Play therapy can be performed in a directed fashion to model and shape behaviours, or in a non-directive manner, allowing children to create their own rules and design a reality where they are in control. This approach allows for processing frightening feelings, traumas, and other problems or insecurities they may be experiencing [94]. A trained play therapist creates a safe environment for the child to express these troubles, and seeks to understand the metaphorical content of a child's play. Insights gained in this way can aid children in expressing their needs, and discovering solutions.

In recent years, some networks have developed the resources of the Internet to provide peer support, play, and diversionary activities for children hospitalized, or confined at home or in a hospice [95–98]. There are concerns regarding the potential for loss of confidentiality and abuse of children online, but many services provide close, online adult supervision and controlled, limited access to the network, in an attempt to minimize the risks. These resources can be helpful in reducing a sense of social isolation. They provide validation of self, and the opportunity to express feelings in a psychologically safe environment, and also perhaps, to explore fantasies which they may not have time to realize.

Prayer

A topic which deserves mention in this section is prayer, both by the patient, and on behalf of the patient [99–101]. Studies in adults suggest that individuals with a personal spiritual practice may live longer [102,103]. Contemporary medical institutions provide chaplain services offering spiritual support to children and their families [104]. As with many other disciplines, the skills, sensitivity and insights of individual chaplains vary greatly. They depend upon the maturity, experience, and comfort with the needs of dying patients, possessed by the chaplain. A family's personal clergyperson may know the family members best, but may be uncomfortable ministering to a dying child benefiting from the support of the palliative care team.

Buddhist and other religious traditions view preparation for death, and the time surrounding death, as an opportunity to assist the soul in completing its life's work and experiencing a peaceful transition out of the body. The term 'soul' has come to have associations with formalised religion, and some families, or even health care personnel, may be uncomfortable with it; but in its essence, it can simply mean 'spirit'—those aspects of a person which are not physical.

Many religious organizations provide support for their members, and hold prayer groups independently of the hospital. Such interventions are referred to as intercessory prayers (prayers on behalf of another), and have received recent attention in the adult medical literature [105–108]. While prospective studies in children are insufficient to determine the benefit of prayer, there can be little doubt of its value to families. Prayer is another activity in which the family can participate actively on behalf of the child, helping offset the sense of helplessness they may feel.

Case B.Z. was a 16-year-old female with an ependymoma who had undergone seven craniotomies over the preceding years, as well as chemotherapy and radiation therapy for tumor recurrence. At the time the Integrative Medicine Service was contacted, she was having persistent, severe, headaches, with poor pharmacologic relief in spite of involvement of the pain service. She had received acupuncture by a pediatric anesthesiologist on the pain service, with little amelioration in her headaches. The family had a very positive attitude about her chances of 'beating' the cancer, and was very optimistic that all would turn out well. She underwent prayer sessions at her synagogue, with her rabbi and mother sitting in front of the ark containing the Torah scrolls (the *Bimah*). She consistently experienced nearly complete relief of her headaches during these sessions, which persisted for several hours. At the recommendation of the acupuncturist, an energy healer from the Integrative Medicine Initiative was requested to provide healing sessions. Nine sessions were provided over several months, each lasting 20–30 min (Figure 31.1). The intention of the healer was to relieve her physical discomfort, and to create a sense of contentment and calm, rather than to cure the tumor. BZ experienced relief of the headaches during the sessions, and fell asleep. Following the sessions, she related that she could feel energy flowing through her like a tingling feeling.

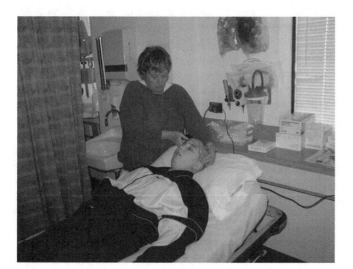

Fig. 31.1 Energy healing session of subject BZ in outpatient clinic setting. Treatment provided for relief of severe headache resulting from recurrent ependymoma.

Cultural diversity

Because they do not depend on inherent physical biological responses, mind-body interventions are reliant on the cultural and ethnic background of patients and their families, and the context in which they are applied [28, 31,109–112]. There may be images, melodies, and linguistic idiosyncrasies of non-dominant cultures that are foreign to many western health care workers. There may be inherent biases and assumptions that are difficult to anticipate without intimate knowledge of cultural norms. The palliative care team is often confronted with important cultural needs, when caring for individuals from unfamiliar religious and cultural traditions. Reliable resources must be identified in each ethnic group one treats, to both avoid unintentional offence and provide optimal care for the life-limited child, in the context of the family and society.

Conclusions

Experience, as well as some research evidence, suggest potential benefits, and occasionally risks, in using complementary therapies in children. It has often been difficult to demonstrate the benefit of complementary therapies using conventional western methods of research. This absence of proof may not represent the absence of efficacy, but rather, imperfect tools of inquiry. For example, outcome measures in scientific medical studies may include tumour size or breathing rate, without evaluating how this affects the individual person, or how it impacts on the quality of his or her life. There are few robust measures of quality of life in children; these are necessary to delineate significant differences which correlate with a better sense of well-being, or with relief from suffering. More powerful tools for evaluating these subjective outcomes should be developed, so that further convincing evidence can be sought regarding the place and timing of complementary interventions in advanced stages of disease.

The families of children who feel they have not been adequately helped by 'conventional' medicine are those most likely to seek out complementary healing modalities, as adjuncts to conventional therapy, or even instead of them. This may include, for example, multiple relapses from cancer, uncorrectable congenital heart disease, and inborn errors of metabolism. Conventional therapies that are oriented towards cure may have little to offer under these circumstances, while some CAM approaches can provide demonstrable improvements in life quality, with little risk of toxicity. Other CAM approaches have very low risks, but data may be too limited to justify unqualified recommendation by allopathic physicians.

Nonetheless, many patients and their families perceive benefit from actively pursuing complementary healing modalities.

Practitioners of allopathic medicine and their colleagues must accept that many patients will seek complementary techniques. Dismissing, or actively opposing, this search risks jeopardising the partnership between family and caregivers. On the other hand, engaging with it can be beneficial in many ways. One goal of contemporary palliative care is to encourage a sense of autonomy, and create a positive attitude towards life in patients and families. By facilitating their contact with trusted CAM therapists, health care workers can empower patients and their families to assume an active role in their own management, and encourage them to abandon the passive, victim role which many feel as the end of life approaches. In so doing, the palliative care team can 'accompany' the family, and reassure the dying patient that care continues even when a cure is no longer possible.

The case histories in this chapter illustrate that CAM therapy can encourage a sense of wellbeing, a reduction in distressing symptoms, and feelings of being cared for and nurtured, resulting in exactly the improvement in quality of life that is the aim of palliative care. Health care professionals are encouraged to explore the options available in their local communities, and to establish a dialogue with practitioners in various non-allopathic fields, who can serve as resources when families ask for complementary therapies.

References

1. Rahe, R. Social stress and illness onset. *J Psychosom Res* 1964;8: 35–44.
2. Kiecolt-Glaser, J. and Glaser, R. Psychological influences on immunity: Implications for AIDS. *Am Psychol* 1988;43:892–8.
3. Cohen, S., DAJ, T, and Smith, A. Psychological stress and susceptibility to the common cold. *N Engl J Med* 1991;325:606–12.
4. Kiecolt-Glaser, J., Marucha, P., Malarkey, W., *et al*. Slowing of wound healing by psychological stress. *Lancet* 1995;346:1194–6.
5. Kiecolt-Glaser, J., Glaser, R., Cacioppo, J., *et al*. Marital stress: Immunologica, neuroendocrine, and autonomic correlates. *Ann NY Acad Sci* 1998;840:656–63.
6. Gilbert, M. Weaving Medicine Back Together: Mind–Body Medicine in the Twenty-First Century. *J Altern Comp Med* 2003;9: 563–70.
7. Dokken, D. and Snydor-Greenberg, N. Exploring complementary and alternative medicine in pediatrics. *Pediatr Nursing* 2000;26.
8. Sanders, H., Davis, M., Duncan, B., *et al*. Use of complementary and alternative medical therapies among children with special health care needs in southern Arizona. *Pediatrics* 2003;111:584–7.
9. Eisenberg, D.M., Kessler, R.C., Foster, C., Norlock, F.E., Calkins, D.R., and Delbanco, T.L., Unconventional medicine in the United States. Prevalence, costs, and patterns of use. [see comment]. *N Eng J Medi* 1993;328(4):246–52.
10. Eisenberg, D., Roger, B., Ettner, S. *et al*. Trends in Alternative Medicine Use in the United States, 1990–1997. *JAMA* 1998;280: 1569–75.
11. Sibinga, E., Ottolini, M., Duggan, A., and Wilson, M., Communication about complementary/alternative medicine use in children. *Pediatr Res* 2000;47:226A.
12. Jansen, L. and Sulmassy, D. Proportionality, terminal suffering and the restorative goals of medicine. *Theoret Med* 2002;23:321–37.
13. Kellehear, A. Complementary medicine: Is it more acceptable in palliative care practice? *MJA* 2003;179:S46–8.
14. Wolfe, J., Grier, H., Levin, S., *et al*. Symptoms and suffering at the end of life in children with cancer. *N Engl J Med* 2000;342:326–33.
15. Zhang, X. Legal Status of Traditional Medicine and Complementary/Alternative Medicine: A Worldwide Review World Health Organization (WHO), 2001; Geneva: Switzerlandhttp://www.who.int/medicines/library/trm/who-edm-trm-2001–2/legalstatus.pdf
16. Zhang, X. World Health Organization Traditional Health Strategy. World Health Organization (WHO), 2002–2005; Geneva: Switzerlandhttp://www.who.int/medicines/library/trm/trm_strat_eng.pdf
17. Technology, S.C.o.S.a., *Complementary and Alternative Medicine*. 2000; London: House of Lords.
18. Simpson, N., Pearce, A., Finaly, F., and Lenton, S. The use of complementary medicine in pediatric outpatient clinics. *Ambulat Child Health* 1998; 3: 351–6.
19. Ernst, E. Prevalence of complementary/alternative medicine for children: a systematic review. *Eur J Pediatr* 1999; 158: 7–11.
20. Lee, A. and Kemper, K. Homeopathy and naturopathy: Practice characteristics in pediatric care. *Arch Pediatr Adol Med* 2001;154:75–80.
21. Kemper, K. Holistic pediatrics = good medicine. *Pediatrics* 2000; 105: 214–8.
22. Fong, D. and Fong, L. Usage of complementary medicine among children. *Aust Fam Physician* 2002;(31):388–91.
23. Kemper, K. Complementary and alternative medicine for children: Does it work? *Arch Dis Child* 2001;84:6–9.
24. Heuschkel, R., Afzal, N., Wuerth, A., *et al*. Complementary Medicine use in children and young adults with inflammatory bowel disease. *Am J Gastroent* 2002; 97: 382–8.
25. Field, T. Massage therapy for infants and children. *J Dev Behav Pediatr* 1995;16:105–11.
26. Jones, J. and Kassity, N. Varieties of alternative experience: Complementary care in the neonatal intensive care unit. *Clin Obst Gynecol* 2001;44:750–68.
27. Neuhouser, M., Patterson, R., Schwartz, S., *et al*. Use of alternative medicine by children with cancer in Washington State. *Prevent Med* 2001;(33).
28. Becera, R. and Iglehart, A. Folk medicine use: Diverse populations in a metropolitan area. *Soc Work Health Care* 1995;21:37–58.
29. Pearl, W., Leo, P., and Tsang, W. Use of Chinese therapies among chinese patients seeking emergency department care. *Ann Emerg Med* 1995;26:735–38.
30. Pachter, L., CLoutier, M., and Bernstein, B. Ethnomedical (folk) remedies for childhood asthma in a mainland Puerto Rican community. *Arch Pediatr Adol Med* 1995;149:982–88.
31. Pachter, L. Practicing culturally sensitive pediatrics. *Contemp Pediatr* 1997;14:139–54.
32. McNamara, B. *Fragile Lives: Death, Dying and Care*. Sydney: Allen and Unwin 2001.

33. Shine, K. A critique on complementary and alternative medicine. *J Altern Comp Med* 2001;7:S145–52.

34. van der Wal, M., Renfurm, L., van Vught, A., and Gemke, R. Circumstances of dying in hospitalized children. *Eur J Pediatr* 1999;158:560–5.

35. Gibbons, M. Psychosocial aspects of serious illness in childhood and adolescence. Armstrong-Dailey and S. Goltzer, eds. In *Hospice Care for Children*, New York: Oxford University Press. 1993, p. 62–3

36. Kemper, K., Cassileth, B., and Ferris, T. Holistic pediatrics: A research agenda. *Pediatrics* 1999;103: 902–9.

37. Kemper, K. and Wornham, W. Consultations for holistic pediatric services for inpatients and outpatient oncology patients at a children's hospital. *Arch Pediatr Adol Med* 2001;155:449–54.

38. Gilmer, M. Pediatric palliative care: *A family-centered model for critical care. Nurs Clin North Am* 2002;14:207–14.

39. Scrace, J. Complementary therapies in palliative care of children with cancer: A literature review. *Paediatr Nurs* 2003;15:36–9.

40. *NIH* Consensus Conference: Acupuncture. *JAMA* 1998;280:1518B4.

41. Berman, B. Clinical applications of acupuncture: An overview of the evidence. *J Altern Comp Med* 2001;7:S111–8.

42. Kaptchuk, T. Acupuncture: Theory, efficacy and practice. *Ann Intern Med* 2002;136:374–83.

43. Ma, S. Enhanced nitric oxide concentrations and expression of nitric oxide synthase in acupuncture points/meridians. *J Altern Comp Med* 2003;9:207–15.

44. Lee, A., Highfield, E., Berde, C., and Kemper, K. Survey of acupuncturists: Practice characteristics and pediatric care. *West J Med* 1999; 171:153–7.

45. Zeltzer, L., Tsao, J., Stelling, C., *et al.* A phase I study on the feasibility and acceptability of an acupuncture/hypnosis intervention for chronic pediatric pain. *J Pain Symptom Manage* 2002;24:437–46.

46. MacPherson, H., White, A. Cummings, M. *et al.* Standards for Reporting Interventions in Controlled Trials of Acupuncture: The STRICTA Recommendations. *J Altern Comp Med* 2002;8:85–9.

47. Kemper, K., Sarah, R., Highfield, E., *et al.* On pins and needles? Pediatric pain patients' experience with acupuncture. *Pediatrics* 2000;105:941–7.

48. Kotani, N., Hashimoto, H., Sato, Y., *et al.* Preoperative intradermal acupuncture reduces postoperative pain, nausea and vomiting, analgesic requirement, and sympathoadrenal responses. *Anesthesiology* 2001;95:349–56.

49. Wang, S. and Kain, Z. P6 acupoint injections are as effective as droperidol in controlling earlypostoperative nausea and vomiting. *Anesthesiology* 2002;97:359–66.

50. Lewis, C., de Vedia, A., Reuer, B., *et al.* Integrating complementary and alternative medicine (CAM) into standard hospice and palliative care. *Am J Hosp Palliat Care* 2003;20:221–8.

51. Rusy, L. and Weisman, S. Complementary therapies for acute pediatric pain management. *Pediatr Clin N Am* 2000; 47(3).

52. Rusy, L., Hoffman, G., and Weisman, S. Electroacupuncture Prophylaxis of postoperative nausea and vomiting following pediatric tonsillectomy with or without Adenoidectomy. *Anesthiology* 2002; 96: 300–5.

53. Agelink, M., Sanner, D., Eich, H., *et al.* Does acupuncture influence the cardiac autonomic nervous system in patients with minor depression or anxiety disorders? *Fortschr Neurol Psychiatr*, 2003; 71:141–9.

54. Benson, H. *The Relaxation Response*. New York: Avon Books, 2000; p. 179.

55. Jacobs, G., The Physiology of mind–body interactions: The stress Response and the Relaxation Response. *J Altern Comp Med* 2001;7: S83–92.

56. Brenner, Z. and Krenzer, M. Using complementary and alternative therapies to promote comfort at end of life. *Crit Care Nurs Clin North Am* 2003;15:355–62.

57. Buckle, S. Aromatherapy and massage: The evidence. *Paediatric Nursing* 2003;15:24–7.

58. Wilkinson, S., Aldridge, J., Salmon, I., *et al.* An evaluation of aromatherapy massage in palliative care. *Palliative Med* 1999;13: 409–17.

59. Pedone, C., Bernabeu, A., Postaire, E., *et al.* The effect of supplementation with milk fermented by Lactobacillus casei on acute diarrhoea in children attending day care centres. *Int J Clin Pract* 1999;53:179–84.

60. Hove, H., Norgaard, H., and Mortensen, P. Lactic acid bacteria and the human gastrointestinal tract. *Eur J Clin Nutr* 1999;53:339–50.

61. Pochapin, M. The effect of probiotics on Clostridium difficile diarrhea. *Am J Gastroenterol* 2000;95:S11–13.

62. Greeson, J., Sanford, B., and Monti, D. St. John's wort: A review of the current pharmacological, toxicological and clinical literature. *Psychopharmcology* 2001;153:402–14.

63. Hammerness, P., Basch, E., Ulbricht, C., *et al.* St. John's wort: A systematic review of adverse effects and drug interactions for the consultation psychiatrist. *Pschosomatics* 2003;44:271–82.

64. Bauer, S., Stormer, E., Johne, A., *et al.* Alterations in cyclosporin A pharmacokinetics and metablism during treatment with St. John's wort in renal transplant patients. *Br J Pharmacol* 2003;55: 203–11.

65. Johne, A., Borckmoller, J., Bauer, S., *et al.* Pharmacokinetic interaction of digoxin with an herbal extract from St. John's wort (Hypericum perforatum). *Clin Pharmacol Ther* 1999;66:338–45.

66. Haller, C., ANderson, I., Kim, S., *et al.* An evaluation of selected herbal regerence texts and comparison to published reports of adverse herbal events. *Adverse Drug React Toxidol Reb* 2002;21: 143–50.

67. Braun, L. Milk thistle (Silybum marianum). *J Comp Med* 2003;2: 60–4.

68. Ernst, E. Serious adverse effects of unconventional therapies for children and adolescents: A systematic review of recent evidence. *Eur J Pediatr* 2003;162:72–80.

69. Woolf, A. Herbal remedies: Do the work? are they harmful? *Pediatrics* 2003;112:240–6.

70. Niggemann, B. and Grueber, C. Side-effects of complementary and alternative medicine. *Allergy* 2003;58:707–16.

71. Oleson, T. Herbal medicine online. *J Altern Comp Med* 2003; 9: 581–4.

72. Styles, J. The use of aromatherapy in hospitalized children with HIV disease. *Complement Ther Nurs Midwifery* 1997;3:16–20.

73. Buckle, J. Use of aromatherapy as a complementary treatment for chronic pain. *Altern Ther Health Med* 1999;5:42–51.

74. Buckle, J. The role of aromatherapy in nursing care. *Jurs Clin North Am* 2001;36:57–72.

75. Anderson, C., Lis-Balchin, M., and Kirk-Smith, M. Evaluation of massage with essential oils on childhood atopic eczema. *Phytother Res* 2000;14:452–6.

76. Goubet, N., Rattaz, C., Pierrat, V., *et al.* Olfactory experience mediates response to pain in preterm newborns. *Dev Psychobiol* 2003; 42:171–80.

77. Fussel, A., Wolf, A., Buter, B., Schrader, E., and Brattstrom, A. Efficient use of sleep pillows in patients suffering from non-organic sleep disorders—a pilot study *Forsch Komplementarmed Klass Naturheilkd* 2001;8:299–304.

78. Oberbaum, M., Yaniv, I., Ben-Gal, Y., *et al.* A randomized, controlled clinical trial of the homeopathic medication traumeel S in the treatment of chemotherapy-induced stomatitis in children undergoing stem cell transplantation. *Cancer* 2001;92:684–90.

79. Vickers, A. and Smith, C. Homoeopathic oscillococcinum for preventing and treating influenza and influenza-like syndromes. *Cochrane Database of Systematic Reviews* 2002;2:p. CD001957.

80. Field, T., Henteleff, T., and Hernandez-Reif, M. Children with asthma have improved pulmonary functions after massage therapy. *J Pediatr* 1998;132:854–8.

81. Hernandez-Reif, M., Field, T., Krasnegor, J., *et al.* Children with cystic fibrosis benefit from massage therapy. *J Pediatr Psychol* 1999; 24:175–81.

82. Lee, A., Li, D., and Kemper, K., Chiropractic care for children. *Arch Pediatr Adolesc Med* 2000;154:401–7.

83. Genuis, M. The use of hypnosis in helping cancer patients control anxity, pain and emesis: a review of recent empirical studies. *Am J Clin Hypn* 1995;37:316–25.

84. Olness, K. Hypnosis and biofeedback with children and adolescents; clinical, research, and educational aspects. *J Dev Behav Pediatr* 1996;17:299.

85. Olness, K. Managing headaches without drugs. *Contemp Pediatr* 1999;16:101–10.

86. Benson, H., *The Relaxation Response.* New York: William Morrow Co, 1975.

87. Meares, A. What can the cancer patient expect from intensive meditation? *Aust Fam Physician* 1980;9:322–5.

88. Marcus, J. and Elkins, G. A model of hypnotic intervention for palliative care. *Adv Mind Body Med* 2003;19:24–7.

89. Liossi, C. and Hatira, P. Clinical hypnosis in the alleviation of procedure-realted pain in pediatric oncology patients. *Int J CLin Exp Hypn* 2003;51:4–28.

90. Stevens, M., Della Pozza, L., Cavalletto, B. *et al.* Pain and symptom control in paediatric palliative care. *Cancer Surv* 1994;21:211–31.

91. Hilliard, R. The effects of music therapy on the quality and length of life of people diagnosed with terminal cancer. *J Music Ther* 2003; 40:113–37.

92. Daveson, B. and Kennelly, J. Music therapy in palliative care for hospitalized children and adolescents. *J Palliative Care* 2000; 16: 35–38.

93. Sahler, O., Hunter, B., and Liesveld, J. The effect of using music therapy wwiht relacation imagery in the management of patients undergoing bone marrow transplantation: A pilot feasibilitiy study. *Altern Ther Health Med* 2003;9:70–4.

94. Krietemeyer, B. and Heiney, S. Storytelling as a therapeutic technique in a group for school-aged oncology patients. *Child Health Care* 1992;21:14–20.

95. Appleby, C. Online. A virtual playground for sick kids. *Hosp Health Networks* 1995;69:57.

96. Lefebvre, A. and McClure, M. Ability OnLine: Children in hospital now in touch with the world. *Leadersh Health Serv* 1995; 4: 26–9.

97. Baldwin, F. The Starbright program showing kids a heavenly good time. *Palliative Med* Supplement(Summer): 2000;11.

98. Holden, G., Bearsion, D., Rode, D., *et al.* The impact of a computer network on pediatric pain and anxiety: A randomized controlled clinical trial. *Soc Work Health Care* 2002;36:21–33.

99. Barnes, L., Plotnikoff, G., Fox, K., *et al.* Spirituality, religion, and pediatrics: intersecting worlds of healing. *Pediatics* 2000;106: S899–908.

100. Kemper, K. and Barnes, L. Considering culture, complementary medicine, and spirituality in pediatrics. *Clin Pediatr* 2003;42: 205–8.

101. Armbruster, C., Chignall, J., and Legett, S. Pediatrician beliefs about spirituality and religion in medicine: Associations with clinical practice. *Pediatrics* 2003;111:e227–35.

102. Helm, H., Hays, J., and Flint, E., *et al.* Does private religious activity prolong survival? A six-year follow-up study of 3,851 older patients. *J Gerontol A Biol Sci Med Sci* 2000;55:M400–405.

103. Townsend, M., Kladder, V., and Ayele, H., *et al.* Systematic review of clinical trials examining the effects of religion on health. *South Med J* 2002;95:1429–34.

104. Feudtner, C., Haney, J., Dimmers, M., Spiritual care needs of hospitalized children and their families: A national survey of pastoral care providers' perceptions. *Pediatrics* 2003; 111: e67–72.

105. Byrd, R. Positive therapeutic effects of intercessory prayer in a coronary care unit population. *South Med J* 1988;81:826–9.

106. Harris, W., Gowda, M., Kolb, J., *et al.* A randomized controlled trial of the effects of remote, intercessory prayer on outcomes in patients admitted to the coronary care unit. *Arch Intern Med* 1999;159:2273–8.

107. Liebovici, L. Effects of remote, retroactive intercessory prayer on outcomes in patients with bloodstream infections: Randomized controlled trial. *BMJ* 2001;323:1450–1.

108. Bernardi, L., Sleight, P., Bandinelli, G., *et al.* Effect of rosary prayer and yoga mantras on autonomic cardiovascular rhythms: Comparative study. *BMJ* 2001;323:1446–9.

109. DeRios, M. Magical realism: A cultural intervention for traumatized Hispanic children. *Cultural Diversity and Mental Health* 1997;3:159–70.

110. Kunin, H. Ethical issues in pediatric life-threatening illness: dilemmas of consent, assent, and communication. *Ethics Behav.* 1997;7:43–57.

111. Field, A., Maher, P., and Webb, D. Cross cultural research in palliative care. *Soc Work Health Care*, 2002;35:523–43.

112. Wissow, L., Larson, S., and Roter, D. Longitudinal care improves disclosure of psychosocial information. *Arch Pediatr Adol Med* 2003;157:419–24.

32 Symptom control at the end-of-life

Dawn Davies and Debbie de Vlaming

Palliative care for children is best thought of as a continuum. Sometimes the management of pain and other symptoms might be relatively unaltered leading up to the child's death. Often in these situations, symptom management at the end of life may involve intensification of management strategies, using higher doses or more frequent administration of previously used medications (please see specific preceding chapters for more details). Not infrequently, though, new symptoms may arise close to the end of life, or symptom progression may be such that symptoms are no longer controlled by previously effective interventions. The following is intended to address symptom control at the very end of life: the hours to days prior to death.

There is a need for caregivers to develop a proactive approach to the 'what ifs...' that families face close to the time of their children's deaths. This anticipatory planning is arguably even more important for families caring for their child at home, and especially for those living in rural areas, or at a distance from their usual health care resources. Contingency plans should be in place for the management of new symptoms. Unexpected or unanticipated symptoms may, in turn, lead caregivers and families alike to rethink the setting in which the child is being cared for. It is often during this period that families that were previously coping very well at home, with in home supports, become frightened, and may wish for admission to hospital, where staff that they know and trust is present.

Because the average parent has very little, if any, direct experience with death, it is our duty as professionals to guide parents honestly through the dying process of their child, anticipating their needs and questions. Well-developed written care plans need to be in place, and provision of ongoing and flexible plans for the changing situation of the child and family is key. Many parents have stated that 'feeling like there's a plan,' and a 'next step,' are crucial to a feeling of coping and control. These plans, in the context of this chapter, need to include a 'next step' for symptom management, and a location for care provision.

As with all human needs, physical needs have to be met as a priority. If the child is in pain, or is distressed by some other symptom, very little can be achieved in enhancing the life of the child and family. Unfortunately, a few landmark papers suggest that uncontrolled symptoms and suffering at the end of children's lives are much too frequent [1,2].

Paradoxically, there is a risk that in pursuing control of symptoms, we can become too interventionist in our approach. For a majority of families, it becomes a priority to avoid hospital admission, where possible. Even turning up for an X-ray may be unwelcome, and most will prefer to avoid blood tests, even if these can be done without attending hospital. In formulating a therapeutic strategy, we need to rely heavily on clinical judgment, rather than investigations, and often, to proceed on the basis of probability, rather than certainty.

Optimum pain and symptom control is the foundation of excellent palliative care, and is the cornerstone that facilitates attainment of all the other goals in care at the end of life. Intensive symptom management, particularly in the last few hours or days of life, is often necessary in order to allow for the peaceful death of the child. It is also crucial for the family and friends that symptoms do not spiral out of control in those last precious moments. The family's feeling that its child did not suffer is paramount, and is the one small comfort that parents often discuss as the only solace to be found, in their monumental loss and devastation. Alternatively, parents have sometimes described being 'haunted' by memories of their child's suffering, when symptom management has been less than optimal. These are the memories that become the family's lasting legacy, and therefore, care of the child and family must be as seamless as possible.

Setting for care in the final phase of life

As the child's condition changes, parents or other caregivers may experience sudden changes of mind as to where and how they want to care for their child, and every attempt should be made to honour these wishes to the extent possible.

Anticipating and planning for sudden hospital re-admission or discharge pre-emptively can be very helpful, thereby allowing maximal flexibility for the child and family (cross ref Place of care chapter, chapter 37, Brook).

Throughout the child's illness, flexibility in approach to care should be optimized such that the child and family lead as normal a life as possible. Having a resource person (also known as a 'key-worker') to coordinate all transitions within the medical system, to home, and back to hospital, has been identified as a crucial part of well-coordinated palliative care. Very often, a 'passport' on which all health care providers record their assessments and treatments, and which is carried by the patient's family through various settings, is helpful. In the absence of such a document, a letter carried by the parents, describing their child's diagnosis and treatment plan (including Do Not Attempt Resuscitation orders, where applicable) is useful. This can facilitate optimal treatment, reflecting the family's wishes, and prevents the family members from having to re-tell their story to yet another practitioner.

Decision-making about the setting in which the child will be cared for, and eventually die, is emotionally charged. Some parents will embrace the opportunity to keep their child at home with the family, in spite of challenges and fears. Others find the dual role of parent and proxy health care provider to be unduly burdensome, or undesirable; they may want to be 'just Mom/Dad.' Some parents, after a period of intensive caregiving at home, will seek help either in a hospice or a hospital setting, at the end of life. Other families fear the impact that a death at home would have on surviving siblings, and many parents have voiced concerns about being able to remain in the family home if their child died there. There is often fear of the unknown, in terms of parents' ability to gauge what their own reaction will be at the time of the child's death, and parents often will state that they cannot bring themselves to even contemplate this in advance. The help of Child Life specialists, social workers, and psychologists can be instrumental in helping families with these issues.

A cautionary note: we, as health care professionals, may sometimes underestimate the ability of families to 'cope at home' in providing palliative care, and we need to refrain from making paternalistic judgments in how we present options to families. Sometimes 'complex' care offered in a hospital, or even in intensive care settings, can be simplified or modified, to allow for safe and comfortable care in the home. The more complicated the situation is, the more advance planning will be needed for a discharge to home. As long as families are aware of the risks, benefits and resources available in various settings, these very personal decisions should be supported, as long as there are no clear medical contra-indications. A good bridge to transitions between hospital and home is a 'trial run.'

The patient may technically remain an in-patient, but has 'passes' to home or an alternate site of care, to see how care in this other setting would work for the child and the family. This also allows time for set-up of the out-patient setting for equipment and pharmacy needs. Some hospitals and intensive care units have care-by-parent units, or 'rooming-in' facilities, in which parents provide all of their child's care, with the benefit of having health care professionals who are well known to them easily available. This often bolsters the confidence of parents upon leaving the hospital.

On the other hand, some families feel that they will want to remain in hospital indefinitely, and may be overwhelmed by the care required by their child. Parents often state that they are afraid to be at home with their child. Often, the further the family lives from immediate medical or nursing assistance, the more this fear is intensified. Over time this may change, as parents first assist in, and then gradually learn to perform independently, the different procedures required. Some parents will eventually master and embrace tasks they initially thought would be overwhelming. In these cases, some families will opt stepwise for passes out of the hospital, evolving to a full discharge home. Appropriate palliative home-care support must be set up in the home as part of a well-constructed discharge plan.

Even in very small towns, palliative care 'teams' can evolve around a particular child; these teams are often composed of local on-call doctors, nurses, pharmacists, and others, who will rally around the family when given the extreme rarity of being called on to perform such a service. Specialized pediatric palliative care teams can be consulted directly by local caregivers as needs change. However, there are rare situations in which the setting decided upon is not ideal, despite everyone's best efforts:

Case Y.K. is a 13-year-old girl who lives in a very remote northern Canadian community of 200 people. There is no road access during winter; access is by flight only. There is a nursing station, with two registered nurses on duty to care for the community at all times, in alternating shifts. The nearest hospital is 700 miles away.

Y.K. has a diffuse brainstem glioma. She is cognitively intact, but has diffuse cranial nerve dysfunction, which has lead to recurrent episodes of aspiration pneumonia. She is cachectic, very weak and bed-bound, and requires total care. Mom is a single parent, and is busy with a job that allows her to be sole provider for her children. Y.K. was residing at home with her Mom and 16-year-old brother until 3 weeks ago. Since then, she has developed Gram-negative bacteremia and urinary tract infection, intolerance of her gastrostomy feeds, vomiting, weight loss, and back pain. She was initially treated in a secondary level center, attended by a pediatrician whom the patient and mother trust. She has now been transferred to a tertiary care center, hundreds of miles from home, for further supportive treatment, and is recovering well. She is much more comfortable, and her deterioration has been slow, over months. But the dilemma for this family is emerging. She is well enough to return to the secondary hospital that referred her, which is much closer to home, and is a place where the family has many psychosocial supports. Mom would like to stay in the secondary hospital with Y.K., but cannot manage this financially, as she has already applied for, and been granted, a year off work to attend to her ill child. There is a 16-year-old sibling who is very close to his dying sister, but the family's relocation for her treatment had a negative impact on him, and the mother is not willing to risk further trauma to him by moving again. It is likely that they will be able to visit Y.K. only for one week of every month from the home community.

Conversely, although aware of her mother's concerns and her own medical situation, Y.K. herself expresses a strong desire to return to her home. This child requires frequent suctioning and attention through the night. There are no professionals to provide in-home assistance, either in her care, or for general respite or homemaking for Mom. Mom is resourceful, dependable, and very aware of their situation. It is very upsetting for her to contemplate being separated from her young daughter at this crucial time, but currently, she feels there is no alternative. She has friends and family in her village, but they all have young children, and she fears that despite people's best intentions, she will be 'on her own' in caring for her child. She states that she is scared by the prospect of taking Y.K. home under such circumstances, and fears for the welfare of her child if she became suddenly ill again, and for her own ability to cope with what may still be a lengthy illness. She is also very concerned about her 16-year-old son, who has been left in the care of relatives much of the time, and Mom states that he is having an increasingly difficult time with separations from her.

However, even in situations like this one, contingency plans to make the best of the situation are still possible. In the above scenario, the patient was able to identify a 'wish list' of things to do in the secondary hospital, and Mom was able to devise a plan, involving friends and relations who could serially spend time with Y.K. A comprehensive plan communicating the patient's desires, dislikes, wants and needs was composed, and there was good nursing and physician transfer of her care. The palliative and oncology teams remained available for consultation, to family and local health care providers alike. Lastly, there was an understanding that if opportunities arose when Y.K. could return home for even short periods of time, they would be availed of, and appropriate equipment would be set up at home in anticipation of such possibilities. Air travel was sponsored by a local airline, in response to requests by the treatment team, to ensure that the child's brother as well as her mother would be able to visit her monthly.

Lines of communication

When a family takes their child home for end-of-life care, it is essential that some sort of continuous on-call coverage be arranged. If a family is not well supported at home, hospitalization is the default position, and this may not be in keeping with its hopes and goals. Different communities will have differing availability of home-health nurses, but some do provide 24-h-a-day on-call service; this service is often the 'first-line' for families' questions or concerns. Regardless of the nursing support available, it is also imperative that a physician or physician group provide continuous on-call coverage as the child's condition changes. In smaller communities, where a family has very close ties to a local general practitioner, that person may elect to be available to the family at all times, given the extreme rarity of the situation. In larger centers, in which caring for a dying child is a less rare occurrence, an on-call group of physicians often shares this responsibility. In many situations, pharmacists, psychologists, clergy, and social workers may be available for home visits. Neighbors, especially those with health care backgrounds, can provide enormous support to families. Regardless of the particular demographics of the health care community, in most cases a system can be devised such that parents know whom to call, day and night, for a variety of concerns. This list should be clearly written and kept handy, as should written care plans, to foster optimal communication.

Changes in the aim of treatment

Periods of transition are difficult for people in general. The transitions involved in redefining the goals of therapy for a child who is dying, then, is often an extremely emotional time for parents and caregivers alike. Often, the end of a child's life is preceded by a period of sometimes quite aggressive efforts to save this child's life. This transition, whether it be over hours, days or months, can be hard to understand. Therapies that were used at an earlier period in the child's illness, or thought to be 'essential,' may no longer have a place in providing a benefit at the end of life, and the new 'essential' medications are often analgesics, anticonvulsants, anxiolytics, antiemetics, and so on.

At the end of life, there are particular issues that recurrently cause distress. Whether, or how, to feed/hydrate their children can cause much distress for families, especially if they are unprepared for the eventuality that the children may either refuse, or become unable, to eat and drink (see also Chpater 4, Ethics; and Chapter 24, Feeding in palliative care). There is a spectrum of responses to this situation, seen in both caregivers and parents. The parents often see the provision of food and drink to their child as the most basic of human comforts, and to be unable to offer this simple type of care is often traumatic. Parents will respond uniquely, with some expressing their view that they 'can't just let him starve', and others seeing this event as a part of the overall picture, in which all of the child's bodily functions are shutting down. It is helpful to explore feelings about this in advance, and to avoid a crisis-oriented approach of solving the problem only when it arises. The evidence suggests that dying persons do not suffer adverse consequences, when they no longer feel like eating/drinking [3]. Patients sometimes complain of adverse effects, such as abdominal pain and distention, when artificially provided hydration or nutrition is given. This knowledge is empowering to parents in their decision making. Similarly, many parents feel that their children's survival might be lengthened if nutrition is artificially provided. For children who have had a long and complicated medical course prior to death, requests for total parenteral nutrition at the end of life are not unheard of. Gently informing the parent that providing nutrition at this stage of the child's illness will not contribute to longer survival is reassuring [4].

Families may seek other 'supportive' treatments very late in the child's illness. For oncology patients, the need for blood transfusions may have become rather routine to the family. Families will sometimes have a hard time letting go of this therapy, especially when they have seen marked improvement in the child's wellbeing at an earlier stage of her illness [5,6]. Parents need to feel that they have done everything that they can to save their child, and in turn, to ensure that they are as comfortable as possible in their dying. As physicians, we recognize that further treatment with packed red cells will have no beneficial effect in the last few days of life. However, we have our medical knowledge, and our practical experience, on which to base this rationale. Families are at a distinct disadvantage in terms of the ability to understand this. When physicians 'deny' their child a therapy that has been routine and previously effective, a negative dynamic can develop in which the parent may fear the team is 'giving up.' Sometimes a 'natural consequences' approach can be helpful in resolving this issue. If it appears that an impasse is being built around issues such as this, it may be most helpful to support the parents in their wishes, with certain provisos built into the administration of the therapy in question. For example, in the case of transfusions, it can be useful to help families understand that the hemoglobin level is no longer relevant, but that the patient's symptomatic relief provided by the transfusion will be the outcome to be evaluated. Most often, it is easier for parents to let go of such therapies, if they can see for themselves that these have become ineffective. The need to feel that they have done everything

possible to ease their child's suffering is immense, and a human, rather than a 'medical' approach to these discussions can have a positive impact.

Alternatively, as the child is seen to be 'dying' by the parents, the situation may suddenly seem intolerable, and parents may ask, indirectly or directly, that the physician end their child's suffering/life. Such requests are not well-reported in the literature. Again, these requests are often borne of a fear or belief that the child is suffering. If the child is suffering from a symptom that has not been controlled, this plea should be taken as an indication that more needs to be done. If the physician feels at his or her limit in offering any further ideas, it behooves that physician to consult with others who may have more expertise, to get this child's symptoms under control.

However, sometimes such a request is made at a stage when the patient appears to be comfortable, but is no longer able to interact. Each physician will have to find his or her own way to explain, as sensitively as possible, that this action cannot be undertaken. In this situation, the distilling of the conversation to a very human level (i.e., 'I as a human being' vs. 'I as her doctor') cannot end her life has been helpful. There is certainly no panacea, and every situation will have individual determinants, which should guide the explanation that makes the most sense to the particular family.

Anticipating likely symptoms

Parents need very specific guidance as to possible and probable symptoms that may emerge, and need to be educated in stepwise plans for control of these. The medical literature suggests that physicians are unable to predict 'how much time is left' for patients in their care, and it is recommended that no guesswork be made regarding specific timelines [7]. If a family expects death to occur at a certain time, anxiety often ensues, whether life expectancy is over-or under-estimated. In any case, families need anticipatory guidance as to how their child may change, with regard to both his or her physical appearance and physical signs of deterioration, as well as possible changes in his or her behavior and interactions. It is common that parents are unaware of what 'dying' may actually look like, and the experience can be devastating, if they are unprepared for the changes that they may see in their child. Parents should be made aware that the child's activity level will decrease, and the time spent sleeping will increase, as will the degree of difficulty in awakening; sometimes, the child will be deeply unconscious for hours to days before his or her death. Similarly, families should be prepared for the physical signs that they may witness, including pallor/cyanosis or mottling of the skin, and progressive cooling of the extremities, usually from distal to proximal. They should know that the child might have noisy respirations as he or she loses control of his or her oropharyngeal muscles and secretions. This should be treated, if distressing to the family, while reassuring them that the child is unaware of and unbothered by the 'death rattle,' as some laypersons know it. Management strategies include positioning the child on his side, with the head slightly lower, by placing the bed in a slight Trendelenberg position. Medications such as glycopyrrolate, hyoscine given parenterally or transdermally, or the use of 1% atropine eye drops given sublingually, can all be helpful. Playing soft music in the background can be a useful distraction.

Management of some particularly problematic symptoms will follow later in the chapter. However, it is essential not just that families are prepared for what is likely to happen today, but also that health care providers be more long-sighted in guiding the families as to what symptoms are probable or possible, as the disease progresses. To that end, advance planning must occur, if the child is to remain adequately managed at home for the duration of his or her illness. A fairly common problem is that of sudden onset or exacerbation of a symptom in 'out-of-hours' periods, such as evenings, nights, or weekends, at the end of life. For children cared for in a hospital or hospice setting, this can be very frightening for a family, if it had not been prepared for such a turn of events. However, in this setting, despite the worry and fear that may have arisen, there will at least be the presence of health care professionals, with immediate access to needed medications.

The same situation occurring in the family home at an inopportune time is much more problematic. Even if the family is well supported by a home health agency or program, accessing needed medication, as circumstances change, is potentially problematic. There are a number of ways to circumvent this problem, but it requires planning. There are situations where the family resides in an urban setting, with physicians, home health nurses, and pharmacies available on a 24 h-a-day, 7 days-a-week basis. However, although access to medications may be 24-h/day, there are the practical problems and inconvenience of dispensing the medication, and having someone pick it up from the pharmacy.

Another approach is that of the 'Emergency Drug Box'. This approach to optimizing palliative care in non-business hours seeks to keep families at home when that is their desire. Certainly, within adult populations, the great majority of patients have indicated that they would prefer to die at home, surrounded by loved ones [8]. It is the wish of many pediatric patients and their parents as well. However, if symptoms suddenly emerge or intensify, hospitalization will likely follow, if adequate resources are unavailable at home. Lack of ready access to new medications is an enormous obstacle to the child experiencing pain, dyspnea, or some other distressing symptom.

Emergency drug boxes can be instrumental in preventing undesired hospital admissions, in the last few hours or days of life (Personal communication: Winnipeg Regional Health Authority, Palliative Care Program; Capital Health Regional Palliative Care Program, Edmonton). These locked boxes are most often released only after consultation of the home health nurse with the most responsible physician. Specific orders should be obtained from the physician before any medication is administered. In turn, medications administered from the emergency drug box are recorded, and education of the family/patient is achieved as new medications are administered.

Emergency drug boxes most often contain sublingual formulations, suppositories, transdermal patches or injectable medications, on the assumption that the patient may no longer be in a condition where oral medications would be practical or possible. The medications contained often include a variety of steroids, benzodiazepines, anti-emetics, anticonvulsants, anti-psychotics and opioids. These are often delivered to the family home by a courier or a taxi company, with whom arrangements have been made in advance, thus freeing family members from having to leave their ill child, at a very distressing time, to go to the pharmacy.

However, many communities are without such programs. In these situations, it is imperative that the treatment team anticipates possible symptoms that may emerge, based on the patient's disease. Medications should be available readily for all the symptoms that are considered possible. It is prudent to ensure that families are given prescriptions for, and receive hands-on education about, the administration of these drugs. The home health nurse is instrumental in reviewing the storage, preparation, and administration of these drugs with the family. If this review doesn't occur, there is a potential for parents to forget, between the time of discharge from hospital and the time the symptom arises, the appropriate medication for each symptom. Safety in a home setting must be reinforced, particularly if there are other small children in the home. All medications should be kept in an easy-to-organize box, such as a tackle or tool box, and be kept locked, whenever not in use.

What follows is specific information in regards to management of a variety of symptoms that often emerge or intensify in the final hours or days of life. There is an intentional emphasis on the practical aspects of how to institute each specific therapy, as the calculations required in mixing parenteral medications in the middle of the night are often vexing, particularly to practitioners who may not be handling these medications routinely. There is an attempt to present a broad range of approaches, recognizing that treatment will be provided in settings ranging from homes in small rural settings to homes in large tertiary centers.

Lastly, parents should be made aware of changes that they will see in their child's body at the time of death, and should be supported through these. They should know that secretions may appear at the mouth/nose, and that the child may be incontinent of stool or urine. They should be reassured that there is no 'right' way to behave, and they should be encouraged to do what they feel is best for them. Families' privacies should be respected, and health care staff should be close at hand, but should not impose. A family may choose to bathe, hold, or dress its child. Other cultural or religious rites may occur around the child's body. The family members should be reassured that there is no rush, and that family members can spend as long as they need to with their child, family, and friends. Families are often very bewildered at this time, and may seek assistance for practical tasks, such as making phone calls to other extended family, selecting a funeral home, etc.

Preparedness through the dying process, and in the immediate period after death, contributes to the parents' sense of control. Their centrality in decision-making empowers them. As devastating as the situation is, knowing what potential problems they may face, having contingency plans, and knowing which people to contact for support, makes it less frightening.

Management of pain exacerbations

This chapter presupposes that the child may previously have been on oral opioids, with good pain control. However, in the final hours and days of life, a sudden crescendo of pain is not uncommon, and must be anticipated; at such times, patients frequently become too ill to manage oral medications. The following describes a step–by–step approach to transition to other forms of analgesia if this occurs, such that physicians less familiar with provision of these medications can administer them with confidence, if their patients require such a change.

Morphine

Of the 'short half-life opioids' (duration of action 3–4 h), morphine is the most commonly used, and is often considered to be 'first line' in treating severe pain, because of availability and familiarity. Starting intravenous and subcutaneous (IV/SC) doses are in the range of 0.05–0.1 mg/kg/dose, typically given every four hours; as an intermittent bolus dose for the opioid naïve child. If the child has previously been on an oral preparation of morphine with well-controlled symptoms, the parenteral dose should be calculated as a half to a third of the oral dose, due to significant first-pass effect of enterally administered morphine through the hepatic circulation.

It is important to note that the child may still need 'rescue' or 'breakthrough' doses of immediate-release morphine in this situation. Generally, the breakthrough dose given is approximately 10% of the total daily morphine requirement, and may be given as frequently as every hour. If the child requires 3 or more doses of rescue medication in a day, the regular dose of medication should be increased by an increment that reflects the total amount of morphine used in the preceding 24-h period. However, if there is rapid escalation of the pain, the regular morphine dose should be increased by 20–50%, and frequent breakthrough doses given to achieve pain control. If such dose–escalation does not achieve good effect, or dose–limiting side effects are encountered, rotation to another opioid may be indicated.

The subcutaneous route means that many children, even without IV access, can be treated with a morphine infusion, avoiding the 'peaks and valleys' of intermitttent boluses. One standard approach to mixing this infusion is to put $1.25 \times$ child's weight (kg) = *dose in mg*, to put in 250 ml of IV fluid. For example, for a 10 kg child:

$$1.25 \times 10 = 12.5 \text{ mg morphine in 250 ml IV fluid.}$$

This is a 5 µg/kg/ml solution. Conventional starting rates for a morphine infusion are 10–40 µg/kg/h. Therefore, using the above formula, the infusion would run at 2–8 ml per hour. It is important that breakthrough doses of analgesia are available. Because the child has a significant systemic level of morphine while on an infusion, boluses should be reduced in magnitude, compared to giving intermittent IV boluses in the absence of an infusion. Therefore, breakthrough doses of 0.02 mg/kg (20 mCg/kg) are considered safe for children on an infusion running at the starting rates above. If the child is requiring more morphine than the range listed previously, then a breakthrough dose equal to the hourly dose, given as a bolus over 10–15 min, is usually adequate.

It is noted that, like all high potency opioids, morphine does not have a ceiling, or upper-limit dose. The amount of drug should be titrated against the pain, providing the minimally effective dose to offer comfort, and the caretakers should against be vigilant for detecting dose–limiting side effects. This applies regardless of the route administered, and regardless of whether it is given as a patient–controlled analgesia (PCA), infusion, or intermittent bolus. It should also be noted that IV access is not necessary, and morphine may also be given subcutaneously, if other routes are not possible or desired, either as intermittent boluses or as a constant infusion. The easiest way to use the same site for multiple doses is to insert an Insuflon™, a small flexible catheter, into the subcutaneous tissue, and fix it in place with a transparent dressing. These may be left in situ for 3–7 days, while vigilance is maintained to catch signs of infection, induration, or medication leakage from the site. Otherwise, a 25–gauge butterfly needle can be secured in place, and repeated doses of medication can be given.

Diamorphine

Diamorphine is not yet available in some parts of the world, including most of North America. Elsewhere, it is one of the main opioids used in palliative medicine. Pharmacologically, it is little different from morphine, into which it is rapidly metabolised. It is no more addictive than morphine, but is 1.5–2 times as potent.

The major advantage of diamorphine is that it is much more soluble in water than morphine. This enables large doses of diamorphine to be prepared in very small volumes of water. Given parenterally, therefore, it is more practical than morphine at very high doses. Current practice in countries where diamorphine is available is often to use morphine for oral medication and diamorphine for subcutaneous or intravenous use. The 24-hourly dose of parenteral diamorphine is calculated from that of oral morphine as follows:

$$\text{Dose of parenteral diamorphine} = \frac{\text{dose of oral morphine}}{1.5 \text{ (potency ratio)}} \times 0.5 \text{ (bioavailability of parenteral formulation rather than oral)}$$

Hydromorphone (Dilaudid™)

An alternative high potency opioid is hydromorphone. Hydromorphone is five times more potent than morphine [9]. Given the preceding, a reasonable starting intermittent parenteral bolus dose is 0.01–0.02 mg/kg/dose. It is also a 'short half-life' opioid, like morphine, and therefore is often given every four hours. If the patient has previously been on oral hydromorphone, the parenteral dose should be calculated as a half to a third of the oral dose, because of first pass metabolism.

If an infusion is desired, it can be prepared using a similar standard formula as used in the preparation of a morphine infusion. Because hydromorphone is five times as potent as morphine, the amount of hydromorphone used is one fifth the amount of morphine, for the same volume of IV fluid. Therefore, 0.25 × weight of the patient (kg) = *amount of drug in mg*, to be placed in 250 ml of IV fluid. Again, in the case of a 10 kg infant:

$$0.25 \times 10 = 2.5 \text{ mg of hydromorphone to be placed in } 250 \text{ ml IV fluid (D5\%W or N/S).}$$

This yields a concentration of 10 mCg/ml, or 1 mCg/Kg/ml. Therefore, running the infusion at 2–8 ml will give a dose of 2–8 mCg/kg/h.

Fentanyl

Fentanyl is an opioid with a half-life that is ultra-short, and for this reason, intermittent dosing is not possible. Therefore, one must use either an IV infusion, or a transdermal form. Regardless of the medication used regularly, the use of a rapid–titration protocol for IV fentanyl has been described, for sudden uncontrolled cancer pain [10]. The more lipophilic nature of this drug, compared to morphine and hydromorphone, yields faster access through the blood–brain barrier, and therefore, a faster onset to peak effect. However, caution for this approach is warranted, given the possibility of respiratory depression in uncontrolled settings.

Fentanyl infusions typically start in the range of 0.5–1 μg/kg/h. As such, perhaps the easiest and safest standardized formula for preparation is:

50 × weight of patient (kgs) = quantity in *micrograms* of fentanyl, to be used to make a total volume of 50 ml of fluid

In the example of a 14 kg patient:

$$50 \times 14 = 700 \text{ μg to a total volume of 50 ml IV fluid}$$
$$= 14 \text{ mCg/ ml}$$

Therefore, for any weight of patient, running the infusion by this method at 0.5 ml/0.5 mL/h equals 0.5 mCg/kg/h, 1 ml/h equals 1 mCg/kg/h, and so on.

The equi-analgesic dose of fentanyl, compared to morphine, has not been accurately determined. In acute use, fentanyl is thought to have 100 times the potency of morphine. However, with prior regular use of opioid medications, fentanyl has been found on average to be 68–85 times more potent than morphine, although the limited studies available, searching for relative potency of these drugs, vary widely. Studies suggest that constipation and laxative use may be less common with fentanyl analgesia [11,12,13].

Transdermal fentanyl

If the patient is of a sufficient size and is not opioid naïve, transdermal fentanyl patches can be a very desirable method of analgesia. Transdermal fentanyl is commercially available as Duragesic™ patches in many countries. This patch is applied to the skin, and works by creation of a reservoir of drug that diffuses at a constant rate into the skin, and then, into the systemic circulation. It can take approximately 12 h to reach a systemic level sufficient to provide analgesia. During the first 12 h of application, regular doses of the opioid being rotated from should be continued. Similarly, when the patch is removed, it takes up to 12 h for plasma levels to decline sufficiently to institute a new regular opioid medication. Rescue doses of breakthrough analgesic should be used through this period of time.

Transdermal fentanyl patches are indicated for stable pain, as fentanyl is not a medication that one can quickly titrate. However, these patches are convenient, and easy to use. Pediatric patients often prefer this modality, because it dispenses with the need to take oral medication, or to be attached to an IV or SC system, normalizing life to some extent [14,15].

Caution is needed if the patient becomes febrile, as the increased skin temperature can increase absorption by up to 30%. The fever should be controlled with anti-pyretics as able. The child should be watched for side-effects of somnolence, and for respiratory depression through this period. The dose should be reduced if these effects are observed, or a different drug, or a different route, should be tried if the child is already on the lowest–dose patch, until the fever subsides.

Currently, fentanyl patches are available in 25, 50, 75, and 100 μg/h formulations. Because the lowest dose patch requires a morphine equivalent of a daily dose of at least 45 mg of oral morphine, this route is often impossible to use in small children. The patches may be used in an additive fashion, to achieve doses higher than 100 μg/h. For example, a patient may wear a 100 mCg/h patch with a 50 mCg/h patch, to achieve a total dose delivery of 150 mCg/h.

Care must be taken in choosing the application site, ensuring the child will not play with, pick at, bite, or eat the patch. Therefore, a position over the middle of the back, between the scapulae, is often a good choice in a small or cognitively-impaired child. The patches are designed such that cutting them disrupts the reservoir and is contra-indicated. There is no good evidence to support the practice of giving 'half-doses' of the smallest patch by placing an occlusive dressing onto the skin, and then placing the patch over this, so that only half of the patch contacts the skin directly.

The patch should be applied to clean skin washed with water only, without soap or detergent. If hair is present, it should be clipped close to the level of the skin, and not shaven, as abrasion can increase the absorption of the medication. To apply, the patch should be placed against the skin, with even pressure from the applicant's hand for 30 s after the protective backing is removed. When the patch is taken off, it should be folded onto itself, skin–side inwards, and placed in a Sharps or other safety container. The hands of the caregiver should be washed with soap and water, to prevent accidental absorption.

Methadone

Methadone is a synthetic long half-life opioid, that differs somewhat from the previously described opioids. It has a *long*

but *unpredictable* half-life, varying from 5–100 h, depending on the individual on whom it is used, with an average half–life, of around 24 h [16]. In Canada, prescribing of methadone is highly regulated, and one must apply for a methadone license through Health Canada. In other countries, methadone is more easily accessible. In the United Kingdom, for example, most general practitioners can prescribe it.

Intractable pain

Patients sometimes experience opioid dose-limiting side effects and severe pain simultaneously, a situation distressing to patient, family, and clinicians alike. In these situations, it is necessary to look quickly for other modalities, that may augment or replace systemic opioid/adjuvant therapy. Examples would be referral to anaesthesiology for consideration of a variety of regional blocks, epidural or intrathecal catheter placement, as deemed necessary.

Another strategy is the provision of low-dose ketamine. Ketamine is a dissociative anaesthetic (certain areas of the brain are affected, while others are unaffected, preserving normal muscle tone and respiration). When ketamine is used as anaesthetic doses, psychomimetic side effects, including hallucinations and nightmares, are described. There are a number of protocols for the use of low-dose, continuous ketamine infusions in refractory cancer pain. However, a recent Cochrane Database Systematic Review of ketamine as an adjuvant to opioids for cancer pain, has concluded that despite broad positive results, there are only two high quality randomized, controlled trials (RCT). The authors conclude that available evidence is insufficient to conclude that ketamine improves the effectiveness of opioid treatment in cancer pain [28,29]. Further studies are therefore required. However, the following clinical experience, and those of others [30–32], suggest consideration of this modality as an alternative, if sequential opioid rotations have been ineffective.

Case A 3-year-old female, with metastatic neuroblastoma, had a known relapse of localized disease in her left femur, which grew visibly over a 10-day period. She was initially given oral morphine, with good effect. Over time, this pain proved recalcitrant to increasing doses, and she was rotated to methadone. This briefly controlled her pain, but she began experiencing dose-limiting side effects. She became very sedated, picked frequently at the air, suggesting visual hallucinations, and her respiratory rate, usually 20–28, dropped to 14. Simultaneously, her pain escalated, interfering with her sleep, and causing her to cry and yell 'owie' frequently through one day. Palliative local radiotherapy was being organized, but the full effect from that would take some days to achieve, and would not help with the immediate pain crisis. Given the lack of efficacy from two types of opioids, and the experience of significant side effects, it was felt that rotation to a third opioid would be unlikely to optimize her pain control. At this point, the help of the anaesthesia service was sought. A continuous ketamine infusion was suggested. The methadone was stopped thereafter, and she was started on a ketamine infusion, at a dose of 0.1 mg/kg/h. She still received boluses of intermittent morphine on the first day of ketamine therapy, but these were needed very infrequently thereafter. Her pain control was greatly improved by this therapy. She was fully conscious, and happy to play in her bed, with improved freedom from incident pain associated with movement of her affected leg. Her sleep was much better, and her interaction with her family 'normal.' As her disease progressed, the ketamine infusion was increased to 0.2 mg/kg/h, and eventually, a morphine infusion was restarted, to a maximum of 60 mCg/kg/h, with good effect. She died peacefully in her sleep, with no signs of toxicity from either the ketamine or the morphine.

Dyspnea

Acute or progressive dyspnea is a relatively common symptom in dying children, particularly those with intrinsic lung disease, such as malignant metastases or cystic fibrosis [33], or those with extrinsic processes, such as neuro-muscular disease, or heart or kidney disease. This may be an increasingly prominent symptom as death approaches, and can signify the beginning of a fairly rapid deterioration of the body's ability to compensate against the disease process.

During the initial assessment of the patient, it may be helpful to start oxygen therapy, to assess for symptomatic relief. If the patient has a disease process in which problematic dyspnea/hypoxemia is anticipated, it is helpful to have oxygen organized for home use before it is actually needed, as getting it into the home requires significant time in many instances. Increased air movement over the child's face, by way of a fan or open window, is sometimes helpful. Another simple measure is to change the patient's position. Trying to sit the child upright, and providing distraction or massage, may relieve some of the associated anxiety. If wheeze is detected, a trial of inhaled bronchodilator is warranted, and easy to provide [34].

Dyspnea is a profoundly anxiety-provoking symptom to patient, family and health care professionals alike. Careful assessment of the cause of the dyspnea must be undertaken, to ensure that treatment of reversible causes such as pulmonary edema, pneumonia, pleural effusions, and ascites, is considered. If treatment of the above conditions with diuretics, antibiotics, chest tubes, or paracentesis respectively is ineffective, medical management should include use of systemic opioids for dyspnea [35]. These should be dosed as per initial doses for analgesia, and titrated to effect, although some patients may require smaller doses than for analgesia.

The use of nebulized opioids continues to be a matter of debate, using current evidence. Since the discovery of opioid receptors in the respiratory tract, opioids have been administered by nebulization. Some case reports reflect a mild beneficial effect on dyspnea [36,37]. The mechanism by which this modality may contribute to the subjective sensation of breathlessness remains unclear [38]. Others have argued that benefit is not a peripheral effect in the respiratory tract, but is a result of systemic absorption. This argument seems to have gained some validity in a study done in which plasma levels of morphine were measured in healthy subjects, after nebulized or oral doses of morphine were administered, demonstrating that nebulization is a rapid, but inefficient, method of administering morphine [39]. A small double–blind randomized placebo controlled study done by Noseda *et al* also concluded that subjects benefited from saline or morphine via a placebo effect, and that morphine had no specific effect on dyspnea [40]. Questions about the possible role of nebulized opioids would likely be better answered by larger, well-constructed clinical studies.

If dyspnea persists despite treatment with opioids, concomitant benzodiazepines or other sedatives should be considered. Co-administration of theses drugs is not extensively reported in the literature, but there are some relevant studies [41,42]. However, in the face of persistent dyspnea, the theoretical risks and benefits of combining these therapies should be evaluated. Ultimately, treating the panicked patient and family will usually override fears of respiratory depression, or misgivings about sedative side effects, in most situations.

If the dyspnea has developed slowly, over days to weeks, anemia may be a contributing factor, and relative risks and benefits of packed red blood cell transfusion should be contemplated, if this is detected [43]. If there is known intrathoracic tumour, initiation of systemic dexamethasone should be considered. In cases of muscle weakness causing dyspnea, referral to a pulmonary physician for evaluation of positive pressure ventilation, using nasal or facial masks, may be considered.

Bleeding/hemorrhage

Bleeding is an extremely distressing symptom to patients and families. Where sudden hemorrhage is thought to be a possibility, families should be counseled about it. In an exsanguinating hemorrhage, be the bleeding internal or external, it is paramount to discuss with the family that the patient will become rapidly unconscious, and will not suffer. This should be reinforced in an anticipatory fashion, and health care providers must ensure they restate this, if they are present during the actual event, to minimize the panic and distress that will arise on the part of those witnessing such bleeding. A simple measure for nursing the child at risk of hemorrhage, is the use of dark fabrics (pajamas, clothing, bedding, towels, etc.), which provides much better camouflage than does light hospital linen.

In the case of brisk, but not exsanguinating, bleeding, the child will no doubt be very panicked and distressed, and a dose of intravenous or intramuscular midazolam will rapidly lead to the patient becoming unconscious, and prevent them from bearing witness to such a distressing event. The possibility of using this modality should be discussed with parents in advance, when time permits, to ensure that they understand that the goal of treatment is not to hasten the death of their child, but to allow them freedom from awareness of what is happening to them. Very often nursing and other staff need this explained in advance, too, to allow time for discussion about concerns and comfort level in providing this treatment.

For patients in whom oozing of blood is a problem, the use of the anti-fibrinolytic drug transexamic acid may be beneficial. If the bleeding is localized to oral mucosa, this can be delivered as a 5% solution mouthwash in which 30 ml is used TID. Dissolving a 500 mg tablet in 5 ml of water yields this concentration. If the bleeding is more widespread (i.e., recurrent GI bleeding) systemic use, giving 20 mg/ kg enterally or intravenously every eight hours, may be beneficial in preventing breakdown of clot. Bleeding cutaneous ulcers may respond to topical application of 1 : 1000 epinephrine.

Seizures

Seizures are extremely frightening to parents, and many will state, after witnessing a first seizure, that they thought their child was dying. Seizures are, unfortunately, not rare as children die. This may be directly related to underlying disease in some cases (e.g., brain metastases or metabolic diseases), or may be related to end-stage hypoxemia, or electrolyte disturbance. It is helpful for the parents to know, first and foremost, that people are not conscious when they have generalized seizures, distressing as they may be to watch. The knowledge that their child is not suffering during this time is helpful to parents. For any patient who has a disease with potential for seizure activity, the parents must be guided through what a seizure would look like, and to have a specific plan in place, should this occur. This would include immediate positioning of the child in a safe place, dispelling of the myth that the child will 'swallow his tongue,' and learning that no foreign objects should be placed in the mouth, in an attempt to open it. The parents should be instructed in the use of either rectal benzodiazepine administration, or in buccal application of a sublingual lorazepam tablet, holding it firmly against the

buccal mucosa until it is dissolved. Rectal diazepam is commercially available in a variety of doses, but unfortunately, the cost can be prohibitive. An alternative is the rectal use of diluted injectable diazepam or lorazepam, given via a 10 ml syringe with the first 5 cm of a small feeding tube (remainder cut away), to deliver the medication rectally. Parents should also know in advance who to call for assistance.

If the seizure does not respond the first dose of medication, parents should be instructed on further doses and dosing intervals when they call for help. In rare instances, the seizure may be refractory to repeated doses of benzodiazepine. For a patient being cared for at home, this situation may require transfer by ambulance to the closest hospital, for further management with IV medications. For a family that lives remotely, and wishes that its child be kept at home no matter what occurs, it may be helpful to include pentobarbital (Nembutal™) in an emergency drug kit. This drug has fallen out of favour, given the genesis of better and safer anti-epileptic/sedative medications, but still has a useful role, given per rectum, or parenterally, in this dire situation [44]. Use of this medication in such a setting would require significant advance planning, discussion, and consultation.

Superior vena cava obstruction syndrome (SVCO)

This complication arises from compression of the superior vena cava (SVC), preventing venous drainage from the head, arms, and upper trunk. Clinical features of SVCO include dyspnea from tracheal edema, headache secondary to cerebral edema, swelling of face, neck, arms and hands, visual changes, and dizziness [45]. It can arise from compression or invasion by tumor, or by the formation of a thrombus around a central subclavian catheter. In the former case, it may occur over weeks or months, allowing collateral drainage to develop. Occasionally, it occurs rapidly over days, and requires urgent treatment. Radiotherapy can be very helpful within the first two weeks of treatment, if the SVCO is caused by extrinsic tumour. In cases where radiotherapy is not possible, or is not efficacious, placement of a stent, as an interventional radiology technique, can also be considered. In the case of a thrombus of the vessel, relief of the obstruction may be obtained by removal of the catheter, although embolization is a risk if the line is left in situ, or as a complication of its removal. For patients receiving palliative care, the risks and benefits of invasive procedures need to be weighed. Factors in the decision would include the burden of suffering arising from the SVCO, the risk of proposed therapy, other comorbidities, predicted length and quality of remaining life, and so on. As a temporizing measure, a course of dexamethasone may be helpful in short–term tumour shrinkage, and this may be particularly pertinent for children in whom this occurs very late in the courses of their lives.

Spinal cord compression

Compression of the spinal cord is a palliative care emergency, as a significant number of patients will survive for a significant length of time after this occurs, and have the added devastation of paraplegia to contend with, if it is not adequately recognized and immediately treated. In adults, the great majority of patients develop this complication secondary to extension of vertebral body metastases into the epidural space [45]. Back pain, often worsened by the Valsalva maneuver, should alert the physician or nurse of this possibility, when caring for a child with cancer. Other warning signs are unpleasant sensations in limbs. Sensory and motor loss occur later, and sphincter disturbance is a late sign. The final stage is cord ischemia, that occurs rapidly over hours. High dose dexamethasone, given immediately, will reduce spinal cord edema, and may temporarily prevent the onset of cord ischemia. Radiotherapy is the definitive treatment, and surgery is indicated for spinal instability in patients who are early in their course. Again, when this symptom occurs very close to the end of life, corticosteroids alone may be employed, provided they do not cause undesired side effects such as emotional lability. The symptoms associated with spinal cord compression can be severe, and intervention with surgery and/or radiotherapy should be discussed with the family, and (where appropriate) the patient, even when he or she is unlikely to survive more than a few weeks. For many, the benefits of such intervention will be outweighed by the possibility of prolonged hospitalisation. Interventions that are commenced more than 48 h after the onset of symptoms of spinal cord compression are highly unlikely to relieve symptoms, and aggressive management should not usually be recommended.

Sedation for intractable distress

Despite the progress made in pain and symptom management over the last few decades, distressing situations still occur, in which symptoms remains uncontrolled in the face of all reasonable efforts to alleviate them. The suffering incurred by patients and families in this circumstance is immense, and the option of providing sedation to the patient, for relief of refractory symptoms, is often entertained at this stage.

Unfortunately, despite descriptions of 'terminal' and 'palliative' sedation in recent medical literature, there remains much confusion about the intended meaning. Descriptions range from mild intermittent sedation at one end of the spectrum, in which patients are able to communicate at least

episodically, to deep continuous sedation, in which the patient is likely to remain unconscious until death, at the other end [46,47]. There has been a recent move to rename this therapy, 'sedation for intractable distress' in the dying patient. Use of the term 'terminal sedation' has been discouraged, because of the misinterpretation of intent (connotation of euthanasia), and because it does not convey the gravity of the severe suffering which this type of sedation serves to lessen. Clearly, when titrated against a particular symptom, this form of sedation can be seen as morally justifiable, as would be the array of potent opioids we bring to palliative care under the auspices of the principle of 'double effect' [48]. In short, provision of relief from a distressing symptom is the morally defensible intent, even if there are foreseeable, but unintended, harmful effects, including respiratory depression, or even the hastening of death. This is in stark contrast to the intent of euthanasia, which is to end suffering by means of ending life. Unfortunately, a class of these sedative agents (barbiturates) is used in Holland for performing euthanasia, and has been recommended for assisting suicide, further adding to the misunderstanding. A recent survey of palliative care experts from eight countries showed 89% agreement that sedation for relief of intractable symptoms is sometimes necessary, and that it was felt to be effective in 90% of cases recalled. Of these experts, 90% were not in support of legalized euthanasia [49]. Importantly, a study in a specialist palliative care unit showed that sedative use was not associated with shorter survival, suggesting that the doctrine of double effect rarely has to be invoked to justify sedative prescribing at the end of life [50].

Before sedation is considered for symptom control, the advice of colleagues with expertise in palliative symptom management and/or anaesthesia should be sought, to ensure that the symptom is truly refractory. In the relatively rare circumstance where this proves to be the case, careful discussions must be held with the parents, involved health care professionals, and the patient, where appropriate. The goal of therapy—relief of suffering from the symptom—must be clearly demarcated from euthanasia. It must be made clear that aside from this alternative, there are no further medical options. It is imperative that the staff attending the family be fully informed about the implementation of this therapy, and related myths dispelled. Otherwise, unhealthy situations can evolve, in which parents are challenged by staff, or equally inappropriately, parents feel the burden of having to help health care professionals 'cope.' Under no circumstance should parents be made to feel that they are choosing between their child's comfort and their child's life—another possible innuendo the parents may feel, if professional caregivers are not well-prepared.

Pharmacologic options for provision of sedation for intractable symptoms include benzodiazepines, neuroleptics, barbiturates and general anaesthetics. Kenny and Frager [51] provide specific guidelines for use of these medications in children at the end of life. Starting doses should be conservative, given the concomitant administration of other centrally acting medications, and can be titrated upwards to effect. A frequently given benzodiazepine is lorazepam, in sublingual (SL), intravenous (IV), or subcutaneous (SC) form. Starting doses of 0.02–0.05 mg/kg are reasonable, and may be given every 6–8 h. Sublingual tablets may be held against the buccal mucosa until absorbed. Diazepam is irritating SC, but may be given IV (0.1 mg/kg), or per rectum (PR) 0.3 mg/kg, in the same time interval.

Neuroleptics, such as haloperidol (0.01 mg/kg), or methotrimeprazine (leromepromazine) (0.1 mg/kg), may be given IV/SC every 8 h.

If symptoms are refractory, despite rapid escalation in 20–50% aliquots from suggested starting doses, advice from anaesthesiologists, regarding use of barbiturates such as pentobarbital, and general anaesthetics such as propofol or ketamine, is suggested.

References

1. Wolfe, J., Grier, H., Klar, N. *et al.* (2000). Symptoms and suffering at the end of life in children with cancer. *N England J Med* 342: 326–33.
2. The SUPPORT Principle Investigators (1995). A controlled trial to improve care for seriously ill hospitalized patients: the Study to Understand Prognoses and Preferences for Outcomes and Risks of Treatments. *JAMA* 274:1591–8.
3. Anonymous (1998). Guidelines for Analgesic Drug Therapy. In: *Cancer pain relief and palliative care in children*, pp. 24–8. World Health Organization, Geneva.
4. Kyriakides, K., Hussain, S.K., Hobbs, G.J. (1999). Management of opioid-induced pruritus: a role for 5-HT3 antagonists? *Br J Anaesth.* 82:439–41.
5. McGrath, P.J., Finley, A. (1996). Attitudes and beliefs about medication and pain management in children. *J Palliat Care* 12:46–50.
6. Schecter, N.L. (1989). The undertreatment of pain in children: an overview. *Pediat Clin North Am* 36:781–794.
7. Liben, S. (1996). Pediatric palliative medicine: obstacles to overcome. *J Palliat Care* 12:24–8.
8. Cantwell, P., MacKay, S., Macmillan, K., Turco, S., McKinnon, S., Read-Paul, L. (1998). Pain. In: Brenneis C., Perry B., Read-Paul L., Bruera E., ed. *99 Common questions (and answers) about Palliative care: a nurses' handbook*. pp. 20. Regional Palliative Care Program, Edmonton.
9. Pereira, J., Bruera, E. (2000). Table of equianalgesic dose's of opioids. *Palliative care handbook*, pp. appendix B. Alberta Cancer Board, Edmonton.
10. Collins, J.J., Dunkel, I.J., Gupta. S.K. *et al.* (1999). Transdermal fentanyl in children with cancer pain: Feasibility, tolerability and pharmakokinetic correlates. *J Pediatr* 134:319–23.
11. Hunt, A., Goldman, A., Devine, T., Phillips, M. (2001). Transdermal fentanyl for pain relief in a pediatric palliative care population. *Palliat Med* 15:405–12.
12. No authors cited (2000). Evidence-Based recommendations for medical management of chronic non-maligant pain. *Reference Guide for clinicians for the treatment of chronic non-malignant pain.* pp. 39–40. College of Physicians and Surgeons of Ontario.
13. Gagnon, B., Bruera, E. (1999). Differences in the ratios of morphine to methadone in patients with neuropathic pain versus non-neuropathic pain. *J Pain Symptom Manage* 18:120–25.
14. Ripamonti, C., Zecca, E., Bruera, E. (1997). An update on the clinical use of methadone for cancer pain. *Pain* 70:109–15.
15. Ripamonti, C., Groff, L., Brunelli, C., Polastri, D., Stavrakis, A., De Conno F. (1998). Switching from morphine to oral methadone in treating cancer pain: what is the equianalgesic dose ratio? *J Clin Oncol* 16:3216–21.
16. Bruera, E., Pereira, J., Watanabe, S., *et al.* (1996). Opioid rotation in patients with cancer pain; a retrospective comparison of dose ratios between methadone, hydromorphone, and morphine. *Cancer* 78:852–7.
17. Wiser, A.W., Miser, J.S. (1985). The use of oral methadone to control moderate and severe pain in children and young adults with malignancy. *Clin J Pain* 1:243–8.
18. Shir, Y., Shenkman, Z., Shavelson, V., Davidson, E., Rosen, G. (1998). Oral methadone for the treatment of severe pain in hospitalized children: a report of five cases. *Clin J Pain* 14:350–53.
19. Zeltzer, L., Bush, J., Chen, E., Riveral, A. (1997). A Psychobiologic approach to pediatric pain: Part II: prevention and treatment. *Curr Probl Pediatr* 27:264–84.
20. Berde, C. (1991). The treatment of pain in children., In: Bond MR, Charlton J.E. and Woolf C.J. ed. *Proceedings of the VIth World Congress on Pain*, pp. 435–40. Elsevier Science Publishers.
21. Collins, J.J. (1996). Intractable pain in children with terminal cancer. *J Palliat Care* 12:29–34.
22. Cooper, M.G., Keneally, J.P., Kinchington, D. (1994). Continuous brachial plexus neural blockade in a child with intractable cancer pain. *J Symptom Manage* 9:277–81.
23. Gurnani, A., Sharma, P.K., Rautela, R.S., Bhattacharya, A. (1996). Analgesia for acute musculoskeletal trauma: low-dose subcutaneous infusion of ketamine. *Anaesth Intensive Care* 24:32–6.
24. Klepstad, P., Borchgrevink, P., Hval, B., Flaat, S., Kaasa, S. (2001). Long-term treatment with ketamine in a 12-year-old girl with severe neuropathic pain caused by a cervical spinal tumor. *J Pediatr Hematol Oncol* 23:616–19.
25. Clark, J.L., Kalan, G.E. (1995). Effective treatment of severe cancer pain of the head using low-dose Ketamine in an opioid-tolerant patient. *J Pain Symptom Manage* 10:310–14.
26. Robinson, W.M., Ravilly, S., Berde, C., Wohl M.E. (1997). End-of-life care in cystic fibrosis. *Pediatrics* 100:205–9.
27. Regnard, C.F., Tempest, S. (1998). Respiratory Problems. In: *A guide to symptom relief in advanced Disease*, Fourth Edition, pp. 32–34. Hochland and Hochland Ltd, Cheshire, England.
28. Kvale, P.A., Simoff, M., Prakash, U.B. (2003). Palliative Care. *Chest* 123:284S–311S.
29. Cohen, S.P., Dawson, T.C. (2002). Nebulized morphine as a treatment for dyspnea in a child with cystic fibrosis. *Pediatrics* 110, e38.

30. Coyne, P.J., Viswanathan, R., Smith, T.J. (2002). Nebulized fentanyl citrate improves patients' perception of breathing, respiratory rate, and oxygen saturation in dyspnea. *J Pain Symptom Manage* 23:157–60.

31. Zebraski, S.E., Kochenash, S.M., Raffa, R.B. (2000). Lung opioid receptors: pharmacology and possible target for nebulized morphine in dyspnea. *Life Sci* 66:2221–31.

32. Masood, A.R., Thomas, S.H. (1996). Systemic absorption of nebulized morphine compared with oral morphine in healthy subjects. *Br J Clin Pharmacol* 41:250–2.

33. Noseda, A., Carpiaux, J.P., Markstein, C., Meyvaert, A., de Maertelaer, V. (1997). Disabling dyspnoea in patients with advanced disease: lack of effect of nebulized morphine. *Eur Respir J* 10:1079–83.

34. Zeppetella, G (1998). The palliation of dyspnea in terminal disease. *Am J Hosp Palliat Care* 15:322–30.

35. Fainsinger, R.L., Waller, A., Bercovici, M. *et al.* (2000). A multicentre international study of sedation for uncontrolled symptoms in terminally ill patients. *Palliat Med* 14:257–65.

36. Gleeson, C., Spencer, D. (1995). Blood transfusion and its benefits in palliative care. *Palliat Med* 9:307–13.

37. Collins, J.J., Devine, T.D., Dick, G.S. (2002). The measurement of symptoms in young children with cancer: the validation of the Memorial Symptom Assessment Scale in children aged 7–12. *J Pain Symptom Manage* 23:10–16.

38. Wilwerding, M.B., Loprinzi, C.L., Mailliard, J.A. *et al.* (1995). A randomized, crossover evaluation of methylphenidate in cancer patients receiving strong narcotics. *Support Care Cancer* 3:135–8.

Section 4

Delivery of care

33 Working as a team

Satbir S. Jassal and Jo Sims

There has been extensive discussion in both business management and health literature surrounding team working, which has clearly been identified as effective, and is advocated by all. Indeed the World Health Organization affirms that primary health should involve all related sectors working together, including education and social services, in addition to health care, and that efforts should be made to co-ordinate these sectors [1]. It is the intention of this chapter to consider the issues around definitions in teamwork briefly and then concentrate on the practical application of team working and how it can be effectively achieved.

Defining teams

Prior to exploring teamworking in paediatric palliative care, it is essential to consider defining 'team'. This may appear to be simple; however, there is still much debate, and there are contentious issues involved [2]. Handy [3] challenges many definitions by demonstrating that they could refer to people who do not even perceive themselves to be part of a group or team; for example, a number of individuals in a pub who are interacting, have a common objective and are aware of each other (often key points that are used in team definitions), by their actions of talking and drinking; however, they do not have the perception of being in a group or team. Others have suggested that following the belief that 'team', and 'teamworking' are aspirational and aiming for co-operation, collaboration and co-ordination, each individual team should define what team means individually to them [2].

Despite difficulties we believe it is helpful and important to have a working definition even if this is viewed as a starting point. We propose to work with West's definition, relevant to the health environment, as 'a group of individuals who share goals and work together to deliver services for which they are mutually accountable' [4]. Team working aims to 'stimulate group cohesion and co-operation towards professional and service objectives' [2]; however a significant omission within these descriptions is the role of the service user, in this case the family and child.

Within health care teams a variety of terms are used relating to the structure and philosophy of the teams; these include multidisciplinary, interdisciplinary, and transdisciplinary. Some use these terms interchangeably, which is inaccurate and therefore confusing. They can be seen, more usefully, as being points on a joint working continuum which goes from professionals working alongside each other, to true partnership between professionals, agencies, the family and the child.

Multidisciplinary teamworking has been described as 'a progressive and beneficial strategy' [5] with many writers demonstrating good practice in the work of multidisciplinary teams [6–10]. Pardess [11] identifies the advantages of multidisciplinary teamwork as reducing bias, enhancing validity and reliability, and offering a source of sharing and support. There are however criticisms of the approach, as it has been argued that multidisciplinary teams tend to concentrate on a specific task, and are often led by professional hierarchy [12].

Inter-disciplinary work is thought to be a development and advance from multidisciplinary working. It is being increasingly introduced in a wide range of settings, including palliative care. It is viewed as being 'unconstrained' compared with the function of a multidisciplinary team, it is inclusive and is not ruled by professional roles, the aims vary over time as appropriate, and there is a continuing sense of working together. This type of working acknowledges the value of involvement of different agencies, including the voluntary and private sectors [12,13].

Transdisciplinary team working is a newer term, still only featured minimally in the literature. This is perhaps because its occurrence in practice is rare. This is where the focus and starting point is with the child and family's needs and how these needs can be met, rather than from the restrictions of existing services. It is believed that this form of working would be welcomed by families [14].

The family in teamworking

Teamwork cannot effectively occur unless the family and the child are viewed by all to be valid members of the team. The concept of family-centred care is fundamentally supported within the paediatric world [15]. However, Taylor [16] identifies that this has not necessarily led to the appropriate discussions with families, and the delivery of individualised care, that may have been presumed. Friction often remains between parents and professionals. Parents continue to cite problems with staff shortages, professional rivalry, numerous separate appointments, difficulty in distinguishing overlapping roles, confused communication of information and difficulty obtaining funding [17]. The professional can perceive parents' reactions to these problems as those of difficult or over-demanding parents. The parents themselves may develop an adversarial attitude toward the professional, by questioning or refuting medical advice, fighting for limited financial resources, or deviousness in identifying what resources they have in fear of losing them. This conflict can be explained in part by the understanding that the family are in fact undertaking a dual role at this time; they are carers for their child and therefore part of the team, however they are also themselves in need of receiving care from other team members. These different roles may conflict and challenge their partnership with others, and certainly adds to the complexity of the situation. Taylor [16] calls for more research within this field to ensure that the obstacles to family centred care are identified and overcome, to enable the development of an equal partnership.

If the family members are included in the team, it follows that some level of teamwork will be required in the care of all children with palliative care needs. It would appear reasonable to presume that a team working together will be more effective and efficient than individuals working independently [18]. The number of professionals and agencies that a family has contact with and the complexity of teamwork needed is dependent on that family's particular needs. On average a disabled child has contact with 10 different professionals and attends 20-clinic visits a year [19]. Equivalent data for palliative care in children has not been collected but it is likely to be of a similar order. This can be expressed diagrammatically, with the child and family firmly occupying the central position (Figure 33.1).

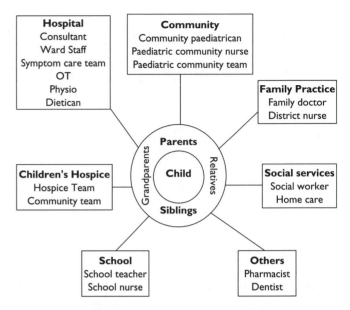

Fig. 33.1 Professional involvement in the care of a child.

As well as each family being different, the range of conditions varies with different patterns of disease progression and palliative care. These will therefore present different challenges to achieving effective teamwork to meet the families' varying needs with time. Reflections on two clinical examples (scenarios 1 and 2) are presented to illustrate this.

Case Jenny is 8 years old, and has Hurlers syndrome. She was admitted to the local district general hospital with a chest infection. Her parents also reported a general deterioration in Jenny's mobility, ability to feed and general condition.

Previously the family members had been eager to limit the number of professionals involved as they felt it was their responsibility to care for their child, and they wished to maintain as much 'normality' as possible. However, they are now clearly very tired, and are expressing that they are unsure how they will cope once they take Jenny home.

Jenny was acutely unwell for a few days, requiring oxygen, suction and intravenous antibiotics. Although her respiratory condition improved, it became evident that she may require some oxygen and suction in the longer term. Also there was little improvement in Jenny's general condition, which led the ward staff and her parents to believe that these skills may not be regained.

In discussion with the parents, it was agreed that there was a need to involve other professionals prior to Jenny's discharge from hospital, as the family's needs had significantly changed. Jenny's parents were keen to keep those involved to a minimum, but appreciated that they would need support in certain areas. These included feeding, seating, mobility, minor adaptations to the home, benefit advice, support with oxygen and suction requirements and potentially respite care.

Invited to the discharge meeting were 12 professionals; however, the family had only met four of them previously.

Case Jamie is 7 years old and has acute myeloid leukaemia, which was diagnosed when he was 5 years old. Jamie relapsed and is now requiring palliative care at home. He and his family have identified that they wish for him to remain at home. However they are concerned about how they will cope.

Jamie has received the majority of his treatment at a tertiary centre that is 30 miles away from his home; the family members have had minimal contact with the local District General hospital, and have not accessed other local services previously.

The specialist nurse at the tertiary centre has been a continuing contact for the family, always on hand with information, advice, and support. However the family members now require other professionals from their locality to become involved so they have support available, close by, 24h a day. The professionals and services in the locality have had experience of this type of palliative care before, but they acknowledge that they do not have the expertise that the specialist nurse has.

Despite the differences, in both these cases there is a sudden increase in the number of professionals the families are introduced to, at a time when they are faced with the deterioration in their child's condition and realisation of their impending mortality. Without careful and effective team work the increase of professional assistance and services will not necessarily have a positive impact on the care of the child and family.

A distinct difference between the scenarios is the expected trajectories of the conditions from this point. Jenny may continue to require palliative care for months to years, whereas Jamie is likely to die within a short time. Therefore in Jenny's case there is a need for the team work to be sustained over a long period of time fluctuating between times of stability and times of need for increase services and support; whereas for Jamie and his family the team has to become effective very quickly, and the care and support may be required to be very intensive throughout the palliative care.

It could be viewed by members of Jamie's family that their main support is becoming distant as others are becoming involved. However a sole worker based some distance away will be unable to meet the needs of the family. Good team working can address the issues of knowledge, time and availability of support that are evident in this scenario.

A particular challenge for members of Jenny's family could be the conflict between realising that they require more assistance and support to care for Jenny and their principles of addressing issues as a family without outside influences; good teamwork in this situation can empower this family members to ensure that they retain control over their lives.

All the children who require palliative care will have different requirements but in common they need everyone to work together and be clear of their roles and responsibilities, to ensure the child's and the family's needs are met in a supportive and timely manner.

Teamworking across agencies

Teamwork to ensure that provision and delivery of care is optimal for an individual child and family is clearly identified, There is also a need to look at joint working at broader levels, including strategic planning and service commissioning [8,11,12].

Consider the situation when, more than one team is involved. To return to both Figure 1 and the clinical scenarios, it is evident that there is a core team around the family, but it is likely that most members of this are also members of other teams. For example, a staff nurse from a hospital ward may be a member of the core team, but will work with the family within a nursing team on the ward, and cannot be present at all times. Also there may be an extended team attached to the ward, for example play specialists, hospital teacher and others so creating another team. These teams within teams are replicated in other services, where even those who appear to be individual workers will have extended teams that may impact on the family. For instance, a family doctor has other doctors in a practice, and also other members of a surgery team (nurses, receptionists). Each of these teams will be required to work effectively, otherwise there is potential for a detrimental effect on the family and child [20]. The requirement for good communication needs to be both within each agency and also between them.

Organizational culture

The carers involved with children with complex needs come from many organisations and each of these have their own way of working, hierarchy, pay, funding, geography and training [14]. This tends to generate different ideologies, culture and attitudes [5]. Organisational rigidity leads to ineffective team working [13]. Different levels of commitment to the care required can lead to frustration and fragmentation of the team. Time factors often mean key personnel not being able to attend meetings and decisions are put off. Linked to this are the personal and organization's perceptions of the value of liaison and communication in team meetings. Differing attitudes towards leadership can mean that the team lacks direction, or conflicts develop as infighting for power within groups. Many team leaders have little or no training in team working or leadership skills. Power struggles develop between organisations, linked to control and funding issues. Funding for equipment is repeatedly seen as an issue between health and social services. Funding for time, and training for team development are overlooked. The issue of justice in the allocation of limited resources can lead to team tension and frustration. Control is often related to how individuals and organisations value their status and who is the 'most important' rather than being held by the key worker on behalf of the family.

Team theory

All those working together in teams need to develop an understanding of how the success of a team can be achieved. Various authors have suggested models for team formation and development (Table 33.1). The key points that emerge from all these papers, are that teams do not magically appear, gel and work immediately. All teams go through stages of development, as individuals learn about each other's skill and knowledge, roles are defined and responsibility is delegated. Conflict appears to be a natural event in the evolution of the team. Role change and mutual respect develops within the team as individuals learn to value the work of their colleagues and the team. The situation is fluid and patterns and aspects of team behaviour may emerge, resolve and then recur with time.

Factors of a successful team

After recognizing that teams do not just occur but take hard work to achieve, many writers have contributed to identifying the factors that can influence the development and work of a team. Handy [3] separates them into *the givens, the intervening factors and the outcomes* (Table 33.2).

Table 33.1 Models for the development of teams

Lowe [21]	Roelofsen [22]	Handy [3]
Becoming acquainted	Process-oriented	Forming
Trial and error	Result-oriented	Storming
Collective indecision	Problem-oriented	Norming
Crisis	Interdisciplinary team	Performing
Resolution		

Table 33.2 Factors for a successful team, Handy [16]

The givens	
The group	Size, member characteristics, individual objectives, and stage of development
The task	Nature of the task; criteria of effectiveness, salience of task, and clarity of task
The environment	Norms and expectations, the leader position, inter-group relations, and the physical location
The intervening factors	Leadership style Process and procedure Motivation
The outcomes	Productivity Member satisfaction

Some of these factors, for example 'productivity', may seem unrelated to teamwork in palliative care and risk being dismissed as irrelevant. However, a family that feels supported and has access to appropriate and timely services should be the 'productivity' that is being sought by all. Madge and Khair [23], writing from a paediatric care perspective, have also identified a number of factors the most important being:

- team membership
- group dynamics, clear objectives
- awareness of colleagues both within and outside the team
- an agreed team philosophy

It is clear that although factors identified by different writers may vary, effective teamwork does not just occur; there are many areas that require consideration and attention. How we take the theory and put it into practice in the real world of organisations, individuals and children with life limiting illness is the great challenge.

The challenges of the team working

Considering the complexity of care that needs to be provided in paediatric palliative care and the emotionally powerful nature of the work, it is perhaps not so surprising that conflicts and problems can occur when people and organizations attempt to work together. The difficulties encountered come in many forms, ranging from conflicts between groups and individuals, to problems of organization within the team. Conflict itself should not be considered a good or bad thing in itself. It is the outcome of the conflict on an individual or group that determines its effect [5]. Thus unchecked conflict can paralyse individuals or divide groups and organizations, whereas providing a forum for expression of differences of opinions can create an environment for shared ideas and openness [24] and in the best of worlds constructive progress.

Interprofessional relationships

Health, education, and social services

The needs of children with life-threatening illness can only be fully assessed and managed by the input of care health, education and social services [25]. However, certainly in the United Kingdom, each of these organizations have different hierarchical structures, management and funding [20,26]. This can lead to differences in service priorities, in aims and objectives of team members, in competing targets for different agencies, disagreement over funding, confusion over accountability, and incompatible exchange of information [13,18]. In addition it has been suggested that the core ideology ingrained in education and training of individuals in the groups is different with medicine founded on a pathophysiological paradigm, nursing on a holistic problem solving framework , and social work on an individual paradigm [5]. Unless individuals from the triad of organisations are able to recognise previously held biases and lay their prejudices to one side and acknowledge each others's strengths conflict is bound to occur [12,27].

Hospital, community, and hospices

The traditional model of care in the United Kingdom of primary care led by family doctors in the community with occasional input from secondary and tertiary centres is inadequate for children with terminal illness. Most family doctors will only look after one or two children with life-threatening illness in their lifetime and therefore most feel they have insufficient training and experience to look after dying children. However, it is generally accepted that most children with life-limiting conditions spend the majority of their time being cared for in the community, and that being at home is the children's and the families' preference. Some of the barriers and prejudices between hospital and community care need to be broken down to enable this to be successful [28]. Some of this has been pioneered very effectively in the care of children with malignant disease through the paediatric oncology outreach nurses and their work in collaboration with children's community nurses. However, the care of children with often more uncommon non-malignant diseases has lagged behind.

The children's hospice movement in the United Kingdom, which developed particularly with these children's needs in mind, has grown greatly in the last ten years. The initial scepticism by hospital paediatricians about their role and value is no longer significant and the benefits of hospice care for children with non-malignant disease are clearly recognised. However their input adds an additional team and approach in the communication network and also difficulties still need solving in relation to issues of competition for staff and resources locally.

Health care professionals

The very interdependency, reliance and need to share information and responsibilities particularly between doctors and nurses, but also other therapists, highlight the need for good close relationships. The belief that one's own profession is superior to the others is the commonest sited obstacle to joint working [12]. Conflict can occur when either party does not complete their expected role and responsibilities or blocks completion of goals set by others [29]. It may result, for example, when doctors assume leadership roles in teams when they may have neither the skill nor the knowledge to lead. Their views may be based on traditional expectations or concern regarding the medico-legal implications for them in cases of complaint or litigation [30]. More often problems occur due to a lack of understanding of the skills and roles of each other's profession [31]. Unfortunately it has been shown that this type of conflict has significant effects, not only on parents' perceptions of the health care professionals [17], but also on patient mortality and morbidity [24].

Communication

Communication at all levels continues to be the most common problem associated with difficulty in team working and little appears to have changed over time [21]. Poor communication can inflict profound, long-term and personal damage on the child and the family [32]. It is particularly relevant as children with life-limiting illness often have complex needs and require support from different agencies. One example of a group which can suffer from poor communication within the wider team is the one involved in a child's education. Health staff often assume that parents act as 'go-between' and convey the necessary information, yet the reality is that teachers may be left in the dark about the needs of the child [20] and are fearful about managing medical problems in the school [25] especially as the child's condition changes.

The way language is used by professionals is often a key to good or bad communication. The use of complex medical terms has the potential to cause confusion for other members of the care team as well as the family. At worst it can be seen as a way of asserting status, power, and knowledge over others [13]. However, the different interpretations of common language by different professionals, for example, 'patient-centred', 'collaboration', or 'advocacy' can lead to an illusion of uniformity of attitude and be just as damaging.

Communication of information still appears to be inadequate between families and children and the healthcare professionals. Families feel that the information they need to arrive at decisions regarding care is lacking. The information they are given is often poor, conflicting, or couched in language they do not understand. There is poor recognition by the professionals of the knowledge and expertise that the families have acquired themselves of looking after their child [25].

The complexity and rarity of the types of medical conditions that children with life-limiting illness have, mean that knowledge about specialist care for the underlying problem may be in the hands of a limited number of experts in tertiary centres who see the child only for short periods of time. Day to day care and ongoing observation of the individual child occurs in the community by general healthcare staff. Both sets of knowledge are essential and unless good communication can occur between the different professionals holding them, through appropriate liaison and discharge arrangements, conflicts and poor healthcare for the family continue to arise [25,28,33].

The family members themselves cross all these geographic and group boundaries and can act as a valuable link between them. However this can also lead to potential problems as the family can have increased stress if they feel too much responsibility is placed on them to support poorly communicating professionals. They can be drawn into taking sides with groups of professionals who are not working and communicating together effectively and occasionally the family themselves can undermine the effective cooperation of other members of the team.

Too many cooks!

Large numbers of professionals can be involved in looking after an individual child and a family, particularly within the first year of diagnosis [17]. The repeated contact by all these workers puts a major strain on family and child in terms of co-ordination, communication, understanding roles, developing relationships and assessing which services are available [34]. Parents will often complain that they feel swamped and suffocated by the number of people from the 'caring professions' they have to meet. The number of people involved can lead to inertia and confusion over care and responsibilities. In contrast, the reverse of this may happen after the death of the child, parents can feel isolated, particularly the prime carer, when their 'social contact' with all the different healthcare professionals finishes abruptly.

Successful teamworking

Planning ahead and careful consideration of the specific issues involved in the needs of children with life-limiting illness and their families is vital when planning a team who will be undertaking care. This falls on the managers of the various organisations who will be contributing so that the design and membership of the team will be appropriate. Time and funds need to be allocated not just for the work of the group, but also for training and development towards team building. The team's location, facilities, resources and the structure and timing of meetings should be planned to reflect the needs of the team and its members. Systems also need to be developed for internal and external audit of the group's work.

Within the team it is essential to develop good leadership, based not on perceived status, but on the skills of the individuals and the role that they play in understanding the needs of the child and the family. The position of 'leader' may need to

change as the needs of the child and the family change. The leader will need to take the responsibility for co-ordinating the individuals from separate organisations and locations, to developing the ways of working across boundaries that is so fundamental [26]. If necessary, team members should attend courses on team work and team management.

Members of the team need to understand their own and other member's roles and respect those with different knowledge and experience. This leads to focused allocation of responsibilities and workload [12]. However it needs to be combined with flexibility and compromise. The balancing act between maintaining professional identity and blurring professional boundaries [13] remains one of the key challenges to team working. If the professionals do not understand each other's role then there is a risk that the parents may also uncertain who to communicate their needs to, and feel clear in their own roles in the team too.

Team meetings require structure and co-ordination [35]. Aims need to be set by formulating clear goals, which are appropriate, specific and measurable. The goals must be in tune with the needs of the parents and the child. Information presented in the meeting should be clear and concise and in a language that is understood by all present [36]. By the end of the meeting, individuals should know what they need to do and in what time frame. Information needs to be given to the parents and the child in a clear manner, sensitive to their culture and language.

Communication both between team members and with families appears to be one of the keys to successful work together. It is important to recognise the need to share professional information between all the individuals looking after the child and the family. This involves dedicated time and good listening skills as well as open, honest provision of information in a form that all will understand.

Service co-ordination and key workers

The identification of an appropriate person to act as key worker and as a coordinator is one suggestion to achieve effective teamwork to meet the palliative care needs of the child and the family. This has been strongly recommended within palliative care documents [37]. It is believed that this role is important to support the family and act as a link and advocate to the rest of the professionals involved. This approach is supported by other writers, in the field of children with disabilities and complex needs (of which many may also have palliative care needs). Recent work in this area is now beginning to address the challenges of implementation of this model [19]. One such model, 'The Team around the Child' [38] is an example concentrating on pre-school children with complex needs which could be extended to all children with palliative care needs.

Some specific roles of a key worker have been identified which include:

- information provision
- identifying and addressing the child and family's needs
- co-ordinating timely services
- emotional support
- acting in the role of advocate.

As with all services, the balance of these roles is dependent on the individual needs of the family and the child [19]. The key worker could be seen as taking on the role of 'team leader' for that child and family.

Some have suggested that a drawback of key working systems is that the key worker tends to co-ordinate current services and is not involved in the synthesis of services which are required in the long term to truly meet a family's needs [14] as demonstrated in transdisciplinary team work; however others believe that effective service co-ordination can lead to changes in systems involved. It also must be anticipated that a key worker is unlikely to be constant. Families' needs may change and professionals will generally not remain in the same role for more than a few years, therefore families need to be prepared for possible changes [39]. Key working appears to be a model worth continuing to explore to enable effective teamwork that is family and child focused. It is believed that key worker systems with good care co-ordination [40] have positive effects [36], but there is still only limited evidence.

Summary

In any discussion of team working in paediatric palliative care it is important to recognize and keep returning to the core concept that the centre to all our work is the family and child [16]. We must look towards the family's concerns and perceptions of need and at the same time recognize the natural expertise the family have acquired [36]. This family centred holistic care will allow interdisciplinary team care to function for the benefit of the life-limited child. Much of this can be achieved through the use of key workers who co-ordinate, advocate and communicate with and on behalf of the family. The enhanced communication this will generate leads to improved relationships between the child, the family and the professionals [41]. Despite all the problems that can potentially arise, the benefits of team working to all concerned are so great that the work involved in achieving an effective team is more than rewarded by the successes that the team can accomplish.

Acknowledgements

We would like to thank Dr Clare Hale for proofreading and correcting our manuscript, and our families for putting up with us whilst we sat endlessly in front of the computer writing this chapter.

References

1. WHO. *Declaration of Alma-Ata*. New York: World Health Organization, 1978.
2. Payne, M. *Teamwork in Multiprofessional Care*. London: Macmillan Press, 2000.
3. Handy, C. *Understanding Organizations* (4th edition). London: Penguin, 1993.
4. Vanclay, L. Teamworking in primary care. *Nurs Stand* 1998;12(20):37–8.
5. Rowe, H. Multidisciplinary teamwork—myth or reality? *J Nurs Manag* 1996;4(2):93–101.
6. Pinkerton, CR. Multidisciplinary care in the management of childhood cancer. *Br J Hosp Med* 1993;50(1):54–9.
7. Esenyel, M. and Currie, D.M. A child with spina bifida, cerebral palsy and juvenile rheumatoid arthritis: rehabilitation challenge. *Disabil Rehabil* 2002;24(9):499–502.
8. Chalkiadis, G.A. Management of chronic pain in children. *Med J Aust* 2001;175(9):476–9.
9. Blake, K.D., Russell-Eggitt, I.M., Morgan., D.W., Ratcliffe, J.M., and Wyse R.K. Who's in CHARGE? Multidisciplinary management of patients with CHARGE association. *Arch Dis Child* 1990;65(2):217–23.
10. Watson, A.R. Strategies to support families of children with end-stage renal failure. *Pediatr Nephrol* 1995;9(5):628–31.
11. Pardess, E., Finzi, R., and Sever, J. Evaluating the best interests of the child—a model of multidisciplinary teamwork. *Med Law* 1993;12(3–5):205–11.
12. Boone, M., Minore, B., Katt, M., and Kinch, P. Strength through sharing: Interdisciplinary teamwork in providing health and social services to northern native communities. *Can J Commun Ment Health* 1997;16(2):15–28.
13. Barr, O. Interdisciplinary teamwork: Consideration of the challenges. British *Nurs* 1997;6(17):1005–10.
14. Norah Fry Research Centre. Working together? Multi-agency working in services to disabled children with complex health care needs and their families. Birmingham: Handsel Trust, 2002.
15. Marshall, M., Fleming, E., Gillibrand, W., and Carter, B. Adaptation and negotiation as an approach to care in paediatric diabetes specialist nursing practice: A critical review. *J Clin Nurs* 2002;11(4):421–9.
16. Taylor C. The partnership myth? Examining current opinions. *J Child Health Care* 1998;2(2):72–5.
17. Bridge, G. A personal reflection on parental participation: How some mothers of babies born with disabilities experience interprofessional care. *J Interprofessional Care* 1993;7(3):263–7.
18. Enderby, P. Teamworking in community rehabilitation. *J Clin Nurs* 2002;11(3):409–11.

19. Sloper, P. National Service Framework for Children, External working group on Disabled Children—Background work on Key Workers. London: *www.doh.gov.uk/nsf/children/externalwgdisabled.htm*, 2002.

20. Mukherjee, S., Lightfoot, J., and Sloper P. Communicating about pupils in mainstream school with special health needs: the NHS perspective. *Child Care Health Dev* 2002;28(1):21–7.

21. Lowe, J. Conflict in Teamwork. *Soc Work Health Care* 1978;3:323–30.

22. Roelofsen, E.E., The BA, Beckerman, H., Lankhorst, GJ., and Bouter, LM. Development and implementation of the Rehabilitation Activities Profile for children: Impact on the rehabilitation team. *Clin Rehabil* 2002;16(4):441–53.

23. Madge, S., Khair, K. Multidisciplinary teams in the United Kingdom: problems and solutions. *J Paediatr Nurs* 2000;15(2):131–4.

24. Forte P.S. The high cost of conflict. *Nurs Econ* 1997;15(3):119–23.

25. Watson, D., Townsley, R., and Abbot, D. Exploring multi-agency working in services to disabled children with complex healthcare needs and their families. *J Clin Nurs* 2002;11:367–75.

26. Hudson, B. Joint working. Prospects of partnership. *Health Serv J* 1998;108(5600):26–7.

27. Lavelle, J. Education and the sick child. In L. Hill, ed. *Caring for Dying Children and Their Families*. London: Chapman & Hall,1994 pp. 87–105.

28. Chambers, E.J. and Oakhill, A. Models of care for children dying of malignant disease. *Palliat Med* 1995;9(3):181–5.

29. Hill, L. The role of the children's hospice. In L. Hill, ed. *Caring for Dying Children and Their Families*. London: Chapman & Hall,1994, pp. 177–183.

30. Robinson, C. and Jackson, P. *Children's Hospices—A lifeline for families?* London: National Children's Bureau, 1999.

31. Nelson, B. Dealing with inappropriate behavior on a multidisciplinary level: A policy is formed. *J Nurs Adm* 1995;25(6):58–61.

32. Dombeck, M. Professional personhood: Training, territoriality and tolerance. *J Interprofessional Care* 1997;11(1):9–21.

33. Nuckles, M. and Bromme, R. Knowing what the others know: A study on interprofessional communication between nurses and medical doctors. *Klin Padiatr* 1998;210(4):291–6.

34. Ledbetter-Stone, M. Family intervention strategies when dealing with futility of treatment issues: A case study. *Crit Care Nurs Q* 1999;22(3):45–50.

35. Hooker, L. and Williams, J. Parent-held shared care records: Bridging the communication gaps. *Br J Nurs* 1996;5(12):738–41.

36. Sloper, P. Models of service support for parents of disabled children. What do we know? What do we need to know? Child. *Care, Health Dev* 1999;25(2):85–99.

37. Yerbury, M. Issues in multidisciplinary teamwork for children with disabilities. Child: *Care, Health Dev* 1997;23(1):77–86.

38. Roelofsen, E.E., Lankhoorst, G.J., and Bouter, L.M. Team conferences in paediatric rehabilitation: Organization, satisfaction and aspects eligible for improvement. *Int J Rehabil Res* 2000;23(3):227–32.

39. ACT. A guide to the development of Children's Palliative Care Services. Bristol & London: Association for Children with Life Threatening or Terminal Conditions and their Families and the Royal College of Paediatrics and Child Health, 2003.

40. Limbrick, P. *The team around the child*. Manchester: Interconnections, 2001.

41. Himid, K.A, Zwi, K., Welch, J.M., and Ball, C.S. The development of a community-based family HIV service. *AIDS Care* 1998;10(2):231–6.

34 Healthcare providers' responses to the death of a child

Danai Papadatou

The myth

In Greek mythology, Chiron was considered the greatest and wiser healer of human suffering. Chiron was a centaur who had the head and torso of a human and the body and legs of a horse. He was a demi-god, born to the union of Cronus (an olympian God) and Philyra (an earthly nymph) who were transformed into horses at the time of his conception. When Philyra gave birth, she realized that she had brought to life a son, who was not a perfect human being. In desperation, she begged the Gods to have pity on her, who then transformed her into a linden tree. Thus, Chiron was left an orphan, until he was found by Apollo, the God of music, light, and poetry, who became his foster parent. Apollo taught him many skills and helped him develop into a talented and charismatic centaur who was highly respected by humans.

Chiron was very different from other centaurs who were forceful, unruly, aggressive, and violent, especially after drinking too much wine. For ancient Greeks, these centaurs represented the wild forces of nature, while Chiron, on the contrary, was perceived as wise, kind, fair, and sophisticated. He became the teacher and mentor of several mythological heroes (Hercules, Achilles, Aesculapius amongst others) and taught them the art of medicine, of ethics, of music, as well as skills of hunting and fighting [1].

One day, Hercules visited his centaur friend Pholos on the mountain of Pelion where centaurs lived. Being a good host, Pholos offered Hercules some good wine, the scent of which attracted the centaurs who lived in the area. They all arrived, quickly got drunk, and began to fight against one another. In his effort to protect himself, Hercules mistakenly wounded his teacher Chiron with one of his poisonous arrows. Being a demi-god, Chiron was half immortal and did not die but was deeply wounded in his knee. Hercules immediately tended to the wound by following Chiron's instructions, but the wound proved to be incurable. From then on, Chiron engaged into a quest to ease his suffering. Progressively, he discovered the healing powers of various herbs and plants and developed an increased empathy for the suffering of others. His wounded knee forced him to direct his attention to the horse-part of his body to which he had given but little importance until then. This lower part of his body was the cause of an earlier psychic wound brought about by his abandonment by his mother. It is, therefore, suggested that both physical and psychic wounds, allowed Chiron to turn inwardly and face his suffering and limitations [2].

In Greek mythology, he is known as the 'wounded healer'. This great healer taught his student Aesculapious that every healer carries a 'wound' to remind him that he is vulnerable. From such a wound, the healer can draw the knowledge that he is not all powerful, all knowledgeable, and invincible, but rather limited, imperfect, and mortal. Such awareness can help any healer develop a deep compassion for others.

The reality

The myth of this wise healer contains three messages, particularly useful for care providers who offer their services to dying and bereaved individuals.

The first message is that we are all vulnerable in the face of illness, dying, and death. These experiences affect us in different ways and to different degrees, and as a result, we often experience suffering. Nevertheless, we hardly ever use the term 'suffering' to describe the emotional, social, and spiritual impact that the care of the dying and the bereaved has upon ourselves. We attribute suffering only to patients and their family members and prefer to define our personal malaise in terms of 'distress', 'burnout', or 'compassion fatigue'.

The second message in this myth is that our vulnerability may bring to the surface, issues related to deeper personal wounds and prior losses, which had never been grieved and integrated into our life. This reactivation of past issues offers a unique opportunity to work through our wounds and examine our fears and anxieties about loss, separation, and death. In addition, it helps us reflect upon our altruistic and egotistic motives for choosing to work in this particular field, and to consider how we seek to satisfy conscious or unconscious personal needs for omnipotence, perfection, control, recognition, or other.

The third message in Chiron's myth is that wisdom and personal growth can stem from recognizing and accepting our vulnerability. According to the Longman Dictionary of Contemporary English [3], 'vulnerable is someone who is easily harmed or hurt emotionally, physically, or morally'. Based on such definition, vulnerability is perceived as a sign of weakness, a negative attribute, a condition we should avoid at all costs because it raises our discomfort and displays our shortcomings and limitations. We mistakenly assume that we should strive towards being invulnerable, in other words, strong, in control, on top of a situation, able to effectively cope, and avoid being damaged, or affected by painful experiences.

The point, which concurrently relates to the myth of Chiron, is that being vulnerable is a necessary and welcome condition when caring for the dying and the bereaved. It entails an ability to remain open to the other and allow the other's experience to enter our personal world. It implies that we are permeable, penetrable, willing to come close and develop an intimate relationship with a patient or a family member who experiences death and separation. This intimacy holds a risk: either to identify totally with the other person and feel that we are dying as well, in which case, we cannot be effective in our helping role, or to identify with aspects of a situation encountered by a person whom we try to understand and support. There is a qualitative difference between these two identificatory processes. The first is total and massive, allowing no differentiation between oneself and the patient or family member. The latter is transitory and comprises an ability to identify with certain aspects of the other's experience (e.g. the fear for the unknown, or the sadness caused by the impending separation, or the need to attribute meaning to one's life and existence), while concurrently maintaining our own perspective of the situation. This form of identification is possible through empathy.

In empathy, we do not equate the person's world with our own, but we try to understand his or her world *as if* it were our own. *As if* is a critical element in this process because it contains both perspectives: the other's and our own. When we fail to be empathic, we become preoccupied with how to display a 'detached concern', and seek to achieve the 'right' distance in our relationships with patients or their relatives. We mistakenly assume that there is an objective, 'perfect' distance that is both close enough and appropriately distant from our patients. We imagine that if we ever manage to obtain it, we will be safe, intact, and unaffected by the pain, loss, and emotional chaos that may unfold around us or within ourselves. In reality, the distance we develop with others changes constantly and varies with the nature of each relationship, and according to the circumstances we encounter. Therefore, a distance that feels right at one time with one person may be uncomfortable at another time with the same or different individual.

It is my belief that the only distance we have power to determine and control is the *distance we choose to maintain from our own selves*. Such distance enables us, first, to recognize how we are affected by our patients, and second, to process the impact that loss and death-related experiences have upon ourselves. Our willingness to turn our gaze inwardly may help us better understand how we invest our relationships with patients and families, and how we are affected when we remain open and vulnerable.

The nature of a care-provider's vulnerability

Vulnerability is not an inherent asset we possess or not possess. We are, more or less, vulnerable at different times in our professional and personal growth and development. The degree of our vulnerability varies on a continuum. At one end of this continuum, we experience ourselves as totally vulnerable, overwhelmed by our experiences, at risk to experience even psychological breakdown. At the other end, we perceive ourselves as invulnerable or invincible by illness, pain, suffering, death, and operate according to the principle of omnipotence. Somewhere in the middle, we experience a vulnerability that is potentially constructive and helpful both to our patients and to ourselves.

The nature and varying degrees of vulnerability become more apparent through the description of different care-providers at three imaginary points on this continuum. First, are presented some characteristics of those professionals who function at either extreme of the continuum, and who are described as 'totally vulnerable' and 'invulnerable'. Then, the characteristics of those, who function effectively and are referred to as 'good enough', are presented (Figure 34.1).

The 'overwhelmed' care-provider

The 'overwhelmed' care-provider is highly permeable in his or her relationships with patients and consequently highly

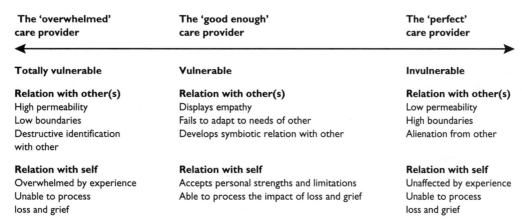

The 'overwhelmed' care provider	The 'good enough' care provider	The 'perfect' care provider
Totally vulnerable	Vulnerable	Invulnerable
Relation with other(s) High permeability Low boundaries Destructive identification with other	**Relation with other(s)** Displays empathy Fails to adapt to needs of other Develops symbiotic relation with other	**Relation with other(s)** Low permeability High boundaries Alienation from other
Relation with self Overwhelmed by experience Unable to process loss and grief	**Relation with self** Accepts personal strengths and limitations Able to process the impact of loss and grief	**Relation with self** Unaffected by experience Unable to process loss and grief

Fig. 34.1 The nature of a care-provider's vulnerability.

vulnerable. By maintaining no boundaries, he or she tends to fully identify with them and, thus, remains unable to hold a personal perspective upon his or her experiences. Totally overwhelmed, he or she is threatened by personal disintegration and is traumatized repetitively, whenever confronted with the suffering of his or her clients which becomes his or her own.

Feeling shame and guilt due to the inability to effectively cope with such experiences, he or she alienates self from patients and colleagues or moves to the other extreme of the continuum and becomes unavailable, emotionally impermeable, or adopts a façade of omnipotence, and overpowering control. This is illustrated in the account of a care-provider who consistently identified with children who had cancer, never gave herself the time to process her experiences and did not seek support:

I think that I age quickly, both biologically and psychologically as a result of this work (with terminally ill children) . . . Now, I experience a pressure upon my heart, a constant weight that does not allow me to breathe.

She later added:

Now, I don't want to be close to any dying child or family. I cannot handle neither their suffering, nor my pain anymore. I cannot even sit by their side, the silence seems very heavy . . . I have nothing to offer . . . words don't come out. . . . I cannot even give this special and tender look I once gave to my patients. If ever I give it, it's filled with despair.

While some highly vulnerable care-providers avoid the suffering of their patients, others on the contrary, choose to cope with their traumatization by repeatedly exposing themselves to death situations in the hope of mastering their trauma. Not infrequently, they engage in repetitive accounts of their suffering—which are hardly ever processed at a deeper level—and elevate themselves into a martyr role in order to overcome their perceived inefficiency and threat of psychic disorganization.

The 'perfect' care-provider

The 'perfect' care-provider does not simply strive for perfection—which is normal and desirable—but is characterized by a compulsive need to prove to oneself and others that he or she is perfect and omnipotent. This obsessive striving serves to hide a latent vulnerability and fear of psychic disorganization in the face of illness, suffering, and death. Since death cannot be conquered and the life of a patient cannot be saved, this palliative care-provider usually fights towards the achievement of a 'perfect death' which is 'beautiful', pain free, with family members gathered in peace around the patient, having settled all their unfinished business. He or she, often displays a behavior described by Speck [4] as 'chronic niceness' which refers to an appearance of being always empathic, understanding, unconditionally accepting and loving towards all patients who are expected, in return, to reward him or her with a 'nice' death to occur in a perfectly organized and healing environment.

Absorbed by such a narcissistic need for perfection, the 'perfect' care-provider remains impermeable and unaware of the individualized needs of patients and families, since he or she foresees their needs, long before they have the chance to voice or express them. Unable to develop authentic and intimate relationships, he or she, often, displays a false self. A latent impermeability exists in the provider's interaction with patients and families along with a defensive lack of introspection. The 'perfect' care-provider fears—and often denies—his or her own vulnerability, limitations or imperfections, and experiences as personal failure any death that is perceived ugly, painful, frightening, or less than perfect.

In summary, being totally vulnerable or acting as if one is totally invulnerable has damaging effects both upon the quality of care itself, as well as upon the mental health of the care-provider. The destructive aspects of one's vulnerability have been the subject of research studies and of interesting debates in the related literature, where different conceptualizations have been offered to delineate various aspects of care-givers' responses at either extreme of the continuum, described above.

Among these conceptualizations, the most commonly used is *burn out*, which is defined as a syndrome of physical, emotional, and mental exhaustion caused by the long-term involvement in emotionally demanding work situations. Care-providers develop negative attitudes towards patients, evaluate themselves negatively, and experience increased dissatisfaction with their work accomplishments [5]. It is often assumed that care providers who are frequently exposed to patient deaths, experience higher levels of burn out by comparison to those who care for patients with less serious health problems. Research findings, however, suggest that although highly stressful, such exposure does not correlate with higher levels of burn out [6–12]. In fact, some studies highlight the rewards derived from caring for dying patients, and the availability of staff support programmes in hospice settings, which seem to counteract the increased levels of distress [13–18].

More recently, Figley [19] proposed the concept of *compassion fatigue* to describe the exhaustion of some professionals who—as a result of being exposed to traumatized clients—are traumatized themselves and exhibit similar characteristics to the people they serve. Figley suggests that those providers who display increased empathy and identify with their clients are at great risk to develop a secondary traumatic stress disorder.

In similar terms, but perceived from a constructivistic theoretical perspective, McCann and Pearlman [20] present the concept of *vicarious traumatization* to highlight the disruption of the provider's beliefs about self and others, causing profound changes in one's sense of meaning, identity, and worldview. They suggest that such disruption may lead to the re-construction of new cognitive schemata, which create new meanings allowing the integration of the cumulative impact of trauma work.

The above conceptualizations have been used to describe extreme forms of vulnerability, which render a provider ineffective and/or impersonal in his or her work. Focus is placed upon the negative outcomes of care giving, rather than upon the process(es) by which trauma and dysfunction develop and are established.

The 'good enough' care-provider

An effective care-provider who is 'good-enough' (Fig. 34.1) has similar characteristics to those proposed by Winnicott [21] who used the concept of 'good-enough' parent to describe the significant role played, particularly, by mothers in creating

an appropriate and safe environment which facilitates the healthy development of their infant. The 'good-enough' provider is characterized by a vulnerability similar in certain ways to that of the mother. By being highly sensitive, he or she is alert to the needs of his or her patients and actively adapts to them to the best of his or her ability. However, part of being good enough implies also, an ability to *gradually fail to adapt* to those needs when the patient becomes independent and self-sufficient, or when the provider gently introduces a reality that the patient avoids to confront. In terminal care, failure to adapt may also entail the ability *to allow the patient to regress into a symbiotic relationship* with the care-provider. This undifferentiated symbiotic relationship reinforces the illusion that both, patient and provider, will face terminal illness together and carry each other beyond the borders of death. So, even though a 'good-enough' care-provider knows that he or she will never be able to complete this journey, he or she, nevertheless, sustains this illusion for the sake of his or her patient. This becomes possible only if the provider is willing to face the threat of loss, tolerate the anxiety and suffering it evokes, recognize that he or she is personally affected, and realize that caring for the dying does not confer any protection against his or her own death [4]. Thus, he or she avoids projecting an image of omnipotence which—consciously or not—reinforces the expectation that he or she is the perfect professional who can ensure a perfect cure or a perfect death. Instead, the 'good-enough' care-provider projects an image of mature acceptance of both his or her strengths and limitations as he or she adapts to the patient's changing needs in a shared journey towards death. With a 'good enough' care-provider on his or her side, the patient is then able to accept his or her carer's vulnerability, imperfection, and deficiencies. In fact, this understanding and acceptance release the provider from the need to be perfect.

Aspects of this form of constructive vulnerability have been described by Benoliel [22], a pioneer nurse in thanatology, who observed that both nurses and physicians display normal grief reactions when caring for patients who die, and by Shanfield [23], a psychiatrist, who underlined the importance of training health-care professionals to recognize their grief responses. It seems, therefore, that grieving is a natural and healthy response, which results when the professional emotionally invests his or her work and relationships with patients. During the last two decades, an increasing number of clinicians and researchers have shed light upon health-care professionals' grieving process, thus recognizing the vulnerable and human aspect of care giving [24–34]. Focus is, therefore, progressively shifted towards the normalization and acceptance of professionals' responses, rather than upon pathology and dysfunction that is caused by the exposure to highly stressful situations.

A model of care-providers' grieving process

To better understand the responses of care-providers who care for dying children, we conducted a series of qualitative studies, in order to explore the experience of those who provide care to dying children in paediatric oncology and critical care units [33,34]. We used a grounded theory methodology according to which, processes and products of research are shaped from data rather than from preconceived and deduced theoretical frameworks [35]. In-depth personal interviews were conducted through consecutive studies in order to identify similarities and differences in health-care providers' responses to childhood death. Professionals' responses were compared with regard to cultural factors (Greek vs. Hong Kong samples) [33], professional backgrounds (physicians vs. nurses) [34], work settings (paediatric oncology vs. critical care units), and needs for support [36]. Findings revealed more similarities than differences and a model was derived from the qualitative analysis of empirical data, which sheds light into the grieving process of providers who care for seriously ill and dying children [37,38]. Five of the most relevant propositions comprising our model (Table 34.1) are:

Proposition 1: The dying process and death of a child is experienced as a loss, which triggers a grieving process

The dying process or death of a child is usually experienced as a loss, which subsequently, triggers in care-providers, a grieving process. This loss, however, is perceived quite uniquely by individual team members. So even though a whole team may be grieving the death of a given patient, in reality each care-provider may be grieving over a different loss. We've identified seven distinct forms of perceived losses (Table 34.2). Death may represent:

(a) the loss of a close personal bond developed with a given child

(b) the loss of a loved person, through the care-provider's identification with the pain and suffering of a particular relative

(c) the non realization of one's professional goals and expectations regarding the ability to cure, to control a life-threatening illness, or to ensure a 'good' death for the child

(d) the loss of one's personal and familiar assumptions about self, others, and life, often disconfirmed since childhood death is commonly perceived as reversing the laws and order of nature

(e) the emergence of a past unresolved or traumatic loss encountered in the care provider's life

(f) the anticipated and fantasized loss of a loved person, who is, not necessarily, in any danger of dying

(g) the sharp awareness of one's mortality.

Each care-provider may experience none, one or more losses throughout the dying process and the actual death of a particular child. The subjective experience of one's loss(es) elicits a natural grieving process that presents some unique characteristics. These characteristics cannot be understood according to traditional grief models, which describe a series of stages, phases that bereaved individuals go through, or according to specific tasks they have to accomplish, in order to adjust to the loss of a loved person. Our findings suggest that care-providers' grief is a dynamic intrapersonal and interpersonal process which presents some unique characteristics as a result of confronting daily situations in which pain, suffering, and death are expected events and part of one's work and chosen career.

Table 34.1 Propositions of a model on care-providers' grief

1. The dying process and death of a child is experienced as a loss which triggers a grieving process

2. The grieving process of care-providers involves a fluctuation process between experiencing and avoiding or repressing grief

3. Grieving involves a process of attributing meaning to childhood death and to one's professional role and contribution in patient care

4. Grieving complications occur when there is persistent lack of fluctuation between experiencing and avoiding or suppressing grief responses

5. The fluctuation of the grieving process is affected by the complex interaction of multiple variables

---

Table 34.2 Nature of perceived losses in relation to patient death

1. Loss of the bond developed with a particular child

2. Loss of a loved person, through identification with a relative's grief

3. Loss though the non-realization of one's professional goals and expectations

4. Loss of familiar assumptions about self, others, life, and death

5. Recurrence of past unresolved or traumatic loss(es)

6. Anticipated and/or imagined loss of a loved person who is not, necessarily, in danger of dying

7. Death of self-realization of one's mortality.

Proposition 2: The grieving process of care-providers involves a fluctuation process between experiencing and avoiding or repressing grief

The grieving process was found to involve an ongoing *fluctuation* between *experiencing grief reactions* by focusing on the loss and *avoiding, suppressing, or repressing grief reactions* by moving away from it.

This fluctuation from one pole to the other which is necessary, adaptive, and healthy is eloquently illustrated in the account of the following male nurse who described his personal experience of caring for a dying child:

> Even though I have tears when a child is dying, I hold them back because I am aware that the child understands everything. However, the moment the patient expires, I cry a great deal . . . I don't know why . . . it's a form of intense release . . . over having been there all night, over the fact that this child has just died . . . I don't know. This emotional release liberates me from a heavy burden, and then I can think, 'What next?'. I am then able to collect myself and get into another psychology (mood): that of my role as a nurse. I then become a leader . . . a leader who must bring everything back to order, who must see to the parents, to the dead child, to the unit, and to all the duties needing to be carried out before dawn . . . Grief does not stop the day after the child's death and is not limited to the confines of the unit. We will always remember some of the things a particular patient did, or some other child will bring back memories of our favourite one. It is as if there is an ongoing relocation of the loss, a stirring that never stops.

This account illustrates how the fluctuation process develops within few hours, yet, it also suggests that grieving is ongoing as the nurse re-thinks, re-constructs the loss experience, and gives new meaning to it before re-locating it in his private world.

A closer examination of both aspects of the fluctuations can help us understand some of the common ways by which care-providers experience and avoid loss and grief.

Experience of grief and loss

When care-providers experience grief by focusing on their loss(es), they display a wide range of affective, cognitive, behavioural, and physical responses. Some describe the recurrence of positive or negative thoughts regarding the child and the dying conditions. Others report feelings of sadness, of depression, of anger, or guilt. Those who cry over various aspects of their perceived loss(es), may experience a cathartic effect, while others report a distressing outcome. The grief, which precedes death may extend over a number of days, as suggested by the following nurse:

> I cry and cry for a week before a death, and after the death. I sometimes dream of the child and light a candle, especially if I have not attended the funeral. At home, I withdraw and I do not want to talk to anybody, not even to my children.

Anger and despair are also common responses as illustrated in the following account:

> It's terrible . . . I sit on my bed and stare at an armchair in front of me. . . . I feel like throwing it out of the window. Some day I will. I sit there with a cup of coffee and I think, think, think of the child, of what happened . . . all by myself, for hours.

While some providers temporarily withdraw from daily activities and grieve in private, others seek support among colleagues and loved ones, while few alternate between privacy and social sharing of their grief. Some report being able to better accept death and experience their grief, if present at the moment a child expires or if at the funeral they participate in rituals, which commemorate the patient. This was evident in the following account of a physician who wished to be present at the death scene and, concurrently, sought a private space for his own grief:

> My role ends when I close the child's eyes and bring the parents into his room. After that, I leave. I go downstairs (to my office) for an hour or so. I sometimes listen to music. I do my grieving, I think about the child's death.

Some care-providers grieve over the death of a patient at times they least expect it, as reported in the following account:

> Sometimes it happens that while I am crying for something personal, I include in my sorrow a second grief about the children who died in our unit, and I cry for those with whom I had shared a special bond.

This indicates that even though grief is often inhibited, it nevertheless, surfaces and becomes conscious later in time. Cook and Oltjenbrun [39] refer to 'incremental grief' in order to describe the additive process of multiple related losses which are grieved and re-grieved over time.

Avoidance, suppression, or repression of grief

Part of the fluctuation process involves an attempt to avoid, suppress or repress one's grief, and move away from the loss experience. This is not, necessarily, maladaptive. Sometimes, it serves as a defence against a stressful and highly threatening situation, but it may also serve as a functional approach to manage work tasks, which need to be carried out when a child is dying or dies.

Other common avoidance responses include a sense of numbness and a 'shut down' of all emotional responses in order to cope with the challenges of terminal care. Under those conditions, care providers often report: 'I feel nothing', 'I am in limbo' or they control their feelings by convincing themselves with statements such as: 'I must be strong', 'I must control my tears, because I wear a uniform', 'I must hide my vulnerability', 'Patients and families have priority and I must support them'. These cognitive, self-reinforcing strategies, seem effective when used temporarily without preventing the provider to recognize and cope with his or her grief and suffering at a later point in time.

Another avoidance response involves the maintenance of distance from dying children and their families, or the active engagement in clinical duties and practical tasks that keep the provider busy, unavailable to patients, and distracted from his or her own pain. To counteract their anxiety and distress, some care-providers adopt an aggressive approach towards symptom management or pursue futile clinical tasks, as reported in the following account:

> I do everything in my power to keep the child alive. I even do useless things and go to extremes so that he does not die before my shift is over.

A temporary distorted perception of reality may protect them from experiencing their losses and grief. Through depersonalisation, they manage to be psychically absent from situations, which are painful and threatening:

> What hurts me most is that I cannot help grieving parents, not even hold their hands or give them a hug. Nothing comes naturally. Sometimes, I catch myself avoiding *to talk* to them. I pass in front of them as if I do not exist, as if I am not there, present.

Occasionally, care providers distort reality by dehumanising the comatose child, and describe him or her as a doll. Alternatively, they humanize a dead child and treat him or her as asleep in order to manage the care of his or her dead body. This process, when temporary, allows them to regulate their grief and respond to the needs of a situation, which is perceived as highly distressing.

Avoiding, suppressing or repressing grief is, sometimes, achieved by plunging into activities that generate a sense of being alive and living (e.g. going out to party, making love, cooking, gardening). These activities provide a symbolic space and a context within which the provider reconnects with self and loved ones. Thus, a new sense of self is construed which expands beyond one's professional role and loss experiences.

In summary, the fluctuation of a natural grieving process is commonly experienced among health care-providers who provide care to dying children. Nevertheless, unique to each professional, team or institution, is the way grief is expressed and the way the fluctuation process is regulated, as evidenced in studies conducted in Greece, Hong Kong, and Canada [31, 32, 33].

Proposition 3: Grieving involves a process of attributing meaning to childhood death and to one's professional role and contribution to patient care

The fluctuation involved in the grieving process helps professionals both to acknowledge their loss(es) and to set them aside in order to function appropriately without being overwhelmed by their grief. Moving in and out of grief, looking closely but also from a distance at the uniqueness of each death, care-providers are helped to attribute meaning to their loss experiences. As a result, death is not forgotten or overcome but, rather, accommodated into one's cognitive framework of life. Meaning attribution is accomplished at two levels:

Meaning is attributed to the death of children

Care-providers try to answer questions such as: 'Why children die?', 'Why did this particular patient die?'. In response, some find meaning in *scientific or biological justifications* (e.g. death is perceived as the inevitable outcome of a fatal and incurable disease). Others find meaning through *philosophical attributions* (e.g. death is perceived as an integral part of life's cycle), while several rely upon their *religious beliefs* to make sense of childhood death (e.g. it is God's will or the fate of the child's karma). Some care-providers develop a *combination of various systems of meanings*, often displaying a maturity towards a reality that is complex as it may hold different, even divergent meanings and interpretations. Finally, few seem to find *no meaning* in childhood death.

Meaning is attributed to one's personal role and contribution with regard to the care of the dying child

Care-providers seek to answer questions such as: 'What is my role in terminal care?', 'What is the quality of care I provided to this particular child or family?', 'How am I affected by his or her death?', 'What did I learn?', 'What did I gain?', 'Why do I suffer?'. For some, care is perceived as meaningful when they succeed—through their knowledge and interventions—to effectively manage the challenges imposed by a difficult disease or the biological process of dying *(disease oriented meaning)*. For others, contribution acquires meaning when the quality of their relationship with a given child and family contributes to an inevitable but, nevertheless, dignified death *(relationship-oriented meaning)*.

Such personal systems of meaning are affected by collective systems of meanings occurring at the level of each team. The social aspect of meaning-making becomes apparent through the exchanges and discussions, which take place among professionals before or after the death of a child. By recounting the patient's passage through the unit, a collective story with meaning is created. In some units, the focus of discussions is primarily on clinical interventions, while in others, it is mostly on the patient's, the family's, and the providers' responses to dying and death. The content of these narratives contributes to the creation of a story that explains the illness, the suffering, the death of a given child, and highlights the role and contribution of individual professionals and of the team as a whole. Each story acquires meaning in relation to the unit's goals and primary task. When professionals remain silent in the face of dying and death or when they are unable to create some coherent story to place a particular death within a meaningful context, then discomfort increases, and grief presents complications or remains disenfranchised.

Proposition 4: Grieving complications occur when there is a persistent lack of fluctuation between experiencing and avoiding or suppressing grief responses

Care-providers who present grief complications, operate at the extreme poles of the vulnerability continuum. Some of them become totally overwhelmed by grief, unable to effectively manage the care of dying children and grieving families, as indicated in the following brief report:

> I don't laugh anymore . . . I feel totally overwhelmed by my own pain that seems endless.

Others, on the contrary, become totally detached and systematically suppress their suffering, avoid to think, feel or process their experiences, as evidenced in these two accounts:

> I close my pain in a little drawer and do not allow myself to think or feel.
> I've learned to simply switch off and avoid all visual images of what I've witnessed.

Unable to process their losses, care-providers at both extremes of the vulnerability continuum, experience a sense of immobilization, of being trapped, and being in an impasse. Their sense of time is suspended. Their experiences are not integrated into a past, present, and future. There is no movement or growth. They become either totally mute or resort to repetitive detailed accounts of traumatic experiences filled with anxiety, helplessness, and hopelessness. Unable to process their suffering, they become traumatized by their own vulnerability or appear invulnerable to avoid further trauma.

Proposition 5: The fluctuation of the grieving process is affected by the complex interaction of multiple variables

It is suggested that grieving is not merely an intrapsychic process understood solely in relation to one's personality, sense of vulnerability, motives to care for the seriously ill, and loss history. Grieving needs to be understood in relation to a number of complex, interactive variables [37,38]. These can be classified in five major categories: (1) *personal variables* (personality characteristics, loss history, professional goals and motives, nature of perceived losses); (2) *patient-family related variables* (personality characteristics, family dynamics, coping with threat or actual death, relationships developed with providers); (3) *situational variables* (illness trajectory, dying and death circumstances); (4) *work-related variables* (unit's primary task, goals of care, rules about professional conduct in the face of death, team-dynamics and functioning in adverse situations); and (5) *socio-cultural variables* (institutional, social, cultural socialization to death and dying, prevailing meaning systems with regard to children, illness and death).

All these variables affect how the death of a child is likely to be perceived, and how grief is likely to be experienced and processed at an individual, as well as, at the level of the team. The death of a child affects in different ways care-providers who work in different settings. Each unit has its own culture that comprises a system of beliefs, values, priorities and primary task(s) with regard to the care of children in illness, dying, and death. The team's culture is governed by a number of *explicit or implicit rules* which determine—among other things—the roles, responsibilities, and expected behaviours of professionals in the face of death. These institutional rules regulate the fluctuation process between experiencing and avoiding grief at a systemic level, and are more or less effective in helping individual care-providers to cope with daily losses at work. Based upon these rules, each team develops group processes, which recognize personal vulnerability and encourage the experiencing of grief (e.g. informal or formal sharing; consultation or stress debriefing sessions; prayer and group rituals following the death of a child). Yet, each team concurrently develops group processes, which reinforce stoicism, grief suppression, and the illusion of invulnerability and omnipotence (e.g. discussions of patients in scientific terms; evaluation of clinical interventions; idealization of the team; avoidance and/or ridicule of personal feelings; death jokes).

The following example illustrates the power of certain unconscious rules, which regulate the grieving process in two different work settings. These rules were uncovered only after interviewing individually all care-providers who worked in these units.

In the oncology unit, the primary task of the team was to strive for a cure and psychologically support the child and the family. Whenever cure proved to be an impossible goal, the primary task shifted to palliation through the active management of the child's pain and other distressing symptoms. During the terminal phase, team members were encouraged to maintain close and supportive relationships with dying children and grieving parents. So, according to one implicit rule, it was accepted and perceived natural to experience and display grief responses when a child was dying or died. However, according to another rule, the intensity and expression of professionals' grief responses should be tempered and controlled. It was expected that grief responses would never be so intense as to impair clinical judgment or lead to emotional breakdown. Another rule implied that the care-providers' vulnerability and suffering should never be apparent to other sick or dying children and to their parents. Team members were expected to publicly display stoicism with regard to their emotions, and to act joyful towards hospitalized children whenever a death occurred on the unit. An additional rule, however, suggested that grieving should remain private and expressed only behind closed doors. Co-workers were expected to support one another and share their personal experiences during specific times of formal or informal gatherings.

In the intensive care unit, the team's primary task was to save the life of critically ill children at any cost. Due to the uncertainty of prognosis, close relationships were discouraged and interactions with family members were kept brief to avoid emotional involvement. Death was perceived as the team's failure to save the child's life, and rules discouraged the display of grieving. The implicit message was: 'Do not grieve, at least not openly. It may be contagious to your colleagues. Be strong and brave in the face of death'. Care-providers helped each other to control their grief responses by limiting discussions to evaluations of medical and nursing interventions, and by sharing cynical death jokes.

It becomes apparent that each unit has its own private code, value system, and norms, which facilitate or hinder the grieving process and allow a more or less constructive sense of vulnerability to develop. Interestingly, some rules can help certain care-providers who are usually overwhelmed by grief, to learn how to contain it, while other rules help those providers who systematically suppress their grief, to acknowledge and express their feelings within a safe and permissive environment.

Reflections about the proposed model

The main message that the model conveys is that part of being vulnerable when caring for children, who eventually die, is to experience and come to terms with a normal and healthy grieving process over one or more perceived losses, which are triggered by the dying process or death of a patient. It is important, however, to differentiate the fluctuation process involved in grief from a similar oscillation process observed by other researchers and clinicians who focused primarily upon the dysfunctional traumatic responses that providers display in the face of trauma, loss, and death. More in particular, Horowitz in his seminal work on trauma [40] identified the antithetical reactions of *intrusion-avoidance* as a person's extreme responses to a traumatic event. He focused on the pathology of intrusion through which, the individual re-experiences feelings and ideas surrounding the event, and the avoidance process by which he or she denies feelings, memories, and thoughts regarding the event. Similar responses were recorded by Raphael [41], Figley [19] and other researchers who studied the effects of trauma—rather than grief—experienced by crisis workers who witness multiple and horrific deaths in disaster situations.

More closely related to the study of grief, is the 'Dual Process Model of Coping with Bereavement', proposed by Stroebe and Schut [42,43]. They describe an oscillation process that individuals experience over the death of a loved person in their attempt to adapt to two types of stressors related to bereavement: (1) *a loss orientation process* (concentration on an aspect of the loss experience—intensive grief work) and (2) *a restoration orientation process* (concentration on secondary stressors resulting from the death of a loved person). This dual process model represents an interesting attempt to integrate existing ideas from a cognitive stress theory and social construction models related to grief [43]. Focus is primarily placed upon the definition of stressors associated with bereavement and the identification of adaptive coping strategies, which facilitate adjustment of the bereaved to these stressors.

Even though our model presents several similarities with Stroebe and Schut's dual process model, differences, nevertheless, exist at a conceptual level, in the terminology used to describe the bereavement process, and in the bereaved populations under study. Our proposed model focuses more upon intrapsychic and systemic processes rather than upon stressors and coping strategies, which promote adjustment to death. Based upon a phenomenological, a systemic, and a social constructivistic approach, we suggest that grieving is affected by how individual care-providers as well as teams recognize and process loss events, experience and avoid subsequent grieving, and attribute meaning to death as well as to their contribution in patient care. One's personal grieving can be understood only in relation to the institutional context in which care is provided, and with regard to the team's primary task, culture, and rules which determine how professionals are expected to function and respond in the face of death.

The functional team

Every death creates a rupture to the bond that exists between individuals. The death of a child threatens the connectedness among family, members but also the solidarity among team members. Sometimes, the team mirrors the suffering of a family, which falls apart. As a result, its cohesion may be seriously compromised. The multiple ways by which a team re-constructs itself after the death of a patient are indicative of how functional it remains in the face of adversity.

It is suggested that a team is functional when it provides a *holding environment* for its members. The concept of the holding environment was first mentioned by Winnicott in a paper entitled 'The theory of the parent-infant relationship' [44]. It refers to the physical act of being held by a mother who expresses love to her infant and offers protection from any danger. This behavior functions as a continuation of the protection her womb previously provided to her unborn child. In addition to protection and safety, such an environment offers a sense of order, predictability, and continuity as the mother introduces in small doses, the external world to her child who progressively accommodates to the external reality. In adulthood, our holding environment is comprised by our family and friends, the network of our colleagues, the social institutions and government policies and services, all of which provide conditions of safety, order, predictability, and continuity in times of trouble. In our daily work with the dying and the bereaved, it is within the team, institution or service we belong to, that we seek this sense of safety, predictability, order and continuity, as well as a coherent cognitive framework to help us attribute meaning to our experiences.

A team that offers a holding environment is able to *contain grief* and to *hold within itself* the suffering of its members without being threatened by it. Such a team allows care-providers to share verbally or symbolically their experiences and to ventilate all kinds of thoughts and feelings—no matter how threatening or painful these may be. Nevertheless, emotional ventilation is not enough by itself, as it may, at times, even prove destructive to some providers. A further cognitive process is necessary in order to help team members to gain deeper insight, attribute meaning and integrate their experiences into a coherent narrative. In reality, it is only within a holding environment that care-providers are able to recognize

Table 34.3 Common dysfunctional patterns in teams dealing with loss

- Scapegoating
- Splitting and rigid sub-grouping
- Avoidance of change
- Team burn out

and explore the threatening realization that all of us, and not only seriously ill patients, eventually die.

Whenever a team is unable to provide this holding environment, then grief is acted out, intense feelings are projected, and dysfunctional patterns of interaction are established. Some common dysfunctional patterns by which teams cope with loss (Table 34.3) are:

1. *Scapegoating* is particularly common in teams which cannot tolerate and work through intense emotions which are, therefore, projected upon a scapegoat. Scapegoats help team members to displace their grief, which is never openly acknowledged and processed.

2. *Splitting* occurs when team members are unable to personally and collectively cope with intense and conflicting feelings evoked by dying and death such as, for example, the need to fight the disease and the need to let go and accompany a child to death; the need to become intimately involved with a patient or family and the need to shun away from close relationships; the need to grieve and the need to remain stoic; the need to be supported and rely upon colleagues and the need to remain independent and self-sufficient. When these conflicting emotional experiences are not recognized, tolerated and integrated, care-providers tend to project them upon others, within or outside their team [45]. Members belonging to the same subgroup project negative qualities to members of another group, while they maintain all the good qualities within their own. Care-providers who find refuge in one of these subgroups, remain unable to integrate the conflicting emotional aspects of their death-related experiences. It is not sub-grouping per se that is destructive to the team, but rather the impermeability of a small group which develops its own private code of values and communication rules excluding other team members from belonging to it. Such splittings are indicative of a team's failure to collectively cope and integrate loss and death in its history and development.

3. *Avoidance of change* reflects, among other things, the team's difficulty to cope with loss and grief since both experiences involve changes and new adaptations. In dysfunctional

teams, members cling to what is familiar and rigidly abide by rules. Nursing, medical procedures, and psychological assessments are standardized and performed in a ritualistic way, while decisions, initiatives are minimized, and projects or new ideas are resented. Whenever problems occur, quick and prescribed solutions are sought. In such teams, collective signs of burn out are displayed through low moral, low quality of care, and chronic disputes among professionals who feel trapped in a job from which they derive little or no satisfaction. Providers become more absorbed by their relationships to the group than by their primary work tasks or goals of care.

An effective way to manage projections, splits, resistance to change, and other non-effective patterns of functioning, is to create the necessary holding environment that recognizes and explores both the destructive as well as the constructive aspects of a team's vulnerability in the face of death and dying. In that respect, 'support', 'consultation', 'exploration' or 'discussion' groups may facilitate the process, if led by an experienced mental health professional or a consultant who has deep knowledge in group dynamics and does not belong to the institution or service which provides care to chronically or critically ill and dying children. Maintaining a stance outside the daily life of an institution makes it easier for such a facilitator to observe, reflect upon his or her observations, communicate them to team members without being caught in the group's dynamics.

Conclusion

The death of a child invites care-providers to confront and come to terms with their strength, limitations, and personal suffering. If these are recognized, accepted and processed, then one's vulnerability may become a source of maturity and growth. If left silent, suppressed, unattended or ignored they may become a source of stress, of alienation and, occasionally, of dysfunction.

We can claim quality in paediatric palliative care, when 'good-enough' care-providers and 'good-enough' teams recognize the risk of being affected but also create the necessary space to experience, reflect, understand, and process their losses, grief, and suffering. This is facilitated when the dying process and death of children are not idealized, romanticized, or shunned away, but rather experienced within a holding environment which helps care-providers to experience and integrate loss into a narrative that is coherent and meaningful, both personally and collectively. A functional team enhances in its members, a sense of belonging to a group, which can tolerate suffering, draw upon its strengths, and learn from experience.

References

1. Kakridis, I. (ed) *Greek Mythology—Vol.II & Vol.IV*. Ekdotiki Athinon, Athens (in Greek language), 1986.
2. Kearney, M. *Mortally wounded: Stories of soul pain, death, and healing,* Marino Books, Dublin, 1996;pp.151–178.
3. Longman Dictionary of Contemporary English (3rd edition) with new words supplement. Pearson Education Limited, Essex, 2001.
4. Speck, P. (2nd edition). Working with dying people: On being good enough. In A. Obholzer and V.Z. Roberts, eds. *The Unconscious at Work: Individual and Organizational Stress at Work*, Brunner-Routledge, London, 2000; pp. 94–100.
5. Maslach, C. *Burnout: The Cost of Caring* Prentice Hall, New Jersey, 1982.
6. Keane, A. Ducette, J., and Adler, D.C. Stress in ICU and non ICU nurses. *Nurs Res* 1985;34:231–36.
7. Foxall, J.M., Zimmerman, L., Standley, R., and Ben, B. A comparison of frequency and sources of nursing job stress perceived by intensive care, hospice and medical-surgical nurses. *J Adv Nurs,* 1990;15:577–84.
8. Bene, B. and Foxall, M.J. Death anxiety and job stress in hospice and medical-surgical nurses. *Hosp J* 1991;7:25–41.
9. Oehler, J.M. and Davidson, M.G. Job stress and burnout in acute and nonacute pediatric nurses. *Am J Crit Care* 1992;2:81–90.
10. Van Servellen, G. and Leake, B. Burnout in hospital nurses: A comparison of acquired immunodeficiency syndrom, oncology, general medical, and intensive care units nurse samples. *J Prof Nurs* 1993;9:169–77.
11. Papadatou, D. Anagnostopoulos, F., and Monos, D. Factors contributing to the development of burnout in oncology nursing. *Br J Med Psychol* 1994;67:187–99.
12. Tummers, G.E.R., van Merode, G.G., and Landeweerd, J.A. The diversity of work: Differences, similarities and relationships concerning characteristics of the organization, the work and psychological work reactions in intensive care and non-intensive care nursing. *Int J Nurs Stud* 2002;39:841–55.
13. Chiriboga, D.A. Jenkins, G., and Bailey, J. Stress and coping among hospice nurses: Test of an analytic model. *Nurs Res* 1983;32: 294–99.
14. Gray-Toft, P. and Anderson, J.G. Sources of stress in nursing terminal patients in a hospice. *Omega* 1986–7;17:27–39.
15. Bram, P.J. and Katz, L.F. Study of burnout in nurses working in hospice and hospital oncology settings. *Oncol Nurs Forum* 1989; 16:555–60.
16. Woolley, H., Stein, A., Forrest, G.C., and Baum, J.D. Staff stress and job satisfaction at a children's hospice. *Arch Dis Child* 1989;64: 114–18.
17. Copp, G. and Dunn, V. Frequent and difficult problems perceived by nurses caring for dying in community, hospice and acute care settings. *Palliat Med* 1993;7:19–25.
18. Vachon, M. Recent research into staff stress in palliative care. *Eur J Palliat Care* 1997;4:99–103.
19. Figley, C.R. (ed.) *Compassion fatigue: Coping with secondary traumatic stress disorder in those who treat the traumatized*. New York: Brunner-Mazel, 1995.
20. McCann, I.L. and Pearlman, L.A. Vicarious traumatization: A framework for understanding the psychological effects of working with victims. *J Trauma Stress* 1990;3:131–49.

21. Winnicott, D.W. Mind and its relation to the psyche-soma. In *Collected papers: Through paediatrics to psycho-analysis, 1958*. London: Hogarth Press and the Institute of Psychoanalysis, 1949; pp. 243–54.

22. Benoliel, J.Q. Anticipatory grief in physicians and nurses. In B. Schoenberg, ed. *Anticipatory grief*. New York: Brunner-Mazel, 1974; pp. 218–28.

23. Shanfield, S.B. The mourning of the health care professional: An important element in education about death and loss. *Death Educ* 1981;4:385–95.

24. Lerea, L.E. and LiMauro, B.F. Grief among healthcare workers: A comparative study. *J Gerontol* 1982;37:604–8.

25. Shread, T. Dealing with nurses' grief. *Nurs Forum* 1984;21:43–45.

26. Harper, B.C. *Death: The coping mechanism of the health professional* (2nd edition). Greenville, South Carolina: Southeastern University Press, Inc., 1994.

27. Saunders, J.M. and Valente, S.M. Nurses' grief. *Cancer Nurs* 1994; 17:318–25.

28. Hinds, P.S., Puckett, P., Donohoe, M., Milligan, M., Payne, K., Phipps, S., Davis, S.E.F., and Martin, G.A. The impact of a grief workshop for pediatric oncology nurses on their grief and perceived stress. *J Pediatr Nurs* 1994;9:388–97.

29. Spencer, L. How do nurses deal with their own grief when a patient dies on an intensive care unit, and what help can be given to enable them to overcome their grief effectively? *J Adv Nurs* 1994;19: 1141–50.

30. Feldstein, M.A. and Gemma, P.B. Oncology nurses and chronic compounded grief. *Cancer Nurs* 1995;18:228–36.

31. Davies, B., Clarke, D., Connaughty, S. *et al.* Caring for dying children: Nurses' experiences. *Pediatr Nurs* 1996;22:500–7.

32. Rashotte, J., Fothergill-Bourbonnais, F., and Chamberlain, M. Pediatric intensive care nurses and their grief experiences: a phenomenological study. *Heart Lung* 1997;26:372–86.

33. Papadatou, D., Martinson, I.M., and Chung, P.M. Caring for dying children: A comparative study of oncology vs critical care nurses' experience in Greece and Hong Kong. *Cancer Nurs* 2001;24:402–12.

34. Papadatou, D., Bellali, T., Papazoglou, I., and Petraki, D. Greek nurses' and physicians' grief as a result of caring for children dying of cancer. *Pediatr Nurs* 2002;28:345–53.

35. Strauss, A. and Corbin, J. *Basics of qualitative research: Techniques and procedures for developing grounded theory* (2nd edition) Thousand Oaks, California: Sage Publication, 1998;pp. 3–14.

36. Papadatou, D., Papazoglou, I., Petraki, D., and Bellali, T. Mutual support among nurses who provide care to dying children. *Illness, Crisis, Loss* 1999;7:37–48.

37. Papadatou, D. A proposed model of health professionals' grieving process. *Omega* 2000;41:59–77.

38. Papadatou, D. The grieving health care provider: Variables affecting the professional response to a child's death. *Bereavement Care* 2001;20:26–9.

39. Cook, A. and Oltjenbruns, K. *Dying and grieving: Lifespan and family perspectives* Ft. Worth, Texas: Harcourt Brace, 1998.

40. Horowitz, M. *Stress response syndromes* New Jersey: Aronson, Northvale, 1986.

41. Raphael, B. *When disaster strikes*. London: Hutchinson, 1986.

42. Stroebe, M.S. and Schut, H. The dual process model of coping with bereavement: rationale and description. *Death Stud* 1999;23:197–224.

43. Stroebe, M.S. and Schut, H. Models of coping with bereavement: A review. In M.S. Stroebe, R.O. Hansson, W. Stroebe, and H. Schut, eds. *Handbook of bereavement research: Consequences, coping, and care*. Washington DC: American Psychological Association, 2001;pp.375–403.

44. Winnicott, D.W. The theory of the parent-infant relationship. In *The Maturational Process and the Facilitating Environment, 1990*. London: Karnac Book, 1960; pp. 37–55.

45. Halton, W. Some unconscious aspects of organizational life. In A. Obholzer, and V.Z. Roberts, eds. *The Unconscious at Work: Individual and Organizational Stress at Work* (2nd edition). London: Brunner-Routledge, 2000;pp. 11–18.

35 Place of care

Lynda Brook, Jan Vickers, and Muriel Barber

Introduction

If we consider the child and family's palliative care journey from the diagnosis of a life-limiting condition, through to death and bereavement we will note numerous problems and challenges along the way. The parents or carers will need help and support in all aspects of palliative care, including symptom management, practical support, psychosocial and spiritual care, at different times and to different extents, in order to achieve the best quality of life for their child.

The primary objective of palliative care is to support the child and family to allow them to maintain resilience and cope, from the time of diagnosis, particularly at times of crisis and at the end of life. The care provided should be tailored to the needs and wishes of the child and family, but inevitably must be delivered within the constraints of available health care staff, facilities and resources. Ideally, care will be delivered with minimal disruption to normal everyday life, such as at home or in school; however, at times care in hospital or hospice will be necessary. The care must be co-ordinated, with emphasis on prompt and effective interprofessional communication, and be flexible enough to adapt to changes in the child's condition and the family's need for support.

This chapter is based upon the models of care in the United Kingdom, but the principles will be applicable widely in the context of different health care systems. We consider the benefits of maintaining structure and normality for the child and family and how these may be threatened by changes in care needs. We examine how care needs are determined, including the wishes of the child and family, and assessment by members of the multidisciplinary team. We then explore how these needs are best met by examining the roles of available carers, including parents and professionals in different care settings.

Maintaining normality

Minimizing disruption

Many families of children with a life-limiting condition will tell you that above all they want their child to be seen as a person first rather than diagnosis [1]. But much of the child's or young person's life is likely to be dominated by their condition and its repercussions on day to day activities. Coping with these problems can be enhanced if the child is cared for at home or in as normal an environment as possible [2]: keeping the disruption of everyday family life to a minimum, and helping the child and family to maintain some sense of being in control [3–7]. However, much can also be done to develop and implement these important coping mechanisms when the child is in hospital or hospice.

Good social networks

Those children and families that have good social networks, with strong family and interpersonal relationships [8], and those that seek social support in times of crisis [9], have greater resilience. There is greater chance for these social networks to develop, if the child is able to be cared for in 'normal' environments such as home and school. These environments also provide structure and nurture stronger social and family relationships.

Family communication and cohesion

Caring for a child with a life-limiting condition puts immense strain on family relationships. But families that are able to communicate openly and honestly are more able to adapt and cope better [10]. Families that have to spend better part of the day travelling to and from hospital experience greater disruption to family life [11]. Communication is more difficult as often one parent stays with the child being cared for in hospital.

Taking control and making choices

Confronting problems [9] and taking control have both been demonstrated as important coping strategies [12]. Families illustrate this in their desire to make choices about the care that the child receives. Taking control and making choices are both facilitated when the child and family are in a familiar environment [6,13].

Flexibility: Changes in condition over time

Maintenance—periods of stability

For many children with life-limiting conditions, especially non-malignant diseases, there are periods of months or even years when they are relatively well and clinically stable. It is entirely appropriate that they should remain at home with minimal trips to the hospital, hospice or clinic as required and take part in more normal activities such as attending school [14,15]. Although the situation may be relatively stable, it is likely that the child and family's needs will change either gradually over time or suddenly. It is therefore essential that the situation is reviewed regularly, keeping all those involved in care up to date, in order to provide a prompt and co-ordinated response to these changes.

The challenge of providing effective care in these 'maintenance' periods is to provide a level of care and support appropriate to the needs of the child and family; avoiding feelings of abandonment [16] but ensuring that multiple appointments do not disrupt normal family life unnecessarily. There may be considerable ongoing needs such as caring for a highly physically dependent child, administering numerous medications and treatments on a daily basis and coping with chronic symptoms such as pain [1] that have an impact on quality of life. These patients can usually be cared for at home but the mental and physical stress on the family is considerable [17] and short (respite) breaks from caring are invaluable in maintaining family resilience.

Gradual deterioration

Many children with life-limiting conditions, for example those with neurodegenerative conditions, experience a gradual deterioration over months to years associated with a corresponding increase in care needs. Home adaptations and provision of special equipment may be needed to cope with increasing physical dependency. Some children may need to change from mainstream school to a school for children with special needs [18]. Key events such as the transition to wheelchair use, or a change in school are particularly distressing for the child and their family as they emphasise the progressive losses that they face [19,20]. These children and families often have an extensive multidisciplinary network of professionals and the input from the different members will vary as the situation changes, making regular reviews and the role of a key worker important.

Changes in the family's needs

Flexibility may be needed to respond to changes in the family's ability to care for their child. With experience some families may be willing to take on new responsibilities [13]. Other families may find that they are unable to continue to provide the same level of care and require additional support. A few families will have more than one family member affected by the same condition [21]. Changes in family dynamics such as a new baby or a parent returning to work have a huge impact [21,22]. Other situations such as illness, bereavement or divorce in the family will also affect the provision of care. These changes maybe transient and the family can resume their normal level of care with additional support over a period of time. However at times the new support offered to care for the child and family will need to be in place indefinitely, or increase further over time with continuing deterioration in the child's condition. This can be a particularly stressful time with parents and other carers experiencing feelings of failure and self-doubt [23].

Sudden changes in condition

Most children with life-limiting conditions experience some periods of stability and others of relatively rapid change in their condition. These may be associated with acute complications, for example chest infections in severe cerebral palsy, or with changes in the underlying disease process, for example a tumour recurrence. There will be a need for rapid assessment and treatment or rehabilitation, usually via hospital-based services. At such times the family and those involved in their care need particular emotional support as they are forced to face the reality of the underlying life-limiting condition again. They may also have to face the possibility that although this change in condition may be successfully treated with a return to stability, it may herald deterioration and a clear step towards the end of life [24,25].

Adjustments in the child's and the family's needs will have to be incorporated in the plans for care and communicated widely to all the health care and other professionals (e.g. teachers) involved. For children who are at risk of a sudden death, for example severe cerebral palsy [26], or congenital cyanotic heart disease [27], anticipatory care will involve talking through this possibility with the family as well as those participating in the child's day to day care. The plan of care will need to identify appropriate actions to be taken in the event of sudden death or sudden life-threatening deterioration in the child's condition. This can help alleviate distress and blame at the time.

Over time, and perhaps with multiple events, each associated with deterioration in the child's condition the aims of treatment are likely to change. It may become clearer that aggressive treatments are now extending life of poor quality, or prolonging dying, and are not in the child's best interest [28]. The focus of care will move further towards an approach aimed at alleviating distressing symptoms and improving quality of life. Again preparation, anticipation and good interprofessional communication are needed so the family's choices are understood and planned for.

End-of-life (terminal) care

The end of life may follow long periods of treatment aimed at prolonging life, failure of curative treatment or may follow a sudden deterioration. It is often not until the 24–48 h prior to death [29] that it becomes absolutely clear that death is imminent. Professionals and families may be reluctant to acknowledge that the patient is dying [30] and consequently defer decisions and the need to anticipate symptoms and emotional needs, so that the most appropriate care may not be provided. Effective provision of end-of-life care poses specific challenges. Symptoms at the end of life can change very rapidly and be difficult to control. Often the family would often like their child to be cared for at home, and there is evidence to suggest that outcomes may be better if this is the case [6,8,31,32]. However to achieve this there may also be an increase in the amount of professional input required.

Assessment of care needs

It is vital that the child and family are involved in decisions related to place and provision of care. Families need a balance so that they are empowered to work in partnership with professionals, taking control and ownership, whilst avoiding feeling pressurised into making decisions about services or issues which they do not wish to be burdened with or about which they have little knowledge [6]. Providing honest and comprehensive information regarding their child's condition and the services available is essential so they can make the most appropriate choices [33]. In addition to detailed discussion with the child and family a more comprehensive multidisciplinary assessment addressing symptom management, personal care including aids and equipment, psychosocial and educational needs will be required to contribute to the development of a detailed care plan [34].

It is important to emphasize that assessment of needs, and provision of care, are parallel and continuous processes. There is a need for careful monitoring and review in order to respond to the inevitable changes in the child's condition, both acute and gradual, and the family's ability to care. If changes in care needs are anticipated and planned for, unnecessary crises, such as emergency admission to hospital because of increasing physical dependency, may be reduced or avoided [35,36].

Individual families are able to cope in different ways and will require very different levels of support [37]. They may have a clear idea of the type and amount of support they require [38]. However, families from ethnic minority groups may not request support and professionals may assume, incorrectly, that needs are being met within the community [39,40]. The needs of the child's brothers and sisters are also important [41] but often not adequately considered [29,42]. Even if the family's expectations or perception of the situation appear unrealistic [13], support that is not provided on the family's terms will not be accepted [43]. Through negotiation the family and professionals need to work towards a mutually acceptable and realistic plan. The family may need help to gain confidence in order to take on new tasks, but also to be able to accept support without feelings of guilt or failure [23].

It is important to discuss openly and ahead of time, the likely changes that will occur as the child's condition worsens and the changes in care needs that this may involve. But talking about possible problems, particularly those leading up to the child's death, is understandably distressing [44,45]. Given appropriate opportunity most children and young adults are able to participate to some extent in decisions relating to their care, even at the end of life [46,47]. However their ability to contribute will depend on the family's coping style and their developmental level. If the family's coping style makes it more difficult to ascertain the child's wishes, demonstrating the child's level of understanding by reflecting on the child's conversation and behaviour can make it easier to gain consent to explore these issues further [48].

What sort of care is needed?

Three dimensions of care have been identified as important for families caring for a child with complex healthcare needs in the community [37].

Information and communication

Both parents and professionals identify the need for open and honest communication. This may involve giving information on a wide range of topics including illness-management, care giving, services, benefits, and equipment [37]. A combination of personal guidance and good quality written information is required [49] both for its intrinsic usefulness and also because it empowers parents to participate in decisions [6]. Unfortunately in many cases parents have to actively seek information and at times the information that is provided is inappropriate, insufficient or even conflicting [37,42,50].

Teaching the parents to understand the child's condition and how to perform practical procedures is an important aspect of specialist nurses' role [37]. The child and family need to understand how to adapt procedures learnt in hospital for the home environment; new procedures may be taught as their child's care needs change. Feedback to the parents or other carers on their skills and coping is important but must be offered in ways that do not leave them feeling pressurised or unfairly criticised when caring for the child [37].

Practical assistance

Professionals will often be involved in organising services and equipment both in preparation for hospital discharge and subsequently as the child and family's needs change. They may act as advocates for the child and family, campaigning on their behalf for services or benefits or acting as an intermediary liasing on their behalf with other professionals [37]. Co-ordination of care can be improved by designating a key worker for the family, from among the network of professionals involved [51]. However, even when professionals take on the role of co-ordination, parents continue to report they often still have to take on much of the co-ordination role themselves [37].

Families may benefit greatly from the opportunity to have a break from the many and often complex tasks that they undertake caring for their child. Short (respite) breaks from caring, and practical help around the home, can facilitate other normal activities like a night-out for the parents as well as allowing families to recuperate or cope with unexpected problems such as family illness [52].

Emotional support

Emotional support is also an essential part of care for children with life-limiting conditions and their families. Families describe the need to feel 'connected' with healthcare professionals and that those healthcare professionals empathise with what is happening to them [5]. Parents describe the need for someone who is familiar with their child and easily accessible for advice and information [37]. Patients, their families and professionals all identify the need for professionals to have good listening and counselling skills [53] to enable children and their families to talk openly, share the burden of feelings and concerns and to help promote parents' self-confidence [6,37]. For some children and families more specialised psychological support is necessary. It will be important to ensure that this need is identified and the child and family are able to access the appropriate services.

The care setting

Care in the home

Most children with life-limiting conditions will spend much of their time at home and care at home has considerable advantages. It is almost always the place where families choose to be [6,31,32,54–56]. Families prefer home care often through the desire to avoid or decrease disruption to family life and normal routines such as school or work. Care at home is also beneficial for siblings [8,57] as well as for increasing the sick child's quality of life. Opportunities to maintain open communication within the family are also greater when the family is at home.

Although care at home offers many benefits for the child and family, it also poses significant challenges. The family will inevitably take on significant responsibility for care. They may have no choice other than to take on these tasks if they are keen to take their child home, but they may also feel pressure from professionals and indirect peer pressure from other families who have already taken on such an extended role [37]. Indeed some parents report significant feelings of ambiguity and indifference particularly with regard to taking on the care of a technology-dependent child at home [58].

As well as their usual parental role, they are likely to be taking on basic nursing tasks including lifting, assistance with washing and dressing, administration of medication [17], and perhaps more complex tasks such as assisted feeding, suction and emergency management of seizures or other acute complications. Families and carers of technology dependent children may take on or assist with care of a highly technical nature, for example changing a tracheostomy tube, which in the past would have been the domain of the professional [13]. Professionals need to encourage parents to attain skills to care for their child and avoid making it seem overwhelming [6]. In some circumstances it may be very difficult for the child, particularly for the technology-dependent child, to get home even though he or she no longer wants or needs to be in hospital. Several barriers that delay the family taking their child home have been identified: attitudes of healthcare professionals, organising responsibility for financing home care, poor management within the health service and collaboration with other agencies, complex social issues, housing problems, and lack of auditing and outcome measures [59].

Caring for a child at home is a 24-h responsibility and may mean months or even years of interrupted sleep with no prospect of a break [17]. There is the additional responsibility of taking on complex tasks knowing that the consequences of a mistake may directly impact on their child's health [13]. Some families may find themselves isolated from family and friends who find the situation distressing and feel powerless or unwilling to help. At times families may also become isolated from professionals. There is a particular risk of this when the child's condition is relatively stable, even if their needs are significant, and professional resources are limited so that children or families with new diagnoses or changing needs are prioritised [50,60]. If care for the child with a life-limiting condition is to be sustained over periods of months to years, the family must remain resilient and able to adapt to changing needs over time. Sharing some of the care and appropriate multidisciplinary support, enabling the child to attend school, short break respite care and occasional holidays can all facilitate the majority of care being provided by the family, in the home environment.

Carers from within the family

Involving members of the family other than the parents in the care of a child with a life-limiting condition is likely to be beneficial for the child, their parents and the family as a whole. The degree to which grandparents become involved with the care of a child with developmental disability and their satisfaction relates both to their attitude towards children with disabilities in general, and their relationship with their children. Involvement with a grandchild with developmental disability appears to strengthen family relationships [61]. Involvement of siblings in the care of their brother or sister has both positive and negative aspects. It can bring closeness, feelings of recognition and appreciation, and may also help long term adjustment [57]. However there may also be feelings of guilt, anger and resentment when the parents have less time for their other children and caring interferes with normal childhood activity [41]. A lack of support for siblings and opportunity to share some of the important issues they face has been recognised [50].

Studies of informal carers (family, friends) of adults have identified high unmet needs. These include the need for information, the opportunity to share experiences, and to be recognised for the care that they are providing. These needs can be met by multi-professional teaching and peer support [62–64].

Trained lay carers

Many families rely on teams of trained lay carers to assist them in caring for their child at home. These carers help with activities such as washing and dressing and are trained to carry out specific nursing tasks, for example administration of medication via gastrostomy. The use of trained lay carers has undoubtedly facilitated many children who would otherwise have remained in hospital being discharged home and attending school. But lack of co-ordination and access to skilled competent carers is a particular problem for some families [50]. The high turnover of carers is a reflection of the significant psychosocial stresses of this role and is a concern for families who have to rely on an inconsistent, frequently changing service [65].

In the United Kingdom parents cannot be paid to carry out care for their own child, although they maybe eligible to receive supplementary benefits. Parents may have to return to work in order to support the family, whilst lay carers are paid to care for their child [66]. Trained lay carers, employed by the local authorities, often work to support a child and their family but the family is not their employer. There may be conflict between the view of the employing authority and the family regarding the role of the carer and the tasks that are appropriate for them to undertake. It can be difficult to work in someone else's home over an extended period whilst maintaining appropriate boundaries. Carers cannot easily escape conflict between family members or they may be inadvertently drawn into an inappropriate counselling role. They risk becoming intensely involved with the child and family and becoming overwhelmed by the situation so that they are unable to cope [65,67]. The impact of these stresses on the trained lay carer, child and family, can be reduced with provision of appropriate clinical supervision [68].

Trained nursing care

Trained nursing staff are frequently the pivotal professionals involved in supporting children with a life-limiting condition and their family at home, often taking on the role of the key-worker. However their availability and role varies considerably depending on the child's diagnosis, location and availability of local resources. Just as professionals assess and make judgements on the child's condition, needs and role of carers, so will parents also assess and judge the level of expertise and knowledge professionals possess [37]. They may preferentially seek advice from those they consider most capable of providing the support they require.

Paediatric outreach nurse specialists are highly trained nurses usually based in a hospital, often as part of a multidisciplinary team caring for a specific diagnosis, for example malignancy or cystic fibrosis, or in a children's hospice. Paediatric oncology outreach nurses have been particularly important in the development of paediatric palliative care as a speciality, and critical in allowing increasing numbers of children with progressive malignancy to die at home [54,69]. As death in childhood is rare, few family doctors, community based children's nurses or adult palliative care nurses will have significant experience of end-of-life care in children. Rather than taking over the care in the home the outreach nurse specialist aims to work in partnership with the family and local health care workers, empowering them to care for the child and facilitating communication between the child and family, primary care team and specialist centre [70]. They provide a combination of informal teaching, expertise in symptom management and psychosocial care, practical advice and support and possibly short periods of respite in the home. They may also take on the role of key-worker and be part of a 24 h on call service to facilitate optimum end-of-life care [71,72].

In contrast to the hospital-based nurse specialists, in the UK many areas have community based children's nurses and more recently some of these teams have developed into multidisciplinary palliative care teams, for example the Diana nursing teams [73,74]. These teams are able to offer much greater co-ordination of care and frequent input at a local level, but are less able to provide disease-specific guidance or advice and support for complex end-of-life care. The most effective care for the child and family can be achieved when these local teams are able to work in partnership with more distantly based specialists with expertise in the child's illness and palliative care.

Although the services provided by children's community nurses are sometimes seen as preferable, there are circumstances where involving other community nursing teams maybe necessary or desirable. In the United Kingdom there are teams of district nurses, usually based at the family doctor's surgery or health centre. These nurses provide a range of services to all patients in the community and this will include children if no specific children's community nursing team is available. Although their experience with children with life-limiting conditions may be limited, their skills and local knowledge with regard to obtaining specialist supplies or equipment can prove invaluable. They may also have considerable experience with providing end-of-life care at home. In this situation additional support and guidance may be required in order to overcome the inherent anxieties of caring for children. However after an initial training period, teams of district nurses will often be able to take on tasks such as daily visits to change a syringe driver and work alongside children's community or outreach nurses in order to facilitate 24 h access to care.

In situations where specialist paediatric palliative care advice is not available, particularly for pain and symptom management at the end of life, it is important that an alternative support of appropriate expertise is identified. Many areas in the United Kingdom have access to community based adult palliative care nurse specialists (Macmillan Nurses). These nurses provide specific expertise in symptom management, psychosocial support and end-of-life care for patients with cancer and work in a predominantly advisory capacity alongside the family doctor and district nursing teams. Although their experience with children may be limited, the principles of symptom management at the end of life are similar to those in adults and the advice they are able to provide for professionals

caring for children, particularly at the end of life at home, can be very helpful.

Doctors

Access to medical advice and support is also essential for the care of the child with a life-limiting condition. Again the provision of such medical support is likely to differ depending on the available expertise, the diagnosis and the needs of the child and family.

All children with life-limiting conditions are likely to be under the care of one or more hospital paediatricians. These may be doctors with specific expertise in the child's condition such as a paediatric oncologist or paediatric neurologist or general paediatricians. These doctors may work closely, particularly with the paediatric outreach nurse specialists to facilitate provision of palliative care to children in the community. In the United Kingdom, the traditional model has been for these doctors to remain hospital-based but some of these specialists have extended their role and are able to visit their patients at home, particularly those with palliative care needs. However clinical workload and other hospital commitments may mean that this service is limited to planned home visits and may not be flexible enough for situations when the child's condition is changing rapidly, for example at the end of life. In many areas of the United Kingdom there are also those who are particularly successfully involved as part of a multidisciplinary team addressing the needs of children with complex chronic conditions [79,80]. However this approach is generally built on a 'well child' model and although undoubtedly very effective in the periods of stability may not be flexible and responsive enough to deal with acute changes in the child's condition such as for end of life care. Both hospital- and community-based paediatricians will need to work closely with the child's community nursing team and family to ensure the best standards of care.

Some children and families retain very close ties with their family practitioner throughout their illness journey. However for others, such as those with cancer, whose care following diagnosis has been lead by hospital based services, the family doctor may have been less involved. The involvement of the child's family doctor is likely to be essential in the provision of good end-of-life care at home [75], visiting the child at home to help provide assistance with symptom management and to support the family. If the family doctor has previously had relatively little involvement in the child's medical care it can lead to tension between him or her and the family [76]. Because of the rarity of the situation family doctors rarely have significant expertise in the care of children dying at home, and will need to work with other professionals such as children's community nurses or outreach nurse specialists for guidance. Sometimes this can also be a source of conflict [77,78] and the family physician may welcome the opportunity to discuss the child's condition and its management with a paediatrician, or paediatric palliative care physician.

At the time of writing there are only a very few paediatric palliative care specialists worldwide. These are paediatricians, often with a general paediatric and paediatric oncology background, who have undergone specific additional training in paediatric palliative care. They offer a tertiary service to children with palliative care needs in hospital, but also in hospice and at home. The small number of paediatric palliative care specialists and the large populations that they serve means that, in addition to offering direct care to their own patients, they must also be available to offer a wider advisory and supportive role to other paediatricians and community teams, as the speciality develops.

The number of other doctors with significant expertise in palliative care for children is increasing. Most paediatric oncologists will have some experience of palliative care for children with cancer and a proportion have considerable expertise in this area. Some general paediatricians are developing an interest in paediatric palliative care and have undertaken additional training in the field and are well placed to support local and community teams. In the United Kingdom many of the children's hospice family doctors have increasing expertise particularly in symptom management and end of life care and again a proportion of them have undertaken additional training in palliative care. Although the work of children's hospice doctors has usually focussed on the needs of inpatients, their increasing expertise, and the rising number of children's hospice outreach teams, certainly in the United Kingdom, suggest that some of these family physicians may also begin to offer their expertise more widely.

Finally adult palliative care physicians who are predominantly based in hospice or hospital may be able to provide advice and support to their paediatric colleagues particularly for symptom management [71,72] and this approach has been particularly evident in where specialised paediatric palliative care is sparse.

Other professions allied to medicine

A number of other professionals are likely to be involved with the child with a life-limiting condition and their family along their journey from diagnosis through to bereavement. As with the key professions already discussed there will be a great variation depending on the child's diagnosis, care needs, care setting, and available expertise.

Social workers may be involved in direct support of the child and family including at the time of diagnosis, during acute crises, at the end of life and during bereavement. Social

workers are most often involved in traditional social work activities such as providing knowledge of community resources and provision of psychosocial support. They may be involved with assessment for grants for adaptations, or continuing care. The role may include facilitating team work and providing psychosocial support for professionals, as well as the child and family [81,82]. Social work involvement as part of the multidisciplinary team can be particularly important when difficult ethical decisions are being discussed. This may include encouraging self-determination, challenging discrimination, being non-judgemental and promoting open discussion. Unfortunately children with complex chronic conditions and high levels of disability are also at increased risk of non-accidental injury and neglect. The social worker may then also have to be involved in child protection work. As with other professions, social worker's experience of palliative care, particularly of end-of-life care, may be limited [83].

Psychologists are a relatively scarce resource and although recognition of psychological needs is an integral part of the philosophy of palliative care, the majority of patients and their families do not need to be under the direct care of a clinical psychologist [84]. Most patients and their families will receive effective informal psychological support from those professionals directly involved in their care such as nurses or social workers. However ideally these professionals will have access to a trained clinical psychologist for supervision, and with whom patients and families can be discussed and if necessary be referred if particular needs are identified, for example particularly challenging cases such as complex collusion, denial or complicated bereavement. Psychologists also have specialised skills in therapy and the use of drawing or play to facilitate communication. In the UK a tiered model has been proposed [85] with patients and families being referred to professionals with increasing levels of expertise in psychological care.

Physiotherapists, occupational therapists, and *speech therapists* may all be involved in the care of children with palliative care needs. Rehabilitation interventions are often overlooked and underutilised despite high levels of functional disability in adult patients with palliative care diagnoses [86–88]. However for children, particularly those with neurodisability, the benefits of physiotherapy, speech therapy and occupation therapy are well recognised for facilitating as normal patterns of development as possible. Often these therapies are delivered as part of a community based programme, via school or nursery or sometimes in the patient's own home. Integral to this approach is working with the child's family in order to teach techniques that can be continued in between therapy sessions. It is important to recognise that in addition to promoting age appropriate developmental patterns the use of techniques such as appropriate positioning, stretching exercises, and the use of aids and adaptations can assist with symptom management. Providing more intensive levels of therapy, such as chest physiotherapy in the community for the end of life [89], or community rehabilitation for a head injured child may prove more difficult if resources are stretched. If care at home is the desired option, it will be particularly important to work with family to teach them appropriate techniques to continue when the therapist is not available.

The role of *the pharmacist* as a member of the multidisciplinary team in adult in-patient palliative care units is well recognised [90]. There is also an increasing recognition of the role of liaison pharmacy in the promoting safe medicines management and effective symptom control for those receiving palliative care in the community [91]. This role may include advice to rationalise inappropriate prescribing regimes, warnings regarding potential drug interactions and advice about therapeutic drug monitoring [92]. Communicating directly with the community dispensing pharmacist gives them confidence if they are not be familiar with drugs and doses used in paediatric palliative care and includes them in the team caring for the family so they can facilitate access to the necessary medications. The importance of safe management of controlled drugs in the community has been highlighted in the United Kingdom following the publication of the report into the case of Dr Harold Shipman [93], with one doctor taking clear lead in prescribing controlled drugs for use in the community and all prescriptions being dispensed at the same pharmacy practice.

Voluntary organizations

In addition to services offered by statutory provider children and their families may be able to access care provided by voluntary, or independent organisations. The services provided are outside those provided by the state medical care system and are usually offered free to the child and family. Such services maybe funded entirely by voluntary donations (charitable organisations) or statutory bodies, such as the state-run health service or social services departments, may contract them to provide services on their behalf. The range of services that can be provided in this way varies immensely and ranges from befriending, help with domestic chores, care for the child or siblings, play-groups and specialist play facilities to bereavement support and counselling. Although these services are often regulated to a certain extent by statutory legislation, their provision is essentially driven by local initiatives and such services may be developed or disappear over a short time scale. This may make it more difficult to establish effective communication with other members of the multidisciplinary team. There is often no substitute for local knowledge to ensure that families are able to access voluntary services, from which they might benefit. Development of local directories of services including voluntary organizations has been advocated as an example of best practice in order to improve access to these and other services [94].

The multidisciplinary paediatric palliative care team

From the preceding discussion it is clear that a vast number of different professionals may be involved in the care of a child with a life-limiting illness, regardless of the care setting. It is important to emphasise that provision of paediatric palliative care is essentially a multidisciplinary approach. The multidisciplinary team caring for an individual child and family needs to be tailored to their individual needs and may change as the child's condition changes and as the child moves into different care settings. Clearly this creates significant challenges for communication, co-ordination and continuity of care (see Chapter 6, Teamwork). At the centre of the team there are likely to be one or more nurses and this is the profession that most often takes on the role of key worker. There are also likely to be one or more doctors and variable provision of support from other professionals. What is important is that the professionals directly involved in the care of the child and family are able to adequately assess the child and family's needs, are aware of their own limitations, and are able to access appropriate advice and support from other professionals where need is identified.

Short break (respite) care at home

Caring for a child with a life-limiting condition can be incredibly demanding both physically and psychologically. Provision of short-break (respite) care can provide an essential break from these demands and ensure resilience so that the family can continue to care for their child. Short break care at home is sometimes seen as the model of choice, as it reduces disruption to the child and their normal routine [23]. Most often this is provided by a team of trained lay carers and children's community nurses. However it may be more difficult to provide short break care in this setting, other than for a few hours at a time, due to resource implications. Furthermore for some children and families, provision of short break care away from home, particularly in a children's hospice (see below), has significant advantages.

School

School is an important part of everyday life providing the opportunity for learning, independence from parents and social interaction [95,96]. Attendance at school provides a natural break from caring for the family. This can be vital in maintaining a family's resilience when caring for a child with complex needs [60]. Although there may be interruptions for acute crises or treatment, most children with a life-limiting condition will be able to attend school during periods when their condition is relatively stable [15,97]. Practical difficulties should not prevent access to school but may require careful planning to ensure that the child is able to participate in school as fully as possible. Parents or other family members should not be the primary source of support in the classroom if the child is to develop independence.

Many children require regular medication during the day as well as treatment for pain or seizures when required. It is not always easy to arrange for school staff to administer medication [60] but careful planning ahead both for routine and emergency care is essential to avoid the parents having to be available to do this [18]. It is important to consider the level of intervention that would be appropriate in the case of a sudden deterioration in the child's condition, such as cardio-respiratory arrest, taking into account the child's prognosis, life expectancy and the wishes of the child and family [18]. Staff can be provided with information about the child's illness and may value contacts with education staff at the hospital and nurse specialists. Families may also appreciate visits from the nurse specialists to the school to educate and support staff and help them in communicating with the other children in the school.

Holidays

When family holidays are planned it is important to anticipate possible changes in the child's condition and also consider adequate holiday insurance [98]. The family will need a covering letter explaining their condition, plans for treatment in an emergency, drugs used, and contact details. Holidays are frequently offered to children and families, particularly toward the end of life and by charities. Although these are greatly appreciated and can be extremely beneficial they may be unrealistic if offered at too late a stage. Participation in school trips may be treated with enthusiasm by children with life-limiting illness, but sometimes less so by their parents [15]. Later, however, such trips are often recognised as being one of the most important events in the child's life.

End-of-life care at home

The majority (78%) of children in the United Kingdom with progressive malignancy will die at home (UKCCSG figures). There are no published figures for numbers of home deaths for children with other life-limiting conditions but data from the UK Association of Children's Hospices suggest that around 36% of hospice users die at home [99].

There is considerable evidence to suggest that families of children who die at home have less difficulty in adjusting and cope better in the medium to long term [8,31,32] but studies in adults have shown home death to be more stressful for families of the deceased [100]. A more recent study [101] in children failed to show any significant difference in short term outcome between parents of children with malignancy dying an acute hospital death and those dying a palliative death, predominantly at home. However a greater proportion of the siblings of the child dying an acute death reported problems compared to those of children who died a palliative death.

End-of-life care at home allows the child and family greater control over their environment with involvement of fewer professionals and increased opportunities for privacy and time together. The family has a clearly defined role in providing the majority of the child's care. It is much easier to include the siblings and to discuss difficult issues [6,57].

If the intention is for the child to be cared for at home during periods of rapid change in the child's condition, including at the end of life, then anticipatory planning is essential. The family, and the involved professionals, will need to be aware of what may be required, and what is available [102,103]. Part of anticipatory planning includes provision of specialist equipment, for example a pressure-relieving mattress, and assistance for physical tasks, for example, lifting and turning also ensuring that appropriate medication for symptom control is available and written up in advance [104]. End-of-life care at home is likely to be difficult, if not impossible, without adequate support but if this is available it is not usually necessary to move a child [103,105]. Such support should include [75] 24 h access to expertise in paediatric and family care, 24 h access to expertise in paediatric palliative care, a key worker to coordinate family and respite care and immediate access to hospital if needed.

Although many families choose home as the place of choice for caring for their child it is important not to underestimate the physical and emotional burden of end-of-life care at home and not to assume that home care is the only choice. Those families that choose death at home are more likely to be self reliant, confident and able to confront problems, all factors that have been shown to be associated with better coping and a better long term outcome [8,106]. However if a family feels isolated and unable to cope at home, the ensuing breakdown of care can result in feelings of guilt and failure [23,107]. Occasionally, difficulties with symptom-control, psychological distress or family wishes mean that the child is transferred to paediatric hospice or hospital [108]. This should not be seen as a failure but as a choice ensuring the best care for the child and family [109,110] and good palliative care can still be achieved.

Care in hospital and intensive care

Much can be done to bring the 'home from home' environment to the child and family in hospital. This may include attention to privacy, involvement in care and decision making [111], stopping intrusive and inappropriate monitoring and keeping the family together, for example by the provision of family accommodation [112,113]. However it is often difficult for siblings to spend much time with their brother or sister in hospital. A system of sharing care where the specialist paediatric hospital works together with a local hospital can enable the child to be transferred and the families to be closer to home [114].

For families of children with prolonged illnesses and complex care needs, admission to hospital can cause particular difficulties. Admission to hospital inevitably involves interaction with a greater number of healthcare professionals than in the community, many of whom may not be familiar with the child and their family. Subtle differences in treatment approach or explanation can result in confusion and lack of trust [42]. Nursing staff may expect parents to both continue day to day to care for their child [13] but at the same time relinquish their control to professionals. Parents report feeling their experience and knowledge is disregarded and their competency questioned [37,115]. These differing, and possibly conflicting, expectations [116] require negotiation of roles between parents and professionals to reflect the differing power balance in the hospital versus home [13].

Short breaks in hospital

Although the acute hospital ward is not generally considered to be a desirable place for short-break care, for some families there are no realistic alternatives. Short breaks in hospital provide reassurance of highly trained staff and a secure environment. A number of purpose-built respite units linked to paediatric units in the United Kingdom have been developed which offer a high standard of home-from-home care with the advantages of close links with the hospital [60].

End-of-life care in hospital

The majority of childhood deaths in the United Kingdom and the United States occur in hospital compared with home or hospice. Of these hospital deaths, around 60% are deaths due to life-limiting (complex chronic) conditions and their complications [117,29]. The majority of childhood deaths from progressive malignancy occur at home, but 40% of children that die of cancer do so following complications of treatment that is intended to be curative [118] and these deaths occur primarily in hospital. Children with complex chronic conditions are more likely to have prolonged hospitalisation and prolonged ventilation prior to their death, when compared to deaths from acute causes [119]. This aggressive treatment of acute episodes in children with ultimately terminal conditions reflects the difficulty in determining short-term prognosis [109] and also the difficulty both for families and professionals in

defining the time when the best interest of the child is to move away from aggressive interventions and focus on symptom management and palliative care.

When it is recognized that the end of life is immanent in hospital, the option of taking the child home for care, particularly if this is something that the child and family would prefer, can help acceptance of the situation [8,120]. The possibility of doing this is not always thought of or offered as proactively as it could be. Some units have pioneered examples of innovative approaches where neonates and children have been taken home from the intensive care unit (ICU) or to a children's hospice and extubated there, to fulfil the family's wishes. Even if it is not possible for the child to die at home the family may be able to take their child home or to a children's hospice after death [121].

The majority of children who die in hospital do so on the paediatric ICU [29,108,119]. Death in these cases is frequently associated with either a 'do not attempt resuscitation order' or withdrawing mechanical ventilation. It is possible to provide effective end-of-life care in the hospital ward or ICU [104]. However evidence suggests that the standard of end-of-life care for children in hospital is still often poor. Aggressive curative treatments may be continued without evidence of benefit and at the expense of recognition of palliative care needs. Families may find it difficult to acknowledge that their child is dying [45], with subsequent long-term difficulties and complicated grief. Families of children dying in hospital [42] continue to identify confusing, inadequate or uncaring communication, oversights in procedures and policies and failure to include siblings. Parents felt that they had little or no control during their child's final days or that they would have liked to make decisions differently [122].

A number of studies have shown that families of children with cancer who die in hospital experience greater guilt [2], anxiety, depression, and interpersonal problems [8] than those of children who die at home. If death does not occur at home, the outcome appears to be better if the family can acknowledge the situation and prognosis, for example by discussing options for hospice care [45].

Children's hospices

Hospice has been described as a philosophy of care rather than a facility [123]. The term is used routinely in this way for all palliative care in the United States and some other projects [124,125] In the United Kingdom the word hospice is more often used to refer to a specialist in-patient facility.

The United Kingdom children's hospice movement began in the 1980s in Oxford [124] with the aim of supporting families who were taking care of their sick child at home most of the time. Inpatient children's hospices are small 'home from home' environments generally providing 8–10 beds with opportunity for the family to stay either in the child's room or in separate family accommodation. Many hospices have excellent recreational and therapeutic facilities that can be accessed by the child and family together including gardens, play facilities, hydrotherapy pools and large living/dining rooms where children, families and staff can socialise and eat together.

Children's hospices have a specialist role for short-break care and for end-of-life care if dying at home is not an option [52]. They maintain links with available community services, provide telephone contact for families and some have outreach and home care services. At the end of life they provide care at the hospice, if that is the family's choice. Families can also use their bereavement suite (with in-built cooling unit) where a child can stay once they have died. The hospice team will continue to provide support following the child's death [110]. The hospice team maintain a strong recognition of psychosocial needs with informal counselling services and often support groups for children and their families. Services aim to be child and family centred and delivered in partnership according to the families wishes [123].

Since the development of the first children's hospice numerous other children's hospices have been established in the United Kingdom and elsewhere [60]. The first children's hospices were nurse-led with support from local family doctors. Most children's hospices in the United Kingdom continue to be nurse-led, but there is increasing involvement of both hospital and community paediatricians [70] as well as an increasing level of specialist skill from the family doctor's involved. The hospices usually have a multidisciplinary team (e.g. physiotherapists, family support workers, play-specialists, teachers, social workers, chaplains) who work closely with their counterparts in hospital and community [127].

Paediatric hospice is not an option chosen by all patients with life-limiting conditions and their families. Unlike adult hospices, relatively few children with cancer will use a paediatric hospice [109]. Instead children that use paediatric hospice more often have slowly progressive irreversible life-limiting conditions such as Duchenne muscular dystrophy, mucopolysaccaridoses and severe static or progressive neurological diseases [70].

Short break (respite) care

The majority of beds in children's hospices are used for short break respite care, in order to give the family a break from routine and stress of caring [23]. The value of this service is demonstrable by the heavy use particularly at weekends and holidays, and the observation that demand has resulted in many children's hospices having to reduce the number of nights they are able to allocate to each family. In addition many hospices offer emergency short-break care at times of crisis such as when a parent is ill or a sibling goes into hospital. This flexibility is particularly important in preventing family breakdown or unnecessary admission to hospital. As qualified nurses staff the children's hospice, short breaks and supportive care can also be offered when the child is unwell, but hospital treatment is not appropriate.

Short breaks can be provided for the child alone, or for the child with family or friends. They provide an opportunity for the family to spend time with the child away from everyday chores and the responsibility of their regular nursing tasks. For young adults short breaks provide valuable independence from family carers and an opportunity to spend time with friends and other young people with similar problems. Short breaks may also allow the family valuable time to do things that simply would not otherwise be possible, knowing that their child is being cared for in 'safe hands', such as a holiday abroad or time to spend with siblings.

Hospice outreach (hospice-to-home) services

A number of paediatric hospices offer a hospice outreach service usually backed up via 24-h telephone advice line. Specialist hospice nurses and other professionals visit the child and family at home. They may also support families during outpatient appointments at the hospital, or visit them when they are admitted to hospital. Although some of these teams offer a short-break service more often the support is aimed at symptom management, psychosocial support, and practical advice in order to enable the family to continue to care for their child effectively [52]. The hospice outreach service needs to work alongside the other health care professionals involved with the family.

Psychosocial support for the child and family

Psychosocial support will be provided as a matter of course by the hospice team during short-break and end-of-life care. In addition informal, one to one counselling services are often available from a family support worker, social worker or counsellor. The opportunity to meet and share experiences with others using the hospice offer the children and their families invaluable support. In recognition of the value of this peer support a number of hospices offer specialist support groups, not just for bereaved parents, but for other family members at any time from diagnosis to bereavement [60]. Hospices can be particularly responsive to the needs of siblings [41].

End-of-life care in hospice

Currently only 20% of children that use a hospice in the United Kingdom will die there [99]. The majority die either at home or in hospital, which partly reflects the difficulty in predicting outcome from acute episodes for many of these children. For those children previously known to the hospice, there is often a period of escalating symptoms and increasingly frequent admissions for short-breaks as their care needs increase. The admission for end-of-life care is the natural sequel to recognition of this irreversible deterioration in the child's condition if it is the family's choice. Sometimes children are admitted to the hospice specifically for end-of-life care for example from hospital. The hospice can offer a much more homely environment with excellent support for a family who prefer not to be at home. The hospice can also be helpful for end-of-life care in families where the parents are estranged, allowing more space for the different parties and a more neutral environment.

Bereavement support

When a child dies within the hospice, the family will be encouraged and supported in spending time with their child and washing and dressing them after death. The bereavement suite (decorated as a bedroom but with inbuilt cooling) is particularly valued by families allowing them to have time with their child, coming and going as they please, until the child's funeral. Families of children who have died in the hospice may wish to continue to stay until their child has left. Furthermore families of children who have died elsewhere, whether they were known to the hospice prior to their death or not, have also used and valued this service [99]. Bereavement support can include helping families planning their child's funeral and then continues with regular follow up and memorial services.

Symptom management

Unlike adult hospices [127], symptom management does not currently constitute a major part of the work of children's hospices. Much of the care provided in children's hospices is in the form of short-breaks and if the children's condition is reasonably stable there is no indication to change management. Most children using a children's hospice will be under the care of one or more paediatricians in hospital and the community who are involved in management of problems such as epilepsy and spasticity. When children receive end-of-life care in hospice symptom management assumes a greater role and a number of hospice family doctors, as well as nursing staff, are now gaining expertise in this area [128]. The increase in numbers of specialists in paediatric palliative care, both paediatricians and hospice family doctors, suggests that symptom management is likely to become more important part of the children's hospice role in the future.

Advantages and disadvantages of children's hospice care

There is no doubt that children's hospice provides an exemplary standard of short-break and end-of-life care for the child and family. In contrast to short-break care provided by other agencies such as social services, care can be provided even when the child is unwell and has significant medical problems but when hospital admission is not appropriate. Although children's hospices endeavour to maintain a 'home from home' they are not the child's home and cannot fully compensate for familiar surroundings and daily routine. Parents may feel a sense of guilt when having to share care with others. Care team members, due to the very nature of their role, can become very involved with the child and family. They too require support to retain appropriate boundaries and continue to empower parents to take the leading role in the care of their child and be involved decision-making. Children's hospice can not provide an acute medical service and at times it will clearly not be appropriate to admit a child to hospice.

All the children's hospices in the United Kingdom are independent and run with charitable donations. They run alongside the relatively under-resourced services provided by the National Health Service. Tensions can arise from this relating to competition for local charitable donations and for staff. Both the hospices and the statutory services need to devote effort to maintaining regular communication over mutual patients and to recognise and acknowledge each others' role in care.

Summary

The primary objective of palliative care is to support the child with life-limiting illness and their family, from the point of diagnosis: enhancing quality of life, maintaining resilience and coping, particularly at times of crisis and at the end of life, and allowing the child and family to achieve as normal a life as possible. Home is where most children and families choose to be and in particular there is evidence that families who provide end-of-life care for their child at home cope better. In order to care for their child at home the family will need help and support from a number of professionals. The optimum configuration for the provision of care will depend on the care setting, the needs of the child and family and the structure and extent of the health care system. However the fundamental role of palliative care remains the same. This will include advice, information, symptom management, emotional and practical support and often short breaks from caring. Successful care will be flexible enough to anticipate and cope with changes in the child and family's needs, communicating effectively and moving seamlessly between home, hospice, hospital or school, wherever the child may be.

References

1. Carter, B., McArthur, E., and Cunliffe, M. Dealing with uncertainty: Parental assessment of pain in their children with profound special needs. *J Adv Nurs* 2002;38(5):449–57.

2. Lauer, M.E., Mulhern, R.K., Wallskog, J.M., and Camitta, B.M. A comparison study of parental adaptation following a child's death at home or in the hospital. *Pediatrics* 1983;71(1):107–12.

3. Grinyer, A. and Thomas, C. Young adults with cancer: The effect of illness on parents and families. *Int J Palliat Nurs* 2001;7(4):162–4, 166–70.

4. Wise, B.V. In their own words; the lived experience of pediatric liver transplantation. *Qual Health Res* 2002;12(1):74–90.

5. James, L. and Johnson, B. The needs of parents of paediatric oncology patients during the palliative care phase. *J Paediatr Oncol Nurs* 1997;14(2):83–95.

6. Vickers, J. and Carlisle, C. Choices and control: Parental experiences in pediatric terminal home care. *J Paediatr Oncol Nurs* 2000;17(1): 12–21.

7. Collins, J.J., Stevens, M.M., and Cousens, P. Home care for the dying child: A parent's perception. *Aust Family Phys* 1998;27(7): 610–4.

8. Mulhern, R.K., Lauer, M.E., and Hoffmann, R.G. Death of a child at home or in the hospital; subsequent psychological adjustment of the family. *Pediatrics* 1983;71(5):743–7.

9. Meijer, S.A., Sinnema, G., Bijstra, J.O., Mellenbergh, G.J., and Wolters, W.H. Coping styles and locus of control as predictors for psychosocial adjustment of adolescents with a chronic illness. *Soc Sci Med* 2002;54(9):1453–61.

10. Hockley, J. Psychosocial aspects in palliative care—communicating with the patient and family. *Acta Oncol* 2000;39(8):905–10.

11. Yantzi, N., Rosenberg, M.W., Burke, S.O., and Harrison, M.B. The impacts of distance to hospital on families with a child with a chronic condition. *Soc Sci Med* 2001;52(12):1777–91.

12. Hechter, S., Poggenpoal, M., and Myburgh, C. Life stories of families with a terminally ill child. *Curationis* 2001;24(2):54–61.

13. Kirk S. Negotiating lay and professional roles in the care of children with complex health care needs. *J Adv Nurs* 2001;34(5): 593–602.

14. Stevenson, R.G. Helping peers to help themselves: The role of peer support in times of crisis. In *What will we do? Preparing a school community to cope with crisis. In R.G. Stevenson, ed. Death Value and Meaning Series*, Amityville NY: Baywood, 1994, pp. 175–81.

15. Bouffet, E., Zucchinelli, V., and Costanzo, P. Schooling as part of palliative care in paediatric oncology. *Palliat Med* 1997;11:133–9.

16. Steele, R.G. Trajectory of death at an unknown time: Children with neurodegenerative life-threatening conditons. *Can J Nurs Res* 2000;32(3):49–67.

17. Roberts, K. and Lawton, D. Acknowledging the extra care parents give their disabled children. *Child: Care Health and Dev* 2001; 27(4):307–19.

18. Ramer Chrastek, Joan. Hospice care for a terminally ill child in the school setting. *J School Nurs* 2000;16(2):52–6.

19. Firth, M., Gardner-Medwin, D., Hoskig, G. *et al.* Interviews with parents of boys suffering from Duchenne muscular dystrophy. *Dev Med Child Neurol* 1983;(25):446–71.

20. Polakoff, R.J., Morton, A.A., Koch, K.D., and Rics, C.M. The psychosocial and cognitive impact of Duchenne's muscular dystrophy. *Semin Paediat Neurol* 1998;5(2):116–23.

21. Dobson. *The Impact of Childhood Disability on Family Life*. York: York Publishing Services, 2001.

22. Kirk, S. Caring for children with specialised health care needs in the community: The challenges for primary care. *Soc Care Commun* 1999;7:350–7.

23. Miller, S. Respite care for children who have complex nursing needs. *Paediatric Nurs* 2002;14(5):33–7.

24. Masri, C., Farrell, C.A., Lacroix, J., Rocker, G., and Shemie, S.D. Decision making and end of life care in critically ill children. *J Palliat Care* 2000;(16 Suppl.): S45–52.

25. Tonelli, M.R. End of life care in cystic fibrosis. *Curr Opin Pulmonary Med* 1998;4:332–6.

26. Reddihough, D.S., Baikies, G., and Walstab, J.E. Cerebral Palsy in Vicoris, Australia: Mortality and causes of death. *J Paediatr Child Health* 2001;37(2):183–6.

27. Wu, M.H., Wang, J.K., and Lue, H.C. Sudden death in patients with right isomerism (asplenism) after palliation. *J Paediatr* 2002;140(1): 93–6.

28. British Medical Association. *Withholding and Withdrawing Life-Prolonging Medical Treatment*—Guidance for Decision Making. London: BMJ Books, 1999.

29. Brook, L., Williams, S., and Farell, M. Paediatric Deaths in Hospital: Scope for palliative care? *Arch Dis Childhood* 2003; 88(Suppl. 1):A61.

30. Davies, B. and Steele, R. Challenges in identifying children for palliative care. *J Palliat Care* 1996;12:5–8.

31. Papadatou, D., Yfantopoulous, J., and Kosmidis, H.V. Death of a child at home or in hospital: Experiences of Greek mothers. *Death Stud* 1996;20(3):215–35.

32. Lauer, M.E., Mulhern, R.K., Schell, M.J., and Camitta, B. Long term follow up of parental adjustment following a child's death at home or in hospital. *Cancer* 1989;63(5):988–94.

33. Kirk, S. and Glendinning, C. *Supporting Families Caring for a Technology-Dependent Child in the Community*. National Primary Care Research and Development Centre, Manchester, 2000.

34. Association for Children with Life Threatening or Terminal Conditions and their Families. *Assessment of Children with Life Limiting Conditions and Their Families: A Guide to Effective Care Planning*. Published by ACT: Bristol, 2003.

35. Levy, M., Duffy, C.M., Pollock, P., Budd, E., Caulfield, L., and Koren, G. Home based palliative care for children—part 1: the institution of the programme. *J Palliat Care* 1990;6(1):11–15.

36. Kopecky, E.A., Jacosbson, S., Joshi, P., Martin, M., and Koren, G. Review of a home-based palliative care programme for children with malignant and non-malignant diseases. *J Palliat Care* 1997; 13(4):28–33.

37. Kirk, S. and Glendinning, C. Supporting 'expert' patents-professional support and families caring for a child with complex health care needs in the community. *Int J Nurs Stud* 2002;39(6):625–35.

38. Witte, R.A. The psychological impact of a progressive physical handicap and terminal illness (Duchenne muscular dystrophy) on adolescents and their families. *Bri J Med Psychol* 1985;58:179–87.

39. Chamba, R. *et al. On the Edge: Minority Ethnic Families Caring for a Severely Disabled Child* for the Joseph Rowntree Foundation, 1999.

40. Firth, S. Wider Horizons: Care of the dying in a multicultural society. *National Council for Hospice and Specialist Palliative Care Services*, London, 2001.

41. Barrell, S. *Brothers and Sisters: How to Held Siblings of Very Sick and Disabled Children*. Published by Sarah Barrell, Oxfordshire, 2002.

42. Contro, N., Larrson, J., Scofield, S., Sourkes, B., and Cohen, H. Family perspectives on the quality of paediatric palliative care. *Arch Paediat Adolesc Med* 2002;156(1):14–19.

43. Beresford, B. *Positively parents: Caring for a severely disabled child*. York: Social Policy Research Unit, 1994.

44. Woolley, H., Stein, A., Forrest, G., and Baum J. Imparting the diagnosis of life threatening illness in children. *BMJ* 1989;298:1623–6.

45. Wolfe, J., Klar, N., Grier, H.E., Duncan, J., Salem-schatz, S., Emanuel, E.J. *et al.* Understanding of prognosis amongst parents of children who died of cancer; impact on treatment goals and integration of palliative care. *JAMA* 2000;284(19):2469–75.

46. Nitschke, R., Humphrey, B., Sexauer, C., Catron, B., Wunder, S., and Jay, S. Therapeutic choices made by patients with end stage cancer. *J Pediat* 1982;101(3):471–6.

47. Thornes R. *Care of Dying Children and Their Families*. National Association of Health Authorities and Trusts, Birmingham, 1988.

48. Purssell Edward. Telling dying children about their impending death. *Bri J Nurs* 1994;3(3):119–20.

49. Mitchell, W. and Sloper, P. Information that informs rather than alienates families with disabled children: Developing a model of good practice. *Health Soc Care the Commun* 2002;10(2):74–81.

50. Parker, D., Maddocks, I., and Stern, L.M. The role of palliative care in advanced muscular dystrophy and spinal muscular atrophy. *J Paediatr Child Health* 1999;35(3):245–50.

51. Mukherjee, S., Beresford, B., and Sloper, P. *Unlocking key working. An analysis and evaluation of key worker services for families and disabled children* 1999; Joseph Rowntree Trust and Community Care. The Policy Press Bristol.

52. Stein, A. and Woolley, H. An evaluation of hospice care for children. In J.D. Baum, *et al.* eds. *Listen my Child has a Lot of Living to do* 1990; Oxford: Oxford University Press.

53. Mari Lloyd Williams ed. *Psychosocial Issues in Palliative Care*. Oxford: Oxford University Press, 2003.

54. Bignold, S., Ball S., and Cribb, A. *Nursing families with children with cancer: the work of the Paediatric Oncology Outreach Nurse Specialists*. Kings College London, Cancer Relief Macmillan Fund & Department of Health 1994.

55. Martinson, I.D., Moldow, D.G., Armstrong, G.D., Henry, W.F., Nesbit, M.E., and Kersey, J.H. Themes from a longitudinal study of family reactions to childhood cancer. *J Psychosoc Oncol* 1986;6:81–98.

56. Mount, B.M. and Mc Harg, L.F. The Montreal children's palliative care assessment committee report. In J.D. Morgan ed. *The Dying and the Bereaved Teenager*. Charles press, 1987.

57. Lauer, M.E., Mulhern, R.K., Wallskog, J.M., and Camitta, B.H. Children's percepton of their sibling's death at home or in hospital: The precursors of differential adjustment. *Cancer Nursing* 1985; 8(1):21–7.

58. Lambrenos, K. Families with a child on PICU-decision and consequences. Presentation to the Northwest Paediatric Palliative Care Forum, Liverpool 2004.

59. Noyes, J. Barriers that delay children and young people who are dependent on mechanical ventilators from being discharged from hospital. *J Clin Nurs* 2002;11(1):2–11.

60. Association for Children with life threatening or terminal conditions and their families and The Royal College of Paediatrics and Child Health. A Guide to the Development of Children's Palliative Care Services. Act, Bristol 2003.

61. Katz, S. and Kessel, L. Grandparents of children with developmental disabilities: perceptions beliefs and involvement in their care. *Issues Comprehens Paediatr Nurs* 2002;25(2):113–28.

62. Harding, R., Leam, C., Pearce, A., Taylor, E., and Higginson, I.J. A multiprofessional short term intervention for informal caregivers of patients using a home palliative care service. *J Palliat Care* 2002; 18(4):275–81.

63. Hudson, P., Aranda, S., and McMuray, N. Intervention development for enhanced lay palliative caregiver support—the use of focus groups. *Eur J Cancer Care* 2002;11(4):262–70.

64. McCorkle, R. and Pasacreta, J.V. Enhancing caregiver outcomes in palliative care. *Cancer Control* 2001;8(1):36–45.

65. McGrath, P. Trained volunteers for families coping with a child with a life-limiting condition. *Child and Family Soc Work* 2001; 6(1):23–9.

66. Putt and McElhill. More needs than most. *Dealing with the family's economic and practical needs when a child has a chronic life-threatening or terminal condition*. London: Whiting and Birch, 1995.

67. Linter, S., Perry, M., and Cherry, D. Continuing care: An integrated approach. *Paediatr Nurs* 2000;12(8):17–18.

68. Horrocks, S., Somerset, M., and Salisbury, C. Do children with a non-malignant life-threatening conditions receive effective palliative care? A pragmatic evaluation of a local service. *Palliat Med* 2002;16:410–16.

69. Martinson, I.M., Armstrong, G.D., Geis, D.P., *et al.* Home care for the child dying from cancer. *Pediatrics* 1978;62(1):106–113.

70. Hain, R.D.W. Paediatric palliative care: The view from a bridge. *Eur J Pallat Care* 2002;9(2):75–7.

71. Finlay, I. and McQuillan, R. Paediatric palliative care: The role of an adult palliative care service. *Palliat Med* 1995;9:179–80.

72. McKeogh, M. Palliative care for children: Role of an adult palliative care service (correspondance). *Palliat Med* 1996;10:51–4.

73. Davies, R.E. The Diana community nursing team and paediatric palliative care. *Bri J Nurs* 1999;8(8):506,508–11.

74. Davies, R.E. and Harding, Y. The first Diana team in Wales: An update. *Paediatr Nurs* 2002;14(2):24–5.

75. Liben, S. and Goldman, A. Home care for children with life-threatening illness. *J Palliat Care* 1998;14(3):33–8.

76. Anonymous. Doctor, help! My child has cancer. *BMJ* 1999;319: 554–6.

77. Seale, C. Community nurses and the care of the dying. *Soc Sci Med* 1992;34(4).

78. Cartwright, A. The relationship between general practitioners, hospital consultants and community nurses when caring for people in the last year of their lives. *Family Prac* 1991;8(4):350–5.

79. Craft, A. Children with complex health care needs—supporting the child and family in the community. *Child: Care Health Dev* 2004;30(3):191–2.

80. Lenton, S. Franck, L., and Salt, A. Children with complex health care needs: Supporting the child and family in the community. *Child: Care Health and Dev* 2004;30(3):191–2.

81. Csikai, E.L. Social worker's participation in the resolution of ethical dilemmas in hospice care. *Health and Soc Work* 2004;29(1):67–76.

82. Sheldon, F. Dimensions of the role of the social worker in palliative care. *Palliat Med* 2000;14(6):491–8.

83. Christ, G.H. Sormanti, M. Advancing social work practice in end of life care. *Social work in Health Care* 1999;30(2):81–9.

84. Payne, S. and Haines, R. The contribution of psychologists to specialist palliative care. *International J Palliat Nurs* 2002;8(8):401–6.

85. NICE. *Improving Outcorners Guidance for Palliative and Supportive Care for Adults with Cancer*. Guidance for Supportive and Palliative Care Services for Patients with Cancer, 2004.

86. Montagnini, M, Lodhi, M., and Born, W. The utilization of physical therapy in a palliative care unit. *J Palliat Med* 2003;6(1):11–7.

87. Santiago-Palma, J. and Payne, R. Palliative care and rehabilitation. *Cancer* 2001;92(4 Suppl.):1049–52.

88. Marcant, D. and Rapin, CH. Role of the physiotherapist in palliative care. *J Pain Symptom Manage* 1993;8(2):68–71.

89. Westwood, A.T. Terminal care in cystic fibrosis: Hospital versus home? [Comment] Pediatrics 102 (2 pt 1); 436; *Pediatrics* 1997; 100(2 pt 1):205–9.

90. Gilbar, P. and Stefaniuk, K. The role of the pharmacist in palliative care: Results of a survey conducted in Australia and Canada. *J Pallia Care* 2002;18(4):287–92.

91. Needham, D.S., Wong, I.C., Campion, P.D., Hull, and East Riding Pharmacy Development Group. Evaluaiton of the effectiveness of UK community pharmacists interventions in community palliative care. *Palliat Med* 2002;16(3):219–25.

92. Lucas, C., Glare, P.A., and Sykes, J.V. Contribution of a liaison clinical pharmacist to an inpatient palliative care unit. *Palliat Med* 1997;11(3):209–16.

93. The Shipman Enquiry-Fourth Report: The Regulation of controlled Drugs in the Community. HMSO, 2004.

94. Every Child Matters: Change for children. HMSO, 2004.

95. Jeffrey, D. Education in palliative care: A qualitative evaluation of the present state and the needs of general practitioners and community nurses. *Eur J Cancer Care* 1994;3(2):67–74.

96. Shelley. *Everybody here? Play and leisure for disabled children*. Contact a family: London, 2002.

97. Lavelle, Education and the sick child. In L. Hill, ed. *Care for dying children and their families*, Chapman and Hall, London, 1994.

98. Myers Kathryn. Flying home; helping patients to arrange international air travel. *Eur J Palliat Care* 1999;6(5):158–61.

99. Association of Children's Hospices. *Annual data collection summary: 1st April 2002–31st March 2003*. Association of Children's Hospices, Bristol 2003.

100. Addington-Hall, J. and Karlsen, S. Do home deaths increase distress in bereavement?. *Palliat Med* 2000;14:161–1.

101. Sirkia, K., Saarinen-Pihkala, U.M., and Hovi, L. Coping of parents and siblings with the death of a child with cancer; death after terminal care compared with the death during active anticancer treatment. *Acta Paediatrica* 2000;89(6):717–21.

102. Bowling, A. Research on dying is scanty [letter]. *BMJ* 2000;320: 1205–6.

103. Lauer, M. and Camitta, B. Home care for dying children: A nursing model. *J Pediatrics* 1980;97(6):1032–35.

104. Ellershaw, John, Foster Alison, Murphy Deborah, Shea Tom, Overill Susan. Developing an integrated care pathway for the dying patient. *Eur J Palliat Care* 1997;46:203–7.

105. Chambers, E.J., Oakhill, A., Cornish, J.M., *et al.* Terminal care at home for children with cancer. *BMJ* 1989;298:937–40.

106. Youngblut, J.M. and Lauzon, S. Family functioning following paediatric intensive care unit hospitalisation. *Issues Comprehens Paediatr Nurs* 1995;18(1):11–25.

107. Reed, S.B. Potential for alterations in family process: When a family has a child with cystic fibrosis. *Issues Comprehen Paediatr Nurs* 1990;13(1):15–23.

108. McCallum, D., Byrne, P., and Bruera, E. How children die in hospital. *J Pain Symptom Manage* 2000;20(6):417–23.

109. Goldman, A., Beardsmore, S., and Hunt, J. Palliative care for children with cancer—Home, hospital or hospice? *Arch Dis Childhood* 1990;65:641–3.

110. Dominica, F. The role of the hospice for the dying child. *Brit J Hosp Med* 1987;(October):335–43.

111. Levetown, M. Facing decisions about life and death—communication with parents. *Bioethics Forum* 2002;18(34):16–22.

112. Ronald Macdonald House Charities. www.rmhc.com/mission/rmhs/index.html.

113. Burns, J.P., Mitchell, C., Outwater, K.M. *et al.* End-of-life care in the pediatric intensive care unit after the forgoing of life-sustaining treatment. *Crit Care Med* 2000;28(8):3060–6.

114. Kisker, C.T., Fethke, C.C., and Tannous, R. Shared management of children with cancer. *Arch Paediatr Adolesc Med* 1997;151(10):1008–13.

115. Burke, S., Kaufamann, E., Costello, E., and Dillon, M. Hazardous secrets and reluctantly taking charge: Parenting a child with repeated hospitalisations. *Image: J Nurs Scholarship* 1991;23:39–45.

116. Hayes, V. and Knox, J. The experience of stress in parents of children hospitalised with long-term disabilities. *J Adv Nurs* 1984;9:333–41.

117. Feudtner, C., Hays, R.M., Haynes, G., Geyer, J.R., Neff, J.M., and Koepsell, T.D. Deaths attributed to pediatric complex chronic conditions: National trends and implications for supportive care services. *Pediatrics* 2001;107(6):E99.

118. Klopfenstein, K.J., Hutchinson, C., Clark, C., Young, D., and Ruymann, F.B. Variables infuencing end-of-life care in children and adolescents with cancer. *J Paediat Hematol Oncol* 2001;23(8):481–6.

119. Feudtner, C., Christakis, D.A., Zimmerman, F.J., Muldoon, J.H., Neff, J.M., and Koepsell, T.D. Characteristics of deaths occurring in children's hospitals: Implications of supportive care services. *Pediatrics* 2002;109(5):887–93.

120. Whittam, E. Terminal care of the dying child: Psychosocial implications of care. *Cancer* 1993;71(10 Suppl.):3450–62.

121. Whittle, M. and Cutts, S. Time to go home: Assisting familes to take their child home following a planned hospital or hospice death. *Paediatr Nurs* 2002;14(10):24–28.

122. Meyer, E.C., Burns, J.P., Griffith, J.L., and Truog, R.D. Parental perspectives on end of life care in the paediatric intensive care unit. *Crit Care Med* 2002;30(1):226–31.

123. Dominica, F. Helen House a Hospice for Children. *Matern Child Health* 1982;355–9.

124. Venables, J., O'Hare, B.A.M., Nalubeg, J.F., Nakakeeto, M., and Southall, D.P. HIV Palliative care: Lessons from and African mobile hospice. *Arch Dis Childhood* 2003;88(Suppl. 1):A62.

125. Brady. Symptom control in dying children. In L. Hill, ed. *Care for Dying Children and their Families*. London: Chapman and Hall, 1994.

126. Association of Children's Hospices. *Guidelines for Good Practice in a Children's Hospice*. Association of Children's Hospices, Bristol, 2001.

127. National Council for Hospice and Specialist Palliative Care Services / The Association for Children with Life-Threatening or Terminal Conditions & their Families (ACT)/Royal College of Paediatrics and Child Health (RCPCH). *Palliative Care for Children—Joint Briefing*, 2001.

128. Amery, J. and Lapwood, S. A study into the educational needs of children's hospice doctors: a descriptive quantitative and qualitative survey educations needs of hospice GPS. *Palliat Med* 2004;18(8):727–33.

36   Intensive care units

Stephen Liben and Tom Lissauer

Introduction

The vision of pediatric and neonatal intensive care is to bring together all the resources of modern medicine, from the latest in high technology equipment to cutting edge treatment protocols in order to fight a common enemy, death. The considerable resources society is prepared to invest in intensive care reflects the high value our society places on saving children from death. Intensive care has succeeded in transforming what was miraculous 20–30 years ago into the commonplace, whether it is supporting extremely low birth weight babies weighing less than 1000 grams, or enabling children with transplanted hearts, kidneys, and livers to survive, or taking over the function of the lungs and heart with innovative technologies.

Given the enormous success of pediatric and neonatal intensive care in saving children from a premature death it may initially appear that palliative care is not needed in intensive care units (ICUs). However, even in the most advanced and well-equipped ICUs death still occurs. Indeed, it is in ICUs, the place where most critically ill children are brought together, that the greatest number of hospitalized children die. It is therefore in ICUs that there is considerable potential for applying the principles of palliative care to both minimize the suffering of children and provide the best possible support to their families. Simply put, if palliative care decreases pain and suffering of dying children and their families, and the ICU is where many children die, then palliative care needs to be in the ICU.

Children dying in intensive care and their families need to be cared for by healthcare professionals who can provide not only everything that modern medicine can deliver to maintain life, but also all that palliative medicine has learned about how to minimize suffering at the end of life. This chapter will outline the ways in which palliative care can be integrated into the care of the critically ill child in both pediatric and neonatal intensive care units.

Development of paediatric and neonatal intensive care

Paediatric intensive care is a relatively recent addition to paediatric medicine. It began in earnest once children who could no longer breathe on their own could be placed on mechanical ventilators. Initially (in the 1950s) these children were cared for in post-anaesthesia units, most often by paediatric anaesthesiologists who were the first 'paediatric intensive care specialists'. During this period the advent of cardio-pulmonary bypass allowed surgeons to operate on the small sized pediatric heart while a bypass machine perfused the remainder of the body. Paediatric intensive care units (PICUs) were developed to manage children following the many types of complex surgery that can now be performed on children, as well as to care for children who have become critically ill from trauma, of from medical illness. Intensive care units are usually located in specialist children's hospitals.

During the 1970s, many of the technological advances used in older children and adults were adapted for newborn babies and neonatal intensive care units (NICUs) were developed. They are more widespread than PICUs as 1–2% of newborn infants require intensive care and 8–10% of all newborn infants are admitted to a special care baby unit.

The widespread use of mechanical ventilation for respiratory failure and the ability to maintain organ perfusion with extracorporeal life support when the heart is no longer beating and the brain is no longer functioning have progressed so far and so fast that at present it is possible to maintain a child in a state somewhere between life and death for a prolonged period. This has created a situation where a child's death can be delayed by intervening with invasive technological support. Along with this ability to delay death has come the need for the intensive care physician to decide whether to withdraw mechanical life-support and allow death to follow. This ability to postpone death has created numerous ethical and moral dilemmas, many of which remain unresolved (see ethics section).

Causes and mode of death in PICU

A medium sized PICU with 800 admissions per year and a 5% mortality rate will experience almost a death per week and in a large PICU there may be as many as 2 deaths per week. A study of all in-patient paediatric hospital deaths showed that the majority are young; with 75% less than 4 years old, most had received invasive therapies such as mechanical ventilation and over 75% died while comatose and sedated in ICUs [1]. In the PICU the most common mode of death is from active withdrawal of therapy (removing a mechanical ventilator, stopping cardiac inotropic and vasopressor medications) or following decisions to not attempt cardio-pulmonary resuscitation [2].

Over half of the children who die in a PICU do so after a very brief illness such as trauma, drowning and infection. Most were previously healthy and the time course to death is incredibly fast with a mean of 3–4 days between admission and death. These families have very little time to come to terms with their child's death. This contrasts with the approximately one third of deaths in children with complex chronic illness such as congenital malformations, neurological problems, cancer, metabolic disease, immune-deficiencies, and respiratory illnesses and whose families have had forewarning that their child may die [3].

Causes and mode of death in NICU

Although the number of deaths in NICUs has fallen markedly over the last 20 years, a medium sized unit will experience about 24 deaths/year. Most, 70%, are because of prematurity, but some are because of congenital malformations or following birth asphyxia [4].

Although 42% of infants died naturally, 40% died following withdrawal of life-support and in 15% following do-not-resuscitate orders. Although life support therapy is often withdrawn when death is inevitable to avoid unnecessary suffering of both infant and family, in others, particularly infants with brain damage relating to prematurity or birth asphyxia, it involves difficult judgments about likely long-term outcome and quality of life. Physician attitude and practices under these circumstances differ markedly in different countries [5].

Decision to withdraw life-support technology

The default treatment mode of intensive care is that all interventions and technologies, no matter the extent of their immediate short-term (and possible medium- and long-term) unpleasantness, are performed in order to sustain life. Decisions to limit life-sustaining therapies range from 'do not escalate orders' that maintain current life-sustaining therapies already in place, to active withdrawal of life-sustaining technologies (most commonly mechanical ventilation). How and why decisions are made to either 'not escalate' or to 'actively withdraw' life-sustaining therapies depends on carefully balanced judgments that include potential for recovery, current and future quality of life, burden of pain and suffering imposed by life-sustaining technologies, and cultural and religious attitudes and beliefs of parents and professional caregivers. This decision making has become more complex because of the:

- Increased number of professional caregivers making co-ordination and agreement in decision making more difficult
- Wish by parents and family to be active participants in decision making rather than relying on healthcare professionals
- Increased reluctance by some parents to accept withdrawal of life-support for religious reasons (Muslim, orthodox Jews, fundamentalist Christians) or unwillingness to accept predictions or advice of physicians
- Fear of litigation or use of the media by parents.

The senior (attending) physician needs to not only co-ordinate decision making between the professionals caring for the child and between the caregivers and the family, but also to manage the timing of the decision making. Nurses, physicians and families may take different lengths of time to reach their decision and may cause considerable tension within the unit.

Where there is disagreement between the physicians and family an independent second opinion may be helpful. Rarely, when agreement cannot be achieved, the case will need to be referred to the Court. Recent high-profile cases in the United Kingdom have included the refusal by parents to agree to withdrawal of mechanical ventilation in an infant with Trisomy 18 who had multiple congenital abnormalities including severe brain damage and a 1-year-old ex-preterm, permanently hospitalized infant with very severe lung disease and several admissions to PICU and where the PICU was refusing to reventilate if respiratory failure developed. These issues are considered further in Chapter 4 on Ethics.

Incorporating palliative care principles in the ICU

Given the very broad range of issues surrounding end-of-life care in the ICU how can the principles of palliative care be applied to ease the burden of suffering for children who die in the ICU and that of their families?

Communication

Good communication between the healthcare team and the parents is crucial. There are a number of key elements for this to be achieved.

Staff communication

Staff communication is an ongoing challenge because of the large number of professional caregivers involved in the child's care. Providing consistent information is problematic but important as parents find even minor differences in information confusing and upsetting. Detailed handovers are therefore required. Parents need to understand the different roles performed by the numerous members of the healthcare team so that they can direct their questions appropriately, for example, details about the day's events are best answered by the nurse caring for their child while questions about management decisions should be posed to the primary physician. This exchange of information is also required to avoid professional caregivers repeatedly asking the family the same questions. A regular weekly multidisciplinary meeting (or round) is helpful to allow the views of team members other than the nurses and doctors to be heard and also because they allow due consideration on aspects of care other than the biological/physiological status of the child.

As the ultimate decision making falls to a senior ICU (attending) physician, it is important that parents have a clear understanding of who is the attending physician for their child. Because the care of a critically ill child may involve many teams of physicians over periods of time (e.g. the separate subspecialty teams involved in a post operative cardiac newborn with renal failure, on total parenteral nutrition, with sepsis and seizures), it can be difficult for parents to consistently identify one physician who assumes the role of primary decision maker and communicator with the family. In some ICU's parents are present during daily medical rounds and get to hear for themselves first hand accounts of what the medical assessment and plans are for their child. In other units parents are not present for rounds and physicians have a separate meeting with parents to ensure communication. Whatever the system used in a particular ICU, it is important that there is a predictable way for parents to communicate with their child's

attending physician. Many units also have an identified nurse who is responsible for co-ordinating nursing care on a long-term basis.

For children or families that have been followed long-term by a primary care physician (or family doctor) it is both important and helpful to ensure that the family is given the option of their continuing input. On admission to the ICU it is helpful to establish whom the family identifies as trusted caregivers in the past and with whom they wish to have an ongoing relationship. Including these non-ICU caregivers in important decision making situations can help to establish trust between the child/family and ICU staff who they may be meeting for the first time.

Communication with children and adolescents

The majority of children who die in the ICU do not have the ability to communicate verbally because they were either pre-verbal due to their young age or non-verbal because of their pre-existing medical condition. For verbal children communication is still very limited during their illness in the ICU because of the illness itself or the life-support technology. This means that these children are often deprived of the opportunity for parents to explain to them about their illness and impending death or for them to talk with their parents about their fears, wishes, dreams, hopes and desires about their life in general and about their possible death in particular.

In the ICU communication between staff and family can become complicated when the patient is a verbal adolescent who has issues he or she wishes to keep private from the parents, and with parents who want medical staff to talk to them first before speaking to their child. Although the legal status of adolescents of a certain age may help clarify rights this does not necessarily reflect nor respect how a family may have managed communication in their own home and according to their own strongly held familial and cultural beliefs. In these difficult situations a careful balance must be made between the patients' rights and respecting individual family dynamics. It can be helpful to have mechanisms in place for patients and families to have designated staff to speak to if they wish to voice their concerns. Some hospitals have an ombudsman or patient representative that may serve to help defuse high-tension situations.

Extended family

Parents may wish healthcare professionals to talk to their extended family, especially grandparents or the parents' brothers or sisters. However, a study that looked at the relative value that parents placed amongst different people involved in important decisions for their children in PICU (staff versus extended family) found that it was the staff that the family found the most helpful and supportive around difficult decisions such as removing life supporting therapy [6]. Parents stated that the only ones who 'really knew what was really going on' were PICU staff and they placed a very high level of trust and power on professional caregivers in decision making even though they had known them for only a short period of time.

Confidentiality

Occasionally a balance has to be struck between the need for communication among many members of the team and the family's need for privacy and confidentiality. It is then best to ensure that family has agreed to what information can be shared.

The unit of care is the child and family

Having a supportive team that is available to focus on the psychological, emotional and spiritual issues that children and families with life-threatening illness face is an essential component of intensive care. The same composition of teams needed to provide psychological, social and spiritual support in hospice care is needed in neonatal and pediatric intensive care units. It should be a basic principle of intensive care that the emotional, psychological and spiritual needs of children and families in crisis need to be addressed on a regular (as opposed to as required) basis. Seen in this light the presence of trained personnel to support the mind and soul of both the child and their family becomes an essential component of intensive care.

While it is important to provide supportive care to family members who are confronted with the possible death of their child, parents also emphasize the importance of the physical environment on their well being and ability to adapt and cope with what is for most of them the most traumatic experience of their lives. Physical facilities for parents such as showers, family rooms for overnight accommodation and kitchenettes together with open visiting policies help to make the point that parents are not 'visitors' but are rather the key people with the most at stake in their child's illness. For parents who are confronted by the possible death of their child for the first time the ICU environment can be a confusing place. The multiple rotating caregivers, lack of privacy, and total disruption of daily life routine coupled with a busy bright physical environment make for a disorienting experience. It can be helpful to have pre-prepared written materials for parents that explain the structure, hierarchy, and options available to them. Another useful resource for families is access to books, videos and web sites that are relevant to their own situation.

Siblings can be helped to cope with their brother or sister's death by being given the opportunity to help with their care in a supervised manner. ICUs can facilitate this by having visiting policies that encourage parents to bring siblings for short visits. For example, a young sibling may be provided with crayons and paper to make a drawing for their sick brother or sister. Older siblings may choose to write a message to be placed with their sibling. Child-life specialists (play-specialists) can be especially helpful in creating the space for siblings to be involved and to assist them express and come to terms with their sibling's illness or possible death.

Whole person/child care

Hospice/palliative care places a high value on care of the *whole* person that recognizes the importance of body, mind, and soul. Traditionally most ICUs have been developed to focus on care of the body with varying degrees of emphasis on other aspects of the child as a whole person.

When cure is no longer possible and the child is likely to die a shift in goals can be helpful for the child and their family as well as for healthcare professionals. Whole-person care is one means to re-establish hope and meaning in their care. While most ICU professionals are adept in reducing pain caused by bodily symptoms, they may have less training in addressing the suffering that results from unresolved existential, psychological, emotional, and spiritual issues. Palliative whole-person care emphasizes the ability to heal even when cure is no longer possible. In adult palliative care there is much literature on how adults can die 'healed' [7]. While dying 'healed' may be an unrealistic goal for many children in the ICU there is still much to be gained by addressing issues related to the child's and the family's emotional and spiritual needs. The beginning of addressing these needs begins with an assessment of the child and the family as whole persons. In practice this evaluation of the whole person means asking questions not necessarily traditionally addressed in paediatric critical care such as:

- What is the most important thing in your life right now?
- What is happening in the ICU that is stopping you from making the most of the time you have with your child right now?
- Are there important celebrations that you would consider having in the ICU very soon, even before the 'real' date? (e.g. birthdays, Christmas, etc . . .)

Establishing the child and family's priorities, what *really* matters to them *right now*, is often a catalyst for ICU staff to align their caregiving in ways that help meet the most urgent needs of the child and family. For example, some families focus on trying to ensure that their ill child survives in order to be present at important milestone holidays. It can be suggested to such families that they consider celebrating an important holiday or birthday now, instead of waiting for the correct chronological date on the calendar. Should the child survive until the 'real' date then families are often more than happy to celebrate the occasion again. This approach of doing whatever the family feels is important to them now, instead of later, can help to relieve pressure.

For some families of children in the PICU it may have always been very important to have a story read to the child at bedtime. Parents can be encouraged to continue this process even in the PICU. Some parents may like the idea of audiotaping themselves either singing or reading a story so that an audiotape can be played to their baby or child when they are absent from the unit.

Pain and symptom management

With some ill neonates and children it is unclear, both to family members and to professional caregivers, when the child is in pain. Meeting together to discuss how parents and staff assess the child's expression of pain in different ways can help to prepare a care plan that respects both professional expertise on pain assessment while acknowledging that parents have unique insights into their own children [8]. Many children in the ICU receive continuous infusions of sedatives and analgesics that were started either post-operatively or at the initiation of mechanical ventilation. Some children are placed on continuous or regular intermittent doses of neuromuscular blockers (NMB) that result in muscle relaxation and paralysis of skeletal muscle without any analgesic or sedative effects. Children on neuromuscular blocking drugs will not move and cannot breathe on their own. In most circumstances it is possible and desirable to interrupt the use of regular neuromuscular blockers in order to assess the level of comfort and sedation of the child [9]. In situations where the child has undergone an acute neurological event it may be difficult for both parents and staff to appreciate the level of neurological function in the presence of high doses of sedative/analgesics. In these circumstances carefully lowering the amount of sedation can allow for a better evaluation of the level of consciousness and amount of pain the child may be experiencing. There is no indication or rationale for increasing sedatives just because the child 'has suffered enough'. Rather the point of sedative/ analgesic administration is to respond to pain by first assessing its cause and intensity and then to selectively apply pain management principles as would be done for any child in pain whether they are 'palliative' or not.

Non-pharmacological pain management techniques can be adapted for use in the ICU. Massage therapy, music therapy, and art therapy for older children who are conscious, and even zoo therapy may sometimes be possible in certain circumstances. Less complex and at no cost but perhaps the most powerful way to help both child and parent are to not only allow but encourage parents to hold their critically ill child in their arms even whilst the child remains connected to a ventilator and many infusion pumps. For parents of ill newborns this may be the only time they get a chance to hold their own child in their arms and may be a powerful experience that would not have happened without the encouragement of the ICU staff.

Setting goals

Acknowledging that a child is terminally ill is especially difficult in an intensive care environment. An advantage of doing so is that all diagnostic tests and therapies are directed towards a common goal: to increase the comfort and quality of life of the child (as opposed to the usual goal of striving to maintain life). For example, a child who suffered an anoxic insult with subsequent seizures will clearly be more comfortable not seizing and therefore the use of anti-convulsants is indicated even if the child is terminally ill, but should the same child develop pneumonia the question of the use of antibiotics is less clear and requires thoughtful and sensitive discussion about benefits and burdens of therapy. However, *one should avoid an order for 'no tests' or 'do not escalate' placed in the chart but rather* do everything possible to ensure maximum comfort and quality of life for the child. Seen in this light a palliative care philosophy is congruent with good medical care and is based on a positive attitude of doing as much as possible to meet agreed goals that serve to make the most of the life of the terminally ill child.

As the time of death approaches

There are children who die in the ICU with little prior warning for parents. Examples are neonates born at term but who die unexpectedly from birth complications, sepsis or have congenital heart or other congenital abnormalities; in older children it may be from severe trauma or sepsis. Another group are children with known conditions that were thought to be stable. For these children there may be little or no time available to plan for how death will occur and palliative care may have more to offer the family survivors after the child has died. In one review of circumstances surrounding end of life in a PICU it was found that decisions to forgo life-sustaining treatment required one or two meetings before consensus was reached [10]. For the many children who die in the ICU after a decision to withdraw life-sustaining therapies it is often possible to guide families as to what to expect and to offer options for different ways that the end of life can happen.

As the time of withdrawal of life-sustaining therapies approaches the family may appreciate being transferred to a private room. For some families it is important that the extended family get to say goodbye and hold the child in their arms before extubation. For other families it may be important to have very few people present in the room at the time of withdrawal. Some ICU's take pictures of the child and family, make footprints of infants, and cut a locket of hair to keep as physical mementos. Some families are keen for the child to go home or to a hospice on ventilator support with removal of the ventilator occurring once the child is at home or hospice [11]. However there are considerable logistic and staffing implications in achieving this and the proportion of children transferred out of intensive care units to the community is small.

For some families it may be important to wait for an important loved one to be present before they die. Many parents find it both hard and at the same time comforting to have their child in their arms before and while the tracheal tube is being removed. Some mothers have commented that they were present for the entry of their child into the world and they want to be present when they leave. The discussion as to what would be the best environment to die is not an easy one for all involved and yet decisions made from this discussion may remain important memories for all those involved for years to come. What is important is to discuss with the family what may be most meaningful to them and not to assume that we know their needs.

An approach to ventilator withdrawal

Once the decision has been made to withdraw mechanical ventilatory support the child and family should be guided through how the process will unfold. It is important to be sure that family, as well as ICU staff, understand that the child is not having *care* withdrawn, but is instead having a treatment removed that no longer has more benefits than burdens. For children on full ventilator support it is important to establish a plan for the control of dyspnoea and secretions upon withdrawal of the ventilator [12]. One approach to ventilator withdrawal is as follows:

1. Carefully titrate opioids and sedatives until the child is comfortable *prior to* changing respiratory settings.

2. Ensure adequate access (intravenous, rectal, subcutaneous) and prepare several doses for the administration of additional opioids and sedatives in the case of increasing pain or distress.

3. Once doses of medications are stable and the child is comfortable (i.e. no pain or dyspnea, secretions easily suctioned) then turn off oxygen saturation and heart rate monitors. There are two reasons for turning off or removing monitors. One is that once the ventilator is withdrawn the alarms will repeatedly go off and become the centre of everyone's focus rather than on being with the child. The second is that the monitors are no longer helpful in managing pain and symptom control as the best gauge of dyspnoea is not a pulse oxymeter but the facial expression and clinical respiratory effort of the child. If parents prefer monitoring to be continued the alarms should be deactivated.

4. Based on previous discussions with the family have all those who wish to be present in the room together and explain what is happening step by step. This is usually the role of the senior attending physician, with the nurse and any key healthcare worker also present. A junior doctor may also be present to learn how to carefully and respectfully withdraw a ventilator and support a family through a very difficult time.

5. Decrease the ventilator settings gradually (respiratory rate and oxygen concentration) while adjusting sedative administration in response to signs of increased dyspnoea or other symptoms. The timing of this decrease in ventilator settings may vary from a few minutes to hours depending on the reasons the child is ventilator-dependent and how they respond to a decrease in mechanical ventilatory assistance.

6. When the child is calm and free of dyspnoea and the ventilator respiratory rate is either at very low rates (e.g. 5 breaths per min) or on continuous positive pressure (CPAP) then the airway should be suctioned and the tracheal tube removed. The ventilator power is then turned off (to avoid alarms ringing).

7. If the child is appropriately medicated to ensure symptom control prior to extubation while on minimal ventilator settings there should not be any sudden change in the child's state of comfort when the tracheal tube is removed. In the rare event of the child's experiencing difficulty breathing with gasping or secretions after extubation the pre-prepared additional doses of sedatives can be administered in doses appropriate to relieve dyspnea.

8. Most children stop breathing within minutes to hours after removal of mechanical ventilation. During this time families may have an opportunity to hold their child without being attached to life-support technologies.

Some children live for unexpectedly prolonged periods once the ventilator is removed. Some may even leave the ICU to the special care nursery or paediatric wards or even go home to live for additional periods of time. Parents must be forewarned about this. Although this rare occurrence is sometimes initially seen as a 'miracle' by parents it may subsequently become a 'burden' for children that continue to live with a poor quality of life.

Some intensivists give extra doses of sedatives just prior to extubation to avoid the possibility of gasping respirations but it is rare for this to occur when taking the stepwise sequence outlined above.

The use of NMBs, which cause muscular paralysis without any effect on sensation, when life support is withdrawn is controversial. There is no role for NMB in symptom control at the end of life, as the child cannot respond to pain. The only way to ensure that a child is not suffering from dyspnoea and pain is by the judicious use of sedatives and analgesics, and occasionally anesthetic agents (e.g. propofol). [13,14]

After the death

(See also Chapter 14, After the child's death, and Chapter 15, Bereavement after death.) Once the child has died families should be allowed to stay with their child in the room until they are ready to leave. Prior to bathing/washing the body ICU staff can remove sutures holding catheters in place and medical devices can be removed. Some parents appreciate being offered the opportunity to clean and bathe the body with staff.

A discussion should take place concerning the possible benefits of an autopsy, which will usually have been considered before death. In some situations an autopsy is mandated by law, otherwise the fact that autopsy examination often reveals additional information needs to be highlighted. Adverse publicity about autopsies regarding the removal and storage of tissue samples and organs has resulted in a marked decline in the autopsy acceptance rate. In the United Kingdom, detailed consent has to be obtained including a description of the procedure and specific agreement obtained about the storage and disposal of tissues and organs and their use for research. Although some parents feel that their child has 'suffered enough' and instinctively want to decline an autopsy, it should be explained that having as complete information as possible is often helpful to fully understand the cause of their child's death and that this may be important for them and their families in the future. This is especially important when the cause of death is uncertain, even though at the time of death they may not appreciate just how much not 'having an answer' may preoccupy them in the future. An autopsy is the only opportunity to settle the question of 'what really happened'. It should be explained that an autopsy does not affect the face

and that when clothed the body's appearance will be unaffected. Parents should be given some time to reflect on the benefits for them and their family of an autopsy before making their decision. Physicians asking for an autopsy should recognize that an autopsy is something that may help to bring some closure to a family and that asking for an autopsy is in the family's best interest. If there is any question of a genetically transmitted disease the results of the autopsy may affect the health of future siblings and generations. For all these reasons, even if parents initially reject an autopsy as they feel that their child has suffered enough, time should be taken to explain again the potential benefits of an autopsy.

Most institutions have a forum for the team to review morbidities and mortalities that happened in the unit. These reviews are often oriented around medical issues pertaining to pathology and symptom control and lessons learnt for the future. They also offer the opportunity to look at the psychological impact of deaths on the families and the healthcare professionals. They also allow staff not on duty at the time of the child's death to be brought up to date and understand the full circumstances surrounding the child's death and to ask questions and consider unresolved issues.

After a child dies there are a number of ways to commemorate the child. One way is for staff to write messages for the family in a card that can be sent to them in the following weeks. This also gives staff who were absent at the time of death the opportunity to offer their condolences to the family. At the same time the staff may wish to create a 'communication book' for the unit in which those who were present at the time of the death can write down what happened as well as their thoughts and feelings about the child. All who knew the child or family can contribute as well.

Another way to commemorate the child is to have a memorial book in the unit, chapel or elsewhere in the hospital. Some families may wish to design a commemorative page in the book, it is an alternative for those families who would like to have a commemorative plaque on the wall but which are usually discouraged as other parents may find this disturbing.

The family needs to be informed of the many different forms of bereavement support available from the hospital or in the community. In addition, all relevant health professionals in the hospital and community need to be informed of the child's death. Some staff may attend the child's funeral. Families are usually appreciative of staff being present. Many units hold memorial services for children who have died in the preceding months. Staff and family attendance and participation can help them cope with their child's death. It can also help staff who were unable to say goodbye to the family after the child's death [15].

The senior physician should arrange to see the family a few weeks after the child's death. It provides an opportunity to review events on the unit and address any unanswered questions about their child's care. Some parents may appreciate telling the 'story' one more time to the doctor who was involved with their child's life at such a vulnerable time. If an autopsy was performed this will need to be reviewed together with an explanation of the significance of its findings. It also allows the physician to review how the family is coping with their bereavement and if additional assistance might be beneficial. [16]

Many families welcome bereavement follow-up from a suitable healthcare professional that knew the family in the intensive care unit. Providing this family counseling requires both training and ongoing support for those who make the often-difficult phone calls and meetings with the bereaved family in the subsequent year or two. Important times to make contact with the family are the child's birthday, anniversary of the death, and during important religious and other holiday periods.

References

1. McCallum, D.E., Byrne, P., and Bruera. How children die in hospital. *J Pain Symptom Manage* 2000;20(6):417–23.
2. Garros, D., Rosychuk, R.J., and Cox, P. Circumstances surrounding end of life in a paediatric intensive care unit. *Paediatrics* 2003;112 (No 5.): e371–e379.
3. Levetown, M., Pollack, M.M., Cuerdon, T.T., Rurrimann, U.E., and Glover, J.J. Limitations and withdrawals of medical intervention in pediatric critical care. *JAMA* 1994;(No 16): 1271–5.
4. Roy, R., Aladangady, N., Costeloe, K., and Larcher, V. Decision Making and Modes of death in a tertiary neonatal unit. *Arch Dis Childhood Fetal Neonatal Ed* 2004;89:F527–F530.
5. Rebagliat, M. *et al.* Neonatal end-of-life decision making: Physicians' attitudes and relationship with self-reported practices in 10 European countries. *JAMA* 2000; 284(2):451–9.
6. Meyer, E.C., Burns, J.P., Griffith, J.L., and Truog, R.D. Parental perspectives on end-of-life care in the PICU. *Crit Care Med* 2002; 30:226–31.
7. Michael Kearney, A. *Place of Healing*, Working with suffering in living and dying. Oxford University Press, 2000.
8. Contro, N., Larson, J., Scofield, S., Sourkes, B., and Cohen, H. Family perspectives on the quality of pediatric palliative care. *Arch Pediatr Adolesc Med* 2002;156:14–19.
9. Hawryluck, L.A., Harevy, W.R.C., Lemieux-Charles, L., and Singer, P.A. Consensus guidelines on analgesia and sedation in dying intensive care unit patients. *BMC Medical Ethics* 2002;3:3.
10. Garros, D., Rosychuk, R.J., and Cox, P. Circumstances surrounding end of life in a pediatric intensive care unit. *Pediatrics* 2003;112(5): e371–e379.
11. Craig, F. and Goldman, A. Home management of the dying NICU patient. *Semin neonat* 2003;8:177–83.
12. von Gunten, C. and Weissman, D.E. Ventilator withdrawal protocol. *J Palliat Med* 2003; 6(5):773–6.
13. Burns, J.P., Mitchell, C., Outwater, K.M. *et al.* End-of-life care in the PICU after the foregoing of life-sustaining treatment. *Crit Care Med* 2000;28(8); 3060–6.
14. Goldstein, B. and Merkens, M. End-of-life in the PICU: Seeking the family's decision of when, not if. *Crit Care Med* 2000;28(8): 3122–3.
15. Macdonald, M.E., Liben, S., Carnevale, F.A., Rennick, J.E., Wolf, S.L., Meloche, D., and Cohen, S.R. Parental persepctives on hospital staff acts of kindness and commemoration after a child's death. *Pediatrics* 2005;116:884–90.
16. Macnab, A.J., Northway, T., Ryall, K., Scott, D., and Straw, G. Death & Bereaevement in a PICU: Parental perceptions of staff support. *Pediatr Child Health* 2003;8(6):357–62.

37 International aspects

Ann Goldman, David Southall, Simon Lenton, and *Nicola Eaton*

Introduction

The global perspective of palliative care, focusing on care for adults, has recently been the topic of two comprehensive reviews [1,2]. These record the expansion of services in the better resourced countries since adult palliative care began in the early 1960s, and strongly emphasize the huge needs remaining in the poorly resourced countries. Comparative information about palliative care in children in different parts of the world is still sparse and preliminary [3–5], though a comprehensive study of hospice and related developments in Eastern Europe, which includes care of children, has recently been published [6]. Current information about the epidemiology of children with life-limiting illnesses has been assessed in Chapter 1.

Many individual paediatric palliative care programmes, in different countries, have been described in the literature, but certainly, even more exist, or are being developed. Currently, the details of many of these individual programmes, and even of the majority of overall situations nationally, are not available. In spite of the additional information generously given through personal communication, the picture we are able to compile here is, without doubt, incomplete. Our apologies to those working on programmes, and in whole countries, whose experiences have not been acknowledged. We would welcome information that will help towards compiling a more comprehensive worldview for the future.

Barriers to care

There is still a very wide variation in awareness and understanding of the philosophy of paediatric palliative care. Even in the countries where there is a growing acknowledgement of its importance, the development of services often lags behind. In those countries where needs seem to have been recognised, services sometimes have evolved primarily in relation to oncology patients, and often, support has only extended to children with other life-limiting illnesses later. As with many new concepts and practices in health care, a determined and persuasive locally based leader in the field, parental pressure and active voluntary organisations have been powerful forces for progress. Home based care, community teams, hospital outreach, respite care, free-standing hospices, and bereavement programmes have all got roles to play. Exactly which evolves in each country, and how quickly paediatric palliative care can move forward, relates to the different barriers formed by culture, geography, health care systems, and, most important of all, resources.

Recognizing the need

Even though the numbers of children dying in resource-rich countries is small compared to adults, this is an insufficient explanation for the lack of acknowledgement of the needs of dying children and their families, both in the literature and in clinical practice. Some professionals and parents can find it difficult to accept the inevitability of a child's death and the need for palliative care; they strive to find further treatment options, sometimes at all costs.

In well resourced countries, the emphasis on technology and the triumphs of medical science have meant that the dying have become, in some ways, a symbol of failure, with their needs neglected. This is particularly so in relation to children. In addition, their care is highly charged emotionally, and brings professionals face to face with their own mortality.

In the majority of poorly resourced countries, despite the fact that there are many children suffering from diseases that are incurable, the concept of palliative care is just not 'awake'. To some extent, this situation relates to the overwhelming need to provide emergency care within poorly funded health systems. Palliative care is still considered a luxury by some.

Understanding the philosophy

Palliative care—an area of medicine on the fringe of the law. (Trethewie, quoting a medical colleague, Personal Communication).

Many professionals still have only a partial or distorted understanding of the current approach to paediatric palliative care. They may hold a very restricted view of its scope as a multidisciplinary holistic practice, and equate it with pain management, opioid use, or even euthanasia. Many do not appreciate how palliative care can benefit the quality of life of children with all life-limiting illnesses, not just cancer. They may not be aware of the flexibility embedded in palliative care, and may not realise that it is not an 'all or nothing' issue, but offers the possibility of running alongside treatments aiming to prolong life, as the situation evolves. Some clinicians may be reluctant to share their patients' care, or discuss the possibilities of palliative care with them. All of these can contribute to lack of referrals, or, to very late referrals, to the detriment of the child's care [7–11].

In some countries, there will be problems with the concept of aiming to relieve suffering, since a number of cultures regard suffering as an important part of living, as something inevitable, and something which should be endured, perhaps to strengthen character, or to ensure a better life in the hereafter. In countries where society accepts heavy corporal punishment in schools, severe physical punishment regimes, and the death sentence, introducing sea changes in attitude to suffering will be a major shift, which may not be welcomed.

Medical supplies and drugs

How will she die if she's not on morphine (Trethewie S quoting a medical colleague, Personal Communication).

Even in resource rich countries where opioids are available, there may be a reluctance to use them appropriately, due to misguided beliefs, ignorance and fear. There is also a lack of understanding about how to use them, with many health professionals still confused about tolerance, physical dependence, and addiction. Others lack even basic knowledge about doses, routes, and side effects.

In many countries, the main problems lie in persuading governments that the drugs used for palliative care, in particular opioids, are inexpensive, and should not only be made available, but provided in a way that is easy to access. Part of the difficulty is related to resources, although many of the essential drugs used in palliative care are not particularly expensive. However, the greatest problem with the provision of drugs relates to attitudes to opioids. Although morphine is the most effective oral and parenteral drug for controlling severe pain, and is recommended by WHO, many countries will not provide the systems necessary to allow it to be used, even in their hospitals, and more particularly, in the community care of patients. Their argument

is that it is a drug of addiction, and therefore, there are potentially major problems in controlling its use. They question whether safe control of the use of these drugs in childhood palliative care is possible. Tragically, many poor countries still have to contend with considerable corruption throughout their systems. When this turns to theft or misappropriation of powerful opioid drugs, there can indeed be serious consequences. However, the processes and systems needed for the introduction of opioids for medical care have been well worked out in many countries, and are not particularly difficult, they just require organisation and acceptance of the importance of making such arrangements. The State has a vital role to play in making it better for children by not restricting or blocking the availability of vital pain-relieving drugs out of security concerns, or outdated and mistaken beliefs about their appropriateness for use in children and the risks of addiction.

Healthcare systems

Many healthcare systems are currently not designed or sufficiently resourced to provide really good palliative care. Governments need to make a formal commitment to develop multidisciplinary care, not only in terms of adequate support for families at home, but also in terms of easy access and excellent communication between hospital and community care. Many countries have not made that decision, and so, although there may be pockets of excellent practice, the truth is that in almost all countries, there is still a heavy reliance on individual initiatives and voluntary organizations, rather than on planned and equitable services.

In addition, some healthcare systems have regulations which seriously limit the practice of good palliative care:

Example 1. There are problems in the United States with reimbursement from insurance systems, as hospice care cannot be funded whilst any curative interventions are still being undertaken. In addition, funding for hospice care is limited rigidly to the last 6 months of life. The current system also acts as a strong disincentive to the provision of palliative care and free-standing children's hospices. [9,12,34]. The lobbying and advocacy of Children's Hospice International is gradually educating the authorities to the special needs of children, enabling more appropriate models of care to be explored.

Example 2. In Canada, home care services in certain provinces are reimbursed according to specific tasks or interventions, and psychosocial care is not viewed or funded as a 'task' (Frager G, Personal Communication).

Lack of education and trained staff

Almost all countries acknowledge that this is a considerable problem. Paediatric palliative care is still a young component of healthcare, and the number of experienced practitioners available as teachers is small. There are few training posts and courses available. In poorly resourced countries, the needs for training are enormous.

Some examples of current practice

From well resourced countries

Australia

Australia has been active in developing paediatric palliative care, with early involvement from oncology services, and also recognition of non-oncology patients' needs [11,13,14]. Some highlights include:

- hospital based specialist teams;
- the development of two children's hospices in Melbourne and Sydney;
- co-operation with adult and community based palliative care at home;
- appointment of specialist paediatric palliative care physicians;
- the establishment of a nurse training programme;
- a physician training fellowship.

Recently an extensive national survey has been undertaken, with wide consultation across all the states, and site visits to 15 different paediatric palliative care agencies [11]. This survey has identified that there are a wide range of models of care across Australia, and that services are unevenly distributed nationally. Families, for the most part, have expressed a preference for children to be cared for, and die, at home. A comprehensive home-based service centred on collaboration, with specialist and hospital-based professionals working together with community and primary care teams, is needed to fulfil a family's wishes. Because of the widely distributed population, it is essential to utilise the already existing adult palliative care network, and strategies are being identified to support this network in working with children and families. For children and families who are cared for in hospital, improvement in appropriate facilities and expertise is needed, to make the experience as comfortable as possible. The review has identified gaps in services, barriers to care, and opportunities for improvements for the future.

Canada

Palliative care has a significant profile in Canada, compared to many countries. Commitment from the Government is evidenced by the Senate's report in 2000, 'Quality End of Life Care: the right of every Canadian' [15]. However, there is still considerable scope for improvement in services for

children, which lag behind adult provisions, particularly for those children with non-malignant life-threatening illnesses. Health care is designated a provincial responsibility, and there continue to be many provinces without formal paediatric palliative care services. Most of the current services are hospital-based consultation teams originating in the major urban centres (for example, Halifax, Montreal, Vancouver, Ottawa, Toronto, Calgary, and Edmonton). These multidisciplinary teams work in the hospitals and liaise and back up local front line services to support families at home. The large geographic areas with scattered population have resulted in some innovative approaches to enable families to be supported at home:

- good collaboration with local paediatric teams and adult palliative care;
- tele-video and audio conference calls;
- site visits requiring overnight stays;
- production of one-to-one videos for teaching specific care for families and local teams;
- Internet network of paediatric palliative care clinicians in Canada.

Canuck Place, Canada's first free-standing residential children's hospice, opened in Vancouver in 1995, and has close links with their hospital team. Further hospices are being developed in Montreal and Toronto.

Germany

The status of palliative care for children in Germany has been assessed through the project PATE (palliative care, therapy and evaluation in paediatric haematology/oncology), which was funded by The German Children's Cancer Fund. It was found that Germany's mortality rate for children from life-threatening illnesses of 1.03/10,000 is similar to mortality rates in the United Kingdom and Poland. The distribution of causes was: cancer, 31%; neuromuscular diseases, 20%; congenital, 16%; cardiovascular, 12%; and metabolic, 9%. They estimate that there are 15,000 children in Germany living with life-threatening illnesses.

There are a range of programmes established in Germany, including hospital-based teams, liaison nurses, home care by nurse-led agencies, and free-standing children's hospices (currently six). The services for children with malignant disease are more extensive, compared to those for children with other illnesses, although even in oncology, comprehensive programmes are not available at all centres. The number of children with malignancy dying at home, if a home care programme was available, was 68%, which compared with a figure of 39% for home deaths in a survey of all children dying from cancer. A comprehensive child- and family-centred model of care for all diagnoses is being introduced at Datteln, with an emphasis on home care and additional aspects of access to paediatric specialists, respite care at a children's hospice, sibling and bereavement programmes, and a consultation service for other health professionals. Access to paediatric nurses, or the few palliative care services, is difficult in rural areas, and adult community and palliative care nurses may be used.

Services are still unequally spread. Barriers come from the lack of recognition of the need, especially for children with non-malignant diseases, and from lack of funding.

New Zealand

Paediatric palliative care was included in a national review of paediatric specialty services in 1998 [16], despite the fact that it did not exist as a speciality at that time. This project, and subsequent work [17], identified that services were patchy, and neither standardised, nor co-ordinated. It also noted lack of respite care, training and bereavement services. The challenge New Zealand has identified is to deliver effective, culturally appropriate palliative care for a relatively small number of children over widespread areas, in an environment of constrained health funding.

The review recommended a cascade model, with a national specialist paediatric palliative care team supporting a network of local regional co-ordinators, who then work with local health care professionals. The networks could then work together to develop and monitor standards of care. Following this review, a small specialist team has now been established at Starship Hospital in Auckland. Other encouraging developments are some excellent examples of collaboration between adult palliative care and child health services, and the opening of video-conferencing facilities at Starship Hospital. However, the establishment of local co-ordinators has been variable, and the awareness of care needs for non-oncology patients and for respite care [18] is still limited.

United Kingdom

Paediatric palliative care began in the early 1980s, with a number of separate initiatives, including outreach nurse specialists in oncology, the first children's hospice, bereavement programmes, and the appointment of the first specialist paediatric palliative care physician. As more programmes developed, the need to work more closely and systematically became apparent. The organisation ACT (Association for Children with Life-Threatening or Terminal Conditions and Their Families) was formed as a charity in 1992. It acts as an umbrella group for professionals and families, who can speak with one voice for children's palliative care. It aims to advocate on behalf of children with life-threatening illness and their families, and campaign for improved provision of care. It promotes good practice, supports professionals through education, and offers an information service. ACT, in association with the Royal College of Paediatrics and Child Health, worked to publish a guide to the development of paediatric palliative care services for children in 1997 (2nd edition 2003); this was followed by a companion document for young people aged 13–24 [19,20]. These have influenced the development of a comprehensive approach to paediatric palliative care in the United Kingdom.

The model advocated is inclusive of all children, and suggests the designation of lead co-ordinators in paediatric palliative care in each health district, working with local multidisciplinary community palliative care teams to support families in day-to-day care. Local community teams work in close co-operation with hospital based care, hospital specialist outreach teams (e.g., oncology), and voluntary organisations, including the children's, and more recently, young people's hospices. Services are becoming more equitable across the country, but gaps still remain. The national government has encouraged development of local teams, and made some contribution in resources towards this (through Diana teams and New Opportunities Fund money), but many services still depend heavily on charity.

The United States

The United States has been involved in promoting hospice programmes (equivalent to palliative care in the United Kingdom and Canada), since the late 1970s. There are a wide variety of programmes in a range of settings; examples are highlighted in the recent report, *When Children Die* [12], and on the Robert Wood Johnson web site [21]. The majority have involved home care, but some are hospital outreach projects, and others are community based. There are relatively few inpatient hospice beds for children, though some are available associated with adult programmes, some in children's hospitals, and some in the first free-standing children's hospices that have opened recently. Programmes have also varied in whether they specifically accept children with malignant diseases, or children with all life-threatening illness. Currently, there are about 450 specifically child-focused hospice, palliative care or home care services, and in addition, almost all of the over 3000 adult hospice programmes in the United States will now accept children. This compares with the availability of only 4 of 1400 programmes to children in 1983 [22].

Since 1983, the organization of Children's Hospice International [22] has been advocating and actively campaigning on behalf of children with life-threatening illness and their families, promoting hospice care, tackling the barriers to its introduction, and promoting education and resources for professionals. Recent years have seen a noticeable increase in awareness of the special needs of children and families as evidenced by:

- The American Academy of Pediatrics Committee on Bioethics and Hospital Care's statement promoting an integrated model of paediatric palliative care in 2000 [23];

- The publication in 2002, and associated publicity of the project and recommendations of 'When Children Die'—improving palliative and end-of-life care for children and their families [12];

- The CHI Programme for All Inclusive Care for Children and their Families (CHI-PACC). This programme co-ordinates a group of demonstration models supported by the government. These promote palliative care from the diagnosis, and support throughout the illness; they allow palliative care alongside disease-directed treatment, and include respite and bereavement care. They have been designed to counter the inappropriate reimbursement system, which has severely limited access to appropriate palliative care in the past. They also offer free training and educational material [22];

- The Initiative for Pediatric Palliative Care (IPPC) funding novel programmes in a number of hospitals; promoting a variety of quality improvement projects in paediatric palliative care [24];

- Increased number of publications and commentaries in high profile journals recently [23, 25–29].

These suggest that a much wider understanding of the philosophy of paediatric palliative care is developing and tackling some of the barriers to its wider use, with optimism for the future. However, recent assessments of the experiences of children and families reveal that problems still exist, and are a salutary reminder against complacency [25,30].

Other European countries

Evidence from the literature and personal communications suggests there is a growing awareness of paediatric palliative care across Europe, but comprehensive services are still not part of most countries' national health plans, and often remain sparse and unequally spread [5,31].

An example where a wider national view has been taken is in France. Following a study there in 1998, a four-year plan was developed to encourage palliative care at home through the setting up of networks to co-ordinate and train professionals, to organise access to home carers and respite, and to develop the roles of volunteers [32,33]. The results of this effort have not been reported yet.

The most active home care programmes in many countries have originated in paediatric oncology units, and this is reflected in the literature [34–39]. In some countries, for example, Belgium and Ireland, some of these initially oncology teams have now evolved a broader brief, and work with all diagnoses.

On the whole, provisions for children with non-malignant diseases are much less clearly recognised as part of palliative care, and tend to depend on individual paediatricians, such as neurologists and their teams.

Adult palliative care teams sometimes contribute to paediatric palliative care, particularly in countries with smaller and widespread populations, however they are more often at home with children with malignancies, and may be reluctant to help with longer terms and rarer conditions.

Educational programmes are helping raise the profile and understanding of the philosophy of paediatric palliative care and training staff in its practice [31,40].

Hong Kong, Japan, and China

Support from the time of diagnosis, palliative care at home, and bereavement follow up for children with cancer and their families, are well established in Hong Kong, provided by multidisciplinary health care professionals in the community, and funded by the Children's Cancer Foundation, working alongside hospital teams [41]. Children with non-malignant life-threatening illness have no structured palliative care service available, but there is evidence of growing interest in recent times [42].

In Japan, paediatric oncologists and nurses have identified a need to develop home-based terminal care [43,44]. There is no mention of palliative care for children in China in the literature, but concerns about pain management in children with cancer have recently been reported [45].

The Middle East

Some programmes have been established in major centres, for example, Saudi Arabia [46], primarily focussed on children with cancer, access to palliative care is not available for the majority of children in this area. The first Middle Eastern Paediatric Palliative Care Meeting is taking place in Kuwait in 2005 and plans for their home care programme and hospice have been launched.

From moderately resourced countries

Belarus

Belarus has a population of 10 million, of which 25% are children, living in an area of 208,000 sq.km. There are currently children's hospice programmes in 4 of the 6 administrative districts.

The Hospice in Minsk was the pioneering programme, and remains the largest [47]. It began in 1994, and now has a multidisciplinary staff, including 2 physicians, and offers:

- a home care service (24 hrs, seven days a week)
- respite care
- a day centre programme
- education for health care professionals.

Palliative care programmes are provided through non-governmental organizations, in close cooperation with the local health authority. The hospices work closely with their local children's hospitals and oncology centres. The projects have developed in the face of difficult political tensions, complex bureaucracy and uncertainty (for example, three different health ministers in less than a year). They are also limited by a serious lack of access to medication such as anti-emetics and analgesics and lack of equipment—both medical, such as oxygen concentrators and syringe drivers, and administrative, for example, mobile phones.

Poland

Poland has a commitment to integrating palliative care into the national health care system. The first paediatric service was founded in Warsaw in 1994, 13 years after the first adult service was registered in Cracow. It was the first dedicated children's hospice programme in Europe, outside of the United Kingdom. Currently, a network of 32 hospice programmes provides care for children, of which 5 are specifically paediatric, and 27, are adult, with in-patient services for children at two [48–50].

Around 1200 children die from life-limiting conditions in Poland each year, which is a death rate of 10.4 per 10,000 children. Between 1985–96, 74% died in hospital and 26% at home, and of those dying at home, 48% had cancer, while the remaining 52% non-malignant diseases [49].

The Warsaw Hospice for Children is the leading children's project and has a multidisciplinary staff, including nursing, medical, psychology, chaplaincy and physiotherapy and it provides:

- a home care service (24 h, seven days a week)
- pain and symptom management
- bereavement support for parents and siblings
- teaching and training programmes
- research.

Apart from providing service to individual children and families, they take an active role in developing standards, evaluation, and advocacy on behalf of all children with life-threatening illness and their families, with both the public and the government.

Romania

Romania, while similar to other European countries with regard to prevalence and incidence of the majority of life-threatening illnesses in children, has the added challenge of having to manage over 50% of all the paediatric AIDS cases in Europe. In 1997, there were 4,376 paediatric AIDS cases registered, and this is probably a conservative estimate.

There are a number of active palliative care programmes for children, which have developed through non-governmental organizations working alongside the national health system [51].

- There are two home care programmes linked to adult hospice projects in Brasov and Oradea, which work with children with all diagnoses. These are able to offer home care, symptom management, psychosocial and practical support, short-term respite care, and bereavement follow up. In addition, there are in-patient beds for children at Brasov, and they run the national education centre for palliative care.
- Two paediatric oncology units also run home care programmes.
- There are several residential facilities, opened by charities, to help children with HIV/AIDS. Initially, these began with the aim of offering terminal care, but as the prognosis for these children has improved, many are now providing more long-term care.

Some of the problems and barriers those working in Romania have identified are:

- Lack of understanding in both professionals and the public, with only 'pockets' of awareness around the country;
- Lack of statistics and databases on children with cancer, AIDS, and other diagnoses because of which identifying the children who might benefit from a palliative care service has been a slow process;
- Legislation regarding the prescribing of opioids, which is very limiting in relation to who can prescribe and how much can be used. Many fears and myths are still present in relation to opioid use.

Other Eastern European countries

Pioneering programmes have been introduced in a number of cities in other countries, such as Bratislava, Slovakia; Riga, Latvia, and Moscow, Russia. These have a common feature in that they involve collaboration between state and non-governmental organisations, and have grown up primarily through the inspiration of innovative and determined local leaders. They have evolved from a hospital base with multi-disciplinary teams and outreach home care, and are leading in their countries in providing a model of care, in education, and in tackling misunderstandings about, and barriers to, paediatric palliative care.

Central and South America

Costa Rica has an active and comprehensive childrens palliative care service, initiated by a determined and energetic leader. It has been functioning since the late 1980s, and is based in the national children's hospital, with outreach across the country. Although initially it served children with cancer, children with all diagnoses have been eligible for care since 1995. It is integrated into the government social security system, with additional support from a national charity. Through education and advocacy, the government has been sensitised to the palliative care needs in the country, and has declared it a constitutional right of every Costa Rican, to die with dignity and with no pain.

Argentina has 4 hospital-based children's services in different stages of evolution, and Mexico has also started a dedicated children's palliative care programme; a number of other countries have some adult services (Colombia, Brazil, Chile, Ecuador, Paraguay, Uruguay), but as yet, nothing specific for children.

From poorly resourced countries

There is a massive lack of palliative care services for children with cancer and other life-limiting illnesses in the poorly resourced countries of the world. Here, more than 90% of such children receive only local remedies, and in addition, there is the devastating problem of HIV and AIDS. This is particularly the case for sub-Saharan Africa, but also for parts of South East Asia.

In these countries, the AIDS pandemic continues unabated, and of the 40 million people currently living with HIV or AIDS, almost 75% are in sub-Saharan Africa [52]. Despite the efficacy of anti-retroviral drugs (ARV's) in reducing perinatal HIV transmission in this population [53], the infrastructure to undertake this relatively straightforward form of treatment does not exist, even though one of the drugs, (nevirapine), and rapid testing for HIV have being made free for eligible countries (Boehringer Ingelheim and Abbott Laboratories, 2003). As a consequence, 2.4 million children aged <15 years of age are living with HIV/AIDS in sub-Saharan Africa. In 2002, there were 700,000 newly infected patients, and 580,000 deaths, or 2,000 deaths per day, as opposed to 500 per year in either the United States or Europe [52]. Between 25–39% of infected African women

transmit HIV to their offspring [54], but the number of children living with HIV/AIDS is lower than one would expect, due their high mortality in early infancy. It is estimated that half of all children infected permanently with HIV die before their first birthday, and most of the remaining die before their fifth birthday [55].

The commonest causes of severe pain in HIV/AIDS are cryptococcal meningitis (requiring fluconazole), oesophageal candidiasis (requiring fluconazole and nystatin), herpes simplex and zoster (some response to expensive acyclovir), and peripheral neuropathies.

Another emerging crisis is the orphan status of so many infected children. It was estimated that by the end of 2001, 880,000 children will have been orphaned as a result of HIV/AIDS in Uganda alone [55]. Given the scale of the problem it is amazing, and a credit to African society, that most of these orphans have been absorbed into extended family networks.

Given the lack of system support, even with donated ARV's, the run-down and poorly equipped hospital services, and the inability to undertake reliable therapy, the need to support this group of HIV positive children by providing care in their homes, and thus supporting their families, is clearly an issue that falls into the category of palliative care.

Africa

Much work in palliative care, particularly with respect to HIV/AIDS, is going ahead in Egypt, Kenya, Malawi, Namibia, South Africa, Tanzania, Uganda, and Zimbabwe. This work is largely concentrated around adult hospices and home care programmes, education of community health workers in the practice of palliative care (for example, in South Africa, more than 30,000 health workers each year are being trained in palliative care), and attempts to persuade governments to make morphine available both for hospital and community care. As a consequence of advocacy, morphine is available nearly throughout Malawi.

Other initiatives that are contributing include:

• The WHO, in close collaboration with its regional office for Africa, has developed a project entitled 'Community Health Approach to Palliative Care for HIV and Cancer Patients in Africa.' In 2002, the 5 countries participating were Ethiopia, Botswana, Uganda, Tanzania, and Zimbabwe.

• A new trans-national association representing palliative care services in Africa (The African Palliative Care Association) has been established [56].

• The United States-based Foundation for Hospices in Sub-Saharan Africa (FHSSA) also generates support and partnership for African home-based hospice and palliative care services caring for those who are dying of HIV/ AIDS [57].

- A most important announcement was the US$15 billion committed by President Bush to HIV/AIDS in key African and Caribbean Nations. 15% of this is for palliative and supportive care, and care for orphans.
- The St. Nicholas Children's Hospice Programme, which has been set up in South Africa.
- A new book for families with AIDS has been written by members of the Association of Women Living with AIDS (NACWOLA) in Uganda.

However, one study from South Africa [58], involving the documentation of 'do not resuscitate' orders and 'comfort care plans,' showed that pain and distress were found in the last 48 h of life in 55% of paediatric patients in the wards of the hospitals. Half of the patients with pain and distress, including 16 with a comfort care plan, received no analgesia. There have also been difficulties in undertaking home based palliative care, which include denial of the prognosis and fear of causing death, exactly the same issues as in rich countries. In hospitals, opposition to palliative care by some senior physicians, who believe that it will accelerate death, has been a major problem.

Uganda

Uganda has made major efforts to address the issues around palliative care, which was first introduced through Hospice Uganda in 1993. In 1998, Mildmay International, in collaboration with the Ministry of Health, opened a centre of excellence, with the President as Patron. This not only provided local care, but also palliative care training for Uganda and for other African countries. Such training is now part of the undergraduate curriculum in Makerere and Mbarara Medical Schools. There are 80 members of the Palliative Care Association of Uganda [59], with much time spent on training. As with most of sub-Saharan Africa, doctors are scarce, one for every 50,000 people, and so, trained nurses and community health workers are essential, including those who provide traditional healing services. One very innovative move has involved a statute that allows palliative care nurse specialists and clinical officers (non-doctors) with palliative care training to prescribe morphine. The aim is to have at least one palliative care specialist in each district. By 2002, morphine had been introduced into 57 districts, with the support of the Ministry of Health [60].

A programme that has been supporting children with HIV/AIDS in Uganda since the beginning of 2001 (run by the charity Child Advocacy International-CAI), provides one potentially sustainable model for the provision of palliative care in a poorly resourced country. At the end of 2001 in Uganda, there were 110,000 children infected with HIV, and very large numbers orphaned as a result of fatal HIV infection in their parents.

- Children are recruited from the out-patient clinics in the main teaching hospital in Uganda, Mulago Hospital. Each child/carer receives pre-HIV-test counseling, and those who are HIV positive then receive care at the clinic, provided the family is able to afford to attend. Antibiotics and anti-fungals are often unavailable, due to their cost.
- To enrol in the CAI programme, the only criteria were that the child has a positive serology result, and is an orphan, that is, he or she has lost one or both parents; in practice, this includes most children who attend the clinic. Many children are enrolled and supported while critically ill as in-patients.
- After enrolling, a monthly home visit is made to every family. Every effort is made to avoid stigmatisation, so a family can enrol without home visits and still receive the same level of support, in terms of food and medication, as do the other families. Families are visited on an appointed day, circled on a calendar when it was rare not to find the families at home.
- The personnel employed are local nurses, trained in counselling, and a driver. Resources include a vehicle, an office, supplies of medication and food, and a database to record each interaction with every child. Drugs and medical supplies were available in a trunk carried in the vehicle.
- Vitamin A is given every 6 months, and mebendazole every 3 months, to all children in each family. The family are supplied with oral rehydration solution (ORS) and paracetamol, and educated in their use. Each HIV infected child is provided with prophylactic co-trimoxazole and multivitamins.
- At each home visit, opportunistic infections are diagnosed and treated, according to guidelines based on the Manual of International Child Healthcare 2002 [61]. Guidelines for treatment are algorithm-based, and are easily followed by nurses and parents.
- Each visit creates an opportunity to give nutritional advice, with particular emphasis on the value of using local produce. The aid agency, with a grant from the Irish Government, has purchased some land, and encourages the caretakers to grow their own food on plots of this land. The World Food Programme provides 75 kg of basic food for each family every month.
- When children are hospitalised, all medication is provided without this assistance, most carers could not afford hospital

care. If children on the programme become sick between home visits, they can attend the office, which is open 6 days a week.

- Psychosocial issues are discussed at monthly carers' meetings, with up to 100 carers present, and monthly child support meetings. Basic health education, education about HIV and its prevention, recognition and management of opportunistic infections, pain control, nutritional advice, and emotional support are discussed. Invited speakers include child psychologists, nutritional experts, and paediatricians. These meetings provide a forum for discussion among carers, and allow the formation of support networks. Carers are also able to discuss concerns with the team nurse in the privacy of their home. If the child is sufficiently mature, disclosure of the diagnosis and its potential implications are considered. If the mother is alive but unwell, discussions about the ongoing care of her children after her death are undertaken.

- A forum for infected children has been developed, called the Children's Club, and is attended by 50 children, who are aware of their diagnoses with the carers' permission. The club is led by a 16-year-old child, with facilitation by an experienced social worker and counsellor.

This programme was established at the beginning of 2001, and by the end of 2003, had cared for 300 children, with a median age of 7 years. The children's primary carers were their sick mothers (48%), fathers (5%), or extended family (47%). The main HIV-related clinical issues experienced by this cohort of children were respiratory failure, severe skin problems, diarrhoea, parotitis, and oral and oesophageal candidiasis.

Over a 10-month period, 15% of the children enrolled died, at an average age of 7.8 years. The causes of death varied, but tuberculosis and wasting, often secondary to oral and oesophageal candidiasis, played a large role. Most patients died after suffering many years of chronic ill health; indications included being too short of breath to walk, much less play. Despite the programme, most children ended their lives in a state of severe malnutrition, partly resulting from oral and oesophageal candida, and chronic diarrhoea.

This type of low cost programme supporting the carers of children with currently fatal HIV infection that is not yet adequately treated with a specific system of effective ARV drugs, can substantially improve the quality of life for children and their carers. It is based in the home, addresses malnutrition through the provision of home grown foods, manages opportunistic infections, supports carers, educates on HIV transmission, and aims to relieve painful and distressing symptoms, and is at least an attempt at palliative care for this disastrous problem. A similar approach can be taken for the care of other life-limiting conditions, such as cancers and severe neurological/developmental disorders in poor countries.

Bosnia and Kosovo

These 2 countries have relatively recently been involved in major armed conflict. As a result, there has been a considerable input of humanitarian medical aid. One of the main problems identified was a minimum availability of pain control, and complete absence of palliative care, for both adults and children. However, like sub-Saharan Africa, the family structures in both of these countries are extremely strong, and can support community (home) based programmes of health care, despite a scarcity of community nursing staff. In both countries, Child Advocacy International was able to introduce palliative care for terminal malignancy in children, by training family members on how to undertake the basic medical components of palliative care for such children in their homes. Thus, parents, grandparents, or siblings were trained to:

- administer oral and subcutaneous infusions of opiate and sedative drugs;

- pass and care for urinary catheters;

- care for pressure areas, for the mouth, and prevent and/or manage constipation;

- manage and pass nasogastric tubes for feeding and fluid administration.

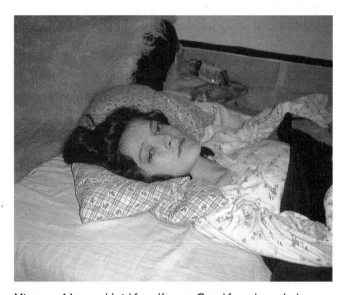

Mimosa, a 14-year-old girl from Kosovo. Cared for at home by her parents, who had been trained to provide palliative care, including morphine and urinary catheterization. She suffered from a rhabdomyosarcoma which led to paraplegia. Permission to publish this photograph was given by Mimosa and her family.

Improving children's palliative care worldwide

The overall goal

Ideally, the goal of children's palliative care is to achieve the best quality of life for patients and their families, consistent with their values, and regardless of their location. In effect, the family is assisted to 'hope for the best, cope with the day-to-day, and prepare for the worst.' A model 'in which the components of palliative care are offered at diagnosis, and continued throughout the course of the illness, whether the outcome ends in cure or death' is widely supported [19,62].

No randomized, controlled trials of interventions for children and families, specifically with life-threatening illnesses, could be found in the literature, although there are examples for chronic illnesses which are likely to be applicable to life-threatening illnesses [63,64]. There are, however, many descriptive studies which conclude that the aims and objectives of a service should be to help the:

Child
by

- maintaining independence;

- providing good symptom control;

- recognising the changing needs of children as they grow and develop;

- improving quality of life;

- involving children in decision-making.

Family
by

- promoting family participation in defining the priorities for care;

- providing accessible information about the condition, prognosis and options available;

- supporting choice over the venue of death, according to family wishes;

- promoting caring and connectedness with health care professionals;

- enabling parents to retain responsibility for their dying child [65];

- reducing the psychosocial impact on parents, siblings, and others;

- providing support for practical problems relating to day-to-day living;

- providing respite care;

- recognizing the child as special, while retaining as much normality as possible within the child and family's lives.

The literature provides many suggestions on how services can best achieve these objectives, and different countries need to plan and develop from these, according to their epidemiology, resources, geography, and healthcare services:

- multi-agency teams, able to deliver care in a variety of settings, but predominantly at home;

- specialist palliative care teams, which support primary and secondary care teams delivering palliative care;

- comprehensive assessment of needs for both child and family members;

- practical and explicit care planning;

- planning ahead for expected complications/crises;

- a key worker to act as a co-ordinator and advocate on behalf of families;

- 24-h access to a service delivered in a setting that is desired and/or appropriate to their needs;

- good co-ordination of care, at any moment in time;

- facilities for respite care;

- continuity of care over the lifetime of child, including transitions, and into the bereavement period;

- easy access to hospital;

- clear standards and quality assurance of services.

Introducing paediatric palliative care in resource poor countries

Rational priority setting in the face of overwhelming poverty and increasing inequalities is extremely difficult. The predominant threats to health in the developing world are malnutrition, infectious disease, social disorder, and economic exploitation. Public health and logic would dictate the need to address these determinants of health, before attempting to develop health services, including palliative care for children. The dilemma is knowing where to invest limited resources to achieve maximum effect.

Whilst few would dispute the aspirations of human rights and palliative care, and nobody would wish to die unsupported and in pain, the reality for the 2 billion people worldwide who are living in extreme poverty is that these ideals are likely to remain out of reach for many years to come.

It is tempting to tackle individual diseases, for example, HIV/AIDS, malaria, tuberculosis, or the major determinants of health, for example, nutrition, water, sanitation, and housing, but even these isolated, targeted approaches are unlikely to have a significant impact in environments of civil unrest, economic exploitation, and corruption. For maximum impact, there needs to be a consistent approach that integrates social, environmental and economic issues, and assesses their impact on health, disease, and health service development. This approach is equally relevant to both the developed and the developing world. It is encapsulated in the sustainable development/agenda 21 movement that was launched in Rio de Janeiro in 1987 [66,67].

Tackling the determinants of health will initially have an overall higher priority than health service development in many poor countries. However, in reality, aspects of both will be addressed simultaneously. In addition, there will be occasions when charitable initiatives, aid or development, or other humanitarian initiatives will promote the development of individual programmes, such as palliative care, within the context of the bigger picture. Where should these initiatives start, and what should their priorities be?

There needs to be:

1. Assessment to define local needs, health system capacity and community preferences;

2. Selection of effective interventions capable of meeting local needs, that can be delivered locally;

3. An appraisal of alternative delivery strategies—is it better to target one condition with great effect, or many conditions with less effect?

4. Implement change, and then check whether the interventions are having the expected effect;

5. Invest in longer term infrastructure—mainly education and training—to maintain and improve on the initial investment [68].

In reality, it is also important to recognize that many aid initiatives have a short life, bringing in new resources that are not normally available locally, and are often dependent on outside agencies, which may have priorities that are not shared by the local community. The sustainability of any project has to be realistically addressed by both the donors and the local people before it starts. Short-lived projects should act as catalysts, enabling local people to achieve their own aspirations with their own resources, rather than imposing goals, values, and ideals that are not owned locally. The absence of evidence-based research is acknowledged [69], and should drive research and evaluation to determine what is effective in the longer term.

Palliative care developments should, therefore, build on existing health services, so one pre-requisite would be some existing health service infrastructure. Education and training in the basic principles of palliative care to increase the capacity, both in terms of numbers and competence, of existing health care workers is a necessary starting place. Use of family members, community volunteers, and using traditional healers/herbalists is better than creating parallel or separate services, and the use of home-based palliative care, wherever possible, reduces capital costs, but is often less appealing to donors [70].

Health workers involved in adult palliative care, and the WHO have identified policies and strategies for developing adult palliative care, using a public health approach [2,71,72]. Many of these organizations and projects have a strong reputation, and have developed networks of communication links and models of good practice. Those of us working to improve paediatric palliative care can learn from these established programmes and work alongside them, highlighting the special needs of children as well as developing specific paediatric projects.

Children's rights

Children have rights that are universal, albeit to very different degrees, depending on where they are living in the world.

The Ottawa Charter 1986 recognises the importance of peace, shelter, education, food, income, stable ecosystem, sustainable resources, social justice, and equity. All of these are initially of a higher priority than the development of health services.

The UN Convention on the Rights of the Child (UNCRC) [73], comprises 54 separate articles setting out the rights of all children. It covers the areas of civil rights and freedom, family environment and alternative care, health and welfare, education, leisure and cultural activities, and special protection measures, for example, child labour, trafficking, juvenile justice, and sexual exploitation. It can act as an important starting point in considering worldwide paediatric palliative care, as all countries except the United States have signed the UN Convention on the Rights of the Child, and therefore, formally agreed with the articles. This argument can help as a lever to ensure that there is at least discussion about the importance of the relief of suffering, the importance of pain control and palliative care, and therefore, the most appropriate services needed to ensure them.

Four principles embody the spirit of the CRC, and are fundamental to the interpretation of all the other rights. They are relevant across the world. They are:

The best interests of the child (Article 3), which establishes that in all actions concerning children their best interest should be a primary consideration;

Survival and development (Article 6), which prioritises not only children's rights to survival and development, but also their right to develop to their fullest potential in every respect, including their personality, talents, and abilities;

Non-discrimination (Article 2), which establishes that children's rights apply to all children without discrimination of any kind, for example, on grounds of gender, disability, ethnicity, religion, and citizenship;

Participation (Article 12), which sets out the principle that children should be listened to on any matter which concerns them, and their views given due consideration in accordance with their age and maturity.

From these general statements, individual services can develop their own philosophies and principles, to guide the development of services when there is an absence of robust evidence. Philosophy generally relates to people, and principles relate to services. Examples are given below:

Philosophy

- Children have rights, which must be respected and promoted, for example, the right to a safe and healthy environment, education, good nutrition, and a secure and loving family life.

- Children should be seen as children first, recognising their changing needs and abilities as they become older, rather than as a disease or problem.

- Parents and children should be actively involved in decisions about the children's care.

- Each child is a unique individual, and racial, linguistic, religious, and cultural background should be respected.

Principles

- Services should be evidence based, and balance both the quantity and quality of provision.

- Services should be both accessible and child-friendly.

- Services should promote and protect the rights of children and families, and be advocates for their needs.

- Services should be well co-ordinated, with continuity over time between the agencies/services involved.

- Services should be delivered as close to home as resources and expertise allow.

- Services should be evaluated regularly, to ensure they are meeting the evolving needs of the child population.

- Services should work within the available resources, taking account of financial, political, and environmental factors.

- Different organisations should seek to influence each other in a positive way, to produce the best possible overall service.

The child-friendly health care initiative

The Child Friendly Health Care Initiative is an example of a project, by a group of agencies, which has incorporated The United Nations Convention on the Rights of The Child. These organizations are Child Advocacy International, the Royal College of Nursing, the Royal College of Paediatrics and Child Health and UNICEF (UK), with technical support from the Child and Adolescent Health Department of WHO in Geneva, and UNICEF in New York. The Child Friendly Health Care Initiative has 12 standards (see below), and for each, a number of defining criteria which outline ways of improving health care for children in all health care facilities.

'Child friendly health care' includes any behaviour, attitude, action, or resource that minimises fear, anxiety, and suffering in children receiving health care, and their families. It must include advocacy and needs to comply with the articles of the United Nations Convention on the Rights of the Child.

Health care workers can practice 'child friendly health care' by acting as advocates for children and families, and by working together to:

1. Keep children out of hospital, unless it is best for the child (UNCRC articles 9,24,25,3).

2. Support and give the best possible health care to pregnant women and children (UNCRC articles 2,6,23,24,37).

3. Give safe care in a secure, clean, child-friendly environment (UNCRC article 3).

4. Give child-centred care (UNCRC articles 5,9,114,37).

5. Share information with the child and family, and enable their participation (UNCRC articles 9,12,13,17).

6. Provide equal care, and treat the child as an individual with rights (UNCRC articles 2,7,8,9,16,23,27,29,37).

7. Recognise and relieve a child's pain and discomfort (UNCRC articles 19,23,24).

8. Provide appropriate emergency care (UNCRC articles 6,24).

9. Enable children to play and learn (UNCRC articles 6,28, 29,31).

10. Recognise, protect, and support the vulnerable or abused child (UNCRC articles 3,11,19,20,21,25,32–37,39).

11. Promote and monitor health (UNCRC articles 6,17, 23,24,33).

12. Support the child's best possible nutrition (UNCRC articles 3,24,26,27).

The supporting criteria for these 12 child-friendly health care standards were developed following wide global consultation with families, health care workers, and organisations involved in children's care. They translate the articles of the UNCRC into everyday practice for all health care workers, whatever type of health care they organise or give.

Standard 7 particularly addresses palliative care, which is defined in the Child Friendly Healthcare Initiative as follows: 'the active total/comprehensive care of a child with an incurable or other life-limiting condition by a multidisciplinary team, to prevent suffering by controlling distressing symptoms, and by providing other general and psychosocial supportive care to the child and family.'

The supportive criteria for Standard 7 in the Child Friendly Healthcare Initiative are as follows:

1. A visible *mission statement*, written in the relevant languages, that includes a commitment to recognising, assessing, and relieving pain and other distressing symptoms;

2. A separate *pain and other symptom management and palliative care service(s)*, with lead health professionals and/or multi disciplinary team(s);

3. Systems of care, guidelines and job aides (for example, tools to relieve pain) to help with *symptom recognition, symptom assessment and restraint for procedures*;

4. *Written guidelines*, evidence-based wherever possible, used by everyone to help with symptom relief, that include advice on the relief of different types of pain and other distressing symptoms, and on how to use non-pharmacological and pharmacological pain relieving strategies in the different age groups;

5. *Material resources* including:
   • a safe, secure supply of free or affordable *essential drugs* for symptom relief, that includes *opioids and non-opioids*;
   • distraction toys and other resources to aid *non-pharmacological* pain and other symptom management;

6. The use of *individual pain* (and other symptom) *plans* made with the children and their parents/carers;

7. *Psychosocial support* for children, families, and health workers;

8. Regular *education/training opportunities* for health workers on the recognition and management of pain and other distressing symptoms, and on the restraint of children;

9. *Keeping records* about use of opioids;

10. *Regular audit* of systems, policies, guidelines, and other job aides.

The pilot project for the Child Friendly Healthcare Initiative, undertaken in 4 poorly resourced countries; Uganda, Pakistan, Moldova and Kosovo, found large numbers of children in the participating countries suffering from uncontrolled pain and other distressing symptoms. Although symptom management was better in some countries than others, experiencing these symptoms is still the unfortunate reality for most of the world's children.

Improved technology and potential advances in care do not always protect or improve the treatment of these distressing symptoms, and can, on occasion, be an additional cause. Routine procedures, such as dressing wounds and taking blood, and other health worker actions, were frequent causes of unnecessary pain and suffering for a child.

The CFHI states that effective relief from pain and other distressing symptoms could be better if health workers:

• were more aware of the suffering and discomfort that all children, including newborn babies, may experience, due to pain and other distressing symptoms;

• always anticipated a child's pain and other distressing symptoms;

• gave a higher priority to relieving each individual child's pain and other distressing symptoms;

• made greater use of pain and symptom-relieving drugs, both non-opiates and opiates;

• understood and used the simple non-pharmaceutical methods that can help (supportive, cognitive, behavioural, and physical);

• knew about and anticipated all the things that can make the experience of pain or other symptoms worse.

To 'make it better', the best practice is for health workers to have core (during initial training) and regular education/training opportunities on the recognition, assessment, and treatment of pain and other distressing symptoms. Best possible practice is also facilitated by having, whenever possible, separate skilled health professionals, who lead and guide the treatment of pain and other symptoms. Having a multidisciplinary team dedicated to symptom relief and other aspects of palliative care, and using standardised guidelines for managing pain and other distressing symptoms, are known to be effective ways of improving care and sharing good practice.

The child's normal health worker, working together with the child and his or her carers, who know the child best, can often reduce pain and other distressing symptoms by:

• planning each individual child's care, as each child responds differently to pain and other distressing symptoms;

• anticipating pain and taking effective measures, and/or giving drugs before the symptoms occur, for example, before a procedure or operation. *Children with recurrent distressing symptoms should not wait for these to re-occur before receiving relief.*

• using pain/symptom assessment tools to help them recognise and assess a child's symptoms and guide the care he or she needs;

• Giving drugs in a way that does not cause more pain and distress. Drugs are often still given in a way that is painful for the child, for example, by intra muscular injection. During the pilot project, many children told us that they would rather pretend that they had no pain or discomfort, than have the medicine given this way. Health workers need to be aware of this, and also that the drugs are frequently available, and equally effective, as intravenous, subcutaneous, or oral preparations, often at a lower cost;

• advocating for the child's needs to be met, if they are unable to meet these needs themselves.

While drugs have an important role to play in the management of pain and other distressing symptoms, there is much that can be done even where drugs are not easily available, to relieve suffering and make an unpleasant experience more bearable, such as:

• being honest with the child, and preparing him or her for what might be a painful experience, can help him or her to cope. Anxiety and mistrust of health workers will make the experience worse;

• using appropriate play, stimulation, and distraction to help in the management of pain and other symptoms;

• using heat, cold, touch, and other comfort measures, as these can sometimes help the distress of pain and other symptoms;

• giving psychological support, simple kindness, and involving parents and other familiar carers where possible.

The CFHI states that it is ethically wrong, and a failure in performance of a health professional's duty, for a child to suffer from uncontrolled pain or other distressing symptoms. This is particularly the case for a child who has a permanent disability that is associated with chronic symptoms, or one who cannot be cured of his or her illness, and may be near the end of his or her life. Relieving pain and distressing symptoms is not always about cure, but is about making the experience of living 'now' more bearable, and so, improving the quality of remaining life.

Access and use of appropriate medications

Control of most symptoms does not require expensive intervention, merely recognition and access to first-line treatments. Continuing powerful advocacy from international organizations, such as WHO, palliative care networks, medical professionals, and the public is needed to educate and encourage governments in the context of their responsibilities to establish national palliative care strategies, and to address the procurement, legislation, and administration processes needed to enable the essential drugs to be used.

WHO recommends that countries should establish an essential palliative care drug list based on the medical needs of their particular population. The WHO Expert Committee on the Use of Essential Drugs has recommended that drugs mentioned in the WHO publication 'Cancer Pain Relief: with a Guide to Opioid Availability [74],' be considered essential.

Encouraging active use of available guidelines

A variety of educational materials and practical guidelines are available, which could be used much more extensively. Some examples include:

• The WHO cancer unit has, since the early 1980's, made major attempts to advocate for pain relief and opioid availability worldwide, in both rich and poor countries. They have produced a number of relevant publications, in particular, 'Cancer pain relief and palliative care in children [75].'

Here is a quote from their web site on this publication:

Almost all children with cancer will experience pain—as a direct result of the disease, as a side-effect of treatments or invasive clinical procedures, or as an aspect of psychological distress. In more than 70% of cases, that pain will at some stage become severe. Although means to relieve pain are widely available, in developed and developing countries alike, their use in children has often been very limited. Fears of drug 'addiction', lack of knowledge of children's perception of pain and illness, use of inappropriate drug doses, and failure to understand the value of supportive, non-drug measures have all contributed to widespread inadequacy in the control of pain in children with cancer.

• WHO provides some excellent general guidelines on opioid and other drug requirements for palliative care in the following publication: 'Cancer pain relief: with guide to opioid availability [74].'

Here is a summary:

This second edition of the WHO guidelines for cancer pain relief presents a simple and practical method to relieve the pain syndromes unique to cancer. After a brief explanation of the physiological and psychological causes of cancer pain,

Part 1 presents a 9-step procedure for pain assessment, including questions clinicians should ask. The most extensive section details how to select and prescribe opioid and non-opioid analgesics, drugs for neuropathic pain, and adjuvant drugs for the treatment of side effects, the enhancement of pain relief, and the management of psychological disturbances. Part 2 describes the international system by which morphine and other opioids are made available for medical purposes. It concludes with the criteria that can be used to regulate the dispensing of opioids by physicians, nurses and pharmacists.

• Child Advocacy International has produced a practical guide to managing common symptoms at the end of life [61].

• WHO, in collaboration with the International Association for the Study of Pain (IASP), has published a power-point presentation entitled 'Cancer pain relief and palliative care in children' on their website.

Education of healthcare professionals

Doctors, nurses, and all members of the multidisciplinary teams involved in providing palliative care can be helped by exposure to existing, well-worked-out local strategies. Paediatric palliative care still needs a critical mass of trainers and practitioners, both to provide the service, and also to train others. A combination of approaches will be needed. Some 'top down' training will be needed for people who are already experienced practitioners in their own field, but need to expand their knowledge, experience, and practice in all aspects of palliative care. In addition 'bottom up' teaching will be needed in the long run, both to train those who will become palliative care practitioners, and to broaden the awareness of all in health care.

One of the most effective ways will be to introduce palliative care into medical, nursing and multi-professional training schools. Palliative care needs to be on the curriculum not only in its own right, but also as a pervasive underlying factor, so that whenever any subject is taught, the palliative care aspects of the treatment plan are considered. Those responsible for setting standards of training need to ensure that parts of the examination syllabus include modules on pain control and palliative care, and that the examinations reflect these modules.

Apart from national and international conferences, some innovative approaches have been undertaken offering training, for example, sponsored places for practitioners in Eastern Europe at the European Paediatric Palliative Care Courses, and individually tailored training programmes with

sponsored places established in Poland [31]. Further, a one-day training programme on pain and control and palliative care was conducted in Uganda in 2001, involving lectures, skill stations, scenarios, and an MCQ test, followed by certification for those who passed. This kind of training might be usefully employed to help team building and practice in the care of children in hospital, and could equally be adapted to include the approaches to be taken in children's homes in other developing countries.

Conclusion

Children's palliative care is a relatively new and emerging specialist with great potential for helping children and families living with life-threatening illnesses in all parts of the world. A range of models of care has been established, particularly in the resource rich countries, but there are also excellent models in some of the less wealthy, and even the very poor, counties. However, the overall picture is still one of immaturity, with unequal services, a lack of evidence base and considerable scope for development.

Broader awareness of the values and philosophy of palliative care, and also of its place in society in relation to children, is needed. It can be a difficult and very gradual process to alter a society's views, especially when some of these are deeply embedded in cultural norms, and rooted in people's own subconscious fears of death. Factual information about the potential benefits of palliative care, about pain relief, and opioids needs to be widely available for the general public, to raise expectations and demands of local health care systems.

Those of us working in paediatric palliative care need to work closely alongside the respected and influential adult palliative care organisations already working across the world, highlighting the special needs of children. As paediatric palliative care increases in size, we will need to enhance the international roles of our own organizations, such as ACT and CHI, and develop more extensive and effective paediatric networks.

Acknowledgements

I am enormously grateful to the many colleagues who have helped inform me with this chapter, with inputs from their experience and services. Thanks to John Collins, Jenny Hynson, and Susan Trethewie in Australia; Sonia Develter in Belgium; Anna Gorchakova in Belarus; Gerri Frager and Hal Siden in Canada; Lisbeth Quesada Tristan in Costa Rica; Stefan Friedrichsdorff and Carla Hassan in Germany; Maria

Bouri and Danai Papadatou in Greece; Florence Chu, Molin Lin and Rosita Lie in Hong Kong; Gudmundur Jonmundsson in Iceland; Maeve O'Reilly and Fiona O'Laughlin in Ireland; Anda Jansone in Latvia; Ross Drake and Adrian Trenholme in New Zealand; Ingeborg Storm Mathisen, Steinunn Egeland and Lise Lotte Hoel in Norway; Tomasz Dangel in Poland; Kirsteen Cowling and Nicoletta Grecu in Romania; Marina Bialik in Russia; Maria Jasenkova in Slovakia; Debbie Norval and Joan Marston in South Africa; Gustav Ljungman in Sweden; Eva Bergstrasser in Switzerland.

38 Quality assurance

Harold Siden

Quality is never an accident; it is always the result of intelligent effort.

John Ruskin (1819–1900)

Case Jessica was a 9-year-old girl with neuroblastoma, initially diagnosed at age five. She underwent bone marrow transplantation, but the disease recurred. Chemotherapy was begun, but had little effect on progression of the disease.

Still, the parents continued to pursue therapies oriented towards another remission and, if possible, cure. Several discussions were held between the parents and the Oncology team. Some members of the team agreed with aggressive therapy, while others recommended a palliative approach.

The idea of meeting the Palliative Care team was introduced, but the parents were not interested. When Jessica was repeatedly hospitalized and began developing pain that was difficult to treat, the parents agreed to involve the Palliative Care team, but only for the purpose of addressing pain.

Over a brief period of time, as Jessica became more ill, the parents developed a better relationship with members of the Palliative Care team, especially the social worker and the chaplain. Jessica's mother was willing to discuss some of her fears and wishes, but her father felt strongly that all discussion should remain hopeful. He refused to discuss a Do Not Resuscitate (DNR) order. Jessica's older half-sister thought that Jessica should be told the truth of her condition. The mother was uncertain about this, but the father felt that it would take away any hope, and further that Jessica 'could not handle it'. Several nurses suspected that Jessica was already well aware of her situation.

Eventually, the family agreed to have Jessica transferred to a paediatric hospice, ostensibly for symptom management. Jessica died two days later. She was receiving oral morphine for pain and had a hyoscine transdermal patch placed to treat excessive secretions. She received intermittent midazolam as well. In the two days before she died she required frequent breakthrough doses of morphine via nasogastric tube, and the nurses' notes commented on 'increasing pain'.

The family was present when she died. Although no DNR order was ever signed because of the parents' lack of agreement, when Jessica stopped breathing no attempt was made at resuscitation, and the family agreed to this when asked by the physician present. After her death a phone call was placed to the Oncology unit at the Children's hospital and to the general practitioner in the community.

The day after Jessica died, the parents spent several hours with the chaplain and the social worker. Members of the Palliative Care and Oncology teams attended the funeral, and the family expressed gratitude to the teams for everything that had been done.

When discussing the case at rounds the week after Jessica's death, the Palliative Care team felt that they had done 'a good job' despite many challenges. Two months later, Jessica's case was reviewed by the Oncology team at a case conference with the pathologist and radiologist. They felt that there was no additional curative therapy that would have been of benefit, and that they would not have changed anything in the original treatment approach 4 years earlier.

The social worker made two bereavement visits in the following months, but could not do more because of staffing issues. She provided information about bereavement and community programs. The social worker reported that the visits went well and the family was coping with their grief.

Introduction

The case described above will sound familiar to anyone involved in paediatric palliative care, whether a nurse, physician, therapist or volunteer. The complexities of care and management are often striking. One of the key challenges both for the team and for the family is communication. Despite these challenges, many times teams and families feel that things 'went well'. In the case described above, the family expressed their satisfaction to the team, and the palliative team acknowledged a sense of success.

Does this case, however, describe quality? Were the communication challenges dealt with effectively—and will there be any improvement the next time? What about the gaps in communication between the oncologists, the palliative team, and the community? Was symptom control ideal? Was there any measurement of symptoms that could provide feedback to medication administration, and will it have an impact on future cases? Was the bereavement and follow-up adequate, despite resource issues? Finally, were the review processes by the palliative team and the oncology team done in the best way possible?

These questions touch on some of the many issues that surround the provision of quality care in paediatric palliative care. The desire to provide high-quality care is inherent in our good intentions in working in this challenging field. A desire to do good—to be empathetic to families in the some of the most difficult circumstances possible—guides many of us. Busy clinicians work hard to stay on top of new literature and attend conferences to stay up to date. Isn't this enough to ensure that we are delivering quality, the best care possible?

Unfortunately, as the saying goes, 'the road to hell is paved with good intentions.' Attention to quality conducted in a systematic manner at the organizational level is now a given within health care, including palliative care. Health care, however, brings special challenges to the application of quality concepts. These challenges are multiplied in the field of palliative care, and multiplied again in paediatric palliative care.

Paediatric palliative care practitioners are no strangers to difficult tasks, and while using quality tools may require effort, it is an undertaking that can be done well. Systems to judge quality are now required as fundamental within health care organizations. Beyond just fulfilling a requirement, organizations that engage in Quality Assurance (QA) and Quality Improvement (QI) processes find that their organizations and team members are better able to carry out their missions—in this case, offering care to children and families living with life-threatening conditions. This chapter will review concepts regarding quality programs and describe how quality-based systems can operate in paediatric palliative care.

Definitions of quality—a review of quality concepts in organizational theory

The term quality, as it has been applied for over 30 years in health care, has acquired a number of overlapping definitions in attempts to make it operational. There is no single definition, but quality can be best thought of as the effort to provide service at the highest possible level, according to the customers' (clients, patients) needs. Specific uses of the term quality within health care will be the subject of this section.

Quality control

Quality measurement and Quality Control were initially industrial concepts, which grew directly out of the experience of mass production in large industrial firms. The Second World War and subsequent economic boom in the United States provided an opportunity to focus on Quality. The war effort required factories to efficiently produce war material in very high volumes. It was detrimental both to the military and to industry to have a high failure rate for equipment. War material was produced according to exacting specifications, so that multiple factories from different companies might all be involved in turning out similar material (e.g. standardized ammunition). For the government, Quality Control meant purchasing standardized items. For the armed forces, it meant having equipment that would function reliably. For the company, it meant increased profits by having fewer defects or rejects in the assembly line.

The resulting approach was Quality Control through inspection. In this scheme, the end product is carefully inspected for defects. Products that do not meet the pre-determined standard are removed at the end of the production line and either discarded or sent back for reprocessing.

In Quality Control, statistical methods measure acceptable defect rates. Companies determine how many defective items can be allowed to roll off the assembly line—usually the 'acceptable' defect rate is on the order of 1–10%. The organizational effort behind quality is put into improving the inspection and control methods available to industry, to ensure that fewer defective products get through the system.

Key features of the Quality Control system are that it accepts a specified error rate, that the standard can be determined by an external source, and that the standard set does not need to be improved upon, only met. In fact, there may be significant cost to exceeding, rather than just meeting, the standard. Finally, Quality Control is done at the end point of the manufacturing process—defects are in the manufacture itself, and are not necessarily thought to relate to design (Figure 38.1).

Accreditation and quality assurance

Within health care, there are parallel systems to the Quality Control approach described above. Some of these health care approaches pre-date or are contemporaneous with the industrial Quality Control developments begun in the 1930s, while others arose later. The two most well known approaches within health care are the closely allied concepts of Accreditation and QA.

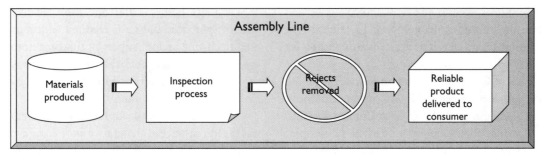

Fig. 38.1 Quality control through inspection.

Accreditation

Initial efforts to introduce quality concepts began with accreditation. External bodies certified—and still do—health care organizations as meeting pre-set standards. The most well known of these in North America is the American Joint Commission for Accreditation of Health Care Organizations (JCAHO). JCAHO started in 1951, and continues to provide standards and benchmarking for health care organizations. Approximately 17,000 organizations undergo the accreditation process through JCAHO [1].

Accreditation involves an agency undergoing review by an external group. The organization wishes to demonstrate that it can meet pre-defined standards in providing care to its patients/clients. Such accreditation, of which the JCAHO is only one example, extends to facilities, care processes, governance, and staffing. Often, such accreditation can be a requirement for licensing by a government body.

There are also accreditation schemes at the individual practitioner level; these include national, provincial, or state licensing bodies overseeing the training, licensure, and conduct of regulated professions. Professional quality begins with accreditation of initial and advanced training, as well as schemes for advanced certification.

One example of an accreditation system functioning at the level of the individual is physician licensing. The most basic licensure programs simply require evidence of completion of a specified medical training program and a minimum of post-graduate training, followed by success on standardized examinations. More recently, both medical school accreditation programs and specialty regulatory systems, such as American Boards of Medical Specialties or the Royal Colleges in many Commonwealth countries, have been requiring evidence of ongoing professional education through approved Continuing Education programs. Lastly, professional accreditation bodies take responsibility for setting and enforcing guidelines regarding professional-ethical behaviour. These approaches to professional accreditation are under scrutiny, both for their effectiveness and for their appropriateness.

Physician certification is only one example of a professional accreditation process, but similar schemes exist for other professionals in the field, including nursing, psychosocial support, expressive therapies and spiritual guidance.

Quality assurance

In the 1960s and 1970s, a broader health care quality effort, beyond accreditation and licensing, was introduced under the rubric of QA programs. An example of this trend is the Peer Review Organizations (PRO) approach, in which an external group of 'peers' or experts examines the quality of health care practices. PROs function mainly within managed health care environments, especially American government systems such as Medicare/Medicaid. Their purpose is to reduce adverse outcomes and, at the same time, to make sure that resources are used efficiently.

Unlike basic accreditation programs, QA systems may focus on quality of care as evidenced through processes and outcomes. QA programs concentrate on using the resources and processes that are in place to ensure that quality standards are being met. These quality standards, however, are still set *a priori* and externally. For QA, as with accreditation schemes, if standards are being met then no further action is taken by the organization until the next review cycle. Features of good QA systems are that they are based on broadly accepted standards, they are usually characterized by voluntary compliance, and they have a functional orientation towards processes or resources. QA reviews should be undertaken regularly to ensure that a specific (usually minimum) standard is met.

The positive aspect of QA systems is that they are designed to reduce error and adverse outcomes, and do so in a way that can examine all aspects of care, not just endpoints. Moreover, because they rely on external standards, what is entailed in meeting those standards is very clear to the healthcare organization.

Finally, while resources need to be devoted to collecting and analyzing data, organizations do not need to reinvent the wheel by developing brand-new internal standards or tools for their evaluation.

The drawback of QA systems is that they are designed to help organizations meet a standard, without any incentive to exceed that standard, just like Quality Control systems. Furthermore, because they embody a pass/fail philosophy, they may be perceived as punitive. It is difficult for staff to generate ongoing enthusiasm for the time and effort required to meet standards that appear to be static and imposed from outside. Finally, accreditation and QA systems are driven by insiders in health care (professionals); there is no inherent linkage to the interests or requests of the consumers of health care—patients and their families.

Quality improvement

Currently, when health care providers think of quality or Quality Control, they are probably thinking of Quality Improvement (QI), which is a distinct approach of its own. In the 1980s and 1990s, QA efforts were superceded in health care by the QI movement. There are a number of quality efforts that fall under this movement, including QI, Continuous Quality Improvement (CQI) and Total Quality Management (TQM). For the purposes of this text, we will simply use the term QI to refer to these efforts.

QI was another direct import from the industrial world into health care, and continues to be the reigning paradigm for quality efforts within the field. In the 1950s a number of industrial innovators improved upon Quality Control methods to help companies improve their processes and turn out better goods. The most well known of these thinkers was W. Edwards Deming who, along with Joseph Juran, introduced advanced quality methods to the Japanese as part of the effort to rebuild their war-torn economy.

While Deming and Juran had differences in their approaches, especially in their use of statistical methods, both—as well as other thinkers, including Kaoru Ishikawa—emphasized the need for quality in each step of the manufacturing process. This emphasis begins right at design in order to produce the highest-quality goods. Consumers would provide feedback to companies by purchasing higher-quality goods, even if they cost more. Deming argued that consumers would focus on high-quality goods, and that if corporations maintained quality, then profits would flow secondarily but necessarily. Orientation towards quality, rather than profits, would actually make companies more successful in the long run.

Deming's name is the one most associated with this quality approach, and he is credited with reforming Japan's manufacturing sector. As part of this breakthrough in thinking, he also promulgated the belief that the standard for a product was not determined at the factory by engineers or managers, but by consumers themselves.

Another critical philosophical piece of Deming's thinking was the importance of an iterative or ongoing cycle of improvement. Not only were the needs of the customer the focus, the process also endeavored to constantly improve quality, thereby seeking higher standards at each iteration.

Therefore the characteristic features of QI are that: (1) The quality standard relies on the customer's assessment, and is not 'externally' determined; (2) Quality needs to be inherent in the business–client relationship; (3) The goal is not just to meet a standard, but to continuously create new standards for the organization (so the quality effort is 'Continuous'); and (4) Quality requires examination of all aspects of the company (is therefore 'Total'). The basic QI process has become identified with the Plan-Do-Study-Act cycle (Figure 38.2).

In practice, it is often found that managers best focus on one aspect of the organization at a time—namely systems (resources and structures), processes (how care is delivered) or outcomes. One cannot focus on any single aspect exclusively, however, as the three are inter-related. For example, processes are often easier to examine, evaluate and quantify than outcomes, especially in health care. It still must be demonstrated that the resulting process evaluation is linked to better outcomes. A method that takes into account all three factors will lead to the most successful implementation of a QI program. This three-part framework of systems, processes and outcomes will be discussed further below.

By the late 1980s, as Japan's economic success took hold, corporations and then health care organizations began to adopt QI methods [2]. The shift from QA to QI in health care

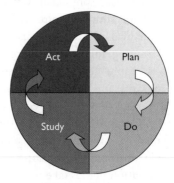

Fig. 38.2 The Deming Cycle: Plan Do Study Act.

may represent not just the influence of the popular image of the Japanese success story, but also fundamental shifts in the nature of health care culture, especially in response to new large-scale managerial structures inherent in both the US managed health care systems and in the UK National Health Service reforms.

In accordance with current thinking, QI methods (CQI, TQM) are well-aligned with the goals of health care in that patient-oriented or family-oriented care is a philosophy that makes the patient's own perception of needs the arbiter of successful care delivery. Quality is therefore aligned with providing the patient with the kind/type of care that they perceive as important for themselves. In some settings, there is close agreement with provider interests; for example, in anaesthesia both parties would likely agree that safe anaesthesia, good pain control, and efficient delivery are important targets. In other areas of health care, determining desirable outcomes is more of a challenge, as will be seen in the discussion of particulars regarding palliative care.

QI and other quality methods found a ready home in certain sectors of health care. These areas are characterized by the routine use of highly standardized procedures where safety is a primary concern. One example already mentioned is anaesthesia, where many patients undergo the same procedure (e.g. the use of inhaled anaesthetics)

repeatedly. While safety and patient outcome are important, so is efficiency because of its impact on operating room schedules. QI approaches are ideally suited to such settings. Therefore, there was a premium on developing standards and measurement tools to improve safety of care, efficiency of care and patient satisfaction. In these settings, resources can be readily delineated and processes described, while outcome measures, such as safe patient anaesthesia, are quantifiable [3].

QI has become so pervasive throughout health care that accrediting bodies, while originally operating from a perspective of QA themselves, are now requiring evidence of QI efforts within health care organizations applying for certification. Both the JCAHO in the United States and the National Health Services (NHS) Trusts in the United Kingdom require that QI processes be in place, in order for a health care organization to qualify for accreditation.

QI efforts should not be confused with cost-effectiveness or other management doctrines. Confusion can exist because of the methods of data collection, the use of the information for program evaluation, and the overlap of purposes; nevertheless, QI efforts specifically address quality issues. Deming saw quality as a fundamental target for organizations to meet, and suggested that other goals, be they profit or effectiveness, would flow from that (Table 38.1).

Table 38.1 Definitions of quality methods

	Quality control	Accreditation	Quality assurance	Quality improvement
Features	Standards determined by an external source	Standards determined by an external source	Standards determined by an external source	Standards determined by feedback provided by consumers
	Accepts a specified error rate	Ensures minimum standards are met at the individual/organizational level	Ensures minimum standards are met at the individual/organizational level	Continually creates new standards for quality (improvement)
	If standard set is met, there is no incentive to improve	If standard set is met, there is no incentive to improve	If standard set is met, there is no incentive to improve	Quality is determined by consumer assessment
	Quality is determined by industry insiders	Quality is determined by industry insiders	Quality is determined by industry insiders	Requires examination of all aspects of an organization
	Takes place at the end point of a process	Requires review by an external group	Focus on processes and outcomes (not just at end points)	Requires examination of all aspects of an organization
	Defect rates measured through statistical methods		Based on broadly accepted standards	
			Characterized by voluntary compliance	
Methods	Inspection	Certification	Peer Review	Continuous Quality Improvement
		Licensing	Organizations	Total Quality management

Challenges of QI

As has been emphasized throughout the literature, implementing QI can be a challenge for organizations, although proponents argue that it has significant rewards. QI represents a fundamental philosophical shift for organizations, especially profit-oriented companies. Engaging in a QI process requires significant and ongoing organizational commitments, including the following:

1. Fundamental orientation for organization.

2. Leadership commitment.

3. Resources, often multi-year—both money and teams [4].

4. Perception of the patient as 'customer' who determines what quality means.

5. Recognition that QI is not the same as accountability for health care managers [5].

6. Acknowledgement that targeted issues/items are fundamental and important to all stakeholders.

It is important that QI mechanisms (e.g. the data collection method) must be easy to integrate into normal practice to enable ongoing support. If the process is difficult, or requires a large block of time episodically, it is less likely to receive continued support. Furthermore, the results of the quality system must be easily accessible, integrated into routine practices, and have an impact on function.

There is some debate regarding the role of a quality system manager—the person responsible in the organization for the quality endeavor. In organizations where there is such a person, both leadership and supervision are embodied in that role. On the downside, all the responsibility for QI is placed on that person. They may begin to play the role of 'police', without other function. Another reason this role often does not work is that QI requires staff input and support—but having a quality manager gives staff the message that quality is someone else's job.

An alternative is to spread QI responsibility throughout an organization, so QI becomes part of everyone's role. In high-functioning organizations, such diffusion enables QI to permeate all relevant groups and improves the opportunity for ground-level support. The challenge then becomes lack of experience in method, lack of commitment by all staff and all managers, and a diffusion of responsibility. This sometimes means that QI is no one's job. Thus, when QI is implemented at the level of managers and line workers, they need sufficient training in the philosophy and processes to allow them to carry out their duties. Furthermore, there needs to be a clear and consistent message from the senior management/ leadership team that QI is an expected component of each of their roles.

Fundamental to either implementation is support for QI at the highest level of the organization. Leadership needs to see QI as fundamental to the organization; these activities cannot be put aside for other considerations, such as temporary crises, lack of time, and other new and exciting initiatives. They need to be seen as part of the day to day processes.

The time required up-front for initial 'buy-in' by line management, and training and support, cannot be underestimated.

Quality initiatives in service organizations

This section will review how quality concepts have been introduced into health care as a general field. It has been noted that the non-profit sector poses different challenges for QI from profit-based organizations. In business, revenues and profit serve as final standards for the success/failure of any given QI activity. Service organizations must choose different bottom-line targets. Peter Drucker and other management thinkers recognize that all businesses have one thing in common—success measured as profit. In contrast, service organizations do not have any such common denominator [6,7].

For both QA and QI activities, the ability to measure outcomes is a core component of the method and a critical feature of evaluation. Since there is no simple common denominator, service organizations must generate their own. There are a number of approaches for this, and unfortunately, no simple answer. That does not mean that service organizations can opt out of undertaking quality initiatives, only that they must be more creative and thorough in their efforts. Measures may be shared by organizations across a field of activity—for example, common outcomes determined for all hospitals. Measures may instead be specific for an individual organization.

The most effective way for organizations to generate these criteria, and to do so in a manner that is internally consistent, is to rely upon mission and goal statements. Missions and goals are generated at the highest level of the organization, usually the Board of Directors, and can thus be thought to represent the fundamentals for the organization, as well as provide some evidence that there is actually backing from leadership for the initiative. Mission and goal statements set out the core targets for the organization, in the same way that profit is the core target of a business. Figure 38.3 shows how mission and goal statements become the foundation of a quality criteria development process.

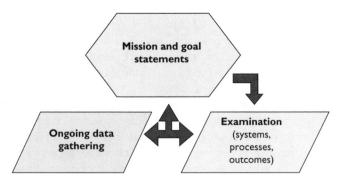

Fig. 38.3 Steps to developing quality criteria in health care.

Quality initiatives in healthcare organizations

Vague terms such as 'serving our clients,' 'improving the environment,' etc., do not generate measurable outcomes. Therefore, generating appropriate mission and goal statements by non-profits is a critical activity that is in turn linked to any QI endeavor. A mission statement and organizational goals document form the basis from which quality approaches can be derived. Boards must take this activity seriously, and commit the organization to working within the framework.

There has been a significant amount of work specifically addressing quality measurement in health care [8–11]. Two of the leading thinkers, Avedis Donabedian and Robert Maxwell have provided a framework for thinking about quality within health care [12,13]. Donabedian proposed that quality in health care is multi-dimensional, and relies upon the 'goodness' of three factors—technical care, interpersonal relationships, and environment.

Technical care encapsulates all the skills of providing care, and is directly related to the effect of care on outcome. The technical component may be more than direct hands-on care for the patient; it may include support items, such as the availability of training for the staff to guarantee clinical excellence. The second factor, interpersonal relationships, is challenging to measure but is a crucial component of satisfaction with care and social concepts of quality. Again, interpersonal relationships is a broad concept, not limited to doctor-patient or nurse-patient interaction. It includes relationships within and between teams, the quality of information-sharing practices, and the warmth and caring experienced by the patient. Finally, there is the environment. Often this is thought of as the physical environment, but may include other aspects, such as technology, that enable care.

For each of these three aspects of care, Donabedian proposed that quality schemes look at systems, processes, and outcomes in a framework that has been widely accepted. These

items became the 'framework', or lens, to examine the dimensions of quality [14]. Systems refers to the underlying resources, programs and administration that enable the organization to function, or enable a particular component of the organization, for example, nursing care, to function. Processes are all of the items and activities involved in providing care. Outcomes are the results of that care, examined in measurable fashion.

These dimensions should not be thought of as rigid—instead there is interplay between them. It is up to the manager or evaluator to determine how an item should be classified in order to enhance an understanding of the impact on Quality. For example, providing safe sedation for painful procedures can be thought of as an outcome in a day treatment setting. Alternatively, it may be examined as a process leading towards another outcome—such as successful endoscopies with earlier diagnosis of cancer.

Robert Maxwell has taken Donabedian's analysis further in examining quality care [13,15]. He has provided six dimensions of quality in health care activities. These dimensions, or questions, expand the concept of quality, and have been used in analysis in the United Kingdom [16]. The dimensions Maxwell uses are:

1. Effectiveness of the treatment based upon evidence.
2. Acceptability—is the treatment acceptable? Is it provided in a manner that patients find acceptable?
3. Efficiency—especially in the use of resources for benefit obtained.
4. Access—what are the barriers and opportunities for using the service?
5. Equity—are all patients and groups being treated in a fair and equal manner?
6. Relevance—how does the service relate to the group of patients and to society as a whole?

As is pointed out by Donald and Sally Irvine, there is a great deal of overlap in these concepts and in quality concepts from other authors and groups [14]. Specific terms may be different, but overall the concepts show great similarity. It is important for health care organizations to use these concepts as broad guidelines, and to assist evaluators in making sure that all relevant dimensions are considered. There is not a cookbook recipe that must be rigidly followed in every given examination of quality.

While the concepts underlying quality are clear, application is difficult. Ideally, one examines systems, processes, and outcomes as a unified entity. Limited resources may tempt one to examine only one of these items, but such isolation does not lead to effective evaluation. For example, evaluating systems alone is challenging in that underlying systems are fundamental components of organizations, and their characteristics may be elusive for insiders to recognize. In turn, there is a natural temptation to evaluate processes alone, as they readily lend themselves to examination—much as manufacturing took the blame in Quality Control where there was an unwillingness to examine design and engineering. Similarly, looking at outcome can have pitfalls. In some areas of health care, it is tempting to isolate outcome as treatment success or improved survival.

Researchers are beginning to examine more sophisticated concepts, such as quality of life resulting from treatment. This is especially true in treatments that may provide longevity, but with the burden of ongoing limitations in activity or health challenges. Improved survival may be an overly simplistic criterion, even in such fields as surgery.

In other specialty areas of health care—for example, those dealing with chronic illness, and especially palliative care—outcomes may be very challenging to measure. Outcome in these areas is generally taken to be at least congruent with patient satisfaction. As will be seen below, it is not always clear that satisfaction is a static concept, or that it is easy to measure.

Taking into consideration the perspectives of the many different stakeholders is a further difficulty. For some time, the opinion of clinicians was assumed to be the relevant data source for quality efforts. This was especially true for QA, where the standards for quality are based upon expert peer opinion. QI, as taken from Deming's work (and in light of health care consumerism) has brought the perspective of the patient to the discussion. Determining who the consumer is (the individual patient, the family, the social group, the health authority); when they should be included (right at the time of treatment, months to years later); and how evaluation should be conducted (quantitative versus qualitative approaches) is a process that is still unsettled.

Despite these challenges, quality efforts in health care have provided positive results. There is now increased thinking about the aims and objectives of health care initiatives. Patient perspectives, albeit difficult to engage, are now taken seriously in discourse. A QI process, with its combination of inductive reasoning and evidence gathering, is well aligned with the scientific approach inherent in modern health care. QI methods enable evaluators to look at the broadest possible picture—from specific treatments to wider questions about resources and goals. A well-functioning quality process may help develop alternative approaches for organizations to achieve their ends, rather than simply trying to eke further benefit from traditional practices.

Case A hospice team in Canada undertook an audit of the use of pain medication. They found that analgesics were frequently prescribed for children during hospice stays based upon pain assessments with standardized tools. Initially the team thought that this represented a satisfactory approach.

Further questioning of families, however, showed that many parents found the system quite cumbersome after discharge, and that there was a delay of several days for getting refills. Often, community pharmacies did not carry the medication in suitable form, and it would have to be specially ordered. Some Family Doctors (GPs) did not have opiate prescribing licenses, or did not feel comfortable prescribing high dose opiates for children.

The hospice team devised a new method, whereby once a stable dose was determined, the hospice physician would order a 30-day supply. In addition, a fax copy of the hospice prescription was simultaneously sent to the family's GP and community pharmacy, to inform them of the drug and dose. This gave the GP immediate information, and provided the local practice and pharmacy with time to make arrangements for refills.

Careful consideration of systems, processes and outcomes, with a focus on end points as defined in missions and goals, reveals that there may be a host of options for fulfilling or achieving those goals, some of which may not be apparent at first.

QA in hospice palliative care programs

Moving from the broad field of health care to the specific area of hospice palliative care reveals important considerations about how to implement quality. Discussion regarding quality emerged within the field of (adult or general) hospice-palliative care by the early 1980s [17–20]. Discussions focused on Quality Assessment and Assurance activities, while initial standards were being developed in hospices [19]. In the United States, the activities of the National Hospice Study establishing cost-effectiveness also enabled an initial determination of standards in order to support the development of Medicare reimbursement policies [21–23].

Currently a number of organizations exercise influence in setting quality-based standards for hospice-palliative care. Some organizations, such as JCAHO, conduct accreditation activities for many types of health care organizations, with hospices considered a sub-set. Accreditation is inherently a QA exercise, but by including a requirement for QI efforts within the standards, the JCAHO has guaranteed that organizations will be functioning at current levels of program evaluation sophistication.

Freestanding hospice accreditation is not, however, equivalent to QA/QI for all palliative care programs, since programs that are hospital- or community-based may not be included in the umbrella. Organizations such as the Canadian Hospice Palliative Care Organization have promulgated

1

national standards for providing care in these settings as well [24]. These standards provide both principles and norms for the provision of hospice-palliative care.

In the United States, standards have been developed specifically for hospices, including those of the National Hospice and Palliative Care Organization [25]. The United Kingdom has established standards through the National Council for Hospice and Specialist Palliative Care Services [26]. Other countries—for example, Australia—have proceeded along similar lines [27]. In all cases the guidelines and standards are voluntary. They begin, however, to establish frameworks and principles that individual hospices/palliative care organizations can refer to when seeking to provide quality care.

QA systems—palliative care professionals

We move next from the level of the organization to the level of the individual professional. Standards are under development for professionals, mainly through Quality Assurance and accreditation approaches. Less stringent requirements have been developed for volunteers, who are the backbone of many palliative care programs, but there are some guides.

Professional quality begins with accreditation of initial and advanced training, as well as schemes for advanced certification. The American Board of Hospice and Palliative Medicine, for example, provides a voluntary system for certification through examination of expertise in the field of palliative medicine. In the United Kingdom, there is now Royal College specialty certification in Palliative Medicine, which requires four years of training in the subject. Similar systems have been developed to include Family Practitioners (e.g. Canadian College of Family Physicians). All of these systems have examination requirements and set standards for ongoing education. Palliative care programs themselves, in lieu of external professional body certification, can establish standards whereby professionals participate in a minimum number of hours of professional development annually.

QI in palliative care

In an ongoing shift, there has been increasing interest among researchers to use QI in palliative care. This has been driven by a number of factors, including increasing sophistication of quality methodology mechanisms. There are external forces at work, including the development of service purchasing in the United Kingdom and managed care in the United States [28–30]. One important conclusion that must be drawn from these initiatives is that quality efforts are often challenging, and those in the field of palliative care especially so. When undertaking quality initiatives, palliative care organizations cannot underestimate the amount of time, money and effort that needs to be devoted to this area. For example, one well-conducted QI effort in pain management in a hospital required a dedicated team, several hundred thousand dollars and many years to complete [4].

Concepts and tools used for quality initiatives in palliative care

Hospice-palliative care programs will find several tools useful in implementing QI programs. As noted previously, quality begins with the development of missions and goals by program leadership. The second step is to determine specific areas in which to implement quality tools. Ideally, all aspects of the program can be evaluated through a quality lens; however, given the resources required, usually only specific, high-impact areas are chosen. However, it is not entirely clear is whether efforts by academic research teams have been replicated in the day-to-day function of typical palliative care programs.

For a palliative care hospice team wishing to undertake a quality effort, several decisions need to be made early on. An initial determination needs to be made regarding the item of concern. Usually this can be gathered through an internal process, whereby staff discuss issues that they feel need to be addressed. This discussion emerges through routine feedback processes, such as staff meetings, and is reviewed at the program leadership level. A less satisfactory approach is to have the item selection imposed externally through an accreditation body or other external agency. The latter method means that the selection is imposed and may not fully engage the staff—it also may not correctly identify the highest-need areas.

A second stage is to more formally assess the area or issue of concern. Typically this takes place with a structured process, sometimes a meeting or retreat, to confirm that the targeted subject is the correct one. Confirmation from program data, a brief literature review, and basic comparison to similar institutions is useful at this step. Because of the resource-intensive nature of quality efforts, it is incumbent upon program leadership to make sure that the focus of the effort be an important one for the program. It must be a core item for the program, worth pursuing and not peripheral.

Because of the nature and focus of palliative care, attention has been focused on two areas: symptom management and interpersonal relationships. These aspects of care are core to the goals of palliative programs and thus have been the focus of evaluative research. Moreover, they are areas where researchers can examine outcomes and then readily correlate these to processes and systems. Examples include pain management [31–36] and professional communication [37,38].

The next stage involves deeper and more focused investigation. Resources within the program need to be devoted to the quality effort, even when an outside consultant is brought in. At this stage a more formal effort is initiated to address the area of interest—examining structures, processes and outcomes. It is often tempting to examine only a single factor (e.g. processes), which seems easy both to measure and to change. That, however, will not fully explain the problem, nor will it guarantee any change in outcome. All three dimensions are linked, and all require attention in the evaluation plan. Another temptation is to focus on outcomes at first. This is problematic if it does not take into account the significant resources that will be required to examine and make changes in systems and processes. Moreover, within palliative care, outcome measures are still problematic, as will be discussed below.

The field of quality in palliative care, while still in its early stages, is now developed enough that there are tools for data gathering—both at the initial stage, when trying to define the problem of interest, and at the subsequent stages of the evaluation cycle when carrying out the QI effort. There is also increasingly better understanding within palliative care as to how these tools can be used together, both quantitative and qualitative, as well as the limitations about the data they gather.

Familiar data-gathering tools include focus groups [28, 37, 39, 40], surveys [32,41,42], clinical audits and report cards [43,44], and mortality rounds and end-of-care debriefings [44,45]. While there is an initial temptation to use surveys, it may be better to start with less structured tools for data gathering, including patient interviews and focus groups. These approaches may yield more detailed information (the term sometimes used is 'rich data') about the program and patient experience. [46]

Qualitative data methods are well accepted, especially for their ability to generate new theory, identify unexpected issues, engage multiple stakeholders, provide highly valid data (but not necessarily data that is reliable or generalizable according to standard psychometrics) and give participants a voice. [47] In palliative care, where so many complex dimensions interact, and where the experience for each subject (patient, family, community, and caregiver) is very personal, qualitative approaches are important tools in quality efforts.

The other tools described above, such as rounds, clinical audits, and end-of-care debriefings, should also be utilized. For example, at one children's hospice a dedicated debriefing round takes place following each death [48]. These sessions involve all members of the care team, and include professionals from the hospital and the community as well. A summary of the child's history is undertaken, as well as a review of management including medicine-nursing, psychosocial, spiritual care and co-ordination of services. Included is a review of care that went well and care that did not, with recommendations for change in the future. Minutes of these sessions are generated and the results are shared with all members of the care team. The full set of these rounds is maintained for periodic review. This is one example of how a clinical audit practice can be incorporated into a QI program.

Quantitative tools can be especially useful in palliative care processes and system resources; however, when it comes to outcomes they are less useful (with the exception of survey instruments). This is due to the fundamental properties of the goals of palliative care, which are oriented towards symptom relief and providing a comfortable and dignified death. In other health care fields, quantifiable outcomes are easier to identify—for example, length-of-stay data, survival data, cure rates, etc. In palliative care, the single common outcome is death, and therefore survival and related quantitative measures are not relevant data items. Surveys and, in some settings, qualitative approaches, can help to access data on outcomes of interest, such as quality of life and satisfaction (Table 38.2). These aspects of assessment and data gathering raise a number of issues for QI in paediatric palliative care that will be discussed further on.

Tools addressing symptoms and satisfaction

Despite these reservations, a number of quantitative tools have been developed within the field of general and adult palliative care to assess symptoms and satisfaction. Of the dozens of tools, some examples include the McGill Quality of Life Questionnaire [49], the Memorial Symptom Assessment Scale [50], and the Quality of End-of-life care and Satisfaction with Treatment (QUEST) scale [51]. Surveys cover all aspects of care, including symptom management, psycho-social care, spiritual care, and bereavement. The Toolkit of Instruments to Measure End-of-Life Care (TIME) provides a current web-based bibliography of numerous tools to measure multiple aspects

Table 38.2 Qualitative and quantitative quality-measurement tools

Qualitative tools	Focus group
	Clinical audit
	Clinical report card
	End-of-care debriefing
	Patient interview
Quantitative tools	Survey
	Measurement scale

of care and of quality of care in palliative medicine. Although survey development can be lengthy and resource-intensive, it is important to remember the imperative of validating the instruments using appropriate techniques [52].

Most of the instruments described above measure either symptoms, quality of life, satisfaction with care, or a combination of factors from each of these domains. In turn, since symptom relief has been used as a proxy outcome measure, these instruments have become important in addressing quality issues within palliative care.

Morita and colleagues developed a 34-item questionnaire in rigorous fashion to explore factors that related to overall satisfaction with care [42]. The assumption is that satisfaction with care becomes the arbiter of quality of care, from the standpoint of the patient and family. This group identified seven dimensions:

(1) Nursing care—warmth, care help, support

(2) Facility—the physical layout

(3) Information—explanations and communication

(4) Availability of hospice care

(5) Family care and support

(6) Cost

(7) Symptom palliation.

For each of these domains, there is a relationship to performance in care, based upon (1) competence, (2) effectiveness, (3) accuracy, (4) attitudes of professionals, (5) the strength of communication, and (6) variables pertaining to the organization.

Tools addressing outcomes and quality

There have been attempts to create scales that address quality and outcome as primary measures, rather than through secondary indices. The tools used in these approaches have undergone testing for reliability and validity, and describe outcomes of value to families and practitioners. Research so far has concentrated on adult palliative care, though there may be some extrapolation possible to paediatrics.

Much of the work in palliative care has been undertaken by Irene Higginson and colleagues in the United Kingdom, and by Joan Teno in the United States. One instrument designed specifically to examine dimensions of quality in palliative care is the Support Team Assessment Schedule (STAS) [53,54]. The STAS is a measure specifically developed to measure key indicators in the delivery of palliative care [53]. It has been used in both community and in-patient settings. The domains in this tool include:

- Pain and other symptoms
- Patient distress

- Family distress
- Communication with health professionals
- Directly obtaining practical aid.

These are measures of patient outcome while participating in hospice care. This schedule needs to be adapted to paediatrics, and some challenges to its reliability will need to be addressed [55]. There are conflicting reports about the ability to use it in different cultural or social settings [56,57]. Nevertheless, the domains are still useful in developing a model of quality.

Another audit tool, currently under development, is the Palliative Outcome Scale, which examines care from the standpoint of both the team and the patient [58].

Challenges and successes in quality efforts in palliative care

There are myriad challenges related to quality efforts in palliative care. The first relates to determining outcomes. While there is general agreement that palliative care addresses comfort and dignity at the end of life, beyond that there is little agreement regarding the tools that enable outcome assessment—both because it is difficult to measure (quantify) these aspects, and because of the multiplicity of subjects (patient, family, providers), whose experiences change over time through the illness-dying-bereavement trajectory. Also, it is difficult to determine when data should be collected—during the entire palliative phase, at end of life, in early or in late bereavement. To summarize, there are challenges in assessing the who, the what and the when of palliative care in order to determine quality of care.

The first problem for either quantitative or qualitative approaches to assessment is determining the recipient(s) of care (patient, close family, extended family, significant others) and in turn who the respondent is to address aspects of that care. Even in the simplest formulation, where the recipient is the patient and care is focused on symptoms, problems arise in evaluating quality. Unlike other areas of biomedicine, the only 'gold standard' for symptom relief is the patient's experience of the symptom (e.g. pain, dyspnoea, anxiety). There are a number of potential respondents who can assess the symptom— the patient, the family, or the professional care provider. Researchers have begun to evaluate the strength of correlation between patient, family (caregivers) and professional assessments of both symptoms and of satisfaction. The literature indicates relatively poor correlation between patients' and caregivers' assessments of symptoms [59]. In this sense, caregivers—even close family members—are not legitimate proxies for patients.

The nature of palliative care requires that the patient experience is a primary outcome of the goals of palliative care.

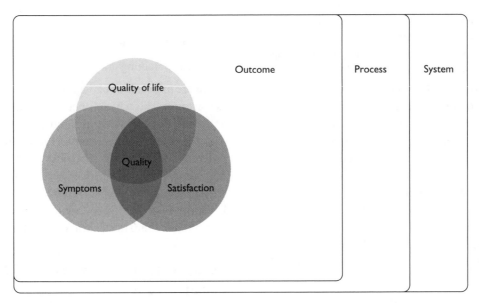

Fig. 38.4 Dimensions of quality of life, symptoms, and satisfaction.

Thus, as researchers have attempted to assess symptoms or satisfaction with care at one of the critical phases of the end-of-life journey, there has been a significant challenge in that other individuals cannot provide valid information for the patient's experience.

For outcome data, determining when data is collected is a second difficulty: during care before death; throughout program involvement or only during inpatient periods; or after death. Patients may be too ill or fatigued to participate in surveys, assessment tools or interviews to provide evaluation data at the end of life [60]. An alternate approach may be to focus on the experience of family and caregivers as they experience the patient's dying and death. For these groups, timing of assessment is an important issue; questions arise as to the best time that grief and bereavement data can be collected. In at least one study, there was a preference by family not to be interviewed until more than six months had passed [39]. The role of grief and the impact it may have on family perception of satisfaction, symptoms and quality requires further exploration.

The next emerging challenge is deciding what to study. There is now recognition that the items of importance to patients regarding palliative care may be distinct for different patient groups. In one study, the goals for palliative care of patients with Chronic Pulmonary Disease were different from those with AIDS and cancer [61]. The implications of this for paediatric palliative care are significant, and challenge any assumptions of using or borrowing tools originally developed in adult palliative care or for cancer-based models of palliative care.

Other interesting findings have come out of this research, including the apparent realization that not only may there be poor correlation between patients' and caregivers' perceptions of symptoms, but more crucially, that patient symptoms may not correlate with satisfaction. In several studies, patients have poorly controlled symptoms and yet express satisfaction with care [32,51,59,62]. The reasons for this require further investigation.

In summary then, there are several overlapping constructs, all of which can be thought to be component parts of 'outcome' for palliative care (Figure 38.4). These constructs include, but are not limited to, comfort and symptom management; care for the family both during the palliative care phase and after death; satisfaction with care for patients and for family; and quality of life. All of these constructs are patient-centred or family-centred. There are other outcomes of relevance to hospice-palliative care organizations at the program level that may be reflected in costs, activity-levels, coordination of care with other agencies, etc. that may be important to study.

Even at the patient-centred level, there is no single construct that can encapsulate outcomes. These constructs interact with each other in complex ways that the quality researcher and program evaluator need to be aware of when establishing a QI program.

The conclusion, therefore, is that measurement of some—but not all—of the key outcomes in palliative care may be challenging, especially during critical phases. Outcome data are not conclusive; because of the methodological challenges it has been difficult to specify the outcomes that best track program success. In turn, this makes overall quality assessment and improvement difficult, but not impossible. Nevertheless, the overall data points to high degrees of satisfaction on the part of patients, family and providers with palliative care. Trends in the field towards comprehensive symptom management, flexibility in care, and care in multiple settings, are all consistent with evidence at this point.

Most of this discussion has emphasized issues regarding outcomes. The framework established by Donabedian and Maxwell, however, included processes and systems. Here the data are much clearer. Processes lend themselves to study because they often have measurable activities, and sometimes external benchmarks. Examples of process evaluation for a hospice-palliative care program include time from referral to first visit, communications (e.g. time to get a letter out), and time for pain medication to be delivered to bedside [38, 63, 64].

One of the single most important process items correlating with satisfaction in care is the nature of interpersonal communications. There are important implications of this work for paediatrics, which will be discussed below [37, 61, 65]. Prognosis information, and symptom management are also critical items linked to satisfaction with care [66]. It should be noted that these items can actually be thought of either as processes or as (intermediate) outcomes. The distinction is not as critical as understanding their link to quality.

There is less information regarding the underlying systems or resources that are required to implement effective palliative care. There are common components of palliative care programs addressing the multiple dimensions of care—for example, physical symptoms, psychosocial issues, and spiritual care.

There are standards and norms documents for hospice-palliative care specifically addressing paediatrics, which shed some light on systems. In the United Kingdom, the National Council for Hospice and Specialist Palliative Care Services has published a set of standards, which apply to all hospice-palliative care programs [67]. Similarly, there is a current norms document set forth by the Canadian Hospice Palliative Care Association [24, 68].

The standards outlined in these documents cover broad areas related to patient and family care:

- Disease management
- Physical issues
- Psychological issues
- Social issues
- Spiritual issues
- Practical issues
- Preparation for death
- Loss, grief and bereavement.

Similarly, there are domains for:

- Process of providing care (e.g. assessment and information sharing)

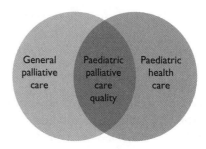

Fig. 38.5 Pediatric palliative care standards.

- Governance and administration
- Program support.

While these documents are an overview for a national approach, and are not specific to paediatrics, they contain specific information regarding items in care provision processes, governance, and administration and program support that may be of value to paediatric programs (Figure 38.5). In assessing and improving quality, programs will likely assess outcomes and process first, and determine whether systems exist to support these.

Quality efforts in paediatric palliative care—evidence base in paediatrics

Moving from the overall area of (adult) palliative care to the more specific area of paediatric palliative care, the evidence base narrows. This is especially true when looking at quality concepts, where relatively little work has been done, and thus there is a need to extrapolate in the first place from the general (adult) palliative literature.

A number of challenges exist to developing quality standards for paediatric palliative care. One is that the field is still relatively young. The first hospice program specifically for children opened in 1982 [69]. Currently, there are almost 40 paediatric palliative care programs/hospices in the United Kingdom, and 10 in Canada [48, 70, 71]. In Poland there is a community-based palliative care program. In the United States, as of 1998 approximately 180 organizations provided some level of paediatric palliative care, across a variety of types of programs. Most of these programs took care of 12 or fewer children per year [72]. There are still only two free-standing paediatric hospice programs in North America at this time, and many programs are hospital-based teams [73]. The field has received increasing attention, but is considered to be in its early stages.

Given that the field is in its early development, one challenge is gathering sufficient data to support the development of quality endeavors. Nevertheless, there are successful developments on two fronts—one being research into the dimensions that are important to families and children in palliative care, and another being the recent publication of initial standards for paediatric palliative care.

Characteristics of paediatric palliative care, described elsewhere in this text, make it quite different from adult care. Notably, the illness models are different. Acute, severe, life-threatening illness makes up a smaller proportion of care for paediatric programs. Longer-term conditions, many of them genetically based, are a large proportion of illnesses. For example, at Canuck Place Children's Hospice in Vancouver, Canada, some 75% of children have diagnoses other than cancer, and similar data is found in the United Kingdom [74,75]. Included are children with neuromuscular diseases, syndromic disorders, neurodegenerative diseases, metabolic disease, HIV/AIDS, inoperable cardio-pulmonary diseases and poorly characterized CNS conditions with Severe Neurological Impairment, which carry a higher mortality risk [76].

A characteristic of these conditions is that prognosis is often difficult to predict, and many children live for many years with these conditions. They therefore require not measures designed to ensure 'death with dignity' but instead 'life-embracing' actions within the context of a shortened life span.

Another crucial feature of all paediatric health care encounters is the developmental nature of child health. Different strategies and approaches need to be used for distinct developmental phases. These approaches require constant revision as the child grows and changes—thus they are not static for a given child. In turn, one must take into account the variation within a paediatric population, from the rapid changes of infancy, the emotional growth inherent in adolescence, and the distinct issues for those children whose development is not typical.

While the challenges for outcome measurement via proxy have already been discussed in regards to palliative care symptom management, there is an additional challenge in paediatrics, namely who is the patient and who speaks for the patient? These are separate but inter-related questions.

Who is the patient? Is it just the child; the child and parents; or the child, parents and siblings? Most definitions go at least this far, although one must also consider the importance of extended family and of close friends. The latter is especially important to adolescents. The issue is not just pertinent in the interpretation of experience for the pre-verbal or non-verbal child. It is also an issue that is developmentally relevant as children only acquire their own 'voice' in establishing autonomous decision making over time. That task is one of the major functions of healthy adolescence, and is only made more complicated within the context of illness.

Thus there are challenges in undertaking quality-related research and evaluation in paediatric palliative care. A modest amount of work has taken place, but at this time there are no reports of comprehensive QI efforts or outcomes research in paediatric palliative care programs, per se; much of the existing research looks at specific symptom management or aspects of care.

In studies that have asked parents directly about their children's care, or have examined the care of children in detail, a number of areas are highlighted where quality measures can have an impact. One is the area of pain management. It is now well documented that pain assessment and treatment is a significant issue in child health. Studies have shown that overall pain management is poor in the paediatric population [77]. Recognition of symptoms and management is a basic foundation and has been highlighted as lacking in the care of dying children [66].

Several dimensions have been found to be very important to families and would be core components of a more global, patient/family-centred quality effort. Studies indicate that the most significant dimension may be good communication with health care providers. In one study, this factor seemed to closely link to satisfaction and had the largest impact on parent's perceptions of the quality of the care for their child [78]. Other factors have been identified as well that link to parent perceptions of quality. These include best-possible prognostic information, respite care, grief-support for losses long before death, coordination of services, equal opportunities for education and recreation, psychological support, sibling support, and efforts to address spiritual concerns [40,79,80].

In a study of satisfaction of parents with hospitalized children (not necessarily palliative), parents noted problems with discharge planning as another important component. It is likely that discharge/transition planning will turn out to be important to families experiencing hospice-palliative care [40]. In an investigation looking specifically at quality in paediatric palliative care, three other issues were identified as linking to family perceptions of quality: meeting the needs of siblings, care for non-English-speaking families, and providing bereavement follow-up [80].

Models and standards for paediatric palliative care

While there is no reliable evidence base regarding systems, processes or outcomes in paediatric palliative care, standards documents have been developed. Usually, these standards are generated through expert consensus and review of best-available evidence. These standards documents can form the basis for an individual program's QI effort by laying out dimensions and targets for quality. These emerging standards will also provide a framework from which evidence-based research and evaluation can be launched.

The existing documents either describe ideals for care, make recommendations, or set forth explicit standards. They are inconsistently evidence-based in their standards and recommendations [81]. At least one of the documents links the promulgated standards to outcomes and indicators, in a US federally funded project for comprehensive children's palliative care [82, 83]. Some of the documents propose broad norms, while others set forth explicit and specific standards [67].

Examples of national and organizational standards for paediatric palliative care include statements by:

1. The Association for Children with Life-threatening or Terminal Conditions and their Families (ACT) in conjunction with the Royal College of Paediatrics and Child Health in the United Kingdom [67].

2. The American Academy of Pediatrics [81].

3. The National Hospice and Palliative Care Organization Administrative/Policy Workgroup on Children's International Project on Palliative/Hospice Services (ChIPPS) [84].

4. The Standards of Care for PACC® (Program for All-Inclusive Care for Children and their Families) developed by Children's Hospice International (Alexandria, Virginia) and the Health Care Financing Administration of the US Department of Health and Human Services [85].

5. The Standards of palliative home care for children in Poland [86].

6. The Association of Children's Hospices.

7. Pediatric Hospice Palliative Care Guiding Principles and Norms of Practice developed by the Canadian Network of Palliative Care for Children and the Canadian Hospice Palliative Care Association [87].

All of these documents share common features and cover a common set of domains, which is not surprising. Domains held in common throughout these documents include:

• Patient- and family-centred care

• Pain and symptom management

• Developmentally appropriate care

• Respite for families

• Bereavement services

• Continuity of care

• Integrated, multi dimensional care

• Professional competence and continuing education

• Research

• Care for caregivers

• Policies and procedures

The various domains addressed in these standards documents are described and compared in Table 3 using Donabedian's framework as an organizing scheme.

In addition to the core domains, additional statements within these standards include:

• Early initiation of symptom management in the course of a disease

• Inclusion of children with any kind of life-limiting condition

• Avoidance of rigid distinctions re cure vs. palliation

• Early discussion of palliative care.

Many of the models of care for palliative care and for paediatric palliative care have not been directly tested [28, 87], and the need to test the individual components is great. Nevertheless, there is a move towards creating standards, both evidence- and consensus-driven, which in turn provide a framework for further QI and research activities. Areas such as team members [88] and spirituality [79] are being addressed.

While most of the standards and norms documents in paediatric palliative care provide high level guidelines for Quality, one program has specifically addressed Quality (via QA) within children's hospices. The Association of Children's Hospices in the United Kingdom recently produced a QA tool designed specifically for children's hospice services. This tool was derived from a wide ranging consultation with users of children's hospice services regarding what they value about children's hospice care, coupled with information provided by staff working in and professionals working alongside the children's hospice services. This consultation generated six key aspects: Access; the Child; the Family; the Staff; the Environment and Communication. The QA package is designed to enable a children's hospice service to self-evaluate their performance against criteria developed from material gathered through the consultation. The toolkit is being readied for publication and dissemination; how it will apply outside of the United Kingdom, and in palliative programs that are not hospice-based, remains to be studied (Table 38.3).

Creating a model of paediatric palliative care quality

Based upon the above documents, one can create a model for paediatric palliative care provided in a quality manner. Each program must undertake this task individually, but at the same time needs to be aware of the significant pitfalls of attempting to do this alone.

Table 38.3 Standards and outcomes in paediatric palliative care

Donabedian[1]	1997 ACT/RCPCH[2]	1998 CHI[3]	2000 American Academy Of Pediatrics[4]	2001 ChIPPS /NHO[5]	2004 Association of Children's Hospices[6]
Technical or clinical care	Flexible service with a care plan based upon individual needs assessment Linked to a local area paediatrician Support for day-to-day management of the child 24-hour care in terminal stages Help for parents and siblings during illness, death and bereavement Respite care Assistance with practical and financial concerns	Pain and symptom management Bereavement program Interdisciplinary team services	Availability of expert assistance 24 h a day Interdisciplinary care team to address physical, psychosocial, emotional and spiritual needs of child and family Respite Bereavement	Relief of physical, social, psychological and existential or spiritual symptom management Supportive and bereavement care should be available as long as necessary Interdisciplinary team Involvement from the time of diagnosis Available to the family 24 h a day, 365 days a year Respite A professional team educated and trained in palliative care.	Pain & symptom control Psycho/spiritual care 24 h access. Respite, emergency and terminal care. Pre and post bereavement care for siblings and close family members for as long as family requires. Care plan worked out with child/family/carers based on needs identification. Interdisciplinary team. Availability of wider multidisciplinary team: clinical, complementary Staff development, Staff support. Advocacy for child and family.
Interpersonal relationships	Keyworker to coordinate care Lead consultant paediatrician who is expert in the child's condition	Access to care Child and family as unit of care Continuity of care	Seamless transition At least one consistent caregiver Care coordinator Support for the caregivers	The unit of care is the child and family Families should be able to refer themselves Child and family are included in designing the priorities of care Enhance the quality of life for the child and family Access to a team of caregivers, or 'keyworker' or care coordinator whose care is seamless Direct caregivers must be provided both formal and informal psychosocial support and supervision Upholds their values, wishes and beliefs	Referral criteria to admit all eligible children. Referral process to ensure all eligible children can access. Referrals from any source. Hospice meets needs of child and family from acceptance, throughout terminal phase, death and after. Seamless and continuous support. Holistic care tailored to meet personal needs of each individual child and family. Knowledge, expertise, emotional,

Table 38.3 (*Continued*)

Donabedian[1]	1997 ACT /RCPCH[2]	1998 CHI[3]	2000 American Academy Of Pediatrics[4]	2001 ChIPPS /NHO[5]	2004 Association of Children's Hospices[6]
					practical support for parents, siblings, wider family, carers. Family values respected. Children's wishes and potential autonomy respected. Siblings supported and included. Staff work in partnership with child and family, leaving choice and control with family. Relationship nurtured and support co-ordinated by key worker. Staff communicate effectively with children and families. Hospice staff work collaboratively with other professionals involved in the child's care.
Environment	Locally based service Single point access for equipment and medications Provision for necessary housing and school adaptations	Policies and procedures Utilization review/ quality Improvement	Explicit and coordination between tertiary care centers and community. Equitable reimbursement for services Improve professional curricula	A setting that is desired and/or appropriate for their needs	Child focused, relaxed atmosphere. Adaptable to age and and condition Personalized according to individual preferences. Facilities and equipment available. Safe. Continuous quality programme

Sources

[1] Donabedian, A. *The Definition of Quality and Approaches to its Assessment.* Ann Arbor, MI: Health Administration Press, 1980.

[2] Anonymous. *A Guide To The Development Of Children's Palliative Care Services.* Bristol, UK: Report of a Joint Working Party of the Association for Children with Life-threatening or Terminal Conditions and their Families And the Royal College of Paediatrics and Child Health, 1997. ISBN 1 900954 06 0.

[3] Anonymous. *Standards of Care for PACC® Programs*: Children's Hospice International, 1997.

[4] Anonymous. American Academy of Pediatrics. Committee on Bioethics and Committee on Hospital Care. Palliative care for children. *Pediatrics* 2000; 106(2 Pt 1):351–7.

[5] Levetown, M., Barnard, M., Byock, I., Carter, B., Connor, S., and Darville, J. *A Call for Change: Recommendations to Improve the Care of Children Living with Life-Threatening Conditions.* Alexandria, Virginia: National Hospice and Palliative Care Organization, October 2001.

[6] Hurd, E. *Are We Getting it Right? A Tool to Measure the Quality of Children's Hospice Services.* Bristol, UK: Association of Children's Hospices, 2004.

The pitfalls are not limited to the expenditure of unnecessary effort where standards and methods have already been recreated—that is, 'reinventing the wheel'. An additional pitfall of developing a quality approach alone is that inadequate tools may be used, generating false answers [52]. The practice of quality in health care is now sufficiently developed that one must be working at a fairly sophisticated level in ensuring that valid and reliable tools are used to measure activity to meet guidelines and standards [13,15].

Another pitfall that must be addressed is integrating the quality effort into the routine of the program or organization. The overall effort that must be devoted to quality endeavors cannot be underestimated [4, 89]. Furthermore, there is a risk of using assessment tools that have been developed in one setting, and assuming they will work in a different one [57]. Lastly, some techniques of assessment and measurement that work well in research settings are not always easily implemented in day to day functioning, and need to be adapted [89].

A working model of quality for paediatric palliative care would have a number of features: first, it would rely on one of the current guidelines/standards as a basic framework. Alternatively, new guidelines may be developed, but the evidence so far indicates that they should include a combination of systems, processes and outcomes.

Systems include a care team with a complement of providers skilled in symptom management, psychological and spiritual support, family support, and a facility or other means to provide respite. In addition, systems include appropriate governance and administration.

Processes include an intake mechanism, assessment of child and family needs, care for those needs, and a communication process for both families and other health care teams. Outcomes should be assessed in a multi dimensional fashion, relying on both the organization's published mission statements and external guidelines. In turn, these outcomes should be assessed taking into account the perspectives of the patient, the family, the palliative care team, and external teams at multiple points in time, both pre- and post-death. Methods should include both quantitative assessments of physical symptoms and satisfaction through surveys, as well as qualitative approaches, including interviews.

A formulation that takes into account multiple aspects of the patient-family experience may yield the best results. This may be especially important in paediatric palliative care, given the added issue of the non-verbal population and developmentally linked assessment. In this formulation, assessment is made of symptoms by patient, family and professionals, of patient satisfaction, of family satisfaction, and of carer perspectives [90].

Second, the items chosen would be consistent with the organization's mission and objectives statements. The systems and processes needed for an in-patient hospice program, a community-based palliative care program and a hospital-based team may be different.

Third, the quality approach would be built into the way that care is provided, with an active feedback loop from the quality system into the care system. The inherent nature of quality is one that has been emphasized. It must have an impact both at the assessment level, as well as at the day to day care level [15].

Case Example of Quality Process—Canuck Place Children's Hospice

One example of an implementation of a quality process is at Canuck Place Children's Hospice, in Vancouver, Canada. While not a complete process, it includes a number of the significant items described above. The quality process is outlined in the basic Strategic Directions of the Hospice program [91]. The quality efforts are overseen by a Quality Council, reporting to the Board of Directors.

The committee meets on a monthly basis. There is representation on the committee from the Board of Directors, program leadership, program staff, and an external member. At the meetings, a number of quality items and their indicators are reviewed. Quality items fall into four broad domains: (1) Responsiveness, (2) System competency, (3) Family/Community expectations and goals, and (4) Quality of work life.

Some items, such as hospice census and acuity, are reviewed at each meeting. Other items—for example, chart audits or professional development, are reviewed on a semi-annual or annual basis, with a different set reviewed each month. This allows staff to be gathering indicator data targeted towards a specific month's deadline. At the next meeting, the Quality Committee reviews the indicators, which are then forwarded on to the Board of Directors.

Items identified for action are then referred back to appropriate individuals, teams, or committees within the hospice program for further study and action.

Conclusion

Quality initiatives, in all their forms as QA and QI, must now be considered fundamental within health care. Quality efforts have the potential to transform health care delivery organizations by providing them with a framework for evaluating their practices. It is no longer sufficient for health care providers to simply assume that they are doing the right things because they are doing them for the right reasons. Quality efforts, especially QI, provide an opportunity for programs and clinicians to use an evidence-based approach for self-evaluation and standards development.

Quality initiatives, however, are not always easy to implement even in the best of circumstances. They require substantial commitment from leadership, both in philosophy and in time and money resources. Undertaking major initiatives without that commitment can leave the organization worse off than before through wasted effort and engendered cynicism. Therefore, the first step in quality efforts is to commit the leadership to the long-term effort and implications of a quality approach. Health care represents a special case for QI, as the outcomes for service organizations are not as easy to measure as those in the commercial world. Palliative care and, even more so, paediatric palliative care present ever-increasing challenges to the researcher and manager who wish to undertake quality initiatives. In addition to the organizational resource challenges, there are issues to be decided regarding outcomes of interest and measurement of those outcomes. These challenges do not, however, exempt paediatric palliative care programs from undertaking quality initiatives. The issues must be addressed head-on regarding the goals of palliative care and the who, what and when to measure questions associated with those goals.

In all likelihood, there is no one single best measurement approach. In the complexities that constitute the paediatric palliative care setting, a mix of quantitative and qualitative approaches to each question will be required. There is also no single best target—symptom management, psycho-social-spiritual care, family care, patient satisfaction, and global quality measures are all valid dimensions that can be looked at in a quality initiative. A successful quality initiative will examine these in combination, creatively and appropriately, to answer questions.

Paediatric palliative care is a relatively young field, and for workers in the field, it is frustrating to be faced with a burden of proof around quality when so much of the basic groundwork to support quality efforts remains to be done. Rather than an obstacle, this should be a spur for each program in the field to undertake the best possible and most practical evaluation approach, and to widely disseminate the results to help the field as a whole.

References

1. Anonymous. Facts about the Joint Commission on Accreditation of Healthcare Organizations [World Wide Web]. Available at: *http://www.jcaho.org/about+us/index.htm.* Accessed 24 April, 2003.

2. Ferris, G.R. and Wagner, J.A. Quality circles in the United States: A conceptual reevaluation. *J Appl Behav Sci* 1985;21(2):155–167.

3. Miller R. (ed.) Anesthesia (5th edition). Philadelphia, PA. Churchill Livingstone, Inc; 2000.

4. Bookbinder, M., Coyle, N., Kiss, M., *et al.* Implementing national standards for cancer pain management: program model and evaluation. *J Pain Symptom Manage* 1996;12(6):334–47; discussion 331–3.

5. Johnston, G.M., Burge, F.I., Boyd, C.J., and MacIntyre, M. End-of-life population study methods. *Can J Public Health* Sep–Oct 2001; 92(5):385–6.

6. Drucker, P.F. Managing the Non-Profit Organization: Principles and Practices (1st edition). New York: Harper Collins; 1990.

7. D'Onofrio C.N. Hospice quality improvement programs: An initial examination. *Topics in Health Inform Manage* 1998;18(4):13–31.

8. Blumenthal, D. Part 1: Quality of care—what is it? New England. *J Med* Sep 19 1996;335(12):891–4.

9. Blumenthal, D. Quality of health care. Part 4: The origins of the quality-of-care debate. *N Eng J Med* Oct 10 1996;335(15): 1146–9.

10. Brook, R.H., McGlynn, E.A., and Cleary, P.D. Quality of health care. Part 2: Measuring quality of care. *N Eng J Med* Sep 26 1996; 335(13):966–70.

11. Chassin, M.R. Quality of health care. Part 3: Improving the quality of care. *N Eng J Med* Oct 3 1996;335(14):1060–3.

12. Donabedian A. *The Definition of Quality and Approaches to its Assessment.* Ann Arbor, MI: Health Administration Press, 1980.

13. Maxwell, R.J. Quality assessment in health. *Br Med J (Clin Res Ed)* May 12 1984;288(6428):1470–2.

14. Irvine, D. and Irvine, S. *The Practice of Quality* Oxford: Radcliffe Medical Press Ltd; 1996.

15. Maxwell, R.J. Dimensions of quality revisited: From thought to action. *Qual Health Care* Sep 1992;1(3):171–7.

16. Armes, P.J. and Higginson, I.J. What constitutes high-quality HIV/AIDS palliative care? *J Palliat Care* 1999;15(4):5–12.

17. Bohnet, N.L. Quality assurance as an ongoing component of hospice care. Qrb. *Qual Rev Bull* 1982;8(5):7–11.

18. Rolka, H.R. Quality assurance for terminally ill. *Hosp Health Services Admin* 1983;28(2):66–80.

19. McCann, B.A. and Enck, R.E. Standards for hospice care: A JCAH hospice project overview. *Prog Clin Biol Res* 1984;156:431–40.

20. Martin, J.P. Ensuring quality hospice care for the person with AIDS. Qrb. *Qual Rev Bull* 1986;12(10):353–8.

21. Greer, D.S., Mor, V., Morris, J.N., Sherwood, S., Kidder, D., and Birnbaum, H. An alternative in terminal care: Results of the National Hospice Study. *J Chronic Dis* 1986;39(1):9–26.

22. Greer, D.S. and Mor, V. An overview of National Hospice Study findings. *J Chronic Dis* 1986;39(1):5–7.

23. Greer, D.S., Mor, V., Sherwood, S., Morris, J.N., and Birnbaum, H. National hospice study analysis plan. *J Chronic Dis* 1983;36(11): 737–80.

24. Ferris, F., Balfour, H., Bowen K., *et al. A Model to Guide Hospice Palliative Care: Based on National Principles and Norms of Practice.* Ottawa, ON: Canadian Hospice Palliative Care Association, 2002.

25. Organization, NHaPC. *Standards of Practice for Hospice Programs.* Alexandria, Virginia.

26. Glickman, M. and Standards, WPo. Making Palliative Care Better: Quality Improvement, Multiprofessional Audit and Standards. Occasional Paper 12, 1997.

27. Committee SaQ. *Standards for Palliative Care Provision* (3rd edition). Deakin Australia: Palliative Care Australia, 1999.

28. Donaldson, M.S. and Field, M.J. Measuring quality of care at the end of life. *Arch Intern Med* 1998;158(2):121–8.

29. Byock, I.R., Teno, J.M., and Field, M.J. Measuring quality of care at life's end. *J Pain Symptom Manage* 1999;17(2):73–4.

30. Higginson, I.J. Accreditation of specialist palliative care: Minimum standards or improved care? *Palliat Med* 1998;12(2):73–74.

31. Braveman, C. and Rodrigues, C. Performance improvement in pain management for home care and hospice programs.[comment]. American *J Hospice Palliat Care* 2001;18(4):257–63.

32. Comley, A.L. amd DeMeyer, E. Assessing patient satisfaction with pain management through a continuous quality improvement effort. *J Pain Symptom Manage* 2001;21(1):27–40.

33. Duggleby, W. and Alden C. Implementation and evaluation of a quality improvement process to improve pain management in a hospice setting. *Am J Hosp Palliat Care* Jul–Aug 1998;15(4):209–216.

34. Higginson, I.J., Finlay, I., Goodwin, D.M., *et al.* Do hospital-based palliative teams improve care for patients or families at the end of life? *J Pain Symptom Manage* 2002;23(2):96–106.

35. McWhinney, I.R., Bass, M.J., and Donner, A. Evaluation of a palliative care service: Problems and pitfalls. *BMJ* Nov 19 1994;309(6965):1340–2.

36. Saunders, J. The control of pain in palliative care. *J R Coll Physicians Lond* Jul-Aug 2000;34(4):326–328.

37. Curtis, J.R., Patrick, D.L., Engelberg, R.A., Norris, K., Asp, C., and Byock, I. A measure of the quality of dying and death. Initial validation using after-death interviews with family members. *J Pain Symptom Manage* Jul 2002;24(1):17–31.

38. Super, A. Improving pain management practice. A medical center moves beyond education to document and manage patient care. *Health Prog* 1996;77(4):50–4.

39. Woodward, C.A. and King, B. Survivor focus groups: A quality assurance technique. *Palliat Med* 1993;7(3):229–34.

40. Homer, C.J., Marino, B., Cleary, P.D., *et al.* Quality of care at a children's hospital: The parent's perspective. *Arch Pediatr Adolesc Med* 1999;153(11):1123–9.

41. Groves, L.E. Preparing for an initial JCAHO survey: One hospice's experience. *Am Jo Hospice Palliat* 2001;18(5):299–302.

42. Morita, T., Chihara, S., and Kashiwagi, T., Quality Audit Committee of the Japanese Association of H., Palliative Care U. A scale to measure satisfaction of bereaved family receiving inpatient palliative care. *Palliat Med* 2002;16(2):141–50.

43. Ingleton, C. and Faulkner, A. Quality assurance. Audit in palliative care: A senior nurse perspective. *Nurs Standard* 1993;7(41 QA):8–9.

44. Johnston, G., Crombie, I.K., Davies, H.T., Alder, E.M., and Millard, A. Reviewing audit: Barriers and facilitating factors for effective clinical audit. *Qual Health Care* Mar 2000;9(1):23–36.

45. Porzsolt, F., Wirth, A., Mayer-Steinacker, R., *et al.* Quality assurance by specification and achievement of goals in palliative cancer treatment. *Cancer Treatment Rev.* 1996;22(Suppl A):41–9.

46. Mahony, C. Interviews with patients better than surveys for generating change. *BMJ* 22 March 2003;326(7390):618.

47. Davies, B., Steele, R., Stajduhar K., and Bruce A. Research in Pediatric Palliative Care. In R.E.B. Portenoy ed. *Topics in Palliative Care*, Vol 5. Oxford, New York: Oxford University Press, Inc; 2003, pp. 355–70.

48. K. Boyer, personal communication, April 1, 2005.

49. Cohen, S.R., Mount, B.M., Strobel, M.G., and Bui, F. The McGill Quality of Life Questionnaire: A measure of quality of life appropriate for people with advanced disease. A preliminary study of validity and acceptability. *Palliat Med* Jul 1995;9(3):207–19.

50. Portenoy, R., Thaler, H., and Kornblith, A. The Memorial Symptom Assessment Scale: An instrument for the evaluation of symptom prevalence, characteristics and distress. *Eur J Cancer Care* (English) 1994;30A:1326–36.

51. Sulmasy, D.P., McIlvane, J.M., Pasley, P.M., and Rahn, M. A scale for measuring patient perceptions of the quality of end-of-life care and satisfaction with treatment: The reliability and validity of QUEST. *J Pain Symptom Manage* 2002;23(6):458–70.

52. Whitfield, M. and Baker, R. Measuring patient satisfaction for audit in general practice. *Qual Health Care* 1992;1(3):151–152.

53. Higginson, I.J., Wade, A.M., and McCarthy, M. Effectiveness of two palliative support teams. *J Public Health Med* 1992;14(1):50–6.

54. Higginson, I. Clinical audit and organizational audit in palliative care. *Cancer Surveys* 1994;21:233–45.

55. Cooper, J. and Hewison, A. Implementing audit in palliative care: an action research approach. *J Adv Nurs* 2002;39(4):360–9.

56. Carson, M.G., Fitch, M.I., and Vachon, M.L. Measuring patient outcomes in palliative care: a reliability and validity study of the Support Team Assessment Schedule. *Palliat Med* 2000;14(1):25–36.

57. Lo, R.S., Ding, A., Chung, T.K., and Woo, J. Prospective study of symptom control in 133 cases of palliative care inpatients in Shatin Hospital. *Palliat Med* 1999;13(4):335–40.

58. Hearn, J. and Higginson, I.J. Development and validation of a core outcome measure for palliative care: The palliative care outcome scale. Palliative Care Core Audit Project Advisory Group. *Qual Health Care* 1999;8(4):219–27.

59. Tierney, R.M., Horton, S.M., Hannan, T.J., and Tierney, W.M. Relationships between symptom relief, quality of life, and satisfaction with hospice care. *Palliat Med* Sep 1998;12(5):333–44.

60. Fakhoury, W.K. Satisfaction with palliative care: What should we be aware of? *Int Jo Nurs Stud* 1998;35(3):171–6.

61. Curtis, J.R., Wenrich, M.D., Carline, J.D., Shannon, S.E., Ambrozy, D.M., and Ramsey, P.G. Patients' perspectives on physician skill in end-of-life care: Differences between patients with COPD, cancer, and AIDS. *Chest* Jul 2002;122(1):356–62.

62. Fowler, Jr F.J., Coppola, K.M., and Teno, J.M. Methodological Challenges for Measuring Quality of Care at the End of Life. *J Pain Symptom Manage* February, 1999;17(2):114–19.

63. Seamark, D.A., Williams, S., Hall, M., Lawrence, C.J., and Gilbert, J. Palliative terminal cancer care in community hospitals and a hospice: A comparative study. *Br J General Practice* 1998;48(431):1312–16.

64. Zwerdling, T., Davies, S., Lazar, L., *et al.* Unique aspects of caring for dying children and their families. *Am J Hosp Palliat Care* Sep–Oct 2000;17(5):305–11.

65. Bookbinder, M. and Romer A.L. Raising the standard of care for imminently dying patients using quality improvement. *J Palliat Med* Aug 2002;5(4):635–44.

66. Wolfe, J., HE, G., Klar, N., *et al.* Symptoms and suffering at the end of life in children with cancer. *N Eng J Med* 2000;342(5):326–33.

67. Anonymous. *A Guide To The Development Of Children's Palliative Care Services.* Bristol, UK: Report of a Joint Working Party of the Association for Children with Life-threatening or Terminal Conditions and their Families And the Royal College of Paediatrics and Child Health; 1997. ISBN 1 900954 06 0.

68. Ferris, F., Balfour, H., Bowen, K., *et al.* A Model to Guide Hospice Palliative Care:. Ottawa, ON: Canadian Hospice Palliative Care Association, 2002.

69. Burne, S.R., Dominica, F., and Baum, J.D. Helen House—a hospice for children: Analysis of the first year. *Br Med J Clin Res* 1984;289(6459):1665–8.

70. Anonymous. Association for Children with Life-Threatening or Terminal Conditions and Their Families. ACT [web site]. Available at: http://www.act.org.uk/pages/start.asp. Accessed 30 April, 2003.

71. Hospices AoCs. Association of Children's Hospices [world wide web]. Available at: http://www.childhospice.org.uk/. Accessed April 30, 2003.

72. Feeg, V. Children's Hospice International 1998 Survey: Hopsice Care for Children. Alexandria, Virginia: Children's Hospice International, 1998.

73. Davies, B. Assessment of need for a children's hospice program. *Death Stud* May–Jun 1996;20(3):247–68.

74. Anonymous. Program Data. Vancouver: Canuck Place Children's Hospice; 15 April 2002.

75. Hunt, A. and Burne, R. Medical and nursing problems of children with neurodegenerative disease. *Palliat Med* Jan 1995;9(1):19–26.

76. Strauss, D., Ashwal, S., Shavelle, R., and Eyman, R.K. Prognosis for survival and improvement in function in children with severe developmental disabilities. *J Pediatr* Nov 1997;131(5):712–17.

77. Schechter, N. The undertreatment of pain in children: An overview. *Ped Clin N Am* 1989;36(4):781–94.

78. Steele, R.G. Trajectory of certain death at an unknown time: Children with neurodegenerative life-threatening illnesses. *Can J Nurs Res* Dec 2000;32(3):49–67.

79. Davies, B., Brenner, P., Orloff, S., Sumner, L., and Worden, W. Addressing spirituality in pediatric hospice and palliative care. *J Palliat Care* Spring 2002;18(1):59–67.

80. Contro, N., Larson, J., Scofield, S., Sourkes, B., and Cohen, H. Family perspectives on the quality of pediatric palliative care [comment]. *Arch Pediatr Adolesc Med* 2002;156(1):14–19.

81. Anonymous. American Academy of Pediatrics. Committee on Bioethics and Committee on Hospital Care. Palliative care for children. *Pediatrics* Aug 2000;106(2 Pt 1):351–7.

82. Anonymous. Standards of Care for PACC® Programs: Children's Hospice International, 1997.

83. American Academy of Pediatrics. The new morbidity revisited: A renewed commitment to the psychosocial aspects of pediatric care. Committee on Psychosocial Aspects of Child and Family Health. *Pediatrics*. 2001;108(5):1227–30.

84. Levetown, M., Barnard, M., Byock, I., Carter, B., Connor, S., and Darville, J. *A Call for Change: Recommendations to Improve the Care of Children Living with Life-Threatening Conditions*. Alexandria, Virginia: National Hospice and Palliative Care Organization, October 2001.

85. American Academy of Pediatrics. Committee on Bioethics and Committee on Hospital Care. Palliative care for children. *Pediatrics* Aug 2000;106(2 Pt 1):351–7.

86. Dangel, T. and Januszaniec, A.M.K. Standardy domowej opieki paliatywnej nad dziecmi. *Nowa Medycyna* 1999;6:43–50.

87. Canadian Network of Palliative Care for Children. Pediatric Hospice Palliative Care Guiding Principles and Norms of Practice [draft]. Canadian Hospice Palliative Care Association. Ottawa: Canada. March 2004.

88. Belasco, J.B., Danz, P., Drill, A., Schmid, W., and Burkey, E. Supportive care: Palliative care in children, adolescents, and young adults—model of care, interventions, and cost of care: A retrospective review. *J Palliat Care* Winter 2000;16(4):39–46.

89. Ingleton, C. and Faulkner, A. Quality assurance in palliative care: Some of the problems. *Eur J Cancer Care* (Engl) Mar 1995;4(1):38–44.

90. Berlin, A., Spencer, J.A., Bhopal, R.S., and van Zwanenberg T.D. Audit of deaths in general practice: Pilot study of the critical incident technique. *Qual Health Care* Dec 1992;1(4):231–5.

91. Kristjanson, L.J. Indicators of quality of palliative care from a family perspective. *J Palliat Care* 1986;1(2):8–17.

92. Strategic Directions. Vancouver: Canuck Place Children's Hospice, Mar 2001.

39 Education and training

Linda M. Ferguson, Susan Fowler-Kerry, and Richard Hain

Introduction

Educational theories in pediatric palliative care practice

Education alone will not ensure the delivery of comprehensive, compassionate, competent, and consistent care. Undergraduate, graduate, and continuing education for health care professionals is, however, necessary to provide the core foundation of scientific knowledge and ethical, attitudinal, and communication skills. For education to sustain and change practice, there is also a need for changes in professional and organizational infrastructures. Without these, educational reform may become more symbolic than consequential.

Objectives and information that are emphasized in the education of health care professionals are important symbols of what these professions should value. Educational reform should be a key element in a comprehensive strategy for improving pediatric palliative care.

Evidence suggests that while some undergraduate medical and nursing educational programs provide a general overview of palliative care, they often include only a brief review of the pediatric specialty [1]. The fact remains that the majority of the undergraduate educational frameworks do not include formal attention to pediatric palliative care [2–4].

Educational strategies directed at pediatric palliative care should begin at the early stages of a health professional's education. These strategies should intensify and gain greater focus during more specialized training, and finally, should be reinforced and updated as needed, throughout a health professional's career [4]. At each stage of an educational program, course objectives should direct student learning toward a core foundation of knowledge, skills, and clinical judgement, which provide a basis for practice expertise that meets the diverse needs and challenges presented by patients and families.

Curriculums in the health sciences are dynamic. Competing interests are constantly lobbying for additional time within the current educational frameworks. Some would argue that with more adults dying than children, pediatric palliative care may only be a peripheral issue. Over the past decade, there has been a growing, concerted effort internationally to develop curriculums to prepare health care professionals to work with dying adults [2], but there has been no similar initiative for children [5].

The inclusion of palliative care in current health science curriculums should not be viewed as a competing special interest issue. The principles of holistic patient care, collaboration, and multi disciplinary teamwork provide a useful template for clinical practice in all content areas. Its principles of whole-patient care and teamwork provide a model for many areas. Furthermore, curriculum change need not be just an expensive addition, but can be an enrichment of established educational content and formats. The use of existing program models, and sharing of information, can reduce the curriculum development burden on any single school. Lastly, the need to look beyond the hospital setting for educational opportunities is not unique to end-of-life care, but can be considered as part of a more general effort to develop non-hospital arrangements for improved training in primary, chronic, and out-patient care [1].

Lack of knowledge and awareness of palliative care

Perhaps the single biggest challenge currently in the field of pediatric palliative care is educating 'palliative care naive' health care professionals, to ensure optimal care for children with life-limiting conditions, and their families [3,6]. Modern medicine has evolved over the decades into a discipline, that often focuses primarily on the investigation, diagnosis, and treatment of diseases. This has led to improved overall survival rates. At the same time, however, it has contributed to a gradual and progressive depersonalization of care [7]. With curative-orientated focus, there has been a growing trend to neglect the care of the terminally ill patient as a whole person belonging to a family, and a failure to address the totality of the human experience of suffering that results from a life-limiting illness [8].

This is particularly true in pediatrics, as a result of the dramatic decrease in child death rates in the developed world, many health care professionals have had limited educational theory, and little or no clinical experience, managing the care of the child and family. In addition, for those working in intensive care settings, a focus on palliative care may appear to contradict the 'culture of high tech [3].' Thus, it is not surprising that the majority of children who die from progressive illness do not receive state-of-the-art end-of-life care [5,8].

The death of a child has long been acknowledged as one of the greatest tragedies that can befall a family. A loss of a life that has not yet been truly lived, and does not follow the natural order in the life cycle, will have psychosocial effects that can be devastating for the surviving family [9]. The expectation that the physician can cure all is never more intense than when a disease is identified as life-threatening [10].

Education for pediatric palliative care

Teaching palliative care and pediatric palliative care is challenging. Pediatric palliative care practitioners have developed practice knowledge that enriches the care of their young patients and the patients' families. This knowledge has developed through their interactions with a large number of dying children and these children's families, and through their thoughtful reflections on the provision of high quality care. These experts provide consultative support to colleagues who care for dying children, often assisting those colleagues in developing their knowledge and skills in the area. Although this manner of education is very effective on a one-to-one basis, educational programs can more efficiently transfer a large amount of knowledge to practitioners in a timely manner. Providing learning and refresher opportunities to existing practitioners through orientation or continuing educational programs, and ensuring that new practitioners have absorbed the knowledge, attitudes, and skills of pediatric palliative care during their educational programs, will raise the quality of care to dying children and their families.

Preparing new practitioners

Educational curriculums

Curriculums for educational programming provide a clear set of goals and instructional outcomes that facilitate learning as well as teaching, and provide a basis for evaluation of learners at the end of the learning process. Curriculums include the processes whereby learners gain knowledge and understanding of the propositional or theoretical aspects, develop skills, and acquire attitudes, values, and beliefs common in the disciplinary practice [11]. Curricular content consists of expected outcomes presented in a pre-designed fashion, and includes learning experiences that assist learners to meet these goals and outcomes [12,13].

In many instances, the curriculum of an institution reflects a philosophical belief about how students learn, including the developmental approach of providing learning experiences that build from simple to complex, concrete to abstract, and general to specific. For pediatric palliative care programs, the intention behind programming is the development of competencies and essential qualities that need to be addressed in basic education, continuing education, or orientation programs [12]. Required content includes critical thinking, cultural competence, managed care, political awareness, ethical and legal concerns, effective communication, collaborative learning experiences, negotiation, and community/family aspects [14–17].

Curriculums for the preparation of health care professionals include formal and informal contents [14,18,19]. The benefit of a formalized curriculum is that all learners are provided with similar experiences, which assist them to learn the expected knowledge, skills, and attitudes [12]. Typically, the curriculums to prepare most health care professionals as generalists are fully programmed. Adding more learning opportunities usually involves extended faculty discussions and negotiations to create a reasonable balance between basic sciences, social sciences, disciplinary knowledge, clinical practice, and self-directed learning experiences. Existing courses are planned to address specific course objectives. Adding new objectives to pre-existing courses is difficult, usually resulting in only cursory consideration being given to such new topics. Curricular modification can successfully be accompanied, however, with the commitment of the whole faculty to the inclusion of such objectives [14,17,19,20].

Much of the content needed for effective practice in palliative care is already included in most preparatory programs for doctors and nurses. Critical areas in communication skills, interdisciplinary collaboration, ethics, symptom management, family and community involvement, and holistic care are common elements in most professional medical and nursing education programs. Since most programs in nurse and physician preparation are generalist in nature, palliative care issues with adults are usually addressed, although not always in depth. The sub-specialty of pediatric palliative care requires a greater commitment to curriculum planning, and is often dependent on the specific experiences of individual learners. Attention must be paid to the inclusion of essential elements, such as family involvement in care, family autonomy, quality of life for pediatric patients, symptom management in dying children, co-ordination of care, and communication among health care professionals.

Unfortunately, much of the content that relates to the values and culture of palliative care, and specifically to pediatric palliative care, falls into the category of the informal curriculum that is not written or formally acknowledged, but addresses the culture of medicine [19]. Because of the lack of formal curriculums in the area of palliative care, learning is inconsistent at best, and at worst, absent. It is often sporadic, and dependent on the clinical experiences of the learner, or on the interests of the teacher. To ensure that content related to palliative care, and specifically to pediatric palliative care, is provided to all learners in a program, the content and learning experiences must be formalized as specific instructional goals and outcomes in the curriculum [17,19].

Cognitive knowledge and psychomotor skills

Curriculums should include cognitive, affective, and psychomotor skills contents that prepare practitioners for practice [12,17]. This content should be stated in terms of expected outcomes of planned learning experiences [21], or of ends-in-view [22]. These educational objectives form the basis for selection of appropriate learning experiences and evaluation of outcomes. Cognitive content relates to knowledge, often explicated through research, which forms the basis for practice. Evidence-based practice adds to the practitioner's cognitive knowledge of the discipline, and provides evidential support for practice decisions. Such knowledge is frequently available in textbooks or journal articles, is easily taught in conventional formats, such as lectures or readings, and is the core of knowledge taught in medical and nursing programs [23]. Facts provide learners with information on which to base practice, and create a non-threatening learning environment within which one can effectively address values in practice [16]. Propositional or theoretical knowledge is essential for safe practice of the discipline; practice or tacit knowledge of the clinician applies it to the individual patient [23–25].

Cognitive knowledge in the areas of symptom management and pain control is the most frequently presented aspect of palliative care [2,8,16,19,26]. This is relatively easily taught; there is a body of knowledge that is research-based, and is available in the scholarly literature [27]. Less easily taught are the values and beliefs that accompany many procedural, assessment, and care management skills. For example, although effective pain control strategies have been demonstrated in practice and reported, nurses and physicians continue to provide analgesia and other pain control measures at less than effective levels [28–30]. This observation is particularly true in general nursing units, where the emphasis is on cure, rather than care, of the dying patient. It is even more apparent in the care of children [23,31]. The same is true for some psychomotor skills that essentially mirror those on general units, but may not be carried out in practice with the necessary degree of commitment to patient autonomy and family preferences, or to compassion [23].

Bloom's taxonomy of objectives in the cognitive domain [32] reflects a belief that knowledge is structured in a hierarchy. Learning progresses through predictable stages, from knowledge of facts and comprehension of information to the application of that knowledge and comprehension in a particular situation. With well-designed learning experiences and sufficient experiential learning, students develop cognitive skills that reflect higher-level thought about a topic, including analysis of factors in a particular situation, synthesis of new ways of approaching dying children and their families, and evaluation of approaches based on particular standards of practice.

Harrow [33] identified a similar progression in the development of psychomotor skills. This progression is generally not affected by the setting of practice. The most important consideration in this setting of pediatric palliative care is the incorporation of family values, preferences, and practices in the performance of skills [34–36]. An example is family control over the provision of care. Good communication among caregivers, and a commitment to quality of care that reflects family preferences, are the most important considerations [23,37]. Family members are frequently primary caregivers, especially in the home, and expect to be part of the team providing care in hospital or hospice [38]. New practitioners in palliative care and pediatric palliative care need good role modeling, to demonstrate how families can be involved in care to the extent that they wish. New learners in the area often need help to create this effective partnership. Rather than a focus on how to learn psychomotor skills for palliative care, new learners need to learn how to *modify* psychomotor skills to better meet the needs of the patient. This needs to be combined with the values, attitudes, and commitment to do so.

Curriculums are designed to emphasize those aspects of professional practice that the faculty considers essential for all practitioners of that discipline, and in doing so, present the values of that discipline. As has been observed, some of the necessary content for pediatric palliative care is already included in medical and nursing curriculums. However, the values of the sub-specialty need to be emphasized by the inclusion of objectives and outcomes that emphasize the 'consciousness of palliation' in the care of dying children and their families. Without the emphasis of these values, the knowledge of content (such as communication skills, growth and development, interdisciplinary team functioning, family dynamics, and community resources) will not be well applied in palliative situations, either in specialist units or at other locations, while caring for dying children. A consciousness of palliation is a predisposition and a commitment to include palliative care concepts in the care of all patients, as may be appropriate.

Teaching the values and beliefs of palliative care

A more challenging aspect of most curriculums is teaching in the affective domain; the values, beliefs, attitudes, and ethics of palliation. This difficulty is reflected in both the challenge of stating expected outcomes, and in the evaluation of the achievement of such objectives. Krathwohl, Bloom, and Maisa [39] formalized the structure of learning in the affective domain, acknowledging the normal progression in learning values. In learning new values, individuals generally progress from the state of being willing to receive the information, to responding with behaviors that are congruent with the desired values, and ultimately, to holding the values and acting in congruence with them. While students are at the stage, of receiving information, or responding in congruence with the stated values, they do not necessarily exhibit commitment to them. Generally, learners need more time in learning interactions, to achieve such a professional commitment.

In palliative care, the values of patient/family autonomy, quality of life, and compassionate care may sometimes be in conflict with those more aligned with curative approaches [23]. Students attain the level of organization when they accept the values of palliation, and create for themselves a meaningful relationship between curative and palliative care. The highest level of the affective domain relates to characterization, wherein the individual practitioner's behavior is consistently characterized by commitment to palliation in care. It may be that faculty members who teach palliative care, or practitioners who advocate for palliation in all relevant aspects of patient care, have attained this level.

The affective aspect of programming often falls into the informal component of curriculums, as educators experience difficulties in defining expected outcomes and determining appropriate ways of teaching and evaluating values, attitudes, and beliefs. A classic example is the focus on compassionate care in palliative care. Although the term is frequently used, educators have difficulty teaching 'genuine caring', and even more difficulty evaluating the level of 'acceptable caring' or

'compassionate caring'. Frequently, educators cannot clearly describe the expected attitudes or values in practice, or the behaviors that learners will demonstrate as evidence of achievement of those values and beliefs. Tacit understanding of how to apply knowledge, or perform technical skills in individual patient situations, develops over time [40]. Unfortunately, educators can more easily identify the absence of the expected attitudes or values, than their presence.

Choosing learning experiences to assist learners to gain the desired values and beliefs requires patience, and a willingness to explore learner thoughts about the proposed values. Today's learners rarely accept or incorporate new values into their existing belief systems, without thorough personal reflection and examination. Teaching in the affective domain is time consuming, requiring teaching strategies such as seminars, group discussion, and case studies that focus on exploration of values and beliefs, emotional responses to patient situations, and clarification of values evident in effective and compassionate patient care. Ethical issues frequently arise for students, as they are socialized into the values of the discipline, and confront their own attitudes about palliative care.

As students enter medical or nursing programs, they generally reflect the values and beliefs of their own societies. This includes beliefs about death and dying. For some learners, the idea of death is a new 'un-experienced' phenomenon that is frightening and unexpected, reflecting the values of a 'death denying society [41].' Billings and Block [14], however, reported that many students in medical education have had significant experiences with those who are dying, among their own families or friends. Entering nursing and medical programs places these learners in situations where they must confront their own beliefs about death and dying, and the cures, or lack thereof, of modern medicine. This process takes time, but can be distributed throughout the curriculum of the professional program.

Unfortunately, the available evidence suggests that very few programs incorporate the necessary time in teaching concepts of palliation. In Britain, by self-report, instruction in palliative care concepts averaged 7.8 h for diploma nursing students, 12.2 h for degree nursing students, and 20 h for medical students [42]. In Canada, Sellick et al. [43] reported that an average of 4.39 h was devoted to education on death in nursing programs, and in Australia, the nursing faculty included an average of 19.25 h on death in its curriculums [44]. In Spain, Zabalegui [45] indicated that formal instruction in end-of-life care is included in most degree programs in nursing, but is inadequate in most diploma programs. In nursing programs, teaching was mainly theoretical, using didactic approaches and small group tutorials. The content was often offered as elective courses or optional clinical modules.

Content on palliation competes with the demands of content in other aspects of nursing or medicine, and often suffers from a lack of advocates for palliative care, especially among faculty or clinicians. It seems the pediatric sub-specialty suffers even more from lack of attention in current nursing and medical curriculums [6].

The process of clarifying values is a challenging one, that is fraught with emotional work by learners, and by perseverance and commitment by educators. Although new learners embrace the concepts of palliative care, they are often challenged to address their own beliefs and issues, while assisting patients and families to address death and dying as realities. Because of these conflicts in values, new learners in nursing and medicine may intellectually embrace the concepts as part of holistic nursing or medical care, but find that because of their own emotional responses, they avoid engagement with patients who are dying.

Attitudes toward death and dying are complex, based on cultural, societal, philosophical, legal, spiritual, and religious belief systems. They develop over the lifetime of the individual, influencing the meaning that individuals ascribe to the process of dying, and to their role in caring for dying patients and their families. New students may have difficulties articulating their own beliefs, and face even more challenges in accepting a professional role in the care of those who are dying. Anxiety around the concept of death is common for students in the health professions. Helping new health professionals, especially younger learners, to explore and clarify their own attitudes and beliefs, may be the single most important aspect determining their commitment to palliation in their later practice [46].

The provision of learning opportunities that allow for the exploration of current beliefs, and the implications of incorporating new beliefs and values, is critical to preparing students for palliative care experiences with patients and their families [4]. While some programs do acknowledge this need, the most frequently used teaching strategy to address palliative care issues is the traditional lecture method, which is probably the least effective way of addressing values clarification [14,47]. More effective strategies include case studies, group discussions, simulations, role-playing, role modeling, questioning, and reflective techniques, such as writing and maintaining a journal.

Souter [48] described a model for structured reflection on palliative care nursing, focused on exploration of the challenges of palliative care nursing. The model was based on 6 types of knowledge or 'ways of knowing [49]:' scientific, personal, socio-political, spiritual, ethical, and aesthetic. The model required nurses to reflect on the aims of the professional interactions, and the sources of the knowledge used for specific types of practice in palliation. It also included questions focused on whether actions were consistent with beliefs of patient autonomy, promotion of quality of life, compassionate care, family involvement, and symptom control. The aim of the process is to assist nurses to critically analyze their own assumptions, values, and beliefs that will influence their actions in practice.

Mazuryk, Daeninck, Neumann, and Bruera [50] described a journal club for family medicine and palliative care residents that met on a regular basis, to discuss critically the clinical application of palliative care articles in current medical literature. Over the course of one year, 252 articles were reviewed and subjected to critique. This strategy had the benefit of reinforcing evidence-based practice in palliative care, and at the same time, raising more diverse topics, such as psychosocial issues.

The aim of these strategies is to assist learners to explore values, interests, attitudes, and beliefs that are foundational to affective behaviors. In palliative care, such strategies help learners to gain a positive attitude toward the care of dying persons and their families, and to learn values that support the incorporation of compassionate holistic care and symptom management in the care of dying persons and their families.

MacDonald [51] described the challenges of 'unlearning' previous beliefs and attitudes before one is able to learn new ways of thinking; she described this process as transformative learning, and emphasized the challenges of the emotional work of unlearning. Many health care professionals have learned particular ways of caring for patients, often with a focus on a curative philosophy. Reconciling a focus on palliation with a curative approach is a challenge for health care professionals, and is often reflected in their care of patients, especially in critical care units [15] and general care units. A safe environment for learning is essential for supporting this transformation. Assessment of death attitudes and beliefs about caring for the terminally ill provide students and educators with a baseline for discussion, and an opportunity to grow both personally and professionally [46]. Case studies and seminars may be useful strategies to raise student awareness of the need for compassionate holistic care of those who are dying. Learning experiences should encourage students to confront their own beliefs and values, and to explore other ways of thinking about palliation.

A strong focus on palliative care in children in the education of health professionals requires faculty who are committed to its values. Sherman, Matzo, Panke, Grant, and Rhome [52] described an approach to strengthening the focus on end-of-life care in educational programs for health professionals. This program, sponsored by the American Association of College of Nursing (AACN), and the End-of-Life Nursing

Education Consortium (ELNEC), focused on educating the educators, based on the premise that nurse educators who are appropriately educated in principles of palliative care will be more likely to incorporate this content into their educational programs. By May 2002, over 900 nursing and continuing education faculty had taken the 3-day training course on didactic and experiential learning experiences. This course consisted of nine modules, addressing topics such as philosophy of palliative care, pain management, symptom management, ethical/legal issues, cultural considerations, communication, grief, loss and bereavement, quality of life, and preparation for death. Strategies such as this one may be required to raise faculty awareness of the importance of palliative care in the education of health care professionals.

Ethical issues

Ethical issues are a daily reality in pediatric palliative care practice. The needs of health care professionals add complexity to the issues of ethics in pediatric palliative care. The aim is 'to enable dying patients to live, until they die, at their own maximum potential, performing to the limits of their physical activity and mental capacity, with control and independence, whenever possible [3].' This imposes specific ethical requirements on palliative care professionals [23].

Health care providers are guided by medical ethical principles, such as justice, beneficence, autonomy and non-malevolence. These ethical principles are frequently challenged by clinical situations, such that health care professionals experience dilemmas in their provision of care. Students in palliative care need opportunities to work through these dilemmas, often through discussion with other health care providers, patients and their families, and their educators. Although, of course, the answers depend on the individual situation, individuals can effectively analyze their own actions and feelings, often in discussion with others who are experiencing similar situations. Many medical and nursing curriculums provide opportunities for students to discuss hypothetical situations that address ethical issues.

Discussions with faculty and other health care professionals may help students understand the complexity of patient and family decision-making. Students need to accept and acknowledge the role of health care professionals [53] in assisting patients or families to understand the information that they have received, and to work through the difficult decisions that they are encountering. Bergum [54] and MacDonald [51] indicate that students must come to a recognition that knowledge needed for ethical care must be constructed jointly by the health care professional and the family, and that both health care professionals and patients try to understand the meaning that the illness or impending death has for the

individual patient and family [55]. Without the opportunity to explore such meanings with families, students are likely to impose their own interpretation and understanding.

In summary, palliative care is an excellent setting in which to develop other professional competencies with an ethical and moral foundation [23]. Its principles of palliative care compel practitioners to provide holistic and compassionate care based on scientific knowledge, incorporating the art of the profession. In these settings, the four aspects of professional competence; knowledge, technical skills, communication and relationships, and affective and moral attitudes, are necessary to provide patient-centered care. Although students may be challenged to integrate all of these concepts in their practice, successful application of the principles of palliative care form an excellent foundation to the professional practice of both nurses and physicians.

Communication skills

Many health care professionals recognize communication difficulties in palliative care in the areas of honesty with patients and caregivers [56,57], and in breaking bad news [58–60]. Research indicates that in reality, communication difficulties are broader than this [15,29]. They include negotiation skills with patients and carers, information gathering (particularly in terms of patient preferences), relationship building, for example, demonstrating empathy, and naming emotions of both patients and professional colleagues.

Basic communication skills are included in professional education programs, but the demands of palliative care are complex and ongoing [15,37,61]. Assuming that students have had opportunities to interact with their patients in therapeutic communication in general patient care, the basic skills should have been mastered by the time students encounter dying patients and their families. Communication skills are a very important element of palliative care, and build on previous learning in a developmental approach. Communication issues that should be addressed in preparation for pediatric palliative care should include breaking bad news, discussion of limits of care or treatment, resolving conflicts among family members, interactions with parents at the child's death, allowing time for questions, exploring options for end-of-life care, pronouncing the death of a child and managing the death certificate, dealing with avoidance of patient and family, exploring patients' cultural practices, and dealing with parents of different ethnic and cultural backgrounds [15]. Students must also learn to deal with their own reactions to the death of a child, and to identify appropriate ways of addressing their own personal issues.

The development of communication skills is based on the theory of effective communication; however, these skills are developed most effectively in the clinical context of the individual patient. Role-playing provides students with 'safe' learning opportunities to practice specific skills and to consider their own performances and those of peers, without repercussions for patient care. DeVita *et al.* [15] describe some scenarios that provide students with opportunities to develop their skills: establishing rapport and wording requests for organ donation, conducting family meetings, and attending to patient emotions. Regardless of the learning opportunities in the classroom, students will still find the actual patient situation challenging and unpredictable, and need the opportunity to debrief and discuss. Particularly challenging are those situations that are anxiety provoking, or that apparently fail to meet patient expectations for empathic and caring interactions. Students also learn a great deal from practitioners who model exemplary communication skills and interactions with dying patients and their families. The opportunity to discuss these interactions simultaneously reinforces the necessity for such skills, and provides the means of improving them.

Symptom management and pain control

Perhaps the least neglected aspects of palliative care involve symptom management and pain control. This content, often presented in a didactic manner, is considered essential content in the preparation of health care professionals. Symptoms that need to be addressed include pain, anxiety, seizures, bowel and bladder problems, and nutrition and fluid management [16]. Research in the area of pain control and other symptom management provides the basis for evidence-based practice. Although this content can be readily addressed in lectures and presentations, health care professionals must have values and beliefs that support use of the knowledge in clinical practice.

Although health care professionals usually acknowledge the importance of this content, it may be difficult to remain up-to-date in this area, as research produces new knowledge [29]. Maintaining current expertise in palliative care is addressed in continuing education programme offerings. Nursing attitudes that demonstrated inappropriate concern for addiction, and lack of knowledge of pain control were influenced by a 40 h continuing education programme [2,3]. Mandatory updates in pain control for all health care professionals have been recommended [59], both to maintain currency, and to support those attitudes and values that facilitate appropriate patient care.

Individual practice expertise

Practice expertise of individual health care professionals determines the quality of pediatric palliative care. Practice expertise has been described as 'humane judgement that, with

scientific judgement, constitutes the clinical judgement of a practitioner' [25], as 'expertise and tacit knowledge in medicine' [62], and as 'embodied know-how or the knowledge embedded in practice' [24]. Each of these authors is referring to the art of the discipline, the aspect of professional health care that individualizes patient care with decisions that are fluid, anticipatory, contextual, skilful, and patient-centred.

In pediatric palliative care, practitioners with this level of expertise have developed it through experiential learning with a large number of patients and their families [24,40,63,64]. This practice knowledge is difficult to describe, and even more difficult to teach, in conventional didactic formats such as lectures.

The most effective way to facilitate student learning is in direct interaction with patients, under the supervision of such an expert practitioner. Prolonged interaction with the family and child over time is necessary to develop this level of engagement. It is time-consuming, but allows new practitioners to acquire experience while observing experienced practitioners, and discussing aspects of care with them.

Preceptored and mentored learning situations are effective in assisting new learners to understand the complexities of decision-making in pediatric palliative care situations. Novices or advanced beginners' typical responses to patient situations are based on theoretical or propositional knowledge, using rules and guidelines for decision-making and care. Learners will usually have already absorbed a breadth of information during their basic programmes. What they lack is the depth of knowledge in pediatric palliative care itself. In working with expert practitioners in the area, they see the depth of knowledge in practice, recognize the multiple sources of patient data that experts respond to, and gain an appreciation of how to work more effectively [24,65,66].

Expert practitioners often have to explain their decision-making, as new learners cannot see the same patient and family cues that experts take into account in their care. Practitioners with experience and expertise often make decisions quickly, using heuristics. Heuristics are 'rules of thumb,' or strategies that simplify decision-making processes. They enable expert practitioners to recognize patterns in patient situations, and respond in predetermined but effective ways [24,40]. Heuristics are based on experiential knowledge, and are meaningful in the context of an expert's practice, but may be difficult to explain [40]; and may even seem meaningless to novices [64].

Expert practitioners interact with children and their families in an engaged and committed manner, and have complete knowledge of patients' usual responses to illness, stages impression of illness, and patient and family issues in palliation. This knowledge is gained through extensive experience with children and their families, and can be modeled in practice and conveyed through stories and narratives of care in past patients. This learning takes time and experience, and are often extracts of emotional toll on learners to one you in the setting [63,67].

In many professional education programs, students are provided with observational experiences in palliative care, as a means of raising their awareness. This brief exposure may not be enough to assist students to learn how to interact with patients and their families, and may not create a pre-disposition to include palliative care concepts in their interactions with patients. Failure to recognize the emotional commitment to caring in palliative care can result in technically focused, depersonalized care [63]. Such brief exposures to palliative care may result in learners who fail to recognize the depth of knowledge and the commitment required. Faculty in professional programs must make judgement about resources, recognizing that a full learning experience for a few students may result in greater commitment to the principles of palliative care, than a brief and superficial experience for many students.

These experiences must be combined with classroom experiences that provide a basis for palliative care for all patients. Involvement of learners in palliative home care situations is important, but challenging [18]. It is further complicated in children by the need for consistency in the care team. Pediatric residents typically have cared for approximately 35 dying children over the first 2½ years of their residency training [16], although very few indicated that they had actually received training in end-of-life care, or felt competent in the care of dying children and their families. Organizing seminars for residents allowed them to explore issues they encountered in these situations with other residents and experts in the field, and facilitated sharing of experiences to broaden the learning horizons of all involved.

Interprofessional or interdisciplinary education

Palliative care requires teamwork among the professionals providing care to the dying child and family [29,68–70], and this is acknowledged in educational recommendations in the field [60,71].

Each team member brings specific skills and competencies [70]. Rather than traditional professional relationships, the focus of teamwork is on patient needs and the needs of the family. Benefits of this focus on patient issues include shared patient focus, improved communication, active involvement with other team members and the patient and family, improved quality of patient care, better understanding of the contributions of other professional groups [72], and a decreased sense of isolation [43].

Team members must perform their specific responsibilities in a timely and responsive manner, and recognize both the autonomy and the interdependence of these members [70]. The roles of various health care professionals are often blurred, as team members focus on meeting the needs of the dying child and his or her family. Family wishes for care, or treatment of complications, must be communicated to other team members, and appropriate referrals made in a timely manner.

Teaching medical and nursing students about interdisciplinary functioning of teams in palliative care and pediatric palliative care requires a commitment to different professions learning together [59,72]. Interdisciplinary education involves learners from different professions learning with, from, and about each other in an interactive process, that results in mutual respect and understanding of the contributions of others. A multi disciplinary teaching team most effectively reinforces and models the concepts of teamwork that they advocate [15,20].

The ideal timing of interdisciplinary experiences is unclear. They should probably occur late enough in the program that students are aware of their professional contributions to the team, but early enough that students are open to working with other professional groups, without the negative effect of traditional hierarchical relationships [72].

Students are able to learn the concept of teamwork most effectively in context, and may have experiences in teamwork in other aspects of their education. However, it is important that their experience in pediatric palliative care should illustrate the benefits of teamwork for the patient and family, and reinforce, through professional modeling, the expectations of interprofessional cooperation. A focus on patient and family issues assists learners to seek creative solutions to complex issues, and to make professional referrals as necessary, to ensure that these issues are addressed in an effective and timely manner.

Cultural implications

Supporting families in the care of their children requires knowledge of their cultural practices around the issues of health and illness, but particularly around death and dying [73]. Doctors and nurses who are unaware of these cultural practices may inadvertently provide care that is inadequate, or culturally inappropriate, for the children and their families. Language differences between patients and families and their caregivers can accentuate these issues [74]. The issue of culturally competent care in all aspects of health services is particularly important in palliative care, where alliances between professional caregivers and families are crucial to the delivery of care that is provided [75].

Medical and nursing students need opportunities to learn about the traditional cultural practices of patients that they will commonly encounter in their practices. Recognizing differences in beliefs and practices, and confronting their own ethnocentrism, are important learning experiences for new practitioners. Providing culturally sensitive palliative care for minority ethnic groups is a challenge [74], particularly in the area of perceptions of illness, care models, traditional practices, and the effects of acculturation. Evidence [76] suggests that culturally sensitive care demands particular attention to six aspects: communication patterns and cues, space needs, social organization of family, implications of time, environmental factors, and biological variations. The ways that individuals express their symptoms and distress, and the ways that doctors and nurses can provide appropriate support, are also important aspects of learning [26]. These factors have implications for how children and families engage in the process of the patients' dying, and how they wish their professional caregivers to be involved.

Educators have the responsibility, and also the opportunity, to assist students to explore the implications of culture on the provision of palliative care. Personal narratives about care, as presentations in formal learning, are often useful in raising awareness of the impact of culturally inappropriate care. Case studies can be helpful, but exposure to the individual cultural practices of patients and their families are most effective. Students need to see practitioners modeling effective means of exploring cultural practices with families, and modifying care to provide it in more appropriate ways.

In summary, the value of culturally sensitive health care needs to be addressed throughout educational programs, and reinforced in practice. Educators can support this learning through appropriate questioning of students, and interactions with patients and families.

Continuing education programming for pediatric palliative care

Health care professionals, in almost every professional pediatric practice, encounter children with needs for palliative care. Although some are referred to palliative care teams or units, many are cared for in a more general clinical environment. While nurses and physicians on general units may not have any specific training in palliative care, their patients nevertheless have needs that require treatment and care based on palliative care principles. Continuing education programs [29,77], are effective in preparing practitioners for the occasional patients needing palliative care.

One of the challenges of continuing education for practitioners [29] is motivating them to attend educational programs, in light of their busy professional schedules. Educators must raise awareness of the need for specific training in pediatric palliative care, since busy health care professionals may not be aware of changes in practice, or more up-to-date evidence-based practice, and may assume that their own practice is current. Most physicians recognize the need for ongoing training in pain management and symptom control [29,78], but may not as easily identify other areas that need continuing professional development, such as working effectively in teams, communication, and family. As has been suggested, palliative care education should reflect palliative care itself; it should be multi-professional, tailored to the needs of individuals, and linked to improving the whole process and outcome [59].

Many physicians and nurses indicated difficulties in attending continuing education sessions, despite being interested in improving their skills in palliative care. Formats that use some distance education methods, such as videoconferencing and teleconferencing, may provide a solution [79,80]. Content in continuing education offerings mirror that offered to nursing and medical students, and to medical residents. Programs that focus on effective communication techniques, involvement of family, team dynamics, and co-ordination of services (rather than symptom control) are very beneficial, but perhaps less well attended. Since many undergraduate programs to date have limited content and experience focused on pediatric palliative care, the ongoing educational needs of practising health professionals are particularly substantial.

Pediatric palliative care program development for nurses

Nursing science is directed toward the development of theories to describe, explain, and understand the nature of the phenomena, and anticipate the occurrence of events and situations related directly or indirectly to nursing care [81]. Nursing knowledge has been described [49] as consisting of four patterns of knowing: ethical knowledge, aesthetics, personal knowledge, and empirical knowledge. The practice in palliative care for nurses generally has focused on understanding and valuing the lived experience of dying as an aesthetic value, as well as advocating for a health care environment that fosters patient and family choice, respects autonomy, and builds from the experience of expert nurses in a wide range of clinical environments [82]. Currently, much of the knowledge about pediatric palliative care is incomplete, or based on best practice, rather than on empirical fact. This reality reflects the fact that palliative care in general, and pediatric palliative care in specific, is a new and emerging specialty.

While there is a growing body of literature devoted to pediatric palliative care, there are few standardized resources, textbooks, manuals, audiovisual aids or websites available currently for educators to use in planning educational programs. In addition, there are a variety of institutions, private and public, that advertize the availability of seminars or training programs on pediatric palliative care. The majority of these courses focus primarily on the needs of children with cancer, which comprise only a small percentage of children who need palliative care [83].

Health care professionals in the area of pediatric palliative care have clearly identified knowledge deficits in this area [2,7,15,84–87]. In addition, the needs of learners may differ: undergraduate students have less of an experiential base in nursing and medicine on which to build new learning in pediatric palliative care. Prior to the development of any course, seminar or program, it is imperative to identify the intended audience of the program. Depending on the audience, program content and teaching strategies will change.

Undergraduate programs

The majority of undergraduate students entering into the health science professions are young and enthusiastic men and women, often with limited personal life experiences. They are influenced and affected by a myriad socio-cultural and personal beliefs and values. Most importantly, modern medicine has had an impact on their attitudes toward death and dying [88]. Thus, many have the inherent belief that modern medicine is cure versus comfort-oriented care. To speak of palliative care in the context of children dying is to step into an area of social discomfort, not only for the students but also for many educators.

Palliative care is a multi-dimensional concept that requires the collaboration of interdisciplinary teams. Subsequently, educational programs should 'practice what they preach,' and develop curriculums that reflect the practice that is proposed.

Pediatric palliative care is a nursing sub-specialty of both pediatrics and palliative care. Any programming in this area must build on the principles and concepts of pediatric nursing and palliative care nursing. Because these areas of nursing are seen as requiring practice experience in the field in general, clinical experiences in these fields tends to be provided later in educational programs. However, pediatric palliative care concepts build on general concepts of nursing care, and should be integrated throughout, covering all the years in the nursing curriculum.

This integration of palliative care and pediatric palliative care into nursing curriculums requires faculty commitment to the values and concepts of palliation. Most educators struggle with the challenges of the over-abundance of content required in professional nursing education, and must set priorities on that content. Many faculties are uncomfortable with the inclusion of concepts of palliative care and death and dying, reflecting a focus on curative care, and the larger societal denial of death [8]. The complexity of palliative care is challenging to deal with in undergraduate programs, especially since clinical experiences in these areas are limited. In addition, nurse educators may deem pediatric palliative care as a sub-specialty of pediatrics and thus, an inappropriate level for a basic nursing program.

In contrast, Olthuis and Dekkers [23] consider competent professional care, with a commitment to a core set of values, to be a prerequisite in palliative care. Palliative care practitioners must integrate knowledge, skills, and judgement, with ethical and moral values. They provide holistic, compassionate, and humanistic care, due to the intense nature of interpersonal interactions. Teaching the principles, concepts, and values of palliative care would assist students to develop the art of medicine. The holistic care required of practitioners in palliative care is necessary for professional competence. The same is true for nursing.

Building the concepts of holistic care, family oriented care, patient autonomy, effective communication, and the good death into nursing curriculums, will assist nurses to develop the art of nursing, and illustrate its importance in holistic compassionate care. Many of these concepts can be integrated early in the curriculums, and are the foundations of more demanding concepts of palliative care and pediatric palliative care. This curriculum development is possible and desired, but is dependent on the commitment of nurse educators and practitioners to the inclusion of these concepts. In some instances, the educators must first be educated [52]. Sixteen principles [14] have been proposed to guide curriculum development (Table 39.1). These principles can be applied to the development of nursing curriculums in pediatric palliative care, either by integration into existing programs, or in the development of new curriculums.

This outline of pediatric palliative care content has been organized into three units: first year, middle year(s), and senior year. Much of it is already addressed in most nursing programs. In order to strengthen nurses' knowledge of pediatric palliative care, however, content needs to be explicitly linked to pediatric palliative care.

First year content

Introduction to the concept of palliative care

Educators should introduce the notion that palliative care is a philosophy, that should influence all areas of clinical practice throughout the professional program. This would include

Table 39.1 Principles for enhancing undergraduate medical education in palliative care

Principles for enhancing undergraduate medical education in palliative care
1. The care of dying persons and their families is a core professional task of physicians. Medical schools have a responsibility to prepare students to provide skilled, compassionate end-of-life care.
2. The following key content areas related to end-of–life care must be addressed in undergraduate medical education:
a. communicating effectively and humanely with the patient and family;
b. skilfully managing pain and other distressing symptoms commonly occurring in end-stage disease;
c. providing accessible, comprehensive, high-quality home and hospice care, as well as other alternatives to acute hospital care;
d. eliciting and implementing patients' end-of-life wishes, and appreciating the limitations of treatment in advanced disease;
e. understanding ethical issues in end-of-life care, and respecting patients' personal values; recognizing and responding to cultural, linguistic, and spiritual diversity, and to varied personal styles;
f. working with an interdisciplinary team to provide comprehensive coordinated care;
g. acknowledging and responding to the personal stresses of professionals working with dying persons;
h. developing an awareness of one's own attitudes, feelings, and expectations regarding death and loss.
3. Medical education should encourage students to develop positive feelings about dying patients and their families, and about the role of the physician in terminal care.
4. Enhanced teaching about death, dying, and bereavement should occur throughout the span of medical education.
5. Educational content and process should be tailored to students' developmental stage.
6. The best learning grows out of direct experiences with patients and families, particularly when students have an opportunity to follow patients longitudinally, and develop a sense of intimacy and manageable personal responsibility for suffering persons.
7. Teaching and learning about death, dying, and bereavement should emphasize humanistic attitudes.
8. Teaching should stress communication skills.
9. Students need to see physicians offering excellent medical care to dying people and their families, and find meaning in their work.
10. Medical education should foster respect for patients' personal values, and an appreciation of cultural and spiritual diversity in approaching death and dying.
11. The teaching process itself should mirror the values to which physicians aspire in working with patients.
12. A comprehensive integrated understanding of, and approach to, death, dying, and bereavement is enhanced when students are exposed to the perspectives of multiple disciplines working together.
13. Faculty should be taught how to teach about end-of-life care, including how to be mentors, and to model ideal behaviors and skills.
14. Student competence in managing proto-typical clinical settings related to death, dying, and bereavement should be evaluated.
15. Educational programs should be evaluated using state-of-the-art methods.
16. Additional resources will be required to implement these changes.

(Adapted from Billings and Block, 1997)

emphasis on the key concepts of holistic, comprehensive, and compassionate care, that are integral to the delivery of palliative care. This approach would build on the ACT/RCPCH definition of pediatric palliative care [89,90]:

Palliative care for children and young people with life-limiting conditions is an active and total approach to care, embracing physical, emotional, social and spiritual elements. It focuses on enhancement of quality of life for the child and support for the family and includes the management of distressing symptoms, provision of respite and care through death and bereavement.

This in turn builds on the WHO definition of palliative care [91]:

Palliative care . . . affirms life and regards dying as a normal process, . . . neither hastens nor postpones death, . . . provides relief from pain and other distressing symptoms, . . . integrates the psychological and spiritual aspects of care, . . . offers a support system to help patients live as actively as possible until death, . . . offers a support system to help the family cope during the patient's illness and in their own bereavement.

Communication skills

Faculty should introduce the concept of therapeutic use of self, and focus on communication skills required for holistic patient assessment. Educators will have to identify varying communication skills for patients at different stages across the life span. For example, how would you initiate an interview with a 6-year-old, as compared to an 86-year-old? To make this model relevant, faculty will need to review and reference the developmental stages, particularly for children.

There must be recognition that communication is more than words, and that tone and quality of voice, eye contact, physical proximity, visual cues, and body language all convey messages. Good communication requires good listening skills. Students should be encouraged to go out to a variety of community agencies, schools, gyms, day care, senior centers to hold dialogue with different groups of people. Such skills are essential to nursing practice. Palliative care is particularly dependent on good communication with patients and their families.

Pain and symptom control

Students need a brief introduction to some of the generic issues regarding symptom control. In practice, symptom control is the area in which the bulk of nurses' time and expertise is spent. It is expected that students will, at this stage of their education, be enrolled in basic anatomy and physiology classes, to provide the foundation to understand the physiological basis of these symptoms and their treatment. Emphasis needs to be placed on the subjective experience of each patient, when he or she is suffering from pain, nausea, dyspnea, sleep deprivation or fatigue, thus recognizing that no two patients will experience any of these symptoms in the same way.

Middle years

Palliative care concepts

Educators need to provide opportunities for more in depth discussions about palliative care and its three main components, namely: supportive, end-of-life care, and bereavement. To do so requires students to explore their own beliefs regarding death and dying. Students should be engaged in dialogue concerning myths and misconceptions surrounding palliative care. Issues addressed should include care versus cure; euthanasia, right to die, living wills, and policies affecting the delivery of palliative care services. Ethical issues and the moral dimensions of palliative care need to be introduced and discussed.

Considering that students will be more comfortable in the health care environment after their first year, students should be encouraged to assess their current clients for palliative care needs. In those situations where dying clients are being cared for in general units, students should be encouraged to provide holistic, compassionate client-centered care, using principles of palliation. Concepts of palliative care should be discussed in all clinical settings, and students should be encouraged to provide palliative care within those settings, where appropriate. Students will need assistance to make referrals to other agencies in collaboration with the patient and family. They should be encouraged to interact with other

health care professionals in meeting the care goals of dying patients and their families.

Issues of pain and symptom control

Theory introduced at this time should build on the basic concepts of the structure and function of the human body. Introductory information on pain and symptom control forms the basis for more advanced exploration of these issues. The context for the discussion is rooted in holistic care concepts introduced in the first year. Because pain is the symptom that causes the most controversy, within and among health care professionals, more detailed discussion of theories of pain control, and nurses' responses, needs to be integrated. Students need to be engaged in discussions of the impact of pain and other symptoms on the lives of their patients and families. Within this context, the concepts of pediatric palliative care should be introduced, whether students have had pediatric clinical experiences to date or not. Students need opportunities to discuss the ethical issues, and their personal responses to pain in children.

Discussions of pain should be more detailed, and in depth. Students need to be introduced to the Gate-Control Theory of Pain [92,93]. Students must become familiar with nociceptive pain pathways, and how pain can be modulated with drugs and non-drug therapies. As has been seen elsewhere in this book (Chapter 8), pain assessment must be presented within the context that pain is a psychological event, making each individual's pain experience unique. A variety of scales can be introduced, including numerical, word anchors, and visual analogue, with an emphasis on developmental issues.

Pain management should emphasize the need for prevention of pain, rather than the crisis management approach. In addition, there need to be dialogue and discussion about the myths and misconceptions of pain management, with special attention to issues specific to the use of narcotics, that is, addiction, tolerance, and dependence. The World Health Organization's [27] 3 Step Ladder Approach to Cancer Pain Management must be introduced; while this approach to pain management is targeted at cancer pain, the theoretical approach inherent in this document is relevant for all patients in pain.

The concept of pain management addressed at this level is relevant to all individuals experiencing pain. The importance of individual assessment of each patient cannot be overstated, as well as the need for evaluation and assessment following each intervention. Students need to be encouraged to develop a professional commitment to the alleviation of pain. The issues of pain in children are particularly difficult for student nurses to manage. To improve this situation, students need to be encouraged to explore their own reactions to caring for children in pain. They need opportunities to engage with children and their families in addressing issues of pain, either through clinical experiences or through vicarious experiences, such as, case studies, patient testimonials, or professional rounds. The key is to engender a consciousness of professional responsibility, in addressing issues of symptom and pain management in collaboration with patients and their families.

Other symptoms, including dyspnea, nausea and vomiting, sleep disturbances, and fatigue need to introduced in more detail, with an emphasis now on prevention of symptoms through both drug and non-drug interventions. Students should be encouraged to explore the nature of these symptoms from a subjective experience of the patient. From a theoretical approach, the use of qualitative research to explore these concepts in depth is particularly useful. However, students need to engage with patients, particularly with children and their families, to explore the personal experiences of these symptoms, and their effect on the quality of life. Such a conceptual understanding of the experience of pain and other symptoms provides the foundation for compassionate and holistic palliative care.

Introduction to pediatrics

Pediatric nursing is considered an essential component of any nursing program, in particular, nursing programs with a focus on community health. Although pediatrics is considered a specialty practice with pediatric palliative care as a subspecialty, the concepts of care of children pervade the practice of nursing. With increasing numbers of children having life-limiting illnesses, and the current commitment to caring for many of these children in the community, many students can anticipate that as graduate registered nurses, they will be pediatric nurses caring for these children as patients in home care or other community agencies. The concepts of health care in children are essential to the concepts of population health and holistic care. Within this concept, the concepts of pediatric palliative care are relevant and essential.

It is essential that students become cognizant of original and landmark documents, such as the United Nations Convention on the Rights of the Child, 1989, asserting healthy child development and the treatment of children as citizens with rights [94], and the ACT Charter (Table 39.2), that forms the philosophical basis for the health care of children. Pediatric nursing concepts are often introduced in the middle years of nursing programs, once students have a foundation in basic nursing care. Certain concepts addressed in pediatric nursing are particularly relevant for pediatric palliative care, including concepts such as family-centered care and Child-Friendly Environment.

Educators need to address communication skills, with special attention to the needs of children and their families. To facilitate holistic care, special attention must be paid to the

---

Table 39.2 The ACT Charter for children with life-threatening conditions and their families

1. Every child shall be treated with dignity and respect, and shall be afforded privacy, whatever the child's physical or intellectual ability.

2. Parents shall be acknowledged as the primary carers, and shall be centrally involved as partners in all care and decisions involving their child.

3. Every child shall be given the opportunity to participate in decisions affecting his or her care, according to age and understanding.

4. Every family shall be given the opportunity of a consultation with a pediatric specialist who has particular knowledge of the child's condition.

5. Information shall be provided for the parents, and for the child and the siblings, according to age and understanding. The needs of other relatives shall also be addressed.

6. An honest, open approach shall be the basis of all communication, which shall be sensitive, and appropriate to age and understanding.

7. The family home shall remain the centre of caring whenever possible. All other care shall be provided by pediatric-trained staff in a child-centered environment.

8. Every child shall have access to education. Efforts shall be made to enable the child to engage in other childhood activities.

9. Every family shall be entitled to a named key worker, who will enable the family to build up, and maintain, an appropriate support system.

10. Every family shall have access to flexible respite care in its own home and in a home-away-from-home setting for the whole family, with appropriate pediatric nursing and medical support.

11. Every family shall have access to pediatric nursing support in the home, when required.

12. Every family shall have access to expert, sensitive advice in procuring practical aids and financial support.

13. Every family shall have access to domestic help at times of stress at home.

14. Bereavement support shall be offered to the whole family, and be available for as long as is required.

impact of developmental and cultural variables on communication skills and techniques. Students need the opportunity to interact with those children and their families, who are experiencing health challenges. This can be achieved in a variety of settings, such as hospital, community, and home.

Communication skills must also focus on interdisciplinary communication as the basis for teamwork within the pediatric palliative care model. Typically, nursing students at this level will require encouragement and assistance to interact professionally with other health care professionals. Although the opportunities for students in the middle years of their programs to interact with dying children and their families in pediatric palliative care may be limited, they will have opportunities to practise their skills with children and families in pediatric units, and within the community. Emphasis on this aspect of the care of children and their families provides a strong foundation for later practice in palliative care situations.

Educators must support students in the involvement of parents in all aspects of their children's care. Since students are generally uncomfortable in providing nursing care in front of individuals other than the patient, they will need support to enable them to see the family as an essential component of the child's care.

Parental involvement in all aspects of the child's care remains a high priority. The importance of the family in the care and well-being of children was recognized in a World Declaration on the Survival, Protection, and Development of Children at the World Summit for Children [95]

The family has the primary responsibility for the nurturing and protection of children from infancy to adolescence . . . and all institutions of society should respect and support the efforts of parents and other caregivers to ensure and care for children in a family environment.

Senior year

The senior year in most programs is an opportunity to address complex and challenging patient situations in a variety of clinical settings. Students will need faculty support to integrate concepts from other aspects of the nursing program. This integration most appropriately occurs in supervized clinical practice. The concepts of palliation can be applied to most clinical settings, but students need faculty support to identify the opportunities for doing so. For students fortunate enough to be placed in these settings during a senior clinical practicum in pediatrics or pediatric palliative care, opportunities to provide holistic and compassionate care will be abundant. However, such opportunities are limited, and students will be stretched to meet the complex needs of their young patients and families. Partnering these learners with nurses experienced in pediatric palliative care is one strategy for supporting them as they learn to apply the challenging concepts of pediatric palliative care. The faculty should anticipate that students will encounter ethical and moral dilemmas in their care, and will need supported learning environments, in order to address their own personal reactions. Interactions with expert nurses in the area will provide a safe environment for the patients and their families while students are learning. The opportunity to develop professional competence under the mentorship of an experienced palliative care nurse will facilitate holistic and compassionate care, and assist students to develop a consciousness of palliation that can be applied to all their patients in any clinical setting. For those student nurses who are employed in pediatric settings, concepts of pediatric palliative care are core foundations for holistic family-centered care.

Theoretical classes dealing with advanced practice, professional issues, case management, and community-based care should involve issues related to pediatric palliative care. The limited number of clinical placements in pediatric palliative care means that only a few students will experience senior clinical placements in this area. At the same time, for it to be an adequate learning experience, there needs to be prolonged engagement in the care of dying children and their families. Observational experiences alone are not usually adequate to learn the complex practice of pediatric palliative care. Therefore, classroom use of case studies, patient narratives, and practice rounds that address the issues of pediatric palliative care can be used to engage students in the issues that dying children and their families encounter.

Pediatric palliative care training for doctors

One challenge facing those who are seeking to provide pediatric palliative care education is that of teaching a wide range of knowledge and skills to a wide range of professionals. There is not always a good match between traditional perceptions of the professionals who need to learn, and the skills they need to be taught. For example, doctors working in palliative care for children will often need to advocate for patients, as nurses have traditionally done, have communication skills more often found among counselors, and have an understanding of holism often found amongst complementary therapists or chaplains. All this is to be achieved without abandoning their understanding of disease and drug management in children.

It is helpful to consider what should ideally be expected from different groups of physicians, who may be called upon to care for dying children [96].

All physicians may encounter occasional children or adolescents with a life-limiting condition. Pediatricians in particular, whether practising in primary care (for example, according to the North American model) or in hospital, will certainly encounter occasional dying children.

Some pediatricians will develop a particular interest in palliative care, but will want to maintain an additional non-palliative practice. In the United Kingdom, this is common in pediatric oncology or neurodisability/'community pediatrics'. In many parts of the world, and increasingly in the United Kingdom, pediatricians with an interest provide medical support for children's hospices. Children's hospice doctors from other backgrounds, usually primary care or general practice, are not usually as trained as pediatricians, and their learning needs may be rather different [97]. A background and training in primary care often imparts particular strengths in some important aspects of pediatric palliative care, for example, in holistic and family-centred understanding and communication skills.

The final category is the tertiary specialist pediatrician, practising full time palliative medicine in children.

The educational needs of these groups are distinct from one another, but are clearly related. The knowledge of those specialising in pediatric palliative medicine should ideally encompass all the other groups. Similarly, a pediatrician with a special interest should be able to draw on knowledge that is greater than that of other pediatricians, and of physicians working outside pediatrics.

All doctors. How much should be taught as part of undergraduate medical training? At first sight, it might seem that pediatric palliative care is too abstruse a subject to be taught to medical students, most of whom will rarely go on to a specialty in which they will be called upon to treat dying children. In fact, however, medical school is an opportunity to teach what is common between the practice of palliative medicine in adults and in children—indeed, as has been seen, core principles that are common to the practice of palliative medicine and that of good medicine generally.

This would include, for example, an understanding of holism, or a bio-psychosocial model, and the philosophical structure it provides for a rational approach that encompasses both evidence base and empiricism. The importance of balancing burden to the patient with benefit is central to good palliative management of children, but is not restricted to it. On the contrary, it is one of the basic tenets of compassionate and ethical medical treatment of any patient, at any stage of his or her disease.

All doctors should have some practical skill in managing symptoms. The two commonest for most patients are pain, and nausea and vomiting, and it would be reasonable to expect newly qualified doctors to have a good understanding of a basic approach to these two symptoms. They should

understand the nature of palliative medicine as a specialty, and the practicality of accessing appropriate specialist skills. This understanding, again, can extend to knowing how to appropriately refer children with symptom control or palliative care needs. This, in turn, means understanding teamwork, the multi disciplinary nature of the specialty, and the value of palliative care skills found outside the medical profession.

A newly qualified doctor, then, should be equipped with an understanding of the 'rules' of palliative medicine in adults or children, and should understand something about basic management of common symptoms and the need for, and availability of, specialist advice in palliative medicine for children as well as adults.

All pediatricians. Although pediatric practice differs in countries across the world, a period of training in medicine among children is mandatory in most countries for those who wish to work full time with children. Most pediatricians will not want to pursue palliative medicine as a special interest. Nevertheless, they are likely to encounter children with life-limiting conditions. Furthermore, even among children whose lifespan is not limited, there will often be the need for palliative care skill. For example, children in a general pediatric ward will often experience pain. What is required at this level is not specialist palliative medicine expertise, but an application of the principle and practice learnt during medical school to the specific case of children.

This would include, for example, developing an understanding of conditions that may limit life in childhood. Many physicians commencing pediatric training will largely see palliative medicine as the management of cancer. It is important that trainee pediatricians should learn the true variety of life-limiting conditions in childhood [83]. They should learn to apply the principle of 'holism' to assessing and understanding the needs of the child and family. There should be an application of fundamental ethical principle to pediatrics. For example, trainee pediatricians should learn about issues of resuscitation, withholding or withdrawing of feeding or life-sustaining treatment, issues of euthanasia, etc. Whilst these are principles of palliative care, they are of relevance to all pediatric practice, and so need to be taught at this level.

Practical palliative care skills that trainee pediatricians need to learn should include basic communication skills, such as active empathic listening, conveying of bad news, and eliciting of fears and beliefs. The trainee pediatrician should be familiar with the basic management of common symptoms, and once again, be aware of the limitation of his or her expertise, and the availability of specialist advice.

Much of the palliative medicine that should be taught to trainee pediatricians will be encountered as part of other training. For example, those who rotate through pediatric oncology may learn something about management of nausea and vomiting, or pain. There remains, however, a need for the pediatric palliative medicine team to assess the learning needs of trainees, and to 'fill in the gaps'.

Pediatrician with an interest. Many pediatricians will want to develop an interest in palliative medicine, without abandoning their general or other specialist pediatric case load. These will be physicians who are already well versed, not only in facts about pediatrics, but also in the culture that surrounds the care of children. They will understand, for example, the need to avoid hospital admission where possible, and what means are available to avoid unnecessary interventions. How should they augment the understanding of pediatric palliative care they have developed during pediatric training?

Pediatricians with an interest are likely to deal with enough children with life-limiting conditions, to maintain basic skills in symptom control and communications. They should feel confident in basic management of most symptoms, including relatively unusual ones such as dyspnoea, depression, or pruritus. They should have an understanding of reflective practice, again recognising when and where to go for more expert advice. They should have good basic counseling skills, and some may choose to develop these to a higher level.

Pediatricians with an interest should also be able to recognize and manage some of the more complex symptoms, such as 'total pain' and neuropathic pain. It would be anticipated that pediatricians with an interest would offer advice to children with malignant and non-malignant conditions, and therefore, would need to be familiar with the possible underlying causes for symptoms that could be reversed in a palliative phase. The learning needs will clearly differ, depending on the individual experience of the pediatrician in question.

Tertiary specialists. Relatively few pediatricians are likely to make palliative medicine their main specialty. However small the numbers may be, though, it is important that at least one such specialist should always be available and accessible [89,90]. According to the adult model, other specialists tend to hand over care of a dying patient to the palliative medicine specialist. In children, this is rarely appropriate. Most children are already well known to their pediatric team, and should not be 'handed over' in the last phase of life. The role of the specialist in pediatric palliative medicine, therefore, is not usually to take over care of the child, but to empower, support and facilitate others in their care. For many families, it may be the oncology outreach and community pediatric nurse who provides most of the hands-on care. This should be made easier by the availability of access to specialist advice.

So what does such a specialist need to know? In a sense, the knowledge base and skill set must always be increasing; one of the roles of any specialist is to keep abreast of new developments. This role will involve considerable familiarity with the adult specialty, in which techniques of good symptom control have been developed. The specialist needs not only to be thoroughly familiar with the principles and practice of symptom control, but also with where to look, if faced with something for the first time.

Good basic communications and counseling skills are mandatory. Many specialists in pediatric palliative medicine have gone on to learn advanced counseling techniques. The ability to distinguish between 'normal' emotional needs of the child and family during the process of losing a child, and the psychopathology that requires advice from others, is an essential skill.

It is imperative that specialists in pediatric palliative medicine have a good understanding of ethical principle, and be well practised in applying it to clinical problems involving children. In addition to understanding of the four basic medical ethical principles, and their scope in application [98], the specialist in pediatric palliative medicine should have a thorough understanding of the principle of double effect [99], and how it relates to appropriate use of interventions in the palliative phase. He or she should be familiar with the issues surrounding, for example, unlicensed medications in children and in palliative medicine [100–104].

Currently, it is difficult for a pediatrician to obtain this kind of specialist experience, except by studying in the adult specialty. Whilst this has its limitations (in general, the 'culture' of pediatrics is not well understood by those working outside it), this is more than offset by the value of exposure to relatively large numbers of patients, and the opportunity to learn advanced symptom control and communication skills. There remain very few 'fellowship programs' in pediatric palliative medicine.

Evaluating competence

Training methods across the world differ considerably. In most places, a doctor is deemed to be competent in a specialty, either because he or she has spent a certain period of time in a recognized training programme, or because he or she is able to demonstrate competency by means of an exam, or both. Increasingly, medical educationalists are putting the emphasis on assessments based on 'competencies'. These are skills that the doctor can demonstrate that he or she has acquired to the necessary level of expertise.

The system works well for some medical skills. Surgical procedures or radiological interventions, for example, can be performed in front of a supervising individual who can then confirm that competence has been achieved. This is much more difficult in pediatric palliative medicine. The nature of the specialty means that the necessary skills do not always lend themselves to this sort of 'tick box' assessment.

Nevertheless, it is important that doctors who wish to train in pediatric palliative medicine are rigorously assessed. In developing a curriculum in pediatric palliative care, the British Society for Paediatric Palliative Medicine drew heavily on the experience of the Paediatric Option of the Diploma in Palliative Medicine, a distance learning qualification based in Cardiff [105]. Here, competencies were assessed using five tools:

1. *Log book.* Trainees are expected to maintain anonymized records on patients they have dealt with. The cases have to illustrate four specified aspects of palliative care in children, such as pain or difficult communication issues. Each account is expected to include references to relevant literature, an account of what was done well, and what could have been done differently with advantage.

   The point of the case books is partly to ensure that the trainee has had exposure to a sample of common palliative care problems in children. More importantly, it is to instil a habit of reflective practice, in which the trainee recognizes the need both to consult external resources, and to think about it afterwards, in order to learn from the experience.

2. *Assignments.* There is a series of four assignments on specific topics, deriving from the taught portion of the course. They include, for example, an assignment to produce a talk on complex pain management, or to draft a consent form to non-invasive ventilation for a boy with Duchenne muscular dystrophy. These demonstrate the trainee's ability to set biomedical and ethical principles into the practical context of palliative medicine for children.

3. *Communications skills assessment.* Good basic communication skills are an essential part of training in pediatric palliative care. Competency assessment is in the form of a semi-structured evaluation of the trainee interacting in a mock patient interview, using a 'scenario' set by the examiners. It can be argued that this is an artificial environment. Communication skills in primary care are taught using video tape recordings of genuine interviews with patients. These are submitted centrally, for semi-structured marking. Perhaps this is an area in which educators in pediatric palliative care can learn from those in primary care, and is something that could be considered in the future.

4. *Examination.* A written examination, or other form of test, can be of limited value in assessing many of the skills needed for palliative medicine. It may, however, have a place in confirming that the trainee has a good grasp of cognitive knowledge, such as the relevant basic clinical science. For example, extended match questions can test the trainee's understanding of opioid conversions, drug side effects, and interactions. These shorter questions can be combined with long 'essay type' questions, that can help assess the trainee's understanding of wider holistic issues, and there is also scope for short answer questions that can test knowledge on a wide variety of relevant topics.

5. *Audit.* Although the term 'audit' is largely restricted to the United Kingdom, it embodies an important concept in improving pediatric practice, which is universally applicable. Its purpose is to compare clinical practice with 'best' practice. In essence, the process of audit is in three stages. The first is to identify the best standard of practice. The second is to compare existing practice with the best standard, and the last is to provide feedback to those providing the service, on the results of such comparison. Designing and carrying out an audit is an important learning tool in pediatric palliative medicine, for a number of reasons. It requires the trainee to become familiar with the process of locating or, if necessary, deriving a set of good standards, based on available evidence. It also encourages a cycle of reflective practice, with reference to external evidence. This is of particular importance for trainees who are going to become tertiary specialists. Because there are very few specialists, there is often little opportunity to compare one's practice with those of peers in the same field. The process of audit also establishes the connection between published research base and clinical practice. This is of particular importance in pediatric palliative medicine, where the evidence base is currently very small.

All of these tools for evaluating competence need to be superimposed on local training assessment structures, such as appraisals, annual feedback, interviews, etc.

How do we provide training?

Pediatrics shares with palliative medicine and primary care the traditions of a holistic approach and of multi disciplinary working. Pediatric palliative medicine is able to draw on the published experience of the adult palliative care movement, which began in the 1960s. The evidence basis may be small, compared with some specialties, but there is evidence there, and we are able to use it to learn and to teach.

Until recently, very few of the text books in pediatric palliative care were of interest or relevance to doctors. This is beginning to change, as chapters on palliative medicine are finding their way into many major pediatric text books, and there even are some text books dedicated to pediatric palliative care [106].

The number of courses and textbooks remains small, however. This is for a variety of reasons. Most of those working with children with life-limiting conditions see a relatively small number in their normal practice. There are few pediatricians doing full time pediatric palliative care, who can accumulate a clinical experience base that allows them to teach trainees confidently. Such specialists as there are, are spread thinly across a large geographical area. In the whole of the United Kingdom, there are only five pediatricians working in full time palliative medicine. Teaching pediatric palliative medicine is likely, therefore, to have low academic priority in any one centre. Interest in teaching and learning pediatric palliative care is often greatest among nurses, so that training programs would need to cross disciplinary and professional boundaries, as well as practical skills.

While none of these difficulties means that training is impossible they do need to be acknowledged and addressed.

The problem of geographical spread can, to some extent, be overcome using distance learning. With the Internet increasingly accessible, some of the basic principles of pediatric palliative medicine can be taught and learnt online. This allows 'pooling' of the expertise of specialists in pediatric palliative medicine from a wide area. As has been explored earlier, this kind of didactic provision of 'cognitive content' is necessary, but by no means sufficient. The Internet may be a less effective tool for more affective content.

A complementary approach is to access the experience of the adult specialist. Roughly seven times as many adults need palliative care as children. It is, therefore, possible to gain a good deal of important experience in some aspects of palliative medicine (particularly aspects of physical symptom control) by working with an adult team. Pediatric programs that allow some time in an adult specialist palliative medicine unit should be encouraged.

Setting up a distance-learning course: The Cardiff experience

The Paediatric Option of the Cardiff Diploma in Palliative Medicine is a distance-learning course for doctors. The Paediatric Option was developed in 2000 [105]. It was based on the existing Adult Diploma in Palliative Medicine, which was well established, having been started in 1988 [107,108]. The course comprised a series of study packs, some with audio tapes, three residential weekends in Cardiff, and a combination of written assignments and exam.

When considering the Adult Diploma, it became clear that the teaching material within it fell into three categories with respect to their relevance to pediatrics.

Much of the written material for the adult course was equally applicable to the pediatric specialty. This included, for example, much of the science of symptom control, the philosophy of palliative medicine, and basic communication skills. A further section became relevant to pediatric palliative care with some modification, often minor. This included many of the legal and ethical issues which were based on adults, but were worked out differently in pediatric practice.

A further proportion of the adult Diploma material had little or no relevance to the pediatric specialty. This included many of the symptoms related to specific adult cancers, such as breast, prostate or lung, and some of the specific non-malignant conditions, such as motor–neuron disease.

Then there was some material, outside the experience of adult physicians and unique to children, that needed to be included in a pediatric qualification. This included some symptoms, for example, muscle spasm, that have received little attention in the adult literature, developmental and communications issues, and some of the wider psychosocial concerns, particularly those relating to school.

The Pediatric Option of the Diploma in Palliative Medicine therefore comprised material that was:

• equally applicable to children and adults

• modified from the adult material to make it relevant to children, and

• generated *de novo* because it was unique to the pediatric specialty.

This approach had a number of advantages. It was efficient, since administrative and educational structures were already in place. Perhaps more importantly, the Pediatric Option was built both on the experience of the adult specialty, and on its high educational profile.

There is potentially, however, a serious disadvantage. Whilst much of the science, and even some of the philosophy, of adult palliative medicine can be extrapolated with apparent validity to children, their application to practice needs to be worked out in a culture and a context that are very different from adults. An educational program in pediatric palliative medicine that is developed from an adult one risks 'missing the point' in children, unless it is continually updated on developments in the pediatric world. Having had a common origin, the two courses must be allowed to diverge as necessary, if the pediatric option is to remain relevant to palliative medicine in children.

Summary

As the important role of doctors in pediatric palliative care is increasingly recognized, so does the need for adequate medical education and training become more apparent. This is complicated by the multi-faceted nature of the specialty itself, and by the geographical and professional diversity of those working with dying children.

Nevertheless, those working with children with life-limiting conditions are linked by a common philosophy, as well as by a number of fundamental scientific and ethical principles that can be taught. Furthermore, technology now means that we can acquire and disseminate such expertise globally. Whilst this can never replace clinical experience, it can provide a valuable complement, and allows 'pooling' of global pediatric palliative medicine knowledge.

Lastly, we have a great deal to learn from what the adult specialty has already achieved. Not only can trainees in the pediatric specialty gain 'distilled experience' by spending time working with adult teams, but as a specialty we need to look to what has been successful, and what has failed, among adult trainees across the decades, and across the world.

References

1. IOM. *Approaching Death: Improving Care at the End of Life*. Washington DC: National Academy Press, 1997.

2. Ferrell, B., Virani, R., and Grant, M. Analysis of end-of-life content in nursing textbooks. *Oncol Nur Forum* 1999;26:869–76.

3. Sumner, L. *Pediatric, Care: The Hospice Perspective*. In B. Ferrel and N. Coyle, ed. Textbook of Palliative Nursing. Oxford: Oxford University Press, 2001.

4. Vazirani, R., Slavin, S., and Feldman, J. Longitudinal study of pediatric house officers' attitudes toward death and dying. *Crit Care Med* 2000;28(37):40–5.

5. Organization NH. Hospice fact sheet. Arlington VA: National Hospice Organization, 1997.

6. Hain, R. and Goldman, A. Training in paediatric palliative medicine. *Palliat Med* 2003;17:229–31.

7. Doyle, D., Hanks, G., and MacDonald, N.N. *Oxford Textbook of Palliative medicine*. Oxford: Oxford University Press.

8. Kane, J.R. and Primono, M. Alleviating the suffering of seriously ill children. *Am J Hospice Palliat Care* 2001;18:161–9.

9. Buckingham, R.W. and Meister, E.A. Hospice are for the child with AIDS. *Soc Sci J* 2001;48:461–7.

10. Brown, E.R. Rockefeller medicine men: Medicine and capitalism in America. Berkely: University Press, 1979.

11. Doll, R.C. *Curriculum Improvement: Decision making and Process*. Ninth edition ed. Boston, MA: Allyn & Bacon; 1996.

12. Billings, D.M. and Halstead, J.A. *Teaching in nursing: A guide for faculty*. Philadelphia, PA: Saunders, 1998.

13. De Young, S. *Teaching Strategies for Nurse Educators*. Upper Saddle River, NJ: Prentice Hall, 2003.

14. Billings, J.A. and Block, S. Palliative care in undergraduate medical education: Status report and future directions. *J Am Med Assoc* 1997;278(9):733–8.

15. DeVita, M.A., Arnold, R.M., and Barnard, D. Teaching palliative care to critical care medicine trainees. *Crit Care Med* 2003; 31:1257–62.

16. Bagatell, R., Meyer, R., Herron, S., Berger, A., and Villar, R. When children die: A seminar series for pediatric residents. *Pediatrics* 2002;110(2):348–53.

17. Ross, D., Fraser, H., and Kutner, J. Institutionalization of a palliative and end-of-life care educational program in a medical school curriculum. *J Pallia Med* 2001;4(4):512–18.

18. Billings, J.A., Ferris, F.D., Macdonald, N., and von Guten, C. The role of palliative care in the home in medical education: Report from a National Consensus Conference. *J Palliat Med* 2001; 4(3):361–71.

19. Block, S.D. Medical education in end-of-life care: The status of reform. *J Palliat Med* 2002;5(2):243–48.

20. Oneschuk, D. Undergraduate medical palliative care education: A new Canadian perspective. *J Palliat Med* 2002;5(1):43–47.

21. Gronlund, N.E. (ed.) *How to Write and Use Instructional Objectives* (5th edition) Englewood Cliffs NJ: Prentice Hall, 1995.

22. Beavis, E.O. and Watson, J. *A Caring Curriculum: A New Pedagogy for Nursing*. New York: National League for Nursing; 1989.

23. Olthuis, G. and Dekers, W. Professional competence and palliative care: an ethical perspective. *J Palliat Care* 2003;19(3):192–7.

24. Benner, P., Tanner, C.A., and Chesla, C.A. *Expertise in Nursing Practice: Caring, clinical judgment and ethics*. New York: Springer; 1996.

25. Downie, R.S., MacNaughton, J., and Randall, F. *Clinical judgement: evidence in practice*. Oxford: Oxford University Press, 2000.

26. Martinson, I.M., Liu-Chiang, C., and L. Y.-H. Distress symptoms and support systems of Chinese parents of children with cancer. *Cancer Nurs* 1997;20(2):94–9.

27. WHO. *Cancer Pain Relief and Palliative Care in Children*. Geneva: World Health Organisation; 1998.

28. Abu-Saad, H.H. and Courtens, A. Pain and symptom management. In H. Abu-Saad, (ed). *Evidence-Based Palliative Care Across the Lifespan*. Oxford: Blackwell Science, 2001; p. 63–87.

29. Barnabe, C. and Kirk, P. A needs assessment for southern Manitoba physicians for palliative care education. *J Palliat Care* 2002; 18(3):175–84.

30. Oakes, L. Reducing pain. In J. Steen RaM, ed. Childhood cancer. Cambridge MA: Perseus Publishers, 2001.

31. McGrath, P.A. *Pain in Children: Nature, Assessment and Treatment*. New York: The Guilford Press; 1990.

32. Bloom, B.S., Englehart, M.D., Furst, E.J., Hill, W.H., and Krathwohl, D.R. *Taxonomy of eduational objectives*: Handbook I, cognitive domain. New York: David McKay, 1956.

33. Harrow, A.J. *A taxonomy in the psychomotor domain*. New York: David McKay; 1972.

34. Duhamel, F. and Dupuis, F. Families in palliative care: exploring family and health-care professionals' belie. *Int J Palliat Nurs* 2003;9(3):113–19.

35. Contro, N., Larson, J., Scofield, S., Sourkes, B., and Cohen, H. Family perspectives on the quality of pediatric palliative care. *Arch Pediatr Adoles Med* 2002;156(1):14–19.

36. Morita, T. and Chihara, S. A scale to measure satisfaction of bereaved family receiving inpatient palliative care. *Palliat Med* 2002;16:141–50.

37. Steele, R. Experiences of families in which a child has a prolonged terminal illness: Modifying factors. *Int J Palliat Nurs* 2002; 8(9):418–34.

38. Mok, E., Chan, F., Chan, V., and Yeung, E. Perceptions of empowerment by family caregivers of patients with a terminal illness in Hong Kong. *Int J Palliat Nurs* 2002;8(3):137–45.

39. Krathwohl, D.R., Bloom, B.S., and Maisa, B.B. *Taxonomy of Educational Objectives: Handbook II, affective domain.* New York: David McKay, 1964.

40. Patel, V., Kaufman, D., and Arocha, J. Emerging paradigms of cognition in medical decision-making. *J Biomed Inform* 2002; 35:52–75.

41. Copp, G. Palliative care nursing education: A review of research findings. *J Adv Nurs* 1994;19:552–7.

42. Lloyd-Williams, M. and Field, D. Are undergraduate nurses taught palliative care furing their training? *Nurs Educ Today* 2002; 22:589–92.

43. Sellick, S., Charles, K., Dagsvik, J., and Kelley, M. Palliative care providers' perspectives on service and education needs. *J Palliat Care* 1996;12(2):34–8.

44. Yates, P., Clinton, M., and Hart, G. Improving psychosocial care: A professional development programme. *International J Palliat Nurs* 1996;2(4):212–16.

45. Zabalegui, A. Palliative nursing care in Spain. *Eur J Cancer Care* 2001;10:280–3.

46. Rooda, L., Clements, R., and Jordan, M. Nurses' attitudes toward death and caring for dying patients. *Oncol Nurs Forum* 1999; 26:1683–87.

47. Bastable, S.B. *Nurse as educator: Principles of Teaching and Learning for Nursing Practice* (2nd edition) Boston, MA: Jones and Bartlett; 2003.

48. Souter, J. Using a model for structured reflection on palliative care nursing: exploring the challenges raised. *Int J Palliat Nurs* 2003;9(1):6–12.

49. Carper, B.A. Fundamental patterns of knowing nursing. *Adv Nurs Sci* 1978;1:13–23.

50. Mazuryk, M., Daeninck, P., Neumann, C.M., and Bruera, E. Daily journal club: An educative tool in palliative care. *Palliat Med* 2002;16:57–61.

51. MacDonald, C. Nurse autonomy as relational. *Nurs Ethics* 2002;9(2):194–201.

52. Sherman, D.W. *et al.* End-of-life nursing education consortium curriculum. *Nurse Educ* 2003;28:111–20.

53. Llewellyn-Thomas, H.A. Patients' health-care decision-making: A framework for descriptive and experimental investigations. *Med Decision Making* 1995;15(2):101–6.

54. Bergum, V. Knowledge for ethical care. *Nurs Ethics* 1994;1(2):71–79.

55. Sherwin, G. A relational approach to autonomy in health care. In S. Sherwin, ed. *The Politics of Women's Health: Exploring Agency and Autonomy.* Philadelphia, PA: Temple University Press, 1998.

56. Georgaki, S., Kalaidopoulou, O., Liarmakopoulos, I., and Mystakidou, K. Nurses' attitudes toward truthful communication with patients with cancer: A Greek study. *Cancer Nurs* 25(6): 436–7.

57. Hu, W., Chiu, T., Chuang, R., and Chen, C. Solving family-related barriers to truthfulness in cases of terminal cancer in Taiwan: A professional perspective. *Cancer Nurs* 2002;25(6):486–7.

58. Arber, A. and Gallagher, A. Breaking bad news revisited: The push for negotiated disclosure and changing practice implications. *International J Palliat Nurs* 2003;9(4):166–72.

59. Dowell, L. Multiprofessional palliative care in a general hospital: Education and training needs. *Int J Palliat Nurs* 2002;8(6):294–303.

60. Rawlinson, F. and Finlay, I. Assessing education in palliative medicine: Development of a tool based on the Association for Palliative Medicine core curriculum. *Palliat Med* 2002;16:51–55.

61. Wilkinson, S., Bailey, K., Aldridge, J., and Roberts, A. A longitudinal evaluation of a communication skills program. *Palliat Med* 1999;13:341–8.

62. Patel, V., Arocha, J., and Kaufman, D. Expertise and tacit knowledge in medicine. In R.H., J.A. Sternberg, ed. *Tacit Knowledge in Professional Practice.* Mahwah NJ: Lawrence Erlbaum; 1999.

63. James, C.R. The problematic nature of education in palliative care. *J Palliat Care* 1993;9(4):5–10.

64. Thompson, C. and Dowding, D. *Clinical Decision Making and Judgement in Nursing.* London: Churchill Livingstone, 2002.

65. Dunniece, U. and Slevin, E. Giving voice to the less articulated knowledge of palliative nursing: an interpretive study. *Int J Palliat Nurs* 2002;8(1):13–20.

66. Rittman, M., Rivera, J., and Godown, I. Phenomenological study of nurses caring for dying patients. *Cancer Nurs* 1997;20(2):115–19.

67. Buller, S. and Butterworth, T. Skilled nursing practice—a qualitative study of the elements of nursing. *Int J Nurs Stud* 2001; 38:405–17.

68. Cowley, S., Bliss, J., Mathew, A., and McVey. Effective interagency and interprofessional working: facilitators and barriers. *Int J Palliat Nurs* 2002;8(1):30–9.

69. Donaghy, K. and Devlin, B. An evaluation of teamwork within a specialist palliative care unit. *Int J Palliat Nurs* 2002;8(11):518–24.

70. Lee, L. Interprofessional working in hospice day care and the patients' experience of service. *Int J Palliat Nurs* 2002;8(8):398–400.

71. Medicine, AAoP. Undergraduate medical education in pain medicine, End-of-Life care, and palliative care. *Pain Med* 2000;1(3):224.

72. Wee, C., Hillier, R., Coles, C., Mountford, C., Sheldon, F., and Turner, P. Palliative care: a suitable setting for undergraduate interprofessional education. *Palliat Med* 2001;15:487–92.

73. Nishimoto, P. Venturing into the unknown: cultural beliefs about death and dying. *Oncol Nurs Forum* 1996;23(6):889–94.

74. Nyatanga, B. Culture, palliative care, and multiculturalism. *Int J Palliat Nurs* 2002;8(5):240–6.

75. Randhawa, G., Owens, A., Fitches, R., and Khan, Z. Communication in the development of culturally competent palliative care services in the UK; a case study. *Int J Palliat Nurs* 2003;9(1):24–31.

76. Gatrad, R. and Sheikh, A. Palliative care for Muslims and issues after death. *Int J Palliat Nurs* 2002;8(12):594–98.

77. Ferrell, B. and Coyle, N. *Textbook of Palliative Nursing.* Oxford: Oxford University Press; 2001.

78. Shipman, C. Addington-Hall, J. Barclay, S. Briggs, J. Cox, I., and Daniels, L. *et al.* Educational opportunities in palliative care: what do general practitioners want? *Palliat Med* 2001;15:191–6.

79. Van Boxel, P., Anderson, K., and Regnard, C. The effectiveness of palliative care education delivered by videoconferencing compared with face-to-face delivery. *Palliat Med* 2003;17:344–58.

80. Regnard, C. Using videoconferencing in palliative care. *Palliat Med* 2000;14:519–28.

81. Meleis, A.I. *Theoretical Nursing: Development and Progress.* New York: Lippincott; 1991.

82. Parker, J. and Aranda, S. *Palliative Care: Explorations and Challenges.* Sydney: Maclennan & Petty; 1998.

83. Hain, R. *Palliative Care in Children in Wales: A study of Provision and Need. Palliat Med* 2005.

84. Dickinson, G.E. Death education in US medical schools. *J Med Educ* 1976;51:34–6.

85. Dickinson, G.E. Changes in death education in U.S. medical schools. *J Med Educ* 1985;12:942–3.

86. Liston, E.H. Education on death and dying. *J Med Educ* 1973:577–8.

87. Smith, M., Sweeney, M., and Katz, B. Characteristics of death education curricula in American medical schools. *J Med Educ* 1980;55:844–50.

88. IOM. *When Children Die: Improving Palliative and End-of-Life Care for Children and their Families.* Washington DC: National Academy Press; 1997.

89. Baum, D., Curtis, H., Elston, S., Goldman, A., Lewis, I., and Rigg, K., *et al. A Guide to the Development of Children's Palliative Care Services* (1 edition). Bristol and London: ACT/RCPCH; 1997.

90. ACT/RCPCH. A Guide to the Development of Children's Palliative Care Services—Second Edition, September 2003. Updated report: ACT/RCPCH; 2003 September, 2003.

91. Organization, W.H. *Cancer Pain Relief and Palliative Care.* Geneva, 1990.

92. Melzack, R. and Wall, P. *Textbook of Pain.* London: Churchill Livingstone; 1994.

93. Melzack, R. and Wall, P.D. Pain mechanisms: a new theory. *Science* 1965;150(699):971–9.

94. Nat U. *The Convention on the Rights of the Child.* New York: United Nations; 1990.

95. United Nations Childrens Fund (UNICEF). *The State of the World's Children.* Oxford: Oxford University Press, 1991.

96. Hain, R. and Goldman, A. Training in paediatric palliative medicine. *Palliat Med* 2003;17(3):229–31.

97. Amery, J. and Lapwood, S. Study into the educational needs of children's hospice doctors: a descriptive quantitative and qualitative survey. *Palliat Med* 2004.

98. Gillon, R. Medical ethics: four principles plus attention to scope. *BMJ* 1994;309:184–8.

99. Fohr, J.D. The Double Effect of Pain Medication: Separating Myth from Reality. *J pall Med* 1998;1:315–28.

100. Atkinson, C.V. and Kirkham, S.R. Unlicensed uses for medication in a palliative care unit. *Palliat med* 1999;13:145–52.

101. Conroy, S., Choonara, I., Impicciatore, P., Mohn, A., Henrik, A., and Rane, A. Survey of unlicensed and off label drug use in paediatric wards in European countries. *BMJ* 2000;320:79–82.

102. Group, M. Using licensed medicines for unlicensed indications. Off-Label Rapid Response 2003.

103. Medicines, RNSCo. The use of unlicensed medicines or licensed medicines for unlicensed applications in paediatric practice. Policy statement produced by the joint RCPCH/NPPG Standing Committee on Medicines (an update of the statement that appears in Medicines for Children, and will appear in the next revised edition. 2000.

104. Twycross, R., Wilcock, A., and Throp, S. *Appendix 7: Using Licensed Drugs for Unlicensed Purposes.* Oxford: Radcliffe Medical Press, 1998.

105. Hain, R., Rawlinson, F., and Finlay, I. A paediatric option? The Diploma in Palliative Medicine 3 years on. *Arch Dis Child* 2004;89 (Suppl. 1):A34.

106. Carter, B.S. and Levetown, M. ed. *Palliative Care* for infants, children and adolescents: A practical handbook. Baltimore, MA: The Johns Hopkins University Press.

107. Finlay, I.G., Stott, N.C., and Kinnersley, P. The assessment of communication skills in palliative medicine: a comparison of the scores of examiners and simulated patients. *Med Educ* 1995;29(6):424–9.

108. Rawlinson, F. and Finlay, I. Assessing education in palliative medicine: development of a tool based on the Association for Palliative Medicine core curriculum. *Palliat Med* 2002;16(1):51–5.

Research

Robert Graham, Veronica Dussel, and Joanne Wolfe

The cart before the horse is neither beautiful nor useful. Before we can adorn our houses with beautiful objects the walls must be stripped ... and beautiful housekeeping ... laid for a foundation.

Henry David Thoreau

No matter what the discipline, medical professionals are either directly engaged in research, or their daily practice is guided by previous research efforts. Anecdotes, clinical experience, and even consensus are not considered to be the optimal basis for informed decision-making. Albeit often unattainable, the prospective, double blind, randomized controlled trial (RCT) has become the gold standard of clinical researchers, and the expectation for critical reviewers. In many settings, evidence-based medicine and clinical practice guidelines are becoming integral parts of medical education, routine care delivery, and hospital quality assurance and improvement efforts. But what of a field with a heterogeneous population, outcomes that are difficult to define and measure, ethical controversies, and charged emotions?

Pediatric palliative care is in its relative nascence within the field of medicine. Care providers have emerged from various backgrounds within pediatrics, including primary care, oncology, critical care, psychiatry, anesthesia, nursing, and from adult practitioners. They are motivated by personal interest and recognized necessity. Not surprisingly, such diversity results in significant variability in palliative care populations, and in the types of services provided. Practice has been adapted from the adult population, and driven by training background, common sense, trial and error, observation, and modeling. Expertise has been established based on eminent domain. Research efforts in pediatrics have lagged behind those for adults, and have been out-paced by a desire to implement clinical programs. As within other fields of medicine, pediatric palliative care providers must show caution in extrapolating from the findings of adult populations.

The preceding chapters have provided a review of the scope of pediatric palliative care. Current methods of symptom management, implementation and withdrawal of technology support, communication strategies, bereavement support, and delivery systems were among the topics discussed. In this chapter, we suggest why research in pediatric palliative care is important, and review its current state. We highlight obstacles to conducting research in children and families affected by life-limiting conditions (LLC), and propose strategies for overcoming these obstacles, in order to systematically advance the field of pediatric palliative care.

Identifying the need for pediatric palliative care research

Millions of dollars and countless hours are spent on refining and developing therapies and techniques to 'treat' disease. Not all patients, however, will respond to treatment. The 'non-responder,' in fact, serves as the impetus for further research into 'cure.' Some care providers, however, recognize the ongoing needs of those 'non-responders,' as well as the needs of their families. Pediatric palliative and end-of-life (EOL) care is not cancer. It is not AIDS. It is not trauma. Rather, it represents a natural end point within all fields of medicine. Palliative care is distinct but not entirely antithetical to the cure paradigm. It is, instead, a complementary and critical part of every disease process. Those interested in providing palliative care would argue that EOL is as important, if not more, than any other aspect of medical care. The necessity for research in EOL and pediatric palliative care is no different than in other fields of study. There are unanswered questions and, presumably, better means of providing care.

As a burgeoning clinical field, some might see expansion of research efforts as a means of solidifying the status of palliative care in clinical fields typically driven by basic science or more definitive outcomes. Ironically, research may also be needed for survival. Practitioners may need to justify their time and, ultimately, salaries. Support for clinical programs from private and government funding sources often relies upon preliminary research findings, or proposed research projects. Subsequent outcome measures and research reports then serve as indices of progress, and may factor into decisions around continued financial or staff support. For the consumer seeking palliative and advanced care services, research may serve as the basis for referral and reimbursement by their primary health care provider, insurers or local and national sponsored agencies.

In areas where resources are scarce, and palliative care for any age group is considered a luxury, pediatric palliative care research has a role in a broader sense. It is difficult to argue that EOL efforts and research should supercede basic preventative medicine interventions, such as immunization, sanitation, nutrition, and access to health care, but underserved does not equate with unworthy. Children within crisis populations, such as those with HIV in sub-Saharan Africa or those in war-torn regions, are entitled to palliative care, and likely have special needs. Research and commitment from the worldwide medical community may demonstrate that some aspects of palliative care can be integrated into routine care systems.

Pragmatics, of course, is not at the heart of most palliative care, nor is it the primary reason to pursue research in the field. Assuring quality and consistent care at the end of life is the goal. Research, itself, may encourage collaboration among care providers who have practiced in relative isolation, learning by individual trial and error. Through research, pediatric palliative care is transitioning from anecdotal, or case-based, medicine to compassionate but evidence-based practice.

Both patient-centered and health services-centered research efforts need to be explored. The former focuses on "the product," or bedside delivery of pediatric palliative care. For example, what medications or techniques best relieve suffering from physical symptoms at the end of life? What is the quality-of-Life (QoL) of families and children experiencing a terminal illness? How can we relieve emotional suffering? Health services research emphasizes and evaluates "the system" of pediatric palliative care delivery. Who, how, and where are services being rendered? Do different settings or care-team compositions promote better palliation? Methodologies differ, but effective and efficient care is contingent upon both approaches.

More communication and critical thinking about pediatric palliative care will refine and optimize practice, broaden the scope of care, and promote system development. Successful research will increase awareness among the general public, as well as in health care providers. A broader advocacy base will promulgate pediatric palliative care as an expectation, rather than an exception, and eventually, bring about more institutional, legislative, and financial support.

The current state of pediatric palliative care research

Pain

The subject of pain in children has been the focus of considerable research efforts. An informal search in Medline carried out by the authors identified that in the period 2000–2004, approximately 12 out of every 1000 publications involving children from birth to 18 years of age concerned pain or analgesia, more than 3 times the papers focusing on AIDS or pneumonia. Pain research exploded in the 1990s. However, it continues to be a growing field. Since 2000, an average of 26 papers per year have been published, about a 30% increase over the 20 papers per year of the past decade.

Arriving at the current concept that children are able to feel [1], remember [2], and manifest [3–5] pain, regardless of their age and cognitive function, took more than 30 years of research, education, and consumer efforts [6]. Between 1960 and the mid 1980s, publications about pain in children were scarce, and mostly limited to dental pain, the so-called functional pains (colic, abdominal and limb pain, and headaches), and congenital analgesia. The prevailing belief was that children did not feel or remember pain, or at best, that they felt it to a lesser extent [7]. In the late 1960s and 1970s, isolated researchers, mainly nurses and psychologists, began to question this conception [8–13], and the first instruments aimed at grasping the child's perception of pain were developed [14–17]. However, it was not until the 1980's, when the landmark studies of Anand and colleagues [18–20] established not only that neonates experienced pain, but also that this could result in deleterious consequences, that the issue of pain in children captured widespread interest. During the last 10–15 years, publications about pain, its evaluation, and treatment have at least doubled in numbers, and in some subgroups, such as newborns and infants, there has been up to a 10-fold increase. As a result, several practice guidelines for the evaluation and treatment of pain have been developed [21–27].

The interpretation of findings has changed dramatically. Thirty-five years ago, the observations that children could be easily distracted [28], did not complain about pain [7,29], received fewer analgesics than adults [7], and, in the case of infants, underwent surgery without anesthesia [30], were all interpreted as evidence supporting the theory that children did not feel pain. Today, easy distraction, and at times, overt manifestations of pain, are seen as some of the distinct ways children use to cope with pain, while abnormal quietness may be an indication of long-term severe pain [23,31,32]. In turn, variability in analgesic provision is understood as a failure of health professionals to capture children's experiences [33].

Early pain assessment instruments used in the 1980's were aimed at gaining insight into children's perception of pain, and facilitated communication about the experience of pain directly from the child [10,15,17,34,35]. They served essentially as a means of establishing that children felt, recalled, and could adequately describe, pain, and ways of relieving it [16, 36]. Yet, the perspective was mainly adult-centered. Many of the findings (e.g., reports of less frequent pain, or lower scores than adults) reinforced the misconception that children experienced less pain, instead of raising the awareness that tools were not capturing the true experience of the child. For instance, Scott [29] in 1977 concluded that measuring pain in children with juvenile chronic polyarthritis was likely to be less useful than in adults, because scores were low, and correlated poorly with measures of disease severity.

Over time, efforts to depict the child's experience have led to the design and validation of several developmentally adapted instruments [37–42]. Assessment in pre-verbal [43,44] (newborns, infants, and toddlers) and non-verbal [5,45–50] (cognitively impaired) children has increasingly become the focus of clinical investigation. Optimal approaches in these patient populations, however, have yet to be clearly established.

Research on pain therapies in children has also evolved. In our informal search, we identified that before 1980, the majority of publications regarding opioids in children concerned toxicity and side effects (specifically regarding the effects of maternal drug addiction on the infant). Only 10% of publications referred to the management of procedural pain, and few addressed management of other types of pain. In the last decade, this relationship has been inverted. In the 1990's, just 20% of pain treatment papers focused on opioid-related toxicity, dealing primarily with nausea, vomiting and pruritus, instead of respiratory depression. In the same period, 40% of pediatric pain treatment papers examined procedural pain, and 30% dwelt on the treatment of other types of pain, mainly cancer. Surprisingly, most studies evaluating opioid side effects have been conducted on newborns and pre-term babies. Only one study was identified that prospectively evaluated morphine side effects in older children [51].

Research methods around the study of pain have also improved. RCT's regarding pain treatments now comprise about 35% of the publications on pediatric pain, as compared to 15% before 1990. The majority of the RCTs address post-surgical analgesia. Fifteen percent concern procedure-related pain, and four percent treatment of sickle cell-related pain. No RCTs evaluating pain related to cancer or other LLCs were found.

Despite advancements in pain as a science, translation into more adequate pain management has yet to occur [52–57]. The reasons for this discrepancy are not well understood. Limitations in nurses and physicians' knowledge [58,59] and attitudes [60–62] towards evaluation and treatment, and the scarcity of widespread standardized treatment guidelines [63] and policies hinders incorporation of research findings into practice. These factors vary widely across countries and regions. In some countries, as many as 90% of physicians surveyed are prepared to provide adequate analgesia [64], while in others, more than 60% do not know methods for pain evaluation, and less than half admit to using opioids [65,66]. Regulatory issues affecting opioid availability and high costs also obstruct progress, especially in developing countries [67, 68]. Introducing change into clinical practice is complex, and driven by scientific, social, and cultural forces [69]. A broader understanding of the barriers to providing adequate pain relief is needed, and international educational and research collaborations should take place, to reduce inequalities in pain management.

Physical symptoms other than pain

Little is known about other symptoms affecting children at the end of life. Studies are mainly retrospective and descriptive in nature. When reported, data about treatment success is collected from caregiver reports and medical charts, rather than with standardized assessment tools, which are scarce [70–78]. However, it has been reported that children with LLC's frequently suffer high distress from more than one symptom [79, 80]. Limited studies have highlighted the prevalence of fatigue [81–84], dyspnea [85], and other symptoms in children with cancer [79,86], chemotherapy-induced [87–91] and postsurgical [92–95] emesis, as well as cholestatic [96] and opioid-induced [97] pruritus.

The Memorial Symptom Assessment Scale (MSAS) is the only multi-symptom scale developed for children [79,86]. MSAS has two versions, one for children aged 10–18 and the other for children aged 7–12 (with 26 and 8 items respectively). It was adapted from the adult MSAS scale, and validated in children receiving cancer treatment. A parental form is now undergoing validation. In addition, several specific symptom scales for fatigue, dyspnea, and cough are currently under investigation [98–102].

Symptom control is an under-researched area. To date, there have been no intervention trials in children with advanced illness, concerning the treatment of non-pain symptoms. Given the fact that children with advanced illness experience unrelieved distress, a better understanding of the pathophysiology, measurement, and treatment of symptoms is imperative.

Quality of life

Thus far, investigation about Quality of Life (QoL) in children has been focused on developing and validating both generic and disease-specific tools. Several reviews have summarized the characteristics of these instruments [103–105].

Children judge their QoL based on the world they know. Their interpretations and experience differ from the adult perspective. Therefore, the direct adaptation of adult tools is not recommended [103]. Instead, instrument developers should collect information directly from children, to identify the domains that are relevant to the different developmental stages. Initially, most QoL instruments were exclusively based on parental reports, especially for children less than 8 years old [106–108]. However, as evidence showed that children were able to reflect effectively about their lives and report on their quality of life [104,109], many instruments have been updated, and now include self-reports from younger children [110–113]. Current research is now focusing on developing tools for very young children, including newborns and infants, and for children with cognitive impairment [112,114–118].

Generic instruments measure QoL as a whole, while disease-specific ones include domains that are particular to a given condition. It is currently recommended that generic and disease-specific tools be used in combination [103]. This allows investigators to ascertain an overall perspective, compare across conditions, and also evaluate the direct impact of the illness [119,120]. Modular QoL tools that contain both generic and disease-specific modules, such as the Pediatric Quality of Life Inventory (PedsQL™) developed by Varni and collaborators [121], are felt to be optimal, although further evaluation would help to validate this approach.

There is no data addressing the impact of life-threatening illness on QoL scores in children. Adults close to death have been found to give more relevance to issues such as meaningfulness and comfort, over physical functioning or social interaction [122]. It is reasonable to presume that children will also value QoL differently when they are ill. More systematic investigations are needed to define which QoL domains become relevant during advanced illness, and if they differ from those of healthier children. This would have important implications, because most of the currently available instruments assume that all individuals define QoL in the same manner and that this conception is constant over time. If illness changes one's values, there is a high risk that these tools will not truly capture QoL. For example, a patient may be bed bound but satisfied with life as a whole, yet her QoL score will be low. Tools that measure the concept from an individual perspective may be more appropriate [122,123].

Individualized QoL instruments that have been validated in adult palliative care populations are the Schedule of the Evaluation of Individual Quality of Life (SEIQoL) [124–126] and the Patient Generated Index (PGI) [127,128]. A similar pediatric tool, the Exeter QoL Scale (Exqol) [129], is still in its validation phase. The underlying theory of Exqol is that QoL is related to the gap between one's expectations and one's reality, and a larger gap corresponds to worse QoL [130]. The tool tries to measure such gaps by using short vignettes, and asking children to rate 'how much they think they are like those kids,' and 'how much they would like to be like them' [129]. Further investigation is needed to define the properties and applications of these instruments in both clinical and research settings. Because of the unique ability to capture individual perspectives, this type of tool seems promising.

The impact of integrating QoL measurement into routine clinical care is currently being investigated in adults with cancer. Preliminary data suggests that systematic collection of QoL data increases patient–provider discussions about QoL issues [131,132], and directly improves patient's QoL [133]. Using QoL assessment as a research tool to assess effectiveness of palliative care interventions, for example, is increasingly encouraged, yet interpretation of results is not straightforward. RCTs evaluating palliative care interventions have failed to demonstrate a significant effect on QoL [123,134]. Whether this means that there is no true effect, or that there is a problem with how the outcome is defined and measured, remains to be determined.

As more valid instruments become available for children, it is foreseeable that many of these issues will soon be better understood.

Evaluation of end-of-life care

To date, evaluation of pediatric palliative care services has been based on a retrospective approach [80,85,135–141], and there have been no intervention trials.

Early studies [85,135–137] served as important milestones in raising awareness about the fact that at least half of the children with advanced diseases had symptoms that require medical treatment. However, their small sample sizes, the use of secondary data sources (clinical records) [85,136,137], and the lack of well-defined populations [135] made the results unreliable and hardly generalizable. Subsequent efforts focused on describing the 'state of the art' of end-of-life care delivered by palliative care programs [140,142] and pediatric centers [80,139,141,143,144]. Their results indicate that many children still suffer from unrelieved symptoms [80,144], and receive highly invasive treatment, with little attention paid to symptom management in their last days of life [139,143].

These findings are most notable when recognizing that pain relief is possible in at least 81% of the children [142], with adequate assessment and treatment. As a result of using larger sample sizes, primary data (parent surveys) in addition to secondary data, and more clearly defined populations, these studies have better validity. Nevertheless, the lack of comparison groups limits conclusions about the impact of offering palliative care services.

The best ways to deliver palliative care have yet to be defined. A complementary model where palliative- and disease-oriented strategies coexist throughout treatment is now recommended [23,145–147]. Yet, integration does not seem to come easy to either providers or families. For example, McCallum et al [139], in their description of end of life care of 72 children whose death was expected, reported that in 70% of the cases, DNR decisions took place only 1 day or hours before the death. Wolfe et al. [148] reported that early recognition of incurability by both parents and physicians led to a significantly earlier introduction of palliative strategies, such as hospice, "do-not-resuscitate" orders, and less use of cancer-directed therapy during the last month of life, suggesting that physician–parent communication strongly influences the type of care delivered. However, the same study indicated that acknowledging that cure is unlikely is also an important factor, which allows for integration of palliative oriented strategies into the plan of care. These findings seem to show that disease- and palliative-oriented strategies are still viewed as mutually exclusive options. Whether this belief is predominantly held by providers, parents, or both still needs to be elucidated, in order to delineate ways of integrating palliative treatments into care.

There is now evidence that both hospital- and community-based services are needed [149–151]. How to best provide these services in an integrated way is still unclear. Pierucci and colleagues [152] were among the first to examine the impact of a pediatric palliative care consult service on the type of care delivered. Through a retrospective case-control study in a neonatal intensive care unit (NICU), they showed that a significantly smaller proportion of infants died in the neonatal or pediatric intensive care unit when a palliative care consult was obtained (68% vs. 97%). Infants of families that received consultations had fewer days in the intensive care units, and less invasive diagnostic and treatment procedures; these families were more frequently referred to chaplains and social services than families not receiving palliative care consultations. The authors concluded that palliative care consultation might enhance end-of-life care for newborns. A cause–effect relationship, however, cannot be inferred: other physician, family, and infant factors may have led to both the palliative care consult and the outcomes achieved. The findings do

suggest that some aspects of care that may affect the child and family's experience are subject to modification.

Recent studies have undoubtedly begun to enlighten the field of pediatric palliative care. The heterogeneity in the definitions and measurement of outcomes, as well as their retrospective nature, however, continue to make findings difficult to interpret, compare, and generalize. Furthermore, large areas remain to be described to any extent. There are virtually no published studies examining the psychological and spiritual needs of children with advanced illness, and their families. Nor are there reports of the differing needs of children and families with diverse backgrounds, including cultural and ethnic differences. Thus, good descriptive multicentered studies are still necessary to establish the "natural history" of advanced diseases, and generate population data that would be useful to design and conduct larger interventional studies. Nevertheless, the already reported high levels of distress make it ethically questionable to conduct only descriptive studies. The data are sufficiently compelling to concurrently develop and pilot interventions aimed at improving the experience of children with advanced illness, and their families.

The experience of palliative care research in adults

Overall, there has been considerably more research regarding adults with advanced illness. The body of literature has grown markedly. The term palliative care was introduced as a Medline heading in 1996, and a Cochrane Group (the Pain, Palliative Care and Supportive Care—PaPaS—Group) was established in 1998 to summarize the available evidence. At least nine journals are now dedicated to palliative care, and the number of clinical trials has also increased over time [153]. RCT's have been used to evaluate interventions related to symptom control, such as pain [154–161], breathlessness [162–170], or cachexia–anorexia [171–176], psychosocial concerns, and decision-making [177–190]. In addition, different palliative care services such as home, hospice, and hospital-based teams, and the coordination of care have also been evaluated, using experimental designs [191–198].

The expansion of adult palliative care research is probably a consequence of multiple forces. Research results, as well as advocacy from consumer and health organizations, such as the World Health Organization (WHO), the National Institute of Clinical Excellence in the United Kingdom, or the Institute of Medicine in the United States, have heightened awareness about patients' unmet needs. As a consequence, palliative care is now a standard of care in many countries. This, in turn, has made more funding available for clinical and research purposes. Additionally, some barriers to research, as described below, are being slowly ameliorated; the development of validated measurement tools [199–201], for example, provides a means of standardizing collection of subjective outcomes, and therefore increases the validity, and thus feasibility, of RCT's. Finally, the current awareness about the many things that can be done to relieve suffering has likely altered health care providers' and Investigation Review Boards' (IRBs') impressions about conducting research in this population. The potential to relieve patient and families' burdens may facilitate the acceptance of research.

One must recognize, however, that more research does not necessarily mean better research. In fact, many of the systematic reviews of symptom control and service delivery effectiveness have been unable to draw strong recommendations [202–212]. This is likely a result of the nature of the subject matter and the marginal quality of reporting [153, 206]. Small numbers of studies for each topic [213–215], limited sample sizes [207], high drop-out rates, few controlled studies [216–218], and insufficiently defined interventions render studies of low validity. In addition, heterogeneity among publications regarding designs, populations, measurement tools, and outcomes also makes the pooling of results challenging [202, 219]. Such problems are potentially unavoidable, but must be acknowledged and minimized, as we discuss in the sections to follow.

Despite the increase in number and sample size seen over time, the quality of reporting in palliative care RCTs has not improved significantly [153]. An analysis of RCTs published before and after the CONSORT statement [220] (CONsolidated Standards Of Reporting Clinical Trials—recommendations to improve the quality of reporting of clinical trials) up to the year 2000, found that more than 70% of the trials were not truly randomized, enrolled less than a 100 subjects, and did not report a power calculation or use intention to treat analysis. Blinding, one of the most important ways of avoiding bias, was used more frequently, yet its use did not increase consistently over time. Most of the leading medical journals now require that authors comply with the CONSORT statement as a means of assuring transparency. A similar initiative to standardize non-RCT health services research reports, the TREND statement (Transparent Reporting of Evaluations with Non-randomized Designs), was proposed early in 2004 [221]. The quality of reporting is an important aspect to research that is usually overlooked, and one that can be improved. Whatever the barriers to research, a thorough report allows the reader to understand the study, assess its validity, and determine which findings are applicable to his or her clinical practice.

Although there is room for improvement, much has been accomplished in the first 40 years of palliative care. Efforts such as the ones supported by the National Institute of Clinical Excellence (NICE) in the United Kingdom, the Institute of Medicine in the United States, or the Palliative Care Association of Australia are on their way to further improve the care of adults with advanced illness. These have helped to pull together the available evidence, identify gaps and drawbacks, and set goals for future research. From a pediatric perspective, we should draw from these experiences and strive to find our own well-connected pathway to advance the care of children.

Barriers to pediatric palliative care research

If the need for research in pediatric palliative care is so evident, then why has it not developed in advance of, or in concert with patient care efforts? The answer, like the subject matter, is not straightforward. Research in this relatively new discipline is subject to the hazards of all clinical investigation. As significant, however, are the additional barriers imposed by the constraints of studying the amalgam of two vulnerable populations, patients at the end-of-life who are children.

Disease and research in children are rare entities

Relative to adult fields, there are few clinical trials throughout all areas of pediatrics [222,223], reflecting, among other issues, the conundrum of good health. Therapeutic sepsis trials, for example, must account for an incidence as low as 0.5 cases per 1000 population per year, with hospital mortality of less than 10% [224], compared to sepsis in adults, where the incidence is greater than 5 cases per 1000 population per year, and mortality reaches nearly 40% [225]. Relative risk reduction of any therapy has a different connotation, given the differing numbers and outcomes. In our roles as care providers, we are fortunate that the incidence of significant illness in children is low. However, as investigators committed to advancing the field of pediatric palliative care, we are ironically unfortunate that the incidence is low.

The challenges of small population studies are further exacerbated when treating children with life-threatening conditions. The Association for Children with Life-Threatening or Terminal Conditions and their Families (ACT) and the Royal College of Paediatrics and Child Health (RCPCH) estimated an annual prevalence of 12/10,000 children, and a mortality rate of 1.5–1.9/10,000 (40% from cancer, 20% from heart disease, and 40% from other LLCs) [146]. As a consequence of this epidemiology, two competing concepts emerge. Issues surrounding death are amplified, while the resources allocated to address them are less plentiful.

Researchers find it difficult to accrue sufficient sample sizes within single care systems, and the logistical obstacles of multicentered trials are not always easily overcome. Dropout rates intrinsic to such a vulnerable, and mortal, population also impact study design. Pharmaceutical industries are less willing to invest in investigation in diseases with small numbers of patients, because the expected return is low [226]. Concerns about liability and malpractice, proper justification, assessment of benefit relative to risk, ability to consent, compensation, and simply, the selection of subjects [227], hinder the growth of pediatric research.

Developmental concerns

Pragmatic barriers and others have promoted a dependence upon adult resources, research, and care experiences. Pediatric practitioners worldwide, however, recognize the limitations and fallacies of extrapolating and adopting such practices. Research in adult palliative care is not a panacea, and the aims of pediatric palliative care may be quite different. Cognitive, psychosocial, and physiologic development affects potential interventions as well as outcome measurement [228–230]. Pain symptoms, as previously noted, are an excellent example. Assessment and treatment depend greatly upon interpretation and communication about the nature and intensity of the pain. Surrogate measures must be used in pre-verbal or non-verbal children. Subsequent treatment options may be limited, due to a smaller armamentarium of pharmacologic agents, narrower therapeutic ranges, and differences in adjuvant therapies. Research in pediatric palliative care must strive to delineate both the similarities and differences between adults and children, with respect to epidemiology, physiology, and psychosocial needs, to determine optimal management strategies.

Heterogeneity among the children

The illnesses contributing to childhood death are immensely diverse. In the United States, for example, cancer and cardiac disease are among the leading causes of non-accidental death in childhood, yet they only account for 4 and 2% of deaths, respectively [147]. With the expansion of clinical pediatric palliative care services come greater heterogeneity in disease states, and a range of practical care issues, which represent considerable and important barriers to practitioners and researchers. Assumptions that death and dying experiences vary between, and even within, subspecialty populations, must consequently be refuted, or be accounted for in study design, recruitment, and interpretation. Advanced pediatric malignancies and the sequelae of therapy, for example, produce an array of symptoms and palliative care needs, depending upon the nature of the underlying condition. Children with

brain tumors are not the same as those with other solid organ tumors, and are, again, different from those with leukemia. It follows that the acute trauma victim, or the child with a chronic neurodegenerative disorder, presumably also has different EOL care needs. Bedside palliative care is tailored to the individual patient and family [231,232], while research interventions are, by nature, less accommodating. Thus, research protocols in pediatric palliative care are challenged to conform to a range of needs, or restrict their focus and address a narrow spectrum of patient needs. Either approach will require a lengthy enrollment period, to attain statistically significant numbers and maximize potential generalizability of the study findings.

Additionally, heterogeneity is not confined to the patient characteristics alone. Pediatric palliative care providers and researchers acknowledge the value of a comprehensive approach to patient care. Thus, developmentally appropriate strategies are devised in the context of the family unit. Is this an only child? Is there concordance between family members regarding the experience of the child? The question arises: who should we study, the patient, parents, and/or siblings? Surrogates for children do not always accurately reflect the condition of the child in question [233], yet this may be the only means available to make assessments.

Heterogeneity among providers

The diversity among children with life-threatening conditions has led to a great diversity in pediatric palliative care providers. The parallel development of services by pediatric oncologists, cardiologists, critical care physicians, ethicists, nurses, social workers and chaplains have met the short-term needs of their patients, but have not fully promoted the long-term development of pediatric palliative care. Explicit or implicit differences between disciplines, institutions, and academic versus community-based programs have promoted a "closed door" phenomenon. Providers from a given subspecialty, and even within a specific care unit, may perceive that they alone understand the needs of the patients and families. For clinical investigators, this perspective limits access to patients and resources, while for the patient, this fragmentation is not necessarily commensurate with optimal care. Tradition and experience are to be respected, but measured hubris will better serve children and their families.

When philosophical differences are resolved, collaborative efforts may still be hampered by differences in care settings, staff composition, and diverse care delivery systems. Comparison or cohorting of patients in the hospice, long-term care facilities, or the variety of acute hospital units may not be valid. Expansion from multidisciplinary to multicenter to multinational collaborations will require standardized nomenclature, data collection methods, and interpretation/data analysis schemes. Researchers will also need to recognize additional confounders, such as language, religion and cultural difference, as well as institutional and governing body regulations.

Temporal boundaries—timing is everything

Regardless of condition, provider differences, resource limitations, and other factors, timing, as a function of disease progression and patient and family receptivity, is a substantial barrier to pediatric palliative care programs and research. The traditional medical model focuses on cure of the underlying illness. Discussions of QoL and palliative, 'comfort-centered' care are thought to be heretical and counter-productive, until all other treatment options have been exhausted.

Prognostic uncertainty limits the delivery of pediatric palliative care and the design, enrollment, and implementation of research studies. Prospective identification of "non-responders" is very difficult. Acute care providers rely upon prediction models, such as the Pediatric Risk of Mortality (PRISM) Score [234,235] or Paediatric Index of Mortality (PIM) [236,237], to identify patients with high likelihood of death. Other subspecialties utilize cell counts, markers of tumor burden, pulmonary function tests, and other clinical indices to help guide the transition to palliation. These are helpful tools when considering a population of patients, but for the individual patient, they provide wide margins of error, and little insight into the exact time or circumstances around death. Reliance on prognostic indices leaves open the possibility that patients who might benefit from palliative care interventions may be excluded [231], however, clinical estimates of life expectancy are often inaccurate [238]. Wolfe and colleagues also found that appreciation of the transition toward palliation differs between parents and physicians [148]. This discrepancy adds to the complexity of identifying a uniform patient population.

High attrition rates

Participant attrition due to death, change in symptom status, and ability or willingness to complete study requirements is inherent to research in palliative care [196]. Studies in adult patients report high levels of attrition (35–80%) [232]. Although such "drop-out," may not be avoidable in this population, the danger of untimely loss of patients or data may significantly compromise study findings. The intent and results of research will vary, depending upon the stage of the disease process and pace of deterioration. Ultimately, pediatric palliative care research is contingent upon subject willingness to participate and the timing of the intervention, relative to disease progression or death.

Lack of appropriate outcome measures

The scope of pediatric palliative care is very broad. Ostensibly, infinite opportunities exist for intervention and study. Developing testable hypotheses and designing research protocols, however, require valid outcomes measures. Survival rates represent an oxymoron in pediatric palliative care, and biologic markers likely have little relevance to our patients. Thus, we focus on symptom control, functional capacity, and general well-being, which are values shared throughout pediatrics [87,199].

Pediatric palliative care is a patient and family-oriented discipline. Investigators must determine what is uniquely important to the population, and develop tools to gauge suffering and satisfaction. The current armamentarium of symptom indices and QoL instruments are useful, but may not be valid or responsive to change at the end-of-life. Table 40.1 outlines several of the instruments available to investigators, and highlights some of the advancements in the measurement of symptoms and health related QoL in children. We selected them based on their psychometric performance, but also tried to include examples of instruments that were developed for, or adapted to, languages other than English. Unfortunately, none of these were developed or validated in children with advanced illness, and therefore, it is not possible at this point to make any recommendation regarding their use in the palliative care setting.

Lack of funding

Clinical programs and researchers all vie for financial support. The number of potential funding sources and the amounts allocated depend upon many factors, including the numbers of people effected, potential extrapolation to other populations, possible financial gains for private sources, and the intangible perception of relevance and importance by the general public, institutions, and policy-makers. By these criteria, pediatric palliative care researchers are at a distinct disadvantage. Despite the critical need and tragic circumstances, childhood end-of-life issues are of relatively low incidence; they have limited application to other patients, and there is minimal direct financial incentive or potential for return. Again, the emphasis on 'cure' is also a substantial barrier in the procurement of research and clinical funding. Pediatric palliative care draws at heartstrings, but not at purse strings.

Ethical barriers

Potentially the greatest barriers to effective research in pediatric palliative care are the intangibles of emotion, spirituality, and ethics. The death of a child is truly tragic. During the dying process, the child, the family, and the care providers may experience anxiety, depression, and the entire spectrum of emotions. Spiritual beliefs may be an invaluable source of

Table 40.1 Examples of available instruments for use in pediatric palliative care

Type of tool	Applicability	Examples*
Generic Quality of Life (QoL) Instruments	Comparison of general QoL across different populations (e.g. cancer vs. cystic fibroses, useful for assessing a palliative care intervention applied to a wide array of conditions)	Pediatric Quality of Life Inventory (PedsQL 4.0)[1] Child Health Questionnaire[2] Quality of Life measure for children aged 3–8 years (TedQL)[3] TNO AZL Children's Quality of Life questionnaire (TACQOL)[4]/(TAPQOL for preschool children)[5] Pictured Child's Quality of Life Self Questionnaire (AUQUEI)[6] Kidscreen[7] KINDL[8]
Disease-Specific QoL Instruments	Comparison of QoL within a given condition (e.g. cancer patients with advanced disease vs. those in active treatment, CF children with advanced lung disease vs. those with moderate disease)	PedsQL 3.0 Cancer[9] Cystic Fibrosis Questionnaire[10] Life Satisfaction Index for Adolescents with Neuromuscular Disorders
Domain Specific Tools	Applicable when research question refers to a specific domain of the illness experience (symptoms, psychological distress, parental distress, etc)	**Unidimensional** (measure only 1 dimension of the domain) Intensity Pain Scales[11] (e.g. Faces Pain Scales, Visual Analog Scales, Numerical Rating Scales, Colorimetric Pain Scales)

* None of the tools mentioned here have been specifically validated in pediatric palliative care populations.

[1] Varni, J.W., Seid, M., and Kurtin, P.S. PedsQL 4.0: Reliability and validity of the Pediatric Quality of Life Inventory version 4.0 generic core scales in healthy and patient populations. *Med Care* 2001;39(8):800–12.

[2] Landgraf, J.M., Measuring health-related quality of life in pediatric oncology patients: A brief commentary on the state of the art of measurement and application (discussion). *Int J Cancer Suppl* 1999;12:147–50.

[3] Lawford, J., Volavka, N., and Eiser, C. A generic measure of Quality of Life for children aged 3–8 years: Results of two preliminary studies. *Pediatr Rehabil* 2001;4(4):197–207.

[4] Vogels, T. et al. Measuring health-related quality of life in children: The development of the TACQOL parent form. *Qual Life Res* 1998;7(5):457–65.

[5] Fekkes, M. et al. Development and psychometric evaluation of the TAPQOL: A health-related quality of life instrument for 1–5-year-old children. *Qual Life Res* 2000;9(8):961–72.

[6] Manificat, S. et al. [Evaluation of the quality of life in pediatrics: How to collect the point of view of children]. *Arch Pediatr* 1997;4(12):1238–46.

[7] Herdman, M. et al. Expert consensus in the development of a European health-related quality of life measure for children and adolescents: A Delphi study. *Acta Paediatr* 2002;91(12):1385–90.

[8] Ravens-Sieberer, U. and Bullinger, M. Assessing health-related quality of life in chronically ill children with the German KINDL: First psychometric and content analytical results. *Qual Life Res* 1998;7(5):399–407.

[9] Varni, J.W., et al. The Pediatric Cancer Quality of Life Inventory-32 (PCQL-32). II. Feasibility and range of measurement. *J Behav Med* 1999;22(4):397–406.

[10] Modi, A.C. and Quittner, A.L. Validation of a disease-specific measure of health-related quality of life for children with cystic fibrosis. *J Pediatr Psychol* 2003;28(8):535–45.

[11] Hain, R.D. Pain scales in children: A review. *Palliat Med* 1997;11(5):341–50.

Table 40.1 (Continued)

Type of tool	Applicability	Examples

Domain Specific Tools	Generic or disease-specific tools may not be able to detect differences regarding specific domains (their goal is to capture the broader picture)	**Multidimensional** (measure >1 dimension of the domain)
		Specific Symptom Scales
		    Pain Scales (e.g. Adolescent Pain Tool[12], McGill Pain Questionnaire for children[13])
		    Fatigue Scales (e.g. Multidimensional Fatigue Scale[14], Fatigue in Cancer[15]
		    Rhodes Adapted Vomiting Score[16]
		    Multiple Symptom Scales (e.g. Memorial Symptom Assessment Scale—MSAS-10–18[17] and 7–12[18])
		Parental Distress
		    General Health Questionnaire[19,20]
		    Kessler-6[21]
		    Impact on Family Scale[22]
		    Pediatric Inventory for Parents[23]
		    General Functioning Scale of the McMaster Family Instrument[24]

[12] Wilkie, D.J, et al. Measuring pain quality: validity and reliability of children's and adolescents' pain language. *Pain* 1990;41(2):151–9.

[13] Abu-Saad, H.H., E. Kroonen, and Halfens, R. On the development of a multidimensional Dutch pain assessment tool for children. *Pain* 1990;43(2):p. 249–56.

[14] Varni, J.W. et al. The PedsQL in pediatric cancer: Reliability and validity of the Pediatric Quality of Life Inventory Generic Core Scales, Multidimensional Fatigue Scale, and Cancer Module. *Cancer* 2002;94(7): 2090–106.

[15] Hockenberry, M.J. et al. Three instruments to assess fatigue in children with cancer: The child, parent and staff perspectives, *J Pain Symptom Manage* 2003;25(4):319–28.

[16] Lo, L.H. and Hayman, L.L. Parents associated with children in measuring acute and delayed nausea and vomiting. *Nurs Health Sci* 1999;1(3): p. 155–61.

[17] Collins, J.J. et al. The measurement of symptoms in children with cancer. J Pain Symptom Manage 2000;19(5):363–77.

[18] Collins, J.J. et al. The measurement of symptoms in young children with cancer: The validation of the Memorial Symptom Assessment Scale in children aged 7–12. *J Pain Symptom Manage* 2002;23(1):10–6.

[19] Banks, M.H. Validation of the General Health Questionnaire in a young community sample. *Psychol Med* 1983;13(2):349–53.

[20] Dockerty, J.D. et al. Impact of childhood cancer on the mental health of parents. *Med Pediatr Oncol*, 2000;35(5):475–83.

[21] Kessler, R.C., et al. Short screening scales to monitor population prevalences and trends in non-specific psychological distress. *Psychol Med* 2002;32(6):959–76.

[22] Stein, R.E. and D.J. Jessop, The impact on family scale revisited: Further psychometric data, *J Dev Behav Pediatr* 2003;24(1):9–16.

[23] Streisand, R. et al. Childhood illness-related parenting stress: The pediatric inventory for parents, *J Pediatr Psychol* 2001;26(3);155–62.

[24] Stevenson-Hinde, J, and Akister, J. The McMaster Model of Family Functioning: Observer and parental ratings in a nonclinical sample. *Fam Process* 1995;34(3):337–47.

buoyancy, but simultaneously, may be called into question when reflecting on the meaning of death in childhood. In a sense, everyone involved is vulnerable. Grieving parents and family may be in conflict amongst themselves, and have limited decision-making capacity, due to the circumstances. Medical care providers are not impervious, and may look to alternative means to provide for the child and his or her family, as they question their own potency at providing 'cure.' The relationship between physician and family may also not allow either side to contradict the requests or suggestions of the other. And, most importantly, as a minor and due to the nature and stage of his or her disease state, the child-patient, by definition, is susceptible to influences from all other parties.

Vulnerability is at the core of ethical conflicts in pediatric palliative care research. A paternalistic perspective would argue against all interventions, suggesting that any intrusion at the end of life places an undue burden, and that any degree of harm may be amplified. The lack of a second opportunity imposes professional biases, making some reluctant to use novel or unfamiliar methods, and potentially hindering quality research [231]. A more liberal vantage might suggest that dying children and their families are entitled to the potential rewards of research, no matter how small. Weighing risks and benefits is the challenge for researchers in study design and for research committees in their support of such research.

Over a half-century of reflection, discussion, and commitment has led to the development and modification of several international codes of conduct surrounding research on human subjects [230]. Beginning with the Nuremberg Code in 1947 [239], the concepts of informed consent and minimal risk, among others, were emphasized. Later, modifications to the Declaration of Helsinki [239] outlined the need for special accommodations when including children as research subjects. Pediatric investigators are held to the same, if not higher, standards as adult researchers. They must simultaneously seek assent from the minor child, as well as informed permission from the parent or guardian. In the United States, protection has been further codified in the Belmont Report [240, 241], and subsequently, the Code of Federal Regulations-45 CFR 46, which state that the potential risk to the child subject must be justified by the potential benefit, and that this balance be at least as favorable as available alternative interventions or their omission. Non-therapeutic trials are permissible in children, assuming that the research poses *no greater than minimal risk* to the subject.

Anecdotal reports suggest that IRB's have a tendency to be overly protective of children receiving palliative care services. Rather than allowing patients and their families to decide for themselves, IRB's have made decisions intended to protect them. In the senior author's study of parents of children who died of cancer, for example, we sought physician permission to contact bereaved parents. A letter of invitation was mailed, with an enclosed *opt-out* postcard. If the postcard was not received within two weeks of the mailing, the parents were called directly to ask about their willingness to participate. This strategy resulted in a 72% response rate. When the study was extended to a second institution, their IRB required that the letter of invitation contain an *opt-in* postcard. This more active step on the part of parents likely contributed to the lower 48% response rate in this second phase. The vast majority of parents who participated at both institutions expressed gratitude for having been invited to "tell their stories." Thus, we believe that the greater stringency of an active *opt-in* requirement imposed an unnecessary barrier to research, shifting the perception of risk–benefit and depriving families of the opportunity to 'tell their stories.'

Some might argue that research at the end of life is by definition "non-therapeutic." Approaching a family at a time of crisis is burden enough to outweigh any potential benefits of research. Families may grant permission out of allegiance to care providers, or because of a sense of altruism, encouraged by assurances that research may benefit other children in similar circumstances. Yet, recent discoveries that children experience undue suffering at the end of life, and that communication with providers is suboptimal, suggest that systematic research is essential to attain much needed improvements. Pediatric palliative care researchers must obviously abide by all accepted standards and regulations, but children who may not survive their illnesses are equally deserving of research aimed at helping them live better. Further, altruism is certainly considered acceptable when the focus of the trial is to discover new disease-directed therapies, such as phase I chemotherapy trials. Altruism should, in turn, be considered an acceptable goal among children with advanced illness, and may be one way that the child and parents find meaning in illness.

Opportunities for improvement

However numerous the barriers described, they should not inhibit research. Nor should they be an excuse for low-quality studies. Rather, being aware of the barriers should assist researchers in designing feasible but rigorous investigations. A combination of flexibility and creativity, as well as drawing experience from related fields is needed to overcome the hurdles.

In this section, we will reflect on the barriers discussed above, and suggest possible solutions based upon established research methods and experiences. Table 40.2 highlights some of this content. An exhaustive methodological discussion is beyond the scope of the chapter, and therefore, we will identify

Table 40.2 Barriers to pediatric palliative care research

Barriers	Consequences	Opportunities for improvement

Small numbers	Low precision in the results
	Low power to detect small or moderate effects
	Causal inference is challenged because of poor ability to control for confounders or modifiers.
	Generalizability is limited
	"Orphan" population
	Lack of advocacy and funding
		Qualitative study design
		Increase study efficiency
		  N-of-1 trials
		  Cross-over RCT
		  Withdrawal designs
		  Data-dependent designs (e.g. sequential, adaptive designs)
		Increase sample size
		  Development of research networks

Developmental concerns	Cannot readily extrapolate from adult data Increases complexity in protocol design Threatens strength of study results	Conduct primary studies in children Studies may have to include family outcomes Design of developmentally appropriate tools

Heterogeneity
  Subjects
  Providers
  Settings
	Decreased study power
	Threatens study generalizability
	Increases complexity in protocol design
		Stratify subjects by "palliative" variables (e.g. models of care, symptom staging systems, age)
		Control variability in the design: randomization, crossover

Prognostic uncertainty	Difficulty in identifying research subjects Selection bias (under-enrollment or over-enrollment)	Use multiple identification strategies (electronic databases, meetings with health care providers) Use of "inclusion promoting" vocabulary in recruitment material
High attrition	Limited sample sizes Decreased study power Selection bias (e.g. the "healthier patients" remain in the study)	Design: Short evaluation periods (e.g. pharmacological interventions), early patient recruitment (e.g. program evaluation) Analysis: Intention-to-treat analysis, estimation of causal effects
Individualized nature of palliative care interventions	Difficulties in evaluation Hard to clearly outline interventions Problems to assess effectiveness	Pilot potential interventions prior to larger scale RCTs Thorough description of interventions
Lack of appropriate outcome measures	Threatens strength of study results Increases random error Measurement bias	Develop partnerships with families to define the relevant outcomes in the field Design and validation of tools that are developmentally adapted Include proxy reports
Poor pediatric palliative care network	Limits ability to conduct multicentered trials	Opportunity to generate a truly interdisciplinary network Need to standardize nomenclature, data collection methods, and data analysis schemes
Lack of funding	Limits possibility of research as a whole	Advocacy efforts aimed at identifying pediatric palliative care as a funding priority
Ethical issues and regulations		

Vulnerability	Children exposed to risky interventions
	Children and parents may feel obliged to accept research
	Health care providers limit patient referral
	IRB limits protocol approval
	Administrative and practical obstacles
		Obtain a valid assent/permission:
		  Use developmentally adapted and gentle assent/permission processes
		  Assess child willingness to participate
		  Separate the researchers' and provider's as much as much as possible
		Improve Risk/benefit ratio:
		  Minimize burden (flexible data collection methods)
		  Minimize risks
		  Evaluate and try maximizing lateral benefits of research
		  Specialized assistance to IRBs

Refusal to do research in subjects which do not have further opportunities for alternate care	Under-enrollment of patients in general Reluctance to randomize	Education of patients and providers Use modified randomized designs (e.g. data-dependent designs, withdrawal designs) or non-randomized designs

specific issues, and refer to more comprehensive texts when appropriate.

Dealing with small populations

As noted above, the lack of patients receiving pediatric palliative care services is fortunate from an epidemiologic perspective, but a conundrum from the research clinical vantage. We strive to provide care tailored to individual patient needs, while simultaneously attempting to glean information from this population as a whole. Using innovative strategies from both qualitative and quantitative research methodologies may help bridge the gap between poignant, but isolated, case reports and an evidence-based practice.

Qualitative methods are being used with increasing frequency in palliative care research, and often involve smaller numbers of subjects. Such studies can be used to explore complex phenomena in depth, such as personal experiences, views, thoughts, hopes, motives, and attitudes. A recent review of the palliative care literature identified 138 qualitative research papers published between 1990 and 1999 [242]. Qualitative research comprises the systematic collection, organization, and interpretation of textual material derived from talk or observation [243]. This methodology has been the subject of scrutiny within the medical community, which has criticized its lack of generalizability and potential subjectivity. Criteria, checklists, standards of scientific rigor [243,244], and guidelines about how to read and interpret qualitative literature were developed by the Evidence-Based Medicine Working Group [245,246], in an effort to increase the acceptance and understanding of the scope, strengths, and limitations of this type of study. Qualitative studies are often hypothesis generating, provide preliminary data, help identify domains for further instrument development, and are often the precursor to the development of quantitative studies. Qualitative methods can also be used in combination with quantitative methods in order to provide larger insight into complex subjective phenomena, a method called triangulation [243, 244]. Given the degree of the unknown, and the extent of complexity of the field, greater use of qualitative research methods may be important to furthering pediatric palliative care research.

Quantitative study designs, whether for analytic or descriptive studies, depend upon the sample size. Measuring outcomes in only a few subjects leads to estimates with a large degree of variability, and therefore, a lack of precision [247]. Results obtained from small studies may not reflect the truth, but rather the role of chance, a Type I error (significance level). Sample size also relates to the size of the effect being studied, and the power[1] desired [248]. The larger the size of the effect (or difference), and the lower the power and precision we aim

for, the smaller the sample size that will be needed. Unfortunately, large effects are uncommon in clinical practice, and therefore, small studies usually have a substantial risk of having false negative results. That is, they fail to find a difference between interventions, when a true difference really exists (Type II error) [248,249]. On the other hand, drawing conclusions based on lower than acceptable levels of significance and/or power would be misleading.

Patients cannot be asked to enroll in a study that in the end will not achieve reliable results. Effect size cannot be modified, however, power and precision may be increased by modifying the design (e.g. reducing variability within the sample), or by increasing the sample size [250]. Designs that use patients as their own controls, such as crossover studies, or those that measure outcomes repeatedly, such as longitudinal studies and enriched RCTs, reduce variability and increase the power of the study. Longitudinal studies reduce random error, and are useful for studying changes over time, or the 'natural history' of a condition. High attrition rates in patients with advanced illness are problematic, but are not irreconcilable, as described in subsequent sections.

Increasing power in small studies may also be accomplished by changing the probability of assignment to a given arm during the course of the study (e.g. sequential or adaptive designs) or the use of some non-randomized designs (e.g. risk-based allocation). The use of decision models in the planning stages of small trials has been encouraged, as a means of helping to model the possible outcomes of a study and then focus on variables that are more sensitive to change, or of greater benefit to study [249].

Two types of crossover designs have been recommended for the palliative care setting, crossover RCTs and N-of-1 trials (see Table 40.3). The crossover RCT is especially useful when the condition is stable, and treatment effect starts readily after administration of the intervention, and ceases rapidly after withdrawal. Therefore, this design is ideal for evaluating symptomatic treatment in chronic conditions [251]. Advantages of crossover RCTs over parallel RCTs include a better ability to control for patient effects, which leads to increased power and smaller sample requirements. Their main limitations are the risks of carry-over and period effects, which should always be ruled out.

Crossover RCTs have been used for evaluating interventions aimed at relieving symptoms, such as neuropathic pain [252], xerostomia [253,254], bowel obstruction [255], opioid-induced sedation [256], and dyspnea [162,163,168], and, in children, mucositis [257–259] and chemotherapy-induced

---

[1] Power: the probability of finding a significant difference when a true difference exists. Power = 1 – Type II error (Pagano & Gavreaux, 2000).

Table 40.3 Cross-over designs

Types	Method and uses	Advantages	Disadvantages
Experimental (Investigator allocates the exposure or intervention)			
Crossover RCT	Patients receive both strategies consecutively. Order is randomly allocated. Wash out periods needed between the control and intervention stages. Best approach for studying cause-effect relationship, since all known and unknown factors are controlled by the patient serving as his/her own control **Useful** for assessment of *short-term* effects and/or *rapid onset* in stable conditions.	Compared to parallel RCTs: • Smaller sample size • >Statistical power • Better for causal inference • Provides data about satisfaction with intervention.	• Expensive • Risk of: • *Carry over effects* (treatment effects persist over the control period) • *Period effects* (changes related to the disease or "practice" rather than intervention) • Long studies result in greater attrition • Blinding difficult if side effects obvious.
N-of-1 trial (see box)	Multiple randomized crossover trials conducted in a single patient over time (ideally double blinded) with the goal of confirming or disproving the effectiveness of treatment in that patient. **Useful** to make treatment decisions for individuals when evidence not available or inappropriate for a particular patient (same conditions as crossover).	• Shorter • Tailored to the patient • Immediate clinical application.	• Identical to cross-over RCTs • Not able to generalize results unless aggregating multiple studies.
Observational (Investigator observes the events)			
Case-Crossover Study	A retrospective non-randomized crossover, or a case-control involving only cases. **Useful** when the exposure is transient and causes immediate change in the risk of an acute disease.	Short Not expensive Self-matching of cases eliminates the threat of control-selection bias and increases efficiency.	Not randomized.

emesis [89,260,261]. With the exception of studies regarding dyspnea and those conducted in children, all other studies failed to show any difference between control and intervention arms. One explanation is that the interventions were not better than placebo or standard practice, which is plausible given the controversies surrounding many of the interventions studied. However, the lack of effect also may be a reflection of the difficulties of studying a small, heterogeneous and very sick population. Compared to the "negative" studies, those that found differences between the treatments under investigation used a short time frame for evaluating outcomes (sometimes as short as minutes) [162,163,168], only included subgroups with high rates of the event under study [261] (e.g. patients receiving highly emetogenic chemotherapy, as opposed to all patients receiving chemotherapy), or those with more severe symptoms [163] (e.g. patients with moderate or severe dyspnea, and not all patients with dyspnea). These strategies resulted in more efficient recruitment and lower attrition rates, increasing the effective sample size and rendering more power to detect differences. It seems as though symptoms that are

clearly limited in duration, such as chemotherapy-induced emesis, or rapidly reversible, such as pain or dyspnea, are better suited for this design than subtle, insidious symptoms, like xerostomia. However, studies with 'positive' results had large effects, which highlights the fact that, although more powerful than parallel RCT's, crossover studies with small samples are still only able to detect differences between arms when the effect size is large. A large sample will always be needed, to confirm that a no detectable effect truly means *no* effect.

N-of-1 trials are conceptually crossover trials conducted in single subjects, and therefore, they share crossover RCTs' requirements and limitations (Table 40.3 and Box 40.1). N-of-1 originated as a decision-making tool, to be used when evidence was not available, or not applicable to a particular, patient. Its use has led to increased satisfaction with medical decisions for both patient and physicians [262]. N-of-1 trials are therefore an appealing tool for the palliative care setting where heterogeneity and lack of sound evidence are pervasive. Furthermore, in N-of-1 trials, intervention and outcomes are

Box 40.1 The N-of-1 trial

In comparing a novel therapy to standard of care, for example, both the investigator and patient are blinded. The patient is randomly assigned to one arm, and then, after a predetermined period of time, is switched to the other arm. This is called a treatment pair. Treatment pairs are continued until both physician and patient are convinced that they have either perceived a difference between the two arms, or are sure that there is no difference between the arms.[1] At that moment the blinding is broken, the results are evaluated using graphs and statistical tests, and a decision to continue or stop the treatment is made.[2] Although the trial can be stopped after any number of pairs, the greater the number of pairs, the stronger the results will be. Analysis after a single treatment pair may lead to false conclusions.

'Individualized cost-effectiveness analysis' may be also included as a useful decision aid when difference between treatments is not striking.[3] Guidelines and extensive descriptions of N-of-1 trials can be found elsewhere.[2,4] Their ultimate contribution is to provide clinicians and patients with a tool that helps make treatment decisions more evidence-based, particularly when evidence is scarce, or not applicable to the individual patient.[5]

[1] Guyatt, G. et al. Determining optimal therapy—randomized trials in individual patients. N Engl J Med 1986;314(14):889–92.

[2] Guyatt, G. et al. A clinician's guide for conducting randomized trials in individual patients. CMAJ 1988;139(6):497–503.

[3] Karnon, J. and Qizilbash, N. Economic evaluation alongside n-of-1 trials: Getting closer to the margin. Health Econ 2001;10(1):79–82.

[4] Cook, D.J. Randomized trials in single subjects: The N of 1 study. Psychopharmacol Bull 1996;32(3):363–7.

[5] Guyatt, G.H. et al. The n-of-1 randomized controlled trial: Clinical usefulness. Our three-year experience. Ann Intern Med 1990;112(4):293–9.

agreed upon by, and tailored to, the patient [263], an ideal of palliative care practice. As with crossovers, this type of study is better suited for chronic conditions that require treatment over a long period of time, and preferably, for rapidly reversible symptoms such as dyspnea [264]. Circumstances that require long washout periods are less likely to be feasible, as the patient may not make it through the study [265]. Many clinicians may be unfamiliar with this methodology, and establishing a coordinating center of n = 1 trials may help to disseminate its use in clinical practice [266].

The role of n-of-1 trials in clinical research needs better delineation. Their ability to measure effectiveness (treatment effect in 'real life'), as opposed to efficacy (treatment effect in a controlled environment), and to differentiate respondents from non-respondents, plus their direct clinical application, makes them attractive [251,267–269]. Yet, because these experiments are conducted in single patients, generalizability has been questioned. There have been both empirical [263, 270] and theoretical [268] proposals for combining multiple n-of-1 studies as a means of providing overall population measures of effectiveness. One way of combining a series of n-of-trials is to make all subjects in the series comply with the same requirements, as if they were joining a group trial. Subjects must meet strict inclusion criteria, and receive uniform treatment procedures, while measurements should be standardized. At study entry, patients are randomized to either enter N-of-1 trial or continue with standard care [271]. Alternatively, patients could be included in an open trial of a new treatment, and those that respond could then be allocated to the n-of-1 design [270]. Zucker et al. [268] proposed a meta-analytic technique to pool the results of published n-of-1 trials. As a means of validating this method, they compared the results obtained by pooling with those of parallel RCT's, and found that the results were similar in both direction and level of confidence. However, these designs are not more powerful than crossover RCT's, and thus, the limitations in finding small or moderate effects still apply.

Another crossover design that hasn't been used so far in palliative care is the case-crossover study, where historical cases serve as their own controls. The exposure rate preceding an event (case) is compared with the exposure rate at a previous but similar moment, when the event did not take place (control) [272]. This design was originally developed to study the role of transient triggers on the risk of acute events [273], such as exercise and myocardial infarction, and the design seems in fact to work better if the exposure is intermittent, the effect on risk immediate and transient, and the outcome abrupt. However, case-crossover studies have also been used to study gradual effects on risk and outcomes with insidious onsets. Some possible applications for palliative care may be to study symptom triggers [274,275], such as the effects of sleep, mood, or physical activity on the development of symptoms, or drug side-effects. Even though not randomized, a case-crossover study could provide valuable information about treatment effectiveness for symptoms that repeat over time with the same intensity, or symptoms that are stable.

The enriched RCT design proposed by Honkanen et al. [276], a three-stage parallel RCT which assesses efficacy three times, theoretically allows for a 20 to 60% sample size reduction, compared to traditional RCTs. This design consists of an initial parallel RCT (stage I), followed by a randomized withdrawal phase for patients who respond to investigational therapy; respondents are randomly assigned to withdraw from or continue the therapy (stage II). At the same time, patients who do not respond to placebo are started on investigational therapy, and entered into a randomized withdrawal phase if they respond (stage III). Similar to crossover studies, the three stage clinical trial requires conditions to be chronic, or at least persist long enough for the patient to advance through the different study stages. Carry-over effects should also be ruled out, but there is less of a need for patients to return to baseline over time. This design is especially appropriate for samples of less than 60, with large effects expected. An additional appealing characteristic is that it offers treatment to all non-responders, reducing the ethical concerns that randomization often raises in palliative care (see below).

An understanding of statistics and research methodology is clearly needed to compensate for limited sample sizes. Collaboration amongst researchers, however, is likely the most robust means of overcoming this barrier, and is encouraged. Multicentered trials may be the only way of accruing a sufficient sample size within a reasonable time frame. For this reason, it is the development of national and international research networks that may have a larger impact on our ability to improve research (see below).

Handling heterogeneity

Ideally, the study population should be similar regarding all characteristics, except the variable(s) under investigation. By controlling variations within the studied groups, differences between groups may become more apparent, increasing the power of the study. Whenever possible, restrictive inclusion criteria should be set, so that subjects are similar at baseline. However, heterogeneity is innate to pediatric palliative care. Therefore, when exploring symptoms, behaviors, or the effectiveness of interventions, it may be important to include a wide range of LLCs, care settings, or individual variability in a sample. The problem is that when variability within a group is very high, real differences between groups may be diluted, leading to weak or even false negative results [277].

One solution regarding the heterogeneous sample is to find common elements within the sample, define what makes the heterogeneous group a group, and be explicit about why one is studying them together. If the groups are analyzed taking into account common characteristics, other differences may be overridden. For instance, children with different LLCs may share palliative care needs as delineated by ACT/RCPCH, who described four groups of LLCs that are likely to share care needs. The four groups include children with: (i) potentially curable diseases which are life-threatening, (ii) incurable diseases, with chances of substantially prolonging life expectancy with the use of intensive treatments, (iii) progressive diseases,

with significant cognitive impairment, and (iv) irreversible conditions, with severe cognitive impairment and risk of premature death [146]. Another way of homogenizing palliative care samples, proposed by Mazzocato et al. [277], is the use of staging systems, which categorize patients into prognostic groups based on a number of symptom characteristics. An example is the Edmonton Staging System for Cancer Pain, which uses five variables (pain mechanism, pain characteristic, psychological distress, tolerance, and history of alcoholism) to categorize patients into good or poor prognostic groups [278]. Finally, when studying children, age is also a relevant way of homogenizing a sample. Children are developing even when they are ill, and at different developmental stages, their needs and responses to treatments are different. Sample stratification, as described above, may be more pertinent when studying palliative care in children with diverse illnesses, and may improve the ability to find effects over classifying by diagnosis or disease stages.

Another way of balancing heterogeneity is by using randomization. The main advantage of randomization is that it balances known and, more importantly, unknown factors between the study groups, so that the 'only relevant difference' between arms is the intervention under investigation [279]. Parallel RCTs, when patients are randomly assigned to either the intervention or control arm, have been rarely used in palliative care [232], and have been limited by a combination of the barriers discussed previously [196,231]. Although the parallel RCT remains the design of choice to evaluate novel interventions, it would be worth learning more about ways to increase the feasibility of such a design.

In the interim, the use of alternative randomized and non-randomized designs should be considered, since these may even be more appropriate to answer some types of questions [251]. For instance, group or cluster randomization trials, randomizing by groups of patients rather than individuals, or even non-randomized trials, may be better when health care interventions are targeted at health care providers or communities. Jordhoy et al. [198] pioneered the use of a group randomized design in palliative care to evaluate a community empowerment program. The main advantage of this design lies in reducing the risk of 'contamination' in the control arm [280]. Its limitation is the inability to do a blind experiment, which may lead to selection bias. Since individuals within a cluster are similar, larger sample sizes are also required to achieve sufficient power [281]. Jordhoy's study failed to find significant improvements in patients' QoL, although a higher rate of home deaths was noted in the intervention group. Nonetheless, it served to further clarify several methodological issues. The investigators found an important selection bias: patients with particular diagnoses were more frequently referred to the study if they lived in an area allocated to the intervention, a consequence of the lack of blinding that is characteristic of this design [282].

Of all the types of randomized studies, crossover studies have the additional attraction of reducing heterogeneity, by using patients as their own controls.

Given that heterogeneity is an unavoidable characteristic, all methods sections should include a thorough description of the study population, in order to allow the reader to interpret whether the results are applicable to his/her patient population.

Managing difficulties in identifying potential research subjects

Subjects included in a study should be representative of the patients for whom study findings might be applied in the future [249]. However, defining who is an appropriate subject for palliative care interventions is challenging.

As mentioned, uncertainty about prognosis may lead to inclusion of subjects who should not be included, and exclusion of those who should be. Even when prognosis can be accurately estimated, controversies about the appropriate moment to introduce a palliative care strategy and the appropriate strategies to test [283], may impair recruitment throughout the study. Doctors' overestimation of survival [284], which is accentuated as patients are healthier and farther away from dying, further affects patient identification. However, because clinicians are able to integrate clinical, emotional, and social factors, clinical prediction is still the best predictor of life expectancy in patients with advanced disease. The use of tools that help clinicians with their estimations may be a way of increasing patient identification. At least two scoring systems [285,286] have been shown to work for adults with a wide array of advanced diseases [287–289]. Unfortunately these only discriminate very short-term survival (classifying patients according to their likelihood of dying within 1 month) limiting their application to research relating to actual end-of-life care. Prognostication modeling techniques that use artificial neural networks have proved to be more accurate than both logistic regression and a scoring system in estimating 1-year survival in patients with cirrhosis, and may be interesting to explore in the palliative care setting [290]. None of these prognostic tools have been validated in children.

Given the current lack of valid prognostication aids, and the hesitation of physicians to refer patients to palliative care studies, researchers should use multiple strategies in order to identify all eligible subjects. Strategies that have been found successful include having regular information sessions with health care providers, assuring the presence of 'project recruiters' in the referring services, permitting referrals from

patients already included, and advertising by means of flyers or public announcements [291]. In addition, consultation of electronic databases, while complying with privacy and confidentiality rules, can increase the ability to identify potential subjects.

Of all the strategies mentioned, educating providers in order to decrease their apprehensions about referring patients to a 'palliative care' study seems to be one of the more powerful tools available to increase identification of potential subjects [291]. If health care clinicians are well educated about the value of early integration of disease modifying and palliative treatments into care, and about the fact that palliative care does not imply giving up hope, but intends to enhance QoL, they may be more willing to refer patients to our protocols.

Coping with high attrition rates

Attrition, the decrease in sample size over time, is inherent to palliative care, and this problem leads to loss of study power. Additionally, attrition leads to bias, since the "healthiest" patients are the ones that remain in the study, resulting in a sample that is not representative of the 'true' population [191, 196,232,292]. Strategies intended to lower attrition rates include the use of short evaluation periods [238,251], which may allow for a larger proportion of the patients to remain evaluable throughout the study, as well as recruiting patients early in the course of the disease [231]. The use of short evaluation periods is a reasonable strategy for interventions that are clearly limited in time, such as pharmacological ones. Early recruitment offers other potential advantages. This strategy increases the number of eligible subjects, and informs about the effects of palliative care interventions during early phases of LLC [147], and, since it allows for researcher and subject to build a relationship, data collection during the advanced stages may feel less intrusive [277].

Since attrition is not avoidable, its occurrence should be carefully described and categorized. Categories that have been included in other research studies are pre-inclusion attrition (refusal to consent), drop-outs at any point during the study, intermittent missing data, and death [123,293]. In RCT's it is important to determine if there is selective drop-out (also called informative or non-random drop-out), if, for instance, death is more frequent in one of the arms of the study. Several approaches have been suggested to deal with attrition in the analysis, the most important being the use of 'intention-to-treat' (ITT) strategies, that is, patients are analyzed in the intervention group to which they were originally assigned, regardless of whether the subjects adhered to it or not [294]. ITT is a way of integrating the specific effect of the intervention with the likelihood of subjects adhering to it over time, and therefore, gives a measure of net benefit. Other alternatives to account for random and non-random censored data involve complex multivariate modeling, and usually would require help from a biostatistician [295,296].

Overcoming difficulties with outlining widely applicable interventions

Health services research focuses mainly on assessing the effectiveness of care interventions or programs. By definition, palliative care interventions are tailored to the individual, thus challenging the whole concept of generalizability. In fact, it has been difficult to prove that palliative care interventions make a difference for patients [232]. A recent systematic review of studies conducted in adult populations concluded that palliative care programs had a positive, but tiny, impact on patients' pain and other symptoms, and failed to show effects on quality of life [134]. In addition to the already mentioned problems with sample size, heterogeneity, and attrition, it has been argued that the difficulty in showing clear effectiveness is also partially due to the great variability and poor definition of the interventions evaluated [231] and outcomes measured.

Every attempt should be made to define the intervention as clearly as possible, administer it in a systematic way, and, when reporting, describe it thoroughly. Pilot studies are an excellent way of better defining interventions, as well as learning about feasibility before embarking on larger projects. When the ideal is not feasible, one may need to redefine the question, or find alternate methods to study the phenomenon of interest. Regarding the delivery of the intervention, two issues are important: first, it should be administered in a comparable way in all subjects; and second, bias associated with measuring outcomes should be minimized. The development of rigorous treatment protocols may help address both concerns. Blinding is also a powerful tool that should be used whenever possible. At the least, the raters should be blinded.

An important consideration that impacts on the systematic delivery of interventions is low adherence rates. The more complex the interventions, the more difficult it is for subjects and providers to comply with them. In order to optimally engage the provider in administering the intervention properly, it should be as simple as possible. There should be extensive education about how to carry it out, as well as guidelines about how to proceed if the intervention fails.

It is common for patients included in all study arms to receive care from other sources (e.g. home care programs, nursing agencies). These may either dilute or inflate the effects of the intervention under study. Thus all types of care provided to patients should be tracked to allow for control using multivariate analysis.

Finally, since pediatric palliative care research is a growing field, it is essential that authors disclose the limits of study findings and report the results of their studies, whether positive or negative. In other words, limited data is better than no data at all.

Defining valid outcome measures

As previously mentioned, there is little consensus about the relevant outcomes to measure for children with LLC's. In the adult setting, there is a lot of work in progress. The 'core of outcome tools' developed by the Palliative Care Core Audit Project Advisory Group in the United Kingdom and the Toolkit of Instruments to Measure End-of-Life Care (TIME) in the United States are examples of what has been achieved [122,200,297]. Each of these two projects proposes to measure three outcomes; the UK project is measuring quality of life, symptoms, and process of care, and TIME is measuring satisfaction with health care, QoL, and survival.

Defining outcomes is, however, not enough. Most of the adult studies have failed to prove efficacy or effectiveness of palliative interventions [216,218,298], even when measuring the appropriate well-defined outcomes. It may be that the outcome tools used are not effective in capturing meaningful changes, or even the underlying concept they are intended to measure. We already addressed the limitations of currently available instruments to portray the individualized and dynamic nature of QoL. No studies that we are aware of have measured the effect of palliative care interventions with an individualized QoL tool. Another explanation is that as death gets closer, the many things that negatively impact QoL may dilute any effect of a given intervention [123]. Finally, the scoring method may also be playing a role. Nordin *et al* reanalyzed RCT data using four different QoL scoring methods, finding that scorings that included some kind of weight or physician input were more responsive to changes than raw scores [299].

In pediatrics, this discussion has not even begun. In addition to defining the relevant outcomes, many other questions need to be addressed in partnership with families. What are the elements of good health care, or of a good quality of life? Does the concept of quality of life change as the disease progresses? What are the best ways of measuring these outcomes? If the patient is unable to report, who is the best proxy? When should outcomes be measured during the illness and/or after death?

Whatever the results of such discussion, the current outcome tools—principally limited to QoL and symptom indices—will probably be part of the armamentarium. Thus, their validation in children with advanced illness is a priority.

Novel instruments, supported by well-grounded qualitative research, are also necessary, and could help to validate, and serve as supplements to, existing instruments.

Ideally, research should advance in a somewhat linear manner, asking meaningful questions (to the patient and investigator), defining measurable outcomes, developing instruments, and proceeding to answer the initial questions. In pediatric palliative care, however, the paucity of data and the unmet needs of children and families compel and oblige us to proceed with all aspects simultaneously.

Considerations when selecting outcomes measurement tools

When faced with choosing a measurement instrument, researchers should consider its psychometric properties, the question at hand, and the population being studied. As stated before, experience with the current inventory of outcome indices is limited in the pediatric palliative care population. Hence, we should proceed with caution, choosing those tools that at least are demonstrated to be valid (measure what they are intended to measure), reliable (measure consistently), responsive to changes, feasible (easily applicable), and interpretable in children [249,300].

Studies looking at a wide array of conditions will benefit from using a generic QoL instrument, while specific tools may be preferable if the question is confined to a particular disease (Table 1). A combination of tools may, in fact, be optimal. Coupling domain-specific tools with more comprehensive measures may give insight into how particular symptoms, such as pain, nausea, or anxiety, are effected by other variables, including coping mechanisms, family distress, or social support. Understanding this interface will allow practitioners to implement tailored palliative care plans.

When children are the subjects of research, additional concerns relate to the role of child's self-report. Both 'objective' (e.g. heart rate for pain, the 15-count for dyspnea, or functional status) and 'proxy' (e.g. parental reports or behavioral checklists) tools have tried to replace children's limited capacity of expression. There is now growing evidence that symptoms and QoL are subjective and multidimensional constructs. Low correlation between objective measures and self-reports [101] as well as between parental and child reports [301], indicates that children have complex, unique, and non-transferable views about their experience. Proxy reports and objective indicators, although necessary in very young or cognitively impaired children, will always be imperfect surrogates. However, since children's judgment is based on their (limited) experience, self-reports alone may not convey a complete picture. Necholaichuk and colleagues reported that when patients, nurses, and relatives rated symptoms simultaneously,

tool reliability substantially increased when compared with just self-reports [301]. Therefore, a combination of objective and subjective, self and proxy, outcomes is currently recommended [104,233,302,303].

In an effort to increase the validity of self-report and direct child measurements, research tools need to have *developmentally adapted versions*. Instruments should account for each stage of child development (e.g. infancy, young childhood, late childhood, and adolescence) [120,304]. The content of domain-specific and generic measures must evolve in parallel with the child, as physical, emotional, cognitive, and social tasks change. Pragmatic considerations, including recognition of different levels of reading and comprehension abilities [305], variable life and cultural backgrounds, and personal experiences, also need consideration. The yield of structured interviews, for example, has improved when interviewers use shorter and simpler questions and response options, adapt items to the child's usual tasks, use pictures, and frame questions within the child's concept of time (e.g. a few days rather than weeks or a month) [86,119,129]. Having a variety of response options available also helps to maintain attention span. With disease progression, investigators also need to recognize the potential for developmental regression, and limitations in compliance [277]. Consequently, there may be a need for severity-adapted versions of a given instrument as well [231].

Because these resources (tools and methods) are scarce, and difficult and time-consuming to develop, new innovations should be shared amongst our research community. The world wide web provides a vector for communication among palliative care reasearchers that is being increasingly used for this purpose.

Lack of funding

Worldwide, research funding comes from public and/or private sources. The decision as to how to allocate these resources is usually based on the alignment of the research topic with national or international priorities, or with a private institution's mission. In addition, the chance of a specific project being awarded a grant rests on its methodological strength, and therefore, its potential to reach reliable and valid results. Given the difficulties already mentioned, palliative care may be trapped in a vicious cycle of not accessing funding because of its 'poor' methodology, which in turn leaves the field without the knowledge necessary to develop better research methods.

There is hope, however. Recent evidence indicating that the needs of children with LLC and their families are far from being met has led national research agencies to identify pediatric palliative care as a research priority in several countries, such as the United States [147], Australia [306], and England [307]. As a consequence, public funding agencies are slowly increasing the allocation of funds to palliative care research in children. As an example, the (US) National Cancer Institute recently released a request for applications for "Reducing barriers to symptom management and palliative care" and the National Institute of Nursing Research (NINR), the National Cancer Institute (NCI) and the National Institute of Child Health and Human Development (NICHD) together cosponsored a program announcement for 'Improving care for dying children and their families'. (See http://www.cancer.gov/researchfunding/announcements/symptommanagement for a list of National Institute of Health funding opportunities in symptom management and palliative care research). In addition, other governmental agencies may also be moved to fund research if they are payers of palliative care services, or if they have a regulating role, and need to set standards of care.

Private foundations are generally moved by altruism, committing funds to topics of interest at their own discretion, regardless of their public health relevance. For this reason, support from private sources may be a great way of generating initial evidence when public funds are not available, as exemplified through the experience of the *Project of Death in America* and the *Open Society Institute* in the United States and Eastern Europe.

In addition, not-for-profit organizations devoted to improve access to care, education and knowledge of specific LLC, such as *Cystic Fibrosis Worldwide*, the *United Cerebral Palsy Research and Educational Foundation (UCP)*, or the several national organizations for *Inborn Errors of Metabolism*, also fund collaborative research initiatives. With the exception of UCP, these organizations have had a greater focus on disease modifying, but public opinion and national/international recommendations may help to expand priorities to include QoL concerns.

Use of research networks

If the main barriers to conducting large collaborative trials in rare diseases are organizational, should we not be investing our scarce resources in overcoming these barriers to collaboration, rather than relying on evidence from trials of inadequate size that may provide misleading?

Although many of the problems discussed may be ameliorated by developing coordinated, multi-centered research efforts, there are virtually no such networks in place today. Table 40.4 summarizes examples of existing collaboratives within palliative care in general, and specifically within pediatric palliative care, though these groups have only been involved in limited

research efforts thus far. Aware that there is an increasing interest in research, the authors informally surveyed members of a pediatric palliative care mailing list (paedpallcare) to uncover any new efforts. Although several single center projects were reported in South Africa, Canada and the United States, we found only one national collaborative from the United Kingdom (Bristol Children's Palliative Care Research Group).

The palliative care community is quite scattered across a wide range of fields, and collaboration may even seem far-fetched. Yet, this limitation can be transformed into a highly productive opportunity—the opportunity of mobilizing the diversity into a genuine interdisciplinary field, where innovative ways of asking and answering questions can take place, and clinical practice can be redefined. For collaborative efforts to be successful, hard work is required. Ideally, well-organized palliative care research networks would be the most effective means to ensure productive research efforts. It would be necessary to establish standardized nomenclature, data collection methods, and data analysis schemes. Input from research methodologists will be needed to account for the complexities of carrying out cross-cultural research across heterogeneous care settings.

The creation of an international research consortium responsible for developing a common research agenda, coordinating activities, and monitoring progress may be the best way of conducting such efforts, while minimizing the risk of duplicating efforts—a risk we cannot afford in a field with limited funding resources. This strategy has already proven useful in pediatrics. The American *Children's Oncology Group* (COG), the *United Kingdom Children's Cancer Study Group* (UKCCSG), the *Société International d'Oncologie Pédiatrique* (SIOP), and the *International Neonatal Network*, among others, are examples of successful research consortiums that are leading to productive research endeavors among small and diverse patient populations.

Initiatives encouraging research in this group of patients, such as the ones promoted by Palliative Care Australia [306] or the Institute of Medicine [147], will promote the creation of collaborations, or influence existing networks to include pediatric palliative care in their research agendas. In addition, other proposals promoting research in children in general—such as the US Food & Drug Administration regulations calling on the pharmaceutical industry to back more research in children [308], may also encourage the development of partnerships, and therefore, improve research efforts.

The benefits of developing research networks cannot be stressed enough. Goss *et al.* [309], reporting the experience with the *Cystic Fibrosis Therapeutics Development Network* (CF-TDN), which has conducted 18 clinical trials in patients

Table 40.4 Examples of existing collaboratives in palliative care

Palliative care collaboratives	Mandate	Contact
Population-based palliative care research network—US	PoPCRN was formed in 1998 as a means for conducting on-going studies of care at the end of life. Specifically, its aim is to facilitate structured and rigorous exploration of issues of importance to patients, families, caregivers, and providers in palliative care and hospice settings.	www.uchsc.edu/popcrn
European Association for Palliative Care Research Network	The Board of Directors of the EAPC consider research a key issue for the future of palliative care, and therefore, decided in 1996 to put together a steering group, with the aim of establishing a research network.	www.eapcnet.org/researchNetwork/ research.asp
The Palliative Care Research Society (PCRS)—UK	The PCRS is dedicated to promoting research into all aspects of palliative care, and to facilitating its dissemination.	www.pcrs.sghms.ac.uk
National Hospice and Palliative care Organization (NHPCO)—US	The NHPCO, a non-profit organization representing programs and professionals committed to improving quality and access to end of life care, has developed collaborative research projects, intending to better define outcomes and evaluate the state of the art.	http://www.nhpco.org
The Association for Children with Life-Threatening or Terminal Conditions and Their Families (ACT)	ACT aims to advocate on behalf of affected children and families by representing their needs, to campaign for the provision of a coordinated network of care and support, to promote models of good care and practice, to support families with a national information service, to enhance the knowledge and skills of professional carers by providing specialist literature and education opportunities.	www.act.org.uk
Children's Hospice International (CHI)	CHI aims to ensure medical, psychological, social and spiritual support to all children with life-threatening conditions, and their families, by providing a network of resources and care. Currently evaluating the Program for All Inclusive Care for Children and Their Families (PACC).	www.chionline.org/
Children's International Project on Palliative/Hospice Services (ChIPPS)	ChIPPS is working to concretely enhance the science and practice of pediatric hospice and palliative care, and to increase the availability of state-of-the-art services to families.	www.nhpco.org/i4a/pages/index. cfm?pageid=34 09
The Initiative for Pediatric Palliative Care (IPPC)	IPPC is dedicated to facilitating improvement in the quality of care for children living with life-threatening conditions and their families.	www.ippcweb.org/index.asp
Children's Oncology Group (COG) Palliative Care Subcommittee	This COG subcommittee aims to facilitate symptom control trials in children with advanced cancer.	hildenj@ccf.org
Bristol Children's Palliative Care Research Group (BCPCRG)	The group's mission is to conduct research to increase the evidence base for the specialty in the United Kingdom. Currently dedicated to evaluate 90 community children's palliative care services. Funded by the New Opportunities Fund (National Lottery charity)	nicola.eaton@uwe.ac.uk

with Cystic Fibrosis in its 3.5 years of functioning, suggested that collaboratives speed the development of specific outcome measures, research methodologies, and also protocol development in itself. A similar experience has been reported by the *Cooperative International Neuromuscular Research Group* (CINRG) [310]. The ability to conduct several studies simultaneously, and to shorten study duration, makes research possible for these populations. In addition, the current availability of internet based software for data entry, monitoring, and communication, facilitates the whole process of research, making data available in real time and allowing for monitoring from a single site, which in turn, results in significant reductions in research costs. Finally, these initiatives may also optimize the ability to secure funding, since they result in better projects and can apply to multiple national and international, governmental and private organizations.

The main difficulties with research collaboratives are the potential for discrepancies in measurements between sites, and false negatives (due to between-site heterogeneity) [310]. Careful training and testing of data collectors is needed to assure good inter-rater reliability. The development of outcomes that focus on the patients' experiences rather than the particularities of their conditions, may also help overcome some of the problems of such heterogeneity [311]. On the other side, heterogeneity supports greater generalizability. When an effect is found, it is much more likely that it will be replicated in other settings, given the similarity of the study populations to 'real life' situations.

Finally, training in research methodology is an impending need for a field that has developed strongly on clinical and compassionate basis. Conferences and symposia focusing on pediatric palliative care research may be a way of stimulating dialogue and collaboration between investigators. To begin, the most efficient strategy may be to organize a pediatric palliative care research symposium, in conjunction with a well-established research meeting. Examples of annual meetings include those organized by the European Society for Pediatric Research (ESPR), Society for Pediatric Research (SPR), or the European Association for Palliative Care (EAPC) Research Network.

Ways to overcome ethical barriers

The ethical concerns surrounding research in patients with advanced disease have contributed greatly to the lack of evidence in the field [238]. Issues such as vulnerability and burden imposed on patients and families have been invoked as impediments for studying this population, both by providers and IRBs. However, it seems as though this is changing. There is some evidence that nurses are now more prone to refer

palliative care patients to studies [312], and that IRBs' main concerns are focused on protocol validity [313].

A recent supplement of the *Journal of Pain and Symptom Management*, dedicated to ethics in research, discussed the relevance and specificity of several ethical topics in the palliative care arena, and made some recommendations about how to resolve them [314]. Similarly, studies such as the one by Ross *et al.* [312], who analyzed the willingness of palliative care patients to participate in clinical trials, may also help providers and IRB's understand better which worries are relevant to patients, and how to better assure a fair balance between respecting patients' rights and advancing their care. In this section we will focus on two ethical problems: vulnerability, and the difficulties related to conducting research in patients who may not have another chance for care, because of their relevance to pediatrics and palliative care.

Vulnerability

Children with LLCs are understandably regarded as a paradigm of vulnerability. As with adults, physical affliction does not necessarily correspond to impaired ability to give a valid informed consent [315]. More important are a child's development and understanding. Ability to provide assent, and certainly consent, is contingent upon appropriate decision-making capacity [316] and a degree of independent thinking; there is no definitive age at which these transitions occur, and thus, each child may be considered separately [317]. In addition, providers must recognize that parents are, in a sense, also a vulnerable population. Their autonomy may be compromised by the child's situation, dependency upon caregivers, and socioeconomic factors. In any case, vulnerability in children with LLC should not be understood as an unequivocal impediment to research, but rather as a multidimensional and dynamic situation, that merits taking appropriate safeguards to assure that an ethical approach is undertaken in designing and implementing clinical trials in this patient population.

There are two essential requirements to involving a vulnerable population in clinical investigation, obtaining a valid consent, and ensuring that the benefit/risk ratio of the study is acceptable.

1. The assent/permission process—In the case of children, there is international consensus [318–321] that consent should be replaced by a dyad of parental permission, which aims to protect the child, and child assent, which allows the child to express his/her preference about participation, a way of showing respect for children's developing autonomy [316].

As described by Agrawal [315], a consent is considered valid if the child is provided with the relevant information, to the best of his/her ability to absorb, about the study, and freely agrees to participate in it, and if the parents or legal guardians give an equally informed and voluntary permission for the child to participate. Therefore, it is paramount that the permission/assent documents and the entire recruitment process be adapted to the different levels of understanding of the target population. As with outcomes assessment, assent information should be written and discussed in a developmentally appropriate way, followed by an evaluation of the child's understanding [316]. This implies having different versions of the assent process for younger and older children. The young child's assent should use concrete examples when explaining the study, and focus on the specific procedures involved, in order to allow the child to state whether he or she agrees to participate. The older the child, the greater the ability to understand study goals, procedures, and the freedom to withdraw [322], and therefore the more an assent document may resemble an adult consent form. In the case of the child who is too young, or unable to assent because of cognitive impairment, parental permission from one or both parents depending on the risk/benefit ratio of the study may suffice [318,321].

In addition to adjusting the content to the subject's understanding, the words used in recruitment material should be carefully considered. For example, material using explicit terms like 'palliative care,' 'end-of-life,' and 'dying,' may only be acceptable to a small number of families, leading to omission of children simply because of the language used in describing the study. Alternatively, words that readily convey similar messages, such as 'advanced illness' or 'relapsed disease,' may not be as difficult for families to bear, and may be preferred.

Besides disclosure and understanding of information, it is also necessary to attend to two sources that may unduly influence willingness to participate. First, a child is naturally influenced by adult opinions, and parents are often the leading authorities in a child's life. The child may logically think that parents 'know better,' and may want to follow their suggestions without much questioning [316]. This 'dependent' behavior may also appear when other adults express their views. Second, the health care provider should be aware that by virtue of inviting a family to become involved in a study, he or she is being coercive, however unintentionally, especially when he or she is the usual care provider. In the case of advanced illness, families may be desperate and more inclined to accept any type of new treatment, regardless of its prospect of benefit. Families may also feel grateful to their clinician and be willing to participate in research as a way of paying them back [315]. For these reasons, it may be better for researchers not to be directly involved in the child's care [312], or if this is not feasible, then health care providers should be trained in recruitment strategies that do not exert inappropriate pressure on patients and families to agree to participation [315].

Given that recruitment and the assent/permission process are challenging, reasons for patient refusal should be carefully tracked. Sharing this information may help to better understand how to approach this understudied population. It is incumbent on investigators to report on successful enrollment strategies, and lessons learned along the way.

2. Difficulties in assessing risks/benefits—An equally important way of addressing vulnerability is by assuring that the risk/benefit ratio of the study is justified. The risk/benefit assessment should consider, among other things, if risks are greater than everyday risks, and if the intervention under study imposes an acceptable burden to patients. Neither of these is easy to evaluate in the palliative care setting.

Everyday, morbidity and mortality risk increase as patients get closer to the end of life. As a result, defining acceptable risks on this basis may lead to either overly permissive or overly stringent criteria. Assessment of burdens is also complicated, because of the rapidly changing nature of advanced disease. Treatment goals change, and the disease itself may cause significant worries in the patient. A survey may be seen as short on one visit and of unbearable length at the next one; what may seem like an innocuous procedure at enrollment, may mean a loss of precious family time when end-of-life is imminent [323, 324]. Researchers need to take these oscillations into account, and design data collection methods that are flexible enough to obtain the maximum information possible at each encounter. As with developmental issues, there may be a need for different versions of an instrument, for different phases of the illness.

One feature that has been frequently underestimated when weighing burden against gains, is the positive effects that may ensue through participation in research. Several studies [141,148,312,324,325] have reported that patients choose to enroll in research because it is right, because it gives them a sense of purpose and meaning. Telling their stories helps them personally. Furthermore, certain data suggest that participation in studies results in better and more comprehensive care. Further research is needed to estimate the relative risks and benefits of participation.

In the end, the IRB is the overarching authority that determines whether the risk/benefit ratio is acceptable. However, IRBs do not have a lot of experience with palliative care studies, and may lack the tools to assess them properly [313]. It has been recommended that palliative care specialists join IRBs, to assist with such situations [314].

Difficulties related to conducting research in patients who may not have other chances for alternate care

When we deal with advanced disease issues, there seems to be less room for error. Any decision made may be the last, or affect an opportunity to do something important. An unwillingness to experiment is thus understandable. However, this perspective ignores the reality that the state of the art is far from optimal, and that as providers, we have a responsibility to improve care.

Randomization is an issue that may be particularly thorny, and that may, in fact, prevent providers from referring patients, and patients from enrolling in trials. Randomization is justified as long as there is a state of equipoise, that is, when there is true uncertainty about whether the benefits or harm of the treatment under study are greater than those obtained with the control treatment. Equipoise might be difficult to define in palliative care, where there is little knowledge about risks and benefits, and there is often a lack of choices. Subjective opinions may then play an important role. Physicians or patients may see an intervention as 'more desirable' because they like it more, for example, home-care vs. hospital care, and therefore refuse randomization because of the risk of not receiving the 'best' treatment option.

There are several ways in which randomization can become more appealing to the patient and providers. For instance, crossover designs or enriched RCT's may be more acceptable, because all or non-respondent subjects are always exposed to the intervention. When the intervention is new, randomization can be made the gateway to the intervention, that is, there is no other access to the intervention other than enrolling in the study [231]. Other options are to vary the randomization process in itself. The easiest way of varying randomization is by increasing the chances of getting the intervention, simply by allocating more patients to the intervention than to the control arm (e.g. 2:1 instead of the classic 1:1), a strategy called *fixed unequal allocation* [326]. Data-dependent designs, such as *sequential* and *adaptive* trials, are more complex ways of altering randomization [249]. In these designs, investigators change the probabilities of allocation while the trial is under way, based on interim analysis results. Adaptive designs favor the best performing intervention, and thus, are especially applicable when there are strong ethical concerns regarding randomization. Another option is to conduct a non-randomized design, such as the *risk-based allocation* trial, which assigns the intervention only to those subjects at higher risk, or with greater severity. This design is well suited for interventions that are already in use and perceived effective; conducting the randomized trial would otherwise be difficult, because subjects may refuse to enroll in a study where they only have a 50% chance of receiving a therapy they believe is useful. As with other issues we discussed, education to both patients and providers regarding the need to randomize and its process, may help more than anything else to increase acceptance.

Lastly, it should be kept in mind that, above all else, it is never justifiable to enroll subjects in a study that has an inappropriate design, or one whose results are predictably invalid.

Setting the agenda

As presented throughout the chapter and book, there is an enormous need for research initiatives in pediatric palliative care.

We already mentioned that government agencies in some developed countries are beginning to consider palliative care in children a research priority. However, this increasing recognition varies greatly. The Canadian Institute for Health Research started to fund several palliative care projects in 2003–2004. The UK National Health Services, in their Cancer Plan, have stated that palliation is one of their research priorities [307]. One of the most comprehensive documents recently published with respect to this issue is the (American) Institute of Medicine Report, 'When Children Die: Improving Palliative and End-of-Life Care for Children and their Families,' which reviews in detail the vast array of needs in pediatric palliative care research. The two main recommendations are to improve the collection of descriptive data at national and regional levels, and for organizations that fund pediatric research related to LLCs to set research priorities in pediatric palliative, end-of-life, and bereavement care [147].

Essential knowledge about the 'natural history' of LLCs is lacking, thus affecting the ability to provide appropriate services to children and their families. Thorough descriptive studies are needed to close this gap, not only regarding clinical care, but also from a psychosocial, financial, and organizational perspective.

In order to reduce suffering, the 'suffering' experience needs to be characterized thoroughly, including a better understanding of what may modulate it. This will help to define the relevant outcomes, and devise appropriate measuring tools. Better knowledge about how children conceptualize QoL during advanced stages of a disease also seems to be crucial, as well as a better understanding of the role of proxy reports when children cannot relay their own experience. In addition, the role of family–provider communication, and its influence on decision-making, needs to be better understood.

Short and long-term impact of a child's illness and death on parents, siblings, and even schoolmates is also an essential research priority, if we are to truly characterize the full extent of the problem. We have stated repeatedly that LLC's are rare in children, contributing to the perception of pediatric palliative care as a small-scale problem. However, there is very little understanding of how the death of a child impacts long-term on siblings, schoolmates and communities. This warrants comprehensive investigation as well.

Other questions that need to be elucidated with sound research are economical issues, such as cost-effectiveness of different models of care, and the financial burden imposed on families caring for a child with an LLC, and the ways to address these needs. There are also particular needs related to regional variations in epidemiology and health system organization. For instance, in South Africa research is mainly devoted to palliative care in AIDS, whereas in Australia, where pediatric subspecialists are sparse, the focus has been on 'integration of child-specific approaches into the palliative care services system, and support of adult-focused services ..' [306].

Though the design of studies in patients with life-limiting illness will have limitations, the challenge to the investigator is to carefully balance methods to achieve meaningful results with the burdens and risks imposed on the patients. However, not doing the research at all poses the greatest risk to this vulnerable patient population. Developing and testing strategies to enhance quality of life and comfort are crucial at a time in life where these constructs have the greatest importance.

Summary

Research in palliative care is necessary for the advancement of the field and of optimal care for our patients and their loved ones. The significant barriers outlined above are daunting, but not insurmountable. Clinicians are encouraged to engage in systematic, rigorous research efforts to support a more evidence-based approach to pediatric palliative care. The immense needs of our patients may compel clinicians to implement untried or unsubstantiated approaches and interventions. While this may prove successful in individual cases, providers should consider the advantages of more methodical strategies. Evidenced-based care is not necessarily insensitive care.

Research is time consuming, and deferred gratification is indisputable. Most of our patients will not benefit from immediate research efforts, but prospects for the future are great. Palliative care practitioners are challenged to better understand the natural history of the experience of children with advanced illness, their families and communities; to develop and validate outcome tools, and at the same time, rigorously evaluate interventions aimed at improving 'bedside' palliation. If thoughtfully designed, these efforts may be most expeditious if done concurrently. Historically, the pediatrics community has overcome numerous obstacles, leading to great discoveries in the care of children with all manner of illnesses. We are, therefore, well equipped to do so for children with advanced illness as well.

References

1. Anand, K.J. and Hickey, P.R. Pain and its effects in the human neonate and fetus. *N Engl J Med* 1987;317(21):1321–9.
2. Puchalski, M. and Hummel, P. The reality of neonatal pain. *Advances in Neonatal Care* 2002;2(5):233–44; quiz 245–7.
3. McGrath, P.A. Pain in the pediatric patient: Practical aspects of assessment. *Pediatr Ann* 1995;24(3):126–33.
4. Coleman, M.M., Solarin, K., and Smith, C. Assessment and management of pain and distress in the neonate. *Adv Neonatal Care*, 2002;2(3):123–36;quiz 137–9.
5. Hunt, A. *et al.* Not knowing—the problem of pain in children with severe neurological impairment. *Int J Nurs Stud* 2003;40(2):171–83.
6. Zisk, R.Y. Our youngest patients' pain—from disbelief to belief? *Pain Manage Nurs* 2003;4(1):40–51.
7. Swafford, L.I. and Allen, D.A. Pain relief in the pediatric patient. *Med Clin NA* 1968;25(1):131–6.
8. Webb, C. Tactics to reduce a child's fear of pain. *AJN* 1966; 66(12): 2698–701.
9. Haslam, D.R. Age and the perception of pain. *Psychosom Sci* 1969; 15:86.
10. Eland, J.M. Children's communication of pain, in Master's Thesis. *University of Iowa*, 1974.
11. Rich, E.C., Marshall, R.E., and Volpe, J.J. The normal neonatal response to pin-prick. *Dev Med Child Neurol* 1974;16(4):432–4.
12. Apley, J. Pain in childhood. *J Psychosom Res* 1976;20(4):383–9.
13. Scott, R. "It hurts red:" A preliminary study of children's perception of pain. *Percept Motor Skills* 1978;47(3 Pt 1):787–91.
14. Eland, J.M. and Anderson, J.E. The Experience of Pain in Children. In A. Jacox, Ed. *Pain: A Source Book for Nurses and Other Health Professionals.* Boston, M.A: Little Brown, 1977.
15. Hester, N.K. The preoperational child's reaction to immunization. *Nurs Res*, 1979;28(4):250–5.
16. Savedra, M. *et al.* How do children describe pain? A tentative assessment. *Pain* 1982;14(2):95–104.
17. Lollar, D.J., Smits, S.J., and Patterson, D.L. Assessment of pediatric pain: An empirical perspective. *J Pediatr Psychol* 1982;7(3):267–77.
18. Anand, K.J. *et al.* Can the human neonate mount an endocrine and metabolic response to surgery? *J Pediatr Surg* 1985;20(1):41–8.
19. Anand, K.J., Sippell, W.G., and Aynsley-Green, A. Randomised trial of fentanyl anaesthesia in preterm babies undergoing surgery: Effects on the stress response.[erratum appears in Lancet 1987 Jan 24;1(8526):234]. *Lancet* 1987;1(8524):62–6.
20. Anand, K.J. *et al.* Does halothane anaesthesia decrease the metabolic and endocrine stress responses of newborn infants undergoing operation? *Br Med J Clin Res* 1988;296(6623):668–72.
21. Cahill, C., Panzarella, C., and Spross, J.A. Oncology Nursing Society position paper on cancer pain. Pediatric cancer pain. *Oncol Nurs Forum* 1990;17(6):948–51.
22. Anon, Clinicians' quick reference guide to acute pain management in infants, children, and adolescents: operative and medical procedures. Pain Management Guideline Panel. Agency for Health Care Policy and Research, US Department of Health and Human Services. *J Pain Symptom Manage* 1992;7(4):229–42.
23. Cancer pain relief and palliative care in children. *Geneva: World Health Organization*, 1998.

24. Anon, Prevention and management of pain and stress in the neonate. American Academy of Pediatrics. Committee on Fetus and Newborn. Committee on Drugs. Section on Anesthesiology. Section on Surgery. Canadian Paediatric Society. Fetus and Newborn Committee. *Pediatr* 2000;105(2):454–61.

25. Anand, K.J. and P. International Evidence-Based Group for Neonatal. Consensus statement for the prevention and management of pain in the newborn. *Arch Pediatr Adolesc Med*, 2001; 155(2):173–80.

26. Larsson, B.A. *et al.* [Swedish guidelines for prevention and treatment of pain in the newborn infant]. *Lakartidningen* 2002;99(17): 1946–9.

27. Rees, D.C. *et al.* Guidelines for the management of the acute painful crisis in sickle cell disease. *Br J Haematol* 2003;120(5):744–52.

28. Poznanski, E.O. Children's reactions to pain: A psychiatrist's perspective. *Clin Pediatr* 1976;15(12):1114–9.

29. Scott, P.J., Ansell, B.M., and Huskisson, E.C. Measurement of pain in juvenile chronic polyarthritis. *Ann Rheumat Dis* 1977;36(2): 186–7.

30. Weiss, C. Does circumcision of the newborn require an anesthetic? *Clin Pediatr* 1968;7(3):128–9.

31. American Academy of Pediatrics. Committee on Psychosocial Aspects of, C. *et al.* The assessment and management of acute pain in infants, children, and adolescents. *Pediatrics* 2001;108(3): 793–7.

32. Gauvain-Piquard, A. *et al.* The development of the DEGR(R): A scale to assess pain in young children with cancer. *Eur J Pain* 1999; 3(2):165–176.

33. Schechter, N.L. The undertreatment of pain in children: An overview. *Pediatr Clin N Am* 1989;36(4):781–94.

34. Unruh, A. *et al.* Children's drawings of their pain. *Pain* 1983;17(4): 385–92.

35. Ross, D.M. and Ross, S.A. Childhood pain: The school-aged child's viewpoint. *Pain* 1984;20(2):179–91.

36. Ross, D.M. and Ross, S.A. The importance of type of question, psychological climate and subject set in interviewing children about pain. *Pain* 1984;19(1):71–9.

37. Tyler, D.C. *et al.* Toward validation of pain measurement tools for children: A pilot study. *Pain* 1993;52(3):301–9.

38. Van Cleve, L.J. and Savedra, M.C. Pain location: Validity and reliability of body outline markings by 4 to 7-year-old children who are hospitalized. *Pediatr Nurs* 1993;19(3):217–20.

39. Joyce, B.A. *et al.* Reliability and validity of preverbal pain assessment tools. *Issues Compr Pediatr Nurs* 1994;17(3):121–35.

40. Stein, P.R. Indices of pain intensity: Construct validity among preschoolers. *Pediatr Nurs* 1995;21(2):119–23.

41. McGrath, P.A. *et al.* A new analogue scale for assessing children's pain: an initial validation study. *Pain* 1996;64(3):435–43.

42. Crow, C.S. Children's Pain Perspectives Inventory (CPPI): Developmental assessment. *Pain* 1997;72(1–2):33–40.

43. Franck, L.S. and Miaskowski, C. Measurement of neonatal responses to painful stimuli: A research review. *J Pain Symptom Manage* 1997; 14(6):343–78.

44. Franck, L.S., Greenberg, C.S., and Stevens, B. Pain assessment in infants and children. *Pediatr Clin North Am* 2000;47(3): 487–512.

45. Soetenga, D., Frank, J., and Pellino, T.A. Assessment of the validity and reliability of the University of Wisconsin Children's Hospital Pain scale for Preverbal and Nonverbal Children. *Pediatr Nurs* 1999;25(6):670–6.

46. Breau, L.M. *et al.* Measuring pain accurately in children with cognitive impairments: Refinement of a caregiver scale. *J Pediatr* 2001;138(5):721–7.

47. Breau, L.M. *et al.* Validation of the Non-communicating Children's Pain Checklist-Postoperative Version. *Anesthesiology* 2002;96(3): 528–35.

48. Carter, B., McArthur, E., and Cunliffe, M. Dealing with uncertainty: Parental assessment of pain in their children with profound special needs. *J Adv Nurs* 2002;38(5):449–57.

49. Stallard, P. *et al.* The development and evaluation of the pain indicator for communicatively impaired children (PICIC). *Pain* 2002;98(1–2):145–9.

50. Voepel-Lewis, T. *et al.* The reliability and validity of the Face, Legs, Activity, Cry, Consolability observational tool as a measure of pain in children with cognitive impairment. *Anesth Analg* 2002;95(5): 1224–9, table of contents.

51. Flogegard, H. and Ljungman, G. Characteristics and adequacy of intravenous morphine infusions in children in a paediatric oncology setting. *Med Pediatr Oncol* 2003;40(4):233–8.

52. Broome, M.E. *et al.* Pediatric pain practices: A national survey of health professionals. *J Pain Symptom Manag* 1996;11(5):312–20.

53. Porter, F.L. *et al.* Pain and pain management in newborn infants: A survey of physicians and nurses. *Pediatrics* 1997;100(4):626–32.

54. Jacob, E. and Puntillo, K.A. Pain in hospitalized children: Pediatric nurses' beliefs and practices. *J Pediatr Nurs* 1999;14(6):379–91.

55. Karling, M., Renstrom, M., and Ljungman, G. Acute and postoperative pain in children: A Swedish nationwide survey. *Acta Paediatrica* 2002;91(6):660–6.

56. Ellis, J.A. *et al.* Pain in hospitalized pediatric patients: How are we doing? *Clin J Pain* 2002;18(4):262–9.

57. Simons, S.H. *et al.* Do we still hurt newborn babies? A prospective study of procedural pain and analgesia in neonates. *Arch Pediatr Adolesc Med* 2003;157(11):1058–64.

58. Caty, S., Tourigny, J., and Koren, I. Assessment and management of children's pain in community hospitals. *J Adv Nurs* 1995;22(4): 638–45.

59. Salantera, S. Finnish nurses' attitudes to pain in children. *J Adv Nurs* 1999;29(3):727–36.

60. Hamers, J.P. *et al.* The influence of children's vocal expressions, age, medical diagnosis and information obtained from parents on nurses' pain assessments and decisions regarding interventions. *Pain* 1996;65(1):53–61.

61. Knoblauch, S.C. and Wilson, C.J. Clinical outcomes of educating nurses about pediatric pain management. *Outcomes Manage Nurs Pract* 1999;3(2):87–9.

62. Halimaa, S.L., Vehvilainen-Julkunen, K., and Heinonen, K. Knowledge, assessment and management of pain related to nursing procedures used with premature babies: Questionnaire study for caregivers. *Int J Nurs Pract* 2001;7(6):422–30.

63. Hain, R.D. and Campbell, C. Invasive procedures carried out in conscious children: Contrast between North American and European paediatric oncology centres. *Arch Dis Childhood* 2001; 85(1):12–5.

64. de Lima, J. *et al.* Infant and neonatal pain: Anaesthetists' perceptions and prescribing patterns. *BMJ* 1996;313(7060):787.

65. Riano Galan, I. *et al.* [The opinion of pediatricians on childhood pain]Opinion de los pediatras sobre el dolor infantil. *Anales Espanoles de Pediatria* 1998;49(6):587–93.

66. Wang, X.S. *et al.* Pediatric cancer pain management practices and attitudes in China. *J Pain Symptom Manage* 2003;26(2):748–59.

67. De Lima, L. *et al.* Legislation analysis according to WHO and INCB criteria on opioid availability: A comparative study of 5 countries and the state of Texas. *Health Policy* 2001;56(2):99–110.

68. De Lima, L. *et al.* Potent Analgesics are More Expensive for Patients in Developing Countries:A Comparative Study. *J Pain Palliat Care Pharmacother* 2004;18(1):59–70.

69. McGrath, P.J. and Unruh, A.M. The social context of neonatal pain. *Clinics in Perinatology* 2002;29(3):555–72.

70. Gregorio, G.V. *et al.* Effect of rifampicin in the treatment of pruritus in hepatic cholestasis. *Arch Dis Child* 1993;69(1):141–3.

71. Airede, A.K. and Weerasinghe, H.D. Rifampicin and the relief of pruritus of hepatic cholestatic origin. *Acta Paediatr* 1996;85(7): 887–8.

72. Trioche, P. *et al.* Ondansetron for pruritus in child with chronic cholestasis. *Eur J Pediatr* 1996;155(11):990.

73. Arai, L. *et al.* The use of ondansetron to treat pruritus associated with intrathecal morphine in two paediatric patients. *Paediatr Anaesth* 1996;6(4):337–9.

74. Johnson, D.L. Intractable hiccups: Treatment by microvascular decompression of the vagus nerve. Case Report. *J Neurosurg* 1993; 78(5):813–6.

75. Johnson, B.R. and Kriel, R.L. Baclofen for chronic hiccups. *Pediatr Neurol* 1996;15(1):66–7.

76. Anso Olivan, S. *et al.* [Chronic hiccups in childhood: Usefulness of baclofen]. *An Esp Pediatr* 1998;49(4):399–400.

77. Janahi, I.A. *et al.* Inhaled morphine to relieve dyspnea in advanced cystic fibrosis lung disease. *Pediat Pulmonol* 2000;30(3):257–9.

78. Cohen, S.P. and Dawson, T.C. Nebulized morphine as a treatment for dyspnea in a child with cystic fibrosis. *Pediatrics* 2002; 110(3):e38.

79. Collins, J.J. *et al.* The measurement of symptoms in children with cancer. *J Pain Symptom Manage* 2000;19(5):363–77.

80. Wolfe, J. *et al.* Symptoms and suffering at the end of life in children with cancer [see comments]. *N Engl J Med* 2000;342(5):326–33.

81. Mock, V. Evaluating a model of fatigue in children with cancer. *J Pediatr Oncol Nurs* 2001;18(2 Suppl 1):13–6.

82. Docherty, S.L. Symptom experiences of children and adolescents with cancer. *Ann Rev Nurs Res* 2003;21:123–49.

83. Hockenberry-Eaton, M. *et al.* Fatigue in children and adolescents with cancer. J Pediatr Oncol Nurs, 1998; 15(3):172–82.

84. Davies, B. *et al.* A typology of fatigue in children with cancer. *J Pediat Nurs* 2002;19(1):12–21.

85. Hain, R.D. *et al.* Respiratory symptoms in children dying from malignant disease. *Palliat Med* 1995;9(3):201–6.

86. Collins, J.J. *et al.* The measurement of symptoms in young children with cancer: The validation of the Memorial Symptom Assessment Scale in children aged 7–12. *J Pain Symptom Manage,* 2002;23(1):10–16.

87. Lebaron, S. and Zeltzer, L. Behavioral intervention for reducing chemotherapy-related nausea and vomiting in adolescents with cancer. *J Adolesc Health Care* 1984;5(3):178–82.

88. Jacknow, D.S. *et al.* Hypnosis in the prevention of chemotherapy-related nausea and vomiting in children: a prospective study. *J Dev Behav Pediatr* 1994;15(4):258–64.

89. Alvarez, O. *et al.* Randomized double-blind crossover ondansetron-dexamethasone versus ondansetron-placebo study for the treatment of chemotherapy-induced nausea and vomiting in pediatric patients with malignancies. *J Pediatr Hematol Oncol* 1995;17(2):145–50.

90. White, L. *et al.* A comparison of oral ondansetron syrup or intravenous ondansetron loading dose regimens given in combination with dexamethasone for the prevention of nausea and emesis in pediatric and adolescent patients receiving moderately/highly emetogenic chemotherapy. *Pediatr Hematol Oncol* 2000;17(6): 445–55.

91. Numbenjapon, T. *et al.* Comparative study of low-dose oral granisetron plus dexamethasone and high-dose metoclopramide plus dexamethasone in prevention of nausea and vomiting induced by CHOP-therapy in young patients with non-Hodgkin's lymphoma. *J Med Assoc Thai* 2002;85(11):1156–63.

92. Figueredo, E.D. and Canosa, L.G. Ondansetron in the prophylaxis of postoperative vomiting: a meta-analysis. *J Clin Anesth* 1998; 10(3):211–21.

93. Henzi, I., Walder, B., and Tramer, M.R. Metoclopramide in the prevention of postoperative nausea and vomiting: a quantitative systematic review of randomized, placebo-controlled studies. *Br J Anaesth* 1999;83(5):761–1.

94. Domino, K.B. *et al.* Comparative efficacy and safety of ondansetron, droperidol, and metoclopramide for preventing postoperative nausea and vomiting: A meta-analysis. *Anesth Analg* 1999;88(6):1370–9.

95. Lee, A. and Done, M.L. The use of nonpharmacologic techniques to prevent postoperative nausea and vomiting: A meta-analysis. *Anesth Analg* 1999;88(6):1362–9.

96. Cynamon, H.A., Andres, J.M., and Iafrate, R.P. Rifampin relieves pruritus in children with cholestatic liver disease. *Gastroenterology* 1990;98(4):1013–6.

97. Gunter, J.B. *et al.* Continuous epidural butorphanol relieves pruritus associated with epidural morphine infusions in children. *Paediatr Anaesth* 2000;10(2):167–72.

98. Iriarte, J., Katsamakis, G., and de Castro, P. The Fatigue Descriptive Scale (FDS): A useful tool to evaluate fatigue in multiple sclerosis. *Multiple Sclerosis* 1999;5(1):10–6.

99. Varni, J.W. *et al.* The PedsQL in pediatric cancer: Reliability and validity of the Pediatric Quality of Life Inventory Generic Core Scales, Multidimensional Fatigue Scale, and Cancer Module. *Cancer* 2002;94(7):2090–106.

100. Hockenberry, M.J. *et al.* Three instruments to assess fatigue in children with cancer: the child, parent and staff perspectives. *J Pain Symptom Manage* 2003;25(4):319–28.

101. Prasad, S.A., Randall, S.D., and Balfour-Lynn, I.M. Fifteen-count breathlessness score: an objective measure for children. *Pediatr Pulmonol* 2000;30(1):56–62.

102. Hamutcu, R. *et al.* Objective monitoring of cough in children with cystic fibrosis. *Pediatr Pulmonol* 2002;34(5):331–5.

103. Eiser, C. and Morse, R. Quality-of-life measures in chronic diseases of childhood. *Health Technol Assess* 2001;5(4):1–157.

104. Wallander, J.L., Schmitt, M., and Koot, H.M. Quality of life measurement in children and adolescents: Issues, instruments, and applications. *J Clin Psychol* 2001;57(4):571–85.

105. Rajmil, L. *et al.* Generic health-related quality of life instruments in children and adolescents: A qualitative analysis of content. *J Adolesc Health* 2004;34(1):37–45.

106. Landgraf, J.M. *et al.* Canadian-French, German and UK versions of the Child Health Questionnaire: Methodology and preliminary item scaling results. *Qual Life Res* 1998;7(5):433–45.

107. Ravens-Sieberer, U. and Bullinger, M. Assessing health-related quality of life in chronically ill children with the German KINDL: First psychometric and content analytical results. *Qual Life Res* 1998;7(5):399–407.

108. Vogels, T. *et al.* Measuring health-related quality of life in children: The development of the TACQOL parent form. *Qual Life Res* 1998;7(5):457–65.

109. Eiser, C., Mohay, H., and Morse, R. The measurement of quality of life in young children. *Child Care Health Dev* 2000;26(5): 401–14.

110. Glaser, A.W. *et al.* Applicability of the Health Utilities Index to a population of childhood survivors of central nervous system tumours in the U.K. *Eur J Cancer* 1999;35(2):256–61.

111. Bullinger, M. *et al.* Pilot testing of the 'Haemo-QoL' quality of life questionnaire for haemophiliac children in six European countries. *Haemophilia* 2002;8(Suppl. 2):47–54.

112. Klassen, A.F. *et al.* Health related quality of life in 3 and 4 year old children and their parents: Preliminary findings about a new questionnaire. *Health Qual Life Outcomes* 2003;1(1):81.

113. Riley, A.W. *et al.* The Child Report Form of the CHIP-Child Edition: Reliability and validity. *Med Care* 2004;42(3):221–31.

114. Manificat, S. *et al.* [Infant quality of life: criteria of parents and professionals. Development of an evaluation instrument]. *Arch Pediatr* 1999;6(1):79–86.

115. Schneider, J.W. *et al.* Health-related quality of life and functional outcome measures for children with cerebral palsy. *Dev Med Child Neurol* 2001;43(9):601–8.

116. McCarthy, M.L. *et al.* Comparing reliability and validity of pediatric instruments for measuring health and well-being of children with spastic cerebral palsy. *Dev Med Child Neurol* 2002; 44(7):468–76.

117. Msall, M.E. and Tremont, M.R. Measuring functional outcomes after prematurity: Developmental impact of very low birth weight and extremely low birth weight status on childhood disability. *Ment Retard Dev Disabil Res Rev* 2002;8(4):258–72.

118. Fekkes, M. *et al.* Development and psychometric evaluation of the TAPQOL: A health-related quality of life instrument for 1–5-year-old children. *Qual Life Res* 2000;9(8):961–72.

119. Varni, J.W., Seid, M., and Rode, C.A. The PedsQL: Measurement model for the pediatric quality of life inventory. *Med Care* 1999; 37(2):126–39.

120. Forrest, C.B. *et al.* Outcomes research in pediatric settings: Recent trends and future directions. Pediatrics 2003; 111(1): 171–8.

121. Varni, J.W., Seid, M., and Kurtin, P.S. PedsQL 4.0: Reliability and validity of the Pediatric Quality of Life Inventory version 4.0 generic core scales in healthy and patient populations. *Med Care* 2001;39(8):800–12.

122. Stewart, A.L. *et al.* The concept of quality of life of dying persons in the context of health care. *J Pain Symptom Manage* 1999;17(2): 93–108.

123. Kaasa, S. and J.H. Loge, Quality-of-life assessment in palliative care. *Lancet Oncol* 2002;3(3):175–82.

124. Hickey, A.M. *et al.* A new short form individual quality of life measure (SEIQoL-DW): Application in a cohort of individuals with HIV/AIDS. *BMJ* 1996;313(7048):29–33.

125. Waldron, D. *et al.* Quality-of-life measurement in advanced cancer: Assessing the individual. *J Clin Oncol* 1999;17(11):3603–11.

126. Joyce, C.R. *et al.* A theory-based method for the evaluation of individual quality of life: The SEIQoL. *Qual Life Res* 2003;12(3): 275–80.

127. Ruta, D.A. *et al.* A new approach to the measurement of quality of life. The Patient-Generated Index. *Med Care* 1994;32(11):1109–26.

128. Camilleri-Brennan, J., Ruta, D.A., and Steele, R.J. Patient generated index: new instrument for measuring quality of life in patients with rectal cancer. *World J Surg* 2002;26(11):1354–9.

129. Eiser, C., Vance, Y.H., and Seamark, D. The development of a theoretically driven generic measure of quality of life for children aged 6–12 years: A preliminary report. *Child Care Health Dev* 2000;26(6):445–56.

130. Calman, K.C. Quality of life in cancer patients—an hypothesis. *J Med Ethics* 1984;10(3):124–7.

131. Taenzer, P. *et al.* Impact of computerized quality of life screening on physician behaviour and patient satisfaction in lung cancer outpatients. *Psychooncology* 2000;9(3):203–13.

132. Detmar, S.B. *et al.* Health-related quality-of-life assessments and patient-physician communication: a randomized controlled trial. *JAMA* 2002;288(23):3027–34.

133. Velikova, G. *et al.* Measuring quality of life in routine oncology practice improves communication and patient well-being: A randomized controlled trial. *J Clin Oncol* 2004;22(4):714–24.

134. Higginson, I.J. *et al.* Is there evidence that palliative care teams alter end-of-life experiences of patients and their caregivers? *J Pain Symptom Manage* 2003;25(2):150–68.

135. Kohler, J.A. and Radford M. Terminal care for children dying of cancer: Quantity and quality of life. *Br Med J* 1985;1985(291): 115–16.

136. Hunt, A.M. A survey of signs, symptoms and symptom control in 30 terminally ill children. *Dev Med Child Neurol* 1990;32(4):341–6.

137. Goldman, A., Beardsmore, S., and Hunt, J. Palliative care for children with cancer—home, hospital, or hospice? [see comments]. *Arch Dis Child* 1990;65(6):641–3.

138. Sirkia, K. *et al.* Terminal care of the child with cancer at home [see comments]. *Acta Paediatr* 1997;86(10):1125–30.

139. McCallum, D.E., Byrne, P., and Bruera, E. How children die in hospital. *J Pain Symptom Manage* 2000;20(6):417–23.

140. Dangel, T., Fowler-Kerry, S., Karwacki, M., and Bereda, J. An evaluation of a home palliative care programme for children. *Amb Child Health* 2000;6(2):101–14.

141. Contro, N. *et al.* Family perspectives on the quality of pediatric palliative care. *Arch Pediatr Adolesc Med* 2002;156:14–19.

142. Sirkia, K. *et al.* Pain medication during terminal care of children with cancer. *J Pain Symptom Manage* 1998;15(4):220–6.

143. Henley, L.D. End of life care in HIV-infected children who died in hospital. *Dev World Bioeth* 2002;2(1):38–54.

144. Hongo, T. *et al.* Analysis of the circumstances at the end of life in children with cancer: Symptoms, suffering and acceptance. *Pediatr Int* 2003;45(1):60–4.

145. American Academy of Pediatrics. Committee on Bioethics and Committee on Hospital Care. Palliative care for children. *Pediatrics* 2000;106(2 Pt 1): 351–7.

146. ACT and RCPCH, A Guide to the Development of Children's Palliative Care Services. (2nd edition), ACT. 53 2003.

147. Field, M.J., Behrman, R.E., and Institute of Medicine (U.S.). Committee on Palliative and End-of-Life Care for Children and Their Families. When Children die: Improving Palliative and End-of-Life Care for Children and their Families. Washington, D.C.: National Academy Press. 2003;xx:690.

148. Wolfe, J. et al. Understanding of prognosis among parents of children who died of cancer: Impact on treatment goals and integration of palliative care. *J Am Med Assoc* 2000;284(19):2469–75.

149. Feudtner, C. et al. Characteristics of deaths occurring in children's hospitals: implications for supportive care services. *Pediatrics* 2002;109(5):887–93.

150. Feudtner, C., DiGiuseppe, D.L., and Neff, J.M. Hospital care for children and young adults in the last year of life: a population-based study. *BMC Med* 2003;1(1):3.

151. Garros, D., Rosychuk, R.J., and Cox, P.N. Circumstances surrounding end of life in a pediatric intensive care unit. *Pediatrics* 2003;112(5):e371.

152. Pierucci, R.L., Kirby, R.S., and Leuthner, S.R. End-of-life care for neonates and infants: The experience and effects of a palliative care consultation service. *Pediatrics* 2001;108(3):653–60.

153. Piggott, M., McGee, H., and Feuer, D. Has CONSORT improved the reporting of randomized controlled trials in the palliative care literature? A systematic review. *Palliat Med* 2004;18(1):32–8.

154. Rimer, B. et al. Enhancing cancer pain control regimens through patient education. *Patient Educ Couns* 1987;10(3):267–77.

155. Cherny, N.I. et al. Opioid responsiveness of cancer pain syndromes caused by neuropathic or nociceptive mechanisms: A combined analysis of controlled, single-dose studies. *Neurology* 1994;44(5):857–61.

156. Syrjala, K.L. et al. Relaxation and imagery and cognitive-behavioral training reduce pain during cancer treatment: A controlled clinical trial. *Pain* 1995;63(2):189–98.

157. Axelsson, B. and Borup, S. Is there an additive analgesic effect of paracetamol at step 3? A double-blind randomized controlled study. *Palliat Med* 2003;17(8):724–5.

158. Small, E.J. et al. Combined analysis of two multicenter, randomized, placebo-controlled studies of pamidronate disodium for the palliation of bone pain in men with metastatic prostate cancer. *J Clin Oncol* 2003;21(23):4277–84.

159. van den Hout, W.B. et al. Single- versus multiple-fraction radiotherapy in patients with painful bone metastases: Cost-utility analysis based on a randomized trial. *J Natl Cancer Inst* 2003; 95(3):222–9.

160. Miaskowski, C. et al. Randomized clinical trial of the effectiveness of a self-care intervention to improve cancer pain management. *J Clin Oncol* 2004; 22(9): 1713–20.

161. Wong, G.Y. et al. Effect of neurolytic celiac plexus block on pain relief, quality of life, and survival in patients with unresectable pancreatic cancer: a randomized controlled trial. *JAMA* 2004; 291(9):1092–9.

162. Bruera, E. et al. Effects of oxygen on dyspnoea in hypoxaemic terminal-cancer patients. *Lancet* 1993;342(8862):13–4.

163. Bruera, E. et al. Subcutaneous morphine for dyspnea in cancer patients. *Ann Intern Med* 1993;119(9):906–7.

164. Booth, S. et al. Does oxygen help dyspnea in patients with cancer? *Am J Resp Crit Care Med* 1996;153(5):1515–8.

165. Poole, P.J., Veale, A.G., and Black, P.N. The effect of sustained-release morphine on breathlessness and quality of life in severe chronic obstructive pulmonary disease. *Am J Resp Crit Care Med* 1998;157(6 Pt 1):1877–80.

166. Mazzocato, C., Buclin, T., and Rapin, C.H. The effects of morphine on dyspnea and ventilatory function in elderly patients with advanced cancer: A randomized double-blind controlled trial. *Ann Oncol* 1999;10(12): 1511–4.

167. Johnson, M.J. et al. Morphine for the relief of breathlessness in patients with chronic heart failure—a pilot study. *Eur J Heart Failure* 2002;4(6):753–6.

168. Bruera, E. et al. A randomized controlled trial of supplemental oxygen versus air in cancer patients with dyspnea. *Palliat Med* 2003;17(8):659–63.

169. Abernethy, A.P. et al. Randomised, double blind, placebo controlled crossover trial of sustained release morphine for the management of refractory dyspnoea. *BMJ* 2003; 327(7414): 523–8.

170. Ahmedzai, S.H. et al. A double-blind, randomised, controlled Phase II trial of Heliox28 gas mixture in lung cancer patients with dyspnoea on exertion. *Br J Cancer* 2004;90(2):366–71.

171. Bruera, E. et al. A controlled trial of megestrol acetate on appetite, caloric intake, nutritional status, and other symptoms in patients with advanced cancer. *Cancer* 1990;66(6):1279–82.

172. Loprinzi, C.L. et al. Controlled trial of megestrol acetate for the treatment of cancer anorexia and cachexia. *J Natl Cancer Inst* 1990;82(13):1127–32.

173. Bruera, E. et al. Effectiveness of megestrol acetate in patients with advanced cancer: A randomized, double-blind, crossover study. *Cancer Prev Control* 1998;2(2):74–8.

174. Loprinzi, C.L. et al. Randomized comparison of megestrol acetate versus dexamethasone versus fluoxymesterone for the treatment of cancer anorexia/cachexia. *J Clin Oncol* 1999;17(10):3299–306.

175. Jatoi, A. et al. Dronabinol versus megestrol acetate versus combination therapy for cancer-associated anorexia: A North Central Cancer Treatment Group study. *J Clin Oncol* 2002;20(2):567–73.

176. Bruera, E. et al. Effect of fish oil on appetite and other symptoms in patients with advanced cancer and anorexia/cachexia: A double-blind, placebo-controlled study. *J Clin Oncol* 2003;21(1):129–34.

177. Hofmann, J.C. et al. Patient preferences for communication with physicians about end-of-life decisions. SUPPORT Investigators. Study to Understand Prognoses and Preference for Outcomes and Risks of Treatment. *Ann Intern Med* 1997;127(1):1–12.

178. McCorkle, R. et al. The effects of home nursing care for patients during terminal illness on the bereaved's psychological distress. Nurs Res 1998;47(1):2–10.

179. Bruera, E. et al. The addition of an audiocassette recording of a consultation to written recommendations for patients with advanced cancer: A randomized, controlled trial. Cancer 1999;86(11):2420–5.

180. Ong, L.M. et al. Effect of providing cancer patients with the audiotaped initial consultation on satisfaction, recall, and quality of life: A randomized, double-blind study. *J Clin Oncol* 2000; 18(16):3052–60.

181. Abbot, N.C. et al. Spiritual healing as a therapy for chronic pain: A randomized, clinical trial. *Pain* 2001;91(1–2):79–89.

182. Ringdal, G.I. et al. The first year of grief and bereavement in close family members to individuals who have died of cancer. *Palliat Med* 2001;15(2):91–105.

183. Wiesendanger, H. *et al.* Chronically ill patients treated by spiritual healing improve in quality of life: Results of a randomized waiting-list controlled study. *J Altern Complement Med* 2001;7(1):45–51.

184. Stroebe, M. *et al.* Does disclosure of emotions facilitate recovery from bereavement? Evidence from two prospective studies. *J Consult Clin Psychol* 2002;70(1):169–78.

185. Bruera, E. *et al.* Breast cancer patient perception of the helpfulness of a prompt sheet versus a general information sheet during outpatient consultation: A randomized, controlled trial. *J Pain Symptom Manage* 2003;25(5):412–9.

186. Flannelly, K.J. *et al.* A systematic review on chaplains and community-based clergy in three palliative care journals: 1990–1999. *Am J Hosp Palliat Care* 2003;20(4):263–8.

187. Kissane, D.W. *et al.* Psychosocial morbidity associated with patterns of family functioning in palliative care: Baseline data from the Family Focused Grief Therapy controlled trial. *Palliat Med* 2003;17(6):527–37.

188. O'Connor, M. *et al.* Writing therapy for the bereaved: Evaluation of an intervention. *J Palliat Med* 2003;6(2):195–204.

189. Ogrodniczuk, J.S., Joyce, A.S., and Piper, W.E. Changes in perceived social support after group therapy for complicated grief. *J Nerv Ment Dis* 2003;191(8):524–30.

190. Flannelly, K.J., Weaver, A.J., and Costa, K.G. A systematic review of religion and spirituality in three palliative care journals, 1990–1999. *J Palliat Care* 2004;20(1):50–6.

191. Kane, R.L. *et al.* A randomised controlled trial of hospice care. *Lancet* 1984;1(8382):890–4.

192. Zimmer, J.G., Groth-Juncker, A., and McCusker, J. A randomized controlled study of a home health care team. *Am J Public Health* 1985;75(2):134–41.

193. McCorkle, R. *et al.* A randomized clinical trial of home nursing care for lung cancer patients. *Cancer* 1989;64(6):1375–82.

194. Hughes, S.L. *et al.* A randomized trial of the cost effectiveness of VA hospital-based home care for the terminally ill. *Health Serv Res* 1992;26(6):801–17.

195. Addington-Hall, J.M. *et al.* Randomised controlled trial of effects of coordinating care for terminally ill cancer patients. *BMJ* 1992; 305(6865):1317–22.

196. McWhinney, I.R., Bass, M.J., and Donner, A. Evaluation of a palliative care service: problems and pitfalls. *BMJ* 1994;309(6965): 1340–2.

197. Grande, G.E.T., Barclay, C.J., and Farquhar, S.I., M.C. Does hospital at home for palliative care facilitate death at home? Randomised controlled trial. *BMJ* 1999;319(7223):1472–5.

198. Jordhoy, M.S. *et al.* A palliative-care intervention and death at home: A cluster randomised trial. *Lancet* 2000;356(9233):888–93.

199. Hearn, J. and Higginson, I.J. Outcome measures in palliative care for advanced cancer patients: a review. *J Public Health Med* 1997; 19(2):193–9.

200. Hearn, J. and Higginson, I.J. Development and validation of a core outcome measure for palliative care: The palliative care outcome scale. Palliative Care Core Audit Project Advisory Group. *Qual Health Care* 1999;8(4):219–27.

201. Caraceni, A. *et al.* Pain measurement tools and methods in clinical research in palliative care: Recommendations of an Expert Working Group of the European Association of Palliative Care. *J Pain Symptom Manage* 2002;23(3):239–55.

202. Hotopf, M., Lewis, G., and Normand, C. Putting trials on trial— the costs and consequences of small trials in depression: a systematic review of methodology. *J Epidemiol Community Health* 1997; 51(4):354–8.

203. Huntley, A. and Ernst, E. Complementary and alternative therapies for treating multiple sclerosis symptoms: A systematic review. *Complement Ther Med* 2000;8(2):97–105.

204. Hurdon, V., Viola, R., and Schroder, C. How useful is docusate in patients at risk for constipation? A systematic review of the evidence in the chronically ill. *J Pain Symptom Manage* 2000;19(2): 130–6.

205. Critchley, P. *et al.* Efficacy of haloperidol in the treatment of nausea and vomiting in the palliative patient: A systematic review. *J Pain Symptom Manage* 2001;22(2):631–4.

206. Goodwin, D.M. *et al.* An evaluation of systematic reviews of palliative care services. *J Palliat Care* 2002;18(2):77–83.

207. Hotopf, M. *et al.* Depression in advanced disease: A systematic review Part 1. Prevalence and case finding. *Palliat Med* 2002; 16(2):81–97.

208. Ly, K.L. *et al.* Depression in palliative care: A systematic review. Part 2. Treatment. *Palliat Med* 2002;16(4):279–84.

209. Bell, R.F., Eccleston, C., and Kalso, E. Ketamine as adjuvant to opioids for cancer pain. A qualitative systematic review. *J Pain Symptom Manage* 2003;26(3):867–75.

210. Harding, R. and Higginson, I.J. What is the best way to help caregivers in cancer and palliative care? A systematic literature review of interventions and their effectiveness. *Palliat Med* 2003;17(1): 63–74.

211. Quigley, C. and Wiffen, P. A systematic review of hydromorphone in acute and chronic pain. *J Pain Symptom Manage* 2003;25(2): 169–78.

212. Booth, S. *et al.* The use of oxygen in the palliation of breathlessness. A report of the expert working group of the Scientific Committee of the Association of Palliative Medicine. *Respir Med* 2004;98(1):66–77.

213. Hirst, A. and Sloan, R. Benzodiazepines and related drugs for insomnia in palliative care. *Cochrane Database Syst Rev* 2002(4): CD003346.

214. Ingleton, C. *et al.* Respite in palliative care: A review and discussion of the literature. *Palliat Med* 2003;17(7):567–75.

215. Jackson, K.C. and Lipman, A.G. Drug therapy for anxiety in palliative care. *Cochrane Database Syst Rev* 2004(1):CD004596.

216. Finlay, I.G. *et al.* Palliative care in hospital, hospice, at home: results from a systematic review. *Ann Oncol* 2002;13(Suppl. 4): 257–64.

217. Salisbury, C. *et al.* The impact of different models of specialist palliative care on patients' quality of life: a systematic literature review. *Palliat Med* 1999;13(1):3–17.

218. Higginson, I.J. *et al.* Do hospital-based palliative teams improve care for patients or families at the end of life? *J Pain Symptom Manage* 2002;23(2):96–106.

219. Higginson, I.J. It would be NICE to have more evidence? *Palliat Med* 2004;18(2):85–6.

220. Moher, D., Schulz, K.F., and Altman, D.G. The CONSORT statement: revised recommendations for improving the quality of reports of parallel-group randomised trials. *Lancet* 2001;357(9263):1191–4.

221. Des Jarlais, D.C., Lyles, C., and Crepaz, N. Improving the reporting quality of nonrandomized evaluations of behavioral and public health interventions: the TREND statement. *Am J Public Health* 2004;94(3):361–6.

222. Campbell, H., Surry, S.A., and Royle, E.M. A review of randomised controlled trials published in Archives of Disease in Childhood from 1982–96. *Arch Dis Childhood* 1998;79(2):192–7.

223. Randolph, A.G. and Lacroix, J. Randomized clinical trials in pediatric critical care: Rarely done but desperately needed. *Pediatr Crit Care Med* 2002;3(2):102–6.

224. Watson, R.S. *et al.* The epidemiology of severe sepsis in children in the United States. *Am J Respir Crit Care Med* 2003;167(5):695–701.

225. Angus, D.C. *et al.* Epidemiology of severe sepsis in the United States: analysis of incidence, outcome, and associated costs of care. *Crit Care Med* 2001;29(7):1303–10.

226. Pediatric Drug Research: Substantial Increase in Studies of Drugs for Children, but Some Challenges Remain. Statement of Janet Heinrich, Director, Health-Care Public Health Issues. In Testimony before the Committe on Health, Education, Labor and Pensions, U.S. Senate. 2001; USGAO. GAO-01-705T: Washington, DC.

227. Grodin, M.A. and Alpert, J.J. Children as participants in medical research. *Pediatr Clin N Am* 1988;35(6):1389–401.

228. Forrest, C.B., Simpson, L., and Clancy, C. Child health services research. Challenges and opportunities. *JAMA* 1997;277(22):1787–93.

229. Hirtz, D.G. and Fitzsimmons, L.G. Regulatory and ethical issues in the conduct of clinical research involving children. *Curr Opin Pediatr* 2002;14(6):669–75.

230. Burns, J.P. Research in children. *Crit Care Med*, 2003;31(3 Suppl):S131–6.

231. Grande, G.E.T., C. J. Why are trials in palliative care so difficult? *Palliative Medicine* 2000;14(1):69–74.

232. Rinck, G.C. *et al.* Methodologic issues in effectiveness research on palliative cancer care: A systematic review. *J Clin Oncol* 1997;15(4):1697–707.

233. Waters, E. *et al.* Influence of parental gender and self-reported health and illness on parent-reported child health. *Pediatrics* 2000;106(6):1422–8.

234. Pollack, M.M., Ruttimann, U.E., and Getson, P.R. Pediatric risk of mortality (PRISM) score. *Crit Care Med* 1988;16(11):1110–6.

235. Pollack, M.M., Patel, K.M., and Ruttimann, U.E. The Pediatric Risk of Mortality III—Acute Physiology Score (PRISM III-APS): A method of assessing physiologic instability for pediatric intensive care unit patients. *J Pediatr* 1997;131(4):575–81.

236. Shann, F. *et al.* Paediatric index of mortality (PIM): A mortality prediction model for children in intensive care. *Intens Care Med* 1997;23(2):201–7.

237. Slater, A., Shann, F., and Pearson, G. PIM2: A revised version of the Paediatric Index of Mortality. *Intens Care Med* 2003;29(2): 278–85.

238. Ling, J., Rees, E., and Hardy, J. What influences participation in clinical trials in palliative care in a cancer centre? *Eur J Cancer* 2000;36(5):621–6.

239. Thompson, I.E., Fundamental ethical principles in health care. *Br Med J (Clin Res Ed)* 1987;295(6611):1461–5.

240. United States. National Commission for the Protection of Human Subjects of Biomedical and Behavioral Research., The Belmont report: ethical principles and guidelines for the protection of human subjects of research. 1978; [Bethesda, Md.] Washington: The Commission; for sale by the Supt. of Docs. U.S. Govt. Print. Off. 20 p.

241. United States. National Commission for the Protection of Human Subjects of Biomedical and Behavioral Research.

Appendix, The Belmont report: Ethical principles and guidelines for the protection of human subjects of research. 1978; [Bethesda, Md.] Washington: The Commission; for sale by the Supt. of Docs., U.S. Govt. Print. Off.

242. Froggatt, K.A. *et al.* Qualitative research in palliative care 1990–1999: A descriptive review. *Int J Palliat Nurs* 2003; 9(3): 98–104.

243. Malterud, K. Qualitative research: Standards, challenges, and guidelines. *Lancet* 2001;358(9280):483–8.

244. Mays, N. and Pope, C. Qualitative research in health care. Assessing quality in qualitative research. *BMJ* 2000;320(7226):50–2.

245. Giacomini, M.K. and Cook, D.J. Users' guides to the medical literature: XXIII. Qualitative research in health care B. What are the results and how do they help me care for my patients? Evidence-Based Medicine Working Group. *JAMA* 2000;284(4): 478–82.

246. Giacomini, M.K. and Cook, D.J. Users' guides to the medical literature: XXIII. Qualitative research in health care A. Are the results of the study valid? Evidence-Based Medicine Working Group. *JAMA* 2000;284(3):357–62.

247. Warlow, C. Advanced issues in the design and conduct of randomized clinical trials: The bigger the better? *Stat Med* 2002; 21(19):2797–805.

248. Pagano, M. and Gauvreau, K. Principles of biostatistics. (2nd edition) Pacific Grove, CA: Duxbury, 1 v. (various pagings), 2000.

249. Evans, C.H., S.T. Ildstad, and Institute of Medicine (U.S.). Committee on Strategies for Small-Number-Participant Clinical Research Trials., Small clinical trials: Issues and challenges. 2001; Washington, D.C.: National Academy Press. 2000 xii, 207 p.

250. Rothman, K.J. and Greenland, S. Modern epidemiology (2nd edition) Philadelphia, PA: Lippincott-Raven, 1998;xiii:737.

251. Mazzocato, C., Sweeney, C., and Bruera, E. Clinical research in palliative care: Choice of trial design. *Palliat Med* 2001;15(3): 261–4.

252. Hammack, J.E. *et al.* Phase III evaluation of nortriptyline for alleviation of symptoms of cis-platinum-induced peripheral neuropathy. *Pain* 2002;98(1–2):195–203.

253. Davies, A.N. *et al.* A comparison of artificial saliva and pilocarpine in the management of xerostomia in patients with advanced cancer. *Palliat Med* 1998;12(2):105–11.

254. Davies, A.N. A comparison of artificial saliva and chewing gum in the management of xerostomia in patients with advanced cancer. *Palliat Med* 2000;14(3):197–203.

255. Hardy, J. *et al.* Pitfalls in placebo-controlled trials in palliative care: Dexamethasone for the palliation of malignant bowel obstruction. *Palliat Med* 1998;12(6):437–42.

256. Wilwerding, M.B. *et al.* A randomized, crossover evaluation of methylphenidate in cancer patients receiving strong narcotics. *Support Care Cancer* 1995;3(2):135–8.

257. Cheng, K.K. and Chang, A.M., Palliation of oral mucositis symptoms in pediatric patients treated with cancer chemotherapy. *Cancer Nurs* 2003;26(6):476–84.

258. Anderson, P.M., Schroeder, G., and Skubitz, K.M. Oral glutamine reduces the duration and severity of stomatitis after cytotoxic cancer chemotherapy. *Cancer* 1998;83(7):1433–9.

259. Collins, J.J. *et al.* Patient-controlled analgesia for mucositis pain in children: A three-period crossover study comparing morphine and hydromorphone. *J Pediatr* 1996;129(5): 722–8.

260. Parker, R.I. *et al.* Randomized, double-blind, crossover, placebo-controlled trial of intravenous ondansetron for the prevention of intrathecal chemotherapy-induced vomiting in children. *J Pediatr Hematol Oncol* 2001;23(9):578–81.

261. Tsuchida, Y. *et al.* Effects of granisetron in children undergoing high-dose chemotherapy: A multi-institutional, cross-over study. *Int J Oncol* 1999;14(4):673–9.

262. Guyatt, G. *et al.* Determining optimal therapy—randomized trials in individual patients. *N Engl J Med* 1986;314(14):889–92.

263. Mahon, J. *et al.* Randomised study of n of 1 trials versus standard practice. *BMJ* 1996;312(7038):1069–74.

264. Bruera, E., Schoeller, T., and MacEachern, T. Symptomatic benefit of supplemental oxygen in hypoxemic patients with terminal cancer: The use of the N of 1 randomized controlled trial. *J Pain Symptom Manage* 1992;7(6):365–8.

265. McQuay, H.J. *et al.* Dextromethorphan for the treatment of neuropathic pain: A double-blind randomised controlled crossover trial with integral n-of-1 design. *Pain* 1994;59(1):127–33.

266. Miller, M.G. and Corner, J. The 'n = 1' randomized controlled trial. *Palliat Med* 1999;13(3):255–9.

267. Bagne, C.A. and Lewis, R.F. Evaluating the effects of drugs on behavior and quality of life: An alternative strategy for clinical trials. *J Consult Clin Psychol* 1992;60(2):225–39.

268. Zucker, D.R. *et al.* Combining single patient (N-of-1) trials to estimate population treatment effects and to evaluate individual patient responses to treatment. *J Clin Epidemiol* 1997;50(4):401–10.

269. Price, J.D. and Grimley Evans, J. N-of-1 randomized controlled trials ('N-of-1 trials'): Singularly useful in geriatric medicine. *Age Ageing* 2002;31(4):227–32.

270. Haines, D.R. and Gaines, S.P. N of 1 randomised controlled trials of oral ketamine in patients with chronic pain. *Pain* 1999;83(2):283–7.

271. Mahon, J.L. *et al.* Theophylline for irreversible chronic airflow limitation: a randomized study comparing n of 1 trials to standard practice. *Chest* 1999;115(1):38–48.

272. Maclure, M. and Mittleman, M.A. Should we use a case-crossover design? *Ann Rev Public Health* 2000;21:193–221.

273. Maclure, M. The case-crossover design: A method for studying transient effects on the risk of acute events. *Am J Epidemiol* 1991; 133(2):144–53.

274. Gonge, H., Jensen, L.D., and Bonde, J.P. Do psychosocial strain and physical exertion predict onset of low-back pain among nursing aides? *Scand J Work Environ Health* 2001;27(6):388–94.

275. Laflamme, L. *et al.* Is perceived failure in school performance a trigger of physical injury? A case-crossover study of children in Stockholm County. *J Epidemiol Commun Health* 2004;58(5): 407–11.

276. Honkanen, V.E. *et al.* A three-stage clinical trial design for rare disorders. *Stat Med* 2001; 20(20): 3009–21.

277. Mazzocato, C., Sweeney, C., and Bruera, E. Clinical research in palliative care: Patient populations, symptoms, interventions and endpoints. *Palliat Med* 2001;15(2):163–8.

278. Bruera, E. *et al.* A prospective multicenter assessment of the Edmonton staging system for cancer pain. *J Pain Symptom Manage* 1995;10(5):348–55.

279. Abel, U. and Koch, A. The role of randomization in clinical studies: Myths and beliefs. *J Clin Epidemiol* 1999;52(6):487–97.

280. Fayers, P.M., Jordhoy, M.S., and Kaasa, S. Cluster-randomized trials. *Palliat Med* 2002;16(1):69–70.

281. Donner, A. and Klar, N. Pitfalls of and controversies in cluster randomization trials. *Am J Public Health* 2004;94(3):416–22.

282. Jordhoy, M.S. *et al.* Lack of concealment may lead to selection bias in cluster randomized trials of palliative care. *Palliat Med* 2002; 16(1):43–9.

283. Edmonds, P. and Lucas, C. A trial that failed because of poor recruitment. *Palliat Med* 2003;17(6):557.

284. Glare, P. *et al.* A systematic review of physicians' survival predictions in terminally ill cancer patients. *BMJ* 2003;327(7408):195.

285. Morita, T. *et al.* The Palliative Prognostic Index: a scoring system for survival prediction of terminally ill cancer patients. *Support Care Cancer* 1999;7(3):128–33.

286. Pirovano, M. *et al.* A new palliative prognostic score: A first step for the staging of terminally ill cancer patients. Italian Multicenter and Study Group on Palliative Care. *J Pain Symptom Manage* 1999;17(4):231–9.

287. Maltoni, M. *et al.* Successful validation of the palliative prognostic score in terminally ill cancer patients. Italian Multicenter Study Group on Palliative Care. *J Pain Symptom Manage* 1999;17(4): 240–7.

288. Morita, T. *et al.* Improved accuracy of physicians' survival prediction for terminally ill cancer patients using the Palliative Prognostic Index. *Palliat Med* 2001;15(5):419–24.

289. Glare, P., Eychmueller, S., and Virik, K. The use of the palliative prognostic score in patients with diagnoses other than cancer. *J Pain Symptom Manage* 2003;26(4):883–5.

290. Banerjee, R. *et al.* Predicting mortality in patients with cirrhosis of liver with application of neural network technology. *J Gastroenterol Hepatol* 2003;18(9):1054–60.

291. Miller, D.K. and Chibnall, J.T. Strategies for recruiting patients into randomized trials of palliative care. *Palliat Med* 2003;17(6): 556–7.

292. Jordhoy, M.S. *et al.* Challenges in palliative care research; recruitment, attrition and compliance: Experience from a randomized controlled trial. *Palliat Med* 1999;13(4):299–310.

293. Zebracki, K. *et al.* Predicting attrition in a pediatric asthma intervention study. *J Pediatr Psychol* 2003;28(8):519–28.

294. Piantadosi, S. Clinical trials: A methodologic perspective. New York: Wiley 1997;xxi:590.

295. Diggle, P. and Kenward, M.G. Informative drop-out in longitudinal data analysis. *Appl Statist* 1995;43(1):49–93.

296. Hogan, J.W. and Laird, N.M. Model-based approaches to analysing incomplete longitudinal and failure time data. *Statistics in Medicine* 1997;16(1–3):259–72.

297. Teno, J.M. *et al.* Validation of Toolkit After-Death Bereaved Family Member Interview. *J Pain Symptom Manage* 2001;22(3): 752–8.

298. Hearn, J. and Higginson, I.J. Do specialist palliative care teams improve outcomes for cancer patients? A systematic literature review. *Palliat Med* 1998;12(5):317–32.

299. Nordin, K. *et al.* Alternative methods of interpreting quality of life data in advanced gastrointestinal cancer patients. *Br J Cancer* 2001;85(9):1265–72.

300. Streiner, D.L. and Norman, G.R. Health measurement scales: A practical guide to their development and use. (2nd edition). Oxford medical publications. Oxford; New York: Oxford University Press, 2001;viii:231.

301. Nekolaichuk, C.L. *et al.* Assessing the reliability of patient, nurse, and family caregiver symptom ratings in hospitalized advanced cancer patients. *J Clin Oncol* 1999;17(11):3621–30.

302. Theunissen, N.C. *et al.* The proxy problem: child report versus parent report in health-related quality of life research. *Qual Life Res* 1998;7(5):387–97.

303. Vance, Y.H. *et al.* Issues in measuring quality of life in childhood cancer: Measures, proxies, and parental mental health. *J Child Psychol Psychiatry* 2001;42(5):661–7.

304. Eiser, C. and Morse, R. The measurement of quality of life in children: Past and future perspectives. *J Dev Behav Pediatr* 2001; 22(4):248–56.

305. Rutter, M. *et al.* Sex differences in developmental reading disability: New findings from 4 epidemiological studies. *JAMMA* 2004; 291(16):2007–12.

306. Palliative Care Australia, Australia's Future in Palliative Care Research. Scoping study to Determine Priorities for Palliative Care Research in Australia., Maddocks, P.I. Ed. 2000; http://www.pall-care.org.au/publications/Future_Research.pdf. p. 44.

307. NHS The NHS Cancer Plan. Investing in the future: Research and genetics, in The NHS Plan 2003–2006. UK: Department of Health, 2002.

308. United States. General Accounting Office., Pediatric drug research: Food and Drug Administration should more efficiently monitor inclusion of minority children : Report to congressional committees. Washington, D.C.: United States General Accounting Office 2003;ii:29.

309. Goss, C.H. *et al.* The cystic fibrosis therapeutics development network (CF TDN): A paradigm of a clinical trials network for genetic and orphan diseases. *Adv Drug Deliv Rev* 2002;54(11): 1505–28.

310. Escolar, D.M. *et al.* Collaborative translational research leading to multicenter clinical trials in Duchenne muscular dystrophy: The Cooperative International Neuromuscular Research Group (CINRG). *Neuromuscul Disord* 2002;12(Suppl 1):S147–154.

311. Carroll, K.M. *et al.* MET meets the real world: Design issues and clinical strategies in the Clinical Trials Network. *J Subst Abuse Treat* 2002;23(2):73–80.

312. Ross, C. and Cornbleet, M. Attitudes of patients and staff to research in a specialist palliative care unit. *Palliat Med* 2003; 17(6):491–7.

313. Stevens, T. *et al.* Palliative care research protocols: a special case for ethical review? *Palliat Med* 2003;17(6):482–90.

314. Casarett, D.J., Knebel, A., and Helmers, K. Ethical challenges of palliative care research. *J Pain Symptom Manage* 2003;25(4): S3–5.

315. Agrawal, M. Voluntariness in clinical research at the end of life. *J Pain Symptom Manage* 2003;25(4):S25–32.

316. Rossi, W.C., Reynolds, W., and Nelson, R.M. Child assent and parental permission in pediatric research. *Theor Med Bioeth* 2003; 24(2):131–48.

317. Kipnis, K. Seven vulnerabilities in the pediatric research subject. *Theor Med Bioeth* 2003;24(2):107–20.

318. United States, Dept. of Health and Human Services. Protection of human subjects. *Code Fed Regul Public Welfare* 1995;Title 45 CFR Part 46.

319. Berglund, C.A. Children in medical research: Australian ethical standards. *Child Care Health Dev* 1995;21(2):49–59.

320. Flagel, D.C. Children as research subjects: new guidelines for Canadian IRBs. *Irb* 2000;22(5):1–3.

321. Gill, D. *et al.* Guidelines for informed consent in biomedical research involving paediatric populations as research participants. *Eur J Pediatr* 2003;162(7–8):455–8.

322. Tait, A.R., Voepel-Lewis, T., and Malviya, S. Do they understand? (part II): assent of children participating in clinical anesthesia and surgery research. *Anesthesiology* 2003;98(3):609–14.

323. Casarett, D.J. and Karlawish, J.H. Are special ethical guidelines needed for palliative care research? *J Pain Symptom Manage* 2000; 20(2):130–9.

324. Addington-Hall, J. Research sensitivities to palliative care patients. *Eur J Cancer Care (Engl)* 2002;11(3):220–4.

325. Fine, P.G. Maximizing benefits and minimizing risks in palliative care research that involves patients near the end of life. *J Pain Symptom Manage* 2003;25(4):S53–62.

326. Palmer, C.R. and Rosenberger, W.F. Ethics and practice: Alternative designs for phase III randomized clinical trials. *Control Clin Trials* 1999;20(2):172–86.

Appendix: Drug doses

Victoria Lidstone

Drug	Indication	Route	Dose	Times daily
Amitriptyline	Neuropathic pain	Oral	500 μg/kg	Nocte
Baclofen	Muscle spasm Start dose	Oral	1–12 yrs: 2.5 mg >12 yrs: 5 mg	3 3
	Muscle spasm Maintenance dose	Oral	1–2 yrs: 5–10 mg 2–6 yrs: 10–15 mg 6–10 yrs: 15–30 mg >12 yrs: 10–20 mg	2 2 2 3
Bisacodyl	Constipation	Oral/Rectal	1 month–10 yrs: 5 mg >10 yrs 5–10 mg	Give tablets at night Suppositories in the morning
Codeine phosphate	Moderate pain/ Diarrhoea	Oral/Rectal	Birth–12 yrs: 0.5–1 mg/kg >12 yrs: 30–60 mg Maximum dose: 240 mg/24 h	4–6 4–6
	Cough	Oral	Use linctus for cough: 1–5 yrs: 3 mg (5 ml paediatric suspension) 5–12 yrs 7.5–15 mg (2.5–5 ml Adult suspension)	 3–4 3–4
Cyclizine	Nausea and vomiting	Oral/Rectal	<1 yr: 1 mg/kg 1–4 yrs: 12.5 mg 4–12 yrs: 25 mg >12 yrs: 50 mg	3 3 3 3
		Subcutaneous/ Intravenous	<1 yr: 3 mg/kg 1–4 yrs: 37.5 mg 4–12 yrs: 75 mg >12 yrs: 150 mg	Continuous over 24 h
		Intravenous	<2 yr: 1 mg/kg 1–5 yrs: 20 mg 6–12 yrs: 25 mg >12 yrs: 50 mg	Single dose
Dantron (co-danthramer)	Constipation	Oral	<12 yrs: 2.5–5 ml of 25/200 >12 yrs: 2.5–20 ml of 25/200	1–2 1–2
Dexamethasone	Raised intracranial pressure: headache	Oral/Subcutaneous/ Intravenous (slowly over 3–5 min)	1 month–12 yrs: 250 μg/kg 12–18 yrs: 4 mg	2 2
	Raised intracranial pressure: other symptoms	Oral/Subcutaneous/ Intravenous (slowly over 3–5 min)	1 month–12 yrs: 125–500 μg/kg 12–18 yrs: 4 mg	2 2
	Spinal cord compression	Oral/Subcutaneous/ Intravenous (slowly over 3–5 min)	2–5 yrs: 2 mg 6–12 yrs: 3 mg >12 yr: 4–8 mg	2 2 2
	Peripheral nerve compression	Oral/Subcutaneous/ Intravenous (slowly over 3–5 min)	Birth–18 yr: 125–500 μg/kg	2
	Nausea associated with chemotherapy	Oral/ Intravenous (slowly over 3–5 min)	<1 yrs: 0.25–1 mg 1–5 yrs: 1–2 mg 6–12 yrs: 2–4 mg >12 yrs: 4 mg	3 3 3 3

Appendix: Drug doses (*Continued*)

Drug	Indication	Route	Dose	Times daily
	Pain	Oral/Subcutaneous/ Intravenous (Slowly over 3–5 min)	Low dose: 2–5 yrs: 0.5–1 mg 6–12 yrs: 1–2 mg >12 yrs: 2–4 mg High dose: 2–5 yrs: 2 mg 6–12 yrs: 3 mg >12 yrs: 4–8 mg	2 2 2 2 2 2
	Bowel obstruction	Oral/Subcutaneous/ Intravenous over 3–5 min	200–500 µg/kg	1
Diamorphine	Severe pain	Intravenous	12.5–25 µg/kg/h	Continuous infusion over 24 h
		Subcutaneous	20–100 µg/kg/h or convert from Oral morphine sulphate	Continuous infusion over 24 h
Diclofenac	Mild/moderate pain, Inflammation	Oral Rectal	6 months–12 yrs: 0.3–1 mg/kg >12 yrs: 25–50 mg Maximum: 150 mg/24 h	3 2–3
Docusate sodium	Constipation	Oral	6-months–12 yrs: 2 mg/kg >12 yrs: 100 mg	2–3 2–3
Fentanyl	Pain	Transdermal	Start with 25 µg/h patch and monitor closely or convert from Oral morphine dose: see notes	One patch every 3 days
		Lozenge	No relationship to dose of background analgesia therefore start at 200 µg and titrate up according to response	
Gabapentin	Nerve pain Starting dose	Oral	10–15 mg/kg	
	Nerve pain Maintenance dose	Oral	24 mg/kg	
Hyoscine butylbromide	Colic (renal/ gastro-intestinal)	Oral/Intravenous/ Subcutaneous	<6 yrs: 5 mg 6–12 yrs: 5–10 mg >12 yrs: 10–20 mg	1–3 1–3 1–4
		Subcutaneous	600–1200 µg/kg	Continuous infusion over 24 h
Hyoscine hydrobromide	Noisy breathing, Hypersalivation	Transdermal	<3 yrs: 1/4 patch 3–9 yr: 1/2 patch >9 yrs: 1 patch	Over 72 h
		Subcutaneous/ Intravenous	1–2 yr: 10 µg/kg >12 yrs: 400 µg	Single dose
		Subcutaneous/ Intravenous	20–60 µg/kg (Maximum 2.4 g/24 h)	Continuous infusion over 24 h
Lorazepam	Anxiety	Oral/Sublingual	25–50 µg/kg (usual max 1 mg)	Single dose
Levomepromazine	Nausea and vomiting	Oral	<12 yrs: 0.25–1 mg/kg (max 25 mg/24 hrs) >12 yrs: 6.25–12.5 mg	1–2 1–2
		Subcutaneous/ Intravenous	<12 yrs: 100–250 µg/kg (max 12.5 mg/24 hrs) >12 yrs: 2.5–6.25 mg	Continuous infusion over 24 h

Appendix: Drug doses (*Continued*)

Drug	Indication	Route	Dose	Times daily
	Terminal restlessness	Subcutaneous/ Intravenous	350 µg–3 mg/kg	Continuous infusion over 24 h
Midazolam	Emergency control of seizures	Intravenous (slowly over 3 mins)/ Subcutaneous	100–200 µg/kg	Single dose
		Intranasal	200 µg/kg maximum dose 10 mg	Single dose
		Sublingual	500 µg/kg maximum dose 10 mg	Single dose
		Intravenous/ Subcutaneous	10–300 µg/kg/hr	Continuous infusion over 24h
	Anxiety, Agitation,	Intranasal	>1 month–18 yrs: 200 µg/kg maximum dose 10 mg	Single dose
		Sublingual	>1 month–18 yrs: 500 µg/kg maximum dose 10 mg	Single dose
		Subcutaneous/ Intravenous	>1 month–18 yrs: 100 µg/kg (slowly over 3 mins)	Single dose
	Terminal restlessness	Subcutaneous/ Intravenous	300–700 µg/kg	Continuous infusion over 24 h
Morphine sulphate	Moderate/severe pain	Oral (starting dose)	1 month–1 yr: 100 µg/kg 1–12 yrs: 200–500 µg/kg >12 yrs: 10–15 mg	Immediate release: 6
Paracetamol	Pain	Oral	Birth–3 months: 10–15 mg/kg (max. 60 mg/kg/24 h)	4–6
			3 months–1 yr: 60–120 mg (max. 90 mg/kg/24 h)	4–6
			1–5 yrs: 120–250 mg (max. 90 mg/kg/24 h)	4–6
			6–12 yrs: 250–500 mg (max. 90 mg/kg/24 h)	4–6
			>12 yrs: 500 mg–1 g (max. 90 mg/kg/24 h)	4–6
		Rectal	Birth–1 month: 20 mg/kg (max. 60 mg/kg/24 h)	1–4
			1 month–12 yrs: 20 mg/kg (max. 90 mg/kg/24 h or 4 g/24 h)	4–6
			>12 yrs: 500 mg–1 g (max. 90 mg/ kg/24 h or 4 g/24 h)	4–6
Phenobarbitone (Phenobarbital)	Seizures	Intravenous (slow over 5 min)	15 mg/kg (max 1 g)	Single dose
		Subcutaneous/ Intravenous	Birth–12 yrs: 5–10 mg/kg/24 h >12 yrs: 600 mg/24 h	Continuous infusion
Tranexamic acid	Bleeding gums and small bleeds	Oral	1 month–12 yr: 25 mg/kg >12 yr: 1–1.5 g	3 3–4
		Topical/mouth wash	See notes	3

Index